Couturier's

Occupational and Environmental Infectious Diseases

Couturier's

Occupational and Environmental Infectious Diseases

Second Edition

William E. Wright, *Editor*

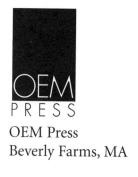

OEM Press
Beverly Farms, MA

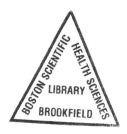

_1990|860_

ISBN 978-1-883595-45-6

Library of Congress Cataloging-in-Publication Data
Couturier's occupational and environmental infectious diseases / William E. Wright, editor. — 2nd ed.
    p. ; cm.
  Rev. ed. of: Occupational and environmental infectious diseases. c2000.
  Includes bibliographical references and index.
  ISBN 978-1-883595-45-6
  1. Occupational diseases.   2. Communicable diseases.   3. Environmentally induced diseases.   I. Wright, William E. (William Evan), 1946–   II. Couturier, Alain J., 1957–   III. Occupational and environmental infectious diseases.
IV. Title: Occupational and environmental infectious diseases.
  [DNLM: 1. Occupational Diseases—prevention & control. 2. Environmental Exposure. 3. Infection Control. 4. Occupational Diseases—epidemiology.
WA 440 C872 2009]
  RC964.O246 2009
  616.9—dc22
                                                                              2008035279

Printed in the United States of America

OEM Press® is a registered trademark of OEM Health Information.

Questions or comments regarding this book should be directed to:

OEM Health Information, Inc.
8 West Street
Beverly Farms, MA 01915-2226
978-921-7300
978-921-0304 (fax)
info@oempress.com
5 4 3 2 1

This book is dedicated to the memory of

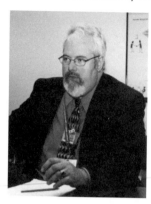

Alain J. Couturier, MD, MS, FACOEM

January 21, 1957–May 25, 2007

Dr. Couturier conceived the textbook, *Occupational and Environmental Infectious Diseases*, and was the editor of the first edition. His work on the second edition was cut short by his unexpected and sudden death. He had a distinguished career that touched many people. Dr. Couturier graduated from the University of Rhode Island with a bachelor of science degree in 1980 and received his doctor of medicine degree from Brown University School of Medicine in 1985. He was awarded a master of science degree in Health Sciences from Purdue University in 1990 and completed a residency in occupational medicine at Boston University Medical Center. His honors included election to Phi Beta Kappa and Phi Kappa Phi. Dr. Couturier was board certified in occupational medicine by the American Board of Preventive Medicine. He became a fellow of the American College of Occupational and Environmental Medicine in 1999 and was active in that organization and in its New England component. During his career he was an assistant professor in the department of family medicine at Wayne State University, served as clinical and executive director in various health networks, published actively in the field of occupational medicine, served as a medical consultant to the U.S. Department of Energy, and was formerly a member of the editorial board of *The Occupational and Environmental Medicine Report* for OEM Press. At the time of his death he was a consultant for the Unum Provident Insurance Company in Portland, Maine. He will be greatly missed by his colleagues and friends. Some will remember him as an avid Boston Red Sox fan. We are proud to carry on his legacy with publication of the second edition. He is survived by his wife, Susan, and two sons, Nicholas and Alexander.

Contents

Contributing Authors

Andrew W. Artenstein, MD
Physician-in-Chief
Department of Medicine
Director, Center for Biodefense and Emerging
    Pathogens
Memorial Hospital of Rhode Island
Associate Professor of Medicine and Community
    Health
The Warren Alpert Medical School of Brown
    University
Providence, Rhode Island
Chapter 15

Shadaba Asad, MD
Clinical Assistant Professor
The Warren Alpert School of Medicine of Brown
    University
Providence, Rhode Island
Chapter 15

Bruce A. Barron, MD, MS
Associate Professor of Environmental Medicine
University of Rochester Medical Center
Rochester, New York
Chapter 25

Karin E. Byers, MD, MS
Assistant Professor of Medicine
University of Pittsburgh Medical Center
Chapter 29

Susan O. Cassidy, MD, JD
CEO, ContourMed
McLean, Virginia
Chapter 6

Marc Croteau MD, MPH
Assistant Professor of Medicine
Division of Public Health and Population Sciences
University of Connecticut School of Medicine
Farmington, Connecticut
Chapter 37

Alain J. Couturier*
Chapter 18, 23

Douglas D'Andrea, MD, MPH
Assistant Professor
Director, Hospitalist Program
University of Connecticut School of Medicine
Farmington, Connecticut
Chapter 8

Roy L. DeHart, MD, MPH
Vanderbilt University Medical Center
Nashville, Tennessee
Chapter 36

John Ellis, MD, MPH
Business Health Solutions
Gainesville, Virginia
Chapter 31

Daymon Evans, MD, MPH
Chief of Occupational Medicine
Preventive Medicine
U.S. Army MEDDAC Headquarters
Fort Knox, Kentucky
Chapter 3, 11B

Jean Spencer Felton*
Chapter 1

Philip E. Fisher, MD
Chapter 19

Paul S. Graman, MD
Professor of Medicine
Infectious Disease Division
University of Rochester Medical Center
Rochester, New York
Chapter 14

Tee L. Guidotti, MD, MPH
Professor of Occupational and Environmental
    Medicine
Department of Medicine
School of Medicine and Public Health
George Washington University
Washington, DC
Chapter 39

*deceased

Gerri S. Hall, Ph.D.
Cleveland Clinic
Cleveland, Ohio
Chapter 2

Harold E. Hoffman, MD, FRCPC, FACOEM
University of Alberta
Edmonton, Alberta, Canada
Chapter 39

Robert P. Hurley, MD, MPH
Medical Director
General Dynamics/Electric Boat Corporation
Groton, Connecticut
Chapter 40

Jeffrey G. Jones, MD, MPH, MS
St. Francis Traveler's Health Center
Indianapolis, Indiana
Chapter 30

Geoffrey A, Kelafant*
Chapter 4

John W. Kephart, MSPH
Research Associate
NEOMA, Inc.
Mill Valley, California
Chapter 22

Ellen R. Kessler, MD, MPH
Associate Medical Director
Comprehensive Health Services, Inc.
Reston, Virginia
Chapter 5

Boris D. Lushniak, MD, MPH
Rear Admiral, USPHS
Assistant Commissioner
US Food and Drug Administration
Rockville, Maryland
Chapter 21

Paul C. Levy, MD
Professor and Vice Chairman
Department of Medicine
University of Rochester Medical Center
Rochester, New York
Chapter 14

Daniel J. Martin, MD
Director ICU/CCU
St Luke's Hospital
New Bedford, Massachusetts
Chapter 12

Jeanne M. McGregor, MD, MPH
Medical Director
Bay Health Center
Plant City, Florida
Assistant Professor and Clinical Instructor
University of South Florida, U.S.F. Health
Chapter 38

Ralph L. McLaury, MD, MPH
OEM\MMSInc.
Baton Rouge, Louisiana
Chapter 17

John D. Meyer, MD, MPH
Associate Professor
Section of Occupational/Environmental Medicine
Division of Public Health and Population Sciences
University of Connecticut School of Medicine
Farmington, Connecticut
Chapter 9

Mary Anne Morgan, MD
Senior Instructor
University of Rochester School of Medicine
Department of Pulmonary and Critical Care
Rochester, New York
Chapter 13

Marina S. Moses, DrPH, MS
Doctoral Program Director and Practicum
  Coordinator
Assistant Professor
The George Washington University School of
  Public Health and Health Services
Washington, DC
Chapter 39

Daniel A. Nackley, MD, MSc
Altoona, Pennsylvania
Chapter 17

Wendell Perry*
Chapter 18

Lou Ellen Phillips-Smith, PhD
Regulatory and Compliance Consulting Services
    (RCCS), Inc.
Vero Beach, Florida
Chapter 2

Marilyn S. Radke, MD, MPH
Director, Office of Scientific Regulatory Services
Centers for Disease Control and Prevention
Atlanta, Georgia
Chapter 4

Robert S. Rhodes, MD
CEO
Global Health Associates
West Bloomfield, Michigan
Chapter 32

Victor S. Roth, MD, MPH
Medical Director
General Motors Powertrain
Toledo, Ohio
Assistant Professor (Adjunct)
Occupational Health
University of Michigan Hospital
Ann Arbor, Michigan
Chapter 7

Jonathan S. Rutchik, MD, MPH
UCSF Division of Occupational Medicine
Private Practice
Occupational/Environmental Neurology
NEOMA.com
Mill Valley, California
Chapter 22

Edward Allen Seidel, MD
The Seidel Group
Ellicott, Maryland
Chapter 33

Gregg M. Stave, MD, JD, MP
Consultant, Occupational Medicine and
    Corporate Health
Assistant Consulting Professor
Department of Community and Family Medicine
Division of Occupational and Environmental
    Medicine
Duke University Medical Center
Durham, North Carolina
Chapter 34

Marian Swinker, MD, MPH
Director of Prospective Health
East Carolina University
Brody School of Medicine
Greenville, North Carolina
Chapter 35

Richard J. Thomas, MD, MPH
Occupational Medicine Physician
National Naval Medical Center
Bethesda, Maryland
Associate Professor Uniformed
    Services University of the Health Sciences
Department off Preventive Medicine and
    Biometrics
Bethesda, Maryland
Chapter 24

Marcia Trapé, MD, FACP, FACOEM
Associate Professor of Clinical Medicine
Medical Director
Employee Health Service
Section of Occupational and Environmental
    Medicine
Division of Public Health and Population Sciences
Department of Medicine
University of Connecticut Health Center
Farmington, Connecticut
Chapter 37

David R. Trawick, MD, PhD
Associate Professor of Medicine
Division of Pulmonary and Critical Care Medicine
University of Rochester School of Medicine and
    Dentistry
Rochester, New York
Chapter 13

Randall L. Updegrove, MD
Warren Alpert School of Medicine
Brown University
Providence, Rhode Island
Chapter 16

Mark J. Utell, MD
Professor of Medicine and Environmental
    Medicine
University of Rochester Medical Center
Rochester, New York
Chapter 25

V.M. Voge, MD, MPH
Gonzales, Texas
Chapter 19

Dorothy J. Wawrose, MD
Medical Officer
US Food and Drug Administration
Rockville, Maryland
Chapter 21

Alan L. Williams, MD
National Institute of Health
Occupational Medical Service
Bethesda, Maryland
Chapter 24

William E. Wright
President, WorkWright, Inc.
McLean, Virginia
Chapters 1, 8, 10, 11A, 18, 19, 23, 26, 27, 28

Carl N. Zenz, Jr., MD
Medical Director
U.O.P. LLC
Des Plaines, Illinois
Chapter 20

Foreword

It is a pleasure and honor to prepare a foreword for my late friend and colleague, Dr. Alain Couturier, for the new edition of his text on occupational and environmental infectious diseases. Alain and I became acquainted nearly 25 years ago when he applied for a residency position in occupational medicine at Boston University Medical Center. Alain performed extremely well in the residency and then went on to his career in occupational medicine. I will always cherish the conversations we had and the enthusiasm and compassion with which he conducted his professional responsibilities. His sense of humor, warmth, and dedication are personal qualities that made our work a pleasure. I am pleased that he developed an interest in writing and publishing and am very proud of his accomplishments, especially the extraordinary effort involved in editing a major textbook. Fortunately, Dr. Will Wright, a former classmate of mine at the Harvard School of Public Health, has stepped in admirably for Alain and has done an excellent job in editing the text and writing a few new chapters as well. Having served as an editor of a number of texts, I realize the amount of work and dedication necessary to develop a successful text such as this one. Dr. Wright should be commended for the accomplishment.

This text should be of great value for infectious disease specialists and occupational physicians with responsibilities for preventing infectious diseases in occupational settings such as medical centers and research operations and in providing advice to travelers to regions of the world in which they may be exposed to infectious agents not customary in the western world. This text offers summaries of infectious diseases—from common types, such as upper respiratory infections, to the esoteric, such as occupational plague—that are not readily available in other sources. Along with fundamentals on epidemiology and immunizations, the text addresses legal challenges, medical surveillance, and influenza, among other topics. What I find particularly valuable in this text is the extensive discussion of infectious diseases associated with business travel. This information is both presented in practical terms and is current. This text will serve as a valuable resource to libraries and physicians who are called upon to evaluate treat and prevent infectious diseases in the occupational setting.

Robert J. McCunney, MD
Boston, MA
August, 2008

Preface to Second Edition

It is an honor and pleasure for me to present this book to you. I came to work on it in gradual, unexpected steps, initially thanks to the editor of the first edition, Dr. Alain Couturier, a friend and colleague. He first asked me to write a chapter, taking a different perspective than was taken in the first edition. Having received that chapter from me and having not found authors for some other chapters, he asked me to do several more. We discussed and carried out some plans for chapter revisions, including expansion of the book's coverage of travel topics. I had a particular interest in this, having traveled to 44 countries on seven continents and overseen workers' health in remote jungle areas worldwide. Unfortunately, during this period, Alain became ill, so he asked me to be a coeditor and help to find additional authors to complete the book. After I took on this activity in early 2007, Alain died suddenly, and I became a coeditor without an editor.

The publisher asked me to carry on as editor and offered to support the project to completion; Alain's family also encouraged me. In picking up the pieces, given the time that had passed during Alain's illness, I asked authors who had submitted chapters in 2005–2006 to provide further updates. They graciously agreed to do this.

Since the first edition was published in 2000, besides Alain's untimely death, to my knowledge, three other first edition contributors have died: Dr. Jean S. Felton, Dr. Geoffrey A. Kelafant, and Dr. Wendell H. Perry. In Alain's draft of a preface, he expressed his sorrow for the loss of these fine colleagues and appreciation for their contributions to the first edition and to our profession. I second Alain's sentiments and extend them to Alain himself, who conceived the first edition and oversaw its creation. In its second edition, this book has been renamed *Couturier's Occupational and Environmental Infectious Diseases* in honor of Dr. Couturier; I have arranged for a proportion of the second edition royalties to go to his school-age children.

The second edition has been entirely updated and has many revisions and additions. There is a greater emphasis on information and resources that the primary care physician, generalist, or occupational health practitioner can use for recognition and management of infectious diseases and their risks and for coworker and employee education. Hence there is an expanded chapter on employer education, a completely new chapter on general travel medicine and prevention of illness, expanded coverage of employee education issues in many chapters, and listings of more Web resources in the chapters and appendices. The book is designed to support the physician reader's own continuing medical education, to help plan education programs and briefings, and to assist with occupational health programs' clinical, preventive, and administrative mandates.

Some readers may use this book as a reference source to look up specific items about diseases. I encourage spending time examining the chapters and resources in depth. The chapters on fundamentals, particularly laboratory methods (Chapter 2), epidemiology (Chapter 3), vaccines (Chapter 5), and legal issues (Chapter 6), are intended to be illuminating and practical. The epidemiology chapter includes important definitions of terms, information on transmission of infectious diseases, explanations of approaches to infectious disease epidemiology and prevention, and background on general principles of infectious diseases. Occupational physicians who are responsible for training employees regarding infectious disease issues will find that these and other chapters have a wealth of well-thought-out, relevant information and useful tools for carrying out their job. The epidemiology chapter is an excellent adjunct to other standard materials used to prepare for the American Board of Preventive Medicine examinations in public health and occupational medicine.

The chapters in the other sections also have been fully updated and enhanced with an eye toward providing well-organized, practical information and education materials rather than emphasizing theory. The travel-related chapters now have their own section in the book, and information on how to stay healthy while traveling is consolidated into an entirely new chapter. Chapter 27 includes new sections related to migrant, immigrant, and refugee health issues, which are becoming increasingly important for travel medicine and occupational health professionals. The sections on diseases and unique problems and settings have an expanded emphasis on globally emerging infections and international health issues, including bioterrorism and disaster preparedness, and resources for sheltering in place, quarantine issues, continuation of operations plans, and business recovery. I've found many of these chapters to be very insightful, and some are downright scary. When one describes what pathogenic microorganisms can do to people, the topics related to pandemics and plagues (e.g., influenza, plague, leprosy, and smallpox) and to topics such as anthrax, protozoans, helminths, rabies, human immunodeficiency virus (HIV), methicillin-resistant *Staphylococcus aureus* with P-VL, hemorrhagic fevers (e.g., Marburg and Ebola), extensively drug-resistant tuberculosis, and others are not for the squeamish. One comes away from immersion in these topics with a deep admiration and even awe for the simplicity, power, and elegance of these opportunistic microorganisms and their abilities to adapt in order to remain successful opportunists.

The emphasis also has been expanded to include more recognition that many infectious diseases are international or global problems and that population pressures; migrations of people, vectors, and germs; human encroachment into previously less settled areas; and climate changes are powerful forces related to infection risks. These perspectives and relevant resources are noted in many chapters, including the travel chapters and those on influenza, globally emerging infections, biological warfare and terrorism, specific disease chapters, and the expanded appendices. The approach is meant to be consistent with the World Health Organization's statement, quoted in several places in this book: "The phenomenon of globalization has altered the traditional distinction between national and international health. Very few urgent public health risks stay solely within national boundaries."

This textbook has been written with this perspective in mind and to remind medical practitioners and the patients, employees, and others we serve of the interrelatedness of humans, our shared interests, and our shared fate.

William E. Wright, MD, MSPH, MS Physiology (Occupational Medicine)
President and Medical Director, WorkWright, Inc.
Fellow, American College of Physicians
Fellow, American College of Occupational and Environmental Medicine
July, 2008

Acknowledgments

I am very grateful for the hard work and support of all my fellow authors who either updated first edition information or wrote anew. Their impressive work was done despite trying circumstances for some, including severe personal illness, job changes, moves, family disruptions, and other life events. I thank all the authors for their kindness, patience, willingness to respond to suggestions, and wonderful dedication.

I am also very grateful to my family, particularly my wife, Dr. Diana Dryer Wright, for wholeheartedly supporting this activity despite the disruptions and time demands that writing and editing entail.

I also extend sincere thanks to the OEM Press Publisher Curtis Vouwie for his guidance and support; to the Production Editor, Marty Tenney, for her expert and unflappable efficiency, focus, and attention to detail; to Dr. Christopher J. Davis, a colleague and friend, for his kind assistance identifying relevant Web-related resources in Great Britain; to Dr. Joseph S. Gots, who piqued my interest in medical school microbiology with his teaching and words to the effect that we live in a sea of feces, and the germs are winning; and to the many coworkers, patients, and clients whom I have served and helped to stay healthy and whose work and travel to remote areas of distant lands sometimes, unfortunately, proved Dr. Gots' view to be correct.

Fundamentals

1

History of Occupational Infectious Diseases

Jean Spencer Felton and William E. Wright

> There are many handicrafts and arts which cause
> those who exercise them certain pains and plagues.
>
> —*Hippocrates*

Populations today are on the move, enabled by advances in transportation and motivated by the many impacts of modern communication. Diseases previously believed to be localized geographically now spread worldwide and affect labor forces everywhere. A look into centuries past reveals the ubiquity of a broad variety of physical disorders occasioned by the inroads into the human body of a diversity of microorganisms.

The rise of terrorism, the fear of biologic warfare, the emergence of new diseases, the resistance of certain pathogens to antibiotics, and the increased frequency of natural disasters have changed the perception of both old and new disease agents. The rise in prison populations, the influx of immigrants from countries where numerous infectious diseases are endemic, and the continuing demands of business travel have fused to a great extent the long-held separateness of occupational and nonoccupational illnesses. The invasion of the business sector by communicable diseases has muddied workers' compensation coverage, often making judgments of job-relatedness extremely difficult.

The Preindustrial Age

Plagues of one disease entity or another have been recorded for centuries, even though their causes were unidentified. Thucydides, considered the greatest historian of antiquity, as early as 430 BC described an epidemic that ravaged Athens, thus strongly influencing the outcome of the Peloponnesian War [1]. The pestilence, presumably starting in Ethiopia, traveled to Egypt and then was carried by ship across the Mediterranean to Athens, bringing death to possibly two-thirds of the population and a disastrous breakdown of the citizens' and military forces' morale, the frequent concomitant of pandemics [2]. A second epidemic struck a military force led by Pericles. This epidemic is believed to have been a highly malignant form of scarlet fever or bubonic plague, typhus, smallpox, measles, or anthrax of extraordinary virulence [3].

Biblical references to individual and mass illnesses are numerous. In Exodus, one learns that the waters of the Nile "were turned to blood," "flies" appeared, as did "lice" and a "cattle murrain," "boils," "hail," "locusts," and "darkness" [4]. The book of Leviticus offers clear diagnoses of leprosy, gonorrhea, and leukorrhea, along with

3

specific directions concerning segregation of the patient, burning of bedclothes, and disinfection [5]. Forewarnings of cholera epidemics, related to polluted water and contaminated foodstuffs, are rife in Leviticus in its references to the dangers of "unclean" cooking vessels, "flying creeping" things, and animal carcasses [6].

Plagues persisted through the years, and the returning Crusaders in the eleventh, twelfth, and thirteenth centuries brought leprosy to Europe, where the disease had always been endemic but at low levels. The number of lepers increased tremendously in Europe during the Middle Ages, although the stigmatization of leprosy was mistakenly attached to a variety of other dermatologic disorders. While not all were contagious, people called *lepers* were completely ostracized from society; distinctive clothing to identify them became mandatory, and their segregation was strictly imposed in places of public assembly or worship [7]. An unwelcome "import" brought back to Europe by the Crusaders was the Black Death, or bubonic plague. Oddly, the fierce Tartars, with some understanding of this scourge's contagion, after attacking a city in the southeast Crimea, on their departure catapulted into the city corpses of soldiers who had died of plague [8].

In the years between AD 540 and 1666, there were three great pandemics: the plague of Justinian in the years 540–590, the Black Death of 1346–1361, and the pandemic that raged in Europe from 1665–1666 and produced the Great Plague of London [9]. At some point during the first and last of these three pandemics, the mode of transmission in pandemics changed from the rat-flea-human cycle of bubonic plague to the predominantly more severe pneumonic form of the disease.

Although the belief that the miasma arising from the earth was the cause of disease was prevalent as late as the seventeenth century, a century earlier, in 1546, Fracastoro identified contagion as the principal factor responsible for the rise and spread of epidemic disease, a conclusion reached after his study of plague, typhus fever, syphilis, and other communicable disorders [10]. His treatise, *De Contagione eet Contagiosis Morbis et Eorum Curatione,* is the first scientific statement on the true nature of contagion and the transmission of diseases by "germs" [11]. This work was translated into English by Wilmer Cave Wright [12], who was later

encouraged to translate Ramazzini's classic work into English, thus making it the standard contemporary reference and Ramazzini the so-called father of occupational medicine. Further, it was Fracastoro who introduced *syphilis* as the first designation given the disease; the term was derived from the name of a shepherd infected with the disease who figured in a medical poem Fracastoro wrote in 1530 [13].

It was Antony van Leeuwenhoek (1632–1723), a linen draper in Delft who developed the microscope, who initially observed bacteria and other microscopic organisms. He described forms known today as *cocci, bacilli,* and *spirilla* [14] but did not make a connection between these "little animals," as he referred to them, and disease. Although there were suggestions concerning this relationship, it was not until the 1830s and 1840s that the germ theory of disease was revived on the basis of new evidence [15]. An early connection between infectious disease and work emerged about the same period. *Fever* was a portmanteau term used for typhoid, typhus, and relapsing fevers. Severe outbreaks of these infections were seen in the early decades of the nineteenth century in Ireland and then in Scotland and England. There was awareness of an economic deficit because these disorders affected workers. Each individual, it was estimated, lost an average of 6 weeks of employment, and for nearly 13,000 patients at the Glasgow Fever Hospital, this totaled £29,004. Added to this sum was the cost of medical and nursing care at £1 per patient. The funeral costs for some and provision for the surviving widows and orphans further raised the debit, all of this stimulating action toward a better public health [16].

Occupational medicine, as a discrete medical discipline in the health care world, was not given substance until 1700, when Bernardino Ramazzini of Modena, Italy, produced the first edition of *Diseases of Workers.* Although sparse writings had appeared earlier, it was this *De Morbis Artificum Diatriba* that offered a view of the work-related illnesses seen in over 50 distinct trades and occupations. As mentioned previously, it was Wright's excellent translation that made this work available to the English-speaking world despite earlier literary appearances in that language [17].

Infectious diseases had yet to be identified in microbiologic terms, but Ramazzini did write of the hazards of military service. "[A]rmies are almost always decimated by some malignant epidemic. Camp fevers . . . and other fatal and contagious diseases are famous or rather infamous" [18]. He cited a Greek military surgeon who, apart from wounds, classifies camp diseases as malignant fever or dysentery and concluded that "the morbific seed of malignity that breeds and fosters camp fever is harbored in corrupt and polluted air" [19]. Sailors and seafarers were subject to "malignant and pestilential fevers" [20], and hunters experienced "day cholera" [21]. Common to many trades, Ramazzini indicated, is terminal "consumption," as seen in glass workers [22], wet nurses [23], stone cutters [24], and silk carders [25]. He cautioned of laundresses' contact with "a thousand kinds of filth from persons . . . polluted with the French disease [syphilis]" and wrote that treatment should "dislodge the gross humors" [26].

It cannot be said that the terms used in Ramazzini's day are the equivalents of today's nosology, but the clinical descriptions of various fevers do parallel some of our current infectious disorders. Not clarified, of course, is the source of the organisms— fellow workers, fomites, the environment, or impaired personal hygiene? In view of the working conditions of the times, it may be concluded that many of the disease states indicated were inherent in these early jobs.

The Industrial Age

Although the calendar marks with stunning accuracy the passage of time, the name given a particular historic era is arbitrary and usually imposed by social historians long after the beginning of the era. In the mid-nineteenth century, at the beginning of what came to be called the *Industrial Age,* many inventions of power machinery, such as Watt's steam engine and Cartwright's power loom, led to changes in the processes used to produce goods. As the eminent British sociologist Arnold Toynbee expressed, "It was by these discoveries that population was drawn out of cottages in distant valleys by secluded streams and driven together into factories and cities" [27]. Or, as stated by his equally famed nephew, Arnold Joseph Toynbee, the period was characterized by "[t]he deliberate application of science to technology" [28].

The term *Industrial Revolution* was coined by the French in the 1830s to describe the change from an agrarian economy to an industrial one in which goods were produced in city factories by machines of mass production. The movement of the masses from farms to cities began in the 1700s in Britain, for the country was then free from wars [29]. The significance of this relocation in regard to infectious disease lies in the sudden congestion in cities of great numbers of persons accustomed to farm living. With the crowding came long hours of work, child labor, the absence of sanitary measures, the creation of slums, the appearance of occupational diseases, and indubitably, the loss of health or life to the invasion of as yet unidentified microorganisms.

The early observers of the interaction of work and health began to see, as did Ramazzini in his day, the devastating effects on workers, whether artisans, laborers, or professionals. One of the first physicians to be concerned with the adverse effects of labor was Charles Turner Thackrah, "born . . . into a society which was distinguished by the profound juxtaposition of wealth and poverty which prevailed at the time" [30]. His work, *The Effects of Arts, Trades, and Professions,* appeared in 1832 [31]. Thackrah died of chronic pulmonary tuberculosis, as did such notable contemporaries as John Hunter and John Keats [32]. The disease was then a common fatal infection of dissecting-room students. Thackrah published early on the subject of cholera and later wrote about sexually transmitted diseases, "I scarcely need advert to the diseases of the genital organs more frequent in soldiers and sailors than in most classes of society" [33]. He also noted that sugar refiners died of tuberculosis [34] and that surgeons and accoucheurs were predisposed in the discharge of their professional duties to the absorption of "syphilitic poison" and its ultimate lethal effects [35]. The latter observation was made long before the identification of the causative *Treponema pallidum* by the microscopist Schaudinn in 1905 [36].

The Factory System and Its Ills

The growth and multiplication of factories continued at a rapid pace during the early nineteenth century, accompanied by the deleterious effects on workers, both adults and children. Although the presence of illness among factory employees was noted by the factory owners and physicians of the day, etiologic clarity was lacking. A practitioner of the period, when asked his opinion concerning the medical effects produced by the hours of labor, responded, "The first effects appear to be upon the digestion, the appetite suffers, the digestion is impaired, and consequent emaciation and debility are induced. Scrofulous diseases are common . . ." [37]. Medical opinions differed as to causation by various exposures in factory settings, some physicians even believing that work in certain plants actually was beneficial and cured disease. Because of the endemicity of so many of the infectious diseases in urban areas, it would be difficult to differentiate an occupational disease from a contagious disorder rampant in the community or to identify "cotton-consumption" or "cotton inflammation of the lungs" [38] specifically as today's byssinosis or byssinosis compounded by tuberculosis. Were the diseases brought into the factories from the totally unsanitary living areas, or were the pneumoconioses that were produced in the manufacturing processes worsened by the endemic "scrofula" of the cities [39]?

A nineteenth-century description of a worker implies a body subject to the invasion of any infectious agent: "These artisans are frequently subject to a disease, in which the sensibility of the stomach and bowels is morbidly excited; the alvine secretions are deranged, and the appetite impaired. Whilst this state continues, the patient loses flesh, his features are sharpened, the skin becomes pale, leaden colored, or of the yellow hue which is observed in those who have suffered from the influence of tropical climates." Following are "the horrors of a disordered imagination, . . . gloomy apprehension, the deepest depression, and . . . despair" [40]. Of the many conditions predisposing to "contagious disease," "extreme labor" and its consequent physical exhaustion were cited [41].

As the nineteenth century approached its close, discerning physicians began to document the afflictions arising in industry. One of the early practitioners concerned with factory medicine was John Thomas Arlidge, whose monograph appeared in 1892 [42]. This magnum opus fell into almost complete oblivion for about 50 years. Like so many dedicated specialists in occupational medicine, Arledge was ostracized "for what was considered to be illegitimate interference with deplorable factory conditions which he had ample opportunity to observe

as a certifying factory surgeon for Stoke, Longton, and Fenton" [43]. In his discussion of organic dust of an animal nature and the manufacture of wool, he wrote of anthrax, then called *wool-sorters' disease*. The rapidity of the disease course was noted; in some instances, death ensued in 19 hours. Of interest also was the case of a mohair sorter's wife, who had not been within half a mile of the mill but developed fatal anthrax of the face [44].

An important tome edited by another British physician, Thomas Oliver, and published in 1902 included an extensive discussion of infectious diseases associated with work [45]. A full chapter was devoted to the diseases of soldiers, including malaria, dysentery, typhoid fever, and cholera. The author of the chapter, John R. Dodd of the Royal Army Medical Corps, pointed out that in the Crimean War, three times as many British troops died of sickness as those who died at the hands of the Russians. Further, because of the accompanying illnesses, he referred to the Ashanti Expeditions into West Africa as *doctors' wars* [46].

Seamen were subject to malaria, yellow fever, dysentery, cholera, plague, and "phthisis." Regrettably, men were allowed to "sign on" as mariners with no inquiry as to their physical fitness for the occupation [47]. Among stable personnel, glanders and its more chronic and constitutional lymphatic form, farcy, were noted, along with tetanus and rabies. Anthrax, vaccinia, tuberculosis, tinea, foot and mouth disease, diphtheria, actinomycosis, and trichinosis were some of the zoonoses to which animal handlers were subject [48].

Upholsterers occasionally had to remake used mattresses, and it was found that when "mattresses have become fouled in places by discharges from patients suffering from infectious diseases, considerable risk is incurred by those who by hand teaze the contents of such bespoiled bedding" [49].

In the late years of the nineteenth century, various legislative actions were taken in England, raising the allowable age at which children could be employed, giving greater power to central authority in the regulation of certain trades, and extending the coverage provided by earlier workers' compensation acts. Oliver, in his 1908 text, expressed some cynicism about the laws passed. He wrote, "In this country industrial legislation is based upon experience and expediency, so that no sooner is an Act in operation than its weak points become apparent and a fresh Act is required to remedy defects and remove flaws, but it too generally ends in introducing controversial matter and in providing employment of lawyers and doctors" [50]. A lengthy chapter was devoted to "Diseases Due to Parasites and Micro-Organisms," much of the discussion relating to ankylostomiasis, particularly because the infestation affected numerous miners in the construction of the St. Gothard Tunnel in Switzerland. In connection with the spread of the illness, Oliver commented that, "Probably one diseased and thoughtless miner is capable of infecting a mine owing to the myriads of ova passed in his stools" [51]. The military were similarly stricken by hookworm disease.

Hospital nurses worked in hazardous conditions because the infirmary wards were poorly ventilated. Many of the nurses suffered from "hospital throat," and those attending patients with infectious diseases could acquire the disorder. Small finger wounds became infected with resulting bacteremia, and tuberculosis was transmitted to the attendant staff through bad handling of the patients' sputum. Physicians ran comparable risks through their "treatment of abscesses and foul wounds in operation" [52].

American Workers

It was noted in the Memorial of Occupational Diseases sent to President Taft in June 1910 by the First National Conference on Industrial Diseases that nearly all the standard reference works on occupational diseases were prepared by English or Continental authorities [53]. To fill this gap, a work was undertaken by Dr. W. Gilman Thompson of Cornell University Medical College in New York. *The Occupational Diseases*, published in 1914, was directed not only to physicians but also to those individuals in various manufactures or trades "in which the health of the workman is closely related to problems of efficiency and humanitarian effort" [54]. Thompson had published extensively before, had established clinics dedicated to occupational disease, and was active on the visiting staffs of New York's largest hospitals.

He, like others, was concerned with tuberculosis and its high mortality among workers [55], and in his discussion of diseases owing to irritant substances, he included a section entitled, "Germs."

Ankylostomiasis, anthrax, foot and mouth disease (aphthous fever), glanders, and farcy were reviewed, as was the "septicemia" incurred by those handling "putrid or decomposing animal products" [56], such as in the making of bone fertilizers from the carcasses of dead horses. Not touched on previously was localized tuberculosis (verruca necrogenica) of the hands and forearms of butchers inoculated through the handling of tuberculous cattle [57]. Thompson advocated the early treatment of syphilis (not necessarily an occupationally acquired disease) because lead poisoning in a patient with syphilis could present "symptoms of unusual gravity" [58].

Dr. George M. Price of New York was closely involved in sanitation controls within the clothing industry and by 1914 believed that tuberculosis was the main end result of the transmission of microorganisms via coughing, sneezing, salivation, and the like in the workplace. He felt that tubercle bacilli were ubiquitous in all industrial plants and that workers already suffering from pulmonary infections or those with dust-laden lungs had no immune resistance to "tuberculous phthisis" [53].

Building on American experience was not easy, for Dr. George M. Kober of Washington, DC, refused a publishers' request in 1911 to produce a book on occupational diseases because "the scarcity of statistical data in reference to disease and accident-hazards in the various occupations in this country, had compelled him in his former writings to get most of his facts from Europe and the State of Massachusetts" [59]. However, 1916 saw the production of Kober and Hanson's nearly 1,000-page volume, which sold for $8 [60]. Anthrax and pulmonary anthrax were reviewed at length [61], and a separate chapter entitled, "Parasites and Occupation," was included. In that chapter, malaria, amebic dysentery, uncinariasis, filariasis, trichinosis, infestation with *Ascaris lumbricoides*, and schistosomiasis were assessed as occupational diseases [62]. The occupational devastation caused by malaria was described as having "been the greatest obstacle to colonization of the tropics by the white race; it has transformed fertile, rich and populous regions into lonely wastes; it has rendered the development of valuable natural resources impossible and by decimating armies has defeated the highest hopes of nations in critical struggles" [62]. The French failure in the construction of a canal in Panama gives substance to this observation. Tuberculosis was discussed as a disease resulting from the continuous and considerable exposure to industrial dust [63].

World War I

Although there had been epidemics of influenza throughout history—in 412 BC, Hippocrates chronicled a flulike disease that obliterated an Athenian army [64]—none manifested the mortality of the scourge of 1918. The disease hit the New World in 1647, coming from Valencia, Spain, and was promptly dubbed *Spanish influenza* (*influence* in Italian). Later, in 1918, the disease had killed more people within days than all the World War I armies in 4 years of fighting. By December, 500,000 Americans had perished, and nearly 20,000,000 had contracted the disease. Attending nurses and volunteers died alongside the patients in their care. The epidemic started on March 11 at Fort Riley, Kansas, and soon after the first patient was stricken, there was an explosive outbreak [65]. Influenza spread throughout Europe after our troops landed in France; 132 cases were reported within 12 days of their arrival. The outbreak was rampant on ships and trains and in army camps and naval hospitals, where people were together in close proximity. An army transport landing troops in England soon had 2,300 ill with influenza, 119 of whom died. Tightly packed troop compartments provided unmatched "culture" conditions for the disease-causing pathogen. After rampaging through the Western world, the disease struck Asia.

In the United States, worker after worker succumbed in the Quincy, Massachusetts, shipyards. Dozens of army camps were affected, and medical care did not alter the spread of the epidemic. Masks were ordered for universal wear; this writer remembers having to don a mask whenever leaving his house in San Francisco, where one-fourth of California's 40,000 cases occurred. All industries were losing employees to influenza: Washington's federal agencies, packing plants, street transportation, East Coast and Gulf Coast shipyards, gold and coal mines, hospitals, and plantations. Public gathering places were closed. All manner of treatment modalities and cures were proffered without effect.

The Navy had been hit badly, with 120,000 of its personnel—one-fourth of its total—being stricken, 5,000 dying. The Army, 10 times the size of the

other service, lost 25,000. Residents of Dublin died at a rate of 250 a day [66]. When the Armistice was signed in November, the siege slackened. At its height, though, one health department was advised, "Hunt up your woodworkers and cabinetmakers and set them making coffins." Later, "[t]hen take your street laborers and set them to digging graves" [67]. With more than 25 million Americans infected, perhaps a billion worldwide, the direct U.S. economic losses were estimated at $3 billion, but it is believed that the epidemic ultimately cost the United States alone 10 million years in productive lives cut off at their prime [67]. Was the pandemic one of occupationally incurred infectious disease because fellow workers transmitted the illness? Was it a community epidemic unrelated to work? Servicemen were workers. Health care personnel were workers. Family members were workers. While the insurance payments going to policyholders were high, no exact data seem to be available that would divide the morbidity or mortality into job-relatedness or nonoccupational illness. It is hoped that no comparable epidemiologic "opportunity" to help answer these questions will arise again.

Between the Wars

In 1920, Dr. Harry E. Mock, a medical officer in World War I and afterward chief surgeon (medical director) of Sears, Roebuck & Company in Chicago, amassed the collective knowledge of occupational medicine current at that time in his book, *Industrial Medicine and Surgery* [68]. By then, the infectious diseases previously described had become common knowledge. In a 15,000-employee company in Chicago, 44 cases of infectious disease were encountered, including mumps (22), scarlet fever (9), diphtheria (6), measles (4), erysipelas (2), and varicella (1) [69]. Typhoid fever and smallpox were discussed, with emphasis placed on preventive vaccination.

Mock indicated that the combating of venereal diseases among employees had been woefully neglected by the majority of physicians in industry. Accounting for this lack of attention were the indifferent attitude that the medical profession always had assumed toward prevention of these diseases and the fact that the employees so affected, when discovered, were discharged. Mock advocated an emphasis on employee education, and some statements selected from a poster used for this purpose are of interest [70]:

- Prevention: (1) Keep away from prostitutes, both professional and non-professional. (2) Sexual intercourse is not necessary to physical and mental health. (3) Antiseptic washes . . . are not always reliable.
- Beware of advertising specialists who claim to cure "nervous debility" and "private diseases of men." Advertising specialists get large sums of money for "diseases" which do not exist.
- What to do (apart from reporting to a physician). Do not worry. Lead a vigorous, healthful life and forget about sex matters. Be consistent and adopt the same standard of sexual conduct for yourself that you expect of women.

In light of contemporary responses by the media to matters sexual and today's advertising emphasis on sex to sell everything and anything, one can conjure up employees' reactions to these precautions of 1920.

Tuberculosis in industry was faced by Mock and other physicians of the period, and they advocated avoiding overcrowding in the workplace, improving ventilation, removing dust, and examining employees. Discussed at length were the industrial pneumoconioses that predisposed to the acquisition of tuberculosis. Frequent examination, provision of sanatorium care, visiting nurse services, and reemployment of the healed employee were strongly advocated [71].

Last, concern was expressed regarding the Americanization of foreign employees and the industrial physician's role in such a program. The same points arise today: standard of living, language barriers, crowding in urban ethnic or national enclaves, inadequate wages, and the like. Mock advised bilingual posters, education, instruction regarding personal hygiene and sanitation, and access to medical care [72].

Sir Thomas M. Legge was Britain's first Medical Inspector of Factories, assuming the post in 1898. Early on, he directed his attention to anthrax [73], but most of his career was devoted to the industrial diseases arising from contact with workplace metals, dusts, organic compounds, and the usual broad variety of other toxic substances. In a work published posthumously, Legge reviewed the hazards of anthrax and tetanus and gave consideration to silicosis accompanied by tuberculosis. He wrote,

"Stress is rightly laid on the fact that the bacillus tuberculosis, whether in the lung before the onset of the damage, during it, or entering after, is of paramount importance in influencing unfavorably the subsequent development of the disease" [74]. In addition, he noted the undue incidence of phthisis among persons employed in brass working [75].

Late in the 1930s, Dr. H. M. Vernon, long identified with occupational medicine, produced a somewhat broader text emphasizing "health" as a goal as well as touching on anthrax in wool sorters [76], the high death rate in laundry workers from tuberculosis [77], and the combination of silicosis and tuberculosis [78, 79].

World War II

The production of armaments and material needed for World War II led to the conversion of many peacetime plants and the construction of new facilities throughout the allied countries. Women, the disabled, and older personnel were added to company rosters, and because of the burgeoning of manufacturing sites, occupational health services were added to worker rosters not only because of the increased labor force—coming from all areas—but also because of the use and production of innumerable toxic materials. By this time, many protective vaccines had been developed, and a broad variety was being administered to military personnel and some to civilian workers. The unidentified plants of the Manhattan District Project focused medical attention on the possible effects of exposure to radioactive sources—"the product"—rather than on specific groups of diseases. In the *Manual of Standard Practices for Industrial Nurses* used at the Hanford Engineer Works in Richland, Washington, however, two of the indicated procedures involved "communicable disease regulations" and "reportable diseases" [80]. No details have remained for review.

Acceptance into the armed services during the early phases of World War II was in keeping with some stringent physical standards. Active tuberculosis in the Army during those years was 1.24 per thousand, about one-ninth that of World War I. Potential Army inductees who had venereal disease (syphilis) were classified as limited service, but none of these were actually inducted until July 1942. Gonorrhea was considered a remedial defect, and such registrants were temporarily deferred until cured. With a liberalization of standards, somewhat over 200,000 registrants with venereal disease were inducted [81]. Men with other acute infectious diseases were deferred until recovery, without disqualifying sequelae. Certain parasitic infections were allowed in registrants, and treatment was initiated, but filariasis, trypanosomiasis, amebiasis, and schistosomiasis were causes for rejection [82].

Many of the immunizations given service personnel predated World War II, but the vaccinations performed also included typhoid-paratyphoid, smallpox, tetanus, yellow fever, cholera, plague, typhus, influenza, and Japanese B encephalitis. Protection for special situations included diphtheria and Rocky Mountain spotted fever immunizations. Human immune serum globulin was used for passive protection against measles and viral hepatitis, and extremely rarely, scarlet fever streptococcus toxin was administered to certain health care personnel [83].

The status of occupational medicine at the time of World War II was expressed by Cook [84] in this manner: "[The] principles of democracy and of economics had integrated industry, labor, and hygiene, at least in the United States, and raised all three to a national level of mutual concern. Research in this area had developed sufficiently for its emphasis to change from inquiry into causes of occupational disease to the anticipation and correction of hazardous conditions."

A wartime publication by Clarence O. Sappington, a prolific writer of the period, was one of the few monographs covering all aspects of occupational medicine until the freshet of monographs appeared after the passage of the Occupational Safety and Health Act in 1970. Sappington remarked that both localized and systemic infections are frequently of occupational origin and listed some 14 disorders and the workers in whom such diseases may be found. For example, he cited psittacosis (bacteriologists and parrot and parakeet handlers) and tetanus (farmers and slaughterhouse and packinghouse workers) [85].

The Postwar Years

During the postwar years, Dr. Rutherford T. Johnstone, a highly respected occupational medicine pi-

oneer in southern California, wrote extensively, producing two textbooks, probably the only ones available to students for many years. In the first, bearing the date of 1948, covering primarily occupationally hazardous materials, tuberculosis was treated as a work-related disease, apart from the disorder in some health care workers and in workers exposed to free silicon dioxide, a relationship alluded to earlier [86].

In Johnstone's second work, an entire chapter reviewed infectious occupational diseases and addressed the question of their rising out of and in the course of employment. The diseases discussed included brucellosis, tularemia, anthrax, erysipeloid, psittacosis, Q fever, equine encephalomyelitis, and mite dermatitis. Those specific infections acquired from a contaminated work environment encompassed histoplasmosis, coccidioidomycosis, blastomycosis, creeping eruption, tetanus, leptospirosis, and schistosomiasis. In summary, Johnstone indicated that "under special circumstances, the infections of ordinary life may become occupational diseases" [87].

The Later Decades of the Twentieth Century

In 1955, the dean of occupational physicians in Great Britain, Dr. Donald Hunter of the London Hospital, produced the first edition of his eponymous classic, the most recent appearing in 1994. Even in the seminal work, Hunter included a heavily illustrated chapter entitled, "Occupational Diseases Due to Infections," naming most of the illnesses described by earlier writers. In recent editions, an entire section is devoted to diseases associated with microbiologic agents (e.g., bacteria, viruses, and biotechnologic hazards), with emphasis on laboratory-acquired infections [88]. While allusions to the infectious diseases potentially acquired by a work force are still touched on in contemporary writings, new fears have arisen throughout the world, occasioned by serious epidemics, contacts with affected populations from endemic areas, and the sequelae of natural disasters. History blends irrevocably into the present as it is learned that infectious disease mortality has been increasing in the United States [89]. These disorders currently are recognized as having an industrial presence, and special attention is now being directed toward health care workers [90–96].

New infectious diseases are emerging, and certain of the once-conquered illnesses are reappearing [97–99]. Some of the determinants in the recrudescence of the old and the arrival of the new are global warming, human migration, population increases, deforestation, poverty, disruption of environmental habitats, the emergence of antibiotic-resistant bacteria, the increase in international travel, and the lack of precautions in many almost-primitive health care facilities [100].

Different work groups, such as the military, the Coast Guard, and international relief personnel, are being exposed to communicable diseases through the extension of aid to refugees and the rescue of migrants [101–103]. The potential for infectious spread is also seen in day-care centers [104], in competitive sports [105], and following natural disasters [106]. The emergence of Ebola hemorrhagic fever, the continuing HIV epidemic, the variant of Creutzfeldt-Jakob disease in the United Kingdom, and the effects of the invasion of hantavirus pale in comparison with the potential for mass casualties through bioterrorism. Biologic warfare technology can involve the use of anthrax spores, botulinum toxin, aflatoxin, or a modified *Yersinia pestis*, the plague bacterium [107]. The medical effects of biologic terrorism can be extreme [108], and as noted by one who conducts studies of agents of terrorism, "Biological weapons are . . . not detected by methods used for explosives and firearms, such as metal detectors and x-ray devices. Moreover, because the first indication of an attack is likely to be hours to days after exposure—when people first begin to develop disease symptoms—the perpetrators can be long gone from the scene before health and law enforcement authorities are aware there is a problem" [109]. American troops have already been given anthrax vaccine in Bosnia [110], Russia has an altered form of anthrax [111], and Iraq reputedly has 2,000 gallons of anthrax [112].

That there is some fear among health care workers of the contagion of infectious diseases—even at the individual, let alone mass, level—is evident in the reluctance of physicians and nurses to perform mouth-to-mouth resuscitation (MMR). Of the physicians, 45%, and of the nurses, 80%, would refuse to do MMR on a stranger. Between 18% and 25% of the two groups would not conduct MMR on a child [113]. In a second study, 82% of the nearly 1,000 persons queried were at least "moderately" concerned about disease transmission in the performance of bystander MMR [114].

Further fear within the United States stems from terrorist activities carried out in the form of the contamination of food with microbiologic agents. Deliberate inoculation of foodstuffs resulted in type 2 *Shigella dysenteriae* infection and salmonellosis in health care workers. The act was initiated by a religious cult in one instance and by someone with laboratory skills in the other [115,116].

The military view is expressed succinctly: "The possibility that biological weapons will be used against us is no longer unthinkable. Until recently, medical officers and other healthcare practitioners may have considered this topic more suitable for academic than practical pursuit. The fact is, however, that biological agents have been used as weapons since antiquity, and the threat that modern weapons will be used is real" [118].

In a summation of bioterrorism, it can be concluded, as set forth in a federal report, that "no government spending priorities for combating terrorism have been set, and no federal entity exists to channel resources where they are most needed and to prevent wasteful spending resulting from unnecessary duplication of effort" [116].

Update for the Second Edition

My now-deceased former colleague, mentor, and friend, Dr. Jean S. Felton, wrote this chapter about 10 years ago. His writing details a number of historic plagues, pandemics, and occupational concerns and foreshadows some of the events, evolution of infectious disease issues, and surveillance activities in occupational medicine that followed publication of the first edition of this book, particularly in reference to biologic weapons, global issues, and the importance of international cooperation.

Since the first edition, a number of noteworthy international activities have occurred related to occupational and environmental infectious diseases, many covered in further detail in the following chapters. The World Health Organization's initiatives and cooperative efforts with a number of nations to address the biblical, medieval, and ongoing scourge of leprosy deserve mention. Surveillance efforts and free multidrug treatment have resulted in elimination of this disease as a significant health problem in 113 nations [119]. A 2003 outbreak of a previously unknown coronavirus resulted in an illness, designated as *severe acute respiratory syndrome* (SARS, caused by SARS-CoV), which originated in China and spread to 29 countries in Asia, the Middle East, Africa, Europe, and the Americas. The syndrome had an about 10% overall case fatality rate and a 50% case fatality rate in elderly victims. It included occupation-related deaths. The outbreak was contained as a result of international cooperation in public health efforts of rapid case detection, contact investigations, patient isolation, and community quarantine. Experience with SARS reinforced and helped to improve standardized methods to protect health care workers, first responders, and emergency personnel from infectious threats. Recently, intense cooperative international efforts have been focused on tracking and containing a new, particularly lethal H5N1 influenza virus (avian flu) in order to avert another pandemic influenza. Unprecedented global surveillance and interventions in cases occurring in humans have been and are being carried out to contain and minimize the threat. These efforts have included improving and increasing capacity to make and distribute protective vaccines for influenza generally, as well as to develop vaccines related to potential pandemics. The world waits to see how effective these efforts will be. In other international efforts, the World Health Organization, the Global Fund to Fight AIDS, Tuberculosis, and Malaria, and many cooperating nations, through a combination of insecticide use, netting, education, early diagnosis, and provision of medications, have made inroads into malaria's widespread morbidity and mortality in African nations, resulting in lower childhood malaria incidence rates in Tanzania, Ethiopia, Rwanda, Zambia, and other countries [120].

In the United States, vaccination efforts have virtually eliminated endemic rubella and congenital rubella syndrome [121], measles case incidence has declined dramatically, and tuberculosis rates that rose in the 1980s and early 1990s have been decreasing. Resurgence of pertussis infections has resulted in modification of immunization protocols, and a 2006 mumps outbreak in 11 states resulted in new guidelines to target susceptible populations. Owing to strides in treatment, estimates of the number of people living with AIDS in the United States are increasing, as well as the number well enough to continue to work; to date, there have been no occupational HIV infectons reported since 2001. However, multiple-drug-resistant tuberculosis, outbreaks of methicillin-resistant *Staphylococcus aureas*, and dengue continue to be of concern. The first edition of this book had no listing of information on West Nile virus. This mosquito-borne disease was unintentionally imported into the United States in New York City in 1999, resulting in bird kills and human illness ranging from a mild febrile illness to meningoencephalitis. Since then, it has spread to birds in every state of the continental United States (with cases of the human neuroinvasive form being reported in about 90% of states) [122] and to Canada.

Despite advances, many of these and other diseases continue to be devastating in countries that lack sufficient infrastructure and resources for treatment and containment. The increases in population migration and travel, including occupational travel, contribute to new case occurrences and outbreaks in the United States and other countries. HIV continues to be an important worldwide problem, as does malaria, tuberculosis, diseases common to childhood, various causes of gastroenteritis/diarrheal disease, other protozoal and helminthic disease, and emerging viral diseases. The World Health Organization reports outbreaks of Marburg virus (The Democratic Republic of the Congo 1998–2000 and Angola 2005) and Ebola (from 2000 to 2007, outbreaks occurred in Uganda, Gabon, the Republic of the Congo, Sudan, and the Democratic Republic of the Congo) with devastatingly high mortality [123].

Since publication of the first edition, several other events deserve mention because of their importance to occupational health and public health. In 2001, the United States sustained an intentional attack by mail with weaponized inhalational anthrax that resulted in occupational and nonoccupational deaths and a need for extensive decontamination of postal facilities and some offices. Thereafter, the United States and other countries have been subject to "white powder" hoaxes and scares, and increasing international resources have been devoted to disaster planning, education of health care providers and the general public about biologic hazards, and research on and protection from biologic weapons, including smallpox, with consideration of revaccination of susceptible populations (see also Chap. 39). The world also has had to deal with mass-casualty situations from deadly large-scale terrorist activities and from natural disasters. In the United States, the 2001 terrorist attacks on New York City's World Trade Center and Washington, DC's Pentagon, which also involved a downed aircraft in Pennsylvania, resulted in thousands of deaths and special infectious disease and other health risks for emergency personnel. Large-scale revamping of surveillance and interventions related to terrorist activity occurred worldwide. Terrorist attacks or bombings in other parts of the world include Iraq, with onset of war that was mounted there in part because of suspected stores of weaponized biologic materials, and other countries throughout the Middle East, Bali (2002), Jakarta (2002–2004), Mumbai (2003), Thailand (2004–2006), Madrid (2005), West Darfur (2008), and others. The natural disaster involving hurricane Katrina in the United States (New Orleans and surrounding areas) in 2005 was devastating but helped raise awareness in the United States of many natural disaster–related health issues, including infectious disease issues for emergency workers and the need for improved disaster preparedness for the general public. Around the world, other prominent natural disasters with similar issues and consequences include the Bolivian earthquake in 1998, the Mt. Papandayan volcano eruption in Indonesia in 2002, the Aceh earthquake and tsunami in Asia in 2004, the Indonesian Java earthquake in 2006, and others. These and other situations have involved cooperative actions to contain occupational and nonoccupational communicable disease risks in the most trying of settings, which include working with severely injured people and animals, dealing with corpses and body parts, and adjusting to damaged medical facilities, disrupted intrastructure and transportation systems, disrupted water/sewage systems, food and water shortages, climate exposures, postevent social disruptions, population displacements, and related challenges to coordination of responses.

In short, the intervening years have been marked by successes, setbacks, and disasters in dealing with communicable disease problems. These affect the occupational setting, capabilities for work, and nonoccupational human activities. The increase in world travel and global trade, human migration and displacements, and further encroachment of higher-density human populations into rural or jungle areas continue to increase the likelihood of communicable disease transmission. The past and current history reflect the power of the unquenchable human spirit and resourcefulness in dealing with communicable diseases and evoke admiration of the simple elegance, power, and adaptability of microorganisms that are such splendid opportunists.

The Future

Concerns about infectious diseases contracted in the workplace have coursed from minimal interest in common disorders brought by workers to their workplaces to an acceptance of some illnesses as concomitants or sequelae of many industrial exposures. While knowledgeable occupational health practitioners can inform or educate those persons whose daily tasks involve contact with pathogenic agents, there are not sufficient professional resources available to reach the solitary, immigrant, or remote workers subject to disease acquisition. The way to the future is clearly through a collaboration among occupational medicine, businesses, public health practitioners, governments, and nations to limit and control infectious disease problems in the workplace and general environment. The World Health Organization in its information on the current revision of the international health regulations stated: "The phenomenon of globalization has altered the traditional distinction between national and international health. Very few urgent public health risks stay solely within national boundaries." In this vein, the director general of the World Health Organization, Margaret Chan, reminded us: "No country can shield itself from invasion by a pathogen incubating in an airline passenger or an insect hiding in a cargo hold" [124]. The old and the new in infectious diseases will remain until an international surveillance system is implemented and fully supported to enable the mobilization of an effective global response when infectious outbreaks occur and when opportunities for control or elimination of serious endemic diseases can be identified. May historic transmittable diseases be eliminated from contemporary worksites and may the fears of world

contamination be replaced by international understanding and cooperation.

References

1. Petersen EA, Mandel RM. Infectious diseases: Old
   diseases return and new agents emerge. *Arch Intern
   Med* 1995;155:1571–2.
2. Cartwright FF. *Disease and History.* New York:
   Crowell, 1972, p 7.
3. *Ibid.,* p 8.
4. Exodus 7–10; Keller W. *The Bible as History,* 2d rev
   ed. New York: William Morrow, 1981, p 124.
5. Leviticus 13–15; Anon. The bible and medicine. *MD*
   1978;22:87–99.
6. Leviticus 11:3–47; Brim CJ. *Medicine in the Bible:
   The Pentateuch.* New York: Froben Press, 1936,
   pp 124–5.
7. Lyons AS, Petrucelli J II. *Medicine: An Illustrated History.* New York: Abrams, 1978, p 345.
8. *Ibid.,* p 349.
9. Ref 2, *supra,* pp 31–2.
10. Rosen G. *A History of Public Health.* New York: MD
    Publications, 1958, p 105.
11. Fracastoro G (Lat. Hieronymus Fracastorius). *Web-
    ster's New Biographical Dictionary.* Springfield, MA:
    Merriam-Webster, 1983. pp 365–6.
12. Fracastorii H. *De Contagione et Contagiosis Morbis et
    Eorum Curatione* [*Contagion, Contagious Diseases,
    and Their Treatment*], Libri III. Translation and
    notes by W. C. Wright. New York: G.P. Putnam, 1930.
13. *Dorland's Illustrated Medical Dictionary,* 28th ed.
    Philadelphia: Saunders, 1994, pp 660, 1646.
14. Ref 10, *supra,* p 107.
15. Ref 10, *supra,* pp 108–9.
16. Ref 10, *supra,* p 212.
17. Ramazzini B. *De Morbis Artificum Diatriba* [*Diseases
    of Workers*]. The Latin text of 1713, revised, with
    translation and notes by Wilmer Cave Wright.
    Chicago: University of Chicago Press, 1940.
18. *Ibid.,* p 359.
19. *Ibid.,* p 363.
20. *Ibid.,* p 465.
21. *Ibid.,* p 473.
22. *Ibid.,* p 65.
23. *Ibid.,* p 195.
24. *Ibid.,* p 249.
25. *Ibid.,* p 261.
26. *Ibid.,* p 255.
27. Toynbee A. *The Industrial Revolution of the 18th
    Century in England.* New York: Humboldt, 1890,
    p 15.
28. Toynbee AJ. *A Study of History,* rev, abridged. New
    York: American Heritage, 1972, p 62.
29. Cooke J, Kramer A, Rowland-Entwistle T. *History's
    Timeline.* New York: Crescent Books, 1981, p 162.
30. Cleeland J, Burt S. Charles Turner Thackrah: A pio-
    neer in the field of occupational health. *Occup Med
    (Oxford)* 1995;45:285–97.
31. Thackrah CT. *The Effects of Arts, Trades, and Profes-
    sions and of Civic States and Habits of Living, on
    Health and Longevity with Suggestions for the Re-
    moval of Many of the Agents Which Produce Disease,
    and Shorten the Duration of Life,* 2d ed, greatly en-
    larged. London: Longman, Rees, Orme, Brown,
    Green & Longman, 1832. Reprinted with a bio-
    graphical essay: Meiklejohn A. *The Life, Work and
    Times of Charles Turner Thackrah, Surgeon and
    Apothecary of Leeds (1795–1833).* London: E&S Liv-
    ingstone, 1957.
32. *Ibid.* (Meiklejohn), p 9.
33. *Ibid.* (Thackrah), p 22.
34. *Ibid.,* p 135.
35. *Ibid.,* p 175.
36. Garrison FH. *An Introduction to the History of Med-
    icine,* 4th ed. Philadelphia: Saunders, 1929, p 708.
37. Noble D. *Facts and Observations Relative to the Influ-
    ence of Manufactures upon Health and Life.* London:
    Churchill, 1843, p 5. Reprinted facsimile by Irish
    University Press, Shannon, Ireland, 1971.
38. *Ibid.,* p 27.
39. *Ibid.,* p 75.
40. Kay JP. *The Moral and Physical Condition of the
    Working Classes Employed in the Cotton Manufacture
    in Manchester.* London: Ridgway, 1832, pp 11–2.
    Reprinted facsimile by Irish University Press, Shan-
    non, Ireland, 1971.
41. *Ibid.,* p 13.
42. Arlidge JT. *The Hygiene Diseases and Mortality of
    Occupations.* London: Percival, 1892.
43. Posner E. John Thomas Arlidge (1822–1899) and
    the potteries. *Br J Ind Med* 1973;30:266–70.
44. Ref 42, *supra,* pp 411–5.
45. Oliver T. *Dangerous Trades: The Historical, Social,
    and Legal Aspects of Industrial Occupations as Affect-
    ing Health, by a Number of Experts.* London: Murray,
    1902.
46. Dodd JR. Diseases of soldiers at home and abroad.
    In *ibid.,* pp 166–81.
47. Collingridge W. Health in the marine service. In ref
    45, *supra,* pp 182–9.
48. Power D. Agriculture; horses; cattle. In ref 45, *supra,*
    pp 232–49.
49. Oliver T. Miscellaneous trades—Upholsterers' occu-
    pation. In ref 45, *supra,* pp 789–90.
50. Oliver T. *Diseases of Occupation from the Legislative-
    Social, and Medical Points of View.* London:
    Methuen, 1908, p xvi.
51. *Ibid.,* p 319.
52. *Ibid.,* pp 345–6.
53. Price GM. *The Modern Factory: Safety, Sanitation
    and Welfare.* New York: Wiley, 1914, p 409.
54. Thompson WG. *The Occupational Diseases: Their
    Causation, Symptoms, Treatment and Prevention.*
    New York: Appleton, 1914, p v.
55. *Ibid.,* pp 53–8.
56. *Ibid.,* pp 449–61.
57. *Ibid.,* p 594.
58. *Ibid.,* p 606. (Interesting relationship.)

59. Kober GM, Hanson WC (eds). *Diseases of Occupation and Vocational Hygiene*. Philadelphia: Blakiston, 1916, p xiv.

60. SDL review of *Diseases of Occupation and Vocational Hygiene* by George M. Kober and William C. Hanson. *Am Labor Leg Rev* 1917;7:226–7.

61. Kober GM, Hanson WC (eds). *Diseases of Occupation and Vocational Hygiene*. Philadelphia: Blakiston, 1916, pp 158–72.

62. *Ibid.*, pp 173–86.

63. *Ibid.*, pp 777–88.

64. Hoehling AA. *The Great Epidemic*. Boston: Little, Brown, 1961, p 4.

65. *Ibid.*, pp 14–5.

66. *Ibid.*, pp 186–9.

67. Fincher J. America's deadly rendezvous with the "Spanish Lady." *Smithsonian* 1989;19:130–45.

68. Mock HE. *Industrial Medicine and Surgery*. Philadelphia: Saunders, 1920.

69. *Ibid.*, p 194.

70. *Ibid.*, pp 196–200.

71. *Ibid.*, pp 429–60.

72. *Ibid.*, pp 769–75.

73. Colis EL. Sir Thomas Morison Legge, C.B.E., M.D., D.P.H. *J Ind Hyg* 1932;14:235–6.

74. Henry SA. Legge's *Industrial Maladies*. London: Oxford University Press, 1934, pp 30, 32, 185–6.

75. *Ibid.*, p 317.

76. Vernon HM. *Health in Relation to Occupation*. London: Oxford University Press, 1939, pp 242–3.

77. *Ibid.*, p 317.

78. *Ibid.*, pp 233–6.

79. Vernon HM. To what extent is the health of industrial workers dependent on occupation? *Occup Psychol* 1939;13:10–24.

80. Cantril ST. Industrial medical program—Hanford Engineer Works. In Stone RS (ed), *Industrial Medicine on the Plutonium Project: Survey and Collected Papers*. New York: McGraw-Hill, 1951, pp 289–307.

81. Coates JB, Hoff EC (eds). *Medical Department, United States Army: Preventive Medicine in World War II*, Vol III: *Personal Health Measures and Immunization*. Washington: Office of the Surgeon General, Department of the Army, 1955, pp 5–7.

82. *Ibid.*, p 5.

83. *Ibid.*, pp 271–341.

84. Cook WL Jr. Occupational health and industrial medicine. In Anderson RS, Hoff EC, Hoff PM (eds), *Medical Department, United States Army: Preventive Medicine in World War II*, Vol IX: *Special Fields*. Washington: Office of the Surgeon General, Department of the Army, 1969, pp 101–201.

85. Sappington CO. *Essentials of Industrial Health*. Philadelphia: Lippincott, 1943, pp 193–4.

86. Johnstone RT. *Occupational Medicine and Industrial Hygiene*. St Louis: Mosby, 1948, pp 402–11.

87. Johnstone RT, Miller SE. *Occupational Diseases and Industrial Medicine*. Philadelphia: Saunders, 1960, pp 252–9.

88. Raffle PAB, Adams PH, Baxter PJ, et al (eds).

Hunters' Diseases of Occupations, 8th ed. Boston: Little, Brown, 1994, pp 545–76.

89. Pinner RW, Teutsch SM, Simonsen L, et al. Increasing U.S. mortality from infectious diseases. *JAMA* 1996;275:1400.

90. Clever LH. AIDS and bloodborne diseases in the workplace. In LaDou J (ed), *Occupational Health and Safety*, 2d ed. Itasca, IL: National Safety Council, 1994, pp 329–44.

91. Gantz NM. Infectious agents. In Levy BS, Wegman DH (eds), *Occupational Health: Recognizing and Preventing Work-Related Disease*. Boston: Little, Brown, 1995, pp 355–79.

92. Garibaldi R, Janis B. Occupational infections. In Rom WN (ed), *Environmental and Occcupational Medicine*, 2d ed. Boston: Little, Brown, 1992, pp 607–17.

93. Garner JS, Simmons BP. CDC guidelines for isolation precautions in hospitals. In *Guidelines for Protecting the Safety and Health of Health Care Workers*. Atlanta: Centers for Disease Control and Prevention, National Institute for Occupational Safety and Health, Division of Standards Development and Technology Transfer, 1988, App 8, pp A8-1–A8-84.

94. Lowenthal G. Occupational health programs in clinics and hospitals. In Zenz C, Dickerson OB, Horvath EP Jr (eds), *Occupational Medicine*, 3d ed. St Louis: Mosby, 1994, pp 875–82.

95. Weeks JL, Levy BS, Wagner GR (eds). *Preventing Occupational Disease and Injury*. Washington: American Public Health Association, 1991, pp 650–2.

96. Williams WW. Guideline for infection control in hospital personnel. In *Guidelines for Protecting the Safety and Health of Health Care Workers*. Atlanta: Centers for Disease Control and Prevention, National Institute for Occupational Safety and Health, Division of Standards Development Technology Transfer, 1988, App 8, pp A8-85–A8-109.

97. Patz JA, Epstein PR, Burke TA, et al. Global climate change and emerging infectious diseases. *JAMA* 1996;275:217–23.

98. Johnson RT. Emerging viral infections. *Arch Neurol* 1996;53:18–22.

99. Peterson EA, Mandel RM. Infectious diseases: Old diseases return and new agents emerge. *Arch Intern Med* 1995;155:1571–2.

100. Stoeckle MY, Douglas G Jr. Infectious diseases. *JAMA* 1996;275:1816.

101. Marfin AA, Moore J, Collins C, et al. Infectious disease surveillance during emergency relief to Bhutanese refugees in Nepal. *JAMA* 1994;272:377–81.

102. Gunby P. Military medicine undertakes peacetime mission, aiding in processing those fleeing from Haiti. *JAMA* 1994;272:191–2.

103. Gunby P. Rescuers of migrants require protection. *JAMA* 1994;22:422.

104. Thacker SB, Addiss DG, Goodman RA, et al. Infectious diseases and injuries in child day care:

Opportunities for healthier children. *JAMA* 1992; 268:1720–6.

105. Goodman RA, Thacker SB, Solomon SL, et al. Infectious diseases in competitive sports. *JAMA* 1994; 271:862–7.

106. Emerging infectious diseases: Coccidioidomycosis following the Northridge earthquake—California, 1994. *Arch Dermatol* 1994;130:555–6.

107. Stephenson J. Confronting a biological Armageddon: Experts tackle prospect of bioterrorism. *JAMA* 1996;276:349–51.

108. Goldsmith MF. Preparing for medical consequences of terrorism. *JAMA* 1996;275:1713–4.

109. Eifried G, cited in ref 107, *supra*.

110. Gunby P. Military stays in Bosnia: Vaccinates for anthrax. *JAMA* 1998;279:260–1.

111. Reichmann D. New Russian anthrax strain might defeat U.S. vaccine. *Press Democrat* (Santa Rosa), February 14, 1998, p A9.

112. Lederer EM. Iraq's arsenal may still include deadly chemicals, countries say. *Press Democrat* (Santa Rosa), February 15, 1998, p A16.

113. Brenner BE, Kauffman J. Reluctance of internists and medical nurses to perform mouth-to-mouth resuscitation. *Arch Intern Med* 1993;153:1763–9.

114. Locke CJ, Berg RA, Sanders AB, et al. Bystander cardiopulmonary resuscitation: Concerns about mouth-to-mouth contact. *Arch Intern Med* 1995; 155:938–43.

115. Kolavic S, Kimura A. An outbreak of *Shigella dysenteriae* type 2 among laboratory workers due to intentional food contamination. *JAMA* 1997;278: 396–8.

116. Torok T, Tauxe T. A large community outbreak of salmonellosis caused by intentional contamination of restaurant salad bars. *JAMA* 1997;389–95.

117. Combating terrorism: Spending on government-wide programs requires better management and coordination. GAO/NSIAD-98-39, December 1, 1997.

118. Eitzen EM Jr, Takafuji ET. Historical overview of biological warfare. In Sidell FR, Takafuji ET, Franz DP (eds), *Medical Aspects of Chemical and Biological Warfare*. Washington: Office of the Surgeon General, 1997, pp 415–23.

119. Leprosy Today and Leprosy Fact Sheet. Geneva: World Health Organization, 2008.

120. World Health Organization (who.org), *Washington Post*, February 19 2008, p A11.

121. Centers for Disease Control and Prevention. *Epidemiology and Prevention of Vaccine-Preventable Diseases*. Atkinson W, Hamborsky J, McIntyre L, Wolfe S, eds. 10th ed. 2nd printing, Washington DC: Public Health Foundation, 2008:163.

122. *MMWR* 2008;57(2):56.

123. Epidemic and Pandemic Alert and Response (EPR). Geneva: World Health Organization, 1998–2007.

124. Perspectives. *Newsweek*, September 03, 2007, p 23.

2

Clinical Laboratory Evaluation of Infectious Diseases

Gerri S. Hall and Lou Ellen Phillips-Smith

The clinical microbiology laboratory plays a key role in aiding internists, family physicians, surgeons, and infectious disease specialists with the diagnosis of infectious diseases in their patients. The role of the microbiology laboratory is more than culturing specimens. It involves the development of guidelines on the appropriateness of specimens for infectious disease analysis and the methods for collecting these specimens, direct microscopic evaluations of specimens, rapid testing for the presence of an infectious disease agent, when available [1], interpretation of results of direct observations, cultures and rapid testing, and when applicable, the susceptibility testing of isolated organisms to determine what antibiotics or other drugs may be appropriate for use—or at best, the ones to which the isolates may be resistant [2–4].

This chapter gives an overview of what assistance clinical microbiologists can provide health care professionals for the diagnosis of infectious diseases. For clinical practicality, the chapter is organized by specimen or body system. In addition, some generalizations about newer, emerging technologies are made.

Specimen Collection

BLOOD CULTURES

When a patient is suspected of having bacteremia or fungemia, the appropriate specimen to collect is a blood culture. The optimal amount of blood to be drawn is 20 mL, which is usually distributed into two different bottles or sources of medium for growth of both bacteria and fungi. The 20 mL is collected using aseptic technique, which requires thorough cleansing of the area around the needlestick with Betadine and alcohol or another disinfectant. The area should not be manipulated after cleansing, but rather the needlestick should be done after the area has been cleaned. Methods for skin antisepsis prior to venipuncture vary from hospital to hospital, but the basic principles are similar. After a vein is palpated, the area around the vein is scrubbed with 70% alcohol for 30 seconds, followed by application of an iodine solution for 30–60 seconds. Application of alcohol alone for longer than 30 seconds may be necessary if a patient is hypersensitive to iodine. The bottle tops are cleansed with alcohol or iodine before venipuncture is performed.

Some labs inoculate bottles of blood culture medium, and the results are read visually by the technologists over a period of 5–7 days. A positive test result is determined by turbidity, hemolysis, or other visible changes. Some laboratories use a lysis centrifugation method (Wampole Isostat/Isolator, Inverness Medical Professional Diagnostics, Princeton, NJ) alone or in conjunction with blood culture bottles. The

Isolator may increase the yield of certain bacteria, such as staphylococci, and fungi. For the culture of blood, most laboratories today use one of the "automated" blood culture systems: BacT/ALERT 3D (bioMerieux, Inc., Durham, NC), Bactec 9240 (BD Diagnostic Systems, Sparks, MD), or VersaTREK (Trek Diagnostics, Cleveland, Ohio). For each of these systems, laboratories determine whether they will inoculate one anaerobic blood culture bottle and one aerobic bottle or place all the blood into two aerobic bottles. In addition, one or both bottles may contain a type of resin—or antibiotic-removal materials—so that organisms may grow even if the patient has already been placed on antibiotics for empirical therapy. When sent to the laboratory, the blood culture bottles are placed onto the appropriate instrument, and for the next 4–7 days, readings are taken to determine growth of an organism in each of the bottles. When a culture is positive, smears are prepared for examination by means of Gram's stain. The smear results are reported to the clinician by phone to give a rapid answer about what might be present in the blood of the patient. For bacteria, blood cultures usually are positive within the first 12 hours or less, and for fungi, within the first 24 hours or less. The blood culture systems used today allow for recovery of most common bacteria and fungi; however, there are some organisms that are not expected to be recovered from routine blood culture, including bacteria such as *Bordetella pertussis, Legionella pneumophila, Fransicella tularensis,* and possibly, *Brucella* and *Bartonella* species. In addition, most of the automated systems may not provide 100% recovery of the dimorphic fungi, especially *Histoplasma capsulatum* or *Blastomyces dermatitidis.* The reason for this may be the length of incubation needed for these fungi to be cultured and not the medium or "system." If any of these agents are suspected, the laboratory should be informed before the blood is collected.

After organisms are isolated from a blood culture, they are assessed for genus and species identification, often followed by susceptibility testing. Laboratories are presently making more of an effort to aid the clinician in detection of possible laboratory contaminants because the cost of identifying and treating potential contaminants is high [2,4]. In general, these contaminants include coagulase-negative staphylococci (CNS), *viridans* streptococci, *Propionibacterium acnes,* and *Bacillus* species. Any one of these organisms may indeed be the true pathogen in certain situations, but its isolation from a single blood culture does not necessarily indicate that the organism is the agent causing illness. After a short period of time, if a blood culture for another organism is positive in the same patient, one needs to reconsider whether the first positive culture truly indicates the pathogen. Generally, fewer than 3% of all blood cultures performed yield these contaminants if proper aseptic technique is employed in the collection process [5–8]. The percentage should be monitored by the laboratory in order to quickly recognize any problems with increased contamination so that efforts to reduce this can be implemented in a timely fashion. Possible reasons for contamination include the improper cleaning of sites before collection of blood, improper disinfection of the ports used to inject blood into blood culture bottles, and improper handling of blood samples once they reach the laboratory. Of all the blood cultures sent to any one laboratory, only about 10% are positive for any bacteria or fungi; most blood samples drawn are negative [5–8].

Transport of blood cultures to the laboratory should be done as quickly as possible, and bottles that contain blood should not be refrigerated before or during transport. If a blood culture is positive and the patient is placed on appropriate antibiotics, the need for subsequent "test of cure" blood cultures is debatable. If further cultures are performed, the blood sample should be drawn at least 4–5 days later, unless the patient does not appear to be responding to treatment, in which case repeat cultures should be performed to be certain another source of bacteremia has not occurred. If the laboratory uses bottles that contain resins, even if the patient is being treated appropriately, the sample may stay positive for a few days longer than anticipated because the resin may inactivate the antibiotic, allowing growth of the organisms in vitro. This appears to occur most often when the pathogen is *Staphylococcus aureus* or coagulase-negative staphylococci [5–8].

Many laboratories incorporate some means of rapid detection of specific pathogens. For example, when gram-positive cocci are seen on Gram's stain, a coagulase determination may be done directly from the blood culture material to establish whether *S. aureus* is the organism [9]; some laboratories may employ a molecular method in these instances, such as a fluorescent in-situ hybridization (FISH) assay to determine if *S. aureus* versus coagulase-negative staphylococci are present or if *Candida albicans* versus another *Candida* species is present when yeast are seen on Gram's stain initially [10–13]. Alternatively, newer commercial assays, along with FISH, are being introduced into clinical laboratories employing polymerase chain reaction (PCR) for detection of *S. aureus* and, more specifically, whether the gram-positive cocci are methicillin-resistant *S. aureus* (MRSA) [14, 15].)

URINE TESTING

The processing of a urine sample for the diagnosis of urinary tract infection is one of the most commonly performed microbiologic assays. Laboratories usually receive more urine specimens than any other single specimen. Collection of urine is believed to be simple; however, its collection can be fraught with many contamination problems. Patients need to be instructed in the proper collection of a urine sample [7,16]. If the area around the urethra is not well cleaned before collection, especially in female patients, then the resulting positive urine culture may contain contaminating skin or normal urethral flora and not the pathogen. Midstream urine collection is ideal and, if done properly, will usually yield the pathogen if one is present in a quantity of about 10^5 CFU/mL or greater [4]. Lesser quantities may be clinically significant depending on the organism and the host. Some laboratories may use one of a variety of screening techniques to determine the likelihood that the urine contains significant quantities of an organism. These include Gram's stain of unspun urine, bioluminescence measurement of bacterial adenosine triphosphate (ATP), and dipstick techniques for determination of the presence of pyuria and/or nitrates. If a screen is used, the samples that screen negative are disposed of and not cultured. If positive, a culture is performed. The culture involves plating 0.001 mL of the urine onto one each of blood agar and gram-negative selective media (Maconkey's agar), incubating for 16–24 hours, and the identifying the resulting colonies. Usually, each laboratory sets up its own guidelines for full identification and susceptibility testing based on the presence of one organism versus more than one in a quantity of 10^5 CFU/mL or greater.

If the patient is catheterized, it is inadvisable to collect the specimen from the Foley catheter bag; rather, it can be collected from the catheter after disinfection of the catheter port. Collection of a suprapubic aspirate from the bladder ensures sterile collection of the urine, and thus anything that grows is considered significant, regardless of the colony count [3, 4].

If urine is being collected for the diagnosis of *Chlamydia trachomatis* or *Neisseria gonorrhoeae* for a patient suspected to have a sexually transmitted disease, the urine tested should be the first-voided urine (i.e., not midstream), without any prior cleaning of the urethral area, and should be collected at least 1 hour after the last urination. Cultures of urine for *C. trachomatis* or *N. gonorrhoeae* are insensitive for detection, but amplification techniques yield sensitivities equivalent to the urethral specimen from a male and nearly as sensitive as a cervical sample from a female.

RESPIRATORY TRACT SPECIMENS
Upper Respiratory Tract

Diagnosis of upper respiratory tract bacterial infection requires the collection of a throat specimen or, for viral isolation or detection, a nasopharyngeal specimen for microscopic examination. Bacterial throat cultures usually are collected only for the detection of group A streptococci or, in specific cases, for isolation of *N. gonorrhoeae* or *Corynebacterium diphtheriae* (when the patient has a pseudomembrane in the throat). Other bacterial organisms often represent only normal oral flora or carrier states and should not be searched for or reported routinely, if found [8, 16].

For the detection of viruses, such as respiratory syncytial virus (RSV), influenza and parainfluenza viruses, adenoviruses, and cytomegalovirus, throat cultures or culture of nasopharyngeal aspirates is appropriate. Often, a panel of the various viral pathogens is searched for by culture or, more commonly, by antigen detection or molecular methods, which provide more rapid results [17–21].

Lower Respiratory Tract

For the diagnosis of pneumonia, sputum for culture is often considered the most appropriate specimen. Unfortunately, sputum collection is problematic. Often patients merely "spit" oral material into the container instead of providing a good specimen that is representative of the lower respiratory tract. Even with a properly collected sputum sample, normal oral flora organisms are likely to be detected because the sputum has to come through the oral cavity during collection. With the use of Gram's stain to determine the quality of the specimen, laboratories should be able to inform the physician of the probability that the specimen is in fact sputum from the lower respiratory tract and therefore should provide adequate and significant clinical information when cultured [22–24]. Gram's stain also may be used to predict the presence of an infectious agent, such as *Streptococcus pneumoniae,* if predominant organisms are of a consistent morphology with this diagnosis. If Gram's stain demonstrates bacteria that are predominantly consistent in appearance with *Neisseria* or *Haemophilus* species, then cultures can be plated appropriately to detect the presence of one of these organisms. If the physician suspects organisms such as *Legionella* species, *Mycoplasma pneumoniae, Chlamydia pneumoniae,* or *Mycobacterium tuberculosis,* specific requests for culture of these organisms need to be made at the time of ordering, before cultures are processed. Likewise, if fungal organisms are suspected, especially *H. capsulatum* or *B. dermatitidis,* the laboratory should be informed of this so that correct media and incubation conditions are used. Requests for anaerobic culturing of the sputum will be rejected because every sputum sample contains anaerobic bacteria owing to the large numbers of such organisms in the oral cavity as part of the normal flora. If anaerobic pneumonia is in the differential diagnosis, i.e., a diagnosis of aspiration pneumonia or empyema is being entertained by the clinician, Gram's stain of the sputum consistent with the presence of anaerobes (i.e., a good-quality specimen with polymorphic bacterial morphologies) should yield the information the clinician needs without having to perform anaerobic culture.

In addition to sputum testing, bronchoalveolar lavage (BAL) to obtain lung secretions for the detection of pneumonia has become very popular [25]. Saline is instilled into the alveolar spaces with a bronchoscope, and then the fluid, along with lung secretions, is removed via an endoscope. Culture of this fluid may increase the yield of the pathogens over that detected by sputum culture. For the diag-

nosis of *Pneumocystis jiroveci (carinii)* pneumonia (PCP), the specimen obtained by BAL is far superior to the sputum sample, even an induced sputum sample [26, 27]. Transtracheal aspirates, if collected appropriately and not merely through a tracheal or bronchial tube, are appropriate samples for determination of the causative agents of pneumonia.

If all the above-mentioned specimens are inconclusive and a definitive diagnosis has not been made, open lung biopsy may be required. Since the lung is a sterile site, any organism detected may represent the pathogen involved in the pneumonia. Again, if organisms such as *L. pneumophila, Mycobacterium tuberculosis* or other mycobacterial strains, dimorphic fungi, or other fastidious organisms are being considered, then the physician should alert the lab and request that specific media be plated for their recovery.

CEREBROSPINAL FLUID

For determination of agents of bacterial, viral, or fungal meningitis, a properly collected cerebrospinal fluid (CSF) specimen is the specimen of choice. To reduce the chance of skin contaminants, usually the second or third collected specimen tube should be sent to the microbiology laboratory [28]. Gram's stain and culture for potential pathogens should be performed and the results of the Gram's stain called in immediately to the physician if they are positive. Requests for bacterial antigen tests (BADs; described in serologic section) should be honored only after consultation with the laboratory. BAD assays are available commercially for the detection of *S. pneumoniae, H. influenzae,* and *N. meningitidis.* These tests may provide additional useful information when the patient has community-acquired pneumonia and has been given antibiotics prior to collection of a CSF specimen, possibly reducing the chance for growth of the pathogen. The sensitivity of most BAD assays is no better than that of Gram's stain and may result in false-positive findings [29]. On the other hand, the request for a cryptococcal antigen assay is appropriate for all cases of suspected fungal meningitis because the sensitivity of this assay for this disease is greater than 90% and its specificity is almost 100% [30].

Diagnosis of aseptic meningitis may be made clinically; if cultures are requested, the most commonly performed test is that for enterovirus. Isolation of herpes simplex virus (HSV) from the CSF has a sensitivity of less than 5%, and if CSF is to be processed for detection of HSV, an amplification assay, such as PCR, should be requested [31]. A PCR assay for the detection of enterovirus in CSF has been developed recently on the GeneXpert System (Cepheid, Sunnyvale, CA) [32].

WOUND SPECIMENS

The sampling of wounds for the diagnosis of wound infections is difficult to perform appropriately. Swabs are not appropriate collection devices [7, 8, 16]. Because of their small size, they sample only a small area for collection of adequate samples; they are not adequate for obtaining samples for anaerobic culturing; and they provide only surface screening of the wound, which often misses the site of the real infection deeper in the wound. Aspirate or biopsy specimens should be obtained, if possible. First, the area needs to be cleaned prior to specimen collection to decrease the amount of normal skin flora in the collection. In areas where aspirates are difficult to obtain, a small amount of nonpreserved saline can be injected into the wound first and then the contents drawn back into the syringe, along with the infected material.

GENITAL SPECIMENS

For patients with suspected sexually transmitted diseases, urethral specimens (from males) and cervical/urethral specimens (from females) should be collected after excess mucus is cleaned from the area [33]. Appropriate transport media for *Chlamydia* include M-4 or 2-SP, and the specimens should be collected with a calcium alginate other than a cotton-tipped swab. The use of wooden swabs should be avoided because these may inhibit the growth of *C. trachomatis* [33]. For isolation of *N. gonorrhoeae,* a culturette type of swab sent immediately to the laboratory after sample collection or plating of the samples onto an appropriate selective medium performed at the clinic office is required. Amplification methods for the diagnosis of these two infectious agents are the preferred method in many laboratories because they have been shown to be more sensitive, especially for the detection of *C. trachomatis.* Each of the manufacturers of amplification assays provides a specific collection and transport kit for their specific assay, and this should be used when applicable [33].

If other organisms are suspected, such as *Haemophilus ducreyi* (chancroid), a specific request needs to be reported to the laboratory. If a chancre is present and *Treponema pallidum* (syphilis) is in the differential diagnosis, the material within the chancre can be sent to the laboratory for dark-field examination, provided it is delivered immediately, before the specimen is allowed to dry. If vaginitis is the clinical diagnosis, *Candida* species and *Trichomonas vaginalis,* if present, can be detected by means of direct microscopic examination for budding yeast, with or without pseudohyphae, or motile trichomonads, respectively. In addition, use of a "scored" Gram's stain for detection of the presence of lactobacilli (as evidence of normal flora) or increased numbers of *Gardnerella vaginalis* (as evidence of bacterial vaginosis) should be performed. There is a nucleic acid probe that can be used for detection of all three entities (AFFIRM, BD Diagnostic Systems, Sparks, MD); this is discussed in a later section of this chapter [34].

STOOL SPECIMENS

Gastroenteritis may be caused by enteric bacterial pathogens, parasites, mycobacterial organisms (in the case of HIV disease), viral pathogens, or the toxins of *Clostridium difficile.* Fungi rarely cause gastroenteritis but may be present in stool specimens if the focus of the fungal disease is gastrointestinal or if the disease is disseminated.

To detect the causative pathogen, a stool sample is sent to the laboratory with specific requests. If an enteric pathogen is being sought, the laboratory will plate the stool for isolation of *Salmonella, Shigella,* and *Campylobacter* species. Many laboratories also provide a means of detection of Shiga toxin and a means of detection of the presence of enterohemorrhagic *E. coli* (*E. coli* O157:H7 and other serotypes) in all stools. A number of antigen methods are available for doing this [35, 36]. Some laboratories look for *E. coli* O157:H7 specifically in bloody stools or on a request basis. If other organisms such as *Yersinia enterocolitica* or *Vibrio* or *Aeromonas* species are being sought, specific requests must be conveyed to the laboratory. The detection of ova and parasites (O&Ps), as evidence of parasitic enteritis, is done by means of direct microscopic examination of unstained and stained preparations or by means of antigen-detection reagents that specifically identify *Giardia lamblia,*

Cryptosporidium species, and/or *Entamoeba histolytica* [37–39]. Processing of stools for enteric bacterial pathogens or parasites should be performed on outpatients and patients who have been in the hospital for fewer than 3 days. After longer hospitalizations, any development of diarrhea or gastroenteritis invariably is caused by other than enteric bacterial pathogens or parasites [40, 41]. If *Mycobacterium avium-intracellulare* is suspected, a specific request must be conveyed to the laboratory, and results may require up to 2–3 weeks. Detection of the toxins of *C. difficile* by means of enzyme immunoassay (EIA) or tissue culture or isolation of the organism and detection of the toxins in the isolates are the way in which *C. difficile* diarrhea is diagnosed in the laboratory. The disease is a clinical disease, and the laboratory merely supports the diagnosis. The request for *C. difficile* detection is appropriate for inpatients and outpatients regardless of their time in the hospital prior to development of diarrhea [42, 43]. For detection of viral agents in stool, direct antigen assays, PCR, or electron microscopy for specific agents is usually employed [44, 45]. For children, antigen assay for the detection of rotavirus is often the initial request for diagnosis of diarrhea [46, 47].

BODY FLUIDS AND TISSUES

Body fluids and tissues need to be collected in a sterile fashion and sent immediately to the laboratory. Routine bacterial cultures detect most bacterial pathogens; fungal and viral cultures need to be specifically requested if a fungus or virus is thought to be a possible pathogen. If the specimen is collected in surgery, that information should be written on the request for culture sent to the laboratory.

ANAEROBES

If the clinician suspects anaerobic bacteria, a specific request for anaerobic culture must be sent to the laboratory. Certain specimens are unacceptable for anaerobic culturing. These include specimens from sites at which anaerobes are part of the normal flora and thus the significance of their isolation could not be interpreted, namely, sputum, throat swabs, vaginal swabs, feces, and saliva [16]. Specimens such as urine or CSF often are not processed for anaerobes because the incidence of anaerobic infections at these sites is very low. Exceptions are

made when all other more common etiologies have been exhausted and in other specific situations after consultation between the laboratory and the clinician. Anaerobic culturing of appropriate sites involves collection of aspirates, tissues, or body fluids, which are transported to the laboratory quickly and in appropriate anaerobic vials or containers. Swabs are inadequate for the isolation of anaerobes and should be discouraged or rejected. Gram staining of the specimens is essential for interpretation of anaerobic cultures and often provides useful information as to the adequacy of the specimen and hence significance of the isolates(s). Most anaerobic infections are polymicrobial, i.e., composed of both aerobes and anaerobes.

Microscopic Identification of Microbial Pathogens

Gram's stain remains the mainstay of microscopic examination of microbial pathogens. It is relatively easy to perform; however, accurate reading and interpretation of the results require a trained technologist or physician. The adequacy of the specimen usually can be judged from the Gram's stain, as well as the quantities and morphology of the organisms seen. An acid-fast bacillus (AFB) smear assists in the rapid detection of mycobacterial organisms. It should be performed on concentrated specimens, and laboratories should be capable of reporting the results of AFB smear within the first 24 hours of receiving a specimen. *Nocardia* species and potentially *Rhodococci* species and some parasites, including *Cryptosporidium* and *Cyclospora* species, are also partially AFB-positive. These stains also require trained personnel for accurate analysis.

Toluidine blue stain, silver stain, calcofluor white fluorescent stain, and Giemsa stain can be used for the detection of *P. jiroveci (carinii)* [48]. In most laboratories, the calcofluor fluorescent wall stain is also used for the detection of fungal organisms, directly in clinical specimens, as a replacement for the KOH or wet mount, but calcofluor white stain provides a more sensitive and often more specific approach to the microscopic examination of fungal organisms.

In addition to microscopic examination of specimens, a number of serologic techniques for the detection of antigens can be used for more rapid detection of bacterial and viral agents. The specimen is homogenized and/or a touch prep is made on a slide, and an antibody tagged with a fluorescent or colored label is added to the specimen. The resulting fluorescent or colored product is read by microscope or colorimeter, respectively. These FISH methods are available for specific pathogen detection in blood culture bottles, as described previously, and may be available for other sites in the future [11, 13, 49]. Serologic detection of antibodies enables the rapid detection of the etiologic agent and may decrease the need for culture depending on the specificity of the antibody and the need to identify polymorphic pathogens. Such antigen-detection methods are discussed in more detail later in this chapter.

Culture

Culture remains the "gold standard" for detection of most pathogenic organisms. Agar and broth bacterial cultures are set up for most clinical specimens and incubated for 24 hours or more depending on the suspected organism. In addition to often being the most sensitive method of detection, cultures also may be necessary for studying the epidemiology of a group of isolates or for performing susceptibility assays to detect resistance. In general, culture takes longer than other rapid molecular methods but may provide the most specific means of identification of the pathogen(s) involved. The media that are used in the laboratory should be planned by the laboratory technologists to provide for isolation of the most common species of bacteria and fungi. In cases in which an unusual pathogen is being considered, clinicians should inform the laboratory of this so that appropriate processing and/or culture medium can be used. An example of this would be a patient in whom *Bartonella* species is being considered. *Bartonella* species may require a nonautomated blood culture method for isolation of the organism and may require longer than the 4–5 days presently required by most laboratories for the detection of agents of bacteremia or fungemia. As molecular methods become commercially available for specific pathogens such as *Bartonella* species, culture may not be the method of choice [50, 51]. If a physician considers *Zygomycetes* in the differential diagnosis, informing the laboratory before processing occurs will ensure

proper specimen handling. *Zygomycetes* may be fragile in specimens, and if it is macerated, ground, or otherwise homogenized, the yield may be low. If the specimen is teased apart and handled gently, the recovery of a *Rhizopus* species or other *Zygomycetes* is more likely [16].

Identification of Bacteria, Fungi, and Viral Agents

Identification of bacteria after isolation on agar or in broth requires use of conventional biochemical and microscopic tests. The biochemical tests may be performed in tubes, on plates, or in microtiter plates. Methods are available for manual or automated procedures, which require hours to days for completion. How far one proceeds with the specific identification is determined by the specimen site and absence or presence of multiple organisms. Most bacterial identifications are complete in fewer than 2 days of isolation. More fastidious bacteria may require longer turnaround times, and in some cases, the isolates may have to be sent out to reference laboratories for complete and specific identification. For mycobacterial isolates, genetic probes are used most often for rapid identification of the more common *M. tuberculosis* complex and *M. avium-intracellulare* complex isolates. For isolates that are probe-negative, more conventional biochemicals or methods of high-performance liquid chromatography (HPLC) or sequencing are used. The latter methods often must be performed at reference laboratories.

Identification of yeast is similar to that of bacteria, requiring microscopic examination and biochemical differentiation. For identification of molds, there are not many available biochemical tools; thus microscopic examination of organisms on a variety of fungal media is required. This usually requires expertise in such identification and/or sending of the isolates to a reference laboratory. Identification of yeast usually requires 4–5 days after isolation; turnaround time for molds differs depending on the species but usually is accomplished, at least to a genus level, in 1–2 weeks after isolation.

Identification of a virus requires determination of the specific cytopathic effect (CPE) in specific tissue cultures or identification of antigens by specific monoclonal antibodies. In many laboratories, molecular techniques using probes, amplification, or in-situ hybridization have replaced more conventional methods of viral identification.

Molecular Methods for Detection or Specific Identification of Infectious Disease Agents

Use of DNA techniques in a wide variety of applications probably represents the major emerging technology in the microbiology laboratory today. There are commercially available culture confirmation probes for the rapid identification of *Mycobacterium* species (e.g., *M. tuberculosis* complex, *M. avium-intracellulare* complex, *M. gordonae,* and *M. kansasii*), fungal isolates (e.g., *H. capsulatum, B. dermatitidis,* and *Coccidioides immitis*), bacteria (e.g., *H. influenzae* and *Campylobacter* species), and viral agents. These probes can be used to confirm the cultural identification of the preceding organisms in less than 3 hours from the beginning of the procedure to completion. However, these probes are not sensitive enough to use directly on clinical specimens [52–54].

A breakthrough in rapid identification occurred when some of the probes that were being developed commercially were applied to detection of organisms directly within the respiratory, genital, or other specimen with a sensitivity approaching the more conventional culture methods. There are commercially available probes for direct detection of *C. trachomatis* and *N. gonorrhoeae* in cervical or urethral specimens (PACE, Gen-Probe, San Diego, CA) [55], for identification of the three most common agents of vaginitis (i.e., *T. vaginalis, Candida* species, and *G. vaginalis*) (AFFIRM, Becton Dickinson, Sparks, MD) [34, 56–58], for direct detection of group A streptococci in throat-swab specimens (Gen-Probe) [59], and for detection of viral agents (e.g., HIV, cytomegalovirus, and Epstein-Barr virus) in clinical specimens. In addition, more probes are available in research formats.

More recently, laboratories have become inundated with developments in the arena of amplification. Amplification techniques enable the laboratory to achieve sensitivities within clinical specimens equal to or better than culture and much more rapidly. Amplification increases the number of nucleic acid copies in a specimen to millions in a very short period of time (often fewer than 5 hours) [60, 61]. With this potential,

at first it appeared that amplification would take over all microbiologic conventional methods. Since its introduction, however, it is obvious that these techniques, although excellent in some areas, may not always be preferable. However, amplification has become very successful in the identification of organisms for which culture methods are long and tedious, for which there may be no available culture methods, or for which the need to know the answer very rapidly overrides the costs that might be involved in the use of molecular methods.

The manufacturing companies that have provided the "kits" that laboratories can use to perform amplification on clinical specimens have done a great job of providing "cookbook" formats for performing these molecular techniques. The detection of *C. trachomatis* (CT) and *N. gonorrhoeae* (GC) in genitourinary tract specimens is done by means of one of three amplification methods: *polymerase chain reaction* (Amplicor PCR or COBAS, Roche Molecular Systems), *transcription-mediated amplification* (TMA, Gen-Probe, Inc.) [23, 43], or *strand-displacement amplification* (SDA, BD Microbiology Systems) [33, 62, 63]. Urine can be the sample for detection of both these sexually transmitted disease etiologies by any of these nucleic acid amplification test (NAAT) systems with sensitivities that approach or equal that of culture [64]. PAP smears collected in Thin-Prep or other transport collection devices also may be validated for use on one or all of the three NAAT systems for detection of CT and GC [65, 66].

For the detection of *M. tuberculosis* complex directly in clinical specimens, two amplification methods are currently available commercially: TMA and PCR [67–69]. Both can be performed on respiratory specimens that are AFB-positive from patients who have never been diagnosed with tuberculosis. The Food and Drug Administration (FDA) put these specific restrictions on their use. The assays require about 5 hours to perform and thus provide a very specific, rapid answer to help clinicians more appropriately treat suspected cases of tuberculosis (TB) and put TB patients in isolation more quickly to prevent further spread of the disease. These assays are expensive to perform, however [53, 70]. Some laboratories employ their own in-house methods for direct detection of *M. tuberculosis* and/or other *Mycobacterium* species in clinical samples, including paraffin-embedded tissue samples [71, 72].

Although not produced commercially, amplification methods are available for a wide variety of agents. They are performed in research laboratories or are offered by commercial companies for detection of, for example, *B. pertussis, C. pneumoniae, M. pneumoniae,* and *Bartonella henselae.* Amplification methods are also available for the detection and determination of the viral load for diseases such as HIV, hepatitis C virus (HCV), cytomegalovirus (CMV), and HSV (in CSF) [31,73–75]. One manufacturer, Digene, provides an assay for human papillomavirus (HPV) that, although not truly an amplification procedure, yields results with a sensitivity equivalent to that of amplification [76].

The use of sequencing to detect and/or identify infectious disease agents from agar or broth cultures or directly within clinical specimens following amplification has become more available to clinical laboratories. Although sequencing is for the most part still in the research arena, in time it may become a more widely available technique in many laboratories.

Genetic typing of isolates by techniques such as pulsed-field gel electrophoresis (PFGE) or rep-PCR (DiversiLab Systems, bioMerieux, Inc., Durham, NC) is being used to determine the relatedness of bacterial or fungal isolates. This is particularly useful in the epidemiologic analysis of outbreaks or cluster cases of unusual organisms. There are a number of hospital and reference laboratories that provide these services [77, 78].

Serologic Evaluation for Diagnosis of Infectious Diseases

The formation of antibodies during the process of infection can be detected in the sera of patients, and this detection can be used as a diagnostic tool for the laboratorian and clinician. In general, two specimens of serum should be submitted to the laboratory for serologic evaluation—one drawn during the peak, or acute, stage of the infectious process and the other during the convalescent phase, which is usually 2–4 weeks or more after the acute serum was drawn. Both specimens should be tested simultaneously to ensure that titer differences are due to the samples and not to variability in testing procedures [79].

Accurate demonstration of a positive serologic response usually requires a fourfold rise or decline in the titer between the acute and convalescent assay results. In addition, demonstration of IgM antibodies with or without IgG antibodies suggests acute infection; presence of IgG alone may indicate present or past infection. Not all infectious disease syndromes have reliable IgM assays that are available, however. Detection of IgG antibodies also may be used to determine the immune status of an individual and hence presumed protection from infection by certain agents. This might include detection of IgG for rubella, CMV, or varicella-zoster virus (VZV). Screening antibody tests also have been developed; their purpose is to screen blood or blood products for the presence of viral agents, including hepatitis viruses, HIV, and CMV.

Many methodologies are available to laboratories for the detection of antibodies specific for a disease. The more commonly employed methods include enzyme immunoassays (EIA), complement fixation (CF), immunodiffusion (ID), indirect immunofluorescence antibody (IFA), indirect hemagglutination assay (IHA), and radioimmunoassay (RIA).

There are some infectious diseases for which serology remains the primary mode of diagnosis because culture is unavailable or requires lengthy incubations or methods not available to most laboratories. This includes the diagnosis of *C. pneumoniae* [80], *M. pneumoniae* [22], and *B. henselae* [81]; Rickettsial diseases [18] such as spotted fevers; *T. pallidum* and *Ehrlichia* species [82]; Lyme disease [83, 84]; and a number of viral entities. For some pathogens, such as *L. pneumophila,* there are culture methods; however, alone, they are often not sensitive enough to provide adequate diagnosis and must be used in combination with serologic studies for maximum efficacy [85].

For the diagnosis of fungal and parasitic disease, detection of antibodies affords a complement to culture and microscopic examinations, respectively. Serologic studies complement culture of the systemic dimorphic fungi *H. capsulatum, B. dermatitidis,* and *C. immitis* [86]. Serology for *E. histolytica* and *Toxoplasma gondii* are often more sensitive than the respective microscopic modalities or culture [87, 88].

Table 2-1 lists some serologic methods and the diseases or organisms for which they are often used.

Table 2-1
Serologic Assays for Infectious Disease Agents

Organism/Disease	Methods	Comments
Bacterial Agents		
Bartonella henselae	IFA, EIA	For diagnosis of bacillary angiomatosis (BA) in HIV or cat-scratch disease.
Borrelia burgdorferi	DFA, EIA; Western blot test	For diagnosis of Lyme disease, CDC recommends confirmation of EIA or DFA with Western blot test; indeterminates are frequent; false-positive results in areas of low prevalence are common.
Legionella pneumophila	IFA	Four-fold rise in titer to 1:128 or single titer of > 1:512 is diagnostic.
Mycoplasma pneumoniae	CF, EIA	Presence of IgM antibodies better than IgG for diagnosis of acute infection. Cold agglutinins often positive but nonspecific.
Streptococcus pyogenes	ASO, anti-DNase B	Used for the diagnosis of sequelae of pharyngitis or group A streptococcal skin infections.
Chlamydia pneumoniae	MIF	IgM > 1:16 or IgG > 1:512; fourfold rise in titer is more specific.
Chlamydia trachomatis, LGV	MIF	IgM > 1:32 and IgG > 1:2,000 is diagnostic.
Chlamydia psittaci	MIF	Fourfold rise in titer most reliable for diagnosis.
Francisella tularensis	Microagglutination	> 1:60 suggestive; fourfold rise in titer most reliable; EIA in development.
Ehrlichia sp.	IFA	Four-fold rise in titer, with baseline of 1:80 is diagnostic; assays not widely available.
Treponema pallidum	VDRL, RPR	Nonspecific screening tests; VDRL preferred for CSF testing.
	FTA-ABA, MHA-TP	Specific treponemal tests; confirmatory assays.
Leptospira sp.	Microagglutination	EIA being developed.
Rickettsia rickettsii	IFA, EIA	> 1:64 positive for Rocky Mountain spotted fever.
	LA	Positive only during acute infection.
Fungal Agents		
Histoplasma capsulatum	ID, CF, EIA	H & M bands on ID; *H* = acute infection; *M* = acute or past.
		CF: > 1:8 suggestive.
		May cross-react with *Blastomyces* or *Coccidioides immitis*.
Blastomyces dermatitidis	ID, CF, EIA	CF: > 1:8 suggestive.
		May cross-react with Histoplasma or *Coccidioides immitis*.
Coccidioides immitis	CF, ID	≥ 1:16 suggestive.
Cryptococcus neoformans		Not usually helpful.
Aspergillus sp.	CF, ID	Number of bands on ID may suggest extent of invasive disease but may be nonspecific for diagnosis.
Candida sp.		Not useful for diagnosis of invasive disease.
Zygomycetes		Not widely available.
Parasites		
Entamoeba histolytica (amebiasis)	EIA, IHA	IHA ≥ 1:256. 95% with extra-GI disease; 70% with GI only.
Ascaris lumbricoides (ascariasis)	EIA	≥ 1:32
Chagas' disease	CF, IHA	≥ 1:8; 1:64
Cysticercosis	IHA	≥ 1:64
Echinococcosis	IHA	≥ 1:256
Fascioliasis	IHA	≥ 1:128
Filariasis	IHA	≥ 1:128
Leishmaniasis	IFA	≥ 1:16

Table 2-1
Serologic Assays for Infectious Disease Agents

Organism/Disease	Methods	Comments
Parasites (continued)		
Paragonimiasis	CF	≥ 1:8
Pneumocystosis	IFA	≥ 1:16
Schistosomiasis	IFA	≥ 1:16
Strongyloidiasis	IHA	≥ 1:64
Toxocariasis	EIA	≥ 1:32
Trichinosis	Bentonite flocculation	≥ 1:16
Toxoplasma gondii	IFA, EIA	IgM = past or present infection.
		IgM = active primary infection.
Plasmodium sp.	IFA	≥ 1:64 for diagnosis of malaria.
Viral Agents		
Adenovirus	CF, EIA	
Arbovirus	IFA	IgM and IgG; CSF and serum.
	CF, HI, EIA	Four-fold rise in titer best for diagnosis.
CMV	CF, IHA, EIA, IFA	
EBV	Heterophile, EIA	IgM and IgG for Viral Capsid (VCA).
	EIA, RIA, CF	For immune status; also for stage of infection.
Hepatitis A	RIA or EIA	IgM anti-HAV = active infection.
Hepatitis B	RIA or EIA	HBsAg, anti-HBs, and anti-HBc donor screening.
Hepatitis C	EIA	
Hepatitis D	RIA	HBsAG, anti-HDV, and IgM anti-HD determines disease state and provides total anti-HEV and IgM anti-HEV.
Hepatitis E	Western blot test, EIA, heterophile agglutination, HI, IFA, CF	
HIV	EIA, Western blot test	Positive EIA: repeat EIA and if still positive perform Western blot test for confirmation.
HSV	CF, IHA, EIA, IFA	Not very useful for diagnosis.
VZV	IFA, FAMA	For immune status; also for stage of infection.
Influenza A and B	CF, HAI	
Measles virus	HI, EIA, IgM by IFA	Four-fold rise for diagnosis.
Mumps virus	IFA, EIA, HAI	
Parainfluenza I, II, III prognostic information	HAI, CF, EIA	
Rabies	IFA, RFFIT	For diagnosis and immune status.
Rubella virus	EIA, IgM by EIA, LA	Four-four rise highly suggestive; Western blot test for diagnosis.

Abbreviations: ASO = antistreptolysin O antibody; CF = complement fixation; DFA = direct fluorescent antibody; EIA = enzyme immunoassay; FTA-= fluorescent treponemal antibody-absorption; HI = hemagglutination inhibition; ID = immunodiffusion; IFA = indirect fluorescent antibody; IHA = indirect hemagglutination antibody; LA = latex agglutination; Microagg = microagglutination assay; MIF = microimmunofluorescence; MHA-TP = microhemagglutination-treponemal; RIA = radioimmunoassay; RPR = rapid plasma reagin; VDRL = Venereal Disease Research Laboratory. Based on data from references 18, 22, 80–88.

Antigen Detection

To provide a more rapid diagnosis than culture provides, detection of antigens of the infectious agent directly in the clinical specimen may be used. There is a urinary antigen that is commercially available for detection of *S. pneumoniae* antigen as a marker for pneumococcal pneumonia. Recently,

the assay has been used successfully in pleural fluid for diagnosis as well [89]. For *L. pneumophila,* use of direct fluorescent antibody stain (DFA) for the detection of antigens of *L. pneumophila* serogroup 1 is available commercially and provides direct examination of, for example, sputum, BAL fluid and cells, or lung tissue for making the diagnosis. The sensitivity of DFA is only about 70–75%, but combined with culture of the organism and sero-logic evaluation, it may provide increased sensitivity for detection of this pathogen. Detection of antigens in urine, rather than in the serum or at a body site, may be effective for diagnosis. Such is the case for detection of urinary antigens of *L. pneumophila* [90] and *H. capsulatum* [91, 92] in the diagnosis of legionnaires' disease and histoplasmosis, respectively. Detection of antigens may denote acute disease; however, with some antigen assays, this detection may indicate prior infection with the specific organism because antigen excretion may extend well past the stage of acute disease. For the detection of *T. vaginalis* in vaginal samples, the OSOM Rapid Test (Genzyme Diagnostics, Cambridge, MA) has been shown to have a better sensitivity than wet mount and compares favorably with recently developed molecular assays [93, 94]. Table 2-2 provides information about some of the available antigen-detection assays. Table 2-3 summarizes the methods for detection of the organisms encountered most commonly occupationally.

Table 2-2
Antigen-Detection Assays for Specific Agents

Agent/Disease	Assay	Specimen	Comments
Bacterial Agents			
Legionella pneumophila	DFA	Respiratory secretions	About 70–75% sensitivity.
	EIA	Urine	
Group A streptococcus	EIA, LA	Throat swab	80% sensitivity; > 100% specificity. Best for serogroup I infections, which are the majority.
	OIA	Throat swab	> 85% sensitivity.
Bordetella pertussis	IFA	Nasopharyngeal specimen	Sensitivity equal to or greater than culture.
Clostridium difficile toxins	EIA	Stool	Sensitivity may be less than that of cytotoxin B assays.
Clostridium difficile antigen	LA	Stool	High predictive value negative. Can be used as a negative screen
Fungal Agents			
Cryptococcus neoformans	LA, EIA	CSF, sera	>90% sensitivity compared to culture.
Histoplasma capsulatum	EIA	Urine, CSF	Good for disseminated histoplasmosis.
Candida sp.	LA	Sera	Specificity for invasive disease: controversial in literature.
Pneumocystis jerovecii (carinii)	DFA	Respiratory secretions	May be more specific than other stains.
Parasites			
Giardia lamblia	EIA, DFA	Stool	More sensitive than direct microscopic examination
Cryptosporidium sp.	EIA, DFA	Stool	More sensitive that direct microscopic examination
Entamoeba histolytica	EIA	Stool	May allow for differentiation of pathogenic vs. non-pathogenic species.
Viral Agents			
CMV	Antigenemia	Sera	Antigenemia assay.
Rotavirus	LA, EIA	Stool	Preferred method.
RSV	DFA, EIA	Nasopharyngeal	Preferred method.
Adenovirus	IFA	Respiratory secretions	Preferred method over culture; often combined in viral respiratory culture.
	LA	Stool	Serotype 40/41.
Influenza	IFA, EIA, LA	Respiratory secretions	Preferred method over culture; often combined in viral respiratory culture. May be less sensitive than PCR
Parainfluenza	IFA, EIA, LA	Respiratory secretions	Preferred method over culture; often combined in viral respiratory panel. May be less sensitive than PCR

Abbreviations: DFA = direct fluorescent antibody; EIA = enzyme immunoassay; LA = latex agglutination; IFA = indirect fluorescent antibody; OIA = optical immunoassay.
Based on data from references 32, 37–39, 46, 90–92, 96–107.

Table 2-3

Methods and Specimens for Some of the Organisms Likely To Be Encountered Occupationally

Agent	Specimen	Culture	Other	Serology
Bacteria				
Bartonella sp. [50, 51]	Blood, skin biopsy	Yes: requires special media	NAAT: may be preferred method when commercially available	Preferred method
Borrelia burgdorferi [83, 84]	Sera	Rarely		
C. trachomatis	Genital discharge	Yes: tissue culture	DFA, EIA, probes, NAAT is preferred method	Preferred method for LGV
Brucella sp	Blood, bone marrow	Yes: requires special media; preferred method		Not specific
C. pneumoniae [80]	Respiratory; sera	Not widely available	NAAT	MIF
C. psittaci	Respiratory secretions	Difficult		Yes: MIF, CF
C. trachomatis	Urine	No	NAAT	
Ehrlichia sp. [82]	Sera	No		Preferred method
F. tularensis				
Legionella pneumophila	Tissue, respiratory secretions, other sites	Yes: requires special media	DFA; PCR	Yes: IFA
Legionella pneumophila	Blood	Yes: rarely		
Legionella pneumophila	Urine		EIA antigen [85]	
Leptospira sp.	Blood in acute phase, urine later	Yes: requires special media	Dark-field exam	Yes: EIA, Agg
M. hominis	Genital discharge, urine, tissue, fluids	Yes		N/A
Mycobacterium sp.	Respiratory secretions, blood, other	Yes: with smear	Amp for MTB [67–72]	Not widely used in U.S.
P. multocida	Wound; blood	Yes		N/A
S. moniliformis	Blood	Yes: requires special media		Yes: agg
Spirillum minor	Wounds, nodes, skin	No	Dark-field exam	
Treponema pallidum	Genital discharge	No	Dark-field exam	Preferred method
M. pneumoniae	Respiratory secretions	Yes: insensitive	PCR	Yes: CF, EIA
Y. pestis	Node, respiratory secretions	Yes		
Fungi				
Aspergillus sp.	Any site	Yes: with stains		Yes: ID, CF; more in development
B. dermatitidis	Respiratory secretions, blood, skin, other	Yes: with smears		Yes: CF, EIA, ID
C. immitis	Respiratory secretions, CSF, skin, other	Yes: with smears	Hazardous to work with in lab	Yes: ID, CF, EIA in development
Dermatophytes	Skin, hair, nails	Yes: with stains		Yes: ID, CF, EIA
H. capsulatum	Bon marrow, respiratory secretions, blood, tissue, fluids	Yes: with smears	Urine and CSF antigen assays [91, 92, 96]	Yes: ID, CF, EIA
Malassezia sp.	Skin, blood	Yes: many species require oil for growth		N/A
Other molds	Any site	Yes: with stains	Must distinguish pathogen from saprophyte on clinical basis	Not widely used, except for *Zygomycetes*

(Continues)

Table 2-3
Continued

Agent	Specimen	Culture	Other	Serology
Fungi *(continued)*				
P. brasiliensis	Skin, respiratory secretions	Yes		Yes: cross-reacts with *B. dermatitidis*
jerovecii (carinii)	Respiratory secretions	No	DFA, toluidine blue, calcofluor, silver stains [26,27]	Yes: IFA
P. marneffei	Blood or any other site	Yes: with smears of tissue	Endemic: Thailand, China, and other countries in Far East	Being developed, as are methods for amp
S. schenckii	Skin, rarely blood or other sites	Yes: smears are insensitive, however		Not widely used
Yeast	Any site	Yes: with stains		Cand-Tec antigen for *C albicans* with questionable specificity for invasive disease
Parasites				
Cryptosporidia	Stool, other	No	O&P with acid-fast stain; antigen detection in stool	N/A
Cyclospora	Stool	No	Acid-fast stain	N/A
E. histolytica	Stool, liver abscess	Not usually used	O&P exam; antigen detection in stool	Yes: IHA, EIA
Echinococcus sp.	Surgical specimen	No	Exam for "hydatid sand" in surgical specimens	Yes: IHA
Giardia lamblia	Stool, string test	No	O&P exam, antigen detection in stool	N/A
Hookworm	Stool	No	O&P for eggs	N/A
Leishmania sp.	Blood, nodes	Yes: not widely available	Exam of tissue for trophozoites	Yes: IFA
Microsporidia	Stool, other sites	No	O&P exam with modified trichome stain	N/A
Plasmodium sp.	Blood smears	No	Exam for ring forms and gametocytes	Yes: IFA
Schistosoma sp.	Stool	No	Exam for eggs	Yes: IFA
Strongyloides sp.	Stool, other sites	Not widely used	O&P for larvae	Yes: IHA
T. canis	Stool, tissue	No	O&P for eggs	Yes: EIA
T. gondii	Blood, CSF, nodes, tissue	Yes: tissue culture not widely available	Giemsa and other stains; amp	Yes: IFA, EIA IgG and IgM
Taenia sp.	Stool	No	Exam for eggs	
Trichinella sp.	Muscle biopsy	No	Exam for cysts	Yes: bentonite flocculation
Trichomonas vaginalis	Vaginal discharge	Yes: but not widely used	Wet mount for motility; probe	N/A
Trypanosoma sp.	Blood, other	No	Exam for trophozoites	Yes: CF, IHA
Viruses				
Arbovirus	Brain biopsy, blood	Rarely done		Preferred: IFA, CF, HI, EIA, IgM and IgG
Adenovirus	Any	Yes: shell vial and conventional	Antigen detection in respiratory specimens	Yes: CF, EIA
	Stool		Antigen detection 40/41	
LCM	CSF, throat, urine, serum	Yes	Biosafety level 4	
CMV	Any	Yes: shell vial and conventional	Antigen detection, probes, amp	Yes: CF, IHA, EIA, IFA

Table 2-3
Continued

Agent	Specimen	Culture	Other	Serology
Viruses *(continued)*				
EBV	Blood	No		Yes: heterophile agg; IgM and IgG VCA, EBNA, EA
Hepatitis A	Blood	No	NAAT (75)	Yes: RIA or EIA, IgM, anti-HAV
Hepatitis B	Blood	No	NAAT	Yes: RIA or EIA
Hepatitis C	Blood	No	NAAT [74]	EIA, Western blot
Hepatitis D	Blood	No		RIA
Hepatitis E	Blood	No		EIA, Western blot
HIV [73]	Blood	Yes but lengthy incubation; may be preferred in neonates	NAAT	EIA with Western blot for confirmation
HSV	CSF	No	Amp preferred method [22]	
	Any other site	Yes: shell vial or conventional	Antigen detection; ELVIS	Available but not specific for diagnosis
Calicivirus, Norwalk virus, astrovirus: gastroenteritis	Stool	No	EM	
Measles	Nasopharynx, throat, other	Not widely used	Direct IFA	Yes: HI, EIA, IgM by IFA, EIA, RIA, CF
Mumps	Blood	No		Yes: IFA, EIA, HAI
Rubella	Throat, tissue, urine	Not widely done		Preferred: EIA, HI, IFA, CF
HPV [50]	Genital	No	Probe, in situ, NAAT	
Rabies	Brain biopsy	Not routine	Direct IFA	IFA, RFFIT: diagnosis and immune status
Influenza A and B	Respiratory secretions	Yes	Direct antigen detection	Yes: CF, HAI
Parainfluenza I, II, III	Respiratory secretions	Yes	Direct antigen detection	Yes: HAI, CF, EIA
	Lesion; vesicle [15]	Yes	DFA	Yes
	NP aspirates	Yes	Direct antigen preferred	N/A

Abbreviations: Agg = agglutination; NAAT = nucleic acid amplification; CF = complement fixation; DFA = direct fluorescence antibody; EIA = enzyme immunoassay; ID = immunodiffusion; IFA = indirect immunofluorescence; IHA = inhibition hemagglutination assay; LGV = lymphogranuloma venereum; MIF = microimmunofluorescence; N/A = not applicable or not available; O&P = ova and parasites; * = research only.

Antimicrobial Susceptibility Testing

Most laboratories perform antimicrobial susceptibility testing routinely or on a request basis. For bacteria commonly isolated from blood, urine, or CSF specimens, for example, each laboratory has the option of performing qualitative assay (Bauer-Kirby) or quantitative assay (MIC or E-Test assay). The choice of assay is often based on the methods available to the laboratory and the demands of the physicians it supports.

The Bauer-Kirby test uses agar plates, onto which selected isolates are inoculated in a "lawn of growth" and on which disks of specific antibiotic concentrations are applied. The plates are incubated, usually overnight, and on the following day, *zones of inhibition* (in millimeters) are recorded for each drug. The larger the zone that is found, the more susceptible the organism is to the drug being tested. There are standard methods for performing the assay with regard to the medium used, inoculation size, and concentration of disks [62, 63].

The minimum inhibitory concentration (MIC) test can be performed in agar plates with varying concentrations of specific drugs, each plate containing one concentration of one drug, or they may be done in large tubes of broth (macrotube dilution) or in small volumes of broth in microtiter trays (microbroth dilutions). Regardless of the manner in which the test is performed, the results are read as the lowest concentration of each drug that inhibits the organism from growing after overnight incubation.

For either the Bauer-Kirby or MIC assay, the results are coded as S = susceptible, I = intermediate, or R = resistant.

In addition to these interpretive criteria, if the MIC is performed, numbers in micrograms per milliliter (μg/mL) are also given to indicate the concentration that actually inhibited the organism.

Some laboratories perform a test called the *E-test,* which employs a strip, rather than a disk, that has been impregnated with a graded concentration of the antibiotic to be tested. These strips are placed on the top of an agar plate that has been seeded with the organism to be tested. When read, the place where the organism's growth crosses a specific concentration of the drug on the strip is read as the MIC. The area of no growth around these strips resembles an ellipse rather than a circle. Use of the E-test is increasing, especially in small laboratories that infrequently perform susceptibility tests and those that test for fastidious organisms, for which the MIC and Bauer-Kirby tests are not available or not rapidly accessible to the laboratory for that specific organism. The Clinical Laboratory Standards Institute (CLSI, formerly NCCLS) has set standard protocols for susceptibility testing procedures and interpretations [95].

The minimum bactericidal concentration (MBC) assay is performed less often in laboratories but, when done, requires determination of not only the inhibitory level but also the actual killing capability of the drug in question. MBCs can be determined only if a prior MIC test has been performed. Samples from the wells or tubes that remain visually negative are plated onto the surface of agar plates and incubated overnight. The next day, colonies are counted to determine which of the visually negative wells actually contains organisms. The well in which no growth occurs after agar plating is considered the MBC. If a drug is "cidal," the MIC and MBC are within one to two dilutions. If the drug is inhibitory and not cidal, then there will

be a more than two-well dilution difference between the MIC and MBC.

Methods have been developed and standardized for the susceptibility testing of *M. tuberculosis* and yeast organisms. For molds and other *Mycobacterium* species, some laboratories may perform susceptibility assays that they have developed in-house or as a part of CLSI evaluation studies. The CLSI is working on a protocol for the susceptibility testing of molds, including dermatophytes. Currently, viral susceptibility testing is in the research stage but probably will be available for clinical use in the future.

Summary of Diagnostic Methods for Parasites, Fungi, Mycobacteria, and Viral Agents

PARASITES

- Stool needs to be submitted fresh or preserved in formalin or PVA. If fresh, they should be sent to laboratory in fewer than 2 hours.
- Specimens are examined microscopically by wet mount; iodine preparations and trichrome-stained preparations are used to visualize trophozoites and cysts (if present).
- Antigen assays also are available for *Giardia, Cryptosporidium* species, and *E. histolytica* [37–39]
- For *Microsporidia,* a modified trichrome called the *Weber stain* is used, and observations are made under oil immersion.
- For *Cyclospora, Cryptosporidium* species, and *Isospora belli,* an acid-fast stain is preferable.
- For *Plasmodium* or *Babesia microtii,* blood is sent to the laboratory, and thick and thin smears are prepared and stained with trichrome stain. Ring forms in red blood cells and the presence of gametes are diagnostic. An immunochromatographic antigen assay for the rapid detection of *Plasmodium* species, in particular, *P. falciparum,* has been introduced recently into clinical microbiology laboratories.
- For leishmaniasis, direct observation of tissue sections, skin snips, or biopsy specimens or culture and serology should be considered to aid in the diagnosis.
- For microfilaria (e.g., *Wuchereria bancrofti, Brugia malayi,* and *Loa loa*), blood smears are used

to see microfilaria; for *W. bancrofti* and *B. malayi,* nocturnal, and for *Loa loa,* diurnal.

- For *Onchocerca,* the presence of microfilaria in skin snips is diagnostic.

- *T. gondii* is usually diagnosed serologically; however, clusters of tachyzoites and, in some cases, cysts can be seen in stained tissue sections. Amplification methods are becoming more the standard for diagnosis.

- For trichinosis, detection of spiral larvae in muscle tissue in conjunction with serologic testing is confirmatory.

- For rapid diagnosis of *T. vaginalis* in vaginal specimens, there is an antigen assay called *OSOM Trichomonas Rapid Test* (Genzyme Diagnostics, Cambridge, MA) that is more sensitive that the wet-mount observation and compares favorably with PCR assays for *T. vaginalis* [93].

FUNGI

- Culture and direct stains by means of calcofluor white or Congo red are standard; amplification is available in research laboratories; serology may be helpful in making some diagnoses.

- For dimorphic fungi, *H. capsulatum, B. dermatitidis, C. immitis, P. brasiliensis, Sporothrix schenckii,* and *Penicillium marneffei,* after isolation in culture, demonstration of the yeast form as a conversion from mold is necessary. Exoantigen or probe tests of the mold form of the organism are needed for definitive identification.

- For *H. capsulatum,* lung, sputum, BAL, lymph nodes, blood, bone marrow, or CSF culture requires up to 6 weeks for isolation and use of specific media; a probe is available for culture confirmation. This requires a special request from the laboratory for isolation of the organism from blood. A *Histoplasma* urinary antigen assay is available commercially and has a very good sensitivity in the diagnosis of extrapulmonary (disseminated) histoplasmosis [91, 92, 96].

- For *B. dermatitidis,* lung, sputum, BAL, skin, bone, or CSF culture is standard; rarely, blood culture is used, but if so, a special request to the laboratory is required. This requires up to 2–3 weeks for isolation of the organism. A probe is available for culture confirmation.

- For *C. immitis,* lung, sputum, BAL, CSF, skin, or rarely, blood culture is done. This requires only 4–5 days for isolation. This organism is a potential hazard in the laboratory, so alert the laboratory if its presence suspected. A probe is available for culture confirmation.

- For *P. brasiliensis,* the approach is the same as for *B. dermatitidis.*

- For *S. schenckii,* skin, lymph nodes, and less likely respiratory or other more systemic sites are cultured; there is no probe because conversion is easy and takes only a short period of time. This requires only about 3–4 days for isolation. Mold is dematiaceous (black).

- For *P. marneffei,* any tissue, blood, or bone marrow can be used; this looks like *H. capsulatum* in tissue and peripheral blood. Conversion from mold (with red diffusible pigment) to a yeast-like form is necessary for confirmation.

- For *Aspergillus* species, isolation can be done from any site; *Aspergillus* may be the pathogen or a contaminate/saprophyte. Antigen assays for detection of galactomannan as a marker for presence of disseminated aspergillosis are available for serum testing [97].

- *Candida* and other yeast usually are easily isolated; any specimen may be used, but *Candida* may be the etiology or part of the normal flora.

- Dermatophytes usually are isolated from specimens of hair, skin, or nails; they may require up to 3–4 weeks for isolation. A genus-level identification is adequate.

- Dematiaceous molds may be soil contaminants in laboratory or saprophytes in patients or may be responsible for clinical disease. They usually require more than 48 hours for isolation. Many genera and species are isolated in human disease; a reference laboratory may be needed for definitive identification.

MYCOBACTERIA

For *M. tuberculosis,* culture and AFB smear of specimens from the respiratory tract, tissue, or body fluids are required. All specimens from nonsterile sites first should be decontaminated and concentrated. Laboratories should use a broth culture supplemented with agar cultures for rapid detection and identification. Testing requires about 10–15 days in broth culture; longer in agar. Once isolated, cultures should be identified by probes, HPLC, or sequencing for rapid identification. Susceptibility testing of all isolates is required. Two amplification assays are available for direct specimen processing, but they should be performed only on respiratory samples that are smear-positive. To meet Centers for Disease Control and Prevention (CDC) guidelines, laboratories should strive to perform AFB smears within 24 hours, isolate and identify *M. tuberculosis* within 21 days, and perform susceptibility testing within 30 days. With the use of probes, the identification of *M. tuberculosis* will be reported as a complex including *M. tuberculosis*, *M. bovis*, *M. microtii*, and *M. africanum* [53, 70, 98].

MOTT (*MYCOBACTERIUM* SPECIES OTHER THAN *M. TUBERCULOSIS*) AND *NOCARDIA* SPECIES

Any specimen sent to the laboratory should be processed as for *M. tuberculosis*. *M. avium-intracellulare* (MAI) is usually isolated within the first 5–7 days and others in varying amounts of time. Rapidly growing *Mycobacterium* species may require variable amounts of time for primary isolation, but on transferring the isolates in the laboratory, fewer than 5–7 days are required. Identification of MAI, *M. gordonae*, and *M. kansasii* can be done with genetic probes. The other species require HPLC, sequencing, or conventional biochemical means of identification. Isolation of a *Nocardia* species or other aerobic actinomycetes is done most often in the mycology or mycobacteria sections of the laboratory. Identification is best accomplished by means of a sequencing method because biochemicals cannot speciate adequately. Susceptibility testing is not thoroughly standardized nor available for all the *Mycobacterium* and *Nocardia* species, although many laboratories will provide MIC testing in-house or as a sendout to a reference laboratory if requested.

VIRUSES

Many viruses can be cultured in the laboratory. For culturing of these viruses, specimens should be transported to the laboratory in an appropriate container/tube that also contains an appropriate viral transport medium and antibiotics. A conventional culture is processed in tubes and incubated for 30 days. Alternatively, a more rapid shell vial technique, requiring 48 hours, may be employed

for some viruses. For some of the viral agents that are responsible for gastroenteritis, such as calicivirus, astrovirus, and Norwalk virus, an electron microscopic examination may be provided; for others, antigen-detection methods can be used on stool specimens. Amplification and probe technology is more and more widely employed for viral diagnosis. Phoning the laboratory with requests often enables the laboratory to search for reference laboratories that do perform the assay if it does not.

References

1. Doern GV, Vautour R, Gaudet M, et al. Clinical impact of rapid in vitro susceptibility testing and bacterial identification. *J Clin Microbiol* 1994;32:1757–62.
2. McLaughlin J. The implementation of cost-effective, clinically relevant diagnostic microbiology policies: The approach. *Clin Microbiol Newsl* 1995;17:70–1.
3. Thomson RB, Peterson LR. The role of the clinical microbiology laboratory in the diagnosis of infections. In Noskin LA (ed), *Management of Infectious Complications in Cancer Patients.* Boston: Kluwer Academic Publishers, 1998.
4. Wilson ML. Clinically relevant, cost-effective clinical microbiology: Strategies to decrease unnecessary testing. *Am J Clin Pathol* 1997;107:154–67.
5. Baron EJ, Wienstein MP, Dunne WM, et al. In Cumitech IC, Sharp SE (eds), Blood Cultures IV. Washington: American Society for Microbiology Press, 2005.
6. Reimer L, Wilson M, Weinstein M. Update on detection of bacteremia and fungemia. *Clin Microbiol Rev* 1997;10:144–65.
7. Wilson ML. General principles in specimen collection and transport. *Clin Infect Dis* 1996;22:766–77.
8. Winn W, Koneman EW, Allen SD, et al. (eds). *Color Atlas and Textbook of Diagnostic Microbiology,* 5th ed. Philadelphia: Lippincott, 2006.
9. Qian Q, Eichelberger K, Kirby JE. Rapid identification of *Staphylococcus aureus* in blood cultures by use of the direct tube coagulase test. *J Clin Microbiol* 2007;45:2267–9.
10. Shephard JR, Addison RM, Alexander BD, et al. Multicenter evaluation of the *Candida albicans/Candida glabrata* peptide nucleic acid fluorescent in situ hybridization method for simultaneous dual-color identification of *C. albicans* and *C. glabrata* directly from blood culture bottles. *J Clin Microbiol* 2008;46:50–5.
11. Hartmann H, Stender H, Schafer A, et al. Rapid identification of *Staphylococcus aureus* in blood cultures by a combination of fluorescence in situ hybridization using peptide nucleic acid probes and flow cytometry. *J Clin Microbiol* 2005;43:4855–7.
12. Forrest GN, Mehta S, Weekes E, et al. Impact of in

situ hybridization testing of coagulase negative staphylococci positive blood cultures. *J Antimicrob Chemother* 2006;58:154–8.

13. Forrest GN. PNA Fish: Present and future impact on patient management. *Expert Rev Mol Diagn* 2007;7: 231–6.

14. Grobner S, Kempf VA. Rapid detection of methicillin-resistant staphylococci by real-time PCR directly from positive blood culture bottles. *Eur J Clin Microbiol Infect Dis* 2007;26:751–4.

15. Stamper PD, Cai M, Howard T, et al. Clinical validation of the molecular BD GeneOhm StaphSR assay for direct detection of *Staphylococcus aureus* and methicillin-resistant *Staphylococcus aureus* in positive blood cultures. *J Clin Microbiol* 2007;45:2191–6.

16. Miller JM. *A Guide to Specimen Management in Clinical Microbiology.* Washington: American Society for Microbiology Press, 1996.

17. Gleaves CA, Hodinka RL, Johnston SLG, et al. *Cumitech 15A: Laboratory Diagnosis of Viral Infections.* Washington: American Society for Microbiology Press, 1994.

18. Lennette EH, Lennette DA, Lennette ET (eds). *Diagnostic Procedures for Viral, Rickettsial, and Chlamydial Infections,* 7th ed. Washington: American Public Health Association, 1995.

19. Marshall DJ, Residorf E, Harms G, et al. Evaluation of a multiplexed PCR assay for detection of respiratory viral pathogens in a public health laboratory setting. *J Clin Microbiol* 2007;45:3875–82.

20. Perez-Ruiz M, Yeste R, Ruiz-Perez MJ, et al. Testing of diagnostic methods for detection of influenza virus for optimal performance in the context of an influenza surveillance network. *J Clin Microbiol* 2007;45:3109–10.

21. Mahony J, Chong S, Merante F, et al. Development of a respiratory virus panel test for detection of twenty human respiratory viruses by use of multiplex PCR and a fluid microbead-based assay. *J Clin Microbiol* 2007;45:2965–70.

22. Sharp SE, Robinson A, Soubolle M, et al. *Cumitech 7B: Laboratory Diagnosis of Lower Respiratory Tract Infections.* Washington: American Society for Microbiology Press, 2005.

23. Murray P, Washington JA. Microscopic and bacteriologic analysis of expectorated sputum. *Mayo Clinic Proc* 1975;50:339–44.

24. Musher VM. The usefulness of sputum Gram stain and culture. *Arch Intern Med* 2005;165:470–1.

25. Baselski V, Mason K. Pneumonia in the immunocompromised host: The value of bronchoscopy and newer diagnostic techniques. *Semin Respir Infect* 2000;15:144–61.

26. Eisen D, Ross BC, Fairbairn J, et al. Comparison of *Pneumocystis carinii* detection by toluidine blue O staining, direct immunofluorescence and DNA amplification in sputum specimens from HIV-positive patients. *Pathology* 1994;26:198–200.

27. Wiwanitkit V. Study of the cost-effectiveness of three staining methods for identification of *P. carinii* in bronchoalveolar lavage fluid. *Trop Doct* 2005;35: 23–5.

28. Gray LD, Fedorko DP. Laboratory diagnosis of bacterial meningitis. *Clin Microbiol Rev* 1992;5:130–45.

29. Perkins MD, Mirrett S, Reller LB. Rapid bacterial antigen detection is not clinically useful. *J Clin Microbiol* 1995;33:1486–90.

30. Antinori S, Radice A, Galimberti L, et al. The role of cryptococcal antigen assay in the diagnosis and monitoring of cryptococcal meningitis. *J Clin Microbiol* 2005;43:5828–9.

31. DeBiasi RL, Kleinschmidt-DeMasters BK, Weinberg A, et al. Use of PCR for the diagnosis of herpesvirus infection of the central nervous system. *J Clin Virol* 2002;25:S5–11.

32. Kost CB, Rogers B, Oberste MS, et al. Multicenter beta trial of the GeneXpert enterovirus assay. *J Clin Microbiol* 2007;45:1081–6.

33. Sharp SE (ed). *Cumitech 44: Nucleic Acid Amplification tests for the detection of Chlamydia trachomatis and Neisseria gonorrhoeae.* Washington: American Society for Microbiology Press, 2006.

34. Briselden A, Hillier SL. Evaluation of ARRIRM VP: Microbial identification test for *Gardnerella vaginalis* and *Trichomonas vaginalis*. *J Clin Microbiol* 1994;32:148–52.

35. Kehl KS, Havens P, Behnke CE, et al. Evaluation of the Premier EHEC assay for detection of Shiga-toxin-producing *Escherichia coli*. *J Clin Microbiol* 1997;35:2051–4.

36. Park CH, Kim HJ, Hixon DL. Importance of testing stool specimens for Shiga toxins. *J Clin Microbiol* 2002;40:3542–3.

37. Schunk M, Jelink T, Weizel K, et al. Detection of *Giardia lamblia* and *Entamoeba histolytica* in stool samples by two enzyme immunoassays. *Eur J Clin Microbiol Infect Dis* 2001;20:389–91.

38. Aldeen WE, Hale D, Robeson AJ, et al. Evaluation of a commercially available ELISA assay for detection of *Giardia lamblia* in fecal specimens. *Diagn Microbiol Infect Dis* 1995;21:1137–42.

39. Weitzel T, Dittrich S, Mohl I, et al. Evaluation of seven commercial antigen tests of *Giardia* and *Cryptosporidium* in stool samples. *Clin Microbiol Infect* 2006;12:656–9.

40. Fan K, Morris A, Reller B. Application of rejection criteria for stool cultures for bacterial enteric pathogens. *J Clin Microbiol* 1993;31:2233–5.

41. Siegel DL, Edelstein PH, Nachamkin I. Inappropriate testing for diarrheal diseases in the hospital. *JAMA* 1990;263:1027–9.

42. Yannelli B, Gurvich I, Schoch PE, et al. Yield of stool cultures, ova and parasite tests, and *Clostridium difficile* determinations in nosocomial diarrhea. *Am J Infect Control* 1988;16:246–9.

43. Peterson LC, Kelly PJ. The role of the clinical laboratory in the management of *C. difficile*–associated diarrhea. *Infect Dis Clin North Am* 1993;7:277–93.

44. Terletskaia-Ladwig E, Leinmuller M, Schneider F, et al. Laboratory approach to the diagnosis of

adenovirus infection depending on clinical manifestations. *Infection* 2007;35:438–43.

45. Lipson SM, Svenssen L, Goodwin L, et al. Evaluation of two current generation enzyme immunoassays and an improved isolation based assay for the rapid detection and isolation of rotavirus from stool. *J Clin Virol* 2001;21:17–27.

46. Sanders RC, Campbell AD, Jenkins AF. Routine detection of human rotavirus by latex agglutination: Comparison with latex agglutination, electron microscopy and polyacrylamide gel electrophoresis. *J Virol Methods* 1986;13:285–90.

47. Logan C, O'Leary JJ, O'Sullivan N. Real-time reverse transcriptase PCR for detection of rotavirus and adenovirus as causative agents of acute gastroenteritis in children. *J Clin Microbiol* 2006;44:3189–95.

48. Stager CE, Fraire AE, Kim H, et al. Modification of the Fungi-Fluor and the Genetic Systems fluorescent antibody methods for detection of *Pneumocystis carinii* in bronchoalveolar lavage specimens. *Arch Pathol Lab Med* 1995;119:142–7.

49. Procop GW. Molecular diagnostics for the detection and characterization of microbial pathogens. *Clin Infect Dis* 2007;45:S99–111.

50. Garcia-Esteban C, Gil H, Rodriguez-Vargas M, et al. Molecular methods for *Bartonella* sp. identification in clinical and environmental samples. *J Clin Microbiol* 2008;46:776–9.

51. Gescher DM, Mallmann C, Kovacevic D, et al. A view on *Bartonella quintana* endocarditis: Confirming the molecular diagnosis by specific fluorescence in situ hybridization. *Diagn Microbiol Infec Dis* 2008; 60:99–102.

52. Hall GS. Probe technology for the clinical microbiology laboratory. *Arch Pathol Lab Med* 1993;117: 578–83.

53. Hall GS. Identifying *M. tuberculosis. Adv Lab Admin* 1995;May:27–34.

54. Tenover FC, Unger ER. Nucleic acid probes for detection and identification of infectious agents. In Persing DH, Smith TF, Tenover FC, et al. (eds), *Diagnostic Molecular Microbiology: Principles and Applications.* Washington: American Society for Microbiology Press, 1993.

55. Iwen PC, Walker RA, Warren KL, et al. Evaluation of nucleic acid–based test (PACE 2C) for simultaneous detection of *Chlamydia trachomatis* and *Neisseria gonorrhoeae* in endocervical specimens. *J Clin Microbiol* 1995;33:2587–91.

56. Petrikkos G, Makrilakis K, Pappas S. Affirm VPIII in the detection and identification of *Candida* sp. in vaginitis. *Int J Gynecol Obstet* 2007;96:39–40.

57. Gazi H, Degerli K, Kurt O, et al. Use of DNA hybridization test for diagnosing bacterial vaginosis in women with symptoms suggestive of infection. *APMIS* 2006;114:784–7.

58. Brown HL, Fuller DD, Jasper LT, et al. Clinical evaluation of Affirm VPIII in the detection and identification of *Trichomonas vaginalis, Gardnerella*

vaginalis, and *Candida* species in vaginitis/vaginosis. *Infect Dis Obstet Gynecol* 2004;12:17–21.

59. Pokorski SJ, Vetter EA, Wollan PC, et al. Comparison of Gen-Probe group A streptococcus direct test with culture for diagnosing streptococcal pharyngitis. *J Clin Microbiol* 1994;32:1440–3.

60. Persing DH. Polymerase chain reaction: Trenches to benches. *J Clin Microbiol* 1991;29:1281–5.

61. Wolcott MJ. Advances in nucleic acid based detection methods. *Clin Microbiol Rev* 1992;5:370–86.

62. Chernesky MA, Jang DE. APTIMA transcription-mediated amplification assays for *C. trachomatis* and *N. gonorrhoeae. Expert Rev Mol Diagn* 2006;6: 519–25.

63. Koenig MG, Kosha SL, Doty BL, et al. Direct comparison of the BD ProbeTecET system with in-house Light Cycler PCR assays for detection of *Chlamydia trachomatis* and *Neisseria gonorrhoeae* from clinical specimens. *J Clin Microbiol* 2005;43:2036–7.

64. Gaydos CA, Theodore M, Dalesio N, et al. Comparison of three nucleic acid amplification tests for detection of *Chlamydia trachomatis* in urine specimens. *J Clin Microbiol* 2004;42:3041–5.

65. Chernesky M, Freund GG, Hook E, et al. Detection of *Chlamydia trachomatis* and *Neisseria gonorrhoeae* infections in North American women by testing SurePath liquid-based PAP specimens in APTIMA assays. *J Clin Microbiol* 2007;45:2434–8.

66. Chernesky M, Jang D, Portillo E, et al. Abilities of APTIMA, AMPLICOR, and ProbeTec assays to detect *Chlamydia trachomatis* and *Neisseria gonorrhoeae* in PreservCyt ThinPrep liquid-based PAP samples. *J Clin Microbiol* 2007;45:2355–8.

67. Eing BR, Becker A, Sohns A, et al. Comparison of Roche COBAS AMPLICOR *Mycobacterium tuberculosis* assay with in-house PCR and culture for detection of *M. tuberculosis. J Clin Microbiol* 1998;36: 2023–9.

68. Gamboa F, Fernandez G, Padilla E, et al. Comparative evaluation of initial and new versions of the Gen-Probe amplified *Mycobacterium tuberculosis* direct test for direct detection of *Mycobacterium tuberculosis* in respiratory specimens. *J Clin Microbiol* 1998;36:684–9.

69. Reischl U, Lehn N, Wolf H, et al. Clinical evaluation of the automated COBAS AMPLICOR MTB assay for testing respiratory and nonrespiratory specimens. *J Clin Microbiol* 1998;36:2853–60.

70. Doern GV. Diagnostic mycobacteriology: Where are we today? *J Clin Microbiol* 1996;34:1873–6.

71. Shrestha NK, Tuohy MJ, Hall GS et al. Detection and differentiation of *Mycobacterium tuberculosis* and nontuberculous mycobacterial isolates by real-time PCR. *J Clin Microbiol* 2003;41:5121–6.

72. Kobayashi N, Fraser TG, Bauer TW, et al. The use of real-time polymerase chain reaction for rapid diagnosis of skeletal tuberculosis. *Arch Pathol Lab Med* 2006;130:1053–6.

73. Yen-Lieberman B. Rapid and alternative specimen

source testing for HIV-1 antibodies. *Clin Microbiol Newsl* 1998;20:133–7.

74. Alte HJ, Sanchez-Pescador R, Urdea MS, et al. Evaluation of branched DNA signal amplification for the detection of hepatitis C virus RNA. *J Viral Hepatitis* 1995;2:121–32.

75. Valsamakis A. Molecular testing in the diagnosis and management of chronic hepatitis A. *Clin Microbiol Rev* 2007;20:426–39.

76. Halfon P, Trepo E, Antoniotti G, et al. Prospective evaluation of Hybrid Capture 2 and AMPLICOR human papillomavirus (HPV) tests for detection of 13 high-risk HPV genotypes in atypical squamous of uncertain origin. *J Clin Microbiol* 2007;45:313–6.

77. Ross TL, Merz WG, Farkosh M, et al. Comparison of an automated repetitive sequence-based PCR microbial typing system to pulsed-field-gel-electrophoresis for analysis of outbreaks of methicillin-resistant *Staphylococcus aureus*. *J Clin Microbiol* 2005;43:5642–7.

78. Healy M, Huong J, Bittner T, et al. Microbial DNA typing by automated repetitive-sequence-based PCR. *J Clin Microbiol* 2005;43:199–207.

79. Detrick B, Hamilton RG, Folds JD (eds). *Manual of Molecular and Clinical Laboratory Immunology*, 7th ed. Washington: American Society for Microbiology Press, 2006.

80. Gaydos CA, Roblin PM, Hammerschlag MR, et al. Diagnostic utility of PCR-enzyme immunoassay, culture, and serology for detection of *Chlamydia pneumoniae* in symptomatic and asymptomatic patients. *J Clin Microbiol* 1994;32:903–5.

81. Raoult D, Fournier PE, Drancourt M, et al. Diagnosis of 22 new cases of *Bartonella* endocarditis. *Ann Intern Med* 1996;125:646–52.

82. Dumler JS, Madigan JE, Pusterla N, et al. Ehrlichiosis in humans: Epidemiology, clinical presentation, diagnosis and treatment. *Clin Infect Dis* 2007;45:S45–51.

83. Coulter P, Lema C, Flayhart D, et al. Two-year evaluation of *Borrelia burgdorferi* culture and supplemental tests for the definitive diagnosis of Lyme disease. *J Clin Microbiol* 2005;43:5080–4.

84. Dumler JS. Molecular diagnosis of Lyme disease: Review and meta-analysis. *Mol Diag* 2001;6:1–11.

85. Waterer GW, Baselski VS, Wunderich RG. *Legionella* and community-acquired pneumonia: A review of current diagnostic tests from a clinician's viewpoint. *Am J Med* 2001;110:41–8.

86. Kwon-Chung KJ, Bennett J (eds). *Medical Mycology*, 3rd ed. Philadelphia: Lea & Febiger, 1992.

87. Garcia LS. *Diagnostic Medical Parasitology*, 5th ed. Washington: American Society for Microbiology Press, 2006.

88. Guichon A, Inzana TJ, Scimeca JM, et al. *Cumitech 28: Laboratory Diagnosis of Zoonotic Infections: Chlamydia, Fungal, Viral, and Parasitic Infections Obtained from Companion and Laboratory Animals.*

Washington: American Society for Microbiology Press, 1996.

89. Porcel JM, Ruiz-Gonzalez A, Falguera M, et al. Contribution of a pleural antigen assay (BINAX NOW) to the diagnosis of pneumococcal pneumonia. *Chest* 2007;131:1442–7.

90. Kashuba ADM, Balows CH. *Legionella* urinary antigen testing: Potential impact on diagnosis and antibiotic therapy. *DMID* 1996;24:129–39.

91. Durkin MM, Connolly PA, Wheat LJ. Comparison of radioimmunoassay and enzyme-linked immunoassay for detection of *Histoplasma capsulatum* var. *capsulatum* antigen. *J Clin Microbiol* 1997;35:2252–5.

92. Wheat LJ, Kohler RB, Tewardi RP, et al. Significance of *Histoplasma* antigen in the cerebrospinal fluid of patients with meningitis. *Arch Intern Med* 1989;149:302–4.

93. Huppert JS, Batteiger BE, Braslins P, et al. Use of an immunochromatographic assay for rapid detection of *Trichomonas vaginalis* in vaginal specimens. *J Clin Microbiol* 2005;43:684–7.

94. Huppert JS, Mortensen JE, Reed JL, et al. Rapid antigen testing compares favorably with transcription-mediated amplification assay for the detection of *Trichomonas vaginalis* in young women. *Clin Infect Dis* 2007;45:194–8.

95. Clinical and Laboratory Standards Institute (formerly NCCLS). *Performance Standards for Antimicrobial Susceptibility Testing: 18th Informational Supplement* (M100-S18). Wayne, PA: CLSI, 2008.

96. Kauffman CA. Histoplasmosis: A clinical and laboratory update. *Clin Microbiol Rev* 2007;20:115–32.

97. El-Mahallawy HA, Shaker HH, Ali-Helmy H, et al. Evaluation of pan-fungal PCR assay and *Aspergillus* antigen detection in the diagnosis of invasive fungal infections in high risk pediatric cancer patients. *Med Mycol* 2006;44:733–9.

98. Cernoch PL, Enns RK, Saubolle MA, et al. *Cumitech 16A: Laboratory Diagnosis of the Mycobacterioses*. Washington: American Society for Microbiology Press, 1994.

99. Baker DM, Cooper RM, Rhodes C, et al. Superiority of conventional culture techniques over rapid detection of group A streptococcus by optical immunoassay. *Diag Microbiol Infect Dis* 1995;21:61–4.

100. Pallavicini F, Izzi I, Pennisi MA, et al. Evaluation of the utility of serological tests in the diagnosis of candidemia. *Minerva Anestesiol* 1999;65:637–9.

101. Furrows SJ, Moody AH, Chiodini PL. Comparison of PCR and antigen detection methods for diagnosis of *Entamoeba histolytica* infection. *J Clin Pathol* 2004;57:1264–6.

102. Visser LG, Verweij JJ, VanEsbroeck M, et al. Diagnostic methods for differentiation of *Entamoeba histolytica* and *Entamoeba dispar* in carriers: Performance and clinical implications in a non-endemic setting. *Int J Med Microbiol* 2006;296:397–403.

103. Jamison RM (ed). *Cumitech 38: Human Cy-*

tomegalovirus. Washington: American Society for Microbiology Press, 2003.

104. Takamoto S, Grandien M, Ishida MA, et al. Comparison of ELISA, indirect immunofluorescence assay and virus isolation for detection of respiratory syncytial virus in nasopharyngeal secretions. *J Clin Microbiol* 1991;29:470–4.

105. Dominquez A, Taber LH, Couch RB. Comparison of rapid diagnostic techniques for respiratory syncytial and influenza A virus respiratory infections in young children. *J Clin Microbiol* 1993;31:2286–90.

106. Reina J, Munar M, Blanco I. Evaluation of a direct immunofluorescence assay, dot-blot enzyme immunoassay, and shell vial culture in the diagnosis of lower respiratory tract infections caused by influenza A virus. *Diag Microbiol Infect Dis* 1996;25:143–5.

107. Caliendo AM, Ingersoll J, Fox-Canale AM, et al. Evaluation of real-time PCR laboratory-developed tests using analyte-specific reagents for cytomegalovirus quantification. *J Clin Microbiol* 2007;45:1723–7

3

Epidemiology and Etiology of Occupational Infectious Diseases

Daymon Evans

Background and History

The central premise of epidemiology is that injuries and illnesses are not distributed randomly. It is the science that estimates the frequency and distribution of injury and illness from accurate knowledge of the frequency and distribution of known risk factors. Epidemiology is the formal study and treatment of populations rather than the linear clinical care of individual patients. It is from the care of the individual that one learns the art of medicine, but it is only from the study of groups that we all find and share the science of medicine. Epidemiology studies the associations, causation, and ultimately, methods of control and prevention of injury and illness and their effectiveness.

The early advancement of medical science depended on the astute individual clinician who was stimulated by a single case, formed a hypothesis of causation, and began a mission of scientific proof. The Henle-Koch postulates formed the basis of the scientific method, and epidemiology was nearly synonymous with communicable disease until the middle of the twentieth century. Epidemiology expanded to other areas such as chronic disease, the behavioral sciences, injuries, and most recently, clinical pathways and outcome analysis collectively now called *evidence-based medicine.* Epidemiology and biostatistics are being used more and more to justify or discredit treatment methods.

Today, there are formal systems of surveillance to look for outbreaks, epidemics, or new associations. Infectious disease, however, remains the number one global cause of death. New infectious agents and diseases are being discovered, most often by a clinician or basic scientist pursuing a premonition. Many familiar chronic and degenerative diseases are now suspected or proved to have microbiotic or immunologic causation. It was only 12 years between the isolation of a strange spiral bacteria from gastric mucosa and the *NIH Consensus Statement on Helicobacter pylori in Peptic Ulcer Disease* [1]. A possible association between infectious agents and coronary artery disease continues to be postulated, debated, and inconclusively studied. Molecular mimicry of infectious agent antigens is theorized to be causative for the growing list of known autoimmune conditions. The postulates of infectious disease have renewed importance in this millennium.

Most occupational and environmental medicine practices in the United States spend more time and effort preventing infectious disease than treating it. This textbook is intended to expand that pattern. It is assumed that the reader has some knowledge of the basic concepts of infectious disease, epidemiology, and cell structure. A review of key definitions that are central to this chapter's and following chapters' topics is presented early in the chapter. Definitions and concepts relative to the epidemiology of infectious disease, totaling over 250, are presented in boldface type throughout this chapter. The first set of 49 definitions is presented in reference to communicable *human* disease, although most have wider applications.

Definitions

Epidemiology: "The study of the distribution and determinants of health-related states and events in populations, and the application of this study to control health problems" [2]. It can be further subdivided into

Descriptive epidemiology: Represents the majority of epidemiologic studies, such as surveys and cross-sectional studies. It is concerned with describing communicable disease with respect to demographic fields such as age, sex, race, occupation, or area of residence. It studies populations "as is" or with "hands off." It is less accurate than experimental epidemiology because it may imply a cause and effect (an **association**) rather than scientifically proving a cause and effect.

Experimental epidemiology: The scientific study, or **control study,** experimentally isolates the factor to be studied prospectively as the main difference in the two groups. The study and control groups are intentionally matched for all factors except that which is to be studied. It is little used in communicable disease, except for clinical trials of antibiotics or vaccines. Withholding available treatment for infections is usually unethical, so the control group is often those receiving the traditional or standard treatment for the infectious disease.

"Shoe leather" epidemiology: A term to describe the hard and menial work of epidemiologic investigation—a reference to John Snow's wearing out his shoes collecting door-to-door information in his epic cholera study. Major U.S. field assignments are often performed by officers or fellows of the Epidemiologic Intelligence Service (EIS), who use the "sole with a hole" emblem.

Infectious agent: Any living or biologic entity (i.e., virus, bacteria, rickettsia, fungus, or multicellular organism) that may cause an infection or illness in a higher life form. This chapter and textbook discuss the agents that may cause human infection.

Host: A human or other animal or insect that is physically supporting or sustaining an infectious agent under natural conditions. A host may or may not be ill or affected by the agent. A **definitive (primary) host** is one in which a parasite attains its sexual or mature stage, whereas an **intermediate (secondary) host** supports or sustains a larval or asexual stage.

Environment: Any part of the universe existing outside a living or biologic entity.

Population: A specified and well-defined group of people, such as residents of a geographic area or employees of a company. This is the usual denominator of epidemiologic study and statistics and represents those who are at some risk of the disease under study.

Rate: The number of cases of an infection (a numerator) occurring in a given population (a denominator) over a specified period of time. Unlike a quotient or percentage, it always must specify a unit of time.

Prevalence: The number of cases of an infectious disease (both new and old) existing or active in or over a period of time. If a period of time is not specified, then it may be a **point prevalence,** or the number or percent infected at a point in time. **Lifetime prevalence** is the percentage of persons who will have a given condition at some time in their life. *Example:* Fifteen percent of the human population will have herpes zoster at some time in their life [3].

Seroprevalence: The percent of a population that has evidence of antibodies to an infectious agent at a point in time, implying a past exposure. This is a very useful statistic in investigating epidemics or clusters of infectious disease in a given area or group. *Example:* In the United States, there is a seroprevalence of 33% for hepatitis A IgM antibody in adults [4]. One of every three adults has evidence of having been exposed to (and recovered from) hepatitis A (HAV). This population seroprevalence may change over time from the now-available hepatitis A vaccines.

Incidence: The number of new cases of an infectious disease that occur over a given period of time. This is the number of persons exposed or at risk who do contract or develop the infectious disease divided by those exposed or at risk who could contract or develop that infectious disease. This is usually presented as a percentage (over a given period of time, an **incident rate**).

Case definition: As with many other diseases, the specific criteria needed to make the diagnosis of the specific infection. This varies from agent to agent and may require specific symptoms, examination findings, laboratory diagnosis, or a combination thereof. The most recent Centers for Disease Control and Prevention (CDC) compendium document of case definitions for infectious disease was in 1997, but updates of case definitions are available at www.cdc.gov/ncphi/disss/nndss/casedef/case_definitions.htm [5].

Historical controls: Comparing the outcome of an infectious disease with that recorded in the past. This could be the same as the natural history of the disease before treatment or prevention was available. *Example:* Historical controls show that nearly 50% of active pulmonary tuberculosis patients died from their disease before twentieth-century controls and treatments.

Epidemic: The incidence of an infectious disease in a specified population over and above that expected from previous experience. Generally found by **surveillance,** this is the formal and organized tracking of an infectious disease's statistics over time. Only two cases can be considered an **outbreak** or epidemic if no cases occurred in that population in the past. An **epizootic** is an epidemic in animals, and an **epornitic** is an epidemic in birds. **Plague** is an older term synonymous with epidemic or pan-

demic but is also specific for diseases caused by *Yersinia pestis.*

Pandemic: An outbreak or epidemic that crosses continents and becomes global. Historically, this has included diseases such as plague, yellow fever, and cholera but more recently has been used with influenza and HIV.

Epidemic curve: The plotting of the number of new cases of an infectious disease (y axis) over a period of time (x axis). The epidemic curve can aid in identification of the infectious agent from determining epidemics (peaks), incubation periods (steepness), and secondary cases (second spikes). Figure 3-1 shows a fictitious epidemic curve.

Endemic: The steady and constant presence (or prevalence) of an infectious agent in a given geographic area or host population. An infectious state that is never cleared from a population and is not typically occurring in epidemics. **Holoendemic** means that most of the population is affected, and **hyperendemic** means than many are infected. *Example:* Plague is endemic in some rodent populations in the western United States. Herpes zoster is holoendemic in adults.

Attack rate: An incident rate or a ratio of those who become infected with a specific infectious agent, calculated from the number who were exposed to that agent. *Example:* Adults living in a home with children during an influenza epidemic have an attack rate of 33% in an average year [6].

Infection: The state of having microorganisms (or parasites) entering, living, and reproducing in or on the physical person. It is not synonymous with disease, which means that the infection is causing symptoms (**apparent illness**). In some cases, an infection is short-lived and causes no symptoms (**inapparent illness**) or persists and causes no symptoms (**colonization**). *Example:* Hepatitis A infection causes apparent illness in only 30% of children under age 6 (therefore, 70% inapparent illness), but 70% of older children or adults have apparent illness [7].

Incubation period: The period of time from being invaded (infected) with an agent until the time that

Figure 3-1
Sample epidemic curve plotting the number of new cases versus time. The initial peak suggests an incubation period of about three to four days, and a second peak suggests secondary cases.

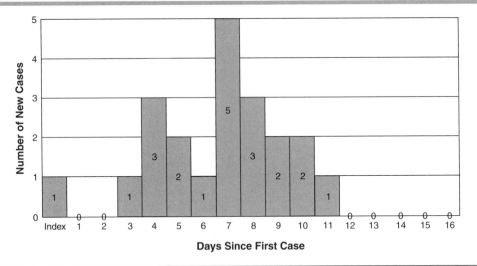

clinical manifestations occur. This is the time during which the agent multiplies or propagates within the infected organism until the time it causes illness. The epidemic curve in Figure 3-1 shows a peak number of persons becoming ill between 3 and 5 days after the first, suggesting an incubation period in this range.

Communicable (or infective) period: Over the course of an infection and illness, the period of time that the person is capable of passing the illness to another. Depending on the infectious agent, it may include periods of time before, during, or after clinical illness.

Case-fatality rate: The percentage of persons infected who will die as a direct result. *Example:* Human rabies has an essentially 100% case-fatality rate.

Flora (normal): The spectrum and balance of microorganisms naturally living on a body surface or within a hollow organ. There is usually some individual differences in flora. Infections can develop when this balance or barrier is disrupted.

Common source: A single person (**index case**), place, or thing responsible for infecting multiple

victims with an infectious agent. A food or a water supply also can be a common source. *Example:* The potato salad served at the Smiths' family reunion in Fairfield, New Jersey, on the afternoon of June 26 was the common source for the food poisoning cases.

Reservoir: The natural habitat of an infectious agent. This is the substrate (i.e., person, animal, plant, insect, water, or soil) where it best survives in either an actively reproducing or dormant state. *Example:* The only reservoir for measles is the human being. When no humans are infected, the disease (rubeola) will be eradicated!

Infestation: The state of having a parasitic organism (generally an arthropod) living on or in the physical surface of the body. Such a person is **infested.** Examples include scabies and head lice.

Immune: The state of being unable to contract a specific infectious disease because one has acquired adequate host defense mechanisms with dedicated killing cells or antibodies. Usually this is through previous exposure (by infection or immunization), followed by an adequate host immune response. Immunity is not always complete because an overwhelming dose of infectious agents (**inoculum**) still could cause some illness (often called a *break-through* infection).

Inoculum: The amount of infectious agent that successfully invades or exposes a host. **Inoculation** is the process of exposing or introducing a host to an infectious agent. An **infective dose** is the number of organisms necessary to cause infection or a measurable host response. An inoculum may be less than the infective dose needed to cause infection or colonization.

Antigen: Any part of an infectious agent (e.g., a protein, polysaccharide, glycolipid, or transplanted tissue) that can induce a specific immune response in the host. If a stable antigen can be reproduced synthetically or separated from its infectious agent, it may be capable of being used as an active vaccine. Antigens of some pathogens such as influenza and HIV can undergo frequent changes and produce essentially new pathogens and essentially new diseases.

Antibody: Proteins (**immunoglobulins**) produced by the body in specific response to microbial antigens that may be efficient in binding to antigen to prevent or fight diseases. In response to some diseases, the human body can produce antibodies that do not seem to be entirely competent in fighting or eradicating the disease. *Examples:* Human immunodeficiency virus (HIV) and hepatitis C virus (HCV). These antibodies may be tested for clinically and used as markers in screening for present disease or past exposure.

Vehicle (of infection): Any mode of transportation for an infectious agent from its reservoir to a person or an inanimate object, including fomites. Food and water can be vehicles.

Fomites: Inanimate objects that serve as surfaces for the spread of infectious agents. *Examples:* Door handles, drinking glasses, toys, keyboards, and medical instruments.

Vector: Any animate object that serves as a carrier of an infectious agent. A **mechanical vector** passively carries the agent somewhere on its body, such as the leg of a fly. A **biologic vector** includes arthropods (insects), which also may serve a role in the replication life cycle of the agent.

Cohort: Any human who may have in common the sharing of a risk and who may be the subject of study for the effect of that risk. Coworkers may be cohorts by virtue of working for the same employer, sharing a workplace risk, or being subjects of a workplace study.

Birth cohorts: All persons born in a given year. Children in the same grade in school are from approximately the same birth cohort. In seroepidemiology, birth cohorts are individuals born at points in time that may define natural exposure to circulating diseases. *Example:* It is published in some guidelines that persons born before 1957 may be assumed to be immune to the wild rubella and rubeola viruses that were in widespread circulation before 1957 [8].

Nosocomial infection: Infection related to or having been acquired while in a health care institution and unrelated to patients' original diagnoses.

Latent infection: Any infection that can remain asymptomatic in the host for long periods of times but with the potential to reactivate. *Examples:* Tuberculosis, syphilis, and many herpesviruses.

Latent period (latency): Classically, the period between the time of invasion and infection until the time of infectivity. However, more recently with HIV, it has come to be used synonymously with *incubation period.* That is, HIV is both latent and infectious at the same time. Asymptomatic diseases with long latency (but high infectivity) can be the most difficult to control.

Carrier: A person or animal that harbors an infective and infectious agent without apparent illness themselves. A carrier can be a short-lived or a **transient carrier** or can become a long-term **chronic carrier**. A person can be a carrier before clinical illness (**incubatory carrier**) or after clinical recovery (**convalescent carrier**).

Susceptible: A person's state of being at risk for infection with an agent because the individual lacks resistance or immunity to that agent.

Susceptible pool: That group of persons in a population who are not immune to a specific infectious agent and therefore are susceptible to infection if exposed. In theory, an epidemic ends when the susceptible pool is exhausted or a high percentage of the population has developed immunity.

Herd immunity: First used in reference to domestic animals, the immunity of a population to a specific infectious agent. Theoretically, there is a percent of immunity (**herd immunity threshold**) at which an epidemic ceases to propagate. This threshold is specific to each disease and is based both on its ability to reproduce and its infectivity [9]. Many mathematical models of vaccine efficacy are based on a target herd immunity.

Seroepidemiology: The use of laboratory studies of infection (antigens) and immunity (antibodies) to study patterns of human infections. **Serosurveys** are a form of observational epidemiology that studies the inapparent infection rates, dormancy, latency, herd immunity, and susceptibility of a natural population. Seroepidemiology is both expensive and time-consuming but provides the most valuable information in investigating epidemics. Blood banks are a valuable resource of population seroepidemiology in the surveillance of such conditions as West Nile virus. Seroepidemiology takes the form of experimental seroepidemiology in highly structured **vaccine efficacy trials.**

Virulence: The degree to which an infectious agent can cause clinical illness, either by its ability to damage tissue and/or by its ability to invade a host. It is best measured by the **case-fatality rate.**

Shedding: The process of a host excreting, exhaling, defecating, or sloughing into the environment infectious agents that are capable of infecting others. Shedding entails an active port of exit from the host. This is the basis for human isolation or quarantine.

Isolation: The process of separating or restricting the movement of an infectious and ill person from those who are well and susceptible. Isolation is imposed for the anticipated duration of the communicable period.

Quarantine: The process of separating a well but exposed person from those who are well and sus-ceptible but not yet exposed for the duration of the anticipated communicable period. Quarantine laws were mainly of historical significance for most diseases before the bioterrorist attack of anthrax immediately after September 11, 2001, Many new quarantine laws have been written in reference to smallpox, drug-resistant tuberculosis, or other potential threats.

Zoonosis: An infection transmitted from vertebrate animals (e.g., rabies and brucellosis) to humans under natural conditions.

Conventions of Reporting and Surveillance

The *International Classification of Disease* (ICD) is a system of cataloging diagnoses that is updated periodically by a committee of the World Health Organization (WHO). Originally used for epidemiologic surveillance, it is now used for financial coding as well. The ninth edition (ICD-9) is the system used in the United States at this time, but a major revision (ICD-10) was written and ratified in 1990. All editions have listed infectious and parasitic diseases first (e.g., in ICD-9, cholera is 001 and typhoid is 002). There are 21 chapters in ICD-10; Chapter 1 is "Infectious and Parasitic Diseases" (A00–B99).

Communicable diseases are also classified as **reportable** or **not reportable.** The status of each disease is determined by the local state, and each licensed physician is responsible for knowing what is reportable and what is not reportable in his or her area and for making individual **case reports.** All states have strict laws of confidentiality governing their public health officers. States then create **collective reports** for their own analysis, which they pass on to the CDC. International communicable disease surveillance is done by the **World Health Organization (WHO).** The WHO's most recent *International Health Regulations* went into effect on June 15, 2007, and are presented graphically on page 50 and Annex II of the regulations [10] (Figure 3-2). The 10 diseases of top concern in these regulations are listed in Table 3-1, and a flowchart of reporting processes is given in Figure 3-2.

Much of the reporting of infectious disease in the United States was inconsistent before 1990. At that time, the CDC and the Council of State and Territorial Epidemiologists (CSTE) established a

Figure 3-2
Triggers for an international health emergency.

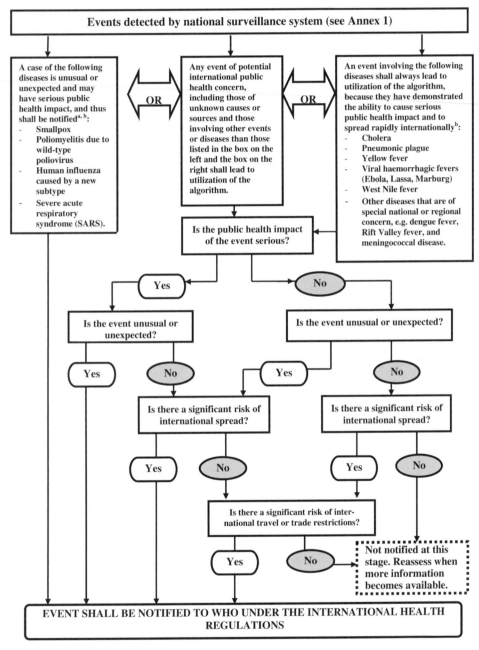

ANNEX 2
DECISION INSTRUMENT FOR THE ASSESSMENT AND NOTIFICATION OF EVENTS THAT MAY CONSTITUTE A PUBLIC HEALTH EMERGENCY OF INTERNATIONAL CONCERN

[a] As per WHO case definitions.
[b] The disease list shall be used only for the purposes of these Regulations.

Source: Annex 2, page 50, of the revision of the International Health Regulations, written by the 58th World Health Assembly in 2005. Available at www.who.int.gb.ebwha/pdf_files/WHA58/WHA58_3-en.pdf.

Table 3-1
Infections That May Constitute a Public Health Emergency of International Concern (Notifiable by WHO International Health Regulations, 2007)

Single Case Report:
    Smallpox
        Poliomyelitis owing to wild-type virus
        Human influenza caused by a new subtype
        Severe acute respiratory syndrome (SARS)
Diseases demonstrating the ability to cause serious public health impact and to spread rapidly internationally:
    Cholera
    Pneumonic plague
    Yellow fever
    Viral hemorrhagic fevers (Ebola, Lassa, Marburg, West Nile fever)
        Other diseases of special national or regional concern
            Dengue fever
            Rift Valley fever
            Meningococcal disease

Available at www.who.int/csr/ihr/contain/en/index.html.

policy that requires state health departments to report cases of selected diseases (Table 3-2) to the CDC's National Notifiable Disease Surveillance System (NNDSS). They also wrote specific criteria for diagnosing each communicable disease (the **case definition**). The list of notifiable diseases is updated or revised annually (www.cdc.gov/ncphi/disss/nndss/phs/infdis2008.htm).

The Epidemiologic Triangle (or Triad)

For an infection to occur, a specific combination of events must occur. There must be an infectious **agent** capable of infecting a human being. The agent must be present in sufficient quantity in the **environment** to cause entry, invasion, and infection of a susceptible human **host.** This triad is called the **epidemiologic triangle** or **triad** (Figure 3-3) and serves as the model and outline for the rest of this chapter. We may think of the agent-environment-host triad as the three points on the corner of the triangle and the concept of **transmission** as the three lines connecting the triangle. The transmission is completed by the existence of a **port of entry,** a **port of exit,** and a **reservoir** for the agent.

This model also can serve as the model for control. That is, a completed triangle is negative, and any and all factors that prevent the triangle from forming are positive. The individual factors of the agent, environment, and host can be studied individually for factors that may remove a corner and thus break the triangle. The sides can be studied for methods of breaking the triangle by blocking transmission. Infection control and preventive medicine must search for the weakest, most practical, and most economical part of the triangle to attack.

THE AGENT

Agents of concern in this text are various infectious microbial organisms or entities with the ability to cause harm to humans. The most basic instinct of infectious agents, as for all living entities, is to survive and propagate their own kind. They are not homicidal by nature because causing rapid death to their human host serves them no purpose. The

Figure 3-3
Epidemiologic triangle displaying the interplay between the host, environment, and agent that produces infection.

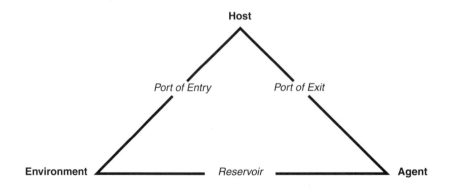

Table 3-2
Infectious Diseases Designated as Notifiable at the National Level, United States, 2008

Acquired immunodeficiency syndrome (AIDS)	Lyme disease
Anthrax	Malaria
Arboviral neuroinvasive and nonneuroinvasive	Measles
California serogroup	Meningococcal disease
Eastern equine encephalitis	Mumps
St. Louis encephalitis	Novel influenza A virus infections
West Nile	Pertussis
Western equine encephalitis	Plague
Botulism	Poliomyelitis, paralytic
Foodborne	Poliovirus infection, nonparalytic
Infant	Psittacosis
Other (wound and unspecified	Q fever
Brucellosis	Rabies (animal or human)
Chancroid	Rocky Mountain spotted fever
Chlamydia trachomatis, genital infections	Rubella
Cholera	Rubella, congenital syndrome
Coccidioidomycosis	Salmonellosis
Cryptosporidiosis	Severe acute respiratory syndrome (coronavirus SARS-CoV)
Diphtheria	Shiga-toxin-producing *Escherichia coli*
Giardiasis	Shigellosis
Gonorrhea	Smallpox
Haemophilus influenzae, invasive	Streptococcal disease, invasive group A
Hansen's disease (leprosy)	*Streptococcal pneumoniae,* drug-resistant, invasive
Hantavirus pulmonary syndrome	*Streptococcal pneumoniae,* non-drug-resistant, invasive (< age 5)
Hemolytic uremic syndrome, postdiarrheal	Syphilis (any stage, stillbirth, congenital)
Hepatitis, viral, acute	Tetanus
Hepatitis A, acute	Toxic-shock syndrome (other than streptococcal)
Hepatitis B, acute	Trichinellosis (trichinosis)
Hepatitis B, perinatal infection	Tuberculosis
Hepatitis C, acute	Tularemia
Hepatitis, viral, chronic	Typhoid fever
Chronic hepatitis B	Vancomycin-intermediate *Staphylococcus aureus* (VISA)
Hepatitis C virus infection (past or present)	Vancomycin-resistant *Staphylococcus aureus* (VRSA)
HIV infections	Varicella (morbidity or deaths)
Adult (over or age 13)	Vibriosis
Pediatric (under age 13)	Yellow fever
Influenza-associated pediatric mortality	
Legionellosis	
Listeriosis	

Available at www.cdc.gov/ncphi/disss/nndss/phs/infdis2008.htm.

most successful viruses are those that can reach the point of being a persistent and latent infection in most humans on Earth (or **holoendemic**). Thus herpes simplex type 1 and varicella viruses are far more successful than rabies or Ebola. Some attributes of infectious agents that can increase their success and survival are listed in Table 3-3.

Agents may come in different varieties of the same species and present symptomatically as different diseases. These are called *subtypes, strains, serotypes,* or *serovars* (serologic variant) depending on the agent. Some agents may have only one pathologic form (e.g., rubella), whereas others may have dozens (e.g., *Shigella, Escherichia coli*, cholera, and adenovirus), hundreds (e.g., rhinovirus), or even thousands (e.g., influenza and *Salmonella*).

THE HOST AND HOST FACTORS

The term *host* in this textbook implies a human being unless otherwise specified, i.e., when the infectious agent may have other hosts in its life cycle. Humans have a great range of factors that can

Table 3-3
Attributes of Infectious Agents Associated with Their Success

Agent must be stable and resistant to physical factors in the environment; is even more successful if it can adapt to changes in the environment.

Agent must exist in sufficient quantity in the environment to cause infection.

Agent must find the proper *vector,* or medium, to use to infect the host.

Agent must have the ability to invade and infect through a host portal of entry.

Agent must be resistant to host-defense factors once it has invaded a host and is more successful if it can actively develop resistance to host defenses.

Agent must have the ability to egress or shed from the host through a portal of exit.

influence their efficiency as a host. Called **host factors,** these include the following:

Age

Young children and adults are very different when it comes to susceptibility and response to infectious diseases. We focus on adults in this text, but an understanding of this difference is essential. A history of childhood diseases is very important, especially for those entering the health care field. A fairly reliable clinical history of varicella during childhood is nearly as sensitive as laboratory confirmation. Many infections are asymptomatic (subclinical) in children but symptomatic (clinical) in adults. Examples include poliovirus, Epstein-Barr virus (mononucleosis), mumps, varicella, *Neisseria meningitidis,* and some types of influenza. Children in their preschool years have maximally efficient immune systems and can form lifelong immunity to all the diseases just mentioned. One study showed that because of exposure to a similar strain when they were children [11], people over age 75 (a birth cohort) had better immunity to the Hong Kong influenza strain during an outbreak than those aged 65–75. The elderly may not be more susceptible to infectious agents in general but are more susceptible to complications and morbidity and mortality from infectious agents.

Socioeconomic Factors

As mentioned earlier, many of the more highly communicable diseases are less severe in childhood. Conditions associated with lower socioeconomic class or poverty (e.g., crowding, poor hygiene and sanitation, and lack of available medical care) seem to protect individuals raised in these conditions from more severe morbidity if an infectious disease is contracted in adulthood. This is most true of the highly endemic or prevalent human diseases that are spread by fecal-oral or direct transmission. However, poor nutrition or poor general health may predispose one to the complications of infection if host defenses are less than optimal. Children living in substandard conditions are more susceptible to a few diseases, such as pulmonary tuberculosis.

Genetics

Like age, inheritance is a biologic factor that cannot be altered. Genetic traits influence susceptibility to certain infections and may determine not only the clinical outcome but also whether the person becomes chronically ill (e.g., chronic hepatitis B or C). Genetics may be a factor in most, if not all, infectious diseases and helps to explain the great variations in human host response. Variations in the human leukocyte antigen (HLA) seem to correlate with both susceptibility and resistance to certain diseases.

Gender

Only a few infectious diseases seem to have a predilection for one gender over the other. Overall, males have slightly more infectious disease risk, and this may be due in part to gender differences in occupation, forms of recreation, or risk-taking behaviors.

Geography

The area of residence is extremely important in individual infectious disease susceptibility. There is tremendous variation in the endemic infectious diseases from continent to continent. One may become exposed and resistant to diseases endemic in the soil of one's homeland but remain susceptible to soil pathogens in another area. In the United States, the best examples of this are cases of histoplasmosis in the Midwest and Ohio Valley and cases of coccidioidomycosis in the Southwest. Adults moving from one area to the other may be more susceptible to developing clinical illness soon after their move, and this may need to be taken into consideration in their pre-employment history.

Immunity

Vaccines can make a host resistant to certain diseases, but we still lack vaccines for many diseases such as the rickettsiae and most bacteria.

Environment

The environment of the Earth's biosphere is extremely delicate and is "colonized" by billions of living organisms, including humans. Each organism has evolved in its own habitat or a place and time where the conditions of temperature, moisture, season, sunlight, and substrate availability are maximal for its survival. Many organisms have evolved life cycles that include other organisms. Humans have a comparatively wide range of habitats because we can ensure our survival almost anywhere on Earth with our technology (e.g., plumbing, energy, clothing, communication, and personal protective equipment). However, most important in our technology is our knowledge of the environments into which we trek or seek to reside and how we can protect ourselves from the biologic hazards we may expect to find in those environments.

Microbiologists and virologists are the primary resource experts on infectious agents, and clinicians are the experts on the host and host responses. Safety, public health, and preventive medicine professionals are the resource experts on the forms of infectious agents in the environment and factors that influence them. Certainly this includes occupational and environmental health professionals. Our occupations and technology take us into environments we would not otherwise visit— i.e., deep in the earth, high in the sky, or under the seas. It may be that our technology has in fact created some of the "new" infections, such as legionellosis. We may become the new and **accidental host** when we have changed the environment or a biologic reservoir in some way. Humans may be accidental hosts for some of the most dangerous infectious agents, such as Ebola virus, hantavirus, rabies, and the plague.

Causality and the Postulates: A Historical Perspective

A **postulate** is an unproven assertion or assumption, a statement or formula offered as the basis of a theory [12]. The postulates for the causation of infectious disease seem simple and logical today, but their hypotheses, written by Jako Henle (1809–1885) in 1840, further modified by his student Robert Koch (1843–1910), and published in 1890 [13], were a major contribution to the medicine of the early nineteenth century. Henle and Koch were aware that many diseases were caused by microbes or bacteria, which they called *parasites*. Their joint hypotheses, known as the *Henle-Koch postulates*, state that

1. The agent must be shown to be present in every case of the disease by isolation in pure culture.
2. The agent must not be found in cases of other diseases.
3. Once isolated, the agent must be capable of reproducing the disease in experimental animals.
4. The agent must be recovered from the experimental disease produced.

Henle and Koch considered postulates 1 and 2 to be essential and postulates 3 and 4 to be further confirmation. The pure postulates may be difficult to adhere to in their entirety because they did not consider that

1. Isolation is not always possible depending on the disease and laboratory techniques available (e.g., there is still no culture technique for some bacteria or viruses).
2. Some individuals may be or have been infected but are or were not ill (inapparent infection).
3. An animal laboratory model does not exist for all human diseases. Some diseases are specific to humans, and therefore,
4. There is no experimental disease or animal model to study.

Rivers questioned the rigidity of the postulates in his presidential address to the American Immunological Society in 1937 [14]. The field of virology was exploding with new knowledge at that time, and viral culture techniques were being perfected. His postulates for the viruses state that

1. A specific virus must be found to be associated with a disease with "a degree of regularity."
2. The virus in the ill person must be proved to be the cause of the disease, not an incidental or accidental finding.
3. Infection is produced with a "degree of regularity" in susceptible hosts by means of inoculating them with material (otherwise uncontaminated) from ill individuals.

However, many other questions remained unanswered in the field of virology. It was found that antibodies to nonpathogenic viruses were often present, some viral infections cleared without stimulating the infected host's production of antibodies, and on occasion, one could be infected (or reinfected) with a virus to which one already had antibodies. Answers to the remaining questions are still elusive, especially since viruses or their specific antibodies increasingly are being suspected of contributing to causation of cancers and other chronic illnesses. Many variations of postulates for causation have been published beyond the topic of infectious disease. Dr. Alfred S. Evans has written many of the more modern postulates, including the 1973 criteria we now associate with the **paired sera** diagnosis of acute viral illness [15]:

1. Specific antibody to the virus is absent in the susceptible person.

2. Specific antibody appears during the illness. Examples are transient specific IgM antibody, persistent IgG antibody, and local IgA at the site of viral multiplication.
3. Specific antibody production is accompanied by the presence of viruses in the infected tissues.
4. Absence of specific IgG indicates susceptibility.
5. Presence of specific IgG indicates immunity.
6. No other virus produces these specific antibodies.
7. Induced production (**active immunization**) of specific antibody prevents disease.

Evans reviewed the history of postulates and the principles of causation in a book published shortly before his death [16]. The concepts of postulates eventually extended far beyond infectious disease. The most up-to-date set of concepts of epidemiologic causation are attributed to British biostatistician Austin Hill (1897–1991) [17]. Hill's criteria for observations that contribute to a valid association are listed in Table 3-4.

In 1964, the U.S. Surgeon General's Advisory Committee accepted Hill's criteria 1, 2, 3, 5, and 7 as the five criteria that should be fulfilled to establish a causal relationship. This was the same year the Surgeon General released his report on the association of tobacco and lung cancer.

Correlates with Other Risks in the Workplace

Hill's criteria for the proof of causation should be very familiar to those trained in occupational and

Table 3-4
Hill's Criteria for a Valid Association

1. **Consistency:** The association is consistent when results are replicated in other studies, or by different methods, or in other locations by other scientists. Also known as *reproducibility.*
2. **Strength:** The association must be of sufficient "size" or magnitude (relative risk) when measured by the *appropriate* tests of statistical significance. Also known as *biostatistic analysis.*
3. **Specificity:** A single risk or cause produces a specific effect. A nonspecific or a variable response to a specific exposure points away from causation.
4. **Dose-response relationship:** An increasing level of exposure or risk (in volume or duration) increases the effect.
5. **Temporal relationship:** Exposure must precede outcome. This is the only absolutely essential criterion. If a risk was not present before or during the time of the effect, it has the most perfect alibi.
6. **Biologic plausibility:** The association agrees with existing knowledge of pathobiologic processes. Also can be called *sensibility.*
7. **Coherence:** The association is compatible with existing theories and knowledge, which may include evidence from previous animal studies. The association must not contradict the principles of science nor the laws of physics.
8. **Experimental evidence:** Experiments or studies designed to interfere or block the risk or exposure will "break" the causation or association: the basic premises of prevention.

environmental medicine or other preventive medicine specialties. Rendering opinions within a scientific basis is the second point of the American College of Occupational and Environmental Medicine's Code of Ethical Conduct [18].

THE HEALTHY-WORKER EFFECT

The **healthy-worker effect (HWE)** states that, in general, employed persons enjoy a higher level of health than the general public such that comparisons of workers with the general public are invalid. The concept is somewhat controversial, but most good occupational studies nevertheless use only employed populations for comparison. Some HWEs may be attributable to infectious diseases because those with genetic or congenital vulnerability to infections may not obtain nor sustain employment. In some cases, the vulnerable may not stay in an occupation that causes them frequent illness. Industries such as health care may conduct screening for vaccine-preventable disease immunity on preplacement examination, and safety training (i.e., bloodborne pathogen training) should begin immediately. Studies have shown that the most dangerous time for injury to workers is their first year on a new job or working for a new employer [19]. This is true for both genders and all age groups. No studies have specifically focused on infections acquired during the first year of employment, but certainly there is a learning curve in many occupations and professions that is a factor in contracting infection (e.g., health care workers and the handling of sharp instruments).

INJURY CONTROL

In the epidemiologic triad for injury, the host is the human, and the agent is energy (e.g., mechanical, electrical, chemical, radiation, or thermal). The environment is those areas where both the agent (e.g., energy) and the host (i.e., the human body) are found in potential conflict.

The classic **Haddon matrix** (Table 3-5) and

model for injury [20] was used initially to study the control of motor vehicle injury [21], in which the agent is kinetic energy. But the matrix model has been expanded to other forms of injury prevention. Haddon's "preinjury" may correlate with the presence of an agent in the environment (the reservoir), creating exposure and a risk of "injury," or with the agent's invasion of the host, and "postinjury" may correlate with the individualized response of the host to the infection or infestation.

The great successes in controlling or eradicating some infectious diseases have been due as much to public sanitation (removing the agent from the environment), improved personal hygiene (removing the risk of transmission through a port of entry), and improved nutrition (improving host response) as they have been due to vaccines or antibiotics (improving host response). Infection or infestation with a pathogenic microorganism may be analogous to an "injury" and may necessitate medical care. Thus the Haddon matrix can be modified as a model of control for biologic hazards as well.

INDUSTRIAL HYGIENE, TOXICOLOGY

The classic four-controls approach of industrial hygiene (i.e., substitution, engineering, administrative, and personal protection) has found application in infection control. In most cases, substitution is not relevant with respect to infectious agents. No techniques are yet developed for substituting drug-sensitive for drug-resistant organisms. But the other controls concepts of engineering, administrative, and personal protection establish an excellent **hierarchy of controls** for infectious agents. The CDC's 1993 Draft Guidelines for Preventing the Transmission of Tuberculosis in Health Care Facilities used the model for the industrial hygiene hierarchy of controls [22]. The Occupational Health and Safety Administration (OSHA) quickly made the guidelines enforceable under the General Duty clause [23]. These guidelines introduced a new concept to infection control—that

Table 3-5
Haddon Matrix

Phases	Human (Host)	Vehicle (Agent)	Environment
Pre-injury	Alcohol intoxication	Utility vehicle instability	Visibility of hazards
Injury	Resistance to energy insult	Sharp/pointed edges and surfaces	Flammable materials
Postinjury	Hemorrhage	Rapidity of energy reduction (decelerate)	EMS response time/quality

tuberculosis is not an infectious disease that can be occupational but rather an occupational disease that can be infectious [24]. Hospitals and the health care industry had been willing to accept that infection control "guidelines" still would allow some occasional worker illness. OSHA was not as lenient in dealing with occupationally acquired fatal infections. Federally mandated infection control was a new and costly concept to health care.

Industrial hygiene focuses on protecting the worker from specific *known* risks by using controls and protection specific to that risk. But protection of workers from communicable diseases usually needs to be more generalized, i.e., based on the assumption that there are multiple unknown pathogens in the work environment. For example, **universal precautions** (now called *standard precautions*) assume that every patient is infected with every bloodborne pathogen. Imposing universal precautions may involve administrative controls, engineering or barrier controls, worker education, protective tasks such as hand washing, and the use of protective equipment. Control of communicable diseases often may require an extensive medical history, a physical examination, laboratory evaluation for immunity, and immunization or postexposure prophylaxis. The occupational health clinician responsible for workers exposed to communicable diseases must assume many of the tasks assumed by other safety or industrial hygiene professionals in other industries. Roles analogous to the industrial hygienist's in industry may be performed by hospital epidemiologists or infection control practitioners and infection control committees in the health care work environment. They use many of the same principles (if not the same hardware) as the industrial hygienist, including routine surveillance and monitoring for nosocomial infections, cumulative reporting of cross-infection between patients and staff, and specific criteria for outbreak analysis. These are not just voluntary activities; they are mandated by accrediting agencies such as the Joint Commission on the Accreditation of Healthcare Organizations (JCAHO) and local and state hospital licensing agencies.

Unlike most other workplace risks, though, workers with communicable illnesses can bring the risk *to* the workplace or take it *from* the workplace. A worker also may acquire disease from (or infect) not only his or her coworkers but also customers and clients. Determining the work-relatedness of an infection can prove more difficult than tracking a specific toxic chemical from a known point of origin.

The classic industrial hygiene approach familiar to safety and occupational health practitioners can be applied easily to communicable disease. In both cases, the emphasis and preferred solution are total removal or eradication of the risk from the work environment. However, this is rarely possible with infectious agents. If the reservoir for the diseases is only the human, then the human body becomes both the host and the environment for the agent. Such diseases may be the most amenable to eradication if a safe and efficacious vaccine can be developed and applied widely (e.g., smallpox). The agent is eradicated by removing the availability of the reservoir, i.e., the susceptibles.

For the occupational physician, the important principles of toxicology have some application in managing patients with infectious diseases. Practitioners who are familiar with chemical and toxic hazards should not be uncomfortable evaluating workers with infectious disease. Many of the same concepts apply to both (Table 3-6).

MATERIAL SAFETY DATA SHEETS
The Public Health Agency of Canada, Office of Laboratory Security, prepares Material Safety Data Sheets (MSDSs) for infectious agents (*www.phac-aspc.gc.ca/msds-ftss/*) The format is similar to chemical hazard MSDSs and was created for laboratory workers who may be exposed to infectious agents in much higher concentration and in different forms than the general public. The format is shown in Figure 3-4, and a list of infectious agents is given in Figure 3-5. The agency attaches the following disclaimer:

> Although the information, opinions, and recommendations contained in this Material Safety Data Sheet are compiled from sources believed to be reliable, we accept no responsibility for the accuracy, sufficiency, or reliability or for any loss or injury resulting from the use of the information. Newly discovered hazards are frequent, and this information may not be completely up to date

These MSDSs provide an excellent reference for quick answers to questions such as what it takes to inactivate an organism, survivability in the envi-

Table 3-6
Comparison of Concepts of Toxicology and Communicable Disease

Toxicology Concept	ID Correlate	Similarities/Dissimilarities
Toxicity of agent	Virulence	Host response may be individualized, especially with IA. Best treatment is avoidance.
Dose	Dose	Question of dose-response relationship. A "threshold" of illness for TA, "infective dose" for IA.
Route of entry	Route of entry	Much the same for both agents. Controls with barriers, behavior, personal protection.
Exposure duration	Exposure duration	Both increase chances of illness; IA might stimulate immunity, and TA stimulate allergy.
Exposure frequency	Exposure frequency	Both increase chances of illness, but IA might stimulate immunity, and TA stimulate allergy.
Absorption	Invasion	May target specific organs and physiology. TA may have more predictable consequences than IA.
Distribution	Systemic/hematogenous	Both may cause generalized multi-organ pathology. TAs decline in concentration, but IAs multiply and increase in concentration.
Metabolism	Host response/immunity	TA metabolites may also be toxic and harmful; IA-antibody complexes may be harmful or stimulate autoantibodies.
Excretion	Shedding	TA excretion of metabolites less likely to be harmful to others than IAs, which are attempting survival by propagation (infectious).

Abbreviations: TA = toxic agent; IA = infectious agent.

Figure 3-4
Format for Material Data Safety Sheets prepared by the Office of Laboratory Security, Public Health Agency of Canada, showing 32 categories under nine headings

Section 1—Infections Agent

Name:
Synonyms or Cross References:
Characteristics:

Section-II—Health Hazard

Pathogenicity:
Epidemiology:
Host Range:
Infectious Dose:
Mode of Transmission:
Incubation Period:
Communicability:

Section III—Dissemination

Reservoir:
Zoonosis:
Vectors:

Section IV—Viability

Drug Susceptibility:
Susceptibility to Disinfectants:
Physical Inactivation:

Section V—Medical

Surveillance:
First Aid / Treatment:
Immunization:
Prophylaxis:

Section VI—Laboratory Methods

Laboratory-Acquired Infections:
Sources/Specimens:
Primary Hazards:
Special Hazards

Section VII—Precautions

Containment Requirements:
Protective Clothing:
Other Precautions:

Section VIII—Handling

Spills:
Disposal:
Storage:

Section IX—Miscellaneous

Figure 3-5
Human infectious agents with MSDSs.

MSDS Sheets for Infectious Agents
on the Internet at *www.phac-aspc.gc.ca/msds-ftss/*
From the Public Health Agency of Canada,
Office of Laboratory Security
All sheets are under current review

Actinobacillus spp.
Actinomyces spp.
Adenovirus (types 1, 2, 3, 4, 5 and 7)
Adenovirus (types 40 and 41)
Aerococcus spp.
Aeromonas hydrophila
Ancylostoma duodenale
Angiostrongylus cantonensis
Ascaris lumbricoides
Ascaris spp.
Aspergillus spp.
Bacillus anthracis
Bacillus cereus
Bacteroides spp.
Balantidium coli
Bartonella bacilliformis
Blastomyces dermatitidis
Bluetongue virus
Bordetella bronchiseptica
Bordetella pertussis
Borrella burgdorferi
Bovine Spongiform Encephalopathy
Branhamella catarrhalis
Brucella spp. (B. abortus, B. canis, B. melitensis, B. suis)
Brugia spp.
Burkholderia (Pseudomonas) mallei
Burkholderia (Pseudomonas) pseudomallei
California serogroup
Campylobacter fetus subsp. fetus
Campylobacter jejuni, C. coli, C. fetus subsp. jejuni
Candida albicans
Capnocytophaga spp.
Chikungunya virus
Chlamydia psittaci
Chlamydia trachomatis
Citrobacter spp.
Clonorchis sinensis

Clostridium botulinum
Clostridium difficile
Clostridium perfringens
Clostridium tetani
Clostridium spp. (other)
Coccidioides immitis
Colorado tick fever virus
Corynebacterium diphtheriae
Coxiella burnetii
Coxsackievirus
Creutzfeldt-Jakob agent, Kuru agent
Crimean-Congo hemorrhagic fever
Cryptococcus neoformans
Cryptosporidium parvum
Cytomegalovirus
Dengue virus (1, 2, 3, 4)
Diphtheroids
Eastern (Western) equine encephalitis
Ebola virus
Echinococcus granulosus
Echinococcus multilocularis
Echovirus
Edwardsiella tarda
Entamoeba histolytica
Enterobacter spp.
Enterovirus 70
Epidermophyton floccosum. Microsporum & Trichophyton spp.
Epstein-Barr virus
Escherichia coli, enterohemorrhagic
Escherichia coli, enteroinvasive
Escherichia coli, enteropathogenic
Escherichia coli, enterotoxigenic
Fasciola hepatica
Francisella tularensis
Fusobacterium spp.
Gemella haemolysans

Giardia lamblia
Haemophilus ducreyi
Haemophilus influenzae (group b)
Hantavirus
Hepatitis A virus
Hepatitis B virus
Hepatitis C virus
Hepatitis D virus
Hepatitis E virus
Herpes simplex virus
Herpesvirus simiae
Histoplasma capsulatum
Human coronavirus
Human immunodeficiency virus
Human papillomavirus
Human rotavirus
Human T-lymphotrophic virus
Influenza virus
Japanese encephalitis virus
Junin virus / Machupo virus
Klebsiella spp.
Kyasanur Forest disease virus
Lactobacillus spp.
Legionella pneumophila
Leishmania spp.
Leptospira interrogans
Listeria monocytogenes
Lymphocytic choriomeningitis virus
Marburg virus
Mayaro virus
Measles virus
Micrococcus spp.
Moraxella spp.
Murray Valley encephalitis virus
Mycobacterium spp. (misc)
Mycobacterium tuberculosis & bovis
Mycoplasma hominis
Mycoplasma pneumoniae
Naegleria fowleri
Necator americanus

Figure 3-5
Continued

Neisseria gonorrhoeae	Rickettsia prowazekii, R.	Taenia saginata
Neisseria meningitidis	Canada	Taenia solium
Neisseria spp. (others)	Rickettsia rickettsii	Toxocara canis, T. cati
Nocardia spp.	Ross river virus	Toxoplasma gondii
Norwalk virus	Rubella virus	Treponema pallidum
Omak hemorrhagic fever virus	Salmonella choleraesuis	Trichinella spp.
Onchocerca volvulus	Salmonella paratyphi	Trichomonas vaginalis
O'Nyong-Nyong virus	Salmonella typhi	Trichuris trichiura
Opisthorchis spp.	Salmonella spp. (others)	Trypanosoma brucei
Parvovirus B19	**Schistosoma spp.**	Ureaplasma urealyticum
Pasteurella spp.	Serratia spp.	Vaccinia virus
Peptococcus spp.	Shigella spp.	Varicella-zoster virus
Peptostreptococcus spp.	Sindbis virus	Venezuelan equine encephalitis
Plesiomonas shigelloides	Sporothrix schenckii	Vesicular stomatitis virus
Powassan encephalitis virus	St. Louis encephalitis	Vibrio cholerae, serovar 01
Proteus spp.	Staphylococcus aureus	Vibrio parahaemolyticus
Pseudomonas spp. (excluding	Streptobacillus moniliformis	West Nile Virus
B. mallei, B. pseudomallel)	Streptococcus agalactiae	Wuchereria bancrofti
Rabies virus	Streptococcus faecalis	Yellow fever virus
Respiratory syncytial virus	Streptococcus pneumoniae	Yersinia enterocolitica & pseudo-
Rhinovirus	Streptococcus pyogenes	tuberculosis
Rickettsia akari	Streptococcus salivarius	Yersinia pestis

Source: Office of Laboratory Security, Public Health Agency of Canada. Available at www.phac-aspc.gc.ca/msds-ftss.

ronment, and worker hazards and controls. Traditional infectious disease textbooks tend to hide such information in context or choose not to mention what is not known (e.g., the infective dose for most agents).

The American Public Health Association publishes the *Control of Communicable Diseases Manual* (edited by David L Heymann) every 5 years [10]. It is an economical pocket reference that presents most of the known human infectious diseases in a standard format: name and synonyms, ICD-9 and ICD-10 codes, identification, infectious agent, occurrence, reservoir, mode of transmission, incubation period, period of communicability, susceptibility and resistance, and methods of control. The methods of control section is further subdivided into preventive measures, control of patient contact and the immediate environment, epidemic measures, disaster implications, and international measures.

Agents of Infectious Disease

The infectious agents responsible for most of the occupational infections in Western civilization are no larger than a single cell. This section presents a basic review of the major classes of infectious agents. The classification and nonclinical characteristics of microbes are disciplines that do not always have relevance to the needs of the busy clinician. Information on the size, shape, taxonomy, and metabolism of infectious agents is not presented in detail. Chapter 2 discusses the principles of laboratory study and diagnosis of the various infectious agents.

This section also reviews attributes of the infectious agents and their products that enable them to cause disease and some of their attributes that enable them to actively develop resistance to treatment.

AGENTS OF OCCUPATIONAL INFECTIOUS DISEASE
Viruses

A virus is among the simplest of all biologic entities but represents the largest class of human pathogens. It is arguable whether viruses meet the full definition of *life form.* They are obligated to infect and reproduce within another organism to complete their life cycle. Specifically, they are obligated to invade the cells of another organism, defining them as **obligate intracellular parasites.** Viruses have limited survival in the free environment and can remain infectious only from minutes to a few weeks at most (e.g., hepatitis B).

Morphology. Viruses have the common characteristics listed in Table 3-7. When a viral agent does have an envelope, it is composed of lipids, proteins, and glycoproteins acquired from the host cell when the virus buds off. The envelope (if present) will protect the virus in the extracellular environment. The outer part of the virus (the capsid or the envelope) contains the structural key to penetrate target cells that have the appropriate receptors for that virus. Part of this ability may be derived from the parts of the envelope that it acquired from a similar cell on its birth. Viruses have been known to infect almost every part of other life forms, including plants, mycoplasmas, fungi, and bacteria (**bacteriophages**).

Subclassifications. There is only a slight tendency for viruses of specific taxonomic classifications to behave in clinically similar manners. Viruses can be classified in several ways. All contain either DNA or RNA of either single (**ss**) or double strands (**ds**) for their genetic core. They also may be classified by size, shape, and the presence or absence of an envelope (Figure 3-6).

Pathogenic DNA viruses are usually double stranded and may be recognized and accepted into the host cell's DNA. Once incorporated, their replication occurs in the nucleus. They can use the cell's RNA polymerases for the creation of their progeny.

RNA viruses are usually single stranded (except for reoviruses and birnaviruses) and must encode for some of their own enzymes. Replication is usually in the cell cytoplasm.

Entry and Invasion. Viruses have been known to infect humans by all portals of entry. They must penetrate either already broken skin or by means of the bite of an arthropod or other multicellular organism or enter through the mucous membranes or epithelium of a body orifice or cavity. Some viruses have adapted multiple methods of entry into the body (e.g., HBV and varicella). **Parenteral** exposure (directly into the bloodstream) is the most efficient port of entry (i.e., **bloodborne pathogens**), but the respiratory route is also efficient and is the most difficult of the natural routes of infection to control.

Once the pathogenic virus obtains entry, it targets specific cells that have the appropriate receptors to allow intracellular invasion. Some examples of specific target cells, their receptors, and invading viruses are listed in Table 3-8.

Once the cell is penetrated, several steps occur:

1. Uncoating of the viral genome (DNA or RNA)
2. Expression of the virus genome
3. Replication of the viral genome by using the cell's stock of nucleic acids and often their polymerase enzymes as well
4. Assembly of **progeny** (children or offspring) viruses
5. Egress from the infected cell, often by lysis, or killing, of the cell.

Clinical Characteristics. Some viruses enter, invade, and predominantly remain within the same organ system. Examples include the viral gastroenteritis caused by the rotavrus and Norwalk virus in the epithelia of the intestines. In most cases, the release of progeny means lysis, or killing, of the host

Table 3-7
Common Characteristics of Viruses

1. A size between 20–300 nm.
2. The structure of:
   a. A genetic *core* of DNA or RNA (but not both), which codes their genetic makeup, or *genome.*
   b. A protein coat enclosing their DNA/RNA (*capsid*).
   c. The core/capsid complex, called a *nucleocapsid,* which in some cases represents the entirety of the virion.
3. May or may not have a surrounding envelope.
4. They infect only:
   a. Specific ranges or types of host cells.
   b. Specific species of higher life forms than them.
   c. Cells that have specific *receptors* on their surface that make them vulnerable to the virus.

Table 3-8
Example of Viral Cell Receptors

Cells	Receptors	Infecting Virus
T4 lymphocytes	CD4	HIV
Skin/membranes	Cell-surface heparin sulfate	Herpes simplex
Oropharynx	CR2	Epstein-Barr

Figure 3-6
Names, shapes, and relative sizes of some vertebrate-animal viruses.

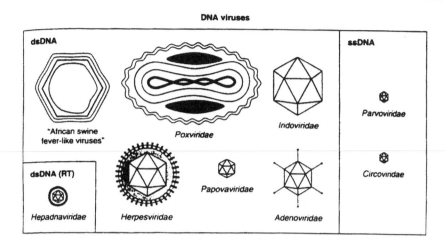

Source: Murphy FA, Fauguet DHL, Bishop SA, et al. *Sixth Report of the International Committee on Taxonomy of Viruses.* Wein: Springer-Verlag, 1995, with permission.

cell, often producing pathologic or clinical (**cytopathogenic**) consequences. The clinical course of a viral infection depends on

1. Virulence of the infecting virus
2. Infective dose
3. Port of entry
4. Type of cells and tissues infected
5. Rate of viral spread and replication
6. Site from which the virus is shed into the environment
7. Nature and magnitude of the immune and host defense responses
8. Acquired or inherited resistance to antiviral medications

These points are addressed in this chapter and in the chapters on specific viral pathogens. Viral infectivity depends in part on the human host's genome. The small variation in human genotypes may explain why some persons are more susceptible to some types of viruses than others. Epstein-Barr virus (EBV), for instance, is fatal to the majority of persons with a specific X-linked defect. There is also variation in the degree of clinical illness, which may be a result of genetics, general health, and the level of preexisting immunity to the causative agent or a closely related virus.

Clinical Outcomes. Viruses are difficult to treat because they reside within the cell during their pathogenic state. The development of drugs that selectively destroy the virus without damage to the protoplasm or genetic material proves difficult.

The exact mechanism by which a virus kills its host cell is not known. Death or impairment of host cell function is responsible for most of the cytopathophysiology of viruses, along with consequences of the host immune responses, which are discussed later. In some cases, the infected host cells and organs are at increased risk for neoplasms. For instance, chronic hepatitis B infection increases the lifetime risk for developing primary liver cancer by a relative risk of 200.

However, not all viruses must kill the host cell to replicate. A virus may infect a cell that does not possess all the factors it needs for replication. If the block occurs early in a replication cycle, the virus genome may be diluted by cell division to the point of viral extinction, and the host may be able to develop immunity to subsequent invasion. If the block occurs later in the replication cycle, the cell

may be lysed but without releasing infectious progeny. Some DNA viruses have evolved the ability to survive in cells that are nonpermissive of viral replication, which may explain latent infection by such classes as the herpesviruses. They still may become active and infectious when conditions change in the cells.

The fate of a virus within the human body is variable. It may fall victim to an efficient immune system and meet with early eradication. Some viruses cause an active infection that leads to death (e.g., rabies) or a slowly progressive chronic illness by selectively damaging cells of a vital organ (e.g., hepatitis B, hepatitis C, and slow viruses). Other viruses may remain in a latent form throughout a normal human life span (e.g., varicella and most of the herpes class of viruses). Specific antibodies may develop to a latent infection but be inefficient in eradicating the disease. Nevertheless, these antibodies can be used as biologic markers or screening tests for diagnosis (e.g., hepatitis C and HIV).

Occupational Considerations. Since viruses have limited survivability in the inanimate environment, the risk of occupational viral infection is higher for those working in health care or in other jobs with close contact with infectious humans (including coworkers) or animals. The great exception is the arboviruses, which are harbored by mosquitos and ticks. Those who may be working outdoors in endemic areas, at specific times of the day or night, and in specific seasons and weather conditions have a higher rate of exposure and risk for arbovirus infections.

Treatment of Viral Infections. RNA viruses must code for their own **RNA polymerase** (called *transcriptases/replicases*). This genome may be specific for that virus. If drugs can be developed that selectively inhibit that genome or enzyme, then viral replication may be inhibited without affecting the function of the host cells. This is the basis for the first generation of antiretroviral (HIV) drugs known as *nucleoside analogues* and *nonnucleoside reverse transcriptase inhibitors.* RNA viruses often also need to code for their own proteases, the enzymes that cleave larger chains of polyproteins to yield the smaller proteins needed to assemble progeny. The protease inhibitors have been the later generation of anti-HIV drugs.

Prevention and Prophylaxis. Despite the advances in antiviral drug therapy, the drug treatment of viral diseases is still in its infancy. Amantadine and rimantadine once helped to prevent or reduce the clinical illness of influenza A (see Chapter 11) before resistance developed. Acyclovir and its precursor drugs may reduce the clinical illness from the herpesviruses but do not eradicate the latent infection.

Prevention by immunization remains the most reliable method of virus control (see Chapter 5). But many viruses undergo rapid genetic variation (e.g., HIV and influenza), and this makes the development of an efficacious vaccine elusive. Other viruses (e.g., adenovirus) have so many pathogenic subtypes that developing a broadly protective vaccine is difficult.

Bacteria

Bacteria is a very broad term for single-cell organisms that may or may not cause human disease (may or may not be pathogenic). They are classified as lower protists, or prokaryotic bacteria. Bacteria are present throughout the biosphere and are highly adapted to specific environments. Only pathogenic bacteria are discussed in this book. Unlike viruses, most bacteria can survive outside hosts. Some common characteristics of human pathogenic bacteria and exceptions are listed in Table 3-9.

Classification. Bacteria are classified in many different ways, not all of which are of clinical significance. These include

SHAPE. Bacteria are classified by their shape as

- **Cocci:** round, spherical, or ovoid in shape. They may be found singularly or in groups or clusters.

- **Bacilli:** basically rod shaped, with square, round, or club-shaped ends.
- **Spirilla:** corkscrew or comma shaped (vibrio and spirochetes).
- **Diplococci:** cocci occurring in pairs.

STAINING. The bacteria with semirigid cell walls are further described by their reaction to the standard **Gram's stain.** Gram-positive organisms stain a purple-black owing to the peptidoglycan and teichoic acid in their cell walls. Gram-negative organisms stain pinkish owing to their thinner layer of peptidoglycan yet thicker and more numerous layers of protein and polysaccharides in their cell walls. All *Spirilla* stain gram-negative.

Two-thirds of cocci are gram-positive, and bacilli are about evenly split between gram-positive and gram-negative. Mycobacteria cannot be demonstrated by Gram staining and are instead stained with acid-fast preparations. All **mycobacteria,** including human tuberculosis, are acid-fast-positive. They lack cell walls but have thick cholesterol-based membranes and are very resistant to most physical forces.

Pathogenic gram-negative bacteria have **pyrogenic,** i.e., fever-inducing, properties. This is due to **endotoxins,** complex phospholipid-polysaccharide macromolecules in the cell walls. Gram-negative bacteria (e.g., *N. meningitidis, Y. pestis,* and *Salmonella typhi*) may be among the most virulent of bacteria and may be responsible for sepsis in about one-fourth of those who develop gram-negative infection in the blood (**bacteremia**). Other gram-negative bacteria that cause sepsis include *E. coli, Klebsiella, Enterobacter, Serratia, Proteus, Pseudomonas aeruginosa,* and *Haemophilus influenzae.*

The incidences of gram-positive bacteremia and sepsis are increasing mainly owing to the use of medical catheters, shunts, and prosthesis, all of which disrupt the natural mucocutaneous barriers and introduce bacteria into the bloodstream (Figure 3-7). Shock and acute respiratory syndromes are less common with gram-positive organisms (e.g., staphylococci, enterococci, and streptococci) than with gram-negative organisms. Many other stains have been used for bacteria, both for clinical indications and for classification.

BIOCHEMICAL ACTIVITY. Most bacteria can be grown in laboratories under a great variety of conditions and using various media. This has led to a

Table 3-9
Characteristics of Pathogenic Human Bacteria

Single-cell organisms:	Exceptions:
Have DNA for their genetic material	—
Do not have a membrane around nucleus	
Reproduce by asexual splitting (or binary fission)	—
Have semirigid cell walls	*Mycoplasma* (no true walls)
	Treponema (thin walls)
	Borrelia (thin walls)
	Leptospira (thin walls)
Are free living	*Rickettsia* (cell parasite)
	Coxiella (cell parasite)
	Chlamydia (cell parasite)

Figure 3-7
Disruptions of the epithelial surfaces that may result in
infection. These include surgery, burns, catheters, and
trauma.

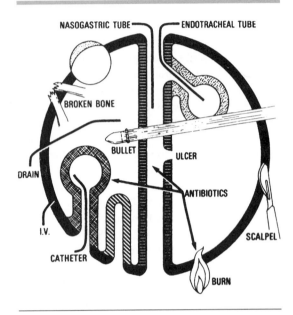

Source: Meakins JL. Host defenses. In: Howard RJ, Simmons RL (eds),
Surgical Infectious Disease, 2nd ed. New York: Appleton-Century-Crofts,
1988, Chap. 11, p. 154, with permission.

classification of bacteria as negative or positive to
lactose, sorbitol, catalase, or coagulase. Bacteria also
can be classified as alpha- or beta-hemolytic on
blood agar. Laboratory methods of bacteriology are
discussed in Chapter 2.

GROWTH PATTERN. Bacteria also are described
by their growth patterns in various atmospheres
using these definitions:

- **Strict (or obligate) aerobic:** Will not grow in the
  absence of oxygen.
- **Strict (or obligate) anaerobic:** Will not grow in
  the presence of oxygen.
- **Facultative anaerobe:** Will use oxygen if present
  but also can grow without oxygen.
- **Microaerophilic:** Requires oxygen concentrations of 2–10% (instead of the atmospheric
  20%). These bacteria also may require higher
  than atmospheric concentration of carbon dioxide.

Anaerobic Infections. Anaerobic bacterial infections usually are due to indigenous (floral)

organisms that are normally found on the low-
oxygen-tension surfaces such as the gingival
crevices of the oral cavity, the distal ileum and
colon, and the endocervix and vagina. Anaerobic
bacteria outnumber aerobic bacteria in the normal
human colon by about 500:1 and are also predominant in the mouth. The study of anaerobes did not
begin until the 1970s because of the difficulty in
obtaining cultures. Some of the most significant
anaerobic organisms are listed in Table 3-10. Facultative anaerobes include Enterobacteriaceae,
staphylococci, and streptococci.

Subclassifications. Several pathogenic groups of
organisms do not meet the classic concept of bacteria but generally are classified with them clinically
because they produce diseases similar to bacteria
and generally are sensitive to the same antibiotics as
free-living bacteria. They are discussed in Chapters
12 and 29.

CHLAMYDIA. Chlamydia are obligate intracellular parasites that can infect mammals, humans,
and domesticated avian species. They are responsible for a prevalent human sexually transmitted disease (STD) but also can cause eye infections,
blindness, and respiratory infections. *Chlamydia
psittaci* can be aerosolized and is responsible for the
occupational disease known as *psittacosis,* or *Parrot
fever.* They are generally susceptible to antibiotics
(see Chapter 12) and are easily treated once recognized.

RICKETTSIAE. Like viruses, rickettsiae are obligate intracellular parasites, but they are also like
bacteria because they divide by binary fission, are
gram-negative, are coccobacillary in shape, contain
both RNA and DNA, have their own metabolism by
electron transport, and use the Krebs cycle. The
four subclasses are *Rickettsia, Coxiella, Ehrlichia,*
and *Rochalimaea.* They are mostly distributed by
arthropod vectors of ticks and lice and are a risk for

Table 3-10
Some Significant Anaerobic Organisms

Group	Organisms
Gram-positive cocci	*Peptostreptococcus, Peptococcus*
Gram-positive bacilli	*Clostridium perfringens* and *Clostridium tetani* (spore formers), *Lactobacillus, Actinomyces*
Gram-negative cocci	*Veillonella*
Gram-negative bacilli	*Bacteroides fragilis* and *Bacteroides bivivus*

outdoor workers. They were named for Dr. H. T. Ricketts, who died from occupational typhus contracted through his research. Rickettsiae require a high level of precautions when handled in laboratories (see Chapter 34) because some types such as *C. burnetii* and *R. rickettsii* (Rocky Mountain spotted fever) also can be inhaled by aerosol.

Nomenclature. The nomenclature for microorganisms is constantly changing (by the International Commission on Microbial Taxonomy) and may confuse clinicians who have learned different names during their training. The reasons for name changes are rarely clinically relevant but are done for taxonomic reasons. Some examples are listed in Table 3-11.

Clinical Outcomes. Bacteria are the only major class of microorganisms that seems to have a vital purpose in survival. We cannot live without bacteria, which are involved in the digestion of food, preparation of food, production of essential vitamins, and debriding of the sloughing tissues of our skin and mucous membranes. A specific bacteria can be either a friend or a foe if it invades outside its habitat on or in our body.

Occupational Considerations. Bacteria are found in almost every square inch of land, water, and sea. Unlike viruses, most bacteria species on Earth can live independent of higher life forms. They are highly adapted to their environment, their hosts, and often both. Many occupations expose humans to bacteria for which they do not have immunity through environmental exposure or by physical trauma and disruption of the flora planes (see Figure 3-7). Consideration of specific occupational environments is discussed in Chapter 4. Chapter 34 is especially important in the handling of all infectious agents, as is Chapter 35.

Prevention and Prophylaxis. Many zoonoses are bacterial or rickettsial in origin: anthrax, brucellosis, leptospirosis, Q fever, bubonic plague, Rocky Mountain spotted fever, salmonellosis, and tu-

laremia. Precautions need to be taken vary with professions; these are explored in Chapters 4 and 36.

Developing vaccines for bacterial disease is considerably more difficult than developing them for viruses. Available live bacterial vaccines are those for tularemia, bacille Calmette-Guérin (BCG) for tuberculosis, and oral live vaccines for typhoid. None has widespread usage in North America. **Toxoids** (inactivated toxin antigen vaccines) are given for diphtheria and tetanus, and both require frequent reimmunizations in adults. Oral vaccines have been developed for diseases naturally inoculated by ingestion (e.g., polio). Most other bacterial vaccines are made from nonviable (dead) cellular components.

Treatment of Bacterial Diseases. Most known bacterial diseases have some available, effective antibiotic or antimicrobial therapy. But drug resistance has been an emerging problem (see Chapter 37) in the treatment of hospitalized patients and is now becoming a problem with the treatment of outpatients. Workers in hospitals and extended-care facilities may be developing colon colonization by resistant species such as vancomycin-resistant enterococcus (VRE) [25]. Although no increased morbidity or mortality has been documented in these workers, they could at some point in later life become septic because of infection with this very difficult to treat pathogen.

Fungi

Fungi are eukaryotic, or possess both plant and animal characteristics. **Yeasts** are defined as spherical organisms that reproduce by budding (like bacteria), and **molds** have branches (**hyphae**) and grow seeds (**spores** or **conidia**), behaving more like plants when they grow into masses (**mycelium**). Some are **dimorphic,** switching between molds and yeasts, depending on the environment and substrate availability. Fungi are present in most parts of the biosphere, living on environmental surfaces and in the soil, contaminating the air with their spores. Thousands of species are known, but only about 100 are pathogenic in humans. Fungi are responsible for causing human allergic reactions (e.g., rhinitis, pneumonitis, and asthma), infections, and toxicity (**mycotoxicoses**). Even dead, or nonviable, parts of fungi can cause allergic reactions and occasionally are implicated in "sick-building syndromes."

Table 3-11
Renamed Bacteria

Current Name	Previous Name
Pneumocystis jiroveci	*Pneumocystis carinii*
Streptococcus pneumoniae	*Diplococcus pneumoniae*
Enterococcus faecalis	*Streptococcus faecalis*
Helicobacter pylori	*Campylobacter pylori*
Morganella morgagni	*Proteus morganii*

Most fungal infections are superficial infections of the skin or nails (**dermatophytosis**). Both are more common in occupations in which bathing facilities may be shared, such as military barracks or athletic gymnasiums. Deep fungal infections of the lung or systemic fungal infections are called *mycoses*. Some human mycoses have a dimorphic form and can switch between being a yeast in tissue and a mold in the environment. Persons who work in occupations in which there is disturbance of the soil or the creation of dust are at risk for infection with aerosolized pathogenic fungi. Histoplasmosis and coccidioidomycosis may result from the inhalation of soil or dust contaminated by bird droppings. Deeper, systemic mycoses occur occasionally in healthy persons but are even more common in immunocompromised individuals. Environmental fungal infections are of great concern as nosocomial infections. Poorly controlled hospital renovation projects have resulted in lawsuits filed by transplant and other immunocompromised patients infected with *Aspergillus*.

Fungi also produce mycotoxins, which have been suspected of being mutagenic, carcinogenic, and teratogenic. *Aspergillus* mycotoxins, known as *aflatoxins,* have direct organ-toxic effects as well. The U.S. Department of Agriculture (USDA) controls conditions under which corn or peanuts must be stored.

Fungemia is the presence of fungi in the bloodstream, becoming a more commonly recognized problem. *Candida* fungemia is the most common and usually occurs in those who are immunosuppressed and in whom mortality is usually high. Fungemia also may originate from the gastrointestinal tract in those who have *Candida* overgrowth from antibiotic treatment. Phagocytic neutrophils and T-lymphocytes are the body's major defense, and infection is more common if there are inadequate host defenses (e.g., neutropenia or cellular immunosuppression).

Parasites

All pathogens discussed in this text are human parasites. But the biomedical disciplines define *parasitology* as the study of the parasitic protozoan, helminthic, and arthropod species, and all these organisms have multiple life-cycle stages and infective forms that can survive outside the body of the human. Most parasitic infections are more signifi-

cant in immunosuppressed hosts. They are all in the subkingdom Protozoa and classified under three phyla: Apicomplexa (the sporozoan), Sarcomastigophora (flagellates and amoebas), and Ciliophora (the ciliates).

Flagellates. Flagellates have one or more whip-like tails (**flagella**) or an undulating membrane (e.g., trypanosomes).

INTESTINAL AND URINARY FLAGELLATES.

Giardia. *Giardia* have four sets of flagella and a double nuclei. They encyst on passing into the colon and may cause illness depending on the infective dose and the health of the host. There is a high inapparent:apparent illness ratio. They are transmitted by fecally contaminated food or water and are treated most easily with metronidazole.

Trichomonas. This parasite has several sets of flagella and an undulating membrane. It is sexually transmitted from the genitourinary tract but may survive short periods on personal fomites. It also has a high inapparent:apparent illness ratio and may be treated with several drugs, including metronidazole.

BLOOD FLAGELLATES.

Trypanosoma. This group of pathogens has an elongated shape and flagella. All pathogenic forms have an intermediate insect host vector. Diseases caused by *Trypanosoma* include African sleeping sickness and Chagas' disease. *Trypanosoma* may be bloodborne and thus transmitted by transfusions. The pathogen's habitats depend on the mosquito species in tropical climates. The disease is hard to treat and may become chronic with cardiac complications.

Leishmania. This infection is spread by the bite of sandflies and can cause cutaneous ulcers. It is also a bloodborne pathogen and was found in some U.S. troops on their donation of blood after returning from the Gulf War.

Amebas. Amebas are large, amorphous moving cells that feed by **phagocytosis** (surrounding and engulfing their meals). An active ameba forms inactive cysts and intermediate precysts. Cysts are found only in the colon or formed stool of humans and some primates and are very sensitive to drying. Amebic infections have a large inapparent:apparent ratio. As many as 5% of U.S. adults harbor *Entamoeba histolytica* asymptomatically. Several therapies, including metronidazole, are available. The disease can cause liver abscesses.

Blood Sporozoans. The plasmodia are ameboid intracellular parasites of vertebrates and are spread by the bite of the female *Anopheles* mosquito. They are responsible for various forms of malaria (see Chapter 25).

Cryptosporidium. Not to be confused with cryptococcosis (torulosis), which is a deep mycosis, cryptosporidiosis is caused by *Cryptosporidium parvum,* a protozoa that is spread by the fecal-oral route between humans and many domestic and wild animals in contaminated food or water. It is a **predictive disease for AIDS** [26] and an occupational risk for farmers, animal handlers, and day-care workers. Also a coccidian protozoan like *Cryptosporidium, Toxoplasma gondii* requires the domestic cat for full completion of its life cycle. Many other animals carry infective stages of the protozoan, which may encyst in their muscle or brain tissue for life. Humans are infected by the fecal-oral route from soil contaminated with cat feces. *Toxoplasma* encephalitis is also a predictive disease of AIDS [26].

Worms. Worms are know as helminths and are multicellular parasites. There are three types of worms: nematodes (roundworms), trematodes (flukes and flatworms), and cestodes (tapeworms).

NEMATODES. Nematodes are an extremely successful phylum that infect almost every species of plant, insect, and invertebrate on the land and in the sea and air. These worms cause a wide range of diseases and conditions that are largely treatable. Infection is usually by ingestion of undercooked contaminated food or vegetables or exposure to contaminated water. The infection has a high inapparent:apparent illness ratio. The current estimated global prevalence of some nematode infections [27] is shown in Table 3-12.

TREMATODES. The flatworms have a very wide variety of life cycles and hosts. The typical flatworms are hermaphroditic, invade by ingestion, and live in the colon. However, the schistosomes have separate sexes and invade through the skin from contaminated water to live in the blood vessels. End-organ damage is common, and flatworms may serve a role in bladder or colon carcinogenesis. Trematodes are more prevalent in tropical climates.

CESTODES. Human cestodal infections include the *Taenia* (taeniasis) species of pork and beef tapeworm. Infection is contracted by eating the poorly

Table 3-12
Global Prevalence of Some Nematode Infections

Nematode	Common Name	Number Infected
Ascaris lumbricoides	Giant roundworm	1 billion
Ancylostoma duodenale or *Necator americanum*	Hookworm	800 million
Wuchereria bancrofti	Filarial worm	hundred millions
Enterobius vermicularis	Pinworm	hundred millions

cooked meat of pigs or cattle that have grazed in human fecally contaminated soil. Humans are the definitive hosts, and swine and cattle are intermediate hosts. Humans are the exclusive hosts for *Mymenolepium nana,* dwarf tapeworms, however. The broad, or fish, tapeworm (*Diphyllobothrium latum*) is the largest of the cestodes, often reaching 30 ft in length. Infection is contracted by eating poorly cooked or raw freshwater fish. Symptoms may include malnutrition and pernicious anemia. This helminth has been found in the colder climates of Alaska and Canada.

ATTRIBUTES OF MICROORGANISMS THAT ENABLE THEM TO CAUSE DISEASE
Toxigenicity

Exotoxins. Exotoxins are antigenic proteins excreted into the environment by bacteria cells (more often gram-positive than gram-negative organisms) that have toxic clinical effects on specific human biologic functions or tissues. Exotoxins derive their name from the fact that they are toxic substances that have been excreted or exited the living bacterial cell. They are found either outside the cells, in the environment, or in bacterial spores. Since they are antigenic proteins, the body can form antibodies, or **antitoxins,** to most exotoxins. Exotoxins generally do not cause fever. Exotoxins may either cause illness by **intoxication** (poisoning) of humans who have either ingested or contacted the exotoxin of a bacteria living outside the human body or by infection when the bacteria is excreting exotoxin within the body (i.e., the intestine or a wound). Exotoxins are toxic to a wide range of cells and tissues that are specific to each exotoxin (Table 3-13).

Clostridium botulinum is an organism that lives in the soil and produces the exotoxin responsible

Table 3-13
Diseases and Exotoxins of the Clostridia and Their Target Tissues

Species and Disease	Exotoxins
C botulinum (botulism)	At least six neurotoxins that cause paralysis
C perfringens, etc. (gas gangrene)	Alpha through zeta exotoxins, which have actions of damaging:
	cells (necrolysis)
	heart muscle (cardiotoxin)
	collagen (collagenase)
	structural protein (proteolytic)
	fatty tissue (lipase)
	blood (hemolytic)
	erythrocytes (lecithinase)
C tetani (tetanus)	Neuromuscular contraction (tetanospasmin)
C diphtheriae (diphtheria)	Cardiac and CNS (diphtheria toxin)

for botulism. Botulism is an intoxication and is the most virulent natural exotoxin known. It is capable of causing death with ingestion of a few thousandths of 1 mg of the exotoxin.

C. perfringens lives in the colon of about 35% of humans and in the urogenital tract of some females. It or *C. septicum* or *C. novyi* may be responsible for gas gangrene. Infection with this exotoxin may be contracted from exposure to contaminated soil or from fecal contamination by injury or perforation of the gastrointestinal or female genital track (e.g., by abortion procedures).

C. tetani also is present in the intestinal flora of humans and domestic animals, and its spores are distributed widely in the soil in crowded or poverty-stricken areas. It is responsible for tetanus, a disease that can be prevented with "toxoid" vaccines made from inactivated toxin. Tetanus killed over 50,000 Axis troops in World War II, whereas Allied troops were spared because they had been immunized.

Staphylococcus can produce a toxin called *toxic shock syndrome toxin 1 (TSST-1)* when *S. aureus* strains colonize mucous membranes. This phenomenon was discovered in the early 1980s in association with the use of superabsorbent tampons. TSST-1 is also a **superantigen,** which means that it stimulates lymphocytes to produce large amounts of interleukin 1 (IL-1) and tumor necrosis factor

(TNF). Toxic shock syndromes also have occurred after influenza infections (see Chapter 11).

Enterotoxin. An enterotoxin is any substance specifically toxic to the cells of the intestinal mucosa. An enterotoxin is a form of exotoxin. Bacterial enterotoxins are responsible for most infectious diarrhea syndromes and may cause illness by either infection or intoxication. Examples of enterotoxin intoxication include botulism and staphylococcal and clostridial food poisoning. Enterotoxin infections include *Salmonella enteritidis,* cholera, and bacillary dysentery (*Shigella*).

The *E. coli* syndromes of enterotoxigenic (ETEC), enterohemorrhagic (EHEC), and enteroaggregative (EAggEC) disease are due to enterotoxins, whereas enteroinvasive (EIEC) and enteropathogenic (EPEC) diseases are not. *Salmonella* has over 2,000 serotypes, and many may cause inapparent illnesses. Humans probably develop progressive immunity to *Salmonella* types over a lifetime. Enteric forms of *Salmonella* infection such as typhoid fever (*S. typhi*) are rare in the United States. The gastroenteritis form is much more common but may require a 10,000-organism inoculum to cause infection. Most *Salmonella* enterotoxins are heat-sensitive and are destroyed by cooking, but a few are heat-resistant.

Shigellosis may occur with a "dose" of as few as 10 bacilli. Both *Shigella* (dysentery) and *Vibrio cholerae* (cholera) produce enterotoxins (Shiga's and choleragen, respectively) that have cytotoxic, neurotoxic, and enterotoxic (inducing fluid secretion) effects.

Species of *S. aureus* may produce a **staphylococcal enterotoxin** while growing in foods not properly refrigerated. There are at least six types, but all are absorbed in the gut and stimulate neural receptors to cause vomiting within a few hours. No other ingested biologic toxin works as quickly. A common-source food poisoning that causes vomiting within a few hours usually proves to be *S. aureus,* although other nonbiologic toxins must be included in the differential diagnosis. Inoculation of the food is often caused by a food worker with an infection on the hand or fingers. Food workers should be restricted from handling open food when they have infections of the exposed upper body.

Most of the enterotoxins are heat-sensitive (except some *Salmonella*) and can be destroyed by a temperature of 140°F (60°C). Exotoxins rarely produce fever.

Endotoxin. Endotoxins are complex phospholipid-polysaccharide macromolecules in the cell wall of gram-negative bacteria that may have virulent properties. The toxin is not released but remains a part of the cell wall of either the living cells or its debris.

Endotoxins derive their name from the fact that they can have toxic effects while remaining part of the wall of the bacterium. They are free only if the cell is destroyed. Endotoxins do not stimulate antibody or antitoxin formation, do not have receptor cells, and are not destroyed by heat or disinfectants. There is variation in the structure and function of the cell wall, and these differences may be important both in virulence and in classification of these bacteria. Endotoxins are **pyrogenic;** i.e., they produce fever. The fever is caused by monocytes' producing **endogenous pyrogen** in reaction to the endotoxin effects on the thermoregulatory center in the hypothalamus.

The **lipopolysaccharide (LPS)** portion of the endotoxin is the most important in determining host tissue reaction. An **O-specific LPS** determines the serologic specificity, and the lipid A portion is responsible for the toxic effect.

GRAM-NEGATIVE SHOCK. Endotoxin can induce tissue inflammation, fever, and shock in those infected; this is known as *gram-negative sepsis.* The LPSs of the endotoxin can enter the bloodstream after death of the cell. This may stimulate the complement system via the alternative pathway (discussed later) and result in the appearance of active effector molecules and inflammatory mediators such as the TNF, cachectin, IL-1, interferon, and cytokines. These can activate vascular endothelium and cause vasodilation and increased blood vessel permeability, which may result in a reduction in blood volume and hypovolemic shock. The **tumor necrosis factor (TNF)** is identical to lymphotoxin produced by activated T cells [28]. Lymphotoxin precipitates the following sequence of events: inflammation, cytotoxicity, cachexia, organ failure, shock, and death. These same biochemicals are also found in some types of cancer. Antibodies can attach to cachectic tumor cells and lymphotoxin, which can inhibit some of the antibody response. Corticosteroids also may help to block reaction to

this cascade, which is possibly why they are effective treatment for some gram-negative shock victims. These agents may be beneficial in small amounts and, when absorbed from the intestinal flora, may serve to stimulate the human immune system during maturation.

CLINICAL EFFECTS. Other oxygen radicals stimulated by endotoxin may cause alveolar damage and acute respiratory distress syndrome (ARDS). Endotoxins also may be responsible for stimulating the biochemical reaction that results in the invasiveness of *H. hemophilus influenzae, Neisseria meningitis,* and other bacteria, causing a break in the bloodbrain barrier and resulting in meningitis and shock. Endotoxin also has been shown to act on macrophages, enhancing their ability to produce oxygen radicals, which have been implicated as mediators of inflammatory tissue damage. Macrophages may stimulate the production and release of collagenase. Endotoxins have been implicated in the destruction of gum tissue in periodontal disease. Gram-negative organisms are the predominant oral flora in those with periodontitis. Endotoxins also may be the agent responsible for **byssinosis,** an occupational illness that can result from the inhalation of the products of gram-negative bacteria contaminating cotton or other vegetable fibers.

Virus-Induced Proliferation of Host Cells. Some DNA viruses have the ability to stimulate division of their host cells, an indirect means of increasing their own progeny. Viral antigens with these properties are called *oncogenes.* They increase the rate of growth of a tissue line or increase the life of individual cells and thus may cause malignancies as a result of latently infected cells. Viruses believed to function as oncogenes include Epstein-Barr, human papillomaviruses, and hepatitis B virus (HBV).

Extracellular Enzymes. Many bacteria produce enzymes that degrade tissue in their vicinity. **Hyaluronidase** hydrolyzes hyaluronic acid from the connective tissue and is produced by many staphylococci, streptococci, and anaerobes. It facilitates their ability to form **abscesses.** *S. aureus* can produce **coagulase,** which coagulates plasma and forms a fibrin mass around the lesion, which helps to protect bacterial abscesses. Many streptococci produce the enzyme **fibrinolysin** (also known as **streptokinase**), which facilitates their growth in coagulated tissue. This enzyme has been synthesized and used to reverse clots in patients with myocardial infarction. Dozens of other tissue-destructive enzymes are known to be produced by bacteria, and some may be considered exotoxins, as described earlier.

Many organisms that invade through the epithelium have the ability to actually cleave the protective secretory IgA antibodies. These are called *IgA1 proteases* and are produced by *N. gonorrhoeae, S. pneumoniae, H. influenzae,* and *N. meningitidis.*

Invasiveness (Infectivity)

The invasiveness of bacteria is partially determined by **adherence.** Adherence can be determined by several factors, including

1. *Surface hydrophobicity.* The more hydrophobic the bacterial surface, the greater is the adherence to the host cell.
2. *Net surface charge.* Both bacteria and host cells tend to be negatively charged, so bacteria gain an advantage if they can move toward being positively charged. Charge can depend on the anions and cations and pH of the local environment.
3. *Binding molecules on the bacteria* (**ligands**) and their ability to adhere to host cell receptors.
4. *Presence of **pili** or **fimbriae.*** These hair-like appendages on bacterial walls may facilitate attachment to host cells receptors such as epithelial cells (e.g., *E. coli* to bowel epithelia and group A streptococcus to buccal epithelia).

Host cells are not always passive, however, because they may be enticed to phagocytize the bacteria after the bacteria have adequately adhered to them. This saves the bacteria the trouble of actively invading. The bacteria is contained in a "Trojan horse" vacuole membrane, which later dissolves. This phenomenon has been seen in vitro with the following bacteria:

1. *Shigella* species, *Yersinia enterocolitica,* and *Listeria monocytogenes* adhere to and are phagocytized by macrophages in the epithelium of the intestine.
2. *Legionella pneumophila* adhere to and are engulfed by pulmonary macrophages.
3. *Neisseria gonorrhoeae* adhere to microvilli of fallopian epithelial cells, are engulfed, and then multiply intracellularly.

METHODS OF RESISTANCE OF THE INFECTIOUS AGENT

All antibiotics work on bacteria either by disrupting their normal biochemical mechanisms or by disrupting the formation of their cell wall. Disruption of biochemical activities involves inhibiting bacteria's synthesis of nucleic acid and/or proteins, disrupting their plasma membrane, or inhibiting their normal enzyme activity in cellular metabolism. Since humans have no cells with walls, cell wall–disrupting drugs—penicillin, cephalosporins, and their synthetic relatives—have been among the most efficacious and least toxic antimicrobials. Some naturally occurring antimicrobial agents, such as the bacitracin from *Bacillus licheniformins,* have been found and synthesized commercially as antibiotics.

Genetic Antimicrobial Resistance

Bacteria and viruses are both **clonal** because they are haploid and produce offspring that are exact replicas of themselves. A clonal line with improved virulence or survivability may gain a competitive advantage over other microorganisms, even of the same species.

Infectious agents may be resistant to antibiotics or disinfectants because of their own constitutional structure or genome or because of resistance they acquire during exposure. Bacteria may develop resistance by the chance mutation and development of enzymes that inactivate antimicrobials. Examples include

1. Enzyme inactivation of aminoglycosides by acetylation, phosphorylation, or adenylation
2. Beta-lactamases that cleave penicillins and cephalosporins
3. Acetylases that acetylate chloramphenicol

Often the resistance itself seems to be contagious, however, more than can be explained by chance single-sequence mutations. Three mechanisms of the moving of larger DNA sequences between infectious agents are known to occur: transformation, transduction, and plasmid transfer.

Transformation. Transformation is a rather inefficient and random event in which an isolated and free DNA fragment is incorporated into the chromosome of a closely related agent. Drug resistance can be transformed into another agent if this sequence codes for resistance.

Transduction. In transduction, the DNA fragment enters the recipient cells by a **bacteriophage.** A bacteriophage is a virus that infects specific bacteria as its host. This mechanism is more efficient than transformation because larger homologous segments may be moved, and it may induce multidrug resistance.

Plasmid (R Factor) Transfer. The most efficient and "sexiest" of resistance transfer is through the plasmids. Many bacteria have nonchromosomal "extra" genetic material not essential to their survival. A physical mating may occur between two widely different bacterial cells, wherein rather large fragments of extrachromosomal DNA is inserted through a hollow **pilus** connecting the mating cells. This DNA is called a **plasmid** or an **R (residence) factor**. This process was first identified during dysentery epidemics in Japan in the 1950s, when *Shigella* species developed antimicrobial resistance factors identical to those of *E. coli* strains from the colons of the same patients.

Biochemical Antimicrobial Resistance

The methods of genetic transfer of resistance factors are better understood than the biochemical mechanisms of this resistance. But several changes in bacterial cells are known to be associated with resistance.

Enzymatic Inactivation of the Antibiotic. Several antibiotics are subject to inactivation by cleaving enzymes produced by bacteria. These include the penicillins and cephalosporins, which are inactivated by **beta-lactamases** into penicilloic and cephalosporic acids, respectively. Aminoglycosides and chloramphenicol are also known to be inactivated by specific bacterial enzymes.

Alterations in Target Site/Permeability. Many pathogenic bacteria are known to alter the coding for their cell wall antibiotic receptor sites. This includes many of the pathogens of concern in the hospital environment, such as **methicillin-resistant S. aureus (MRSA)** and penicillin-resistant *Streptococcus pneumoniae*. Bacteria also may change the permeability of their cell walls to antibiotics, especially the gram-negative bacteria, which have a cell membrane outside their wall. This may be responsible for their resistance to tetracycline and sulfa drugs.

Unblocked Metabolic Pathways. Many antibiotics work by blocking critical metabolic pathways. Plasmids, or R factors, may code for changes in bacterial enzymes that are either less sensitive to blocking or are able to bypass the block through an alternative pathway.

Viral Drug Resistance. The development of antiviral therapeutic agents lags decades behind that of antibacterial agents. Nevertheless, viruses seem to have developed resistance to antiviral drugs just like bacteria to antibacterial drugs. Influenza A's resistance to amantadine and rimantadine can develop in a matter of days or even hours, and resistance of HIV to any and all antiretroviral drugs has been seen. Less is known about antiviral-drug resistance, which simply may be due to antigenic changes.

The Antibiogram

Health care organizations must track drug sensitivities of microorganisms cultured within their facilities and share these results, in written form, with prescribing physicians and clinical pharmacists. This document is called an *antibiogram*. An example of an annual antibiogram for three hospitals is shown in Table 3-14. The document can show the pattern of emergence of resistance over time. Antibiograms serve several purposes. They may help the clinician to prescribe more effective drugs to seriously ill patients between the time of their presentation and obtaining culture and sensitivity results. Antibiograms also can be used to control costs by serving as guideposts to the use of the least expensive but effective drugs. Hospitals can use antibiograms to establish clinical pathways and to control the development of new drug resistances. Matching antibiogram patterns of sensitivity also may have epidemiologic utility because they may point toward a common source during a nosocomial outbreak.

The Host and Host Response

HOST RESPONSE TO INVASION
The Biologic Gradient

A host's clinical responses to invasion by infectious agents may vary greatly, ranging from rapid tissue destruction and death of the host to no clinical, or apparent, effect. Advances in microbiology and serology have led to the **iceberg concept** of infectious disease (Figure 3-8). The base of the iceberg is

Table 3-14
Antibiogram from Community Hospital

PERCENT SENSITIVITY INFORMATION FOR THE TOP ISOLATES*   1/97–12/97   ICU

Community Hospital East (ICU)

Group	ORGANISMS		AMK	GEN	TOB	CFZ	CTN	CXM	CTX	CTZ	AMP	A/S	PEN	PIP	AZT	CIP	I/C	TET	T/S	ERY	CLN	VAN
GRAM NEG.	Pseudomonas aeruginosa	66	96	85	100					80				91	71	85	76					
	Escherichia coli	44	100	100	100	96	100	93	98	97	61	58		71	100	100	100		93			
	Klebsiella pneumoniae	38	100	100	100		100	100	100	100	0	78		83	100	100	97		97			
	Enterobacter cloacae	22	100	100	100		20	8	36	33	0	8		48		100	100		100			
	Stenotrophomonas maltophilia	14	42	38	46					15				15		46	0		60			
	Klebsiella oxytoca	12	100	100	100		100	100	100	100	0		100	80	100		100					
	Serratia marcescens	12	100	100	100		100	0	100	100	8	25		100	100	75	100		100			
	Proteus mirabilis	11	100	100	100		100	100	100	100	82	90		90		90	100		73			
	Morganella morganii	8	100	100	100		100	19	100	100	0	20		100		63	88		63			
	Enterobacter aerogenes	5	100	100	100	0	60	50	80	80	0	67		100		100	100		100			
GRAM POS.	Staphylococcus aureus (MSSA)	69				95					5	95	11			96	100	100	100	77	97	100
	Enterococcus species	59									75		86					26	59	31	55	86
	Staphylococcus epidermidis	51				25					0	21	2			45		63	59	12	29	100
	Staphylococcus aureus (MRSA)	42				0					0	0	0			7		82	73			100

Community Hospital North (ICU)

Group	ORGANISMS		AMK	GEN	TOB	CFZ	CTN	CXM	CTX	CTZ	AMP	A/S	PEN	PIP	AZT	CIP	I/C	TET	T/S	ERY	CLN	VAN
GRAM NEG.	Escherichia coli	27	100	100	100		100	89	100	95	85	81		86	100	100	100		100			
	Pseudomonas aeruginosa	20	100	95	100					85	0			90	53	45	85					
	Klebsiella pneumoniae	14	100	100	100		100	100	100	100	0	60		93	100	86	100		86			
	Proteus mirabilis	5	100	100	100			100	100	100	100	100		100	100	100	100		100			
	Enterobacter cloacae	5	100	100	100		40	10	80	80	0			80		100	100		100			
GRAM POS.	Staphylococcus aureus (MSSA)	29				100					0	100	0			90		91	100	76	100	100
	Staphylococcus epidermidis	15				30					10	20	7			27		93	60	33	53	100
	Enterococcus species	12									92		92					58				100
	Staphylococcus aureus (MRSA)	9				0					0	0	0			0		78	33	22	22	100

Community Hospital South (ICU)

Group	ORGANISMS		AMK	GEN	TOB	CFZ	CTN	CXM	CTX	CTZ	AMP	A/S	PEN	PIP	AZT	CIP	I/C	TET	T/S	ERY	CLN	VAN
GRAM NEG.	Escherichia coli	26	100	96	100	100	100	98	100	100	77	79		74	100	100	100		92			
	Pseudomonas aeruginosa	10	100	90	100					100	10			100	78	70	100					
	Klebsiella pneumoniae	10	100	100	100	100	100	100	100	100	10	67		100	100	100	100		90			
GRAM POS.	Enterococcus species	18									94		89			18		6				94
	Staphylococcus epidermidis	11				13						27	9					82	36	27	73	100
	Staphylococcus aureus (MSSA)	8				100						100	0			100		86	100	100	100	100
	Staphylococcus aureus (MRSA)	6				0					0	0	0			0		100	100	67	83	100

BOXES CONTAINING NO NUMBERS INDICATES THE ANTIBIOTIC WAS NOT TESTED FOR THAT PATHOGEN
*Sensitivities reported for antibiotics where at least half the isolates were tested

ABBREVIATIONS

AMK=AMIKACIN
AMP=AMPICILLIN
A/S=AMPICILLIN/SULB.
AZT=AZTREONAM

CFZ=CEFAZOLIN
CIP=CIPROFLOXACIN
CLN=CLINDAMYCIN
CTN=CEFOTETAN

CTX=CEFTRIAXONE
CTZ=CEFTAZIDIME
CXM=CEFUROXIME
ERY=ERYTHROMYCIN

GEN=GENTAMICIN
I/C=IMIPENEM/CILASTATIN
PEN=PENICILLIN
PIP=PIPERACILLIN

TZP=PIPERACILLIN/TAZOBAC.
TET=TETRACYCLINE
TOB=TOBRAMYCIN
T/S=TRIMETHOPRIM/SULFA.

VAN=VANCOMYCIN

Figure 3-8
The "iceberg concept" of host responses to infectious agents. Most intrusions of infectious agents into the host do not result in clinical symptoms.

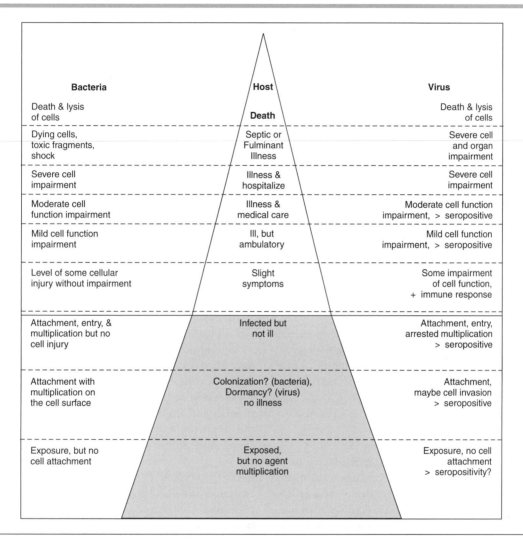

Bacteria	Host	Virus
Death & lysis of cells	**Death**	Death & lysis of cells
Dying cells, toxic fragments, shock	Septic or Fulminant Illness	Severe cell and organ impairment
Severe cell impairment	Illness & hospitalize	Severe cell impairment
Moderate cell function impairment	Illness & medical care	Moderate cell function impairment, > seropositive
Mild cell function impairment	Ill, but ambulatory	Mild cell function impairment, > seropositive
Level of some cellular injury without impairment	Slight symptoms	Some impairment of cell function, + immune response
Attachment, entry, & multiplication but no cell injury	Infected but not ill	Attachment, entry, arrested multiplication > seropositive
Attachment with multiplication on the cell surface	Colonization? (bacteria), Dormancy? (virus) no illness	Attachment, maybe cell invasion > seropositive
Exposure, but no cell attachment	Exposed, but no agent multiplication	Exposure, no cell attachment > seropositivity?

Source: Modified from Evans AS, Kaslow RA (eds), *Infections of Humans: Epidemiology and Control*, 4th ed. New York: Plenum, p. 26.

the majority of host exposures, which will not result in attachment or invasion. A smaller number may result in the development of immunity, as detected by laboratory studies, and an even smaller number may result in infection with no clinical symptoms. Only those infections with clinical symptoms appear above the waterline, and the very peak represents fatal host infections.

Clinical infections can be called *apparent,* whereas asymptomatic infections can be called *sub-clinical,* or *inapparent.* Inapparent infection can be diagnosed only by laboratory studies that detect the presence of persistent antibodies or isolate the agent. The **inapparent:apparent ratio** (i.e., sub-clinical:clinical ratio) is considerably wider for viruses than for other infectious agents. The ratio for human rabies is 0:100, whereas paralysis from wild poliomyelitis virus may be over 1,000:1. Other examples are measles, 1:99; influenza, 1.5:1; and rubella, 2:1. Because of the limits of serology testing, less is known about ratios for bacterial, fungal, and parasitic infections.

Inapparent:apparent ratios also can vary greatly depending on the age of the human host at the time of exposure. Most viral diseases have less morbidity in those who are young at the time of exposure. Hepatitis A has a ratio of 20:1 at age 5, 11:1 at 5–9, 7:1 at 10–15, and 2–3:1 after age 15. Many of the herpesviruses (e.g., EBV, cytomegalovirus, and varicella) cause more severe illness when they infect susceptible adults. There is great individual variation in how humans respond to specific infectious agents, especially fungi and viruses. Even when correcting for age, sex, general health, infective dose, and method of transmission, there are great individual differences in human host responses. This variation is called the *biologic gradient.* With some agents (such as *N. meningitides*), only rarely does an infected individual become ill and succumb; the majority have inapparent infection or even colonization. With other agents (such as HIV), it is rare that an infected person does not have progressive illness.

These differences stem from both Mendelian and multifactorial genetics and may have a very significant role in human evolution. One-third of all people who were exposed to the great plagues were not clinically ill, and this "surviving genome" may explain in part why plagues have not recurred.

Colonization and Carriage

Some bacteria and fungi seem well adapted to adhere and grow in "colonies" on human skin, mucous membranes, or other epithelial surfaces. This **colonization** may be due to a combination of inadequate or permissive host immunity and/or properties of the infectious agent that allow them to attach to lectins (adhesins) on the epithelial cell surfaces. Some bacteria have appendages called *pili* or *fimbriae* that allow them to attach to specific epithelial cells. These bacteria may colonize for only a short period of time, depending on seasons, host conditions, or host behaviors. If a host is infected with an agent that it can communicate to others, the term *carriage* is used. Carriage can exist before (**incubatory carrier**) or after (**convalescent carrier**) illness. In some cases, the host may never be symptomatic from carriage of the agent (**healthy carrier**). The host may be either a **transient carrier** or an indefinite **chronic carrier**.

While bacteria and fungi tend to colonize humans, some viral infections (e.g., varicella, poliomyelitis, herpes simplex, and cytomegalovirus) can remain subclinical (**latent,** or **dormant**) for the lifetime of the host. Infections with some mycobacteria species (e.g., tuberculosis) also may remain latent (inapparent). Disease (apparent infection) may be reactivated by immune deficiency or other stressors or factors not fully understood. Among the diseases most difficult to control are those with a long latency period (i.e., time between infection and clinical illness) that remain infectious to others (e.g., HIV).

Biologic Interference: Normal Flora

Resident, or normal, bacterial flora of the skin or mucous membrane may competitively inhibit more pathogenic organisms from establishing infections in the host. This phenomenon is called *bacterial interference,* although the mechanism is not fully understood. Bacteria may compete for binding sites on host cells, compete for the nutrient substrates from expired host cells, or produce substances toxic to other organisms.

The suppression or deletion of normal bacterial flora often results in other microbial agents becoming opportunistic. Clinical examples include the **superinfection** of Candida vaginitis after oral antibiotics and antibiotic-associated colitis caused by the opportunistic colonization of the colon by *Clostridium difficile* (**pseudomembranous colitis**).

Invasive Flora: Attack from Within

Not all normal flora remain forever harmless to their host. Many can cause infections under conditions of immunosuppression of the host or in situations in which a disruption of anatomic planes introduces the infectious agent into other tissues (see Figure 3-7), e.g., disruption by penetrating wounds or surgery. Examples include *Peptostreptococcus*' establishing vegetation on heart valves (infective endocarditis) after tooth extraction. Penetrating injuries of the bowel were nearly universally fatal before the advent of antibiotics. Anaerobic bacteria may compromise up to 30% of the mass of normal feces but an even higher percentage if there is peristaltic stasis or ileus. An increase in bacterial mass (as high as 10^{11} organisms per gram), along with inflammation of the bowel, may cause bacteremia and sepsis. The most serious new nosocomial infection has been **vancomycin-resistant enterococcus (VRE).** Hospitalized patients may become colonized with VRE, although the organism may be clinically apparent only when it invades an organ or vascular space other than the bowel or gastrointestinal tract. The mode of transmission most often suspected is the unwashed hands of health care workers. It is reasonable to expect that a high percentage of hospital workers are being colonized with VRE.

Host immunosuppression also may cause normal flora to become opportunistic. This suggests that flora organisms are at least partially policed by a healthy host's immune system.

HOST RESISTANCE: THE NONSPECIFIC (INNATE) IMMUNE SYSTEM

Nonspecific (innate) immunity is the combination of inborn and natural host factors that serves to prevent the establishment of foreign invaders, including infectious agents. Innate immunity comprises barriers such as skin and mucous membranes and nonspecific physiologic and immune responses by white blood cells (**leukocytes**), blood proteins, and scavenger cells in the tissues. The host reactions of fever and inflammation are also functions of innate immunity.

Skin

The skin is the largest organ of the body and the most important barrier to infectious agents. It is constantly growing and shedding the outer cornified epithelium (epidermis), which contains most of the indigenous bacteria. The skin's normal bacterial flora do not seem to be essential for survival because animals have been raised experimentally in microbe-free environments. Skin varies in its properties of thickness, rate of growth, and flora depending on the part of the body it covers.

Traumatic skin breaks such as abrasions, lacerations, and bites cause susceptibility to infections and may represent a large proportion of work-related infections. "Natural" breaks in the skin barrier occur at the hair follicles and sweat and sebaceous glands. These glandular secretions have an acidic pH and a high content of long-chain fatty acids with antimicrobial activity to pathogenic organisms such as fungi. Prepubescent children have more susceptibility to ringworm and other dermatophytes before the sebaceous glands are fully developed. Lipophilic and anaerobic bacteria such as *Propionibacterium acnes* live deep in the sebaceous glands and are not exposed to surface controls. These organisms are frequently found in blood cultures, cerebrospinal fluid (CSF) cultures, bone marrow aspirates, and any other procedures that involve puncturing the skin and underlying sebaceous glands and are deemed contaminants.

Sweat glands also secrete **lysozyme (muramidase),** an enzyme that can dissolve the bacterial cell walls of some gram-positive organisms. Normal flora of the skin (Table 3-15) have evolved the

Table 3-15
Normal Flora of the Skin[a]

Infectious Agent	Incidence	Comments
Staphylococcus epidermidis	+++	Coagulase-negative
Propionibacterium acnes (corynebacteria)	+++	Anaerobic near sebaceous glands
Diphtheroids	++	Aerobic corynebacteria
Clostridium perfringens	++	Especially groin and legs
		Gas gangrene
Lactobacilli	++	
Staphylococcus aureus (*S albus*)	+	Coagulase-positive nostrils, perianal area
Moraxella sp.	+	
Streptococcus pyogenes (Gr A)	+	
Candida albicans	Rare	
Other *Candida* sp.	+	
Enterobacteriaceae	Rare	
Mycobacterium sp.	Rare	

[a]Predominantly gram-positive cocci and rods, with some gram-negative bacteria in moist areas of skin (under clothing, groin). Many transient organisms can also reside temporarily.
Key: +++ = most humans; ++ = many humans; + = some humans at times.

ability to colonize the skin and to inhibit more pathogenic bacteria in the competition for substrates living on the skin (bacteriologic interference). For instance, some gram-positive organisms have enzymes that break down complex lipids produced by sebaceous glands to unsaturated fatty acids with antimicrobial activity against gram-negative organisms or fungi. It is the fatty acids of the skin that cause odor, and commercial deodorants are selectively gram-positive bactericidal. These products may shift the floral toward gram-negative predominance and toward gram-negative infections. The more serious bacterial infection of the skin (e.g., gangrene or necrotizing fasciitis) often represent combinations of aerobic and anaerobic organisms and may be very difficult to culture.

The skin is quite resistant to viruses but may be contaminated with viral pathogens at times. True viral or rickettsial colonization of the skin is not believed to occur. Viruses that can penetrate small abrasions in the skin include poxviruses, papillomavirus, herpes simplex, and possibly other herpesviruses. The bites of arthropod vectors transmit arboviruses and rickettsial infection. The bites of vertebrates transmit rabies and herpes type B (Simian) infections. Human-made punctures of the skin (e.g., intravenous drug use, transfusions, and needlesticks) may be the mode of transmission for many viral **bloodborne** infections.

Since the outermost layer of the skin is devoid of blood vessels or nerves, very few viruses cause local infection (exceptions are molluscum contagiosum, papillomaviruses, and rarely, herpes simplex). Most viral lesions of the skin are from hematogenous spread and are from other ports of entry, such as the respiratory tract. Cutaneous manifestations of viral infections are called *exanthems*. Exanthematous diseases have a great range of severity, prevalence, and patterns of lesion morphology and distribution. These include the "usual" childhood disease of rubeola, rubella, varicella, roseola, and erythema infectiosum. With the possible exception of varicella, exanthems are generally not infectious. Skin lesions serve as portals of exit (are infectious) for only very few viral skin infections, including poxviruses, herpes simplex, and herpes zoster. But even with acute varicella, the viruses in oropharyngeal secretions may be more important than skin in disease transmission.

Skin lesions of rickettsial infections (e.g., Rocky Mountain spotted fever, rickettsial pox, typhus, and trench fever) are due to vasculitis in the blood vessels of the skin; they are not portals of exit and are not infectious.

Nose and Nasopharynx

Normal flora of the nose and nasopharynx (Table 3-16) may be highly variable, even in the same individual over periods of time. The rim of the nares has a transitional zone with facial skin and a predominance of *Staphylococcus epidermidis*. But the nose and nasopharynx also contain a large number of anaerobic diphtheroids, which rarely causes host infection. Cultures of the posterior nares or na-

Table 3-16
Normal Flora of the Nose and Nasopharynx

Infectious Agent	Incidence	Comments
Staphylococcus epidermidis	+++	At margins of narcs
Staphylococcus aureus	+++	At margins of narcs
Haemophilus parainfluenzae	++	Rarely pathologic; lack LPS in walls
Diphtheroids (anaerobic corynebacteria)	++	Rarely pathologic species
Haemophilus influenzae	++	May cause otitis media
Branhamella catarrhalis	++	
Group A *Streptococcus pyogenes*	+	
Streptococcus pneumoniae	+	Rarely pathologic; lack LPS in walls
Enterobacteriaccae	+	
Moraxella nonliquefaciens	+	
Neisseria meningitidis	+	
Alpha-nonhemolytic streptococcus	Rare	

Key: +++ = most humans; ++ = many humans; + = some humans at times.

sopharynx pose special problems because of contamination from the outer area. The area is very difficult to culture, requiring special swabs and techniques. This area is also important as an origin of infections of the sinuses and the middle ear. Outbreaks of nosocomial MRSA have been attributed to nasal-colonized health care workers. The membranes of the nose and nasopharynx have their own lysozymes and secretory IgA.

Respiratory System

The respiratory system is one of the most efficient routes of entry for infectious agents, just as it is for chemical hazards. Nasal hairs provide some filtration, but their primary function is to produce turbulence of inspired air to trap particles on mucous membranes of the respiratory tree. The nasal and sinus turbinates present a large surface area of mucous membranes that are lined with special ciliated epithelial cells. Trapped particles are moved along the surface by the cilia (the **mucociliary elevator**) toward the oropharynx. There, the trapped agents are periodically swallowed and digested. The smaller particles may get past the nasopharynx or oropharynx but then may be caught by the mucociliary elevator of the lower pharynx or tracheal tree and moved to the oropharynx for swallowing.

The mucous membranes of the respiratory tract have more than just mechanical defenses. The cells have lysozymes and mucopolysaccharide inhibitors and phagocytic cells. The secretions also contain specific antibodies (IgA) to prevent bacteria adherence and viral penetrance and to aid in phagocytosis. The resident flora of the respiratory tree also may suppress pathogens by bacterial interference.

The smallest of infectious agents (i.e., some viruses, spores, and infective nuclei) of approximately 5 μm (microns) or less may reach the alveoli. There, they may be phagocytized by alveolar macrophages, but they also may cross the alveoli to cause infection by entering the lymphatic system or blood vessels. A few bacteria and many viruses invade the respiratory epithelial cells or alveolar macrophages directly and may cause clinical illness (Table 3-17).

Other viral agents that have routes of entry through the respiratory epithelial cells include varicella, rubella, mumps, measles (rubeola), arenavirus, and hantavirus. Many bacterial infections

Table 3-17
Some Viruses Responsible for Respiratory Illnesses

Viruses responsible for the upper respiratory infections
    Adenovirus, common cold
    Rhinovirus, common cold
    Coronavirus, common cold
    Myxovirus, parainfluenza and respiratory syncytial
    Orthomyxovirus, influenza
Viruses responsible for mononucleosis syndromes
    Epstein-Barr (human gamma herpesvirus 4)
    Cytomegalovirus (human beta herpesvirus 5)
    Roseola infantum (human herpesvirus 6)
    Human immunodeficiency virus (seroconversion illness)
Viruses responsible for sore throats (oropharyngitis)
    Adenovirus
    Herpes simplex, type 1
    Enteroviruses (coxsackieviruses, echoviruses)
    Orthomyxovirus, influenza
    Myxovirus, parainfluenza and respiratory syncytial

of the lower lungs (Table 3-18) may be associated with oropharyngeal flora (Table 3-19).

Factors of general health and behavior have great influence on host responses of the respiratory system. Smoking damages the mucociliary function and alveolar host defenses. Acute and chronic alcoholism may be associated with colonization of the upper airway by aerobic gram-negative bacilli. Chronic use of alcohol may diminish the gag reflex and impair tracheobronchial ciliary function. All these factors are associated with increased risk for aspiration pneumonia. Stomach acids can further damage the bronchial system and increase the risk for pneumonia owing to infection of the lungs by gastrointestinal flora.

General poor health or debilitation increases the prevalence of gram-negative organisms in the gastrointestinal and respiratory systems and the risk of

Table 3-18
Lower Respiratory Bacterial Infections

Disease	Pathogens
Empyema	Group A streptococcus, *Streptococcus pneumoniae*
Bronchiectasis	*Pseudomonas aeruginosa,* other aerobic and anaerobic bacteria
Lung abscesses	Many bacteria
Aspiration pneumonia	Many aerobic and anaerobic bacteria

Table 3-19
Normal Flora of the Oropharynx

Infectious Agent	Prevalence	Comments
Streptococcus (alpha-nonhemolytic)	+++	
Other *Streptococcus* sp.	+++	*S viridans*
Branhamella catarrhalis sinusitis	+++	May cause pneumonia or otitis
Aerobic *Corynebacterium*	+++	Diphtheroids
Staphylococcus aureus	++	
Streptococcus epidermitis	++	
Streptococcus pneumoniae	++	
Bacteroides sp.	++	
Haemophilus influenzae	++	
Haemophilus parainfluenzae	++	
Neisseria meningitidis	+	
Aerobic streptococci	+	
Anaerobic micrococci	+	
Pyogenic group A streptococcus	+	Up to 9% of adults
Campylobacter sputorum	+	
Gram-negative bacteria	Rare	Causes serious illness

Key: +++ = most humans; ++ = many humans; + = some humans at times.

aspiration and decreases the ability to initiate protective cough responses. The use of antacids and H_2 blockers, administered through a nasogastric tube, to prevent stress-related gastric ulcers may lower pH and contribute to pathogens' colonizing the pharynx and infecting the lungs.

Mouth and Oropharynx

The mucosa of the oropharynx and mouth have the widest range of flora of the human body (Tables 3-19 and 3-20). They are sterile at birth but are contaminated by passage through the birth canal and by exposure to the mother and other humans. The various alpha-hemolytic and nonhemolytic streptococcal species (formerly called *viridans*) are established as the predominant organism of the flora within a few hours of birth and remain so throughout life. Various aerobic and anaerobic staphylococci, gram-negative diplococci such as *Neisseria, Moraxella catarrhalis,* diphtheroids, and *Lactobacillus* are added soon afterward. After the teeth erupt, various spirochetes and fungi (e.g.,

Table 3-20
Normal Flora of the Mouth and Surface of Teeth

Infectious Agent	Prevalence	Comments
Streptococcus (alpha-nonhemolytic)	100%	Also known as *S. viridans*
Anaerobic micrococci	100%	On caries
Veillonella alcalescens (anaerobic)	100%	On caries
Staphylococcus epidermidis	+++	Coagulase-negative
Lactobacillus sp.	+++	
Fusobacterium nucleatum	++	
Enterobacteriaceae	++	
Bacteroides sp.	++	
Peptostreptococcus	++	May cause endocarditis
Treponema sp.	++	On caries
Staphylococcus aureus	+	Coagulase-positive
Candida albicans	+	Opportunistic in the immunosuppressed
Mycobacterium sp.	+	

Key: +++ = most humans; ++ = many humans; + = some humans at times.

Candida and *Actinomyces*) colonize the mouth and tonsillar tissues. Some of these organisms may be implicated in sinus, ear, and lung infections. Many of the throat flora are known to be antagonistic to group A streptococci, yet up to 9% of people remain colonized with pyogenic forms. The mouth and oropharynx may develop a predominance of gram-negative organisms during periods of very serious illness, which can have positive associations with multiple antibiotic usage and length of hospital stay. This may contribute to gram-negative sepsis in the critically ill.

Several viral groups can cause lesions of the mouth or oropharynx, including herpes simplex virus and coxsackievirus group A types 1–24. Fungal infections of the mouth and upper respiratory systems usually are caused by normal flora in immunosuppressed individuals.

Teeth

The flora of the mouth may have great individual variation depending on the presence of teeth and the presence of caries. Much of this variation involves the streptococcal species. *S. sanguis* and *S. mutans* colonize the tooth surface, whereas *S. salivarius* attaches to gingival and buccal epithelium. The combined presence of certain bacteria contributes to the formation of plaque, which results in a lower oxidation-reduction potential at the level of the tooth surface. This may stimulate the growth of strict anaerobes, such as various *Bacteroides* species and *Veillonella alcalescens*. There is also a high association of *S. mutans* with dental caries. *S. mutans* produces glucans (carbohydrate polymers) and results in a strong acidic demineralizing (**cariogenic**) force on the enamel. Those with extensive active caries have a higher number of both anaerobic bacteria and oral treponemes. They are at higher risk of anaerobic pulmonary infections after aspiration of oral secretions. Extractions or adequate dental care can reduce this risk and greatly change the mouth flora. Human bites are frequent occupational injuries in law enforcement, child care, and mental health workers, and any of these factors can increase the likelihood of anaerobic infections from human bites.

Stomach and Small Intestines

The major defense of the lower gastrointestinal tract is the low pH. Bile and pancreatic secretions of the duodenum also have strong antimicrobial properties. Very few microorganisms survive in this environment even for short periods of time (Table 3-21). Susceptible organisms survive the stomach only if there is a rapid transit or if the pH is above normal. Neonates, those taking antacid medications, and those who have had surgical gastrectomy have lower acidity (**achlorhydria**) and may have different flora of the stomach and upper intestine. Achlorhydria may increase exposure to some infectious agents.

With achlorhydria, the flora are more like the flora of the mouth and oropharynx and may include anaerobic and gram-negative aerobic bacteria. The bile and pancreatic ducts are normally sterile, but infection with *Salmonella* (including *S. typhi*), *Enterococcus*, *Bacteroides*, or *Clostridium* species is then more likely.

Distally in the small intestine, there is an increase in the number of colon-type organisms, including anaerobic bacteria and enterococci. Any disruption of the normal small or large intestine motility (e.g., surgery, obstruction, or ileus) may produce an overgrowth of facultative anaerobes of the small intestine with clinical consequences.

Large Intestine

Like the mouth and oropharynx, the colon is sterile at birth but soon harbors the largest microbial population of the body (Table 3-22). There are up to 10^{11} organisms per gram—even higher if colon motility is decreased below normal. Children who

Table 3-21
Normal Flora of the Stomach and Small Intestine

Infectious Agent	Prevalence	Comments
Stomach, if pH 2–3	Near sterile	with pH
Jejunum		with pH
Enterococci	+	
Lactobacilli	+	
Diphtheroids	+	
Anaerobics	Rare	
Ileum		with pH
Enterobacteria	+	
Anaerobic gram-negative bacteria	+	
Candida albicans	++	Opportunistic in immunosuppressed

Key: +++ = most humans; ++ = many humans; + = some humans at times.

Table 3-22
Normal Flora of the Large Intestine

Flora	Prevalence
Bacteria	
Anaerobic gram-negative:	
Bacteroides	
fragilis	100%
oralis	100%
melaninogenicus	100%
Fusobacterium sp.	100%
Anaerobic gram-positive:	
Clostridium	
perfringens	++
innocuum	++
tetani	+
septicum	+
ramosum	+
difficile	3%
Lactobacilli	+++
Bifidobacterium bifidum	+++
Eubacterium limosum	+++
Peptostreptococci	++
Peptococci	+
Facultative gram-negative aerobic:	
Enterococci	100%
Escherichia coli	100%
Klebsiella	++
Enterobacter sp.	++
Proteus spp	+
Salmonella (2000+)	+
Pseudomonas aeruginosa	+
Shigella	Rare
Salmonella typhi	Very rare
Gram-positive aerobic:	
Enterococci	100%
Staphylococcus aureus (with nasal)	++
Streptococci (non-A)	+
Fungi	
Candida albicans	++

Key: +++ = most humans; ++ = many humans; + = some humans at times.

are breast-fed seem to have a predominance of lactobacilli, but the flora pattern changes rapidly after weaning.

The flora of the adult colon are predominantly anaerobic (99%) and represent over 100 species. There is also a great range of virulence of the species that does not correlate with their prevalence in fecal flora. Facultative aerobic bacteria such as *E. coli* represent 0.06% of fecal organisms but are frequent causes of clinical infection from fecal conta-

mination of the urinary tract or surgical wounds. Variations in the virulence of the many *Bacteroides* species are related to the great variance in the toxicity of capsular polysaccharides.

The gram-positive spore-forming bacilli (e.g., *Clostridium perfringens, C. difficile,* and *C. tetani*) are present in the colon of about half of humans and are responsible for the global spore contamination of soil and water. Bacterial interference is very complex in the colon, but it is known that *Shigella, Salmonella,* and *Cholera* pathogens are inhibited by the short-chain fatty organic acids produced by anaerobes. Specific IgA in intestinal mucosa may prevent many infections, including cholera.

The flora load of the intestine increases with conditions that slow motility. Likewise, the flora load is greatly reduced by diarrhea, which may be stimulated by many infectious agents or their enterotoxins or by intoxication from the ingestion of exotoxins. Diarrhea may be either a toxin reaction, a defense mechanism to rid the body of harmful agents, or both. In children, diarrhea is the world's leading cause of death from infectious disease. Most clinical protocols involve treating the dehydration and malnutrition associated with diarrhea rather than trying to suppress the diarrhea itself.

Other Host Defenses

The host defenses described are by no means complete. Because of the theme of occupation-related disease in this text, the genitourinary, maternal-neonate-placental, and sexually transmitted aspects of host defenses are not presented.

Phagocytosis. In addition to the nonspecific host responses discussed thus far, a major part of nonspecific immunity is the defense offered by cells dedicated to ingesting and destroying foreign matter, including infectious agents. These cells are collectively called *phagocytes.*

DEFINITION OF PHAGOCYTE. A cell possessing the ability to ingest bacteria, other infectious or foreign agents, and other cells is a *phagocyte. Phagocytosis* is the process of engulfing foreign material. Phagocytes include several different types of cells, all of which have their origin in bone marrow precursor cells (Figure 3-9). Phagocytes receive signals from foreign microorganisms, from antibodies, or from parts of the complement system. These "opsins"

Figure 3-9
The development pathways of immunoactive cells, from a common stem cell.

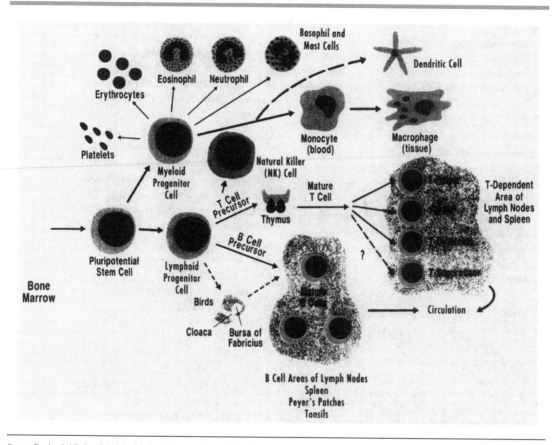

Source: Benjamini E, Sunshie G, Leskowitz S. *Immunology: A Short Course,* 3rd ed. New York: Wiley-Liss, 12996, p. 21, with permission.

prepare the microbe to be a target for a phagocyte.

TYPES OF PHAGOCYTES.

Monocytes and Macrophages. Monocytes circulate in blood and become larger (macrophages) when they move into tissue or organs. These long-lived cells then become a stationary part of the body's reticuloendothelial system. The kidneys, spleen, peritoneum, lungs (alveolar macrophages), liver (Kupffer cells), and brain (microglial cells) all have specialized macrophages. As part of the reticuloendothelial system, the tissue macrophages are also the local housekeepers and assist in ridding the body of older cells and cellular debris. Other portions of the reticuloendothelial system perform the same function throughout the body, filtering the blood and lymphatic system of microorganism and other organic debris. The tissue-bound macro-

phages also can work in concert with the T cells of the acquired immune system, to which they are closely related. T cells and tissue macrophages communicate chemically by cytokines.

Granulomas are the scar tissue structures that may form owing to long-term phagocytosis of some infectious or foreign agents. Granulomatous meningitis may result from tuberculosis or *Cryptococcus* infection. Granulomas also can be seen in the lungs owing to tuberculosis or other infectious disease, as well as chronic workplace exposures to some synthetic fibers.

Leukocytes. Leukocytes are the white blood cells that constitute the plasma of circulating blood. Their primary function is one of immunity. Lymphocytes are involved primarily in acquired immunity, whereas the granulocytes are involved primarily in nonspecific immunity. Leukocytes work together as a team in the face of adversity.

Granulocytes. These are circulating mature white blood cells that appear as granules on staining (i.e., neutrophils, basophils, and eosinophils) and are involved in functioning of the immune system.

Neutrophils [polymorphonuclear leukocytes (PMNs)]. These are mature circulating phagocytic granulocytes that stain neutral. The cytoplasmic granules contain biochemicals that degrade and digest ingested cellular matter.

Eosinophils. These are mature circulating granulocytes that stain acidic and contain cytoplasmic granules that can degranulate into immunoactive substances.

Basophils. These are mature circulating granulocytes that stain basic and contain cytoplasmic granules that can degranulate into immunoactive substances. **Mast cells** are twins of basophils and are found in the lungs, skin, tongue, and linings of the nose and intestinal tract; they are responsible for many of the symptoms of allergy.

Granular leukocytes are part of the nonspecific or innate immune system and have shorter lives than tissue macrophages. Neutrophils adhere to infectious agents and phagocytize them, forming **phagosomes.** Neutrophils then discharge their hydrolytic and other antimicrobial agents (**degranulation**) into the cell now called a **phagolysosome.** These agents may include hydrogen peroxide, peroxidase, chlorine, oxygen radicals, cathepsin, lysozyme, lactic acid, and acid hydrolase. Some individuals may have a deficiency in fighting catalase-producing organisms and thus have chronic *S. aureus,* fungi, and aerobic gram-negative bacterial infections.

NATURAL KILLER CELLS (NK CELLS). Unlike the T-lymphocyte cells, which have specific target cells, NK lymphocytes may have a wider range of nonspecific target cells. They do not kill by phagocytosis but rather by releasing very potent biochemicals in the vicinity of and in response to a target cell. This is also called *extracellular killing.* The NK cells respond to soluble mediators such as **interferon** and the **interleukins.** They are manufactured by various leukocytes, fibroblasts, activated T-lymphocytes, and even infected cells themselves. All are a call for NK cells. This system also may play a large roll in the natural control of cancer cells.

THE INFLAMMATORY RESPONSE

Inflammation is a very nonspecific protective response to a wide variety of noxious stimuli, including infectious agents. Inflammation also can be a response to mechanical, thermal, or chemical trauma. Overreaction of the inflammatory response may be a large component of allergic, hypersensitivity, and autoimmune conditions. Specific types of responses depend on the stimulus.

The complement system may be triggered by **C-reactive proteins** in response to specific infectious agents or antigen-antibody complexes. This trigger may come from the acquired (or memory-mediated) immune system and will result in inflammation in the area "requested." Explanations of the complement and acquired immune system follow.

Direct tissue injury releases the **kinin system,** a complex system of local smooth muscle, nerve, membrane, clotting, and tissue reactions that stimulate healing, inflammation, and perceptions of pain. The trigger is activation of **Hageman factor,** or factor VII, of the clotting cascade.

Cytokines are released by activated tissue macrophages and **monokines** by monocytes. Cytokines can induce coagulation, stimulate other phagocytes and leukocytes to enter the area and bind to vascular endothelial cells, and increase vascular permeability. Macrophages enter the area a few hours later to destroy antigens and help defend the area.

The study of these complex biochemical and tissue reactions has helped to explain the historical and physical findings of inflammation, which are

pain	*dolor*
heat	*calor*
redness	*rubor*
swelling	*tumor*
and loss of function	

The inflammation system may be overly efficient. In many cases, inflammation remains in a tissue or joint much longer than seemingly necessary, and inflammation becomes the chief complaint. The standard treatments (i.e., ice, elevation, and nonsteroidal or even steroidal anti-inflammatory medications) offer some symptomatic relief, but there is little evidence that they modify or improve the body's reaction.

THE FEBRILE RESPONSE

Fever generally is associated with the presence of and reaction to infectious agents, although some drug reactions (e.g., neuroleptic malignant syndrome), hot environmental conditions, or overexertion also may cause fever. The thermostat for controlling body temperature is located in the anterior hypothalamus. This mechanism is driven by endocrine and metabolic controls, the selective control of blood flow to tissues, and sweating or shivering.

The cause of fever in the face of an infectious agent is the cytokines produced by macrophages, the same process that initiates local inflammatory response. Several cytokines have been found to cause febrile responses: IL-1, macrophage inflammatory protein 1 (MIP-1), and TNF. These same cytokines have other roles, such as improving the efficiency of T-lymphocytes, stimulating fibrinogen, and increasing normal erythrocytes aggregation (the reason for elevated sedimentation rates in persons with fever).

Animal studies have shown that antibody production and T-cell proliferation are more efficient at higher body temperatures than at normal body temperature and may be the natural reason for fever. Known harmful effects of prolonged high fever however include cerebral cortex damage, stress on the heart and great vessels, and negative nitrogen balance. However, the suppression of fever by medication (e.g., aspirin or acetaminophen) has not been shown to diminish favorable outcome of infections. These drugs do alleviate symptoms and make febrile patients more comfortable, however.

ACQUIRED (ADAPTIVE OR SPECIFIC) IMMUNITY

Acquired, or adaptive, immunity is that acquired after exposure to a specific antigen of an infectious agent. The average adult may have acquired immunity for as many as 10^6 to 10^8 antigens. If all this immunity were innate, the human would need about 50 sets of chromosomes instead of the bequeathed 23.

Acquired immunity is mediated by either lymphoid tissues or specific antibodies. Acquired immunity can be either active or passive. **Passive immunity** is tantamount to "borrowing" the antibodies of another human for a temporary period.

Maternal antibodies are passive immunity but are not discussed in this chapter. **Passive immunotherapy** is the administration of human blood products after exposure to a specific infectious agent or toxin. It may be thought of as an available "antidote" or "antitoxin." Passive immunization is discussed in Chapter 5. The remainder of this chapter discusses **active immunity**, the "immunization" that is acquired from the natural exposure to one of the Earth's thousands of infectious agents.

Role of the Lymphatic System

Most of the immune system's assets are derived from **stem cells,** multipurpose precursor cells derived from the bone marrow [9]. These cells are the first stage of all circulating blood cells. **Erythroid cells** develop into red blood cells, **myeloid** into granulocytes, and **lymphoid** into the lymphocytes.

Some of the lymphoid cells are now known to develop in the fetal liver before migrating to the bone marrow. These cells were originally called *bursal cells* because they were found to originate from bursae in birds. The human **B cells** are now known to function from bone marrow, a **primary lymphoid organ** (which conveniently starts with a *B*). They are the antibody-producing cells that mediate our **humoral immunity** (or *B* for blood). They are transported by the blood to **secondary lymphoid organs,** where they remain.

Some of the lymphoid cells migrate into the thymus gland and mature into **T-lymphocytes** (*T* for thymus). The thymus is a gland in the upper thorax (also a *T*) that atrophies after puberty. It is also a primary lymphoepithelial organ. After migrating to the thymus gland, T-lymphocytes then move to secondary lymphoid organs, where they are stored indefinitely.

The secondary lymphoid organs are the spleen, lymph nodes, appendix, tonsils, some small patches in the small bowel (**Peyer's patches**), and very small patches in other mucous membranes. The lymphatic system is both an anatomic and physiologic entity that is not discussed in detail in this text. These glands and nodes have complex anatomies and physiologies because they maintain the red and white blood cells and foreign antigens and filter them from the blood. Lymphocytes are strategically located along lymphatic vessels.

Humoral Immunity

It is in these secondary lymphoid organs that B-lymphocytes respond to specific antigens by making specific antibodies. For the purpose of this text, antigens are infectious agents but also may be other "foreign" or nonhost antigens such as toxins, cancerous cells, transplanted tissues or organs, and free allergens.

The B-cell lymphocytes secrete soluble antibodies into both vascular and extravascular body fluids, which is defined as **humoral immunity.** They work only on extracellular antigens and cannot attack intracellular antigens (in **target cells**). Each lymphocyte is programmed for a specific antibody. When a B cell encounters its triggering antigen, it gives rise to many large cells known as **plasma cells.** The plasma cells then manufacture specific antibodies for circulation in the bloodstream.

Each antibody is an **immunoglobulin,** a protein with a globular structure and a specific immune function. Antibodies fall into one of several structural and functional classes (Ig "X"). Each immunoglobulin has a basic structure of four polypeptide chains and two identical heavy (**H**) chains and two identical (**L**) chains. There are some fundamental differences and some consistent similarities between the immunoglobulins of different species that can be used in some laboratory studies. The immunoglobulin classes (isotopes) are named after the heavy chain.

IgA Immunoglobulin Antibodies. These are the major antibodies of external secretions and concentrates in body fluids, tears, saliva, and secretions of the respiratory, digestive, and genitourinary tract. They establish the guarding, or "surface," immunity at the port-of-entry sites of infectious agents. They are also the major immunoglobulin of mothers' milk and may help to protect and establish the proper gastrointestinal flora in infants. Quantitatively, they are the largest class of human antibodies. Some oral active vaccines stimulate IgA immunity (e.g., typhoid, oral polio, and rotavirus vaccines).

IgG Immunoglobulin Antibodies. These are the major antibodies of the "internal" body fluids (e.g., blood, lymph, CSF, and peritoneal fluid). They coat the infectious agents once they are recognized and stimulate their uptake and actions by other parts of the immune system. They provide the more long-term immunity, and their presence in laboratory studies usually can be interpreted as past exposure. They are the only antibodies that pass through the placenta and are responsible for all passive immunity.

IgM Immunoglobulin Antibodies. These are directly effective in killing bacterial cells and are manufactured acutely in response to new infectious agent antigens. Their presence in laboratory studies usually can be interpreted as recent exposure. They are the largest of the antibodies and do not cross the placenta or blood-brain barrier. Children may be more susceptible to gram-negative infections because of their lower levels of IgM.

IgE Immunoglobulin Antibodies. These provide incomplete protection against parasites but also are responsible for most of the symptoms of allergic reactions owing to their ability to degranulate mast cells. They have the smallest concentration but the most dramatic actions.

IgD Immunoglobulin Antibodies. These are found on antigen receptors in the more mature B cells of the gut and respiratory system. Their true function is less understood.

Cellular Immunity

It is the T-lymphocytes that control **cell-mediated immunity,** the immunity that combats intracellular antigens. It may be the more recently evolved part of the immune system. Humoral immunity and antibodies can function only outside cells. Like B cells, T cells have receptors for antigens. However, they do not produce antibodies but rather secrete **cytokines,** specifically **lymphokines.** These agents can

- Bind to target cells.
- Stimulate and mobilize other immune system cells or "direct traffic" for the
  - Destruction of target cells.
  - Arousal of **phagocytes** (monocytes and macrophage).

Immature T-lymphocytes can develop into one of two types of mature lymphocytes. They can become mature **helper T-lymphocytes** (with CD4 receptors), which regulate cellular immune response. It is this binding site that is vulnerable to the HIV virus, and these lymphocytes that are destroyed during the latent period of HIV infection. The other T cells are the **cytotoxic T-lymphocytes** (with CD8 receptors), programmed to destroy **target cells** that are infected (or cancerous).

The Complement System

The complement system is an important part of both the humoral immune response and inflammatory reactions. It is a system of at least 20 circulating or membrane proteins that work to "complement" the actions of antibodies. It also helps to clear the body of antibody-coated antigens (**antigen-antibody complexes**). Complement is responsible primarily for the inflammatory response previously described.

Activation of the first protein by an antibody-antigen complex starts a cascade of activation of the C1–C9 proteins in the **classical complement pathway.** Components C3 or beyond trigger the release of physiologically active substances at the site of the reaction. This results is a cylindrical complex's insertion into the cell wall and eventual destruction of the target cell. Some of the proteins of the cascade (e.g., C4a, C3a, and C5a) may stimulate anaphylaxis (**anaphylatoxins**), which induces tissue mast cells and serum basophils to degranulate and release histamine. Histamine increases capillary permeability and the smooth muscle contraction responsible for anaphylactic allergic reactions, vascular dilatation, and damage to the endothelium caused by neutrophil adhesion. Complement also can cause **opsonization,** preparation of the microbe to be phagocytized by macrophages.

The **alternative complement pathway** is a more primitive (evolutionarily older) system that is activated by the LPSs (lipopolysaccharides of the bacterial cell wall) of endotoxin. The cells of some yeast also trigger the alternative pathway, as can some venoms from poisonous reptiles. The alternative pathway begins at C3 but may work with the classical pathway to amplify both the antibody-dependent and antibody-independent activity starting at C3.

Components of the complement systems are manufactured by liver hepatocytes, epithelial cells of the gastrointestinal tract, blood monocytes, and tissue macrophages. Components are encoded on at least eight chromosomes (1, 4, 6, 9, 11, 12, 19, and X). Genetic defects have been found for most of the components of the complement system. Individuals with a heterozygous defect of a single allele have half as much of that component and may be susceptible to some infections. Homozygous defects in the complement system are very rare. Specific genetic defects in one or more of the complement proteins may be responsible for individual susceptibility to specific infections. The complement system also may have played a role in genetic selection and evolution in the face of epidemics. At least one deficit (C3) seems responsible for vulnerability to *Neisseria* species. Meningococcal infections (*N. meningitides*) can become "invasive" or septic in a small percentage of the population, whereas most individuals develop inapparent infection and immunity or asymptomatic colonization (see Chapter 23). Overactivity of some components are believed to be contributory to some autoimmune diseases such as systemic lupus erythematosis.

ABNORMALITIES OF IMMUNITY
Allergy

Allergic or **hypersensitivity reactions** are also mediated by the immune system and are defined as an exaggerated or overreactive response to a seemingly harmless antigen (renamed an **allergen**). They are divided into four classes by the Gell-Coombs system:

- *Type I:* The **sensitization phase** is the production of specific IgE to an allergen, which binds to the basophils or mast cells (**sensitized**). They are triggered to degranulate on reexposure to the antigen (**activation phase**). They release histamine, leukotrienes, heparin, and substances that activate other leukocytes. In the **effector phase,** these substances can produce an **anaphylactic reaction,** with an influx of eosinophils, increases in vascular permeability, and constriction of smooth muscles. Local cutaneous reactions at the site of the allergen can cause reactions within minutes (**wheal and flare**). If the allergen is systemically distributed, a life-threatening **systemic anaphylaxis** can occur. This type of immunity likely has its origins in providing protection from parasites.
- *Type II:* When a specific IgM or IgG antibody binds to a cellular surface allergen (target cell), it may trigger an activation of the complement cascade and result in cellular destruction. This is the **cytotoxic reaction.** These reactions may be seen with blood transfusion ABO group

incompatibility, Rh factor incompatibility, and drug reactions. Drugs that cause agranulocytosis or hemolytic anemia are usually phagocytic or cytotoxic (type II) reactions. Many autoimmune diseases may be chronic cytotoxic reactions.

- *Type III:* These are the **immune-complex reactions**, a triggering of the complement cascade with antigen-antibody (allergen-antibody) complexes. Granulocytes are attracted to the local area and degranulate, causing lytic reactions within a few hours. Local reactions historically have been called the *Arthus reaction* and may be the pathogenesis of some venom reactions. Systemic reactions have been called *serum sickness.* Type III pulmonary reactions are responsible for many occupational pulmonary diseases.
- *Type IV:* These reactions are mediated by the T-lymphocytes, not antibodies. Type IV reaction has been called *delayed-type hypersensitivity* or *cell-mediated immunity.* It also has been called the *tuberculin reaction* because it is responsible for purified protein derivative (PPD) and other positive skin tests showing local induration or redness. The allergen-activated T-lymphocytes release cytokines. Cytokines attract monocyte and macrophages, which are not specific for this allergen. Type IV reactions are delayed 24–48 hours. **Contact sensitivity** is a form of delayed hypersensitivity in which the target cells and organ is the skin. Naturally occurring oils (such as the urushiol of poison ivy) or industrial oils can penetrate skin because of their lipophilic properties.

Autoimmunity

For reasons that are poorly understood, the immune system may malfunction and develop immune reactions to its own tissues. Antibodies become **autoantibodies.** Autoantibodies have been implicated as the cause of hemolytic anemias, Graves' disease, and myasthenia gravis. Dozens of other conditions are suspected of being autoimmune. Suspected T-cell-mediated autoimmune diseases include type I diabetes mellitus, Hashimoto's thyroiditis, and multiple sclerosis.

Most of these diseases have **multifactorial** causes, combinations of multiple genetic (**polygenic**) factors and environmental conditions. Environmental conditions may include exposure to infectious agents or occupational risks, although definitive causation is lacking.

Immune-Complex Diseases

Immune complexes (antigen-antibody complexes) from infections may fail to be cleared at times and may be due to abnormalities in complement receptors. Complexes become trapped and cause direct damage to the kidney (e.g., poststreptococcal glomerulonephritis), the liver (e.g., viral hepatitis), skin, joints, or blood vessels.

Immunodeficiency

The **primary immune deficiency disorders** are those that are hereditary or develop as primary diseases. Much of what we know of the normal immune system comes from studying the illnesses and infections of those with specific deficits. These disorders are rare—on the order of 1:10,000 persons. Their approximate prevalences by percentage are listed in Table 3-23.

The B-cell disorders are called *hypogammaglobulinemias,* but excess disorders (**monoclonal gammopathies**) and B-cell cancers also occur. Those with T-cell deficits also may develop malignancies. Excesses in the complement system also can occur if one of the inhibitor enzymes is absent. The absence of C1 esterase is one cause of persistent angioneurotic edema.

Secondary immune deficiency disorders are much more common and are the result of malignancies of leukocytes (leukemias) owing to medical chemotherapy or deliberate immunosuppression such as that performed with transplantation. The immune system also may fail in the face of overwhelming bacterial infections and sepsis, which usually results in death.

Table 3-23
Primary Immune Deficiency Disorders, by Percent

Disorder	Percent (%)
B-cell antibody mediated	50
Both B- and T-cell mediated	20
Phagocytes and/or killer cells	18
T-cell mediated	10
Complement cascade	2

The Environment and Reservoirs of Infectious Agents

THE ENVIRONMENT

There will always be infectious agents in the environment, and for most diseases, there will remain susceptible hosts. The triangle is complete only when the human host is invaded through a **portal of entry**. For human-to-human diseases transmitted directly or indirectly through the environment, the **portal of exit** is just as important in the life cycle and survival of the agent. The portal of exit of an infectious agent from its host is its portal of entry into the environment, the port of exit from the environment is its portal of entry to the host.

For many agents, the human is not the natural host and is infected by "accident." This is especially true for workers who, in the course of their duties, interrupt the environment and the triangle of other natural cycles. Diseases that occur by "accident" include anthrax, brucellosis, leptospirosis, Q fever, plague, Rocky Mountain spotted fever, salmonella, tularemia, and dozens of others. Workers may use technology to enter new environments or environmental conditions and thus be exposed to new biohazard challenges to human host defenses. Workers also may, in the course their duties, travel to foreign environments and be exposed to infectious agents to which they are susceptible.

Exposure to the Environment

The width and breadth of one's exposure to infectious agents are positively related to the width and breadth of one's exposure to the environment and to their behavior patterns in that environment (Figure 3-10). Risk can be reduced by an awareness of the environmental hazards and the use of vaccination, chemoprophylaxis, personal protective equipment, engineering, and education on safe behavior. Each is discussed in the other chapters of this text.

The relative number and the danger of infectious agents in our environment are increasing for several reasons:

1. As the last wilderness areas of the Earth are invaded by working humans using technology in the search for resources, we may be unearthing the reservoir of some virulent infectious agents for which we have not evolved innate resistance or other defense mechanisms. This may be the case for the hantavirus, HIV, and Ebola virus.
2. New forms of infectious agents, such as the drug-resistant strains of bacteria found in hospitals, may arise from our technology. Legionellosis may be a disease that has arisen from our heating, cooling, and air-conditioning technology. Natural human *Legionella* infection from the disturbance of natural or non-manmade environments has yet to be proved.
3. Because of the increasing prevalence of immunosuppressed persons in our society, dozens of bacteria, virus, fungi, and parasite species once considered to be harmless have been added to the list of pathogens. A dozen of these agents were included in the 1987 CDC definition of the AIDS diagnosis (**"AIDS-Predicting Illness"** [26], later called "AIDS-Defining Illnesses").

Infectivity from the Environmental Reservoir

For an infectious agent to cause human infection from the environment or reservoir, it must

1. Be stable and resistant to the physical factors and stressors of that environment. The more it can adapt to changes in its environment, the wider its range and longer it may survive.
2. Have a port of entry into the human host.
3. Exist and enter in sufficient quantity to cause infection (the **infective dose**).
4. Have a means of reproduction to replace the natural death or loss of viability of infectious agents in the environment or the host.

Ecology of Microbes in the Environment

The total number of microorganisms in the biosphere is nearly constant. Knowledge of the growth patterns, nutritional needs, and optimal environmental conditions for various infectious agents comes from observational studies of their growth in the laboratory. The growth patterns of bacteria and some fungi in specific substrates is a principal means of identifying them in the clinical microbiology laboratory. The growth equations, curves, and mathematical models of microbial growth on media in the laboratory are of little use in the study of disease in the host or their persistence in the environment.

The interrelationships between the bacteria, fungi, and viruses in the natural environment are still poorly understood. Attempts to make objects sterile or to alter their flora patterns in the natural environment by and large have failed. Any manufactured void of microbial life is filled eventually by another microbe, and even later, the original "extinct" microbe may return to the original balance of flora.

Viruses are inert in the extracellular environment. They may survive and remain infective for short periods, but they do not reproduce. Viruses are known to infect all higher life forms, even down to single-cell mycoplasmas, bacteria, and algae. Neither the origins of viruses nor their true function in nature are known. But because of their reaction of pilfering and plundering genetic material, they may be a major component of Darwinian evolution. Besides sabotaging and, in rarer cases, "improving" the genome of various species, viruses may cause human epidemics that reduce the population but "improve" the human genome through the survivors. It is known that as many as 5% of persons living with the HIV infection do not seem to progress to clinical disease (AIDS) and are often called *nonprogressors*. These individuals may be infected with a less virulent strain, or it is possible that they possess some genetic advantage inherited from ancestors that survived a similar virus.

THE RESERVOIRS

Both Heymann [10] and Last [2] give the same definition for a *reservoir* of infectious agents: "Any person, animal, arthropod, plant, soil, or substance (or combination of these) in which an infectious agent normally lives and multiplies, on which it depends primarily for survival, and where it reproduces itself in such a manner that it can be transmitted to a susceptible host." Last adds, "the natural habitat of the infectious agent."

The known natural prevalence of a potentially infectious agent in a reservoir is called **endemicity.** For occupational and environmental health professionals, this should be considered a "risk." The presence of a potentially infectious agent in the reservoir should be approached no differently than the kinetic injury of a punch press, the carcinogenic property of vinyl chloride gas, or the consequences of a maturing cataract in the eye of an airline pilot. One must assess the risks of the environment

(reservoir) and take appropriate preventive action. Evaluating and estimating which potentially infectious agents have reservoirs or infective forms in the work environment should be a routine part of any job risk evaluation. Even the physical proximity of workers to one another may help to predict the incidence and prevalence of upper respiratory infection (see Chapters 11 and 14).

All human infectious agents are derived from at least one of three reservoirs: humans, other living creatures, or the environment (see Figure 3-10).

The Human Host as the Reservoir

Many infectious agents are exclusively human and have little or no survivability outside the human host (Table 3-24). For these agents, the environment is removed from the equation. The human body *is* the environment, and the agent persists only as long as a single human is infected and infectious and another human remains susceptible. The agent may travel through a life cycle from human host to human host with no carrier, colonization, or dormant state. Such an agent would require very efficient routes of entry and exit and adequate infectivity to "leapfrog" from one susceptible human to another (e.g., measles, mumps, and rubella). The infected human's portal of exit is the susceptible human's portal of entry. Most of the

Figure 3-10
Only a small portion of all potentially infectious agents are pathogenic to humans. These agents may be of inanimate, invertebrate, vertebrate, or human origin.

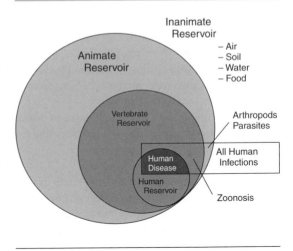

Table 3-24
Human-Specific Infectious Agents (No Significant Animal or Environmental Reservoir)

Disease	Agent	Transmission	Vac[a]	Erad[b]	Problems
AIDS/HIV	Virus	Parenteral	No	No	Long latency
		Sexual			Unstable antigen
					Attacks immune system
Actinomycosis	Bacteria	Oral	No	No	Endogenous flora
Candidiasis	Fungus	Oral	No	No	Endogenous flora
Chancroid	Bacteria	Sexual	No	No	Tracing contacts difficult
Coxsackievirus	Virus	Sexual	No	No	Many forms, difficult diagnosis
		Oral/MM[c]			
Cytomegalovirus	Virus	Oral/MM[c]	No	No	Lifelong latency
					Reactivation?
Diphtheria	Bacteria	Direct	Yes	Yes	Adult immunity decay
Epstein-Barr virus	Virus	Direct/MM	No	No	Many chronic carriers
Genital chlamydia	Chlamydia	Sexual	No	No	Male carriage/high inapparent illness rate
Gonorrhea	Bacteria	Sexual	No	No	High inapparent illness rate
Granuloma inguinal	Bacteria	Sexual	No	No	Rare in U.S.
Haemophilus influenzae B	Bacteria	Droplet/MM[c]	Yes	Yes	Variation in host response
Helicobacter pylori	Bacteria	Direct?	No	No	Unknown mode of transmission
Hepatitis B	Virus	Sexual	Yes	Yes	Chronic carriers
		Parenteral			
Hepatitis C	Virus	Parenteral	No	No	High prevalence
					High inapparent illness rate
Herpes simplex	Virus	Direct/MM[c]	No	No	High prevalence
		Sexual	No	No	Exacerbations
Influenza	Virus	Airborne	Yes	No	Many antigenic forms
		Direct/MM[c]			Highly prevalent
					Global circulation
Lymphogranuloma venereum	Chlamydia	Sexual	No	No	High inapparent illness rate, especially in females
					Long latency and incubation
Measles	Virus	Airborne	Yes	Possible	Highly contagious
Mumps	Virus	Droplet/MM[c]	Yes	Yes	Unimmunized children
Mycoplasma	Bacterilike	Droplet/MM[c]	No	No	High inapparent illness rate
Neisseria meningitides	Bacteria	Direct/MM[c]	Yes	No	High inapparent illness rate, floral
Pertussis	Bacteria	Droplet/MM[c]	Yes	Yes	Fail immunity as adults
Parvovirus-19 (Fifth's disease)	Virus	Direct	No	No	High inapparent illness rate
Rhinitis	Virus	Airborne	No	No	Many serovars
		Direct/MM[c]			
Rubella	Virus	Airborne	Yes	Yes	One serovar!!
Streptococcus pneumoniae	Bacteria	Droplet/MM[c]	Yes	No	Many carriers, high inapparent illness rate
Smallpox	Virus	Airborne	Yes	GONE!	Security of culture stock and global populace susceptibility
Varicella	Virus	Droplet	Yes	No	Lifelong latency
		Contact			
		Oral/MM[c]			

[a]Vaccine available?
[b]Potential for eradication within a generation?
[c]Mucous membrane contact or secretions.

sexually transmitted diseases (STDs) are human-specific (e.g., HIV, herpes simplex, syphilis, gonorrhea, genital chlamydia, and trichomoniasis). Some infectious agents may change their antigenic properties frequently and therefore make the previously infected susceptible again (e.g., influenza).

The agent may be able to establish a long latent period of communicability and even inapparent infection (e.g., HIV, HCV, and HBV). The agent may be able to establish lifelong infections with infectivity only during periods of exacerbations (e.g., varicella, herpes simplex, EBV, and cytomegalovirus). The agent may be able to colonize the healthy person and cause infections only under certain conditions such as trauma or immunosuppression (e.g., actinomycosis, *C. albicans* infection, *M. tuberculosis* infection, and vancomycin-resistant *Enterococcus*).

The colonization of human organs or surfaces and all types of human carriers (healthy or asymptomatic, incubatory or convalescent, temporary or transient, and active or chronic) should be considered reservoirs that represent risk to susceptible humans.

The Animate Reservoir

Insects (arthropods) or animals may serve as a reservoir for about half the known human pathogenic infectious agents of significance. Humans, animals, and arthropod hosts may inject, excrete, exhale, defecate, or slough infectious agents into the environment that are capable of infecting others. This process also may be called *shedding*. The environment also may be contaminated by infectious agents remaining in the body of dead plants and animals.

Diseases spread by vertebrate animal hosts to humans are called *zoonoses*. Vertebrate animal vectors can be wild, livestock, or pets. Workers who handle any of these classes of vertebrates (live or dead) should take the appropriate methods of protections and prevention (see Chapters 4 and 36).

Many human infectious diseases occur in predictable seasonal patterns (e.g., arbovirus encephalitis in warmer months and upper respiratory tract viruses in cold months). Seasonal patterns suggest that the source of infection is related to the seasonal life cycles of plants or animals, seasonal environmental conditions, or seasonal human recreational or occupational behaviors that increase exposure. The reservoir remains unknown

for only a few infectious agents (e.g., Ebola virus and Kawasaki agent).

The arboviruses were named for their association with arthropods (i.e., mosquitoes, mites, ticks, and flies). By definition, arboviruses propagate in arthropods. Arthropods are infected by biting infected vertebrates (especially small mammals and birds) during a period of viremia. Horses were once considered to be the reservoir for some of the encephalitis viral diseases found in the United States, and thus the disease was named *equine*. Horses, as well as humans, may be affected, but they are not the reservoir. Nor are the living arthropods the true reservoir because most live only part of the year. They may pass the infection to their offspring vertically or through the **transovarian route.** The virus also may live through the winter in birds or small mammals, a reservoir method known as **overwintering.**

The reservoir of the seasonal respiratory viruses also has been a mystery as to where they reside during the "off-season." For influenza, it is believed that the opposite hemisphere serves as the reservoir because mutating influenza strains constantly circle the Earth. Animals are suspected reservoirs for several diseases. The section entitled "Swine Flu" in Chapter 11B describes the dramatic 80-year-long suspicion and investigation of a possible dormant domestic animal reservoir for the agent responsible for the twentieth century's most deadly epidemic.

The Inanimate Reservoir

The presence of infectious agents in or on inanimate objects in the environment is termed *contamination*. It differs from **pollution**, the presence of noxious or toxic chemical or noninfectious agents in or on inanimate objects of the environment. Inanimate reservoirs include food and water (the human substrates). Essentially all food and water contains bacteria and fungus or their spores and may contain some viruses and parasites as well. The oral and gastrointestinal host defenses have been discussed previously. Some organisms are capable of actual multiplication within the environment of soil, plants, food, and milk. An organism will grow in the presence of the proper and sufficient nutrients and substrates. Climatic conditions also affect the relative balance of microorganisms in the biosphere and may be influenced by global climate change.

Physical Factors in the Inanimate Reservoir.
TEMPERATURE AND SEASONS. The law of Brownian
motion states that molecular motion increases with
temperature and slows with cooling. Living creatures are much the same, becoming more active in
warmer weather. Most infectious agents of concern
to humans are **mesophilic,** or survive best at or just
below human body temperatures. **Thermophilic**
("heat loving") or **psychrophilic** ("cold loving")
agents are less frequently pathogenic. Human behavioral patterns change with the temperature.
Recreational activity in warmer climates increases
the risk of exposure to pathogens from swimming
in natural bodies of water and sewage, the risk of
skin wounds and infection, and the bites of arthropod vectors.

In colder climates, humans tend to gather inside
and thus share seasonal increases in the communicable respiratory infections (see Chapters 11B, 13,
and 14). Many animals and insects that serve as
hosts have life cycles that depend on the seasons
and cause human seasonal epidemics of diseases
(e.g., viral encephalitis from mosquito-borne arboviruses). Occupational infectious diseases contracted from crops peak with harvesting (e.g.,
sporotrichosis), and diseases contracted from domestic livestock occur in seasonal slaughters or
shearing (e.g., Orf with the shearing of sheep).

HUMIDITY, WATER, AND FLOODING. Periods of
draught, high humidity, or flood can change the
growth pattern of bacteria and especially fungi. *El
Niño* is an episodic variance of weather in which
warm winds blow easterly rather than the usual
westerly direction across the Pacific. Although dis-
puted among climatologists, it may be responsible
for widening the extremes of weather patterns,
which could affect natural disease patterns through
the changes in humidity and as a consequence of
weather-related disasters.

The lack of moisture in an environment is a
powerful stimulus for some microorganisms to initiate species-preservation defenses. Many fungi
make spores or conidia, which can survive desiccation in the soil yet remain viable and virulent.
Other spore-forming organisms and diseases are
the clostridia (e.g., botulism, tetanus, gas gangrene,
and pseudomembranous colitis) and bacilli (e.g.,
anthrax and food poisoning). Bacterial endospores
are the most resistant of all living entities, requiring
sterilization of surgical instruments and the boiling

and/or canning of preserved foods. Endospores for
C. tetani have survived in a viable state in soil for 2
years, and those for *C. perfringens* have survived in
frozen meat for 1 year. Drought also may increase
the amount of dust in the air and serve as a vehicle
for infection. Starvation from drought may lower
host immunity and defenses and stimulate the occurrence of an epidemic.

Flooding is the natural disaster with the greatest
impact on infectious diseases. Sanitation systems
fail when clean water mixes with contaminated
sewage water in reservoirs and wells. Food stocks,
crops, and building structures also may be contaminated with dozens of infectious agents transmitted
by the fecal-oral route. In addition, fungi thrive on
the wet wood and environmental surfaces of homes
and other structures. Cleanup procedures should
adhere to the latest flood disaster guidelines for decontamination, disinfection, and disease prophylaxis [29]. The recent Indonesian tsunami and
hurricane Katrina disasters have greatly expanded
knowledge in disease reduction.

LIGHT AND RADIATION. Bacteria have varying
degrees of sensitivity to ultraviolet (UV) radiation
and direct sunlight. But the spores of the bacilli and
clostridia are highly resistant to light and drying.
UV radiation is defined as that part of the electromagnetic spectrum of wavelengths from 100–400
nm (UV-A is 320–400 nm, UV-B is 290–320 nm,
and UV-C is 100–290 nm). Commercial units ad-
mitting a wavelength of 253.7 nm have been used to
control *M. tuberculosis* in the venting or upper
room air of health care facilities. Tubercles have remained viable in sputum for 6–8 months if kept in
a cool, dry location. Relative humidity has been
noted to have an adverse effect on UV germicidal
irradiation [30].

UV radiation, x-rays, and high-energy particles
all can inactivate viruses. Lethal dosage varies by
the type of virus. Infectivity is the most radiosensi-
tive property of viruses because their entire genetic
content is needed for their successful replication.
Damage to any part of the genome prevents replication, although some pathogenicity still may be
expressed in the host cell.

GEOLOGIC BOUNDARIES (AND TRAVEL). Natural
habitats are separated by natural geologic boundaries of oceans, rivers, or mountain ranges. Plants,
animals, and infectious agents have adapted to local
conditions and may not be able to survive outside a

geographic location or to cross a natural boundary. This is best exemplified by the hundreds of species of arbovirus, each confined to a specific reservoir area by the geologic requirements of their arthropod host. Island isolation may protect a population from a disease (e.g., rabies is eradicated in Scandinavia) but could make it vulnerable to disease for which it has no acquired immunity. If an infectious agent is taken out of its natural habitat, it may find a sustaining reservoir devoid of natural enemies. Even humans seem to have some geographic and ethnic differences in disease susceptibility. For instance, some native Africans seem to have a natural resistance to some forms of malaria indigenous to their native area. The geographic high prevalence of this genetic trait may be a result of the natural selection of this population to survive in this malaria-endemic area. Again, global climate may change natural habitats and reservoirs.

The speed of modern air travel negates the natural boundaries. A traveler can spread an infectious agent across the globe in a matter of hours—well less than the incubation period for most infectious diseases. The worker who is to travel to a foreign area requires both an assessment of the local reservoirs and his or her own susceptibility. Likewise, a traveler may become an index case to a native population with no acquired immunity. The usual childhood diseases of the European conquerors may have triggered high mortality epidemics in the adults of Native American tribes in North America. The principles of travel medicine are covered elsewhere in this text.

Divisions of the Inanimate Reservoir. SOIL (AND DUST) RESERVOIRS. The soil is the largest and most important inanimate infectious agent reservoir (for **geophilic species**) and the most important inanimate source of occupational infections. The soil reservoir is dynamic. It seeds infectious agents into the air through dust or digging and into the bodies of water (including groundwater) by rain and gravity. It constantly receives agents falling from the atmosphere from gravity or precipitation, from overflowing bodies of water, and from the excretory system of higher life forms. It also receives and processes the remains of dead plants and animals. But the soil is also nature's filtering agent for infectious disease, greatly reducing the contamination of water as it seeps from the surface to the more pure groundwater.

Tens of thousands of fungi and bacterial species perform the useful function of breaking down and recycling decaying organic matter. The term *saprophytes* was defined originally as "plants that live on decaying organic matter." However, because bacteria and fungi are no longer classified as plants, the term *saprobe* has been used for any microorganism living on decaying organic matter from the soil in the inanimate reservoir.

Many soil microorganisms have a useful purpose. Some bacteria species grow in the nodules of the roots of legume plants and perform **nitrogen fixation,** an anaerobic process performed below ground. This process converts nitrogen gas from the air into a usable form for plants and animals and is an essential function of the biosphere and food chain.

The soil (and water) also serves as the "toilet" for all creatures. Hundreds of infectious agents have adapted their life cycle to the "soil–gastrointestinal tract cycle" of higher organisms. The soil is a reservoir of infectious agents "hibernating" in soil substrates in various inactive spore or cyst forms, which lie in wait to be ingested or inhaled. Only a few examples are discussed in this chapter.

Gram-Positive Soil Pathogens. *Aerococcus* species (viridans) are soil saprobes found throughout the biosphere. These organisms are opportunistic in immunocompromised individuals if they are ingested or in healthy individuals with trauma. They live in both fresh water and saltwater and are responsible for a disease fatal to lobsters. In addition, they are airborne contaminants and are responsible for the greenish color that reliably forms on pickled or cooked meats (e.g., cold cut ham slices).

Nocardia species, which cause nocardiosis, are transmitted by the inhalation of contaminated dust and can cause abscesses of the brain or other organs. These are saprobes of decaying vegetation and pose a risk to farmers in Mexico and tropical parts of Africa and Asia.

Several gram-positive cocci (e.g., *Peptococcus* and *Peptostreptococcus*) found in normal oral flora can survive in the soil. Newborns may be colonized early. These organisms also can cause wound infections after soil-contaminated trauma. *S. aureus* is another gram-positive cocci that can cause food poisoning by the ingestion of an enterotoxin or wound infections from broken skin. *S. aureus* is a saprobe that can live in an animal carcass for 42 days or survive or grow in meat products for up to 60 days. The streptococcal species are not believed to cause infections from soil exposure, although some have been found to live in soil for weeks to months.

Bacillus Species. *Bacillus* species form spores that can remain viable in the soil for many years and also can contaminate from dust. *B. anthracis* causes anthrax or woolsorters' disease. Almost all domestic and grazing mammals can be infected with *B. anthracis* and contaminate the soil in populated or agricultural areas. Besides ingestion, the organism can infect by inhalation of contaminated dust or direct contamination of skin or wounds. It also may be spread mechanically by biting flies. Anthrax is among the most deadly diseases and could be used in biologic warfare or bioterrorism. The U.S. military began immunizing some troops for anthrax in 1998 and more after the 2001 anthrax attacks by mail.

B. cereus causes food poisoning by a toxin. Food is probably infected from floating spores landing on food kept at ambient temperature, but the organism also may contaminate crop foods such as rice directly. Spores may survive boiling up to 10 minutes.

Clostridia Species. Clostridia are colon bacteria that also form spores that can survive for long periods in the soil and require long boiling to inactivate in food. About 2–3% of humans are colonized with *C. difficile*, which can overgrow in antibiotic- or cancer chemotherapy–associated colitis. *C. difficile* is an important nosocomial pathogen transmitted via the fecal-oral route that can superinfect patients after antibiotic usage. *C. perfringens* is also found in the gastrointestinal tract of healthy persons and those of livestock, fish, or poultry. It can cause an enterotoxin poison in food contaminated by soil or feces or in inadequately cooked meat. Only 10 organisms per gram can be infective. Tetanus is caused by *C. tetani,* producer of a potent exotoxin. Spores are concentrated in animal feces and the soil in populated or agricultural areas.

Gram-Negative Soil Pathogens. Gram-negative bacteria are primarily responsible for the decomposition of plant products. Workers exposed to plant or vegetable products, especially in dry environments, are at risk for illness from the inhalation of endotoxins. Symptoms may include a dry cough,

tightness in the chest, headache, chills, malaise, and fever. Symptoms may peak a few hours after exposure (**Monday fever**), but chronic pulmonary damage and disease may occur with long-term exposure. Bacteremia does not seem to occur by inhalation. The effects may be due to a combination of toxicity and allergenicity to organic plant dusts. *Byssinosis,* or *brown lung,* is the name given to occupational cotton-dust reaction. This syndrome and the spectrum of illnesses attributable to endotoxin inhalation are yet to be well named, however. There is also the potential for endotoxin to be weaponized by terrorists.

Aeromonas hydrophilia is a gram-negative rod that survives in soil and in both fresh water and saltwater; it forms both spores and exotoxins and is a common pathogen found in both marine and freshwater animals and amphibians. In humans, *A. hydrophilia* can cause wound infections and many other organ infections and sepsis. The human incidence is increasing dramatically and is most often misdiagnosed as coliforms.

Yersinia enterocolitica produces a very heat-stable enterotoxin that causes an enteric lymphadenitis mimicking appendicitis. The organism is spread by fecal-oral contamination of food or water. It can survive in water for 20 days and in soil for up to 2 years. *Y. pestis* (plague) is a "forgotten" saprobe that can survive in a human body up to 9 months after death. A human carcass is probably not directly infectious to humans but may infect rodents and their arthropod vectors and thus sustain an epidemic.

Coxiella burnetii, the rickettsia that causes Q fever, has been shown to survive in dust up to 120 days. Viable organisms have been shown to travel a half-mile downwind from sites infected by domestic livestock. The rickettsiae are very resistant to physical inactivation and require biosafety level 3 (described later) when their cultures are handled.

Viral Soil Pathogens. Viruses rarely survive in dry environments and generally do not cause human infections through exposure to soil or dust. Some exceptions may be the rare hanta, machupo, and lymphocytic choriomeningitis viral infections from the very recent contamination of dust by rodent excreta.

Fungal Soil Pathogens. Many fungi are soil saprobes (or saprophytes) and live on plant vegetation, wood, and other organic matter in the soil for months to years. Most are not pathogenic to humans. Fungal spores also contaminate some types of wood and may be responsible for some of the extrinsic allergic alveolitis from sawdust (**aeroallergens**) that afflicts woodworkers. *Aspergillus* species (**farmers' lung**) are associated with the decay of grains, hay, and plant material. They are distributed throughout nature and are dangerous to immunosuppressed persons. Toxins from *Aspergillus* (aflatoxins) have been associated with primary hepatocellular cancer in Africa and Asia.

Coccidioides immitis is responsible for coccidioidomycosis (valley and desert fever), which is caused by its endospores found in the soil around rodent burrows in the southwestern United States and in Central and South America. Cryptococcosis occurs mainly in immunosuppressed individuals and is due to a yeast saprobe of pigeon droppings. The various **dermatophytoses** (skin infections) caused by fungi (e.g., *Epidermophyton*, *Microsporum*, or *Trichophyton* species) can remain infective for years in fomites contaminated with desquamated epithelium from humans or animals.

H. capsulatum (histoplasmosis) is a saprobic endemic mold found in soil around the world but most concentrated in the eastern and midwestern U.S. river valleys. Most people in these areas have positive skin tests confirming past exposure. *H. capsulatum* spores can remain viable for long periods in almost any soil but are most concentrated in soil contaminated by bird or bat excreta. This pathogen is discussed further in Chapter 13. *Sporothrix schenckii* is a soil saprobe that not only causes pulmonary disease (sporotrichosis) but also wound infections. High-risk professions include farmers and gardeners.

Parasitic Soil Pathogens. *Ascaris lumbricoides* (roundworm) eggs can remain viable in favorable soil conditions for many years. An infection that occurs only in humans, it is a pure example of the agent-host-environment model with a fecal-oral route of transmission and a soil reservoir. Symptoms also positively correlate with the volume of ingested eggs (**worm load**). The eggs of various tapeworms (i.e., *Echinococcus* or *Taenia*) species may survive for months in the soil under a wide range of temperatures and conditions. *Giardia lamblia* (giardiasis) is a protozoan with a cyst that can survive for long periods in food, water, or soil. It is transmitted by the fecal-oral route and has great resistance to chlorination

Leptospirosis, or swineherd's disease (*Leptospira interrogans*), is a generalized illness caused by a spirochete that contaminates the soil from the urine of a wide range of domestic, pet, and wild animals. It can remain infective in soil for weeks. A wide range of occupations, including farmers, pickers, veterinarians, miners, and laboratory workers who handle infected dogs or rodents, have been infected.

The incidence of toxocariasis (*Toxicari canis* and *T cati*) is increasing worldwide. The pathogen is a nematode with eggs that can live for months in the soil. It is transmitted by the fecal-oral route through contact with soil contaminated with pet dog or cat feces. It is the cause of visceral larva and ocular larva migrans. Toxoplasmosis (*T. gondii*) also can be transmitted by the fecal-oral route through contact with soil contaminated with cat feces.

WATER RESERVOIRS. Bacteria, fungi, and algae contaminate water and are active in the decay and recycling of organic mater. Fortunately, most of these organisms are inactivated by commercial water-treatment methods. However, protozoa and helminths also contaminate bodies of water and are harder to inactivate. Giardiasis and cryptosporidiosis have been responsible for some very large outbreaks in municipal water supplies. Some viruses are present in water even after treatment, including poliovirus and other enteroviruses.

Water is not homogeneous in temperature nor flora but exists in levels called *thermal stratifications*. Seasonal changes "turn over" strata and can change the microbial content at the surface. Bodies of water differ in their oxygen content. Methane is produced by bacteria at the lower levels of bodies of water with heavy organic contamination (**biologic oxygen demand**).

Drinking Water. In the United States, 90% of drinking water is from ground sources. But 36% of tap-water samples contain one or more bacterial contaminants that exceed the regulation limits. Treated drinking water should have about 0.4 ppm of available chlorine.

Bacteria are removed from water in drinking supplies by several methods. Chlorine combines with the nitrogen of ammonia to form chlorine compounds that have biocidal properties. Chlorination should occur after most of the organic sediment has been removed. The mixing of high levels of chlorine and hydrocarbons is suspected of making **chloramines,** which have germicidal but possible carcinogenic properties. In water treatment, anaerobic microbes may be killed by aeration and/or the use of ozone to oxidize the water. UV light and/or chlorine dioxide may be used in commercial water-treatment facilities.

WATER AND OTHER RESERVOIRS. Some of the waterborne infectious agents also infect soil and have been already discussed. These include gram-positive agents (e.g., *Aerococcus* and *C. difficile*) and gram-negative agents (e.g., *A. hydrophilia* in fresh water and saltwater, *Enterobacter* species, and *Y. enterocolitica*).

Gram-Positive Bacterial Waterborne Pathogens. Listeria monocytogenes is gram-positive bacillus with the rare ability to survive and actually grow in cold water near the freezing point. It also survives well in soil, water, mud, food, feces, and the tissue of many wild and domestic animals. It is opportunistic in the immunosuppressed, the very elderly, the very young, and pregnant women. It crosses the placenta and can cause serious neonatal infections or stillbirth. Up to 5% of humans are colon carriers. *Listeria* can be a serious threat after flooding. Few other waterborne infections are associated with gram-positive bacteria.

Gram-Negative Bacterial Waterborne Pathogens. Enterotoxigenic *E. coli* cause one form of **traveler's diarrhea,** a disease usually caused by ingestion of at least 100 million food-borne or waterborne organisms. It is more common in underdeveloped countries and more pathogenic to visitors exposed to the toxins for the first time.

L. pneumophila has its reservoir in water, including treated drinking water. It may survive for months in tap water and even distilled water. It is not infective by ingestion but from aerosol transmission with rapid drying of contaminated water in air-conditioning or evaporation units. It also may aerosolize from hot showers and cause nosocomial pneumonia. It requires a higher level of chlorination to control.

Typhoid fever is a human disease that can result from the ingestion of food or water contaminated with *S. typhi*. Besides fecal contamination, it also may infect through urine. A single chronic carrier may contaminate a water source or any food that he or she handles. The best known carrier was **"Typhoid Mary,"** a cook in New York City responsible for typhoid epidemics [31]. This moniker is used to describe any unknowing index case of any disease.

There are over 2,000 serotypes of other *Salmonella* species that cause millions of cases of foodborne or waterborne infections in the United States each year. Both animal and plant foods have been implicated in *Salmonella* infections, but most often infection is caused by contamination of poultry products. Pet reptiles, especially pet turtles, also have been implicated. Up to 5% of children and 1% of adults may excrete organisms for over a year, making direct human-to-human fecal-oral transmission possible.

Shigella species are also spread by food and water through fecal-oral transmission. Humans are the only significant host and may become ill from less than 200 organisms. *Shigella* remains viable in water for only a few days, so human carriers may be the more important reservoir. Also known as **bacillary dysentery,** the infection is endemic to some tropical areas and is another travel-related enteritis.

Cholerae causes the prototype human enteric disease associated with human feces-contaminated water. Cholera is disease 001 in all 10 ICD classifications, and *V. cholerae* has been responsible for many pandemics throughout history. Cholera has a 50% mortality if untreated but less than 1% if treated. Cholera is a frequent consequence of flood or war, most recently occurring in Iraq after the first Gulf War.

Viral Waterborne Pathogens. More and more viruses are being recognized as waterborne agents. Hepatitis A was among the first recognized and can survive in water and sewage for very long periods. *Rotavirus* is the world's leading cause of gastroenteritis in children and can survive for a month in water as cold as 4°C (40°F). Norwalk virus is a recently recognized class of waterborne pathogen that causes gastroenteritis. It can live in water supplies, but the reasons for outbreaks remain a mystery.

Coxsackieviruses cause a range of human conditions and are spread primarily by direct human-to-human contact, but the virus can be isolated and remain viable in stool specimens for several weeks.

It may have some waterborne spread. The echoviruses are enteric cytopathogens that can survive weeks in the environment; their transmission is believed to be directly by the fecal-oral route.

Fungal Food- and Waterborne Pathogens. Water and food are both contaminated with various forms of fungal species, but disease caused by their ingestion has not been described. Fungi seem very sensitive to digestive enzymes and gastric pH. *Candida* species can cause thrush, moniliasis, and lesions in the gastrointestinal organs in immunocompromised hosts. But *Candida* are part of the normal flora, and infection is probably endogenous in origin.

Parasitic Waterborne Pathogens. Some of these parasites were discussed in the section on soil parasites, including *Cryptosporidium*, the tapeworms, *Giardia, Leptospira*, and *Toxoplasma*.

Balantidium coli (balantidial dysentery) is a ciliated protozoa found in water contaminated by human or swine feces. It is relatively rare but has caused epidemics. *Entamoeba histolytica* causes a prototypical amoebic infection that occurs only in humans and often because of an asymptomatic **cyst-passer** index case. It has a fecal-oral mode of spread from food or water, and individual reinfection is rare. It causes another form of dysentery that may be associated with travel. *Naegleria fowleri* is an ameba that invades the brain and meninges through the nasal mucosa. It is associated with swimming in contaminated pools, hot tubs, or stagnant natural bodies of water.

One Asian trematode (*Fasciola hepatica*, or sheep liver fluke) is acquired by eating undercooked water plants contaminated by human, pig, or dog feces. But the most prevalent waterborne parasites are the *Schistosoma* trematodes (blood flukes). These trematodes directly penetrate the skin of humans who work or wade in water contaminated by animal excrement. They are found around the world in warmer climates and may infect hundreds of millions of humans while bathing or working. Some nonhuman species can penetrate the skin to cause **swimmer's itch,** although they do not mature further. In the United States, these have been found on beaches, including those of the Great Lakes. The skin irritation resulting from *Schistosoma* infection is often confused with **sea bather's itch,** caused by jellyfish larvae.

FOOD-BORNE INFECTIOUS AGENTS. Food poisoning is a general term that means contamination of food by any of the infectious agents or their toxins or by chemicals, metal, or radionucleotides.

Bacterial Food-Borne Infections. Bacteria with specific metabolic properties are used in food processing. Such processes include the production of butter, cheese, yogurt, buttermilk, pickles, sauerkraut, olives, wine, and beer. *Actinobactor* is used in the production of vinegar. *Lactobacillus* has been cultured from 100-year-old cheese and is an essential colonic flora bacteria. The bacteria of the gastrointestinal tract of humans and ruminants (i.e., cattle and sheep) can synthesize vitamin K and most of the B-complex vitamins.

Almost all human foods are also "enjoyed" by bacteria. Commercial food processing and packaging attempt to inhibit the growth of bacteria in food. Most bacterial food contaminants grow best near room temperature. Specific food controls are covered later.

Because of the lack of direct relevance to occupational infections, milk is not discussed. It is the best single food medium for infectious agents and is worthy of chapter status in most other textbooks on infectious disease.

Some food-borne infectious agents are discussed under soil or water, including *Aerococcus* species, *B. cereus, C. perfringens, Listerella, Salmonella, Shigella*, and *Y. enterocolitica*.

Gram-Positive Food-Borne Infections. *S. aureus* is an important organism in occupational medicine. Commercial food handlers with suspected staphylococcal wound infections of the upper body should be removed from the handling or preparation of open food until their wounds are treated or healed. Likewise, health care workers with noninfected open wounds of the hand(s) or arm(s) should be relieved from work in patient care areas. Methicillin-resistant *S. aureus* (MRSA) can infect and colonize health care workers. Other than the enterotoxin of *Staphylococcus*, gram-positive bacteria do not generally cause food-borne disease in healthy individuals with intact immune defenses.

Gram-Negative Food-Borne Infections. Immunosuppressed persons may become ill from *Citrobacter* species and develop severe diarrhea or septicemia. They also may become ill from various *Proteus* species (e.g., *P. mirabilis* or *P. vulgaris*) found in food. Hospital patients seem to be susceptible to *Proteus* urinary tract infections, bacteremia, or pneumonia after antimicrobial therapy. The oral reintroduction of a normal intestinal floral organism seems to present a risk of invasion of other organs in these patients.

E. coli, either the enterotoxigenic (ETEC) or the enterohemorrhagic (EHEC) form, can cause infection. The first causes a watery diarrhea, and the second causes a bloody diarrhea. Serotype O157:H7 is an ETEC that causes severe illness and is increasing in incidence.

Viral Food-Borne Infections. The Norwalk group of viruses has been linked to institutional epidemics in camps, schools, nursing homes, and even cruise ships. Contamination of raw shellfish and vegetables is the common mode of spread. While rotavirus seems to occur more in children, Norwalk virus is more common in adults. The disease caused by both has been called by a number of names, including *epidemic viral gastroenteritis.*

Fungal Food-Borne Infections. Mycotoxins are toxic metabolites of molds (fungi) that contaminate food. They may be produced by *Aspergillus, Fusarium,* and even *Penicillium* molds. The mycotoxins of most concern are the aflatoxins, the most powerful biologic carcinogens known. They may be found in grains, nuts, and some dairy products if cattle are fed mold-contaminated foods. Aflatoxins can form from the wet storage of seeds and grain. Storage of these is now under strict Food and Drug Administration (FDA) regulations.

Parasitic Food-Borne Infections. Most of the parasites that infect food were discussed previously under soil and water, including *Ascaris, C. parvum,* the *Echinococcus* tapeworms, *E. histolytica, F. hepatica, Giardia, Leptospira,* and the *Taenia* tapeworms.

Opisthorchis species are trematode liver flukes that encyst in fish and may cause human infection if fish is improperly cooked. Symptoms may include biliary tree inflammation and obstruction and cholangiocarcinoma. These species are endemic to some parts of Southeast Asia and eastern Europe and the former Soviet republics. The cysts may be killed by freezing and thawing of fish.

The *Trichinella* species are nematodes that cause trichinellosis (trichinosis), a disease acquired from the ingestion of the raw or undercooked flesh of pork or other mammals. Symptoms stem from massive invasion of muscle and can vary from inapparent to fatal if cardiac and neurologic complications develop. Eosinophilia is a consistent finding. Gamma radiation or 1 month of deep freezing may be necessary to kill the cysts. *Toxoplasma* (an obligate intracellular sporozoan) causes a similar disease acquired from cysts in undercooked pork, mutton, or beef. The definitive host is cats, but many other domestic animals may serve as intermediate hosts. It has a high association with immune suppression and is an AIDS-predicting disease [26] in the form of an associated encephalitis.

Other Food-Associated Infectious Agents. The agent for **scrapie** is the most recently discovered infectious organism. It has been called a *prion* and is a filterable self-replicating agent that may cause slowly progressive neurologic diseases. Scrapie may be contracted by the ingestion of infected animal tissues, although this has not been proved to occur in humans at the present time.

THE NOSOCOMIAL RESERVOIR. Hospital and health care facilities are worthy of a section heading equal to that of food, water, or soil. These facilities are "meeting places" for the most virulent, infective, and drug-resistant infectious agents shed from the most ill hosts into the environment or onto environmental surfaces and medical equipment and instruments, exposing the most susceptible of human people (the very young, the very old, the immunosuppressed, and those with broken skin or other compromised defenses).

Many gram-negative organisms are nosocomial threats. Over two-thirds of all cases of *Klebsiella* pneumonia are acquired during hospitalization. The organism has been found to grow in bronchodilator solutions, surviving for several days. Other gram-negative water bacteria such as *P. aeruginosa,* some nontuberculous mycobacteria such as *M. avium,* and *Legionella* can live and multiply in a hospital's warm-water supply. *Legionella* can aerosolize from hot showers and be responsible for nosocomial pneumonias. *Pseudomonas* also has been found to grow in the water in vaporizing respiratory equipment. *Enterobacter* species are gram-negative rods with a history of nosocomial fecal-oral spread. These organisms caused a nationwide epidemic of septicemia from intravenous solutions in 1971. *Enterobacter* species may survive in the water reservoirs of medical equipment (e.g., nebulizers and incubators) for 21 days.

Mechanical vector arthropods also have been found in hospitals. *Streptococcus pyogenes* (responsible for many infections, including impetigo, erysipelas, puerperal fever, strep throat, and necrotizing fasciitis) has been cultured from the legs of flies caught in hospitals. Most hospitals are required to have double sets of entry and exit doors and sealed windows to protect patients and workers from insect vectors.

The Transmission of Infectious Agents: The Triad Completed

MODELS OF TRANSMISSION

Some models of infection have added a fourth component to the agent-host-environment model—the **vehicle.** The definition for *vehicle of infection transmission* is "the mode of transmission of an infectious agent from its reservoir to a susceptible host. This can be person-to-person, food, vector-borne, etc." [2].

The four-component model conceives of transmission as one in a blend of four nouns. The triangular model uses three nouns connected by the action verb *transmission.* The triangular model concept is preferred in this text on occupational infections because much of infectious disease transmission is related to human behavior and tasks, and much of it can be prevented by teaching, learning, and training, all verbs denoting *control.*

TYPES OF TRANSMISSION

An infectious agent must be transmitted, either directly or indirectly, from one place to another. A standard system of nomenclature for classifying transmission has been accepted. The practical interpretation of this nomenclature comprises favorite questions on tests and board examinations. Standard terms and new definitions not yet covered in this text are presented in boldface type, and examples of some of the more common diseases are given, although not all are directly relevant to the workplace. Unless otherwise specified, all hosts are human. The section after that on the types of transmission reviews the portals of entry and exit and is followed by a section on means of controlling transmission.

Direct Transmission

Direct transmission means the transference of infectious agents directly and rather immediately into the portal of entry of a susceptible host. There is **no vehicle, vector,** or **"floating" to the host,** either actively or passively. For most diseases, direct contact means that between humans or their gravity-sensitive body fluids. Examples of direct transmission are listed in Table 3-25.

Droplet Spread. Examples of bacteria transmitted by droplets (the vehicle) are group A beta-hemolytic streptococci, *Mycoplasma pneumoniae, S. pneumoniae,* pneumonic plague, and *N. meningitidis.* Examples of viruses spread by droplets are rubella, adeno-, rhino-, corona-, and coxsack-

Table 3-25
Examples of Direct Transmission

Skin to skin
• By touching or embracing (staphylococcus, enterococcus, scabies, pediculosis)

Percutaneous
• By biting (rabies, cat scratch, hepatitis B, encephalitis)
• Wound contamination with an environmental contaminating infectious agent (tetanus, sporotrichosis, *Staphylococcus aureus,* aeromonas)

Mucous membrane to mucous membrane
• By sexual intercourse (syphilis, gonorrhea, chlamydia, HIV, HBV)
• By kissing (Epstein-Barr virus, CMV, mycoplasma)

Maternal-fetal
• *Transplacental transmission* is the passage of an infectious agent from mother to unborn fetus across the placenta. Examples of agents with this route of transmission are rubella, HIV, and cytomegalovirus. This route is also called *vertical transmission,* although vertical transmission may also include infection of the infant by agents that colonize the birth canal (e.g., *Listeria,* HIV, Group B streptococcus).

ieviruses, mumps, parvovirus, EBV, and cytomegalovirus (CMV) and other herpesviruses.

Droplet spread is the transmission by the gravity-sensitive or "falling" body-fluid projectiles from coughing, sneezing, singing, spitting, or talking. Various texts list this distance as anywhere from 3 ft (1 m) [2] to 6 ft [32]. In droplet spread, the portal of entry is the mucous membrane surfaces of the lungs, nose, mouth, throat, or conjunctivae. Not all infectious agents with this respiratory-nasal-oral portal of exit must be considered direct transmission, however. An infectious agent that can be spread by "floating" a greater distance is considered to be *indirectly* transmitted.

Indirect Transmission

Indirect transmission occurs when an infectious agent is removed from its reservoir and carried to the susceptible host over a distance of at least several feet and up to many miles. The type of indirect transmission is further defined by the mechanism of that transmission.

Vehicle (Vehicle-Borne) Spread. This is the meeting of an infectious agent and a susceptible host through contact with *contaminated inanimate objects.* Commonly used objects or articles such as environmental surfaces, clothing, bedding, toys, or money can serve as fomites (vehicles). Infection by ingestion (of food or water) is also a form of indirect transmission. The transmission of a blood-borne pathogen by transfusion, needlestick, or tissue transplantation is considered indirect; the respective vehicles in these examples are the blood unit, the needle, and the tissue specimen.

The infectious agent may contaminate only the vehicle (e.g., EBV in saliva on a child's toy), or it actually may live and multiply in the vehicle (e.g., *S. aureus* in a jar of unrefrigerated mayonnaise).

Vector (Vector-Borne) Spread. This is defined as the indirect transmission of an infectious agent to a susceptible host by an animate or living entity. Vectors generally are small species that move intentionally in the cycle of their own survival but infect incidentally. Vectors can be subdivided further.

MECHANICAL VECTORS. Mechanical vectors move the agents to the host via their own contaminated body organs or surfaces. An insect such as a fly that carries on its legs infectious bacteria (e.g., *S. pyogenes*) as it moves from a fecal meal to a human

wound is an example of mechanical vectorization. Fleas, cockroaches, and flies have been shown to be mechanical vectors for the transmission of *Pasteurella* to open wounds and *Salmonella* and *Shigella* to food. These insects also may carry the infectious agent in their gastrointestinal tracts. Mechanical vectors are not a natural part of the life cycle of infectious agents; the vector just happens to be "contaminated" or "colonized" with the agent, which causes it no harm.

BIOLOGIC VECTORS. These are the classic insect (arthropod) vectors that serve a role in the life cycle of the infectious agent. The agent passes through one or more life cycles in the arthropod before it can become infective to humans by its bite. For example, the female *Anopheles* mosquito spreads malaria to humans, and the *Plasmodium* parasite that causes malaria needs the mosquito as part of its life cycle. The agent may or may not cause harm to the arthropod.

Biologic-vector transmission is further divided into **transovarial transmission,** the passing of the infection "vertically" from a female arthropod to her offspring, and **transstadial transmission,** the continuation of the infection in the arthropod host as it moves from one life-cycle stage to another (i.e., from a nymph to an adult).

Airborne Spread. This is the movement of infectious agents into the susceptible host by the air. Infectious agents in this class can be inhaled directly into the alveoli of the lungs, past the mechanical host defenses of the nose and throat. Airborne indirect transmission is further divided into two vehicle classes.

DUST. Dust is any organic or inorganic material capable of floating in the air for any distance. The dust particle itself is the vehicle and may carry spores or exotoxins. Exposure to infections from dust is a risk in any profession exposed to wind, dryness, or the mechanical disturbance of soil. It also may be a risk to laboratory workers.

DROPLET NUCLEI. Droplet nuclei are the smallest of infective vehicles, generally less than 5 μm in size. They can be produced naturally by the evaporation of droplet body fluids from infected hosts and float long distances to cause infections. They are the most difficult diseases to prevent but fortunately are relatively few in number. They include tuberculosis (and other mycobacterial infections), influenza (orthomyxoviruses), rubeola (measles), and varicella (chickenpox). Droplet nuclei also may be produced unnaturally by mechanical devices in laboratories or abattoirs (slaughterhouses). Note that some organisms that cause infection by droplet nuclei also can cause disease by direct droplets. For example, influenza can infect not only indirectly by droplet nuclei but also closer by the direct droplets dispersed in the air by a sneeze or cough.

IMPORTANCE OF THE TRANSMISSION CLASSES

The classifications of transmission may seem rather didactic and confusing, but they are important to understand in order to design and use methods of controls. They are not just rigid definitions left unchanged out of respect for the original writer. Knowing the differences in the definitions of the transmission classes and why spread of airborne droplets is direct and that of airborne droplet nuclei is indirect will help in the understanding and classification of controls. In the hospital isolation system, the former can be prevented by wearing a simple surgical mask near the patient's bedside in the regular semiprivate room, whereas the latter requires the wearing of a high-efficiency particulate-air (HEPA) respirator everywhere in a negative-ventilated private room with the door closed.

Transmission systems should not be confused with the portal-of-entry and portal-of-exit concepts discussed next. These are entirely different but equally important. For instance, *fecal-oral* describes routes of entry and exit, not the method of transmission. Fecal-oral transmission can be direct, in cases of oral-anal sexual transmission, or indirect, in cases of food or water contamination. Although an organism may be the same agent, transmitted by the same portal of entry and the same port of exit, one cannot *control transmission* without knowing the *type of transmission*. Safe sex practices will not prevent hepatitis A food poisoning, nor will safe food handling prevent sexual transmission of hepatitis A.

If it is learned how an agent is transmitted, its transmission may be prevented or blocked years before its identity is known. Thanks to John Snow's work on discovering the mechanism of transmission of cholera, it could be prevented a century before its etiology was identified. The risk factors for AIDS transmission were identified a few months after the disease's existence was recognized and several years before the infectious agent was isolated or named. Perhaps the best examples for this text are, however, the dozen or more infectious diseases that were named after occupations, implying that the risk factors of transmission were known years or even centuries before the respective agents were named.

Infectious agents do not always have a single port of entry, exit, or method of transmission. The most successful (i.e., difficult to control) infectious agents have more than one method of transmission. The varicella-zoster virus (VZV), for instance, can be transmitted directly by contact with vesicular fluid (zoster) or by airborne droplet (varicella). However, it also can be spread indirectly by droplet nuclei from respiratory secretions (varicella) or by fomites (varicella or zoster). Note that this agent produces two separate disease forms, infects for life, and can reactivate randomly. The weakness of the virus is that it infects only humans, has no other reservoir, and survives only a few minutes outside the human body. Despite there now being an effective vaccine, though, the disease still may take a century to eradicate. It will not be eradicated until the last human with latent VZV dies and/or all humans on Earth have immunity.

PORTALS OF ENTRY

For infection to occur, there must be a portal of entry into a susceptible host. Often the portal of entry and the portal of exit are in the same organ system and are also the organs affected. For example, if an individual releases an agent into the air by coughing, another may acquire it by inhaling, and the respiratory tree and lung suffer the pathogenicity of the agent. But many infections are far from being this simple.

The Respiratory System as a Port of Entry

As with chemical and toxic occupational and environmental risks, the respiratory route is the most important and efficient natural means of entry for harmful agents. Infections contracted by the respiratory route are the most difficult to control because humans obligatorily take "sample specimens" of their immediate atmosphere (air) 12–20 times a minute in breathing. Most of the great pandemics in history (e.g., the plague, Spanish influenza, and leprosy) have been acquired primarily by the respiratory route. Most of the "usual" childhood illness (e.g., measles, rubella, varicella, and mumps) also are acquired by inspiration or by direct contamination of the upper respiratory system from the respiratory secretions of cohorts. More than any other pathogens, respiratory-acquired infections do not spare the healthy.

The mechanical and immunologic host defenses of the respiratory system were described earlier in this chapter, and controls are discussed later. Infectious agents are transmitted to the respiratory system in one of the following ways:

- Directly by gravity-influenced droplets from a human or other vertebrate in the immediate vicinity
- Indirectly by dust (a vehicle) from a source of any distance
- Indirectly by a floating droplet nuclei from a human or other vertebrate beyond the immediate inspiration zone

Bacterial agents known to cause infection from some distance include *M. tuberculosis, C. burnetti* (Q fever), and *Legionella;* viral agents include influenza, rubeola, and rubella. Outbreaks of all these agents have been reported in the workplace or in military units.

Not all human-specific diseases acquired by inspiration have the respiratory system as the portal of exit, however. The poxviruses (e.g., varicella, vaccinia, and monkeypox), for instance, can be aerosolized from vesicles. And some animal respiratory secretions can aerosolize to cause infection in animal researchers. This was documented to have occurred in two laboratory workers doing research on swine influenza [33].

Gastrointestinal System as a Port of Entry

The term *fecal-oral spread* is not synonymous with a gastrointestinal portal of entry. It implies a gastrointestinal exit *and* an oral route of entry as a means of transmission of an agent. Fecal-oral spread may be direct or indirect from mechanical vectors or on vehicles such as food, water, or fomites. Orally acquired bacterial infections also may be called *enteric fevers* (see Chapter 1). Some enteric fevers may be humans-only diseases transmitted by the fecal-oral route and spread predominantly by the hands of humans (e.g., *Shigella*),or by

water (e.g., cholera and typhoid). However, others may be transmitted by ingestion of food contaminated by the infected feces of domestic animal hosts (e.g., *Y. enterocolitica, Salmonella,* and *Campylobacter*).

Most fecal-oral viral infections are classified in the genus *Enterovirus* (echovirus) or *Reovirus* (rotavirus). A large percentage of these are subclinical and inapparent, especially in adults. Norwalk-like viruses occur infrequently as an epidemic of adult diarrheal illness contracted by ingestion of feces-contaminated food or water. Hepatitis A virus (HAV) is a fecal-oral agent that infects food more often than water.

Not all orally acquired infections are of fecal origin. Many viruses and bacteria may be acquired orally, nasally, by direct droplet, or in some combination. This includes most of the herpes class of viruses (e.g., CMV, EBV, herpes simplex, influenza virus, and rhinovirus), as well as bacteria, such as group A beta-hemolytic streptococci, *Corynebacterium diphtheriae,* and *Mycoplasma.*

Skin as a Port of Entry

The skin is very important as a portal of entry, especially for occupationally acquired infections. The normal flora and host defenses of the skin were discussed previously. Work-related skin infections include not only those associated with the trauma of cuts and abrasions but also those associated with occupationally acquired contact dermatitis or other rashes, which may serve as a source of wound infections or a route for bloodborne pathogens or other serious exposures. Skin and wound infections are of special consequences in health care workers not only because of the possible exposure to body fluids and drug-resistant organisms but also because of the cost of restricting caregivers from working.

A full discussion of all infections that gain entry through the skin or wounds is beyond the scope of this chapter. Some of the more common agents of wound infections were discussed in the previous section on the inanimate reservoir and soil.

Percutaneous Entry. Percutaneous infections are those acquired by penetration of the skin, including trauma (e.g., cuts or abrasions), penetration by instruments (e.g., needlesticks), and bites of animals or arthropods. Needlesticks are covered in more detail elsewhere in this book. Blood transfusions also may serve as indirect percutaneous sources of infectious agents. Besides the more common pathogens of HIV, HBV, and HCV, rare transfusion-related bloodborne pathogens include CMV, arboviruses, HTLV-1, *Babesia*, EBV, the prion causing Creutzfeldt-Jakob disease, *Brucella, Leptospira, Plasmodium, Borrelia, Treponema palladium,* and most recently West Nile virus. These infections legally could be considered work-related health problems that fall under workers' compensation if they occur as complications of a transfusion given in the course of treating a work-related injury.

ARTHROPOD BITES. The arboviruses are defined as viruses that replicate in both vertebrates and arthropods (e.g., mosquitoes, ticks, midges, and sandflies) during their life cycle and transmit disease between vertebrates by arthropod bites. Thousands of arboviruses have been identified and recorded by the *International Catalogue of Arboviruses* [34], and some are listed in Table 3-26.

Rickettsia akari (rickettsialpox) is spread by the bites of ticks and has as its reservoir house mice and rats. *Rickettsia. rickettsii* (Rocky Mountain spotted fever) has as its reservoir dogs, rodents, and other small mammals. Lyme disease (*Borrelia burgdorferi;* see Chapter 26) is the most recently recognized of the tick-borne diseases and can have a chronic course. Animal hosts vary according to the stage of the *Ixodid* ticks. The malarial parasites, which are spread by mosquitoes, are covered in Chapter 25.

Table 3-26
Major Classes of Arboviruses and the Diseases They Cause

Togaviridae family, *Alphavirus* genus (horses, birds)
    Eastern equine encephalitis (mosquitoes)
    Western equine encephalitis (mosquitoes)
    Venezuelan equine encephalitis (mosquitoes)
Flaviviridae family (birds, groundhogs, monkeys)
    Yellow fever (mosquitoes)
    West Nile (mosquitoes)
    St. Louis encephalitis (mosquitoes)
    Japanese B encephalitis (mosquitoes)
    Powassan encephalitis (ticks)
    Dengue fever (mosquitoes)
Reoviridae, *Orbivirus* genus
    Colorado tick fever (ticks)
Bunyaviridae family
    California encephalitis (mosquitoes)
    LaCrosse encephalitis (mosquitoes)
    Jamestown Canyon encephalitis (mosquitoes)
Rhabdoviridae family, vesiculoviruses (domestic animals)
    Vesicular stomatitis (sandflies, mosquitoes, blackflies)

ANIMAL BITES. Wound infections are the most common complications of animal bites and are covered in parts of the text. *Pasteurella* species of bacteria can cause localized infections and osteomyelitis from cat or dog bites, especially in colder weather. *Streptobacillus moniliformis* can cause a serious systemic illness and multiple organ abscesses after rat bites and may have a mortality up to 7% in the United States. Most cases are related to laboratory rat bites. Both *Pasteurella* and *S. moniliformis* are very sensitive to penicillin and its derivatives. *Herpesvirus simiae* is a close relative of herpes simplex and has its reservoir in the mouths of macaque and other Old World monkeys. Thirty-one cases have been reported, with a 68% fatality rate. Most deaths have been occupationally related. This virus should be handled only under laboratory biosafety level 4.

PORTALS OF EXIT

To survive, infectious organisms must have a portal of exit from a host, either directly into another susceptible host or into the environment to await indirect entry into a susceptible host. Surprisingly few infectious diseases enter, exit, and cause disease all in the same organ systems. Examples include some respiratory diseases (e.g., tuberculosis, influenza, and rhinovirus infection) and some of the diarrheal illnesses spread by the fecal-oral route. There are five classic portals of exit from a human or animal reservoir, but for occupational infectious diseases, one might add a unique sixth. **Bleeding wounds** may be considered a portal of exit for those exposed to human blood in the course of their employment.

Respiratory Portal of Exit

Factors influencing the efficiency of the human respiratory system as a portal of exit include

- Intensity and propulsion of discharge of secretions from the system. This can range from drainage and direct contact or contamination of fomites, to coughing, to the most efficient means, which is sneezing.
- Size of the droplets being exited, which generally ranges from 1–20 μm. The size of the droplets also can be influenced positively by ambient humidity and negatively by ambient temperature.
- Wind currents in the local area.

- Concentration of viable and infective units. Infective doses by inhalation can be as low as 7 virions for an adenovirus in the weightless environment [35], to 10 bacilli for *M. tuberculosis*, to 1,300 bacteria for anthrax.

It is well established that many respiratory viruses (e.g., influenza, respiratory syncytial virus, and rhinoviruses) can be spread by direct contact of mucous membranes with hands and other fomites. There may be nearly 2 million particles extruded from a sneeze, compared with fewer than 100,000 from a cough [36]. But more infective particles may be released in a cough because of the deeper origin in the lungs [37].

Many studies of the infectivity of respiratory viruses have been conducted by Knight's group [37] and include mathematical theories and models of the infectivity of viruses in zero gravity [35]. Knight and colleagues also have theorized that some respiratory diseases may be more infectious in space travel because larger drops float longer and further. All U.S. space modules, starting with Apollo, have used HEPA air filters. Table 3-27 summarizes the behavior of spherical objects in still air.

Gastrointestinal Portal of Exit

Very few infectious organisms are known to be spread by vomiting. However, bloody vomitus should be considered a bloodborne pathogen risk, especially in patients with hepatitis B. Oral secretions may transmit many viruses, as discussed previously, including most of the "usual" childhood illnesses and the herpes family of viruses. Respiratory and oral secretions may be mixed, especially in ill children. Rabies can exit the body via saliva and be infective by a bite.

Many fecally excreted infectious agents can persist in the soil and water for long periods, and examples are given in Table 3-28.

Skin as a Portal of Exit

Organisms in superficial lesions such as the lesions of impetigo, syphilis, and chickenpox can be dislodged easily. Other organisms (e.g., plasmodia and HBV) exit the body via the percutaneous route through breaks in the skin, insect bites, and needles.

Genitourinary Tract as a Portal of Exit

The sexually transmitted diseases are not discussed but serve as an important portal of exit (and entry) for many diseases that also may be acquired occupationally, including HIV, HBV, and HSV infection. A careful sexual history and possibly a genitourinary examination may be needed for the

Table 3-28
Fecally Excreted Infectious Agents and Their Environmental Survival

Bacteria
- *Bacillus cereus* spores may survive for years in environment of soil or water, including surviving cooking.
- *Clostridium* spores may survive in soil for months to years and in meat for 330 days.
- *Aeromonas, Listeria,* and *Salmonella* have long survival in water or soil.
- *Citrobacter* species and cholera survive well in water.
- *Escherichia coli* (enterotoxigenic) survives 84 days in soil or stool.
- *Yersinia enterocolitica* can survive in soil for 540 days, water for 20 days, and cold seawater for up to 105 days.
- *Salmonella typhi* can survive in ashes for 130 days, dust up to 30 days, and feces for 60 days. One human carrier can expel billions of infectious units and infect many others.

Viruses
- Echoviruses (enteroviruses) may survive pH as low as 3, and can survive in stool for three weeks at room temperature.
- Hepatitis A (an RNA picornavirus) can survive long periods in water and sewage.
- Rotavirus can live for months in water near freezing.
- Norwalk virus' survival conditions are unknown.

Parasites
- *Ascaris* (roundworm) and *Toxocara* eggs can live months in soil.
- *Balantidium* protozoan cysts can survive months and possibly years in soil.
- *Cryptosporidium parvum* oocysts and *Giardia* and *Amoeba* cysts can survive several months in moisture or water.
- Almost all tapeworm cysts can live months in the environment.

Table 3-27
Behavior of Spherical Infectious Particles (in Still Air)

Diameter	To Fall 3 Meters	Transmission
100 μm	10 seconds	Very direct only
40 μm	1 minute	Direct only
20 μm	4 minutes	Direct
10 μm	17 minutes	Some indirect?
≥6 μm	May float	Caught by nasal hair
0.6–6.0 μm	Floats	Into lungs

differential diagnosis of a work-related illness. *S. typhi* is shed from human urine and can contaminate food or water, causing typhoid fever.

A few zoonotic diseases are known to be shed from urine. *Leptospira* species can be shed from the urine of animals for up to 11 months after initial infection and from the urine of infected humans for up to 1 month. Rodent urine contamination of the soil and dust may be a method of transmission of Lassa fever and hanta, junin, and machupo viral infections.

Principles of Controlling Occupational Infectious Disease

This chapter has described the concepts of the agent-host-environment triad and their linkage by transmission. This section addresses the principles of control of occupational infectious disease risks at these four levels using the classic industrial hygiene (IH) approach of *recognition, evaluation,* and *control.*

For most workplace risks, the goals are to quantitatively contain the risk at a safe level. For infectious agents, the goal is to prevent or at least control exposure of the susceptible worker host to a less than infective dose of an infectious agent. Despite the great advances made in the treatment of infectious disease during the last century, such treatment remains a large part of clinical medicine.

The tools and methods to control or prevent infectious diseases at the level of the infectious agent, the susceptible host, or the environment are rather limited. All infectious agents from the environment cannot be eliminated, nor should they be. Nor can all workers be rendered immune to all infectious agents. The weak link is transmission. The spread of cholera was controlled a century before the agent was identified because the method of transmission was learned (fecal-oral) and the reservoir (contaminated water) identified by John Snow. Avoiding the drinking of potentially human feces–contaminated water controlled the disease, and this behavior also controlled dozens of other diseases with identical reservoirs for transmission.

The first step in the classic IH evaluation of a health hazard is to acquire knowledge of the existence of the threatening agent and then knowledge of the workplace process. In evaluating infectious diseases, knowledge of the workplace and the work process and its environment often precedes evaluation of risks for specific infectious agents, which, in turn, first must be known so that they can be controlled at the source, pathway, and/or worker. The classic IH method, however, may be translated to evaluation of risks for transmission of occupational infectious agents:

Classic IH Evaluation	Evaluation of Occupational Infectious Agents
Control at the Source	*Transmission* at the Agent
Pathway	Environment
Worker	Host

IH professionals can obtain area or personal samples for many nonbiologic hazards. But the culturing or isolating of all possible infectious agents in a work environment is rarely practical. Workers in only a few occupations may be constantly exposed to a single known infectious agent, e.g., laboratory, food, or pharmaceutical workers who handle or use a potentially infectious agent as an inherent part of their job. Most workers who are exposed to infectious agents are exposed to a variety of agents in a less predictable, random pattern. Examples include hospital workers and those who work in the wilderness. Their protection and job precautions may be "generalized" and relate to behavioral patterns (e.g., washing hands or using insect repellents) but also may be agent-specific (e.g., HBV vaccination or rabies vaccination).

The hierarchy of classic industrial hygiene controls, in order of importance, is

1. **Substitution** (of the agent)
2. **Engineering controls**
3. **Administrative controls**
4. **Personal protection controls**

Since infectious agents are rarely of value to the workplace, **avoidance** or **eradication** of them can "substitute" for classic IH substitution. Most methods of control involve more than one level, or **integrated controls.** For instance, the control program for tuberculosis in a health care facility may involve the use of negative-pressure rooms and UV lighting (i.e., engineering controls), may require that all employees screen patients for tuberculosis symptoms and risk factors at the time of entry into the health care system (i.e., administrative controls), may require that medical staff have special training in the recognition of tuberculosis (i.e., administrative controls), and may require that staff be trained to use N-95 respirators when in contact with potential tuberculosis patients (i.e., personal protection). No one level of control alone will suffice.

CONTROLLING THE AGENT
Substitution

Use of the concept of substitution for infectious agents has limited applications. Live, attenuated vaccines are a form of substitution of a less virulent agent (antigen) to stimulate immunity (see Chapter 5). The less virulent oral poliovirus (an enterovirus) vaccine may "substitute" for the wild virus found in municipal sewage [38]. When the wild virus has been completely substituted in the environment and in the human host, it will be eradicated. The rare cases occurring presently are due to mutation of the vaccine virus "back" to a pathogenic or paralytic strain.

The ability to use a true in vivo substitution of one less virulent infectious agent for another may be less difficult than attempting eradication, especially for organisms that are normal residents of human flora. In the early antibiotic era, there were outbreaks of the penicillin-resistant S. aureus 80/81 phagotype transmitted from mothers to infants in newborn nurseries and later from infant to infant. After that, newborns were deliberately colonized with S. aureus 502A, a less virulent organism that inhibited the virulent form by **bacterial interference.**

Eradication (Extinction) of an Infectious Agent

The complete extinction of a human infectious agent from the planet is the ultimate goal of infection control because only a few seem to serve an otherwise essential role in the biosphere. Smallpox was eradicated in 1979. The goal of eradication of wild poliomyelitis before 2000 was a failed goal, and the remaining hurdles are cultural and political rather than technical. Very few other infectious agent extinctions are expected in our lifetime. Some factors that may contribute to the possibility of eradication of a human infectious disease and agent are presented in Table 3-29.

The most difficult diseases to eradicate are those with a wide and well-protected "endemic" reservoir.

Table 3-29

Factors Contributing to Eradication of an Infectious Agent

- The disease exists only in humans (see Table 3-24), with no animal or insect hosts or vectors and no environmental survival (reservoir). That is, the entire reservoir is approachable and treatable if the agent is only transmitted directly human to human.
- The disease has a very low inapparent:apparent ratio: Cases do not escape diagnosis because they do not have "silent" symptoms.
- The disease has a rather distinct clinical presentation, narrow differential diagnosis, and therefore a reliable clinical diagnosis and accurate case reporting. An example is the characteristic clinical course and presentation of mumps (parotitis).
- The incubation and communicable period is short, with little to no carriage, colonization, or latency states. Measles, with its short incubation and infective period, is easier to eradicate than varicella-zoster virus or latent tuberculosis, both of which may persist for life and become reactivated.
- A highly efficacious vaccination or other highly reliable prevention exists and is widely delivered. The susceptible population is reduced (herd immunity), or the susceptibles are so isolated and remote from the active cases that the infectious agent is routed to a dead end.
- The disease has only a single serotype or strain. Rubella has only one form, whereas influenza and Salmonella have thousands.
- The cost of eradication also should be cost-effective. Rubella would not have been worthy of vaccine research or been on the International Task Force for Disease Eradication list had it not been for the discovery of the costly congenital rubella syndrome (CRS). Rubella is otherwise a mild disease of rare clinical consequence.

Human rabies is rare in most parts of the world, and adequate vaccines are available for both humans and animals, but vaccination of all wild animals in the global reservoir is impossible. The best hope is, at least, eradication of "urban rabies."

Eradicating the Agent within the Host. Treatment, or chemotherapy, for illness of human infectious disease represents a large portion of general clinical practice. The many classes and mechanisms of action of antimicrobials are beyond the scope of this chapter. The development of new classes of antimicrobial agents barely keeps pace with the development of resistance. Antiviral resistance is now seen with amantadine and rimantadine for influenza (see Chapters 11A and 11B) and antiretroviral medications for HIV (see Chapter 24). Many parasites also have developed resistance to previously effective treatments.

At rare times there may be indications for treating asymptomatic workers, especially those in health care, or groups of workers colonized with bacteria that pose a risk to their patients or clients. Health care personnel who were carriers of group A streptococci (GAS) have been linked infrequently to sporadic outbreaks of surgical site, postpartum, and burn wound infections [39–45] and food-borne transmission of GAS-caused pharyngitis [46]. Investigations of nosocomial infections have shown a link between methicillin-resistant *S. aureus* (MRSA) and health care workers [47–54]. However, CDC guidelines do not advise "routine" culturing of specimens from health care workers unless they have been linked epidemiologically to infected patients [8]—i.e., not unless they have been common caregivers to two or more patients who have been positive for the condition. Epidemics of diseases among workers at non–health care facilities also have been reported. One study reported 165 of 232 workers at a textile plant who tested PPD-positive after exposure to an undiagnosed coworker with an especially virulent strain of active pulmonary tuberculosis [55].

Eradicating the Agent in the Environment. Complete eradication of an infectious agent in inanimate reservoirs (i.e., air, soil, or water) is rarely possible. Even eliminating an infectious agent in animate reservoirs is challenging.

However, one major reservoir of very serious infectious agents is approachable by controls, i.e., health care facilities and their patient care equipment. Here, the goal is eradication of infectious agents or at least a reduction of the **bioburden** of agents to a level below the infective doses. The eradication or reduction of infectious agents in the health care environment has developed into a field of study generally termed *sterilization and disinfection.*

STERILIZATION AND DISINFECTION. Research in this field has contributed most of the available information on the physical and chemical sensitivities of all infectious agents and life forms. The research for new technology and products is very competitive and driven by commercial interests. Toxicity and workers sensitization are barriers to developing usable products. Three major problems have evolved, and these have been addressed only recently.

1. *Terminology.* A confusing vocabulary has developed in the field [56]. The public, health professionals, and even manufacturers have deviated from the true dictionary definitions. Different classification systems also have evolved.
2. *Regulations.* Several agencies have been involved in the regulation and testing of germicides, leading to conflicts, inconsistencies, and gaps in control.
3. *Safety issues.* Both patients and health care workers may suffer harmful effects from the chemicals and hardware used in sterilization and disinfection. Some germicidal agents have been found to damage delicate instruments, or the instruments' lumina have not been adequately drained and have caused injury to patients [57].

TERMINOLOGY AND CLASSIFICATION: GERMICIDAL TERMS

Cleaning: In the health care environment, the removal of *visible* dirt, debris, soil, or any organic or inorganic material from the surface of objects. It is a very crude but major reduction of the bioburden and potential substrates. It *must* precede all disinfection or sterilization procedures because effectiveness is inversely related to the amount of initial debris.

Bioburden: The sum total of the number and range of biologic contamination on or in an inanimate object. This is analogous to the flora count on an animate surface.

Antibacterials: Germicidal chemicals that may counteract, inhibit, and to some limited degree destroy some bacteria. These include many over-the-counter products for household cleaning, dishwashing, and bathing. The sale of such products greatly increased throughout the 1990s and may contribute to some development of resistance.

Antiseptics: The relatively mild antimicrobial germicides used to reduce microbes on the skin or living tissues. Applies only to agents meant for direct contact on *biologic surfaces* as opposed to environmental surfaces (disinfection).

Disinfectants: Germicidal agents used to destroy or inhibit the growth of most pathogenic bacteria and some viruses on environmental or *nonbiologic sur-*

faces. Some bacteria (mycobacteria and endospores) and some viruses may survive some disinfectants.

Disinfection: Any process that reduces pathogenic infectious agents. Does not imply the complete destruction of all pathogenic infectious agents.

Spores: A small dormant or inactive single-cell reproductive body produced by some bacteria, fungi, or lower plants as a means of surviving adverse conditions. **Endospore** is the inner layer of the wall of a bacterial spore. Spores are the most difficult of all infectious agents to kill (Figure 3-11).

Bacteriostat(ic): Chemical products intended to retard or inhibit the *growth* of bacteria, including bacteriostatic chemical polymers used in the manufacturing of building materials surfaces (e.g., restaurants or hospitals) or medical products.

Bacteriocide: Germicide used to *kill* pathogenic bacteria rather that just inhibit or retard their growth.

Sterilization: The highest level ("gold standard") of germicidal processes; the killing or inactivating of all living entities and their by-products, including endospores.

Sterility assurance level: The probability of a microorganism surviving on an object of less than 1 in 1 million (10^6). Used as a definition for level of sterilization.

Decontamination: A less desirable term (than *sterility assurance level*) that implies only that some effort was used to make an object reasonably free of microorganisms and thus reduce the risk of disease transmission. The word alone does not imply the degree to which that risk has been reduced, however.

CLASSIFICATION SYSTEMS FOR GERMICIDAL PROCESSES

One of the standard systems for classifying inanimate surfaces in the hospital environment was developed by Spaulding in 1972 [58] and involves three germicidal levels:

1. **Critical.** Instruments or devices that are to contact normally sterile body cavities (including vascular) must be sterilized.

2. **Semicritical.** Instruments or devices that touch mucous membranes may be either sterilized or disinfected.

3. **Noncritical.** Instruments or devices that touch skin or the patient only indirectly can be cleaned and then disinfected with an intermediate-level disinfectant, sanitized with a low-level disinfectant, or simply cleaned with soap and water.

Spaulding also classified the chemical germicidal agents by "activity" level:

1. **High-level disinfection.** Kills vegetative microorganisms but not necessarily a high number of bacterial spores when it is used for contact times of 10–30 minutes. These agents are capable of sterilization only with contact times of 6–10 hours. These qualify for the current Environmental Protection Agency (EPA) designation "sterilant/disinfectants" and include the glutaraldehyde-, chlorine dioxide–, hydrogen peroxide–, and peracetic acid–based products.

2. **Intermediate-level disinfection.** Kills vegetative bacteria, including *M. tuberculosis,* all fungi, and most viruses. These agents are the iodophors, phenolics, and chlorine (bleach) compounds. A 1:10 dilution of household bleach (sodium hypochlorite) will inactivate HBV and HIV in a blood spill.

3. **Low-level disinfection.** Kills all vegetative bacteria, with the exception of *M. tuberculosis,* some fungi, and a few viruses. Does not kill spores. These are EPA registered as "hospital disinfectants" or "sanitizers" and include the quaternary ammonium compounds, some iodophors, and some phenolics.

REGULATION OF CHEMICAL GERMICIDES

In the United States, two different agencies regulate chemical germicides: the Environmental Protection Agency (EPA) and the Food and Drug Administration (FDA). Agents formulated as sterilants or disinfectants had been regulated by the EPA, but both agencies agreed that agents used on specific medical devices fall under the purview of the FDA. The FDA also regulates all sterilization devices, such as autoclaves and dry-heat ovens, and any products to be used in direct contact with human tissues. The FDA also oversees manufacturers'

Figure 3-11
Levels of infectious agent survival from categories of germicidal agents, from the most resistant to the least resistant. Sterility implies the absence of all infectious agents, including bacterial spores. This survival order is approximately the same to heat, light, salinity, and pH.

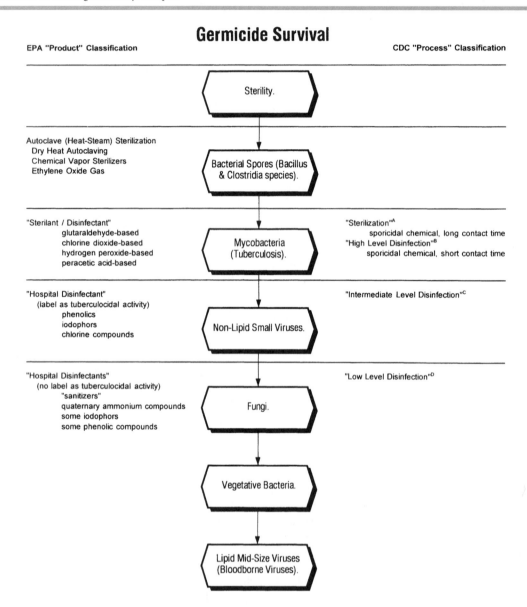

A	Appropriate only for critical or semi-critical instruments that are damaged by heat and can not be autoclaved (i.e., laparoscopes). Not capable of being biologically monitored and requires cumbersome post exposure manipulation such as rinsing, drying, and wiping with sterile towels. Less than true sterilization.	
B	Appropriate only for semi-critical instruments that are damaged by heat and cannot be cleaned by autoclaving (i.e., colonoscopes). Requires washing with sterile water before next use.	
C	Appropriate for between-patient processing of certain noncritical instruments or devices or for environmental surfaces, such as spills of blood or microbial cultures.	
D	Appropriate for between patient processing of certain noncritical instruments/devices or for routine cleaning and housekeeping.	

Source: Benjamini E, Sunshie G, Leskowitz S. *Immunology: A Short Course,* 3rd ed. New York: Wiley-Liss, 1996, p. 21, with permission.

recommendations and the compatibility of devices and germicides. The agency still oversees the manufacturing and testing of sanitizers, disinfectants, hospital disinfectants, and sterilant/disinfectants (sporicides), including testing for potency, stability, and toxicity to humans. The CDC does not have regulatory powers but only makes recommendations for infection control for each infectious agent or process category. OSHA has the responsibility for insuring worker safety and controlling exposure to germicides and germicidal processes.

METHODS OF STERILIZATION

Infectious agents can be classified by the temperatures needed to inactivate them, which comprise a spectrum from the bacterial endospores (*Bacillus* and *Clostridium*), which require high temperatures and are the hardest to kill, to the medium-size lipid viruses, which can be killed at lower temperatures (see Figure 3-11). Fortunately, HIV and the other bloodborne viruses are at the lowest level on the spectrum, and relatively few virulent organisms are at the highest.

Although the other methods of sterilization seem to follow the same kill chart, heat remains at least three orders of magnitude superior to the best liquid-chemical sterilization process. Monitoring is done with a **spore test** using harmless spore-forming organisms such as *Bacillus. stearothermophilus*. Quality is also controlled with heat-change tapes and slow-change chemical indicator strips. Steam under pressure is the "gold standard." Methods of sterilization for medical instruments include

- **Autoclaving:** Temperature of 250°F (121°C) at 15–20 lb/in^2 of pressure for 30 minutes. The timer should not be set until the necessary temperature and pressure are reached. Errors include overloading, overcrowding, leaving organic debris, using nonporous wrapping, and failure in settings. Other errors may include autoclaving materials such as plastic. Serious steam burns can occur with malfunctioning units, but otherwise the units are safe for workers. Many smaller clinical facilities today find the use of disposable sterile products preferable to on-site sterilization.
- **Dry heat:** Most autoclaves can be converted to dry-heat sterilization, which is more suitable for powders, oils, and some fine instruments used in dental offices. Dry-heat sterilization must reach 325°F (163°C) for 1 hour. Instruments must cool before being used.
- **Chemical vapor sterilizers:** These have the advantages of leaving cutting instruments free of corrosion, of being faster, and of requiring no cooling time. Chemical vapor sterilization requires 270°F (132°C) for 20 minutes at 25 lb/in^2. These sterilizers are more expensive, and noxious gases may develop if the proper sterilizing bags are not used or certain metals are sterilized. Excellent ventilation is required.
- **Ethylene oxide:** This gas is the first choice for sterilizing fine heat-sensitive instruments. It has a broad killing spectrum but requires many hours of contact. It is also explosive at over a 3% concentration and can cause burns if traces are left on gloves or clothing. It is also very toxic, possibly carcinogenic, and falls under a full OSHA standard. Many facilities have found alternatives to ethylene oxide (an example of the IH control approach of **substitution**).
- **Chemical sterilants:** Chemical sterilants fall into two classes: the chlorine compounds and the glutaraldehydes. They should be used in closed units and in excellent ventilation. Goggles and gloves should be worn, and instruments should be well cleaned before contacting the chemicals. These solutions can disinfect in a few minutes, but it usually takes 6–10 hours for sterilization. More dilute solutions are used for disinfection.

Very few chlorine-based compounds are accepted as a sterilant. Such compounds contain sodium chlorite, which releases nascent oxygen on contact with cell surfaces and leaves harmless residues. It is a noxious chemical that also damages many metal surfaces on instruments. The glutaraldehydes are used in acidic, neutral, and alkaline forms. A 2% alkaline solution is used most widely. All chemical sterilants should be used according to FDA-approved manufacturers' recommendations.

CONTROLLING THE ENVIRONMENT (RESERVOIR)

The success of attempting to control the environment or reservoir of infectious agents is generally limited to controlling that environment in the near proximity of susceptible hosts and their ports of entry. Means of controlling infectious agents by removing them near their source of origin is known as *source-control technique*. The appropriate safety and industrial hygiene techniques depend on the nature of the work, the risks associated with infectious agents, and the nature of the source of the infectious agents. Appropriate techniques may include regular culturing of a reservoir for harmful infectious agents (e.g., hospital hot-water systems for levels of *Legionella* and *M. avium*).

Controlling the Airborne Environment

Outdoors. Control of infectious agents in the outdoor air is impossible. Dust can be locally and partially controlled by the spraying of water or oil. A 3% formaldehyde solution can be used in some areas of suspected heavy contamination by *Histoplasma capsulatum* or *Coccidioides immitis* fungus. This concentration requires an EPA permit. Those doing the work should wear particulate respirator masks and ideally should be native to the area. A 1% hypochlorite spray can be used for suspected viral dust contamination, such as hantavirus.

Indoors. Attempts to completely sterilize indoor air by filtration, propylene glycol, and UV light all have met with failure. There are limits on the infection control afforded by ventilation [59]. The best controls generally involve controlling directions of indoor airflow. The size and viability of bioaerosols may depend on their electric charge, moisture content, hygroscopicity, density, cell composition, and shape. Naturally occurring viable bioaerosols (i.e., droplets or droplet nuclei from coughing or sneezing) have been discussed.

Source-control techniques have had some success in health care facilities. **Negative-pressure ventilation** is achieved by having the exhaust-air velocity exceed the intake in an area that contains and encloses the source. No air should escape the enclosure (e.g., patient's room), and directional flow can be measured with smoke tubes as a quality control. Exhaust air is passed through a **HEPA filter,** defined as one capable of filtering out 99.97% of particles 0.3 µm or less in diameter. If HEPA filters are not used, then the exhausted air should be discharged well above the reentry zone. High-power UV lighting (with eye protection) and laminar airflow are used in surgical suites with some success for high-risk cases, such as total joint

replacements.

General ventilation can be one of two types. **Single-pass ventilation** systems take 100% of exhausted air out of the structure and obtain 100% of intake fresh air from outside the structure. This is the desirable system for infection control but is expensive because the fresh air must be controlled to the proper temperature and humidity. Most structures use **recirculated ventilation,** in which only a portion of the exhausted air is replaced by fresh.

Viable bioaerosols of infectious agents not naturally infectious by bioaerosols theoretically could be produced by laboratory spills or centrifuge accidents. The infectivity of such agents also would depend on the method of aerosol generation, the nature of liquid that surrounds the microorganism, and the size or weight of the organism itself. Laboratory safety protocols for most infectious agents call for allowing 30 minutes for aerosols to settle before beginning cleanup.

Another concern is the possibility of aerosolized bloodborne or tissue-borne pathogens generated by laser plumes or by high-speed high-energy surgical "power" tools. This was a concern for hepatitis B patients even before HIV was described, but studies showed that high-speed dental drills did not produce particles small enough for inspiration [60]. Note that HBV infections have been spread by direct splatter of infected body fluid onto mucous membranes; however, transmission by aerosolization has not been proven. Experimental studies have shown that aerosols produced by surgical instruments can culture HIV [61]. Other experimental studies have shown that surgical drills have produced inspirable particles of bone or tendon of 5 µm or less, laser plumes have produced particles between 0.3 and 100 µm, and electrocautery has produced particles of 0.7 µm [62–64]. It is unlikely that a paper mask would offer protection from particles this small, but several serosurveys of dentists and orthopedic surgeons [65] who use these instruments regularly show no increased risk of HIV infection in these groups. No cases of HIV transmission from aerosolized tissue or blood have been confirmed. The source-control devices being used perform suctioning near the aerosolization of plumes by **smoke evacuators.** These consist of a vacuum pump, a HEPA filter, a hose, and an inlet nozzle. A **capture velocity** of 100–150 ft/min, with the inlet nozzle held within 2 in of the surgical site

[66,67], is recommended.

Control of the Water and Soil Environment

Water is a dynamic resource cycling between bodies of fresh water, the ground, the sea, and evaporation into the atmosphere and precipitation from the atmosphere. This is called the *hydrologic cycle*. Water can be contaminated at any point in the cycle but is most likely to be contaminated by the lower atmosphere during precipitation and on contact with (and runoff from) the soil. The least contaminated water is that found in **groundwater,** the zone of saturation deep in the soil and earth. The upper portion of this zone is the **water table,** which must be penetrated by wells in order to use groundwater sources. Thus the purest and most contaminated and polluted water on Earth may be separated only by a relatively thin layer of soil. This layer is nature's water filter, which **percolates** or **recharges** groundwater. It is at the mercy of humans and civilization and is violated by septic tanks and wells. The outermost layer of soil, which can generate dust, is called the *surficial level.*

Preschool-age children usually eat a certain amount of soil and dust purposefully or during play. This averages a few hundred milligrams per day, more in children with nutritional deficiencies or pica. Gardening, some turf sports, and many occupations pose a risk for swallowing or inhaling dust and soil. Pollutants such as metals and organic toxins may be of greater concern than microorganisms, however. Soil, of course, is a major route of entry of infectious agents for many animals and grazing livestock.

"Night soil" is the historical, polite name for human excreta, which may contaminant soil or spill into wells or other water sources. The protection of water involves both the treatment of drinking water and the control and containment of human garbage and fecal waste (**sewage**).

The reader is referred to other sources [68,69] for in-depth discussions of water treatment, sanitation technology, and regulations. Chlorination and other treatments of drinking water have been the most important technologies in reducing infectious disease in the last century. The time-tested yardstick of fecal contamination of drinking water is the **coliform determination,** or culturing of those organisms found most frequently in the colon of human and other warm-blooded animals. Col-

iform bacteria serve as the **indicator organisms** of fecal contamination. High coliform counts on cultures signify inadequate treatment of water or point contamination after treatment. Various enteric viruses (e.g., HAV, polioviruses, and coxsackieviruses), as well as echo-, reo-, rota-, and Norwalk viruses, may contaminate water. Standard or economical tests for quality control of viral contamination have not been developed, nor do practical tests exist for the protozoans of concern (*Giardia lamblia, Cryptosporidium,* and *Cyclospora*), which were responsible for very large outbreaks in the 1990s.

The 1989 Surface Water Treatment Rules (ESWTRs) established stricter baseline filtration, disinfection, and pathogen-removal requirements for surface water in response to *Giardia* and viral infections. They also created a schedule of new contaminants and pollutants to be regulated over the turn of the millennium. ESWTRs did not specifically cover groundwater drinking sources nor adequately address *Cryptosporidium* or more heavily contaminated water. We have entered a new era of conflict between the microbial rules for drinking water and concern with the **microbial and disinfection by-products (M-DBPs).** These include trihalomethanes such as chloroform, haloacetic acids, bromates, chlorite, and other by-products of water treatment that may be toxic and/or carcinogenic.

The greatest single threat to the water supply is flooding because of the resulting mixing of sewage with drinking water supplies. For rescue agency workers or contractors working in postflood areas, it also may pose the greatest occupational threat from water contamination.

In an emergency, any water suspected of being contaminated with bacteria may be treated with any of the following treatments:

1. Vigorous boiling for 20 minutes
2. Chlorine tablet, 1 per quart
3. Chlorine bleach, 2 drops per quart, then letting the water stand for 30 minutes
4. Iodine tablets, 1 per quart, and then letting the water stand for 30 minutes
5. Tincture of iodine, 2% USP, 5 drops per quart, and then letting water stand for 30 minutes (water should be cool)

Note that these processes are for the treatment of water contamination by infectious agents. They will not reduce chemical or metal pollutants. More information on waterborne infections is presented elsewhere in this book.

Control of Food Vehicles

It is important for occupational and environmental health clinicians to be familiar with infection controls for food processing and preparation for the following reasons:

1. Although few domestic cases of food poisoning are adjudicated as workers' compensation, they may be covered by workers' compensation if a worker travels in the course of employment. The clinician should be familiar with the principles of protection from food-borne contaminants and have the knowledge to serve as a resource for employers and workers.
2. Infectious-agent poisonings may be considered in the differential diagnosis for the evaluation of acute illness in workers.
3. Agriculture and food services is the largest industry in the United States and most other nations. Occupational physicians should have a basic understanding of food workers' roles and be members of the team needed to deliver safe produce and food products.

The protection of food from contamination by infectious agents should be practiced at every stage in the planting, growth, harvesting, processing, packaging, distributing, displaying, and preparing of food. The surfaces of foods can be contaminated by soil, insects, rodents, and aerosols from coughing or sneezing and by the hands or body fluids of food handlers. Almost all diseases caused by the ingestion of soil or water also can contaminate food. Milk is the food vehicle that has been most difficult to control and thus has been regulated progressively for well over a century. Milk and dairy products rightfully should be considered "body fluids" and a superb culture media. About two dozen diseases, including brucellosis, tuberculosis, and Q fever, have been associated with diseased cattle or milk. Milk is also very susceptible to contamination after pasteurization. Mastitis of cows has been caused by various streptococci, staphylococci, *Pasteurella* species, and *Listeria monocytogenes*. Traces

of antibiotics used to treat mastitis may become milk pollutants or allergens. *Campylobacter* and various *Salmonella* species are found in high concentration in cattle, pigs, chickens, and the agricultural environment. Controlling these agents so that livestock, milk, and dairy products are not infected has proved difficult and sometimes impossible.

All foods contain some bacteria, although most are not pathogenic. Bacteria are used in the processing of many foods, including *Lactobacillus* for sauerkraut, *Acetobacter* for vinegar, and various yeasts for bread and beer, but many pathogenic bacteria can grow in foods at or around room temperatures. Even refrigerated foods eventually spoil owing to the psychrophilic organisms that can grow at 32–40°F (0–5°C).

The solute content of food also can affect growth. For instance, the microbial cells must compete with solutes such as sodium chloride for the **available water (a_w)** in food. With the exception of *S. aureus,* bacteria are rather poor competitors, whereas molds are excellent. Table 3-30 shows the decrease in water activity with salinity. Most infectious agents have a specific range of a_w that will support their growth. Greater solute content may not kill bacteria, only inhibit or halt its growth. Processed foods such as canned soup tend to be very high in salt content and may require the addition of water before preparation.

However, temperature and a_w have an inverse relationship because more heat is required to inhibit bacteria as the a_w becomes lowered. But the pH also affects growth. The interplay between these factors can be used in food-preservation technology. *Clostridium. botulinum* will not grow in a food with a pH below 5.0 *and* an a_w of less than 0.935, although it would grow without the two in combina-

Table 3-30
Salinity and Water Activity in Food (Available Water)

Percent NaCl	Water Activity (a_w)
0.9	0.99+
1.7	0.99
3.5	0.98
7.0	0.96
10.0	0.94
13.0	0.92
16.0	0.90
22.0	0.86

tion. This is called the *hurdle effect* and is a basic concept of food processing. It requires experimentation to determine the properties of each food and the processing needed to inhibit microbial growth in it and preserve its quality.

The use of disinfectants and sanitizers on food-preparation surfaces is also important and is similar to the medical disinfection and sterilization technology previously described. The personal hygiene and training of food workers are just as important, however.

An in-depth discussion of food-protection technology is available in other texts [68,70]. There are also many excellent food-safety resources available on the Internet, including the *Bad Bug Book* (Figure 3-12) published by the FDA (available at *http://vm .cfsan.fda.gov/~mow/intro.html*). This website lists the most prevalent infectious agents in food and gives a detailed description of each. An excellent table of the onset, duration, and symptoms of food-borne illness is available for use in the differential diagnosis of suspected food-borne illness *http://vm.cfsan.fda.gov/~mow/app2.html*). Recent well-publicized adverse food events, such as deaths from *E. coli* 0:157, *Salmonella* content of chickens, and the "new" pathogenic protozoa *Cyclospora cayetanensis* found in imported strawberries, all have heightened public interest in food safety. One example of a conjoint public and private food-safety campaign is the Fight BAC! program by the Partnership for Food Safety Education (Figures 3-13 and 3-14).

Training programs and certifications for food service professionals have expanded with the **Hazard Analysis Critical Control Points (HACCP) courses.** A list of training courses is available at www.haccpalliance.org/alliance/training.html. There is very little controversy concerning the principles of food-poisoning prevention at the consumer level. The 10 basic principles are presented in Table 3-31. Employer- or company-sponsored picnics or "pitch-ins" may reduce liability and other losses owing to food poisoning by posting warnings about this problem before such events.

Global Food Status. According to the Food and Agriculture Organization (FAO) of the United Nations, 25% of all global food production is lost to insect infestation, rodents, bacteria, molds, and premature germination. Food-borne bacteria are responsible for 9,000 deaths and up to 80 million

Table 3-31

Ten Principles of Food Poisoning Prevention

1. Keep hot foods hot, and cold foods cold. Refrigerated food should be well below 40°F (5°C) and cooked food above 165°F (74°C).
2. Do grocery shopping trips last, on the way home. Pick cold and frozen foods last. Most groceries now have these items last in the market loop aisles.
3. Keep thermometers visible; and set at under 40°F (5°C) in the refrigerator and under 0°F (−18°C) in the freezer.
4. Thaw meat in the refrigerator or in water-tight bags in water, and never let it sit out (unrefrigerated) more than two hours.
5. Refrigerate leftovers immediately. Reheat them to high temperatures.
6. Keep ice chests cold on picnics and camping trips. Both have high associations with food poisonings.
7. Pay special attention to creams, custards, mayonnaise, pudding, yogurt, or any dairy products left sitting out or open.
8. Cutting boards and counter tops in contact with raw foods should be cleaned with bleach and hot water to avoid cross-contamination.
9. Wash hands before and after eating or preparing meals.
10. When in doubt, throw it out!

cases of diarrheal illness in the United States alone. Data are less accurate globally, but diarrhea is the leading cause of infant death. The inability of nations to satisfy each other's food quarantine and health regulations is often a barrier to trade. Food laws are often misused for political agendas.

Food Irradiation. The irradiation of food was first performed in 1905, but it was perfected in the 1940s and 1950s. Health and safety officials from 39 countries have approved the irradiation of some 40 types of foods. This technology has helped address many long-standing and global food problems. The people of the United States are far behind most nations in their acceptance of irradiated products because of myths and fears regarding nuclear technology. The first international acceptance was the 1983 **Codex Alimentarius Commission** issued by a joint expert committee of the FAO, the World Health Organization (WHO), and the International Atomic Energy Agency [72]. The Codex declared that irradiation up to 10 kGy (106 rads) posed no toxic, nutritional, or microbiologic hazards and that no further testing was needed.

Most irradiation of food employs gamma rays and the cobalt-60 radioisotope. Cobalt-60 is produced by neutron bombardment of cobalt-59 and then is double encapsulated into "pencils" for use at irradiation plants. It has a half-life of only 5.3 years. No other source of radiation has proved as

Figure 3-12
The FDA "Bad Bug Book"

This handbook provides basic facts regarding foodborne pathogenic microorganisms and natural toxins. It brings together in one place information from the Food & Drug Administration, the Centers for Disease Control & Prevention, the USDA Food Safety Inspection Service, and the National Institutes of Health.

Some technical terms have been linked to the National Library of Medicine's Entrez glossary. Recent articles from Morbidity and Mortality Weekly Reports have been added to selected chapters to update the handbook with information on later outbreaks or incidents of foodborne disease. At the end of selected chapters on pathogenic microorganisms, hypertext links are included to relevant Entrez abstracts and GenBank genetic loci. A more complete description of the handbook may be found in the Preface

PATHOGENIC BACTERIA
Salmonella spp.
Clostridium botulinum
Staphylococcus aureus
Campylobacter jejuni
Yersinia enterocolitica and Yersinia pseudotuberculosis
Listeria monocytogenes
Vibrio cholerae O1
Vibrio cholerae non-O1
Vibrio parahaemolyticus and other vibrios
Vibrio vulnificus
Clostridium perfringens
Bacillus cereus
Aeromonas hydrophila and other spp.
Plesiomonas shigelloides
Shigella spp.
Miscellaneous enterics
Streptococcus

ENTEROVIRULENT ESCHERICHIA COLI GROUP (EEC Group)
Escherichia coli—enterotoxigenic (ETEC)
Escherichia coli—enteropathogenic (EPEC)
Escherichia coli O157:H7 enterohemorrhagic (EHEC)
Escherichia coli—enteroinvasive (EIEC)

PARASITIC PROTOZOA and WORMS
Giardia lamblia
Entamoeba histolytica
Cryptosporidium parvum
Cyclospora cayetanensis
Anisakis sp. and related worms
Diphyllobothrium spp.
Nanophyetus spp.

Eustrongylides sp.
Acanthamoeba and other free-living amoebae
Ascaris lumbricoides and Trichuris trichiura

VIRUSES
Hepatitis A virus
Hepatitis E virus
Rotavirus
Norwalk virus group
Other viral agents
NATURAL TOXINS
Ciguatera poisoning
Shellfish toxins (PSP, DSP, NSP, ASP)
Scombroid poisoning
Tetrodotoxin (Pufferfish)
Mushroom toxins
Aflatoxins
Pyrrolizidine alkaloids
Phytohaemagglutinin (Red kidney bean poisoning)
Grayanotoxin (Honey intoxication)
Gempylotoxin (Gastrointestinal illness from consumption of Escolar and Oilfish)

OTHER PATHOGENIC AGENTS
Prions

APPENDICES
Infective dose
Epidemiology summary table
Factors affecting microbial growth in foods
Foodborne Disease Outbreaks, United States 1988–1992
Additional Foodborne Disease Outbreak Articles and Databases.

Source: http://vm.cfsan.fda.gov/~mow.intro.html, with hyperlinks to more information on foodborne pathogens microorganisms.

Figure 3-13
Four general principles for the consumer to avoid cross-contamination of food.

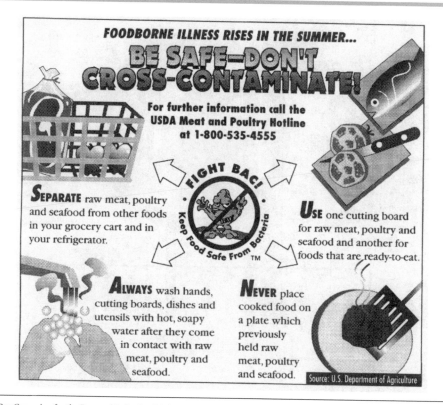

Source: Fight-Bac Campaign for the Partnership for Food Safety Education.

economical, safe, or effective. The food is passed by conveyor belts through the energy field; dosage, belt speed, and energy are specific for each food. The food receives energy but does not itself become radioactive. The main purpose of food irradiation is to kill bacteria that may be in a growth cycle. DNA is far more sensitive to radiation energy than nutrients such as nucleoproteins, carbohydrates, fats, enzymes, and vitamins. Even damage of only a few percent of bacterial DNA will stop replication. Irradiation with dosages of up to 10 kGy is called *radurization* or *radicidation* and is the upper limit currently approved. This dosage is sufficient to kill *Salmonella, Campylobacter, B. cereus, S. aureus*, fungi, and protozoal cysts. *C. botulinum* may survive, but the number of organisms is reduced, and the pathogen becomes more sensitive to heat, pH, and salt. Complete sterilization using much higher doses is called *radappertization.*

Irradiation of food produces **radiolytic products.** These are mostly natural metabolites such as acetaldehyde, carbon dioxide, glucose, peroxide, and formic acid. They are also naturally present in foods and may be generated by heat processing or cooking. Irradiation causes the formation of unstable and reactive free radicals but in less volume than that resulting from toasting, frying, and freeze drying [73]. In any case, the free radicals are inactivated by liquids such as saliva. No mutagenic effects have been found in animals fed heavily irradiated food.

Food irradiation is not meant to substitute for **good manufacturing practices (GMPs).** Food is still subject to surface contamination after treatment, and irradiation cannot make spoiled or bad food into good food. Furthermore, radiation does not kill all preformed bacterial toxins nor all viruses.

112

Figure 3-14
Front and back side of brochure on the four simple steps to food safety.

Fight BAC!™

Four Simple Steps to Food Safety

Apply the Heat...and *Fight BAC!*™

Cooking food to the proper temperature kills harmful bacteria. So *Fight BAC!*™ by thoroughly cooking your food as follows:

Raw Food	Internal Temperature
Ground Products	
Hamburger	160°F
Beef, veal, lamb, pork	160°F
Chicken, turkey	165°F
Beef, Veal, Lamb	
Roasts & Steaks	
medium-rare	145°F
medium	160°F
well-done	170°F
Pork	
Chops, roasts, ribs	160°F
medium	160°F
well-done	170°F
Ham, fresh	160°F
Sausage, fresh	160°F
Poultry	
Chicken, whole & pieces	180°F
Duck	180°F
Turkey *(unstuffed)*	180°F
Whole	180°F
Breast	170°F
Dark meat	180°F
Stuffing (cooked separately)	165°F
Eggs	
Fried, poached	*Yolk & white are firm*
Casseroles	160°F
Sauces, custards	160°F

This chart has been adapted for home use and is consistent with customer guidelines from the U.S. Department of Agriculture (USDA) and U.S. Food & Drug Administration (FDA).

Be a BAC Fighter

Although an invisible enemy may be in your kitchen, you have four powerful tools to *Fight BAC!*™: washing hands and surfaces often, avoiding cross-contamination, cooking to proper temperatures, and refrigerating promptly. So, be a BAC Fighter and make the meals and snacks from your kitchen as safe as possible.

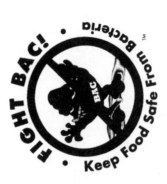

FIGHT BAC!™ • Keep Food Safe From • Bacteria™

For More Information About Safe Food Handling and Preparation

USDA's Meat and Poultry Hotline
1-800-535-4555

FDA's Food Information and Seafood Hotline
1-800-332-4010

Partnership for Food Safety Education Web Site
www.fightbac.org

Or contact your local cooperative extension office.

Right now, there may be an invisible enemy ready to strike. He's called BAC (bacteria) and he can make you and those you care about sick. In fact, even though you can't see BAC — or smell him, or feel him — he and millions more like him may have already invaded the food you eat.

But you have the power to *Fight BAC!™* and to keep your food safe from harmful bacteria. It's as easy as following these four simple steps:

Clean:
Wash hands and surfaces often

Bacteria can spread throughout the kitchen and get onto cutting boards, utensils, sponges and counter tops. Here's how to *Fight BAC!™*

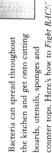

■ Wash your hands with hot soapy water before handling food and after using the bathroom, changing diapers and handling pets.

■ Wash your cutting boards, dishes, utensils and counter tops with hot soapy water after preparing each food item and before you go on to the next food.

■ Use plastic or other non-porous cutting boards. These boards should be run through the dishwasher — or washed in hot soapy water — after use.

■ Consider using paper towels to clean up kitchen surfaces. If you use cloth towels, wash them often in the hot cycle of your washing machine.

Separate:
Don't cross-contaminate

Cross-contamination is the scientific word for how bacteria can be spread from one food product to another. This is especially true when handling raw meat, poultry and seafood, so keep these foods and their juices away from ready-to-eat foods. Here's how to *Fight BAC!™*

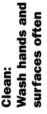

■ Separate raw meat, poultry and seafood from other foods in your grocery shopping cart and in your refrigerator.

■ If possible, use a different cutting board for raw meat products.

■ Always wash hands, cutting boards, dishes and utensils with hot soapy water after they come in contact with raw meat, poultry and seafood.

■ Never place cooked food on a plate which previously held raw meat, poultry and seafood.

Cook:
Cook to proper temperatures

Food safety experts agree that foods are properly cooked when they are heated for a long enough time and at a high enough temperature to kill the harmful bacteria that cause foodborne illness. The best way to *Fight BAC!™* is to:

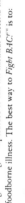

■ Use a clean thermometer, which measures the internal temperature of cooked foods, to make sure meat, poultry, casseroles and other foods are cooked all the way through.

■ Cook roasts and steaks to at least 145°F. Whole poultry should be cooked to 180°F for doneness.

■ Cook ground beef, where bacteria can spread during processing, to at least 160°F. Information from the Centers for Disease Control and Prevention (CDC) link eating undercooked, pink ground beef with a higher risk of illness. If a thermometer is not available, do not eat ground beef that is still pink inside.

■ Cook eggs until the yolk and white are firm. Don't use recipes in which eggs remain raw or only partially cooked.

■ Fish should be opaque and flake easily with a fork.

■ When cooking in a microwave oven, make sure there are no cold spots in food where bacteria can survive . For best results, cover food, stir and rotate for even cooking. If there is no turntable, rotate the dish by hand once or twice during cooking.

■ Bring sauces, soups and gravy to a boil when reheating. Heat other leftovers thoroughly to at least 165°F.

Chill:
Refrigerate promptly

Refrigerate foods quickly because cold temperatures keep harmful bacteria from growing and multiplying. So, set your refrigerator no higher than 40°F and the freezer unit at 0°F. Check these temperatures occasionally with an appliance thermometer. Then, *Fight BAC!™* by following these steps:

■ Refrigerate or freeze perishables, prepared foods and leftovers within two hours or sooner.

■ Never defrost food at room temperature. Thaw food in the refrigerator, under cold running water or in the microwave. Marinate foods in the refrigerator.

■ Divide large amounts of leftovers into small, shallow containers for quick cooling in the refrigerator.

■ Don't pack the refrigerator. Cool air must circulate to keep food safe.

Source: Fight-Bac Campaign of the Partnership for Food Safety Education.

For most foods, the color and odor produced by bacteria are the warnings of spoilage. However, studies by European and Scandinavian countries have shown no increased risk of food spoilage after bacteria have been irradiated. Note that pasteurization, freezing, and preservatives used in food processing also destroy some bacteria. Although the shelf life of produce may be prolonged, the look and smell of spoilage are the same in irradiated food as those in nonirradiated food. Other theoretical advantages of food irradiation are less dependence on insecticides, fumigants, preservatives, or other pollutants of food and lower energy costs for refrigeration. In reality, however, these methods of control are still used in conjunction with irradiation.

Control of the Animate Reservoir. ARTHROPOD CONTROL. The largest attempts to control animate vectors of infectious agents (e.g., viruses, parasites, and rickettsiae) in their natural environment has involved arthropods. Although some good control of arthropod-transmitted diseases has occurred, human-made changes in the environment or wars often promote their resurgence. Arthropods that are associated with human diseases include fleas, flies, lice, mites, roaches, mosquitoes, and ticks. Flies and roaches can transmit infectious organisms mechanically, especially enteric fecal-oral pathogens such as those causing typhoid, *Shigella*, and *V. cholerae.*

Most of the science of controlling arthropods is related to their ranges, climactic requirements and preferences, geologic boundaries, and seasons. Routine surveillance and surveys of mosquito populations are conducted in most areas by trained and licensed public employees or contractors. Studies of larval samples from artificial or still bodies of water also are conducted. Various traps are available for capturing adult mosquitoes. Arthropod **vector abundance** is measured several ways, such as the number of mosquitoes caught per **light-trap night.** Measured overabundance of a specific vector species may predict human outbreaks of the disease it causes.

Larvicides, fogging units, and mists are used in specific areas of **harborage** of mosquitoes, and these efforts are increased when populations and thus the risk for transmission of infection increases. However, these **chemical controls** are the least preferred because of environmental concerns and the development of resistance to the chemicals. Other controls have included **biologic controls,**

such as introducing arthropod parasites, natural insect predators, and minnow fish to eat larva. Building reservoirs and ditches that maintain some movement of water (**mechanical control**) to prevent stagnation is the best single prevention because larvae must have still water to complete their life cycle. Migrating birds play a role in distributing viruses associated with mosquitoes and encephalitis. Only a few species of birds suffer illness from mosquito bites and viremia. Trying to control the arboviruses in their wild primary host would prove most difficult.

Human vaccines have been developed for only a few of the arthropod-vector diseases, but horses are immunized routinely for Venezuela (VEE), eastern (EEE), and western (WEE) equine encephalitis. The majority of arthropod-borne viral infections do not have vaccines or effective therapies. Other forms of control and prevention of arthropod-associated infections are covered in the chapters of the text on malaria (see Chapter 25), meningitis (see Chapter 23), and travel (see Chapters 27–32).

RODENT CONTROL. **Murine rodents** are those that live and feed on the fringes of the human habitat—the house mouse, roof rat, and Norway rat. Wild rodents are the principal hosts of many tick (larval and nymphal stages) diseases, including some forms of tick-borne encephalitis and other illnesses (e.g., Kyasanur Forest and Crimean-Congo hemorrhagic fever and Powassan and Colorado tick fever). Adult ticks more often bite large animals, including humans. Rodents can serve as reservoirs for hantavirus and leptospires, transmitting infection through their dried urine and feces. Fortunately, rodents have a rather limited local range and a predictable environment. Methods of rodent control include isolation, substitution, treatment, shielding, and prevention. Prevention involves the removal of food sources, places of harborage, and adequate maintenance. It often involves training of humans to control rodents' food stores and wastes, including pet foods. Structural integrity and the removal of debris or supplies that may serve as harborage areas for rodents should be part of the eradication process and ongoing preventive maintenance. Community and local resident education is essential to ongoing prevention in residential areas.

The safest rodent poisons are the anticoagulants. They take several days to work, and the rodents rarely learn to associate the bait with the illness. Some rodenticides are too toxic to be used inside. In areas where the presence of hantavirus is suspected, cleanup should be done with personal protective equipment (PPE), including HEPA-filter respirators, disposable coveralls, and shoe covers. All PPE should be decontaminated or destroyed after use.

ZOONOSIS CONTROL. Most animals on Earth have their own pathogenic infectious agents. Relatively few also can infect humans. One disease— brucellosis—can serve as an excellent, nearly ideal model for the control of zoonotic diseases. Brucellosis (also known as *Mediterranean, Malta,* or *undulant fever*) is a complex of diseases caused by small gram-negative rods that infect a wide range of domestic and wild mammals. Besides the wide range of animals, it can infect a wide range of tissues and organs through a wide range of portals of entry, portals of exit, and modes of transmission. The differential diagnosis for brucellosis is further complicated by its relatively long and variable incubation period, range of symptoms, and spontaneous relapses and remissions. Doubtless thousands of human cases remain undiagnosed and untreated around the world.

Brucella species include *B. abortus* (cattle), *B. suis* (swine), *B. canis* (cats and dogs), and *B. melitensis* (sheep and goats). Besides animal-to-animal, sexual, and other routes of transmission, the pathogen is transmitted between domestic and wild animals (e.g., cattle, caribou, dogs, and coyotes). Humans may be infected by handling infected tissues, aborted fetuses and placentas, blood, urine, discharges, and other body fluids, as well as by ingestion of contaminated milk or cheese. There is a high association of the infection with occupations that involve handling animals or animal products and with hunting, in which dead game is handled. The bacteriologist Alice Evans, who did most of the pioneering studies of the disease, was occupationally infected and suffered brucellosis relapses for 20 years. Humans can contract the infection by ingestion, mucous membrane or sexual organ contact, the bloodborne route, and by minor percutaneous injuries. Hundreds of clinical laboratory workers were occupationally infected before the use of biologic safety cabinets was introduced, suggesting aerosol transmission as well. Completing brucellosis's claim to being the "perfect" zoonotic disease is the fact that it can remain viable and infectious in the environment (soil) for up to 125 days and in carcasses for 135 days.

Brucellosis also serves as a superb model for infection control at the agent, host, environment, and transmission levels. Where research, regulation, and other intervention efforts have been implemented, the disease has become rare. Less than 100 cases occur in the United States each year. Some of the methods and principles of control for brucellosis are presented in Table 3-32. Brucellosis should rank high in the differential diagnosis for any fever of unknown origin in a worker with occupational risks for the disease.

Levels of Control for Zoonotic Diseases. Most nations have their own restrictions and quarantine laws for handling animal species. Many have specific holding areas and mandatory inspections. Regulations may be imposed to protect local livestock, pets, and native species from infectious agents. All municipalities in the United States have rabies vaccination laws for pets (see Chapter 20).

HIGH-TECHNOLOGY APPLICATIONS FOR ANIMATE RESERVOIR CONTROL. The National Aeronautics and Space Administration (NASA) and the National Institute of Allergy and Infectious Diseases (NIAID) have cooperatively funded grants for the development of remote sensing and geographic

Table 3-32
Brucellosis as an Example of Integrated Controls

1. Eradication of the agent
   - By antibiotics (tetracycline, streptomycin, rifampin) at the level of the human host or the animal host after definitive or presumed diagnosis.
   - By laws requiring pasteurization, of the animal body fluid known as milk.
2. Eradication of the host(s):
   - By slaughtering the infected host herd (swine or cattle).
3. Control of the environment
   - By establishing and enforcing aggressive control laws, the disease is eliminated from the host and eventually from the environment (i.e., placental or body fluid contamination of the pasture's soil is eliminated after a four-month quarantine of the unused pasture). This may be done by fencing (a barrier or a containment).
   - By totally eliminating the disease from the environment through the use of administrative controls and regulation (e.g., those of the Scandinavian countries).
4. Control of transmission
   - By immunizing domestic animals and thus making them nonsusceptible if exposed to soil, wild animals, or infected cohorts. An adequate vaccine does not exist for humans.
   - By use of personal protective equipment (e.g., long-arm rubber gloves while delivering cattle).
   - By education. Training animal and agricultural workers on the risks for the disease and how to prevent transmission. Also by basic training of physicians and veterinarians about the disease and how to recognize cases.

information system (RS/GIS) technologies to control infectious diseases [75]. The purpose is to predict future disease outbreaks and identify areas where specific control programs should be concentrated.

Projects have included using aerial multispectral videography to detect electromagnetic radiation from ground objects in the Ohio Valley. Known tire dumps and their infrared "fingerprints" are used to detect the location of other tire dumps from aerial studies. This technology is used to estimate the size of dumps, which can be up to 50 million tires in size. Water remaining in tires serves as a breeding ground for mosquitoes. Tire dump cleanups pose risks for cleanup workers when they are abated. Satellites have been used to study ocean height, temperature, and phytoplankton and zooplankton blooms in the Indian Ocean off India and Bangladesh both before and after the 2005 tsunami. These blooms can harbor cholera, and measurable variables of the blooms have been correlated with outbreaks. Other RS/GIS grantees have included [75]

- Yale grantees' study of specific vegetation and landscape patterns in residential Westchester County, New York, the major hot spot of tick-borne Lyme disease
- Studies of hantavirus host (rodent) habitats in the Southwest
- Studies of Brazilian environmental factors that correlate with leishmaniasis and schistosomiasis
- Studies of the distribution of helminthic diseases in China
- Studies of the epidemiology of malaria in Mali

CONTROLLING HOST RESPONSE

Controlling the human host response to infectious disease is the domain of clinical medicine. Unfortunately, infectious disease still represents a large proportion of the practice of medicine. Specific antimicrobial treatments and prophylaxis are discussed in other chapters.

Wellness and Susceptibility

Two of the most rapidly expanding fields of interest and knowledge in clinical medicine are the human immune system and the effects of physical activity. The 1996 release of the Surgeon General's Report on Physical Activity and Health summarizes, by organ system, the positive relationship between activity and health [76]. The effects of various forms of stress on the human immune system are irrefutable. A PubMed search for review articles associating stress with immunity published just in the English language since 1990 retrieves over 300 reviews averaging nearly 100 references each. Every known part of the human immune system response is significantly affected by stress. The veterinary literature confirms the same associations in animals studies. It may be that the improved life span of AIDS patients may be due in part to increased social acceptance of the disease.

This is not surprising to experienced corporate-based occupational health practitioners. Workplace stressors such as mandatory overtime, layoffs, management changes, mergers, military base closures and realignments, and even the rumors of such have an impact on absenteeism and illness owing to infectious diseases. These adverse health effects are too often dismissed as "blue flu," "mass psychogenic illness," or "well-disguised job actions." The associations between workplace stress and immunity have been inadequately studied.

The better studies of the relationship between stressors and infectious diseases have come from college health services. A large serial study of one class of cadets attending the U.S. Military Academy at West Point correlated many factors with the risk of development of clinically apparent infectious mononucleosis in cadets first infected with EBV [77]. Illness was significantly predicted to occur in cadets who had overachieving fathers and a strong personal motivation and commitment to and identification with a military career, coupled with a relatively poor academic performance. The study corrected for all other socioeconomic and demographic data.

CONTROLLING TRANSMISSION: INTERRUPTION

> The bugs are many; but your doors and windows are few.
>
> —*Daymon Evans (I just made it up.)*

Despite the thousands of known infectious agents contaminating almost every square inch of the Earth and with essentially every multicellular organism in life serving as a host, humans can be protected by adherence to a few basic principles. Transmission is the weakest point in the epidemiologic triad and is broken by any blockage of the portal of entry, the portal of exit, or another break in the transmission of viable infectious agents into a susceptible host or from an infecting host. Controlling the agent within the host or environment is much more difficult than controlling the transmission.

Transporting Infectious Agents

Several agencies regulate the movement of infectious agents and vectors of human disease. These include the Public Health Service Foreign Quarantine Regulations and the Department of Transportation. The U.S. Department of Agriculture regulates the importation and interstate shipment of animal pathogens and prohibits the importation, possession, or use of certain exotic animal disease agents that pose a serious disease threat to domestic livestock and poultry. Figure 3-15 shows the required packing and labeling of etiologic agents [78].

Models of Transmission Control

This chapter presents two models for preventing transmission of infection, although both are covered elsewhere in this book. These models reflect the principles of **containment** and **isolation,** as demonstrated and practiced by **laboratory biosafety levels (BSLs)** [79] and the CDC's **hospi-**tal isolation categories [80]. Both sets of principles govern the safety of workers and the general public.

Containment (Biosafety). The best model for the containment (rather than destruction) of infectious agents is the microbiology laboratory and shipping laws regarding infectious agents. **Primary containment** is the protection of personnel and their immediate environment from exposure to infectious agents. **Secondary containment** is the protection of the environment external to the laboratory. The three elements of laboratory containment of infectious agents are (1) laboratory practice and technique, (2) safety equipment, and (3) facility designs. Each is covered in Chapter 33.

Biosafety is defined as the application of specific safety protocols to the handling of biologic risks, both specimens of infectious agents and animals that may be infected. The full force of biosafety levels includes a combination of engineering controls, administrative controls, work practices and procedures, and on occasion, medical interventions.

All infectious agents are classified by risk into **biosafety levels** 1 through 4 (BSLs 1–4) for microbiologic and biomedical laboratories (Table 3-33). Four categories of risk also are used for the

Figure 3-15
Proper biosafety packaging and labeling of an etiologic agent for transport.

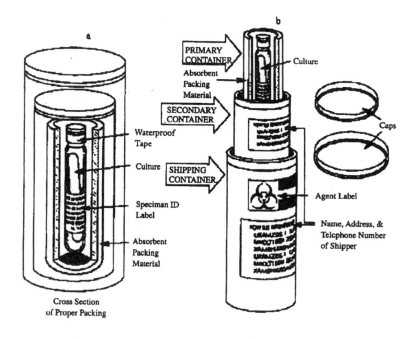

Source: Available at www.cdc.gov/od/ohs.biosfty/brnbl/fig4/gif.

Table 3-33
Summary of Biosafety Levels (BSLs)

Biosafety Levels (BSLs) for Infectious Agents

BSL	Agents	Practices	Safety Equipment (Primary Barriers)	Facilities (Secondary Barriers)
1	Not known to cause disease in healthy adults	Standard microbiologic practices (SMP): Wash hands before/after; no eat, drink, smoke, or cosmetics; no mouth pipetting; clean surfaces; splash spill precautions; biohazard disposal.	None. Biologic Safety Cabinet (BSC) not required.	Open Bench top sink.
2	Associated with human disease, a hazard of auto-inoculation, ingestion, or mucous membrane exposure	SMP plus "Limited Access, Biohazard" signage, sharps precautions, biosafety manual (BSM) defining needed water decontamination or medical surveillance.	BSC 1 or 2, containment of all devices with potential splash or aerosolizing capacity. PPEs of lab coats, gloves, face protection.	BSL 1 plus autoclave or other sterilization available.
3	Indigenous or exotic agents with potential for aerosol transmission; disease may have serious or lethal consequences	BSL 2 plus "Controlled Access"; decontamination of all waste and clothing before laundering; baseline serology on worker.	BSC 1 or 2, all manipulations done with containment devices. PPE: protective lab clothing, gloves, respiratory protection as needed.	BSL 2 plus physical separation from access corridors; self-closing double doors; exhausted air (not recirculated). Negative airflow into laboratory.
4	Dangerous/exotic agents that pose high risk of life-threatening disease. Aerosol-transmitted lab infections or related agents with unknown risk of transmission.	BSL 3 plus clothing change before entering; shower on exit. All material decontaminated on exit from facility.	All primary barriers plus all procedures in a BSC 3, or ½ with full-body air-supplied positive-pressure personnel suit.	BSL 3 plus separate building, or isolated zone. Dedicated supply/exhaust vacuum and decontaminated systems.

Vertebrate Animal Biosafety Levels (ABLSs) for Infectious Agents

BSL	Agents	Practices	Safety Equipment (Primary Barriers)	Facilities (Secondary Barriers)
1	Not known to cause disease in healthy human adults	Standard animal care and management practices, including appropriate medical surveillance programs.	As required for normal care of each species.	Standard animal facility nonrecirculation of exhausted air; directional air flow recommended.
2	Associated with human disease. Hazard: ingestion, percutaneous and mucous membrane exposure	ABSL-1 practices, limited access; biohazard warning signs; sharps precautions; biosafety manual; decontamination of all infectious wastes and of animal cages prior to washing.	ABSL-1 equipment, primary barriers; containment equipment appropriate for animal species; PPE: lab coats, gloves, face and respiratory protection as required.	ABSL-1 facility plus autoclave available; hand-washing sink available in the animal room.
3	Indigenous or exotic agents with potential for aerosol transmission; disease may have serious health effects	ABSL-2 practices, controlled access; decontamination of clothing before laundering; cages decontaminated before bedding removed; disinfectant foot bath as needed.	ABSL-2 equipment, containment equipment for housing animals and cage dumping, class ½ BSCs for procedures (inoculation, necropsy) that may > infectious aerosols. PPEs: appropriate respiratory protection.	ABSL-2, facility, physical separation from access corridors; self-closing double doors, access sealed penetration; sealed windows autoclave available in facility.
4	Dangerous/exotic agents that pose high risk of life-threatening disease; aerosol transmission, or related agents with unknown risk of transmission	ABSL-3 practices, entrance through change room where personal clothing removed and lab clothing on. Shower on exiting, all water decontaminated before removal from facility.	ABSL-3 equipment, maximum containment equipment (i.e., class 3 BSC or partial containment equipment with combination with full-body air-supplied positive pressure suit used for all procedures and activities.	ABSL-3 facility, separate building or isolated zone; dedicated supply/exhaust zone; vacuum and decontamination systems. Floor drains with traps and disinfectant. Windows sealed.

handling of animals (ABSLs 1–4) [81]. The principal piece of safety equipment in the laboratory is the **biologic safety cabinet (BSC).** The cabinet serves as an excellent model for the prevention of all types of transmission. These cabinets are the ultimate invention for local source-control, or containment, techniques. These techniques include

- *Air transmission* by the use of controlled directional flow away from workers' respiratory portals of entry and through HEPA filtration to be exhausted outside. BSCs use negative pressure as local source control.
- *Direct transmission* by the use of solid and see-through barriers that prevent exposure of workers' skin or mucous membranes to splashes or aerosolization. The surfaces are nonporous and can be cleaned easily. Direct transmission also requires various levels of personal protective equipment (e.g., gloves, goggles, and gowns).

BSCs are governed by regular inspection and maintenance schedules. Class 1 BSCs provide a basic barrier as well as splash protection and air-flow in the front and out of the top. Class 1 BSCs are not intended to protect the specimen or product. Levels 2, 3, and 4 are intended to protect the product/specimen and contain several subclasses, which are differentiated by design and airflow pattern. Class 3 is gas-sealed or airtight and exhausts externally through at least two HEPA filters.

Standard safe-laboratory practices and behavior are learned in training, which helps to prevent accidental transmission by the oral, mucous membrane, or percutaneous route. Protocols also exist for the disposal of cultures and other laboratory wastes in the secondary containment program. Only some viruses currently fall under BSL 4, and they are listed in Table 3-34. Only about 30 BSL 4 laboratories exist, including 8 in the United States. BSL 5 is referenced only in science fiction because BSL 4 represents maximum available technology.

Isolation and Quarantine. Isolation and quarantine are not synonymous. **Quarantine** is the restriction of the activities or habitat of well persons or animals (i.e., contacts) who have been exposed to a communicable agent. Quarantine should be for no longer than the maximum known period of incubation or infectivity of the specific pathogen. The purpose of quarantine is to protect the well and susceptible.

Table 3-34

Infectious Agents Requiring Biosafety Level 4 Containment

Bacteria
None
Fungi
None
Parasites
None
Viruses
Arenaviridae
Lassa, Junin, Machupo, Sabia, Guanarto
Bunyaviridaea
Genus *Nairovirus:* Crimean-Congo hemorrhagic fever
Filoviridae
Ebola
Marburg
Flaviviridae[a]
Tick-borne encephalitis complex
Russian spring-summer encephalitis
Kyasanur Forest
Omsk hemorrhagic fever
Herpesviridae
Alphaherpesviridae
Herpes simplex virus
Herpes B (monkey, simian)
Poxviridae
Orthopoxivirus
Variola
Monkeypox

[a]Arthropod-borne viruses.

There are quarantine laws for immigrants and imported animals in most countries. Authority to place U.S. citizens in strict or complete quarantine (usually only for tuberculosis) had been left to the states until 2005. In response to the anthrax attacks of 2001 and the fear of influenza or another global pandemic, federal regulations were enacted [82]. U.S. citizens are very rarely confined involuntarily. However, workers may be the subjects of "modified quarantine" from their workplace to protect patients in health care facilities. Terms such as *furlough, reassignment,* and *leave of absence* are used as synonyms for *modified quarantine* in these guidelines. An example is the removal of a health care worker with known or possible susceptibility to varicella from days 10–21 after an exposure or removal of a food service worker with HAV until 1 week after jaundice has subsided [8]. With the varicella and HAV vaccines now available, such removal should occur less frequently.

HISTORY OF HOSPITAL ISOLATION. The first recommendations for hospital isolation precautions were published in 1877 and ultimately resulted in special infectious disease hospitals. But nosocomial infections continued to occur because patients were not segregated by disease. By 1910, some aseptic practices were developed and the "cubicle," or multibed wards, were built to replace single open rooms in hospitals. This crude isolation system was called *barrier nursing.* It was not until the 1950s and 1960s that infectious disease hospitals and tuberculosis sanatoriums closed. Acute-care hospitals began developing isolation wards and rooms.

The first official manual of isolation precautions was published by the CDC in 1970 [83] and was revised for the first time in 1975 [84]. There were seven categories based on the existing knowledge of transmission. These were *strict isolation, respiratory isolation, protective ("reverse") isolation, enteric precautions, wound and skin precautions, discharge precautions,* and blood precautions. Color-coded stickers and signage were made for each category. However, the system did not protect against the development of nosocomial infections, nor was the effectiveness of the system studied empirically.

The next guidelines, written by interdisciplinary panels of experts, were published in 1983 [85]. They allowed hospital infection control committees to have some flexibility and clinicians to customize precautions to the specific disease and patient. *Protective isolation* was deleted because of lack of efficacy. *Blood precautions* was expanded to include other "body fluids." There were four categories of isolation—*strict, contact, respiratory,* and *tuberculosis/AFB*—and three categories of precautions—*enteric, drainage/secretion,* and *blood and body fluid.* Many questions and controversies persisted regarding diseases such as measles, rubella, respiratory syncytial virus, and influenza. All of these were inadequately isolated by the respiratory precautions.

Many addenda and other guidelines were published for specific diseases, including HIV **universal precautions (UPs)** (1985), hemorrhagic fever precautions (1988), parvovirus B-19 precautions (1989), and tuberculosis precautions (1990, 1993, 1994). Some nongovernment-affiliated experts initiated a **body substance isolation (BSI)** system that was adopted by many hospitals. It had the advantages of both ease and implementation but the disadvantage of being weak on precautions for airborne diseases, and it did not recommend routine hand washing if gloves had been worn. Thus the OSHA Bloodborne Pathogen Standard was implemented in 1991 [86], but confusion and conflict continued over the use of UPs versus BSI. Hand

washing (Table 3-35) is basic to all isolation principles.

PRESENT ISOLATION SYSTEMS. The most recent guidelines [80] have simplified the UPs and BSI principles into a single level called *standard precautions* (SPs). SPs simultaneously reduce the risk of both bloodborne and other pathogens. All the other previous categories of isolation and precautions are collapsed into a single set of **transmission-based precautions.** The three major types of hospital transmission (i.e., airborne, droplet, and contact) are recognized as more important than specific diagnoses or infectious body substances (Table 3-36). These precautions are consistent with the most recent thinking—that the mode of transmission is indeed the weak link in the epidemiologic triad.

Besides the airborne, droplet, and contact modes of transmission, however, one must not forget the common-vehicle and vector-borne modes of transmission. These modes of transmission are not generally considered nosocomial because they are covered by the "business as usual" or "institutional infrastructure" of general housekeeping, as well as insect and other vermin control. Common-source controls include the safe handling of food and water and the disinfection and sterilization of surfaces and equipment. These things are taken for granted by clinicians in U.S. hospitals. However, with the increasing prevalence of immunosuppressed patients and drug resistance in U.S. hospitals, they may be the subject of increasing clinician scrutiny and control in the future.

1996 and 2007 Transmission-Based Precautions. Standard precautions (SPs or Ss) synthesize the major features of UPs and BSI and apply them to all patients who receive care in hospitals regardless of

Table 3-35
Principles of Hand Washing in Health Care

1. Hands should be washed before and after gloving.
2. Gloves should never be substituted for hand washing.
3. Disposable gloves must not be reused.
4. Nonlatex and powder-free alternatives should be available for workers (and patients) with sensitivities to latex and/or powder.
5. Fingernails should be kept short to avoid soiling and to prevent glove tearing.
6. Petroleum-based lotions and hand treatments should not be used, since they threaten the integrity of latex.
7. Hands should be dried completely, either by hand blowers or papers towels that are beyond the splash range of other hand washers.

Table 3-36
1996 CDC Isolation Categories, Updated in 2007 for Hospitals: Examples by Disease

Standard precautions (body fluids)
- Use for the care of all patients, alone and with all other categories below

Airborne precautions
- Measles
- Varicella (includes disseminated varicella-zoster virus)
- Tuberculosis (includes special N-95 respirators)
- SARS (newest addition)

Droplet precautions
- Invasive *Haemophilus influenzae* type B (meningitis, pneumonia, epiglottitis, sepsis)
- Invasive *Neisseria meningitides* (meningitis, pneumonia, sepsis)
- Diphtheria
- *Mycoplasma* pneumonia
- Pneumonic plague
- Group A streptococci (pharyngitis, pneumonia, scarlet fever)
- Adenovirus
- Influenza
- Mumps
- Parvovirus B19 (Fifth's disease)
- Rubella

Contact precautions
- Gastrointestinal, respiratory, skin, or wound infection or colonization with a multidrug-resistant bacteria judged to be of clinical or epidemiologic significance, i.e., vancomycin-resistant enterococci (VRE) or methicillin-resistant *Staphylococcus aureus* (MRSA)
- *Clostridium difficile*
- Diapered or incontinent patients; *Escherichia coli* 0157:H7, *Shigella,* hepatitis A, or rotavirus

their diagnosis or presumed infection status. SPs apply to

- Blood
- All body fluids, secretions, and excretions except sweat, regardless of whether or not they contain visible blood
- Nonintact skin
- Mucous membranes

and consist of

- Hand hygiene
- Gloves, gowns, and masks
- Eye protection or face shield depending on anticipated exposure

In the updated 2007 guidelines, three more components were added:

- Respiratory hygiene/cough etiquette (in response to the SARS outbreak)

- Safe injection practices
- Use of masks for insertion of catheters or injection into spinal or epidural spaces

SPs are included within all the other transmission-based precautions [80] (Figure 3-16). These precautions are designed for patients proven or suspected to be infected with highly transmissible or epidemiologically important pathogens for which additional precautions, beyond SPs, are needed to interrupt transmission in the hospital.

Airborne Precautions (A). These are designed to reduce transmission of infectious diseases spread by droplet nuclei (≤ 5 μm in size) that may remain suspended in air for long periods of time and may be infective for some distance. They should be used in combination with special air handling such as negative pressure and with personal protection.

Droplet Precautions (D). These are designed to reduce transmission of infections diseases spread by droplet nuclei (>5 μm in size) through coughing, sneezing, or talking or during the performance of procedures on the airway from a distance of about 3 ft or less. One becomes infected by droplet nuclei from an infected individual coming into contact with respiratory surfaces or the mucous membranes of the mouth or eyes.

Contact Precautions (C). These are designed to reduce the risk of transmission of epidemiologically important microorganisms by direct skin-to-skin contact and physical transfer of microorganisms to a susceptible host from a colonized or infected person. They also protect against indirect transmission from intermediate or inanimate objects.

Some diseases, such as varicella (A and C), may require more than one form of isolation. A complete list of recommended precautions and their duration is found in Appendix A of reference 80; it is too extensive for publication in this chapter. Table 3-36 lists isolation categories by example, and Table 3-37 lists recommended categories of isolation based on clinical syndromes pending confirmation.

Gloving

There are three indications for gloving in the health care environment [80]:

1. To provide a protective barrier and prevent gross contamination of the hands when touching blood, body fluids, secretions, excretions,

Figure 3-16
Four categories of "transmission-based" hospital isolations, per the 1996 CDC Recommendations.

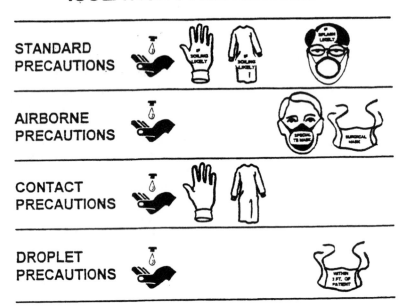

Source: Adapted from Centers for Disease Control. Guidelines for isolation precautions in hospitals. Hospital Infection Control Practices Advisory Committee (HICPAC). *Infect Control Hosp Epidemiol* 1996;17:24–52.

Table 3-37
Clinical Syndromes Warranting Additional Precautions to Prevent Transmission of Epidemiologically Important Pathogens Pending Confirmation of Diagnosis

Clinical Syndrome	Potential Pathogen	Precautions
Diarrhea		
Incontinence or diaper	Enteric pathogens	C
Adult, recent antibiotic use	*Clostridium difficile*	C
Meningitis	*Neisseria meningitides*	D
Rash or exanthems		
Petechial/fever	*Neisseria meningitides*	D
Vesicular	Varicella	A, C
Mac-pap, coryza, fever	Measles (rubeola)	A
Respiratory infections		
Cough/fever/upper lobes/HIV-/any lobes/HIV+	Tuberculosis	A
Paroxysmal or severe cough	Pertussis (epidemic)	D
Infant or child, croup	Respiratory syncytial virus or parainfluenza	C
Multidrug resistance risk		
Previous history of resistant organisms	Resistant agent?	C
Skin, GI, or wound nosocomial infection	Resistant agent?	C
Skin or wound abscess or drain not coverable	*Staphylococcus aureus,* or group A streptococcus	C

Abbreviations: A = airborne; D = droplet; C = contact.

mucous membranes, and nonintact skin. Gloving in these situations protects the worker and is mandated by OSHA [86].

2. To reduce the likelihood that microorganisms present on the hands of personnel will be transmitted to patients during invasive or other patient care procedures that involve touching a patient's mucous membranes or nonintact skin. This protects the patient.

3. To reduce the likelihood that the hands of personnel contaminated with microorganisms from a patient or a fomite can transmit these microorganisms to another patient. In this situation, gloves must be changed between patient contacts and hands washed after the gloves are removed. This protects other patients but also serves to protect the worker.

Wearing gloves does not replace the need for hand washing because gloves may have small, inapparent defects or may be torn during use. Gloves also can become contaminated during removal and therefore are to be used only once.

Hand Washing

Hand washing (see Table 3-35) is the single most important procedure for preventing nosocomial infections [87,88]. It is just as important in preventing the spread of infection in the child care and food industries. Multiple agencies and organizations, including OSHA, the CDC, the FDA, the Association of Operating Room Nurses (AORN), and the Association for Practitioners of Infection Control and Epidemiology (APIC), have published guidelines on hand-washing techniques. Hand washing is included in all categories of hospital isolation in the CDC guidelines.

OSHA 29 CFR 1910.1030, Section (d)(2)(III–IV) do not address hand-washing agents or technique. They do address the availability of hand-washing facilities and recommended frequency as well as "alternative" methods of hand washing such as antiseptic towelettes if workers subsequently wash hands with soap and water as soon as feasible. This is to cover field workers in emergency medical services, law enforcement, and mobile blood collection units. All fixed health care facilities must have hand-washing facilities available. Passing through stairs or doors and thus making environmental contamination possible is a

violation of Section (d)(2)(III). OSHA also requires adequate training in hand washing.

Hand washing serves two main purposes:

1. Removal of gross contamination by organic and inorganic debris by the friction of rubbing the hands together and the "degreasing" properties of soap and lather.
2. Removal of some microorganisms from the skin depending on the soap or hand-washing solution.

Bar soap should be kept on a draining rack to prevent contamination. Fresh soap products should not be added to old dispensers; disposable dispensers are recommended. Lotions should be in small personal containers because *Pseudomonas. aeruginosa* has been associated with infections in refillable lotion containers.

CDC and APIC guidelines for general patient care call for application of nonantimicrobial soap followed by vigorous rubbing together of lathered hands for 10–15 seconds. Antimicrobial soaps *should* be used in caring for newborns and the immunosuppressed and in performing invasive procedures. Preoperative hand washing should be done for 120 seconds, or 20 seconds if using an alcohol-based product. Hot water traditionally has been recommended but may increase drying and be associated with the development of rashes and dermatitis in health care workers or others who wash frequently. When harsh soaps are required, such as in hospital units, workers should wet their hands before applying soap to avoid skin contact with undiluted, full-strength soap and the possible resulting irritation.

In non–food and non–health care workers, hand washing is part of general personal hygiene (see below). Hands should be washed before preparing food for consumption by others. They also should be washed after defecating or urinating and after handling items that may be contaminated.

Commercial training programs and products are available to teach hand-washing techniques. Glo-Germ [89] is a commercial company that makes a fluorescent dye that is applied and then black-lighted after hand washing for quality control.

General Personal Hygiene

No topic can serve as a better conclusion to this large and complex chapter than the topic of

Table 3-38
Principles of Personal Hygiene

1. Wash hands in soap and water immediately after urinating, defecating, or touching any mucous membranes. This is especially important before eating, drinking, or preparing food for others or after handling fomites such as money or tickets.
2. Keep hands and any unclean personal articles (e.g., toothbrush, hairbrush, nail clippers) away from the mouth, nose, eyes, ears, genitalia, and wounds of others.
3. Keep fingernails trimmed and clean.
4. Avoid using common unclean eating utensils, drinking cups, linen, handkerchiefs, combs, or brushes of others.
5. Avoid exposing others to spray from the nose or mouth when coughing, sneezing, laughing, or talking.
6. Keep body and clothing clean and nonoffensive to others.

personal hygiene. *Personal hygiene* is defined as those protective measures and behaviors under the responsibility of the individual that maintain his or her own health and prevent the spread of disease. Personal hygiene is most important for preventing direct transmission. Workers in health care, food, and some manufacturing industries may work under more specific guidelines, regulations, or employer policies. Regardless of the industry or regulations, all employers should have either written policies or at least a "company culture" that includes the principles listed in Table 3-38.

References

1. NIH Consensus Statement. *Helicobacter pylori in Peptic Ulcer Disease.* Bethesda MD: National Institutes of Health, 1994.
2. Last JM (ed). *A Dictionary of Epidemiology,* 3rd ed. New York: Oxford University Press, 1995, pp 55–6.
3. Hope-Simpson RE. The nature of herpes zoster: A long-term study and a new hypothesis. *Proc R Soc Lond* 1965;58:9–20.
3. *Third National Health and Nutrition Examination Survey (NHANES III).* DHHS 94-1308. Hyattsville, MD: U.S. Department of Health and Human Services, National Center for Health Statistics, 1994.
5. Centers for Disease Control and Prevention. Case definitions for infectious conditions under public health surveillance. *MMWR* 1997;46:1–56. Individual conditions updates available.
6. Glezen WP, Couch RB. Influenza viruses. In Evans AS, Kaslow RA (eds), *Viral Infections of Humans: Epidemiology and Control,* 4th ed. New York: Plenum Press, 1997. p 482.
7. Centers for Disease Control and Prevention. Prevention of hepatitis A through active or passive immunization: Recommendations of the Advisory Committee on Immunization Practices. *MMWR* 1996;45:1.
8. Centers for Disease Control and Prevention. Draft guidelines for infection control in health care personnel. *Fedl Reg* 1997;62:47275–327.
9. Fine PEM. Herd immunity: History, theory, practice. *Epidemiol Rev* 1993;15:265–302.
10. Heymann David L (ed). *Control of Communicable Diseases Manual,* 18th ed. Washington: American Public Health Association, 2005 (also available on CD-ROM).
11. Houseworth WJ, Spoon MM. The age distribution of excess mortality during A2 Hong Kong influenza epidemics compared with earlier A2 outbreaks. *Am J Epidemiol* 1974;94:348–50.
12. *Stedman's Pocket Medical Dictionary* (abridged from 24th ed). Baltimore: Williams & Wilkins, 1987, p 602.
13. Koch R. Uber bacteriologische Forschung. *Int Med Cong (Berl)* 1891;1:35.
14. Rivers T. Viruses and Koch's postulates. *J Bacteriol* 1937;33:1–12.
15. Evans AS. Causation and disease: The Heenle-Koch postulates revisited. *Yale J Biol Med* 1976;49:175–95.
16. Evans AS. *Causation and Disease: A Chronological Journey.* New York: Plenum Press, 1993.
17. Hill AB. The environment and disease: Association or causation? *Proc R Soc Med* 1965;58:295–300.
18. Code of Ethical Conduct, American College of Occupational and Environmental Medicine. Washington. Adopted by ACOEM Board of Directors, October 15, 1993.
19. Suskind F. Another look at the link between work injuries and job experience. *Month Labor Rev* 1982; 105:38.
20. Haddon W Jr. The changing approach to the epidemiology, prevention, and amelioration of trauma: The transition to approach etiology rather than descriptively based. *Am J Public Health* 1968;58:1431–8.
21. Haddon W Jr. A logical framework for categorizing highway safety phenomena and activity. *J Trauma* 1972;12:193–207.
22. Centers for Disease Control and Prevention. Draft guidelines for preventing the transmission of tuberculosis in health-care settings, 2nd ed. *Fed Reg* 1993;58:52809–54.
23. Memorandum for Regional Administrators (letter). Re: Enforcement Policy and Procedure for Occupational Exposure to Tuberculosis. Roger A. Clark, Director of Compliance Programs, Occupational Health and Safety Administration, Washington, October 8, 1993.
24. Gerberding JL. Occupational infectious diseases or infectious occupational diseases? Bridging the views on tuberculosis control (editorial). *Infect Control Hosp Epidemiol* 1993;14:686–8.
25. Recommendations for preventing the spread of vancomycin resistance. Recommendations of the Hospital Infection Control Practices Advisory Committee (HICPAC). *MMWR* 1995;44:RR-12.
26. Revision of the CDC surveillance case definition for acquired human immune insufficiency virus. Conference of State and Territorial Epidemiologists,

Center for Disease Control, Atlanta. *MMWR* 1987; 36:1S.

27. Brooks GF, Butel JS, Morse SA. *Jawetz, Melnick, and Adelberg's Medical Microbiology*, 21st ed. Stamford, CT: Appleton & Lange, 1998.

28. Urbaschek B, Urbaschek R. Introduction and summary: Perspective on bacterial pathogenesis and host defense. *Rev Infect Dis* 1987;9:S431–6.

29. Center for Disease Control and Prevention. Emergency Preparedness and Response—Floods; available at http://emergency.cdc.gov/disasters/floods/ (20 downloadable guideline files, plus hyperlinks).

30. Riley RI, Kaufman JE. Effect of relative humidity on the inactivation of airborne *Serratia marcescens* by ultraviolet radiation. *Appl Microbiol* 1972;23:1113–20.

31. Soper GA. The curious career of Typhoid Mary. *Bull NY Acad Med* 1939;15:698–712.

32. Cassens BJ. *Preventive Medicine and Public Health*, 2nd ed. Philadelphia: Harwal Publishing, 1992, p 6.

33. Wentworth DE, McGregor MW, Macklin MD, et al. Transmission of swine influenza virus to humans after exposure to experimentally infected pigs. *J Infect Dis* 1997;175:7–14.

34. Karabatsos N (ed). *International Catalogue of Arboviruses*. San Antonio, TX: American Society of Tropical Medicine and Hygiene, Subcommittee on Information Exchange, 1985.

35. Knight V, Couch RB, Landahl HD. The effect of the lack of gravity on airborne infection during space flight. *JAMA* 1970;214:513–8.

36. Gerone PJ, Couch RB, Keefer GV, et al. Assessment of experimental and natural viral aerosols. *Bacteriol Rev* 1966;30:576–88.

37. Knight V (ed). *Viral and Mycoplasma Infections of the Respiratory Tract*. Philadelphia: Lea and Febiger, 1973.

38. Kelly S, Winsser J, Winkelstein W Jr. Poliomyelitis and other enteric viruses in sewage. *Am J Public Health* 1957;47:72–7.

39. Mastro TD, Farley TA, Elliott JA, et al. An outbreak of surgical-wound infections due to group A streptococcus carried on the scalp. *N Engl J Med* 1990; 323:968–72.

40. Viglionese A, Nottebart VF, Bodman HA, et al. Recurrent group A streptococcal carriage in a health care worker associated with widely separated nosocomial outbreaks. *Am J Med* 1991;91:329–33S.

41. Paul SM, Genese C, Spitalny K. Postoperative group A β-hemolytic streptococcus outbreak with the pathogen traced to a member of a healthcare worker's household. *Infect Control Hosp Epidemiol* 1990;11:643–6.

42. Ridgeway EJ, Allen KD. Clustering of group A streptococcal infections on a burns unit: Important lessons in outbreak management. *J Hosp Infect* 1993; 25:173–82.

43. Berkelman RL, Martin D, Graham DR, et al. Streptococcal wound infections caused by a vaginal carrier. *JAMA* 1982;247:2680–2.

44. Schaffner W, Lefkowitz LB Jr, Goodman JS, et al. Hospital outbreak of infections with group A streptococci traced to an asymptomatic anal carrier. *N Engl J Med* 1969;280:1224–5.

45. Richman DD, Breton SJ, Goldmann DA. Scarlet fever and group A streptococcal surgical wound infection traced to an anal carrier. *J Pediatr* 1977;90: 387–90.

46. Decker MD, Lavely GB, Hutcheson RHJ, et al. Foodborne streptococcal pharyngitis in a hospital pediatrics clinics. *JAMA* 1986;253:679–81.

47. Boyce JM, Opal SM, Byone-Potter G, et al. Spread of methicillin-resistant *Staphylococcus aureus* in a hospital after exposure to a health care worker with chronic sinusitis. *Clin Infect Dis* 1993;17:496–504.

48. Sherertz RJ, Reagan DR, Hampton KD, et al. A cloud adult: The *Staphylococcus aureus*–virus interaction revisited. *Ann Intern Med* 1996;124:539–47.

49. Belani A, Sherertz RJ, Sullivan ML, et al. Outbreak of staphylococcal infection in two hospital nurseries traced to a single nasal carrier. *Infect Control* 1986;7: 487–90.

50. Kreiswirth BN, Kravitz GR, Schlievert PM, et al. Nosocomial transmission of a strain of *Staphylococcus aureus* causing toxic shock syndrome. *Ann Intern Med* 1986;195:704–7.

51. Boyce JM. Methicillin-resistant *Staphylococcus aureus* in hospitals and long-term care facilities: Microbiology, epidemiology, and preventive measures. *Infect Control Hosp Epidemiol* 1992;13:725–37.

52. Boyce JM, Landry M, Deetz TR, et al. Epidemiologic studies of an outbreak of nosocomial methicillin-resistant *Staphylococcus aureus* infections. *Infect Control* 1981;2:110–6.

53. Walsh TJ, Standiford HD, et al. Randomized, double-blinded trial of rifampin with either novobiocin or trimethoprim-sulfamethoxazole against methicillin-resistant *Staphylococcus aureus* colonization: Prevention of antimicrobial resistance and effect of host factors on outcome. *Antimicrob Agents Chemother* 1993;37:1334–42.

54. Mulligan ME, Murray-Leisure KA, Ribner BS, et al. Methicillin-resistant *Staphylococcus aureus*: A consensus review of the microbiology, pathogenesis, and epidemiology with implications for prevention and management. *Am J Med* 1993;94:313–28.

55. Valway SE. An outbreak involving extensive transmission of a virulent strain of *Mycobacterium tuberculosis*. *N Engl J Med* 1998;338:633–9.

56. Glaser ZR. A dictionary for central sterilization. *Infect Control Steril Technol* 1998;4:14–46.

57. Durante L. Investigation of an outbreak of bloody diarrhea association with an endoscopic cleaning solution and demonstration of lesions in an animal model. *Am J Med* 1992;92:476–80.

58. Spaulding EH. Chemical disinfection and antisepsis in the hospital. *J Hosp Res* 1972;9:5–31.

59. Nardell EA, Keegan J, Cheny SA, et al. Airborne infection: Theoretical limits of protection achievable

by building ventilation. *Am Rev Respir Dis* 1991;
144:302–6.

60. Petersen NJ. An assessment of the airborne route in hepatitis B transmission. *Ann NY Acad Sci* 1980;353:157–66.

61. Johnson GK, Robinson WS. Human immunodeficiency virus-1 in the vapors of surgical power instruments. *J Med Virol* 1991;33:47–50.

62. Jewett DL, Heinsohn PA, Bennett C, et al. Blood-containing aerosols generated by surgical techniques: A possible infectious hazard. *Am Ind Assoc J* 1992;53:228–31.

63. Heinsohn PA, Jewett DL. Exposure to blood-containing aerosols in the operating room: A preliminary study. *Am Ind Hyg Assoc J* 1993;54:446–53.

64. Heinsohn PA, Jewett DL, Balzer L, et al. Aerosols created by some surgical power tools: Particle-size distribution and qualitative hemoglobin content. *Appl Occup Environ Hyg* 1991;6:773–6.

65. Tokars J, Chamberland ME, Schable CA, et al. A survey of occupational blood contact and HIV infections among orthopedic surgeons. *JAMA* 1991;268:489–94.

66. Evaluation of a smoke evacuator used for laser surgery. *Lasers Surg Med* 1989;9:276–81.

67. NIOSH Health Hazard Evaluation and Technical Assistance Reports. HETA 85-126-1932 (1989) and HETA 88-101-2008 (1990). Also available at www.cdc.gov/niosh/hc11.html.

68. Koren H, Bisesi M. *Handbook of Environmental Health and Safety*, 3rd ed. Boca Raton, FL: Lewis (CRC) Publishers, 1996, Vol 2, Chaps 3–7, pp 233–608; Vol 1, Chap 2, pp 107–201.

69. Okun DA. Water quality management. In Last JM, Wallace RB (eds), *Maxcy-Rosenau-Last Public Health and Preventive Medicine*, 13th ed. Norwalk, CT: Appleton & Lange, 1992, pp 618–48.

70. Frank JF, Barnhart HM. Food and dairy sanitation. In Last JM, Wallace RB (eds), *Maxcy-Rosenau-Last Public Health and Preventive Medicine*, 13th ed. Norwalk, CT: Appleton & Lange, 1992, pp 589–618.

71. U.S. Food and Drug Administration. *Bad Bug Book: Foodborne Pathogenic Microorganisms and Natural Toxins Handbook* (online textbook); available at http://vm.cfsan.fda.gov/~mow/app2.html, Table: Onset, Duration, and Symptoms of Foodborne Illness.

72. *Codex General Standard for f Irradiated Food.* Codex Alimentarius. *Codex Stan* 106–1983, rev. 1–2003; available at www.codexalimentarius.net/download/standards/16/CXS_106_2003e.pdf.

73. Merritt C. Radiolytic products: Are they safe? In *Safety Factors Influencing the Acceptance of Food Irradiation Technology*. TECDOC-490. Vienna, Austria: International Atomic Energy Commission, 1989.

74. U.S. Food and Drug Administration. Final rule. *Fed Reg* 1989;55:18538–44.

75. *Satellites Help Scientists Focus on Emerging Diseases* (Factsheet). Bethesda, MD: Office of Communications, National Institute of Allergy and Infectious Diseases, National Institutes for Health, 1998. Available at www.niaid.nih.gov/publications/dateline/0997/shsfed.htm.

76. *Physical Activity and Health: A Report of the Surgeon General.* Atlanta, GA: U.S. Department of Health and Human Services, Centers for Disease Control and Prevention, National Center for Chronic Disease Prevention and Health Promotion, 1996.

77. Kasl SV, Evans AS, Niederman JC. Psychosocial risk factors in the development of infectious mononucleosis. *Psychosom Med* 1979;41:445–66.

78. Figure 4, Packing and Labeling of Etiologic Agents, graphic, U.S. Government. Available at www.cdc.gov/od/biosfty/bmbl/fig4.gif.

79. Richmond JY, McKinney RW. *Biosafety in Microbiological and Biomedical Laboratories*, 3rd ed. Washington: U.S. Department of Health and Human Services, 1993; available at www.cdc.gov/od/ohs/biosfty/bmbl/bmbl3toc.htm.

80. Centers for Disease Control and Prevention. Guideline for isolation precautions in hospitals—2007. Hospital Infection Control Practices Advisory Committee (HICPAC); available at www.cdc.gov/ncidod/dhqp/pdf/guidelines/Isolation2007.pdf.

81. *Guide for the Care and Use of Laboratory Animals.* HEW (NIH) 86-23. Rev 1985 and Laboratory Animal Welfare Regulations 9 CFR Subchapter A, Parts 1, 2, 3, 1985.

82. Title 42—The Public Health and Welfare, Chapter 6A—Public Health Service, Subchapter II—General Powers and Duties, Part G—Quarantine and Inspection, Section 264. Regulations to control communicable diseases. Available at www.access.gpo.gov/uscode/title42/chapter6a_subchapterii_partg_.html.

83. National Communicable Disease Center. *Isolation Techniques for Use in Hospitals.* PHS No 2054. Washington: NCDC, 1970.

84. Centers for Disease Control. *Isolation Techniques for Use in Hospitals*, 2nd ed. HHS No 80-8314. Washington: CDC, 1975.

85. Garner JS, Simmon BP. *CDC Guideline for Isolation Precautions in Hospitals.* HHS No 83-8314. Atlanta: U.S. Department of Health and Human Services, 1983. Also in *Infect Control* 1983;4:245–325 and *Am J Infect Control* 1984;12:103–63.

86. Occupational exposure to bloodborne pathogens: Final rule. Department of Labor, Occupational Safety and Health Administration. *Fed Reg* 1991;56:64175–82.

87. Centers for Disease Control and Prevention. Guidelines for handwashing and hospital environmental control, 1985. *MMWR* 1987;36 (No. 2S):1S-18S.

88. Hart PD. Current recommendations for handwashing compliance in the clinical setting. *Infect Control Steril Technol* 1996;2:1.

89. Glo-Germ, P.O. Box 189, Moab, Utah 84532, 1-800-842-6622; www.glogerm.com.

4 Occupations at Risk

Marilyn S. Radke and Geoffrey A. Kelafant

Until recently, infectious disease has played a significant role in the health of individuals, populations, and even the course of history. Improvements in hygiene and technology have greatly reduced the burden of suffering in many developed areas. Despite these advances, much of the world is still at risk from infectious diseases, which have significant morbidity and mortality.

As the world shrinks, the possibility of being confronted with unfamiliar diseases increases. Infected individuals can travel farther and faster than ever before. The classic definition of occupational disease blurs in cases of work-related infectious disease because the occupational risk is in merely being present in an area rather than just working in a particular job. Since some of these diseases are virtually unknown to many health care practitioners, it is crucial to maintain a high index of suspicion to recognize infections when they occur.

Diseases Affecting Those Who Work with People

HEALTH CARE WORKERS, PERSONAL CARE WORKERS, AND DAY-CARE WORKERS

In some countries, health care workers face the greatest risk of acquiring occupational infectious disease. In the United States, health care workers continue to be at risk from hepatitis B virus, HIV, *Mycobacterium tuberculosis,* and other infectious agents. Concern for health care workers has involved health care facilities and systems in the regulatory milieu as never before. Entire industries have been created over the last 20 years to address this single problem.

Health care workers may acquire diseases via airborne, fecal-oral, bloodborne/ percutaneous, or direct contact routes. Although in theory a huge number of diseases may be spread to health care workers (and from health care workers), the most commonly cited are found in Table 4-1. Diseases known to have been contracted from percutaneous injuries in laboratory and research facilities are listed in Table 4-2.

PUBLIC SAFETY AND EMERGENCY RESPONSE WORKERS

Public safety and emergency response workers face risks similar to those faced by health care workers. In addition, depending on the particular job, they also may be at risk for zoonotic disease (e.g., from animal bites or contact), water-borne disease (e.g., in divers and rescue personnel), arthropod-borne disease, and soil-borne disease. Because of the diverse and sometimes odd nature of the tasks these workers often are asked to perform, persistent or unusual infections require a thorough investigation. Zoonotic, water-borne, arthropod-borne, and soil-borne diseases are discussed elsewhere in this chapter.

Table 4-1
Infectious Diseases Affecting Health Care Workers and Routes of Transmission

Airborne	Fecal-Oral	Percutaneous/Bloodborne	Direct Contact
Adenovirus	Hepatitis A	AIDS/HIV	Dermatophytoses
Influenza	Norwalk virus	Crimean hemorrhagic fever	Herpetic whitlow
Measles	Polio	Ebola virus	Scabies
Meningococcal disease	Salmonellosis	Hepatitis B	Tinea corporis
Mumps	Shigellosis	Hepatitis C	Warts
Parvovirus B19		Lassa fever	
Pertussis		Marburg virus	
Respiratory syncytial virus			
Rubella			
Severe Acute Respiratory Syndrome (SARS)			
Tuberculosis			
Varicella			

Table 4-2
Diseases Acquired Percutaneously

Blastomycosis	Malaria
Brucellosis	Mycoplasmosis
Cryptococcosis	Rocky Mountain spotted fever
Creutzfeldt-Jakob disease	Scrub typhus
Diphtheria	Sporotrichosis
Ebola virus	Staphylococcal disease
Gonorrhea	Streptococcal disease
Herpes simplex	Syphilis
Herpes B virus	Toxoplasmosis
Japanese encephalitis	Tuberculosis
Leptospirosis	Yellow fever

Diseases Affecting Those Who Work with Animals

Although advances in hygiene and technology have made zoonotic diseases a curiosity in some countries, there remain dozens of diseases that can spread from animals to humans (Table 4-3). Numerous occupations (Tables 4-4 and 4-5) involve extensive contact with animals, animal tissues, animal waste, and animal products. Ticks, fleas, and mites may be closely associated with some animal species. These diseases may be acquired via airborne spread; the fecal-oral route; contact with blood, secretions, or fluids; or direct contact or bites. Some are spread via multiple routes.

Diseases Affecting Those Who Work Outdoors

Numerous occupations involve outdoor work (Table 4-6). The two potential exposures presenting

Table 4-3
Occupational Zoonotic Disease by Animal

Animal Group	Diseases
Amphibians	*Edwardsiella tarda*
	Salmonellosis
	Sparganosis
Armadillos, sloths, anteaters	Leprosy
Bats	Duvenhage virus
	Histoplasmosis
	Kasokero virus
	Lyssavirus
	Mokola virus
	Rabies
	Salmonellosis
	Yuli virus
Birds	Campylobacteriosis
	Cryptococcosis
	Erysipeloid
	Histoplasmosis
	Newcastle disease
	Ornithosis
	Pasteurella multocida
	Salmonellosis
	Tuberculosis
	Yersiniosis
Camels, llamas	Brucellosis
	Campylobacteriosis
	Plague
	Q fever
	Salmonellosis
Cats	Campylobacteriosis
	Capnocytophaga
	Cat-scratch disease
	Cutaneous larval migrans
	Dermatophytosis
	Leptospirosis
	Plague

Table 4-3
Continued

Animal Group	Diseases	Animal Group	Diseases
Cats *continued*	Q fever		Salmonellosis
	Salmonellosis		Tularemia
	Strongyloidiasis		Vibriosis
	Toxoplasmosis		Warts
	Visceral larval migrans	Horses	Anthrax
	Yersiniosis		Brucellosis
Cattle	Anthrax		Cryptosporidiosis
	Brucellosis		Dermatophilosis
	Campylobacteriosis		Eastern equine encephalitis
	Cowpox		*Equine Morbillivirus*
	Dermatophilosis		Glanders
	Erysipeloid		Leptospirosis
	Leptospirosis		Salmonellosis
	Milker's nodules		Venezuelan equine encephalitis
	Mycobacterium bovis		Western equine encephalitis
	Psuedocowpox		Yersiniosis
	Q fever	Lizards	Salmonellosis
	Salmonellosis	Marsupials	Anthrax
	Streptococcosis		Dermatophytosis
	Yersiniosis		Leptospirosis
Dogs	American trypanosomiasis		Melioidosis
	Blastomycosis		*Mycobacterium bovis*
	Brucellosis		Pasteurellosis
	Campylobacteriosis		Q fever
	Capnocytophaga		Salmonellosis
	Cat-scratch disease		Scabies
	Cutaneous larval migrans	Pigs	Anthrax
	Dermatophytosis		Brucellosis
	Echinococcosis		Erysipeloid
	Ehrlichiosis		Influenza
	Giardiasis		Leptospirosis
	Leptospirosis		*Pasteurella multocida*
	Lyme disease		Salmonellosis
	Pasteurellosis		Streptococcosis
	Plague		Yersiniosis
	Q fever	Primates	Amebiasis
	Rabies		Ascariasis
	Rocky Mountain spotted fever		Campylobacteriosis
	Salmonellosis		Cestodiasis
	Strongyloidiasis		Dengue
	Trichostrongylosis		Dermatophilosis
	Visceral larval migrans		Giardiasis
	Yersiniosis		Hepatitis A
Fish	*Aeromonas hydrophila*		Herpes B virus
	Cercarial dermatitis		Leprosy
	Cholera		Marburg virus
	Erysipeloid		Measles
	Mycobacterium marinum granuloma		Monkeypox
	Nanophyetiasis		Salmonellosis
	Pseudomonas aeruginosa		Shigellosis

(continues)

Table 4-3
Continued

Animal Group	Diseases	Animal Group	Diseases
Primates (continued)	Strongyloidiasis	Sheep, goats (continued)	Q fever
	Tanapox		Salmonellosis
	Trichostrongylosis		Yersiniosis
	Tuberculosis	Snakes	Aeromonas hydrophila
	Yaba virus		Edwardsiella tarda
Rabbits, hares	Campylobacteriosis		Escherichia coli
	Derematomycosis		Mesocestoidiasis
	Dermatophilosis		Morganella morganii
	Erysipeloid		Mycobacterium ulcerans
	Leptospirosis		Proteus vulgaris
	Plague		Providencia
	Q fever		Q fever
	Salmonellosis		Salmonellosis
	Tularemia		Sparganosis
	Yersiniosis	Turtles, tortoises, terrapins	Campylobacteriosis
Raccoons	Edwardsiella tarda		Edwardsiella tarda
	Rabies		Salmonellosis
	Salmonellosis	Whales, dolphins, porpoises	Erysipeloid
Rodents	American trypanosomiasis		Mycobacterium marinum
	Babesiosis		Seal finger
	Cestodiasis		
	Colorado tick fever		
	Dermatophytosis		
	Hantavirus		
	Leptospirosis		
	Listeriosis		
	Lyme disease		
	Lymphocytic choriomeningitis		
	Murine typhus		
	Plague		
	Powassan encephalitis		
	Rabies		
	Rat-bite fever		
	Relapsing fever		
	Rickettsialpox		
	Rocky Mountain spotted fever		
	Salmonellosis		
	Scrub typhus		
	Yersiniosis		
Seals, sea lions, walruses	Erysipeloid		
	Influenza A		
	Seal finger		
Sheep, goats	Anthrax		
	Brucellosis		
	Campylobacteriosis		
	Cryptosporidiosis		
	Dermatomycosis		
	Erysipeloid		
	Leptospirosis		
	Orf		
	Plague		

Table 4-4
Occupational Groups at Risk for Zoonotic Disease

Agricultural workers

Animal handlers	Pest control workers
Animal husbandry workers	Primate handlers
Butchers	Ranchers
Cannery workers	Research laboratory workers
Cattle breeders	Sewer workers
Cooks	Sheepherders
Dairy farmers	Slaughterhouse workers
Fishermen	Stockyard workers
Forestry workers	Trappers
Hunters	Travelers
Livestock handlers	Veterinarians
Meat and poultry workers	Weavers
Miners	Zookeepers
Packing house workers	

Table 4-5
Occupations at Risk and Specific Zoonotic Diseases

Occupations	Diseases
Bird handlers	Cryptococcosis
	Histoplasmosis
	Newcastle disease
	Ornithosis
	Pasteurellosis
	Tuberculosis

Table 4-5
Continued

Occupations	Diseases
Butchers, slaughterhouse workers	Anthrax
	Brucellosis
	Campylobacteriosis
	Leptospirosis
	Listeriosis
	Q fever
	Streptococcosis
	Tuberculosis (cutaneous)
	Tularemia
	Warts
Fishermen	Erysipeloid
	Nanophyetiasis
	Swimming pool granu-loma
Livestock handlers	Anthrax
	Brucellosis
	Cryptosporidiosis
	Dermatophilosis
	Dermatophytosis
	Leptospirosis
	Listeriosis
	Q fever
	Streptococcosis
	Salmonella (cutaneous)
	Tuberculosis
Pest control workers	Hantavirus
	Leptospirosis
Poultry workers	Cryptococcosis
	Erysipeloid
	Newcastle disease
	Ornithosis
	Pasteurellosis
Primate handlers	Giardiasis
	Hepatitis A
	Herpes B virus
	Marburg virus
	Measles
	Monkeypox
	Shigellosis
	Tuberculosis
	Yabapox
Sheep handlers	Anthrax
	Brucellosis
	Dermatophilosis
	Echinococcosis
	Orf
	Q fever
Veterinarians, animal handlers	Anthrax
	Brucellois
	Cat-scratch disease
	Dermatophytosis

Table 4-5
Continued

Occupations	Diseases
Veterinarians, animal handlers *continued*	Erysipeloid
	Leptospirosis
	Listeriosis
	Milker's nodules
	Newcastle disease
	Q fever
	Rabies
	Salmonella (cutaneous)
	Toxoplasmosis
	Tuberculosis (cutaneous)
	Tularemia
	Warts

Table 4-6
Outdoor Workers at Risk

Agricultural workers	Landscapers
Construction workers	Lumberjacks
Excavators	Miners
Foresters	Surveyors
Geologists	Travelers
Hunters	Wildlife and parks workers

the greatest risk to outdoor workers are soil-borne and arthropod-borne disease (Table 4-7). Soil organisms, predominantly fungi, may cause infection through inhalation or direct inoculation through the skin. Arthropod-borne disease, which may be viral, rickettsial, protozoal, or bacterial, is acquired through contact with mosquitoes, ticks, fleas, and mites. The spectrum of arthropod-borne disease is staggering, with well over 200 arboviral infections alone.

Diseases Affecting Those Who Work Around Water

Diseases are easily transmitted by water. Some occupations, such as diving or working with sewage or biohazardous waste, entail significant exposure to water. Additionally, agricultural work and construction work may involve exposure to water. Many diseases, especially those that are transmitted via the fecal-oral route, may be acquired during work activities involving water exposure (Table 4-8). Other diseases may involve only the skin.

Table 4-7
Diseases Affecting Those Who Work Outdoors

Arthropod-borne Diseases	Soil-borne Diseases	Other Diseases
Viral		
California encephalitis	Anthrax	Amebiasis
Colorado tick fever	*Ascaris lumbricoides* infection	Hantavirus infection
Crimean-Congo hemorrhagic fever	Blastomycosis	Rabies
Dengue	Chromomycosis	
	Coccidioidomycosis	
	Cryptococcosis	
Eastern equine encephalitis	Cutaneous larval migrans	
Japanese encephalitis	Dermatophytosis (geophilic)	
La Crosse encephalitis	Histoplasmosis	
	Hookworm infection	
Powassan encephalitis	Maduromycosis	
Rift Valley fever	Melioidosis	
Russian spring-summer encephalitis	Mycetoma	
Sandfly fever	Nocardiosis	
St. Louis encephalitis	Paracoccidioidomycosis	
Venezuelan equine encephalitis	Sporotrichosis	
Western equine encephalitis	Strongyloidiasis	
Yellow fever	Tetanus	
Many others	*Trichuris trichiura* infection	
Rickettsial		
Ehrlichiosis		
Louse-borne typhus		
Murine typhus		
Rickettsialpox		
Rocky Mountain spotted fever		
Scrub typhus		
Trench fever		
Bacterial		
Lyme disease		
Plague		
Relapsing fever		
Tularemia		
Protozoal		
African trypanosomiasis (Sleeping sickness)		
American trypanosomiasis (Chagas' disease)		
Babesiosis		
Dirofilarial infections		
Leishmaniases		
Malaria		

Diseases Affecting Travelers

Travel-related occupational infectious disease is a relativistic field. It depends on the observer's frame of reference. Many of the diseases mentioned in this book may be of concern to a traveling worker, depending on point of origin, destination, and type of work performed. Some are vaccine-preventable, and some have chemoprophylaxis and/or treat-ment available. Table 4-9 lists vaccine-preventable diseases. Please note that availability and effectiveness of vaccines vary widely.

Diseases Affecting Those Who Work Indoors

Many building-related illnesses are respiratory in nature, usually presenting as asthma or hypersensitivity pneumonitis, and do not represent true infec-

Table 4-8
Diseases Affecting Those Who Work Around Water

Aeromonas hydrophila infection	Leptospirosis
Amebiasis	*Mycobacterium marinum* granuloma
Amebic meningoencephalitis	Nanophyetiasis
Aspergillosis	Polio
Candidiasis	*Pseudomonas aeruginosa* infection
Cercarial dermatitis	Schistosomal dermatitis
Cholera	Schistosomiasis
Dermatophytosis	Shigellosis
Escherichia coli infection	Tularemia
Erysipeloid	Typhoid
Hepatitis A	Vibriosis
Hepatitis E	Warts
Legionellosis	Other diseases spread by fecal contamination

Table 4-9
Vaccine-Preventable Diseases

Anthrax	Pertussis
Cervical cancer (Human Papillomavirus)	Pneumococcal disease
Diphtheria	Polio
Haemophilus influenzae type b (Hib)	Rabies
Hepatitis A	Rotavirus
Hepatitis B	Rubella
Influenza	Shingles (Herpes Zoster)
Japanese encephalitis	Smallpox
Lyme disease	Tetanus
Measles	Tuberculosis
Meningococcal disease	Typhoid
Monkeypox (Note: There is *no* monkeypox vaccine. The smallpox vaccine is used for this disease).	Varicella
Mumps	Yellow fever

tions. Infectious organisms (e.g., bacteria, fungi, viruses, and protozoa) may reside in heating, cooling, and ventilation systems or be introduced into the indoor environment via water, carpets, plants, animals, birds, pillows, bedding, dust, wet or damp materials, outside air, and humans. Organisms implicated in infectious building-related illness are listed in Table 4-10.

Table 4-10
Organisms Affecting Those Who Work Indoors

Aspergillus
Coccidioides immitis
Cryptococcus neoformans
Histoplasma capsulatum
Influenza and other airborne viruses
Legionella pneumophila
Mycobacterium tuberculosis
Naegleria fowleri
Pneumococcal and other airborne bacteria

Diseases Affecting Those in Food Production

Although many disease outbreaks associated with food involve consumers of contaminated food products and not workers, there are occupational infectious disease risks associated with employ-ment in the food industry (Table 4-11). Most of these diseases are associated with the processing of raw food products, mainly affecting those who slaughter and butcher livestock and poultry.

Table 4-11
Diseases Affecting Those Who Work Around Food

Anthrax	Nanophyetiasis
Brucellosis	Ornithosis
Erysipeloid	Q fever
Leptospirosis	Streptococcosis
Listeriosis	Tuberculosis (cutaneous)
Milker's nodules	Tularemia

Bibliography

Calisher CH. Medically important arboviruses of the United States and Canada. *Clin Microbiol Rev* 1994;7: 89–116.

Casey KR. Atypical pneumonia and environmental factors. *Clin Chest Med* 1991;12:285–302.

Centers for Disease Control and Prevention. *Epidemiology and Prevention of Vaccine-Preventable Diseases*, 5th ed. Atlanta: CDC, 1999.

Centers for Disease Control and Prevention. *Health Information for International Travel 2008*. Atlanta: CDC, 2008.

Centers for Disease Control and Prevention. Immunization of health care workers: Recommendations of the Advisory Committee on Immunization Practices (ACIP) and the Hospital Infection Control Practices Advisory Committee (HICPAC). *MMWR* 1997;46:1–42.

Cohen R. Occupational infections. In LaDou J (ed), *Occupational Medicine*. East Norwalk, CT: Appleton & Lange, 1990.

Fang G, Araujo V, Guerrant RL. Enteric infections associated with exposure to animals or animal products. *Infect Dis Clin North Am* 1991;5:681–701.

Ferson MJ. Infections in day care. *Curr Opin Pediatr* 1993;5:35–40.

Fox JG, Lipman NS. Infections transmitted by large and small laboratory animals. *Infect Dis Clin North Am* 1991;5:131–61.

Garibaldi R, Janis B. Occupational infections. In Rom WN (ed), *Environmental and Occupational Medicine*, 2nd ed. Boston: Little, Brown, 1992.

Gerberding JL, Holmes KK. Microbial agents and infectious diseases. In Rosenstock LR, Cullen MR (eds), *Textbook of Clinical Occupational and Environmental Medicine*. Philadelphia: Saunders, 1994.

Kelafant GA (ed). *Guidelines for Employee Health Services in Health Care Facilities* (hypertext document). Chicago: American College of Occupational and Environmental Medicine, Medical Center Occupational Health Section, 1998. Available at www.occenvmed .net/ehsg.

Kligman EW, Peate WF, Cordes DH. Occupational infections in farm workers. In Cordes DH, Rea DF (eds), *Health hazards of farming. Occup Med State Art Rev* 1991;6:429–46.

Lanphear BP. Transmission and control of bloodborne viral hepatitis in health care workers. In McDiarmid MA, Kessler ER (eds), The health care worker. *Occup Med State Art Rev* 1997;12:717–30.

Madkour MM. Occupation-related infectious arthritis. *Baillieres Clin Rheumatol* 1989;3:157–92.

Seltzer JM. Biologic contaminants. In Seltzer JM (ed), Effects of the indoor environment on health. *Occup Med State Art Rev* 1995;10;1:1–26.

Sepkowitz KA. Occupationally acquired infections in health care workers, parts I and II. *Ann Intern Med* 1996;125:826–35, 917–28.

Snashall D. Occupational infections. *Br Med J* 1996; 313:551–4.

Udasin IG. Biologic agents. In Brooks SM, Gochfeld M, Herzstein J (eds), *Environmental Medicine*. St. Louis: Mosby, 1995.

University of Maryland Farm Safety Database. *Occupational Diseases* (hypertext document), 1997. Available at www.inform.umd.edu/EdRes/Topic/AgrEnv/ndd/occsafe/INFECTIOUS_DISEASES.html.

Internet Sources

Centers for Disease Control and Prevention. Access to information on hospital occupational health, immunizations, travel medicine, and infectious diseases. Also provides access to an electronic version of the *Morbidity and Mortality Weekly Report* and List of Vaccine-Preventable Diseases. Available at www.cdc.gov/. Most recent used for this chapter: CDC List of Vaccine-Preventable Diseases found online at http://www.cdc .gov/print.do?url=http://www.cdc.gov/vaccines/vpd-vac/vpd-list.htm last modified on July 19, 2007

National Library of Medicine. Free Medline searches; links to a wide variety of medical topics. Available at www.nlm.nih.gov/.

Occupational and environmental medicine resources. Access to the Guidelines for Employee Health Services in Health Care Facilities (Medical Center Occupational Health Section of the American College of Occupational and Environmental Medicine); home page for the Medical Center Occupational Health Section; information on the Medical Center Occupational Health Mailing List and archives of the list; links to hundreds of general medical as well as occupational and environmental medicine resources. Available at www.occenvmed.net/.

Duke University Occupational and Environmental Medicine. Access to information on the Occupational and Environmental Medicine Mailing List and archives of the list; compilation of recent government (e.g., CDC, NIOSH, and EPA) documents pertinent to occupational and environmental medicine; links to many occupational and environmental medicine resources. Available at http://152.3.65.120/oem/.

5

Vaccine-Preventable Diseases in Occupational Medicine

Ellen R. Kessler

Immunization programs play a key role in the prevention of disease by protecting the individual receiving the vaccines and by reducing spread of the disease in the community. Vaccine schedules for children and adults are vital to public health strategy and have resulted in a dramatic decline in or even elimination of some diseases. Certain occupations or work environments place individuals at a greater risk of exposure to infectious diseases. Therefore, employers have both a legal and an ethical duty to provide a safe work environment for their employees and those who visit their workplaces. They also have a major business interest in supporting employees' health and welfare, maximizing their satisfaction and productivity, and preventing needless corporate financial burdens owing to absenteeism. Because of these imperatives, employers have an obligation to protect the work force from occupationally acquired infections and diseases by making available an ongoing employment-based immunization program.

This chapter addresses current immunization guidelines for the prevention of incidentally and epidemically acquired infections and suggests strategies for increasing compliance with these guidelines. Additionally, the Centers for Disease Control and Prevention (CDC) website (www.cdc.gov/) is an excellent resource for published recommendations from the major vaccine policymaking committees, such as the Advisory Committee on Immunization Practices (ACIP). Subsequent chapters address exposure prevention and postexposure prophylaxis for work-related infectious diseases for which there are no available immunizations. Later chapters also provide more detailed information regarding the signs and symptoms and epidemiology of diseases that can be prevented through comprehensive workplace immunization programs.

There has always been an obvious need for infectious disease prevention programs within health care facilities, and more recently, there is a growing awareness of similar needs among other industries. Employers' ever-expanding responsibilities and opportunities to protect their employees from occupationally acquired diseases are evidenced by the increased numbers of employees traveling to foreign countries and the development of engineered vaccines such as the hepatitis A vaccine. Unfortunately, the effectiveness and cost-efficiency of adult immunization programs as tools for preventing disease are often overlooked. The underutilization of vaccines capable of preventing diseases and decreasing their morbidity and mortality remains a reality. The case of an unfortunate cardiovascular surgical resident who had not been immunized against hepatitis B and, despite adherence to infection control practices, contracted the disease and then transmitted the infection to 19 patients is a stark reminder of this underutilization [1].

Fortunately, there are nationwide campaigns in progress to ensure compliance with childhood vaccination programs, and there is increasing participation on the part of medical insurance providers in offering preventive services, including immunizations. However, the hesitancy of much of the adult population to participate in immunization programs warrants close attention and points out the need for more concentrated efforts to increase compliance. Reasons (or rationales) for noncompliance include

- Denial of need for protection
- Resistance or lack of interest
- Inconvenience, time, and pain associated with vaccine administration
- Misunderstandings regarding the need, effectiveness, and safety of vaccines
- The variances in indications for vaccinations and administration schedules based on age, medical conditions, and work environments
- Inconvenience and costs associated with vaccine availability

To overcome these obstacles, employers and occupational health professionals must address employees' misconceptions and concerns directly. This requires active physician support and an in-depth understanding of the importance and efficacy of the vaccines appropriate for specific work environments. It also requires ongoing educational efforts to inform potential vaccine recipients of the importance of acquiring immunity to certain vaccine-preventable diseases. Continuous highlighting of other workplace hazard controls, such as the observance of administrative and workplace health and safety procedures and the use of appropriate personal protective equipment, is also warranted and should be an integral component of the employee education process. For many companies, computerized tracking systems are instrumental in evaluating the progress of their immunization efforts, as well as in identifying specific departments or employee groups that require more targeted educational programs or other strategies to improve compliance.

Recommended Vaccines for Adults

The U.S. Public Health Service Advisory Committee on Immunization Practices (ACIP) regularly publishes the most recent recommendations regarding specific immunizations for adults and children in the journal *Morbidity and Mortality Weekly Report*. Discussion of every available vaccine is beyond the scope of this chapter, but immunization recommendations for certain occupational groups, including travelers to foreign countries, are ad-

Table 5-1A
Recommended Adult Immunization Schedule by Vaccine and Age Group: United States, October 2007–September 2008 [22]

Vaccine	Age Group		
	19–49 years	50–64 years	≥65 years
Tetanus, diphtheria, pertussis (Td/Tdap)[1,*]	1 dose of Td booster every 10 years		
	Substitute 1 dose of Tdap for Td		
Human papillomavirus (HPV)[2,*]	3 doses for females (0, 2, 6 months)		
Measles, mumps, rubella (MMR)[3,*]	1 or 2 doses	1 dose	
Varicella[4,*]	2 doses (0, 4–8 weeks)		
Influenza[5,*]	1 dose annually		
Pneumococcal (polysaccharide)[6,7]	1–2 doses		1 dose
Hepatitis A[8,*]	2 doses (0, 6–12 months or 0, 6–18 months)		
Hepatitis B[9,*]	3 doses (0, 1–2, 4–6 months)		
Meningococcal[10,*]	1 or more doses		
Zoster[11]			1 dose

For all persons in this category who meet the age requirements and who lack evidence of immunity (e.g., lack documentation of vaccination or have no evidence of prior infection)

Recommended if some other risk factor is present (e.g., on the basis of medical, occupational, life style, or other indications)

Table 5-1B
Vaccines That May Be Indicated for Adults Based on Medical and Other Conditions

Indication / Vaccine	Pregnancy	Immuno-compromising Conditions (Excluding HIV), Medications, Radiation	Human Immunodeficiency Virus (HIV) Infection[3,12,13] CD4+ T-Lymphocyte Count <200 cells/µL	≥200 cells/µL	Diabetes, Heart Disease, Chronic Pulmonary Disease, Chronic Alcoholism	Asplenia[12] (Including Elective Splenectomy and Terminal Complement Component Deficiencies)	Chronic Liver Disease	Kidney Failure, End-Stage Renal Disease, Recipients of Hemodialysis	Health Care Personnel
Tetanus, diphtheria, pertussis (Td/Tdap)[1,*]	Substitute 1 dose of Tdap for Td	1 dose of Td booster every 10 years							
Human papillomavirus (HPV)[2,*]		3 doses for females through age 26 years (0, 2, 6 months)							
Measles, mumps, rubella (MMR)[3,*]		Contraindicated	Contraindicated	1 or 2 doses					
Varicella[4,*]		Contraindicated	Contraindicated	2 doses (0, 4–8 weeks)					
Influenza[5,*]				1 dose of TIV annually					1 dose of TIV or LAIV q yr
Pneumococcal (polysaccharide)[6,7]					1–2 doses				
Hepatitis A[8,*]			2 doses (0, 6–12 months or 0, 6–18 months)						
Hepatitis B[9,*]			3 Doses (0, 1–2, 4–6 months)						
Meningococcal[10,*]					1 or more doses				
Zoster[11]	Contraindicated						1 dose		

For all persons in this category who meet the age requirements and who lack evidence of immunity (e.g., lack documentation of vaccination or have no evidence of prior infection)

Recommended if some other risk factor is present (e.g., on the basis of medical, occupational, life style, or other indications)

Note: Approved by the Advisory Committee on Immunization Practices (ACIP), the American Academy of Family Physicians, the American College of Obstetricians and Gynecologists, and the American College of Physicians. Complete statements from the ACIP are available at www.cdc.gov/vaccines/pubs/acip-list.htm.

*Covered by the Vaccine Injury Compensation Program.

[1] Tetanus, diphtheria, and acellular pertussis (Td/Tdap) vaccination. Tdap should replace a single dose of Td for adults aged <65 years who have not previously received a dose of Tdap. Only one of two Tdap products (Adacel; Sanofi Pasteur) is licensed for use in adults. Adults with uncertain histories of a complete primary vaccination series with tetanus and diphtheria toxoid–containing vaccines should begin or complete a primary vaccination series. A primary series for adults is 3 doses of tetanus and diphtheria toxoid–containing vaccines; administer the first 2 doses at least 4 weeks apart and the third dose 6–12 months after the second. However, Tdap can substitute for any one of the doses of Td in the 3-dose primary series. The booster dose of tetanus and diphtheria toxoid–containing vaccine should be administered to adults who have completed a primary series and if the last vaccination was received ≥10 years previously; Tdap or Td vaccine may be used as indicated. If the person is pregnant and received the last Td vaccination ≥10 years previously; administer Tdap during the second or third trimester; if the person received the last Td vaccination in <10 years, administer Tdap during the immediate postpartum period. A one-time administration of 1 dose of Tdap with an interval as short as 2 years from a previous Td vaccination is recommended for postpartum women, close contacts of infants aged <12 months, and all health care workers with direct patient contact. In certain situations, Td can be deferred during pregnancy and Tdap substituted in the immediate postpartum period or Tdap can be administered instead of Td to a pregnant woman after an informed discussion with the woman. Consult the ACIP statement for recommendations for administering Td as prophylaxis in wound management.

[2] Human papillomavirus (HPV) vaccination. HPV vaccination is recommended for all females aged ≤26 years who have not completed the vaccine series. History of genital warts, abnormal Papanicolaou test, or positive HPV DNA test is not evidence of prior infection with all vaccine HPV types; HPV vaccination is still recommended before potential exposure to HPV

(continues)

Table 5-1B
Continued

through sexual activity; however, females who are sexually active should still be vaccinated. Sexually active females who have not been infected with any of the HPV vaccine types receive the full benefit of the vaccination. Vaccination is less beneficial for females who have already been infected with one or more of the HPV vaccine types.

A complete series consists of 3 doses. The second dose should be administered 2 months after the first dose; the third dose should be administered 6 months after the first dose.

Although HPV vaccination is not specifically recommended for females with the medical indications described in Table 5-1B, "Vaccines that might be indicated for adults based on medical and other indications," it is not a live-virus vaccine and can be administered. However, immune response and vaccine efficacy might be less than in persons who do not have the medical indications described or who are immunocompetent.

[3] Measles, mumps, rubella (MMR) vaccination. *Measles component:* Adults born before 1957 can be considered immune to measles. Adults born during or after 1957 should receive ≥1 dose of MMR unless they have a medical contraindication, documentation of ≥1 dose, history of measles based on health care provider diagnosis, or laboratory evidence of immunity. A second dose of MMR is recommended for adults who (1) have been recently exposed to measles or are in an outbreak setting, (2) have been previously vaccinated with killed measles vaccine, (3) have been vaccinated with an unknown type of measles vaccine during 1963–1967, (4) are students in postsecondary educational institutions, (5) work in a health care facility, or (6) plan to travel internationally. *Mumps component:* Adults born before 1957 generally can be considered immune to mumps. Adults born during or after 1957 should receive 1 dose of MMR unless they have a medical contraindication, history of mumps based on health care provider diagnosis, or laboratory evidence of immunity. A second dose of MMR is recommended for adults who (1) are in an age group that is affected during a mumps outbreak, (2) are students in postsecondary educational institutions, (3) work in a health care facility, or (4) plan to travel internationally. For unvaccinated health care workers born before 1957 who do not have other evidence of mumps immunity, consider administering 1 dose on a routine basis and strongly consider administering a second dose during an outbreak. *Rubella component:* Administer 1 dose of MMR vaccine to women whose rubella vaccination history is unreliable or who lack laboratory evidence of immunity. For women of childbearing age, regardless of birth year, routinely determine rubella immunity and counsel women regarding congenital rubella syndrome. Women who do not have evidence of immunity should receive MMR vaccine on completion or termination of pregnancy and before discharge from the health care facility.

[4] Varicella vaccination. All adults without evidence of immunity to varicella should receive 2 doses of single-antigen varicella vaccine unless they have a medical contraindication. Special consideration should be given to those who (1) have close contact with persons at high risk for severe disease (e.g., health care personnel and family contacts of immunocompromised persons) or (2) are at high risk for exposure or transmission (e.g., teachers, child-care employees, residents and staff members of institutional settings, including correctional institutions, college students, military personnel, adolescents and adults living in households with children, nonpregnant women of childbearing age, and international travelers). Evidence of immunity to varicella in adults includes any of the following: (1) documentation of 2 doses of varicella vaccine at least 4 weeks apart, (2) U.S.-born before 1980 (although for health care personnel and pregnant women, birth before 1980 should not be considered evidence of immunity), (3) history of varicella based on diagnosis or verification of varicella by a health care provider (for a patient reporting a history of or presenting with an atypical case, a mild case, or both, health care providers should seek either an epidemiologic link with a typical varicella case or to a laboratory-confirmed case or evidence of laboratory confirmation, if it was performed at the time of acute disease), (4) history of herpes zoster based on health care provider diagnosis, or (5) laboratory evidence of immunity or laboratory confirmation of disease. Assess pregnant women for evidence of varicella immunity. Women who do not have evidence of immunity should receive the first dose of varicella vaccine on completion or termination of pregnancy and before discharge from the health care facility. The second dose should be administered 4–8 weeks after the first dose.

[5] Influenza vaccination. *Medical indications:* Chronic disorders of the cardiovascular or pulmonary systems, including asthma; chronic metabolic diseases, including diabetes mellitus, renal or hepatic dysfunction, hemoglobinopathies, or immunosuppression (including immunosuppression caused by medications or HIV); any condition that compromises respiratory function or the handling of respiratory secretions or that can increase the risk of aspiration (e.g., cognitive dysfunction, spinal cord injury, or seizure disorder or other neuromuscular disorder); and pregnancy during the influenza season. No data exist on the risk for severe or complicated influenza disease among persons with asplenia; however, influenza is a risk factor for secondary bacterial infections that can cause severe disease among persons with asplenia. *Occupational indications:* Health care personnel and employees of long-term-care and assisted-living facilities. *Other indications:* Residents of nursing homes and other long-term-care and assisted-living facilities, persons likely to transmit influenza to persons at high risk (e.g., in-home household contacts and caregivers of children aged 0–59 months or persons of all ages with high-risk conditions), and anyone who would like to be vaccinated. Healthy, nonpregnant adults aged ≤49 years without high-risk medical conditions who are not contacts of severely immunocompromised persons in special care units can receive either intranasally administered live, attenuated influenza vaccine (FluMist) or inactivated vaccine. Other persons should receive the inactivated vaccine.

[6] Pneumococcal polysaccharide vaccination. *Medical indications:* Chronic pulmonary disease (excluding asthma); chronic cardiovascular diseases; diabetes mellitus; chronic liver diseases, including liver disease as a result of alcohol abuse (e.g., cirrhosis); chronic alcoholism; chronic renal failure; nephrotic syndrome; functional or anatomic asplenia (e.g., sickle cell disease or splenectomy; if elective splenectomy is planned, vaccinate at least 2 weeks before surgery); immunosuppressive conditions; and cochlear implants and cerebrospinal fluid leaks. Vaccinate as close to HIV diagnosis as possible. *Other indications:* Alaska natives and certain American Indian populations and residents of nursing homes or other long-term-care facilities.

[7] Revaccination with pneumococcal polysaccharide vaccine. One-time revaccination after 5 years for persons with chronic renal failure or nephrotic syndrome; functional or anatomic asplenia (e.g., sickle cell disease or splenectomy), or immunosuppressive conditions. For persons aged ≥65 years, one-time revaccination if they were vaccinated ≥5 years previously and were aged <65 years at the time of primary vaccination.

[8] Hepatitis A vaccination. *Medical indications:* Persons with chronic liver disease and persons who receive clotting factor concentrates. *Behavioral indications:* Men who have sex with men and persons who use illegal drugs. *Occupational indications:* Persons working with hepatitis A virus (HAV)–infected primates or with HAV in a research laboratory setting. *Other indications:* Persons traveling to or working in countries that have high or intermediate endemicity of hepatitis A (a list of countries is available at www.n.cdc.gov/travel/contentdiseases.aspx) and any person seeking protection from HAV infection. Single-antigen vaccine formulations should be administered in a 2-dose schedule at either 0 and 6–12 months (Havrix) or 0 and 6–18 months (Vaqta). If the combined hepatitis A and hepatitis B vaccine (Twinrix) is used, administer 3 doses at 0, 1, and 6 months.

[9] Hepatitis B vaccination. *Medical indications:* Persons with end-stage renal disease, including patients receiving hemodialysis, persons with HIV infection, and persons with chronic liver disease. *Occupational indications:* Health care personnel and public safety workers who are exposed to blood or other potentially infectious body fluids. *Behavioral indications:* Sexually active persons who are not in a long-term, mutually monogamous relationship (e.g., persons with more than one sex partner during the previous 6 months), current or recent injection-drug users, and men who have sex with men. *Other indications:* Household contacts and sex partners of persons with chronic hepatitis B virus (HBV) infection, clients and staff members of institutions

for persons with developmental disabilities, international travelers to countries with high or intermediate prevalence of chronic HBV infection (a list of countries is available at www.n.cdc.gov/travel/contentdiseases.aspx), and any adult seeking protection from HBV infection. Settings where hepatitis B vaccination is recommended for all adults: STD treatment facilities, HIV testing and treatment facilities, facilities providing drug-abuse treatment and prevention services, health care settings targeting services to injection-drug users or men who have sex with men, correctional facilities, end-stage renal disease programs and facilities for chronic hemodialysis patients, and institutions and nonresidential day-care facilities for persons with developmental disabilities. *Special formulation indications:* For adult patients receiving hemodialysis and other immunocompromised adults, 1 dose of 40 μg/mL (Recombivax HB) or 2 doses of 20 μg/mL (Engerix-B) administered simultaneously.

[10]Meningococcal vaccination. *Medical indications:* Adults with anatomic or functional asplenia or terminal complement component deficiencies. *Other indications:* First-year college students living in dormitories; microbiologists who are routinely exposed to isolates of *Neisseria meningitidis*; military recruits; and persons who travel to or live in countries in which meningococcal disease is hyperendemic or epidemic [e.g., the "meningitis belt" of sub-Saharan Africa during the dry season (December–June)], particularly if their contact with local populations will be prolonged. Vaccination is required by the government of Saudi Arabia for all travelers to Mecca during the annual Hajj. Meningococcal conjugate vaccine is preferred for adults with any of the preceding indications who are aged ≤55 years, although meningococcal polysaccharide vaccine (MPSV4) is an acceptable alternative. Revaccination after 3–5 years might be indicated for adults previously vaccinated with MPSV4 who remain at increased risk for infection (e.g., persons residing in areas in which disease is epidemic).

[11]Herpes zoster vaccination. A single dose of zoster vaccine is recommended for adults aged ≥60 years regardless of whether they report a prior episode of herpes zoster. Persons with chronic medical conditions may be vaccinated unless a contraindication or precaution exists for their condition.

[12]Selected conditions for which *Haemophilus influenzae* type b (Hib) vaccine may be used. Hib conjugate vaccines are licensed for children aged 6 weeks to 71 months. No efficacy data are available on which to base a recommendation concerning use of Hib vaccine for older children and adults with the chronic conditions associated with an increased risk for Hib disease. However, studies suggest good immunogenicity in patients who have sickle cell disease, leukemia, or HIV infection or who have had splenectomies; administering vaccine to these patients is not contraindicated.

[13]Immunocompromising conditions. Inactivated vaccines generally are acceptable (e.g., pneumococcal, meningococcal, and influenza—trivalent inactivated influenza vaccine) and live vaccines generally are avoided in persons with immune deficiencies or immune suppressive conditions. Information on specific conditions is available at www.cdc.gov/vaccines/pubs/acip-list.htm.

These schedules indicate the recommended age groups and medical indications for routine administration of currently licensed vaccines for persons aged ≥19 years, as of October 1, 2007. Licensed combination vaccines may be used whenever any components of the combination are indicated and when the vaccine's other components are not contraindicated. For detailed recommendations on all vaccines, including those used primarily for travelers or those issued during the year, consult the manufacturers' package inserts and the complete statements from the Advisory Committee on Immunization Practices (available at www.cdc.gov/vaccines/pubs/acip-list.htm).

Report all clinically significant postvaccination reactions to the Vaccine Adverse Event Reporting System (VAERS). Reporting forms and instructions on filing a VAERS report are available at www.vaers.hhs.gov or by telephone at 800-822-7967. Information on how to file a Vaccine Injury Compensation Program claim is available at www.hrsa.gov/vaccinecompensation or by telephone at 800-338-2382. To file a claim for vaccine injury, contact the U.S. Court of Federal Claims, 717 Madison Place, N.W., Washington, D.C. 20005; telephone 202-357-6400. Use of trade names and commercial sources is for identification only and does not imply endorsement by the U.S. Department of Health and Human Services.

Table 5-2
Recommended Postexposure Prophylaxis for Exposure to Hepatitis B Virus

Vaccination and Antibody Response Status of Exposed Person[a]	Source HBsAg[b] Positive	Treatment Source HBsAg[b] Negative	Source unknown or not Available for testing
Unvaccinated	HBIG[c] x 1; initiate HB vaccine series	Initiate HB vaccine series.	Initiate HB vaccine series.
Previously vaccinated			
Known responder[d]	No treatment.	No treatment.	No treatment.
Known nonresponder[e]	HBIG x 2[f] or HBIG x 1 and initiate revaccination	No treatment.	If known high-risk source, treat as if source were HBsAg positive.
Antibody response unknown	Test exposed person for anti-HBs[g] 1. If adequate,[d] no treatment is necessary. 2. If inadequate,[e] HBIG x 1 and vaccine booster	No treatment.	Test exposed person for anti-HBs: 1. If adequate,[d] no treatment. 2. If inadequate,[e] administer vaccine booster and recheck titer in 1-2 months.

a. Persons who have previously been infected with HBV are immune to reinfection and do not require postexposure prophylaxis
b. Hepatitis B surface antigen.
c. Hepatitis B immune globulin; dose 0.06 mL/kg intramuscularly.
d. A responder is a person with adequate levels of serum antibody to hepatitis B surface antigen (i.e., anti-HBs $\geq$ 10 IU/mL).
e. A nonresponder is a person with inadequate response to vaccination (i.e., serum anti-HBs $\geq$10 mIU/mL).
f. The option of giving one dose of HBIG and reinitiating the vaccine series is preferred for nonresponders who have not completed a second 3-dose vaccine series. For persons who previously completed a second vaccine series but failed to respond, two doses of HBIG are preferred.
g. Antibody to HBsAg
Adapted from: Updated U.S. Public Health Service Guidelines for the Management of Occupational Exposures to HBV, HCV, and HIV and Recommendations for Postexposure Prophylaxis. MMWR 2001; 50(RR-11), 22.

Table 5-3
Rabies Preexposure Immunization

Risk Category	Nature of Risk	Typical Populations	Preexposure Regimen
Continuous	Virus present continuously, often in high concentrations. Aerosol, mucous membrane, bite, or nonbite exposure possible. Specific exposures may go unrecognized.	Rabies research lab workers.* Rabies biologics production workers.	Primary preexposure immunization course. Serology every 6 months. Booster immunization when antibody titer falls below acceptable level.*
Frequent	Exposure usually episodic, with source recognized, but exposure also may be unrecognized. Aerosol, mucous membrane, bite, or nonbite exposure.	Rabies diagnostic laboratory workers,* spelunkers, veterinarians, and animal control and wildlife workers in rabies epizootic areas.	Primary preexposure immunization course. Booster immunization or serology every 2 years.†
Infrequent (greater than population-at-large)	Exposure nearly always episodic with source recognized. Mucous membrane, bite, or nonbite exposure.	Veterinarians and animal control and wildlife workers in areas of low rabies endemicity. Certain travelers to foreign rabies epizootic areas. Veterinary students.	Primary preexposure immunization course. No routine booster immunization or serology.
Rare (population-at-large)	Exposure always episodic, mucous membrane, or bite with source recognized.	U.S. population at large, including individuals in rabies epizootic areas.	

*Judgment of relative risk and extra monitoring of immunization status of laboratory workers are the responsibility of the laboratory supervisor (see U.S. Department of Health and Human Services Biosafety in Microbiological and Biomedical Laboratories, 1984).
†Preexposure booster immunization consists of one dose of HDCV, 1.0 mL/dose IM (deltoid area). Acceptable antibody level is 1:5 titer (complete inhibition in RFFIT at 1:5 dilution). Boost if titer falls below 1:5.
Source: Centers for Disease Control and Prevention. Human Rabies Prevention—United States, 1999: Recommendations of the Advisory Committee (ACIP). *MMWR* 1999;48:1–21.

Table 5-4
Rabies Vaccine Schedule

Vaccine or Toxoid	Indications	Schedule	Major Contraindications	Comments
Rabies, human diploid cell (HDCV)	See Tables 5-3, 5-5	Three doses (0.1 mL ID) on days 0,7, and 21 or 28	See Table 5-5	Boost after two years or test serum for antibody level. Must not use chloroquine for malaria prophylaxis until three weeks after completion of third ID dose of vaccine
Rabies, human diploid cell or rabies vaccine absorbed (RVA)	See Tables 5-3, 5-5	Three doses (1 mL IM in deltoid area) on days 0,7, and 28	See Table 5-5	Boost after two years or test serum for antibody level

dressed in this chapter. Tables 5-1 through 5-5 outline the most commonly used vaccines for adults in occupational settings.

INFLUENZA VACCINE

Outbreaks of type A or B influenza typically peak in the winter and cause community-wide epidemics every 1–3 years. Each year, the virus undergoes an antigenic drift that precludes complete natural or vaccinated immunity from the previous year. In some years, there is a total antigenic shift in which the virus is entirely dissimilar from previous years and subsequently is responsible for pandemics or worldwide epidemics.

Influenza outbreaks occur explosively, and one person can infect many others. An epidemic usually peaks 2–3 weeks following the first reported cases in a community and continues for approximately 5–6 weeks. School-age children typically have the highest attack rate (50%), but theirs is generally a mild illness of fever and upper respiratory tract infection.

Mortality rates are significant for residents of long-term care facilities, for those who have underlying medical conditions, such as cardiac and pulmonary disease, and for newborns and the elderly.

The trivalent inactivated influenza vaccine (TIV), which is composed of two A subtypes and one B subtype of the influenza virus, is the mainstay for prevention of the spread of disease. Viral subtypes that have been identified from the previous year go into the formulation of the vaccine for the upcoming year. A live, attenuated influenza vaccine (LAIV) was approved for use in the United States in 2003. LAIV is administered as a nasal spray and contains the same three influenza viruses as the inactivated version. LAIV is approved by the U.S. Food and Drug Administration (FDA) for use among healthy persons 5–49 years of age who want to reduce their risk of influenza. Among this group are those with close contacts to people at high risk for complications of influenza, with the exception of immunosuppressed individuals. Health care workers and employees of long-term care facilities who have contact with immunosuppressed persons should receive the TIV. Ideally, all health care workers should receive the influenza vaccine on an annual basis. Groups that should be targeted include physicians, nurses, and other personnel in hospitals and outpatient settings, including home care, who have contact with patients of all ages at high risk of developing complications from influenza [2].

Many occupational health services provide annual influenza vaccination programs for their employees. The employer recognizes that there is an easily attainable reduction in costs related to absenteeism during the flu season when the vaccine is both encouraged and provided, especially if vaccination is available at the worksite.

Sporadic human cases of infection with highly pathogenic avian influenza A (H5N1) viruses have been identified in Asia, Africa, and the Middle East, primarily among individuals who have had close contact with sick or dead birds. To date, no evidence exists of genetic reassortment between human influenza A and H5N1 viruses, but the potential does exist.

Although the influenza vaccines do not provide protection against avian influenza A viruses, the reduction in seasonal influenza risk may reduce the theoretical risk of recombination of both viruses

Table 5-5
Vaccines for Foreign Travelers

Vaccine or Toxoid	Indications	Schedule	Major Contraindications	Comments
Hepatitis B	Those at risk of Blood or body fluid exposure	See Tables 5-1A, 5-1B		
Hepatitis A	See Tables 5-1A, 5-1B			
Poliovirus	Health care workers and laboratory workers who may be in close contact with patients excreting wild poliovirus or who handle specimens from such patients. Travelers to developing countries outside the Americas—OPV available only for control of outbreaks.	*Unimmunized adults:* IPV. Two doses at 4–8-week intervals, third dose 6–12 months after second (can be as soon as 2 months). Dose: 0.5 mL SC. *Partially immunized adults:* Complete primary series with IPV above.	Pregnancy Anaphylactic Allergy to neomycin or streptomycin	
Japanese encephalitis	Travelers should check wwwn.cdc.gov/travel for current recommendations.	Three doses given days 0, 7, and 30.	Pregnancy Severe illness Previous serious reaction to vaccine	
Plague* (available for military, police, and first responders only)	Not available commercially	First dose (1 mL IM); second dose (0.2 mL IM) 4 weeks later; third dose (0.2 mL IM) 3–6 months after dose 2.		Antibiotics (e.g., doxycycline, tetracycline) in epizootic or endemic areas.
Yellow fever*	Travelers should check wwwn.cdc.gov/travel for current recommendations.	One dose (0.5 mL SC). Booster every 10 years.	Thymus disorders or dysfunction, symptomatic HIV, egg allergy with anaphylaxis.	
Meningococcal polysaccharide (tetravalent A, C, W135, and y)	Travelers to sub-Saharan Africa during December through June.	See Tables 5-1A, 5-1B		
Typhoid vaccine IM and oral	Travelers to South Asia and developing countries in Asia, Africa, the Caribbean, and Central and South America.	IM vaccine: One 0.5-mL dose, booster 0.5 mL every 2 years. Oral vaccine: Four doses on alternative days. The manufacturer recommends revaccination with the entire four-dose series every 5 years.	Severe local or systemic reaction to a previous dose. Ty21a (oral) vaccine should not be administered to immunocompromised persons or to persons receiving antimicrobial agents.	Vaccine should not be considered an alternative to the use of proper procedures when handling specimens and cultures in the laboratory.
Rabies	Travelers planning to be more than 30 days in an area of the world where rabies is a constant threat.	See Table 5-3	Known reaction[†] Neomycin allergy[†] Thimerosal allergy[†]	

Abbreviations: ID = intradermal; IPV = inactivated poliovirus vaccine; OPV = oral poliovaccine; PO = orally; SC = subcutaneously.
*See manufacturer's package insert for recommendations on dosage.
[†]Not major contraindication.

within a human host. Therefore, the CDC has recommended that all individuals responsible for investigating avian influenza outbreaks among poultry should receive seasonal influenza vaccinations [3]. The Occupational Safety and Health Administration (OSHA) also has issued an advisory notice recommending that poultry workers in facilities with a suspected or confirmed avian flu outbreak receive the influenza vaccination [4].

TETANUS TOXOID AND PERTUSSIS

Tetanus is an often fatal disease characterized by severe muscle spasms that typically occur in the neck and trunk muscles. These manifestations are caused by an exotoxin produced by the *Clostridium tetani,* an anaerobic or microaerophilic bacillus that proliferates at the site of injured tissue—typically a crush or puncture wound. The disease is most likely to occur in rural settings, where there is a greater exposure to animals and contaminated soil. Employee populations most at risk are those in agriculture and forestry industries.

Essentially all working-age individuals who were born in or have resided in the United States received the completed series of tetanus vaccinations as a prerequisite for enrollment into school. However, it is essential that previously vaccinated employees receive booster vaccinations with the tetanus and diptheria vaccine (Td) at least every 10 years. Therefore, it is important to determine the Td vaccination status of all employees, particularly foreign-born individuals from rural areas of Africa, Asia, and South America, where immunization programs may not be routine.

Pertussis, or whooping cough, an upper respiratory infection caused by the *Bordetella pertussis* bacterium, remains endemic in the United States despite long-standing routine childhood pertussis vaccination. Immunity to pertussis wanes approximately 5–10 years after completion of childhood vaccination, leaving adolescents and adults particularly susceptible to infection. Since the 1980s, the number of reported pertussis cases has increased steadily, and outbreaks have been documented regularly in both the community and workplace settings. In 2005, a tetanus toxoid, reduced diphtheria toxoid, and acellular pertussis vaccine (Tdap) formulated for use in adults and adolescents was licensed in the United States. In the same year, the ACIP recommended the routine use of Tdap among adults aged 19–64 years [5].

MEASLES, MUMPS, AND RUBELLA VACCINE (MMR)

In the United States, the incidence of measles declined considerably after the introduction of the live, attenuated MMR vaccine in 1963. In 1983, only 1,493 cases were recorded; however, this trend reversed dramatically in the years 1989–1991, with a peak of 27,786 recorded cases in 1990. After this brief period, the downward trend resumed, and in 2002 and 2003, only 44 and 56 cases, respectively, were documented, which are the lowest numbers of annual cases ever recorded [6].

Worldwide, measles infection continues to be problematic. Each year, there are an estimated 36.5 million cases and 1 million deaths caused by the disease, most of them in Africa. Since 2001, most of the recorded cases in the United States have been imported from China and Japan.

Health care workers and other employees who may have contact with measles carriers should be required to show evidence of immunity. This is particularly true for individuals who travel to countries where measles is poorly controlled. The ACIP defines immunity as physician documentation of infection, serologic evidence of immunity, or documentation of two doses of the MMR vaccine administered after 16 months of age. Individuals born before 1957 are considered to have natural immunity; however, serologic sampling of hospital workers has indicated that approximately 5% of those born before 1957 were not immune to measles. Because nearly 30% of all health care workers who acquired measles at work between 1985 and 1989 were born before 1957 [7,8], the ACIP recommends that consideration be given to vaccinating an individual if there is reason to believe the person, regardless of age, is not immune.

In both children and adults, rubella virus presents as a mild febrile disease accompanied by a maculopapular rash. However, rubella can cause intrauterine death or devastating congenital abnormalities in the developing fetus. A single dose of live, attenuated rubella vaccine as part of the MMR will elicit an adequate antibody response in nearly 99% of susceptible individuals. In the United States, two doses of MMR are recommended as part of the childhood vaccination program. Medical personnel and all nonpregnant women of childbearing age who are likely to come in contact with individuals who have rubella or with patients in prenatal clinics should have serologic proof of immunization or physician-written documentation of at least one rubella immunization at the time of or after the first birthday. Ideally, all susceptible health care workers and women of childbearing age who are not pregnant or plan to become pregnant in the next 4 weeks should be immunized. As a result of intense public health efforts in 2005, the CDC was able to declare the elimination of rubella and congenital rubella in the United States. The number of reported cases in the United States was 11 in 2006 and 10 in 2007. Since 2002, all cases have been traceable to foreigners who carried the virus in from abroad [9,10].

Mumps, an RNA virus in the Paramyxoviridae family, is spread either from person to person by saliva droplets or by direct contact with objects contaminated with infected saliva. The more common features of this disease include parotid gland swelling and orchitis in adolescent and adult males; however one of seven people shows signs of central nervous system involvement. Approximately 15–20% of adults infected with the disease remain asymptomatic [11].

In 2006, a mumps epidemic in the central United States was cause for significant public concern. A total of 2,597 mumps cases were reported in 11 states, representing a marked resurgence of the disease in a single year. Most of these cases occurred in college students between the ages of 18 and 25 years.

The mechanisms for mumps vaccine failure in the 2006 U.S. outbreak most likely resulted from a combination of factors: high viral burden in close settings such as college campuses, suboptimal vaccination in high-risk populations, poor storage and handling practices, and waning immunity in previously vaccinated individuals. In response, the CDC issued new guidelines to specifically target susceptible populations such as college students, health care workers, and international travelers.

PNEUMOCOCCAL VACCINE

In the United States, pneumococcal infections are responsible for approximately 40,000 deaths per year—i.e., more deaths than any other vaccine-preventable infection [12]. Individuals at risk who should be vaccinated include those age 65 or older and individuals with chronic diseases such as cardiovascular disease, pulmonary disease (excluding asthma), diabetes mellitus, chronic liver disease, alcoholism, and asplenism.

The Americans with Disabilities Act (ADA) of 1990 laid the foundation for more individuals with chronic illnesses to enter the work force. In addition, more and more individuals age 65 or older are remaining in or returning to the workplace. While the employee's primary care provider generally is responsible for providing the pneumococcal vaccine, the occupational health center may play an invaluable role by identifying employees at risk and directing them to their primary care provider or their company's occupational health service for appropriate vaccination.

VARICELLA VACCINE AND HERPES ZOSTER VACCINE

Varicella (chickenpox) and herpes zoster (shingles) are clinical manifestations of the varicella-zoster virus (VZV). Varicella, the primary infection, is extremely contagious but generally is regarded as a benign, self-limited infection of childhood. However, varicella can be life-threatening for premature infants, individuals who are immunocompromised, and patients with chronic lung or skin afflictions. Any person over the age of 13 who has active infection also may suffer serious and sometimes fatal complications.

Approximately 9% of individuals older than age 15 are considered to be nonimmune, but a higher percent is found among people raised in the tropics or subtropics. Herpes zoster, the localized reactivation of the primary infection, occurs in all age groups but most commonly in the elderly.

In the workplace setting, VZV vaccine is underutilized. This is true particularly among health care workers who do not have a positive history of immunity to the disease. VZV vaccine has proved to be safe in healthy nonpregnant individuals and can reduce the costs of a hospital VZV control program [13]. Concerns have been raised regarding the risk of transmission of virus following vaccination, particularly if the individual develops a varicella-like rash following immunization. To date, the benefits have far outweighed the theoretical risks; thus susceptible health care workers should receive the vaccine. Nonimmune staff members in institutional settings, employees who are likely to travel to countries where VZV is prevalent, and workers who have exposures to nonimmunized children, as in a child care or classroom setting, also should consider vaccination.

The Zoster vaccine has been recommended recently by the ACIP for all immunocompetent adults age 60 and older. The pain and discomfort of herpes zoster infection and postherpetic neuralgia bring about substantial morbidity in this age range. It is estimated that 1 million or more cases occur each year in the United States, a number that is likely to increase as the population ages. The Zoster vaccine has been shown to reduce the overall incidence of herpes zoster by 51.3% and significantly reduce the pain and discomfort among subjects in whom herpes zoster developed [14].

HEPATITIS B VACCINE

Hepatitis B vaccine, which was first made available in 1976, has been a significant factor in the decline of transmission of hepatitis B virus (HBV) among health care workers. At one university hospital, the incidence of clinical HBV decreased from 82 cases per 100,000 between 1980 and 1984 to 0 cases between 1985 and 1989 [15].

Although hepatitis B vaccine—a highly purified viral antigen manufactured initially from pooled donor serum and later genetically engineered—has proved to be safe, the rate of acceptance among health care workers is strikingly inadequate. Many health care workers and other employees who come in contact with blood and other potentially infectious material (OPIM) believe that they are not at risk for contracting the disease. One study demonstrated that 22.5% of participating transplant surgeons were inadequately vaccinated against HBV and 35.7% failed to seek evaluation following possible exposures to HBV [16]. Although the OSHA Bloodborne Pathogen Standard mandates that employers offer potentially exposed employees the vaccine series at no cost, aggressive immunization campaigns are often lacking.

Prevaccination serologic screening for prior infection is not warranted for individuals receiving the vaccine series. Postvaccination testing for antibodies may be advisable if the individual is likely to have ongoing risk of injuries from sharp instruments or needlesticks. Testing should be performed 1–2 months after completion of the vaccine series. Knowledge of the individual's antibody response after completion of the hepatitis series aids in determination of the need for immediate postexposure prophylaxis in the event of an accident.

In a significant percentage of individuals, antibodies to HBV following vaccination decrease gradually over time. However, studies have shown that despite waning antibody titers to HBV, vaccine-induced immunity persists and probably will prevent clinical hepatitis or viremia [17]. Therefore, booster doses generally are unnecessary [18] (see Table 5-2).

HEPATITIS A VACCINE

Hepatitis A continues to be one of the most frequently reported vaccine-preventable diseases in the United States despite the licensure of two hepatitis A vaccines, Havrix (GlaxoSmithKline) and VAQTA (Merck & Co., Inc.). Twinrix (GlaxoSmithKline), a combination of both hepatitis A and B vaccines, is also available commercially. The ACIP has published recommendations for the prevention of hepatitis A virus (HAV) infection [19].

Employees who travel to or work in countries that have high or intermediate HAV endemicity should be vaccinated before departure. U.S. travelers to other countries in North America (except Mexico and Central America), western Europe, Japan, Australia, or New Zealand are not considered to be at greater risk than those who travel within the United States.

Employees who work with HAV-infected primates or with HAV in a research laboratory are the only occupational groups shown to be at increased risk for HAV infection because of occupational exposure. Although outbreaks of hepatitis A have been documented in other work settings, such as food handling, health care centers, sewage treatment facilities, and child-care centers, preexposure immunization is not routinely recommended. Individuals who have been exposed to HAV recently and who have not had the hepatitis A vaccine previously should be given a single intramuscular (IM) dose of immunoglobulin (0.02 mL/kg) as soon as possible but not more than 2 weeks after the last exposure. Those who have been administered one dose of hepatitis A vaccine at least 1 month before exposure to HAV do not need immunoglobulin.

POLIOVIRUS VACCINE

In the United States, control of poliomyelitis has essentially been achieved because of the success of the polio vaccination program that began in the 1950s. Since 1980, fewer than 150 cases of paralytic poliomyelitis have been reported, most of which were associated with vaccination; a handful of cases has been due to importation of the wild poliovirus into the United States. Prevention of epidemics owing to imported virus can be sustained only by ongoing early childhood vaccination programs. Routine vaccination of adults who reside in the United States is not recommended because of the low probability of exposure and the high probability of immunity in the adult population.

Adults should receive the poliovirus vaccine only if they have a high risk of exposure to the virus. All health care workers and laboratory workers who are in close contact with patients excreting wild poliovirus or who handle specimens from those patients should receive the vaccine. Travelers to developing countries outside the Americas are also candidates for vaccination against polio. In July 1999, the ACIP recommended that the use of inactivated poliovirus vaccine (IPV) instead of the oral poliovirus vaccine (OPV) to reduce the risk of vaccine-associated paralytic paralysis (VAPP). As of 2000, OPV is no longer routinely available in the United States [20].

LYME DISEASE VACCINE

Lyme disease is a tick-borne infection caused by the spirochete *Borrelia burgdorferi*. It is the most common tick-borne disease in the United States. There were 64,382 cases reported to the CDC during 2003–2005 [21]. The disease occurs primarily in the northeastern, mid-Atlantic, and upper north central regions of the United States, as well as in the northwestern regions of California. The transmission of the spirochete from the tick occurs after 24–48 hours of attachment to the individual. Transmission peaks from April through July, when the nymphal stages of the tick vectors of Lyme disease, *Ixodes scapularis* and *I. pacificus,* are actively seeking hosts.

Approximately 85% of individuals with symptomatic Lyme disease have the typical erythema migrans rash. If untreated, the infection can cause arthritis or neurologic symptoms such as radiculoneuropathy or encephalopathy. Antibiotics usually are effective in eradicating the disease completely.

A Lyme disease vaccine, LYMErix, had been approved in 1998 by the FDA for use and was available in the United States until 2002. GlaxoSmithKline, the maker of LYMErix, pulled the vaccine off the market in 2002, blaming poor sales. Factors including the recommendation for vaccine use in high-risk regions only, the lack of FDA approval for use in children, and the limited duration of immunity and protection contributed to its poor commercial success. Although research is ongoing in both the United States and Europe for a more effective vaccine, there are no available vaccines against Lyme disease at this time.

RABIES VACCINE

Rabies is a fatal viral disease of the central nervous system that can infect most mammals. The most susceptible animals are bats, raccoons, skunks, coyotes, foxes, wolves, and unvaccinated dogs, cats, and livestock. Occupational groups such as veterinarians, veterinary technicians, animal control officers, wildlife workers, and other animal handlers who are frequently exposed to these animals are at particular risk of viral transmission, and exposures may be inapparent. Laboratory workers who work with the live rabies virus, spelunkers (cave explorers), certain construction workers, and travelers to foreign countries where canine rabies is a problem also should be considered at risk for exposure to rabies. All these workers should undergo the three-dose preexposure series with the rabies vaccine. This is particularly necessary if the individual is working in a remote area where the vaccine is not readily available. If a rabies exposure takes place, postexposure immunization with two doses of the vaccine is still necessary, even if the exposed individual has received the preexposure series.

The newer rabies vaccines have proved to be safe and better tolerated than the earlier formulations. Most of the symptoms (i.e., fever, rash, and muscle aches) have been due to preservatives in the vaccine; the most recently approved preservative-free vaccine may decrease these side effects significantly. The recommended vaccine schedules for various risk categories of rabies exposure are covered in Tables 5-3 and 5-4.

Vaccines for Health Care and Laboratory Workers

Health care and laboratory workers are exposed to a variety of infections in the occupational setting. Most of these exposures are in some manner representative of exposures from the community that these workers serve. However, because of the increased diversity of communities, the types of infectious disease exposures have become more varied. In addition, laboratory workers are more likely to encounter a greater variety of infectious agents when handling cultures or infected animals for research purposes.

Health care workers have been added to the Adult Immunization Schedule in an effort to facilitate assessment of the vaccination status of health care workers and administration of needed vaccinations [22]. It cannot be overemphasized that sound preventive measures such as standard precautions, thorough hand washing, and the use of personal protective equipment are the most important methods for reducing the risk of transmitting nosocomial infections to other patients and health care workers. Vaccines that are safe and effective in reducing nosocomial infections must be promoted and made easily available to all employees, including those working night and weekend shifts. Extended clinic hours and on-site vaccination programs help to increase employee participation in employers' vaccination campaigns, especially at certain times such as during the annual influenza season.

Vaccines for Travelers to Foreign Countries and Endemic Areas

It has become more commonplace for employees in both the public and private sectors to have work duties that require either frequent travel or temporary assignment outside the United States. In addition, international agencies recruit health care workers to volunteer their time to reconstruction efforts in countries devastated by war, natural disaster, or poverty. The possibility of exposure to malaria, yellow fever, typhoid, polio, hepatitis A, meningitis, and other infectious diseases must be evaluated prior to travel abroad. Not infrequently, these assignments occur unexpectedly and preclude adequate time for optimal vaccination. For workers whose jobs entail travel, particularly in certain endemic areas, all possible health and safety measures must be taken, which necessitates having the most current information on infectious disease outbreaks in a particular area. The CDC's Traveler's Health Hotline (phone: 877-394-8747; fax: 888-232-3299; website: wwwn.cdc.gov/travel/default.aspx), as well as most travelers' clinics, may be instrumental in providing necessary information on recommended immunizations and schedules. Table 5-5 categorizes the most frequently required immunizations for individuals who travel abroad.

Future Vaccines

The research and development of several new vaccines such as malaria vaccine and Ebola virus vaccine hold considerable promise. In addition, major research has been launched to develop new tuberculosis vaccines [23]. Scientists are also developing unique delivery symptoms for vaccines. For example, a National Institute of Allergy and Infectious Diseases (NIAID)–supported study of an edible potato vaccine demonstrated that such a vaccine could stimulate an immune response. By eating genetically engineered raw potatoes containing a section of a strain of *E. coli*, the volunteers developed antibodies against the bacteria.

Role of Employers and Occupational Health Professionals

Over the past decade, significant progress has been made in dealing with work-related infectious disease exposure and prevention. Legislative directives, most notably OSHA's Bloodborne Pathogen Standard, broke new ground on the prevention front by mandating employer responsibility for at-risk employees. Compliance with this standard resulted in HBV vaccination campaigns. Unfortunately, employees' acceptance of this and other safety-proven vaccines sometimes has been disappointing, and the occurrences of preventable work-related infectious diseases continue to be of concern. Employers, particularly in the health care industry, generally have assumed responsibility for providing the appropriate immunizations according to recommended guidelines, but this becomes an increasingly difficult task when, for example, hospitals merge to become complex hospital systems, and outpatient services and physician practices are purchased by these systems.

Besides employers, occupational health professionals also play a major role in influencing employees and increasing their understanding and acceptance of preventive procedures such as vaccinations. Providing employees with immunization programs not only supports workers' health and safety but also saves dollars for the organization over the long term—namely, through decreases in lost workdays and thus increased productivity, as well as decreases in workers' compensation costs. However, to realize the long-term gains, employers must be willing to bear the costs associated with the administration of vaccines, as well as the costs associated with ongoing employee education and efforts to gain increased employee acceptance of them.

References

1. Harpaz R, Von Seidlein L, Averhoff FM, et al. Transmission of hepatitis B virus to multiple patients from a surgeon without evidence of inadequate infection control. *N Engl J Med* 1996;334:594–95.

2. Prevention and Control of Influenza: Recommendations of the Advisory Committee on Immunization Practices (ACIP). *MMWR* 2007;56;1–54

3. CDC. Interim Guidance for Protection of Persons Involved in U.S. Avian Influenza Outbreak Disease Control and Eradication Activities. Atlanta: U.S. Department of Health and Human Services, CDC, 2006. Available at www.cdc.gov/flu/avian/professional/protect-guid.htm.

4. Occupational Safety and Health Administration. OSHA Guidance Update on Protecting Employees from Avian Flu (Avian Influenza) Viruses. Washington: U.S. Department of Labor, Occupational Safety and Health Administration, 2006. Available at www.osha.gov/OshDoc/data_AvianFlu/avian_flu_guidance_english.pdf.

5. Preventing tetanus, diphtheria, and pertussis among adults: Use of tetanus toxoid, reduced diphtheria toxoid and acellular pertussis vaccine. Recommendations of the Advisory Committee on Immunization Practices (ACIP). *MMWR* 2006;55;1–33.

6. Centers for Disease Control and Prevention. Epidemiology of measles—United States, 2001–2003. *MMWR* 2004;53;713–6.

7. Braunstein H, Thomas S, Ito R. Immunity to measles in a large population of varying age. *Am J Dis Child* 1990;144:296–8.

8. Smith E, Welch W, Berhow M, et al. Measles susceptibility of hospital employees as determined by ELISA. *Clin Res* 1990;38:183A.

9. Achievements in public health: Elimination of rubella and congenital rubella syndrome—United States, 1969–2004. *MMWR* 2005;54:279–82.

10. Notifiable diseases/deaths in selected cities—Weekly information. *MMWR* 2008;57:16–28.

11. Kancherla V, Hanson C. Mumps resurgence in the United States. *J Allergy Clin Immunol* 2006;118:938–41.

12. Prevention of pneumococcal disease: Recommendations of the Advisory Committee on Immunization Practices (ACIP). *MMWR* 1997;46:3.

13. Nettleman M, Schmid M. Controlling varicella in the healthcare setting: The cost effectiveness of using varicella vaccine in healthcare workers. *Infect Control Hosp Epidemiol* 1997;18:504–8.

14. Oxman MN, Levin MJ, Johnson, M.S. et al. A vaccine to prevent herpes zoster and postherpetic neuralgia in older adults. *N Engl J Med* 2005;352:2271–84.

15. Lamphear BP, Linneman CC Jr, Cannon CG, et al. Decline of clinical hepatitis B in workers at a general hospital: Relation to increasing vaccine-induced immunity. *Clin Infect Dis* 1993;11:10–4.

16. Halpern SD, Asch DA, Shaked A, et al. Inadequate hepatitis B vaccination and post-exposure evaluation among transplant surgeons. *Ann Surg* 2006;244:305–9.

17. Hadler SC, Margolis HS. Hepatitis B immunization: Vaccine types, efficacy and indications for immunization. In Remington JS, Swartz MN (eds), *Current Topics in Infectious Diseases*. Boston: Blackwell Scientific, 1992, pp 282–308.

18. Centers for Disease Control and Prevention. Hepatitis B virus: A comprehensive strategy for eliminating transmission in the United States through childhood immunization. Recommendations of the Advisory Committee on Immunization Practices (ACIP). *MMWR* 1991;40:1–25.

19. Centers for Disease Control and Prevention. Prevention of hepatitis A through active or passive immunization: Recommendations of the Advisory Committee on Immunization Practices (ACIP). *MMWR* 1999;48:1–37.

20. Poliomyelitis prevention in the United States: Updated recommendations of the Advisory Committee on Immunization Practices (ACIP). *MMWR* 2000;49:1–22.

21. Centers for Disease Control and Prevention. Lyme disease—United States, 2003–2005. *MMWR* 2007;56:573–6.

22. Centers for Disease Control and Prevention. Recommended adult immunization schedule—United States, October 2007–September 2008. *MMWR* 2007;56:Q1–4.

23. Centers for Disease Control and Prevention. Development of new vaccines for tuberculosis: Recommendations of the Advisory Council for the Elimination of Tuberculosis (ACET). *MMWR* 1998;47:1–6.

6 Legal Challenges

Susan O. Cassidy

Managing employees with health problems is an increasingly complex legal challenge. Prior to 1990, workers' compensation and state disability laws determined employers' duties and workers' benefits. The explosion of laws providing new protections and benefits for workers has led to confusing and often conflicting duties for employers. The primary reasons for this confusion are the diversity of purpose and the lack of common goals of the laws and regulations governing employer duties.

Workers' compensation provides compensation for lost wages (indemnity costs), medical expenses, and financial compensation for permanent impairment, but only if an individual has a work-related injury or illness. Under the workers' compensation system, workers who are injured or who become ill as a result of their job generally are entitled to specified benefits without regard to the duration or permanency of the impairment.

The Americans with Disabilities Act (ADA) was enacted to facilitate the integration of disabled individuals back into the workplace and into society. The ADA does not provide financial benefits but rather seeks to level the playing field for impaired individuals whose disability is substantial and of significant duration. Under the ADA, workplace accommodations are required if they will enable a qualified individual with a disability to perform the essential functions of a job for which they are otherwise qualified.

The Family Medical Leave Act (FMLA) provides covered individuals with unpaid time away from work to recuperate or care for an ill family member. Unlike workers' compensation, the ADA and FMLA apply to specified disabled or medically ill individuals regardless of whether or not their illness or injury is job-related. While certain short-term illnesses may be covered under workers' compensation and the FMLA, they are expressly excluded from ADA protections.

Managing exposure and communicability issues associated with infectious disease in the workplace adds substantially to the complexity of the legally mandated employer duties. The potential for significant effects on business productivity and for exposure to huge financial losses makes it imperative that employers and health care professionals have a firm grasp of the areas of conflict and overlap and of the scope of employee protections under these laws. Further complicating this complex interplay of medicine and employment protections are privacy and confidentiality concerns, as well as the laws regulating the collection and release of medical information. In addition to federal laws such as the Health Insurance Portability and Accountability Act (HIPAA), there is a patchwork of state statutory and case law that differs across state borders.

Workers' Compensation

HISTORICAL OVERVIEW

Common law imposed employer duties such as the provision of a safe place to work, safe tools and equipment, and the need to give adequate warnings when a "servant" (employee) could not appreciate a danger. Further, employers were expected to train "fellow servants" (workers) to minimize workplace accidents and injuries [1]. Common law permitted an injured employee to bring legal action against his or her employer for breach of these duties, but the remedies for injury or death were inadequate owing to the "unholy trinity" of common-law defenses. These three employer defenses—fellow-servant doctrine, contributory negligence, and assumption of risk—left many workers without recourse or compensation for work-related injuries or illnesses. In this way, courts, reflecting societal desires to encourage and support continued industrial growth and expansion, shielded employers from much of the financial burden for worker injury. Many of these same defenses continue to exist in one form or another in the current American tort system.

Fellow-Servant Doctrine

In the absence of an express written contract, a "master" (employer) was not liable to an employee for the injuries caused by the negligence of a "fellow servant" (another employee). Such negligence was a risk incident to employment and was assumed by the employee. It was believed that this would lead to coworkers being careful and watchful of each other. The harshness of this doctrine was mitigated by several well-recognized exceptions—situations in which "fellow servants" did not have a "common master," those in which "servants" were not engaged in the same enterprise, and those wherein injury was caused by the negligence of a vice principal acting as the employer's agent or supervisor [2].

Contributory Negligence

Under common law, employees had a duty to exercise reasonable care for their own safety. Where an employee failed to exercise reasonable care or take prudent safety precautions, the individual was barred from recovery from the employer under a contributory negligence defense. This defense was weakened with the enactment of statutes expressly imposing worker safety requirements for certain categories of employees and creating comparative negligence defenses.

Assumption of Risk

Under common law, employees were deemed to have voluntarily assumed certain risks incident to working. Such risks included those that a mature worker was presumed to know even if the individual worker did not have actual knowledge and also included extraordinary or substantial risks of which the worker had actual knowledge. In contrast to the contributory negligence defense, grounded in tort theories of duty and breach of such duty, assumption-of-risk theory was contractual in nature. Consequently, the presence or absence of fault had little role in raising or mitigating an assumption-of-risk defense. However, even when an employee could prove that he or she did not assume the risk of the danger that caused his or her injury, he or she could be barred from recovery if the employer could show contributory negligence [3].

In the nineteenth century, rising industrial injury and death rates prompted enactment of employer liability legislation. The "fellow servant doctrine" defense was eroded in 1855 when the state of Georgia enacted provisions for railroad worker protections for workers injured by the negligence of a fellow worker. By the early 1900s, almost every other jurisdiction in the United States had enacted statutes providing similar protections [4]. In 1908, Congress passed legislation that covered interstate railroad workers, and later seamen, under an employer's liability act system. These protections soon proved inadequate because workers continued to have the burden of invoking the legal system to obtain recovery from employers for workplace injuries.

European counties were struggling with their own forms of compensation for injured workers. Both the German and British systems of compensation greatly influenced the ultimate form of workers' compensation in the United States. In 1884, Germany enacted the first workers' compensation act when it passed legislation establishing a compulsory system of accident insurance for employees in the manufacturing, mining, and transportation industries [5]. Great Britain enacted the Workmen's Compensation Act of 1897, which served as the template for the legislation passed in the United

States in the early 1900s [6]. The British act set forth limitations on the scope of coverage "arising out of and in the course of employment" [7]. This enduring phrase is still found in state workers' compensation statutes throughout the United States. While the Workmen's Compensation Act of 1897 provided coverage for hazardous jobs, it did not contain insurance provisions, leaving that burden on employers as a cost of doing business.

While it is beyond the scope of this chapter to cover all employee protection legislation, it is important to recognize that once legislative rule-making began in this arena, many laws providing protections to certain worker groups were passed. Such early legislation included the Federal Employees' Compensation Act, the Federal Employers' Liability Act, the Jones Act, the Long Shore and Harbor Workers' Compensation Act, the Federal Coal Mine Health and Safety Act of 1969, and federal black lung benefits legislation.

GENERAL PROVISIONS

While the provisions and policies of workers' compensation statutes have evolved over the intervening years, general themes continue to characterize this system of legal recovery for work-related illness and injury. The elective nature of workers' compensation coverage gave way to presumptive coverage, wherein a worker was presumed to be covered by his or her employer unless coverage was contractually waived and subsequently provided for the compulsory coverage system used in a majority of states. Constitutional objections to such state action have been overcome by amending state constitutions to grant the state the necessary legislative power to enact workers' compensation laws [8].

Generally, a "covered employer" is an employer with at least one employee. Covered employees are those incurring an injury that arises out of and in the course of the employment relationship. In most states, an employee with a preexisting condition aggravated or accelerated by the workplace is also covered under workers' compensation. In addition to compulsory coverage, a key component of all workers' compensation systems is the exclusive coverage provision. Exclusivity provisions enable an ill or injured worker or his or her dependents legal recovery regardless of fault; they also provide for financial compensation to the worker and ensure coverage of the costs of medical treatment without

the necessity of bringing suit against the employer. The price for these employee protections was employer protection from negligence suits brought by their employees. Much controversy and uneasiness continue to surround exclusivity provisions. Employee advocates argue that such provisions eviscerate the due process rights of injured individuals by limiting recovery to modest compensation for injuries and illness without the ability to sue to recover for employer negligence. Under this no-fault system, employers have lost the right to assert contributory negligence, assumption of risk, and "fellow servant" defenses but can limit their financial exposure and get fixed costs by insuring the liability. Despite no-fault provisions, certain employee actions—e.g., self-inflicted injuries and intoxication—can preclude financial recovery. Workers' compensation systems operate by spreading the cost of workplace illness and injuries across society because the costs to employers are then incorporated into the price of products and cost of services.

BENEFITS

Employee benefits under workers' compensation vary by state and are based on a wage-loss rationale, a medical-loss rationale, or a combined scheme. A wage-loss approach compensates an individual who suffers a loss of wages or diminished earning capacity, whereas a medical-loss approach provides for compensation for a medical loss—e.g., loss of vision or an extremity—without regard to loss of wages or diminished earning capacity [9]. Regardless of the approach, the system generally provides only modest compensation to the injured or ill worker, and the standardized schedule of awards in some states results in inadequate and inequitable remedies for some individuals.

THIRD-PARTY LIABILITY

While workers generally are barred from bringing suit against their employer and must accept workers' compensation as their sole remedy if they sustain a work-related illness or injury, they are not prohibited from seeking legal redress from third parties. Increasingly, affected employees are initiating suit against coworkers, including physicians employed by the company. While coworkers may have immunity for nonintentional acts under state workers' compensation statutes or under case law, a few states permit actions to be brought against anyone other than the employer. In these states, a worker or his or her dependents may bring legal action against a coworker whose negligence results in injury or loss of life [10].

Affected employees are not prohibited from suing employers and others for property damage. In addition, employees may sue the involved third party if injury is the result of negligent inspection or performance by company vendors. Employers and their insurers also have been sued successfully by employees who can demonstrate bad faith in the processing or administration of a workers' compensation claim [11]. Such actions create an opportunity for large monetary awards for relatively minor injuries.

Claimants also have used product liability statutes when injury has occurred as the result of a specific product or instrument. Courts increasingly have embraced strict liability in many product liability suits against product manufacturers, opening the door for substantial monetary awards. Dual-capacity liability may be claimed, in addition to the workers' compensation claim, if a worker is injured while using a product manufactured by his or her employer. Private physicians treating employees for workers' compensation claims are liable for medical malpractice under the usual tort statutes of duty and breach of that duty with resulting harm. Physicians who are employed by the company may escape liability for negligence under coworker immunity provisions of the workers' compensation statutes, but it could be argued that they are independent contractors and therefore subject to tort liability as a third party.

INTENTIONAL TORTS

Workers' compensation immunity does not extend to employers' intentional torts against workers. Employers have been sued successfully for intentional infliction of emotional distress [12], retaliation and discrimination [13], and sexual assault [14]. Increasingly, courts are permitting claims of intentional torts to be filed as part of workers' compensation claims. In such instances, employees have received enhanced awards without the necessity of separate tort actions against their employers. Additionally, employers may face criminal liability if serious injury or death has resulted from an employer's failure to remediate a known hazard or in instances in which an employer knew or should

have known of employee exposure to highly hazardous materials or operations.

Most states permit discharged employees to sue for retaliatory discharge if there is evidence that an employee was fired for filing a workers' compensation claim. In addition, workers' compensation legislation does not preempt federal law, thus permitting claims for age, gender, or disability discrimination or other federal discrimination claims to be brought against employers. Furthermore, state actions, including but not limited to harassment, libel, slander, and false imprisonment, are not barred by workers' compensation laws.

COVERAGE

Workers' compensation coverage hinges on employee status, employment relatedness, and the medical condition at issue. Compensation is available only if there is a reasonable nexus between the injury and the job. States have enacted specific exclusions, such as commuting to and from work and employer recreational activities, as well as specific inclusions and criteria, such as cardiac injury. As a general rule, coverage is available if the accident occurs on company premises, during travel between company sites, or during travel required as part of the job. Home offices are also considered company premises for purposes of workers' compensation coverage if the employee regularly performs work for the company there. Most state workers' compensation laws require claimants to demonstrate that they sustained their injuries or illnesses *during the course of their employment* and that their *condition arose out of their employment* [15]. The course of employment inquiry considers time, location, and circumstances of the incident, whereas the "arising out of" inquiry involves evaluation of the underlying cause of the claimant's injuries.

In the area of work-related infectious diseases, courts generally have limited coverage to workers who can demonstrate that their employment exposed them to increased risk of infection compared with that of the general public [16]. Historically, such workers have been health care workers exposed to infected patients, corrections and law enforcement officers, and workers who, by the nature of their jobs, are required to work in unsanitary conditions. Unlike accidents or acute injuries when infectious diseases are involved, it is more difficult to prove causality for purposes of workers' compensation. Reasons for this include the long latency period of many infectious diseases prior to the development of clinical symptoms and/or signs, the prevalence of certain infections in the community, and the lack of specific markers to track the source of infection. When infections develop suddenly owing to sudden exposure to infectious agents in the workplace, there is generally little difficulty demonstrating work-relatedness. However, some states permit claimants legal recovery under workers' compensation if they can prove that their job placed them at increased risk for their illness. In a Connecticut case, a dental hygienist was awarded workers' compensation after the court concluded that "it is more likely than not that Claimant's infection with hepatitis arose out of and in the course of her employment" [17]. To be compensable, a disease is not required to be one that arises solely out of the particular kind of employment in which the employee is engaged, nor must it be due to causes in excess of the ordinary hazards of that particular type of employment [18].

Further, it is now not always necessary to actually contract an illness or disease to recover under workers' compensation. In *Doe v. Stamford* [19], the state's highest court recently held that a police officer who, during the course of restraining a prisoner, was exposed to but had not contracted a potentially fatal contagious disease was entitled to recover the reasonable expenses that he incurred for medically appropriate testing and treatment. The claimant police officer was exposed to HIV and tuberculosis during two separate incidents 3 months apart. The HIV exposure was the result of his thumb, which had an open wound, coming into contact with medical pads contaminated with bodily fluids from a criminal suspect who was HIV-positive. The tuberculosis exposure resulted from repeated close physical contact with another criminal suspect who, it was later learned, had active disease [20]. The court held that these exposures constituted compensable "injuries" within the definitional boundaries of the state's workers' compensation act.

HIPAA, Confidentiality, and Release of Medical Information

Lack of national standards and requirements for the release, storage, and use of medical records, resulted in the passage of the Health Insurance Portability and Accountability Act of 1996 (HIPAA). Congress directed the Department of Health and Human Services (HHS) to establish national standards for electronic health care transactions and national identifiers for providers, health plans, and employers. Further, under the Administrative Simplification provisions of HIPAA, HHS must address privacy and security issues relating to health data.

HIPAA took effect on April 14, 2003, and established federal privacy standards to protect patients' medical records and other health information provided to health plans, doctors, hospitals, and other health care providers. Under HIPAA, patients have access to their medical records and more control over how their personal health information is used and disclosed. HIPAA includes provisions encouraging electronic transactions and heightened safeguards to protect against unauthorized disclosures of health information. Final regulations promulgated by HHS cover health plans, health care clearinghouses, and providers who conduct financial transactions such as eligibility verification, enrollment, and billing electronically. These provisions include physicians, health insurers, pharmacies, and other health care providers. Failure to implement or comply with these standards may under certain circumstances trigger the imposition of civil or criminal penalties. While these privacy rules establish a foundation of federal protection of the privacy of protected health information, they do not replace federal, state, or other laws that grant individuals even greater privacy protections. Further, covered entities are free to adopt or retain more stringent policies or practices [21].

HIPAA was in large part due to the expanded collection of individual health data and the increasing public concern about the uses and potential misuses of personal health information. Computerized recording of medical data and technologic advances in diagnostic testing and genome identification and mapping have left workers increasingly concerned that employers' knowledge and access to such data may negatively affect their employment status. It is against this backdrop that heightened care must be exercised in the collection and release of medical information regardless of the setting or payment system.

It has been generally recognized that workers seeking payment for medical expenses and wage replacement waive confidentiality of the medical information related to the work-related injury or medical condition. In addition to provisions of HIPAA, specific laws governing medical records vary by state, and there has been an increasing tendency to narrow the scope of the medical information available to payers without express release by the claimant. Several states limit this access to the treating physician or curtail the content and scope of discussions between employers and their agents and the claimant's physician. Further, the ADA sets forth confidentiality requirements for the protection and release of employee medical information. The ADA's express intention to provide protection of employee medical data must be considered when releasing any type of employee medical data. Even where state laws purport to give greater freedom to release medical information, they are not a defense to a wrongful disclosure claim under federal legislation such as HIPAA or the ADA. While states are free to require greater protections for employee medical information, they cannot provide less protection than outlined in the ADA, HIPAA, or other laws. This aspect of the preemption of state laws by federal laws, such as HIPAA and the ADA, has not received the attention it deserves, particularly with regard to the use and disclosure of medical information in the workers' compensation setting. Currently, it is not uncommon for employee medical information related to a workplace incident, including symptoms and diagnosis, to be freely shared with numerous individuals within the company or insurance environment. Equal Employment Opportunity Commission (EEOC) enforcement guidance documents provide clarification regarding employer confidentiality duties [22].

An employer must keep any medical information on applicants or employees confidential with the following limited exceptions:

- Supervisors and managers may be told about necessary restrictions on the work or duties of the employee and about necessary accommodations;
- First-aid and safety personnel may be told if the disability might require emergency treatment;
- Government officials investigating compliance with the ADA must be given relevant information on request;

- Employers may give information to state workers' compensation offices, state second injury funds or workers' compensation insurance carriers in accordance with state workers' compensation laws;
- Employers may use the information for insurance purposes. For example, an employer may submit medical information to the company's health insurance carrier if the information is needed to administer a health insurance plan in accordance with §501(c) of the ADA.

EEOC guidelines on release and disclosure of medical information clearly specify that such information is lawfully disclosed within the company only on a strict *need-to-know basis* and stipulate that employee medical information must be kept separate from personnel records. This applies to workers' compensation information, such as diagnosis or symptoms, as well as to non-work-related medical conditions. Documents containing medical information that need to be put into the personnel file must have all medical information removed prior to placement in that file [23].

While many state workers' compensation forms signed by claimants authorize release of medical information and records to the payer and the state, it has become increasingly important for health care professionals to obtain a signed, specific release prior to disclosing any medical information to anyone besides the claimant. It is imperative that HIPAA-compliant medical releases be obtained prior to release and/or discussion of an individual's medical condition even in the scope of handling workers' compensation issues or ADA requests or duties. Such releases at a minimum must contain the reason for request or release of the diagnosis or medical condition, identity of the facility and/or individuals receiving the information, duration of the authorized release interval, the scope of the medical information being released, the purpose for which the medical information will be used, and a prohibition against redisclosure of the information.

Special care must be exercised not to exceed the scope of the release, and if sensitive medical information such as substance abuse, psychiatric information, or HIV/AIDS data are involved, it is imperative that specific federal and state laws regarding the process and procedures for lawful release are followed. Many states have specific laws regarding HIV/AIDS testing and information release—e.g., New York State requires that a special state form be used to lawfully release such information. Connecticut, while not requiring a special form, has a statute-prescribed paragraph that must be included on the medical release form. As of July 1998, 32 states have enacted HIV/AIDS reporting requirements for revealing the identities of individuals so diagnosed. Such reporting requirements have rigid confidentiality and release protections.

In the workers' compensation setting and in general, even if lawful consent can be obtained, it is prudent not to release or discuss any medical information that is not relevant to the narrow scope of issues at hand. Physicians have been sued successfully for release of HIV data that they received during the course of treating a workers' compensation injury. A New York court ruled that a physician who had released medical records that included HIV status had violated the law because she had not used the state-required consent form. In this case, the physician treating the claimant for a workers' compensation injury had released the medical records to the Pennsylvania workers' compensation board pursuant to a subpoena [24]. When releasing medical information relevant to the workers' compensation claim to anyone, including the employer or the state, specific consent by the claimant for the release should be obtained. If an overriding public health consideration or a demand for medical information pursuant to a subpoena arises, it is prudent to obtain legal advice to frame the issues, ensure that the most conservative approach is taken, and provide for a defensible position in the event of future legal scrutiny.

The Family and Medical Leave Act

In addition to workers' compensation benefits, employees with occupationally related infectious diseases are also likely to be entitled to unpaid FMLA leave [25]. FMLA was enacted to provide workers with time to recuperate from a health condition or, in certain circumstances, to provide care for others. An employee receives up to 12 weeks of unpaid leave per 12-month period in any of the following circumstances:

- Child care following the birth of a child or placement of a child for adoption or foster care.

- The employee's need to care for a spouse, child, or parent who has a serious health condition.
- A serious health condition that makes the employee unable to perform the essential functions of his or her position.

Serious health condition is defined as
- Inpatient care or any period of incapacity or any subsequent treatment in connection with such inpatient care
- Absence from work plus treatment by a health care provider
- Pregnancy
- A chronic condition requiring treatment
- Permanent or long-term condition requiring supervision
- Multiple treatments for a nonchronic condition

It is likely that most employees who contract an occupationally related infectious disease will be entitled to FMLA leave, as well as paid time off, for the time they are rendered unable to work owing to their illness. Exceptions to FMLA entitlement occur when an employee has not been employed long enough to be eligible or has previously exhausted his or her FMLA benefits within the same benefits year. FMLA leave can run concurrently with paid time off under workers' compensation, the employer's sick-days program, or short-term disability, provided the employer notifies the employee that the paid time off is also being counted against the 12 weeks that the individual may be entitled to under the FMLA.

Americans with Disabilities Act (ADA)

In 1990, Congress passed landmark legislation to address inequities faced by individuals with disabilities. In the employment sector, this federal law trumps state legislation, including workers' compensation laws. While states are free to provide greater protections to its citizens under workers' compensation statutes, they cannot enact laws that violate or narrow protections provided under the ADA. Individuals with an illness or injury may be covered by one, both, or neither law. In addition, FMLA and state disability laws may come into play and must be reconciled with the rights, duties, and benefits of workers' compensation and the ADA.

Title I of the ADA prohibits employers from discriminating against qualified individuals because of disability in all aspects of employment [26]. This contrasts with workers' compensation law, which provides a scheme for prompt and fair settlement of employees' claims (for lost wages, lost earning capacity, and medical expenses) against employers for occupational injury and illness. An employee with an occupational injury or illness generally has a "disability" for workers' compensation purposes but may not have a "disability" for purposes of the ADA [27]. Further, ADA proscriptions temper or invalidate states' worker exclusion laws. In its guidance document, the EEOC expressly addresses the apparent conflict of the ADA with state health and safety laws, which permit or require an employer to exclude individuals with certain disabilities from employment. The ADA does not allow such exclusion except where the employer can demonstrate that the individual is a "direct threat" [28]. Further, even if an individual poses a "direct threat" to himself or herself or other employees, the employer has a duty to investigate whether the threat can be reduced or eliminated by reasonable accommodation. If an employer cannot show that an individual is a direct threat or that reasonable accommodation is not possible, exclusion of an employee based on a state law is not a defense to a claim of ADA discrimination by a covered individual.

Return-to-Work Issues

FULL-DUTY REQUIREMENTS

In addition to invalidating state exclusionary laws, the ADA impacts "return to full-duty requirements." Many workers' compensation schemes permit an employer to require that an injured employee be able to return to "full duty" before returning to work. If an employer uses the term *full duty* to apply to job functions that are "marginal" in nature, it is in violation of the ADA if the individual can perform the *essential* functions of the job with or without reasonable accommodation. Unlike workers' compensation systems, in which the treating physician releases an individual to return to work, under the ADA, the employer bears the ultimate legal responsibility for deciding whether an employee with a disability-related occupational injury or illness is ready to return to work [29].

DIRECT-THREAT ANALYSIS

Under the ADA, the return-to-work decision about an employee who has a communicable or potentially communicable disease should trigger a direct-threat analysis. The provisions of the ADA come into play if an individual with such a condition desires to return to work in a setting that causes the employer concern about the individual's medical condition relative to the safety of that individual or coworkers. Under the ADA, the direct-threat standard must be satisfied before an employer can lawfully prevent a covered individual from returning to his or her job. It is important to remember that not all workers with an occupationally related infectious disease are covered by the ADA. Those with self-limited infections of short duration, regardless of their severity, may not be covered unless the employer causes protections to attach by "regarding the individual as disabled" [30].

EEOC regulations define *direct threat* as one that presents a significant risk of substantial harm to the health or safety of the individual worker or other workers and that cannot be eliminated or reduced by reasonable accommodation. An individualized assessment of the worker's present ability to perform the essential functions of the job is required. The standard must be applied uniformly, and reasonable medical judgment based on current medical knowledge and/or the best available objective evidence with respect to the infectious disease must be used. Further, the specific behavior or condition that would pose a threat must be identified. If a significant risk of substantial harm is identified, then reasonable accommodations that may reduce or eliminate the risk must be considered. ADA regulations, as promulgated by the EEOC, define the factors to be considered when assessing whether an individual presents a direct threat. These factors are [31]

- Duration of the risk
- Nature and severity of the potential harm
- Likelihood that the potential harm will occur
- Imminence of the potential harm

A direct-threat analysis also should include a determination of the likelihood and imminence of the danger. Similar to the concerns and issues raised if an individual has a mental condition, factors such as failure of prior treatment, treatment noncompliance, and evaluation of recent and past behavior are relevant to the assessment of likelihood of harm. For example, in the infectious disease setting, a health care worker's failure or refusal to use universal precautions or other protective equipment is a crucial piece of the behavioral assessment of that worker. As noted earlier, even if an employee, by nature of his or her medical condition, does not meet the "disability" impairment threshold for ADA protection, the individual can become covered under the provisions of the ADA if the employer reacts to and treats the person as if such an impairment existed. This is an important consideration in the infectious disease setting, in which the risks of disease transmission (to coworkers, customers, and patients) must be balanced against the rights of the affected individual to be in the workplace as long as he or she can perform his or her job.

Prior to enactment of the ADA and the plethora of HIV and AIDS cases in which legal action was taken by individuals seeking disability protections and financial remuneration, perhaps the best-known case involving infectious disease and employment rights was *School Board of Nassau County v Arline*. This case was brought under Section 504 of the 1973 Rehabilitation Act after a school teacher who had been treated for tuberculosis was denied the right to return to her teaching job despite her lack of contiguousness with other people at work. In *Arline*, the U.S. Supreme Court ruled that a teacher with reactivation of tuberculosis was protected under Section 504 of the Rehabilitation Act and that the relevant inquiry was whether or not she was "otherwise qualified." To answer this, the court held that an individualized inquiry as to whether or not she posed a threat of infection to the students must be conducted. Based on the public health authorities' contention that she had been treated and did not pose a threat of infection, she was reinstated in her job. In *Arline*, the American Medical Association (AMA) submitted an amicus brief that articulated the standards for conducting the appropriate inquiry as to threat of infection [32]. The AMA's position, largely adopted by the court, focused on facts based on the state of medical knowledge and reasonable medical judgments drawn from these facts concerning

- Nature of the risk (how the disease is transmitted)
- Duration of the risk (how long the carrier is infectious)
- Severity of the risk (the potential harm to third parties)
- Probability that the disease will be transmitted and will cause varying degrees of harm

The Court then touched on the employer's duty to reasonably accommodate workers when appropriate [33].

The majority of the infectious disease cases under the ADA have involved HIV-positive individuals (with or without AIDS) alleging denial of employment owing to their disease status. These cases provide a template for the standards and assessment process required in managing the employment status of employees with infectious diseases. A recent U.S. Supreme Court decision broadened the scope of ADA protection for HIV-positive individuals, ruling that HIV-positive status alone invokes ADA protections [34]. This effectively negates the need for an HIV-positive individual to be substantially impaired in one or more major life activities to be considered disabled under the ADA.

Direct threat and safety concerns have been raised successfully by employers, with courts declining to follow the EEOC's interpretation of the direct-threat standard. In *Doe v. University of Maryland*, the U.S. district court upheld the right of the hospital to exclude an HIV-positive neurosurgery resident from its training program because the individual presented an appreciable risk of catastrophic harm [35]. Courts also have upheld hospitals' rights to reassign HIV-positive individuals to other jobs if they present appreciable risk of catastrophic harm in their present jobs. In a Texas case, the U.S. district court ruled that it was permissible for the employer to reassign an HIV-positive surgical technician [36]. In another case in which a surgical technician was suspected of being HIV-positive, a Michigan court ruled that while infrequent, there was some contact (hands in direct contact or in the immediate vicinity of an incision) that was essential to the success of a surgical procedure and that this was an essential job function. The hospital was not required to restructure the essential functions of the job by providing another person in the operating room [37].

Decisions about employees' ability to work should be based on sound scientific knowledge as to the nature of the infectious agent, its infectivity and invasiveness, the mode of transmission, the host status, and the susceptibility of coworkers and others working near or in close contact with the affected individual. Currently, aside from the bloodborne pathogen standard and the general duty clause, there is little OSHA or state statutory guidance regulating the return to work of an individual being treated or recently treated for an infectious disease. The proposed OSHA tuberculosis standard does, however, provide some clarification regarding employer duties in the infectious disease setting [38]. Medical removal protection requirements provide for employees with suspected or confirmed infectious tuberculosis to be kept out of the workplace until they are determined to be noninfectious. The proposed standard outlines benefit and wage provisions as well as job modification guidance and employee/employer notification requirements.

In managing an employee with an infectious disease, the initial step is evaluating the individual's recent ability to perform essential job duties. Attention to the physical and emotional job demands should be evaluated and documented. If there is no issue regarding the employee's ability to perform the essential job tasks, the inquiry then should focus, if appropriate, on the safety of others in the workplace. This involves an evaluation of the affected individual's proximity to coworkers and customers/clients and an assessment of contagiousness. As stated previously, current scientific medical literature and accepted sources should be consulted. Prior to exclusion of an infected individual from returning to work, public health officials should be contacted for their input. All steps in the evaluation process should be documented carefully—specifically, the nature of the infectious disease in question, the status of the affected employee, including his or her compliance with treatment and job-required protective equipment, and the type of work the employee performs. Such documentation also should include the reasoning behind the decision making. Care should be taken not to generalize based on the virulence of the infectious agent because disease stage, ease of transmission, and coworker/patient/customer issues and job requirements are also important factors to consider in the individualized assessment. If it is established that there are legitimate reasons for concern about the individual's presence in the workplace relative to safety, attention then must shift to consideration of available means to mitigate or reduce the likelihood of harm. These may include modification or change of job duties or even reassignment of the individual to a vacant position.

In *Bragdon v Abbott,* a recent case involving an HIV-positive claimant who, under the ADA, brought legal action against a dentist who refused to treat the individual in his office, the U.S. Supreme Court held that the patient's disease status must be assessed to determine whether or not it poses a significant threat to the health and safety of others and, if a health risk was shown to exist, whether or not it could be eliminated by safety procedures. In *Bragdon,* this objective inquiry was held to be required under the ADA to justify the dentist's refusal to treat the patient in his office [34]. This type of individualized assessment will be required when evaluating employees with infectious diseases if they desire to return to work.

Historically, the causality issues associated with infectious diseases have resulted in many exposures and infections being handled outside the workers' compensation system. Articles in the legal and public health literature have highlighted the difficulty of proving causation of infectious disease by work-related factors if the disease is prevalent in the community [3]. Additionally, for ease of management or financial reasons, many workplace incidents and exposures have been handled on-site at the company's premises or through the employer's group health plan. Prior to prophylaxis after HIV exposure and other expensive testing and treatments, many workplace needlestick exposures were handled in the hospital's employee health department. Given the inconsistent reporting and causation issues surrounding work-related infectious diseases, it is likely that their true magnitude has been unappreciated.

There is a strong likelihood that infectious diseases will become a greater issue in the workers' compensation arena, presenting special workplace safety concerns and ADA compliance challenges.

The severe acute respiratory syndrome (SARS) and avian flu outbreaks are two recent examples. Technologic advances in molecular epidemiologic analysis, improved diagnostic testing, the advent of new infections, better identification of common disease agents, and the resurgence of infections once thought to be controlled or eradicated will lead to an increased number of workplace infectious disease challenges. In addition, employee protection laws, such as the ADA, which have paved the way for individuals with chronic diseases to remain in the workplace, will further compound the challenges. These laws will drive demographic changes in the health status of the "typical" American worker. Changes in employee medical benefit, retirement, and disability plans also will lead to an increased number of individuals with medical conditions remaining at work. Such changes will lead to a greater number of employees who are immunocompromised by virtue of age, organ transplantation status, steroid use, cancer, or other chronic diseases working alongside a greater number of employees with acute and chronic infections. Further, there will be an increase in the number of employees who are chronic infectious disease carriers or have acute but undiagnosed infectious disease, e.g., hepatitis or HIV [3].

The increased globalization of U.S. businesses has resulted in an explosion in employee travel on company business to remote places where food preparation, water safety, and general sanitation frequently are substandard and constitute significant health hazards from infectious disease. While most companies comply with the immunization requirements for foreign country entry, few prepare their employees adequately for the challenges they will encounter. Further, the ADA has significantly limited companies in denying overseas work assignments based on the presence of significant medical conditions in employees or their dependents. Employees with complex and serious medical conditions now may accept an overseas assignment despite the absence of adequate medical resources or exposure concerns present in the foreign country.

The availability of vaccines and immunizations for diseases such as hepatitis B has led to increased employer responsibilities in preventing work-related infectious disease. While the Occupational

Safety and Health Administration (OSHA) requires employers to provide hepatitis B virus (HBV) vaccine for all employees who are at risk of infection, employers should consider providing other immunizations at no cost to employees [3]. This has both public health and employer productivity benefits. If an employee has not had a childhood infectious disease or immunization for that disease, contracting the disease secondary to a workplace exposure not only results in costs and morbidity for the individual employee but also opens the door to a widespread workplace outbreak of the disease. Additionally, the company may incur third-party liability for dependents of the employee who become infected, particularly if they suffer serious sequelae.

The resurgence of multidrug-resistant tuberculosis has led OSHA to address occupational tuberculosis exposure and develop tuberculosis standards addressing medical surveillance for the disease [39]. OSHA standards interpretation letters (2006 and 2007), while not mandating annual fit testing of respirators used for protection against tuberculosis owing to appropriations restrictions, reiterated the respiratory protection standard's requirements, including annual fit testing for respirator use against other hazards, such as SARS or other bioaerosols [40].

The role of occupational medicine professionals in the management of infectious disease issues in the workplace continues to expand. In addition to medical treatment issues, the ADA's direct-threat standard and OSHA general duty clause [41] will shape and guide decision making in striking the delicate balance between an infected individual's right to be in the workplace and the employer's duty to protect the safety and well-being of coworkers and others. The ADA provides a clearly articulated legal mandate stating that the direct-threat standard requires an individualized assessment based on current, objective scientific evidence about the medical condition and consideration of reasonable accommodations that may mitigate any threat to workplace safety and health. While pre-employment medical examinations became extinct after enactment of the ADA, the need for occupational medicine physicians with strong clinical, public health, and legal knowledge has never been greater.

References

1. Hood JB, Hardy BA, Lewis HS. *Workers' Compensation and Employee Protection Laws.* St. Paul, MN: West Publishing, 1990, p 1.
2. *Ibid.,* p 2.
3. *Ibid.,* p 4.
4. *Ibid.,* p 5.
5. *Ibid.,* p 7.
6. *Ibid.*
7. *Ibid.*
8. *Ibid.,* p 27.
9. *Ibid.,* p 29.
10. *Ibid.,* p 35.
11. *Simkins v Great West Cas. Co.,* 831 F2d 792 (8th Cir 1987).
12. *Childers v Chesapeake & Potomac Tele. Co.* (1989).
13. *Smolarek v Chrysler Corp.* (1989).
14. *Paroline v Unisys Corp.* (1989).
15. Rothstein MA, Craver CB, Schroeder EP, et al. *Employment Law.* Westlaw School Hornbook, Thompson West, St. Paul, MN: 1994.
16. Rothstein MA, Craver CB, Schroeder EP, et al. *Employment Law.* Westlaw School Hornbook, Thompson West, St. Paul, MN: 1994.
17. *Hansen v Gordon,* 221 Conn 29 (1992).
18. *Ibid.,* p 36.
19. 241 Conn 692 (1997).
20. *Ibid.,* p 694.
21. www.cms.hhs.gov/HIPAAGenInfo/.
22. Equal Employment Opportunity Commission. *ADA Enforcement Guidance: Pre-employment Disability-Related Questions and Medical Examinations.* Washington: EEOC, October 15, 1995.
23. 42 USC §12201(c); 29 CFR 1630 app. §1630.14(b); 29 CFR. 1630 app. §1630, p 3.
24. *Doe v Roe,* 190 A2d 463, 599 NYS2d 350 (1993).
25. 29 USCA §§2601–54.
26. 42 USC §12112(a); 29 CFR §1630.4.
27. Equal Employment Opportunity Commission. *ADA Enforcement Guidance: Workers' Compensation and the ADA.* No 915.002. Washington: EEOC, September 3, 1996, p 7.
28. *Ibid.,* p 9.
29. *Ibid.,* p 14.
30. 42 USC 12102–13 (1994).
31. *Ibid.*
32. Richards EP, Rathbun KC. *Law and the Physician: A Practical Guide.* Boston: Little, Brown, 1993, Chap 23.
33. *School Board of Nassua County v Arline,* 107 SCt 1123 (1987).
34. *Bragdon v Abbott,* 8 AD Cases 239, US, No 97-156, 6/25/98.
35. 50 F3d 1261 (4th Cir 1995).
36. *Bradley v University of Texas M.D. Anderson Cancer Ctr.,* 3 F3d 922, 925 (5th Cir 1993).
37. *Mauro v Borgess Medical Ctr.,* 886 F Supp 1349 (WD Mich 1995).
38. Occupational Exposure Rule for Tuberculosis Standard (g)5(i)(ii)(iii)(iv).
39. www.osha.gov/SLTC/tuberculosis/standards.html.
40. www.osha.gov/pls/oshaweb/owadisp.show_document?p_table=INTERPRETATIONS&p_id=25843.
41. OSH Act 1970, Sec. 5. Duties:
    (a) Each employer
        (1) Shall furnish to each of his employees employment and a place of employment which are free from recognized hazards that are causing or are likely to cause death or serious physical harm to his employees;
        (2) Shall comply with occupational safety and health standards promulgated under this Act.
    Each employee shall comply with occupational safety and health standards and all rules, regulations, and orders issued pursuant to this Act which are applicable to his own actions and conduct.

7 Medical Surveillance of Workers

Victor S. Roth

Fundamentals of Medical Surveillance

Depending on potential hazards present in the workplace and to comply with federal and state regulations, the employer has an ethical and legal responsibility to provide a medical surveillance program for its workers. It is important to understand the general principles that are the foundation for medical surveillance. Medical surveillance for infectious diseases plays a major role in health care facilities and also has a place in general industry. Two types of surveillance programs in which it plays a larger role are highlighted in this chapter: programs for animal handlers and those for health care workers.

Merriam-Webster's Online defines *surveillance* as a "close watch kept over someone or something". To develop a sound medical surveillance program, an understanding of primary, secondary, and tertiary prevention is necessary. Primary prevention is aimed at preventing disease. This involves (in order of preference) material substitution, engineering controls, administrative controls, and personal protective equipment [1]. This sequence of measures attempts to eliminate or control exposure. If the hazard cannot be eliminated or controlled, then attempts are made at limiting exposure through work practices or protective equipment. Personal protective equipment is the least desirable of control strategies because failure at this level results in immediate exposure of the worker to the hazard. Secondary prevention is detection of disease at a subclinical stage or at an early stage such that progression is reversible or can be stopped. Strictly defined, medical surveillance falls under secondary prevention. Tertiary prevention is the medical treatment of disease once it is clinically present and not reversible.

In a properly functioning medical surveillance program the overriding goal is to maintain the absence of disease with the secondary goal being the early detection of disease at a reversible stage. In other words, when a medical surveillance program fails in the primary prevention of disease, secondary prevention complements primary prevention efforts. Workplace professionals such as industrial hygienists, safety professionals, and occupational medicine specialists generally perform primary prevention efforts. A well-designed medical surveillance program has occupational medical professionals actively participating in implementing primary prevention controls in the workplace along with other occupational health and safety professionals (industrial hygiene and safety).

Fundamentals of Medical Surveillance Programs

REASONS FOR MEDICAL SURVEILLANCE PROGRAMS

The most common reasons for employers to establish surveillance programs are concern for the health and fitness of employees and the need to comply with governmental regulations [2]. Good employee health promotes good business and productivity [3]. Quality medical surveillance programs have many benefits [4]. A medical surveillance program should be complementary to the existing industrial hygiene, safety, and occupational health programs. The occupational medicine provider who serves as director of the surveillance program can alleviate the job demands placed on the industrial hygienist and other health and safety professionals. Regulatory compliance issues can be addressed as a team, drawing on the expertise of diverse health and safety professionals.

BARRIERS TO ESTABLISHING PROGRAMS

There may be barriers to establishing a medical surveillance program [4]. A major obstacle is the existence of an institutional or corporate culture that deemphasizes safety. This could be the result of either employer or employee attitudes or both. For a safety culture to exist, top management must "buy into" and champion safety. Usually, employees will either rise or fall to the safety performance level expected and rewarded. The success or failure of a medical surveillance program depends on the support of top management. The employer must emphasize to employees the reasons for surveillance and allow them adequate time to participate in the surveillance program. Employees' mistrust of the employer's motives render many surveillance programs ineffective. It should be clearly stated that the medical surveillance program is not intended to identify employees for punitive reasons Employers should have a policy that incorporates work accommodations or job transfer for employees discovered to have a medical condition by medical surveillance that adversely affects that medical condition as a result of a workplace exposure on the offending job.

PROGRAM COMPONENTS

Most medical surveillance programs use a computer tracking system that provides a database of surveillance activities [5–8], assists in identification and timely scheduling of needed examinations, and serves as a communication tool between medical and other health and safety professionals and management. Epidemiologic analysis of the database can assist in identification of workplace problems. Early identification of workplace trends allows for more effective preventive measures and gives added value to the provision of medical surveillance services.

The confidentiality of workplace information has undergone an unprecedented assault from advances in information technology. Confidentiality of medical information obtained as a result of the surveillance process must be protected and not compromised. The ethical and legal questions raised by these workplace confidentiality issues will continue to evolve through debate in the professional arena and in the courtroom [9–18]. The American College of Occupational and Environmental Medicine's (ACOEM) *Code of Ethical Conduct* sets a standard for professional ethical conduct regarding confidentiality. It requires the physician to "keep confidential all individual medical information, releasing such information only when required by law or overriding public health considerations, or to other physicians according to accepted medical practice, or to others at the request of the individual." Also stated in the code is that the physician should "recognize that employers may be entitled to counsel about an individual's medical work fitness, but not to diagnoses or specific details, except in compliance with laws and regulations." Similar issues are addressed in ACOEM's Confidentiality of Medical Information in the Workplace and in the Association of Occupational and Environmental Clinics (AOEC's) Patient Bill of Rights [15].

Appropriate training is a regulatory requirement when hazardous work is being done. The Hazard Communication Standard, 29 CFR 1910.1200, imparts to employees a "right to know" about workplace hazards and entitles them to training that will protect them from the hazard [2,19,20]. The training program should be generated and supervised by the departments involved in the actual training. The occupational medicine services unit should be involved as an information resource and actively participate when needed. The occupational medicine provider's objective and scientific opinion will serve to give added weight to a health or safety issue.

The initial and periodic medical evaluations are important to the medical surveillance program. The preplacement medical examination or periodic examination is a good time for the occupational medicine provider to discuss with the employee ways to reduce risks. Evaluations for injuries or illnesses are a time to discuss workplace practices with the goal of minimizing work-related illnesses. An illness event should prompt an incident evaluation. This should include a walk-through of the workplace by the occupational medicine professional and an in-depth discussion with the affected employee. This allows the occupational medical service unit to learn more about the workplace and interact with the employees and the actual job duties that are performed.

AMERICANS WITH DISABILITIES ACT

The Americans with Disabilities Act (ADA) has reshaped the legal landscape of the workplace and the duties of the occupational health professional. The ADA prohibits discrimination against the disabled individual seeking employment. Although simple in its intent, it has proved difficult in interpretation. The inherent ambiguity of the ADA definitions of *disability, qualified individual, reasonable accommodations, direct threat,* and *undue hardship* requires case-by-case analysis when applying the law. For additional guidance, one should refer to the U.S. Equal Employment Opportunity Commission (EEOC) and the U.S. Department of Justice (DOJ), both of which have excellent Internet sites at www.eeoc.gov and www.usdoj.gov, respectively. The medical surveillance process affects the employment process and is subject to the ADA.

Knowledge of the ADA and its protections is essential if the occupational medicine provider is to appropriately make decisions to assist with job placement. Individuals diagnosed with either preexisting chronic infectious disease or infectious disease acquired while already employed (whether or not the disease is work related) must be evaluated carefully for the presence of disability, as defined by the ADA, and whether or not there is a need for reasonable accommodations. To quality for ADA protection, a disabled person must be qualified for the job. Although an employer has no legal obligation to hire unqualified people, an employer is obligated to provide reasonable work accommodations for a disabled individual who is otherwise qualified to perform the job. Reasonable accommodation entails an employer's provision of flexibility in job structure or work environment or of special equipment without imposing undue hardship on the employer. The ADA covers all aspects of the employment process. A job applicant is protected from having to divulge any medical information or submit to any medical examination prior to being offered a job. The employer may not ask any question to which the answer may reveal information about the existence of a disability. However, the employer is allowed to ask the applicant if essential job functions can be performed with or without reasonable accommodations. The ADA requires that if an employment entrance examination is performed, it be required for all new employees in the same job category.

The ADA has had a major impact on the periodic examination of current employees. If periodic examination is mandatory for employment, it must be job-specific in its scope. Employees may voluntarily participate in periodic medical surveillance examinations offered by their employer. Still, only job-related information may be released to the employer.

RELATIONSHIP TO HAZARD EVALUATION

The need for medical surveillance is a function of exposure. For workplaces with no potential for exposure to hazardous agents, there is no need for medical surveillance. Proper risk/exposure assessment is a prerequisite for planning and implementing an appropriate medical surveillance program [4,21]. Industrial hygiene, safety and health, and occupational medicine professionals function as a team to anticipate, recognize, evaluate and control hazards. Communication among these professionals is essential in achieving the goal of prevention of occupational illness and injury.

Risk assessment as a process has taken on increasing importance owing to an increasingly complicated workplace environment. Biologic research continues to expand in scope and present new types of exposure risks. Risk is a probability determination of an adverse outcome. A formal risk assessment process is the characterization of the probability of an adverse health effect from exposure to an agent. The risk assessment process is systematic and scientific in its approach [22]. Sequential steps detailed by the National Academy of Science include hazard identification, dose-response assessment, exposure assessment, and risk characterization [23].

Risk communication is conveying information about the elements of risk inherent in the workplace and work process to all involved parties. Timely and accurate risk communication is essential to preserve the institutional good-citizen image [24].

The risk assessment process should drive the medical surveillance process. Some might argue that if the risk assessment and risk management processes work correctly, there would be no need for medical surveillance. Medical surveillance is a method of monitoring or measuring the controls put in place to manage risk. As pointed out previously, there are some inherent limitations in the risk assessment process. Without medical surveillance, some workers, especially the most susceptible, would succumb to occupational illnesses. In these cases, the medical surveillance process may be able to spur the risk assessment process, limiting and controlling institutional risk. For example, if during the periodic medical examinations workers reported high rates of symptoms to indicate a possible infectious disease or exhibited objective signs of an infectious disease illnesses, this would be communicated to safety and occupational medicine personnel. It is expected that this would be the impetus to initiate an exposure assessment to evaluate for a potential source of exposure. The medical surveillance process provides needed redundancy to ensure worker safety [25].

Activities of Occupational Health Professionals

The occupational medicine provider must be proficient at performing an occupational medical history and a focused physical examination and obtaining information pertinent to the workplace. Standard occupational medicine textbooks can be used to formulate a working guideline for incorporation into the medical surveillance program. An exposure history template was developed by the Agency for Toxic Substances and Disease Registry (ATSDR) and National Institute for Occupational

Safety and Health (NIOSH). This template, which is comprehensive, is available from ATSDR [26].

As in any type of medical encounter, the history obtained from the employee provides the most important information for decision making in occupational medicine. It is important to understand exactly what the employee does in his or her job, how he or she performs the job, what personal protective equipment is used (or should be used) in the performance of the job, and what the current workplace environment is. In this regard, the employee's job description should be made available to the medical provider. Likewise, it is important to know the employee's past job history, workplace exposures, and any leisure activities or hobbies that could have an impact on health.. Many times an employee does multiple tasks outside his or her job description. It may be tasks outside of work and not a workplace exposure that is causing the employee's symptoms or illness. To facilitate the interview process, most occupational medicine providers formulate a health questionnaire covering general medical and specific occupational information. The questionnaire is typically a combination of check-off-type questions, a listing of specific items, and then room for descriptive elaboration by the employee. Typically, the employee fills out the questionnaire prior to the interview and reviews it with the medical professional during the interview and examination. The length of the interview and examination is directly proportional to the complexity of the situation. Young healthy employees with no symptoms or signs of disease and a very brief work history can be evaluated quickly, whereas employees with symptoms or signs of disease or with a complex work-exposure history may need a very time-consuming evaluation.

In the medical surveillance process, the occupational medicine provider's initial encounter with a worker is typically the preplacement examination. At this point in the employment process, the individual has been offered a job on the condition that he or she undergo a medical examination. Up to this point, the employee has not had to provide any medical information to the employer, as governed by the ADA. The employer has deemed the applicant qualified for the job, and the medical examination is done to assess if the applicant can perform the essential functions of the job with or without reasonable accommodations. The applicant is required to provide a complete medical history to allow for this determination but is provided confidentiality in its disclosure.

In essence, the preplacement examination is a risk assessment process during which the medical professional is attempting to determine if the individual can work safely, based on knowledge of the individual and knowledge of the workplace. Such issues as employee susceptibility and direct threat come into consideration. Certainly, some medical conditions present a direct threat to the individual and his or her coworkers. The ADA defines *direct threat* as a reasonable probability of substantial harm to self or others. For example, an individual with a well-controlled seizure disorder cannot be considered a direct threat even though it is possible that he or she could have a seizure on the job. The ADA does not allow speculation on all possibilities but only on what is a reasonable possibility.

Current employees may voluntarily participate in periodic medical surveillance examinations that may be comprehensive in nature, similar to the preplacement examination. In institutions in which periodic examinations are mandatory for continued employment, they must be job-specific in scope. Any periodic examination participant is entitled to medical information confidentiality and ADA protection. The employer is only entitled to job-related information.

Episodic examinations will be driven by the occurrence of symptoms and diagnosed illnesses. All patient interactions should be seen as a chance to measure how well the occupational safety and medical surveillance programs are functioning. They present an opportunity for the occupational medicine provider to learn more about any work process changes or any hazards that have recently been identified in the workplace. Episodic examinations serve as a two-pronged relationship builder through (1) providing care for the employees and (2) working with other occupational health professionals in the provision of a safe workplace.

An employer may offer an exit examination to an employee leaving the institution. In general, exit examinations are not well received by employees. Once the decision has been made to change jobs, most employees will not schedule an exit examination unless some overriding health concern exists.

Medical Surveillance of Occupational Infectious Diseases

OVERVIEW

Animal handlers and health care workers have the greatest occupational exposure risk for infectious disease. Thus the following will deal primarily with medical surveillance in these two occupational groups. The special exposure situations that can occur during occupational travel are covered in other chapters.

ANIMAL HANDLERS

Medical surveillance plays an important role in the protection of the health and safety of animal handlers. Medical surveillance programs should be provided for all personnel involved in care and research use of animals [27]. The surveillance is exposure-driven through environmental monitoring performed by the workplace health and safety professionals. In an animal care facility, the institutional veterinary staff is usually the principal source of exposure information. Medical surveillance needs vary among institutions, and it is critical for occupational health professionals to work closely with the animal care facility professionals to ensure that an effective program exists. It is crucial that the occupational health professional involved in the program have a clear understanding of the institution's surveillance requirements coupled with sensitivity for the budgetary constraints faced by the animal facility managers. Approximately 90,000 workers in the United States have direct contact with animals in research or industrial facilities[28].The medical surveillance program for animal handlers monitors the effectiveness of engineering controls, work practices, and use of personal protective equipment [29]. The scope and duties of a medical surveillance program depend on the needs of the animal care center. Services provided should be based on an adequate risk assessment of the animal care facility. This assessment should consider:

- Animal handler's contact with animals
- Exposure intensity of the contact
- Exposure frequency of that contact
- Physical and biologic hazards presented by the animals and their husbandry activities

- Hazardous nature of the agents and protocols used in the research
- Individual susceptibilities of the animal handlers
- Occupational history of the animal handlers and the experience of other animal handlers in other settings [27]

Assessment of risk involves evaluating the worksite for work activities that create risk of occupational illness. Such risks include animal handlers' direct handling of macaques leading to potential herpes B virus exposures or handling and removing soiled litter from cages with increased exposure to specific agents [27]. It is important for all involved in administering the program that adverse health outcomes are quickly recognized and evaluated to determine whether the adverse outcome was the result of a failed program [27]. It is essential for the facility to have a policy statement regarding animal handler selection, medical evaluations and medical surveillance, and relocation and dismissal plans. During preplacement medical evaluation, animal handlers should be informed about potential hazards that will be encountered while performing their jobs and about safe work practices required to avoid those hazards. Information about reporting procedures and the medical surveillance program also should be covered at this time [29].

A narrowly focused surveillance program better serves the needs of most facilities. A comprehensive animal care program may appear to require a comprehensive surveillance program but may only need a focused surveillance program specific to the identified inherent risks and the needs of animal handlers. Most comprehensive animal research centers are located or associated with academic centers that have access to an academic occupational medicine service capable of meeting all their needs and requirements and serving as a resource for specific issues and questions. If this is not the case, access to a primary care service or occupational medicine service, with an interest and willingness to assume the duties and responsibilities is required.

Primary contacts/persons from both the occupational medical service unit and the animal care program should be designated to facilitate communication. The contact person from the occupational medical service unit should develop a working knowledge of the exposures and risks involved at the animal care facility, especially in the area of zoonoses. This individual must be willing to make worksite visits and be capable of developing a medical surveillance program based on the exposure risk assessment.

REGULATIONS AND GUIDELINES THAT AFFECT PROGRAMS

Animal care and research facilities are subject to numerous regulations. These regulations and guidelines can be federal, state, local, and institutional. Federal regulations include Occupational Safety and Health Administration (OSHA) standards and guidelines, the Centers for Disease Control and Prevention (CDC) recommendations, and the National Institutes of Health (NIH) guidelines. OSHA's general duty clause requires employers to provide a safe and healthy workplace free from recognized hazards. The OSHA Bloodborne Pathogens Standard (29 CFR 1910.1031) requires the employer to provide hepatitis vaccination if there is a risk of exposure. The OSHA Occupational Exposure to Hazardous Chemicals in Laboratories Standard (29 CFR 1910.1450) requires medical surveillance if exposures routinely occur above the action level. Other OSHA standards that could apply are the OSHA Hazard Communication Standard (29 CFR 1910.1200), the OSHA Ethylene Oxide Standard (29 CFR 1910.1047), and the OSHA Formaldehyde Standard (29 CFR 1910.1048). CDC guidelines are applicable if institutions receive federal funding. *The Public Health Service Policy on Humane Care and Use of Laboratory Animals* and the *Biosafety in Microbiological and Biomedical Biotechnical Laboratories* guidelines require that institutions provide occupational health services to animal handlers [30–32]. The *Biosafety in Microbiological and Biomedical Laboratories* is being revised at this time. The current edition was published in 1993. It is directed at research programs involving experimentally or naturally infected vertebrates and has recommendations regarding serum banking that are no longer believed to be necessary because other approaches are now used. The guidelines recommend limiting access of individuals who would be highly susceptible or who would likely have more complicated courses of illness if infected. It is now recommended that serum banking of a baseline sample be secured for specific agents under biosafety level (BSL) 2. This applies if a substantial risk of infection exists and there is a reliable method to measure immunologic response to the specific infectious agent. BSL 3 agents require serum banking if the previously mentioned criteria are met. Immunizations should be given when safe and effective vaccines exist and there is a clearly identified risk for employees. Such vaccines as hepatitis B, yellow fever, rabies, polio, and diphtheria/tetanus would be considered applicable. It is also recommended that a tuberculosis (TB) surveillance program be in place [27].

The NIH Guidelines for Research Involving Recombinant DNA Molecules requires occupational health services for employees working with viable recombinant DNA containing microorganisms that need BSL 3 or greater. One of the requirements is to keep a record of agents handled by the individuals involved. Another requirement is the maintenance of serial serum samples (serum banking) for monitoring of serologic changes [27].

HAZARDS AND RISK ASSESSMENT

Medical surveillance is a means of measuring the effectiveness of risk assessment and control of hazards and risk of exposure. One needs to understand what the hazards are in an animal handing facility and use appropriate methods to assess risk of exposure [32]. Animal handlers may encounter any of the following type of hazards: physical hazards, chemical hazards, or biologic hazards [27,33]. Physical hazards can be classified as animal bites, scratches, and kicks and may result in exposure to infectious agents from the animal, a contaminated work environment, or secondary infection. Biologic hazards can be divided into zoonotic infections, allergens, and research protocol infections. Since these hazards are potentially present in animal care and research facilities, risk assessment efforts should be directed at detecting those hazards [27, 33–42]. The occupational health professional must be familiar with all workplace hazards and be comfortable interfacing with the animal care professional about the workplace assessment. Substantial contact with an animal is not a sufficient indicator of risk. A determination should be based on the nature of hazards associated with the care and use of research animals and the intensity and frequency of employee exposure to these hazards [27]. Safety procedures can minimize the potential risks of exposure to zoonotic infections. These procedures include [1]:

- Purchase of pathogen-free animals, if possible
- Use of a holding facility for quarantine of newly acquired animals and animals suspected of being infected; in such a facility the animals can be evaluated for pathogens and treated appropriately
- Vaccination of animal handlers
- Use of specialized containment caging or chemical restraint and protective clothing

The risk of animal handlers acquiring a zoonotic disease has declined, especially for those handling small animals. The major reason is that, currently, these animals are more often bred in barrier facilities [1]. Large animals still pose considerable risk because they are frequently obtained from the wild or from facilities that are not true barrier facilities [1]. Animals used as models in infectious disease studies pose a threat regardless of where they were bred [4, 14]. Transmission of zoonotic agents to animal handlers is either by direct contact with infected animals or indirectly by exposure to contaminated equipment or supplies [1]. Aerosolization of infectious agents is considered the main way most zoonotic diseases are transmitted [1]. Bites, scratches, and exposure to contaminated equipment, resulting in direct inoculation, are other means of transmission [1, 27].

Animal handlers need to be continually reminded of the importance of reporting all wounds and accidents. This enables the occupational medicine services unit to initiate appropriate follow-up measures. Animal handlers need to be educated about the importance of reporting any gastrointestinal, respiratory, or dermal conditions with symptoms that are similar to those occurring in the animals they are tending. This helps surveillance program personnel to decide if control measures are working correctly and effectively. The following is a brief overview of some zoonoses that may affect animal handlers. They are presented according to general animal groupings. The groupings are rodents and rabbits, carnivores, ungulates, and nonhuman primates.

Rabbits and Rodents

Zoonotic diseases associated with modern rodent- and rabbit-research holding facilities are infrequent. However, there are reports of cases of lymphocytic choriomeningitis virus, Korean hemorrhagic fever caused by hantavirus, leptospirosis, the tapeworm *Hymenolepis nana*, and ringworm that purportedly were acquired in laboratory facilities. Most infections acquired by animal handlers from rodents and rabbits are via direct contact with the animals or the animals' excretions or indirectly via aerosolized contaminants. Proper handling of rabbits and rodents is the most effective measure of preventing bites and scratches from these species [43]. Other potential infections from this group of animals include brucellosis, *Yersinia* infection, and some parasitic diseases.

Carnivores

Dogs, cats, and ferrets are the most common carnivores used in laboratory settings. Rabies is the most important zoonotic disease associated with carnivores, because carnivores are not likely to have come from barrier breeding facilities. Bites and scratches are the most common source of zoonotic disease transmission to animal handlers with these animals [43]. Other potential infections from this group of animals include *Pasturella multocida* infection (drug of first choice penicillin G: alternatively, doxycycline or amoxicillin/clavulanate [44] and infection from the more common bacterial pathogens (*Streptococcus* and *Staphlococcus*) from cat or dog bite wounds, toxoplasmosis, leptospirosis, Q fever, *Yersinia infection, Mycobacteria* infection (various strains), *Cryptococcus neoformans* infection, echinococcosis, visceral larva migrans, dipylidiasis (dog tapeworm found in cats and dogs), coenuriasis, and other parasitic diseases.

Ungulates

Ungulates (i.e., sheep and goats) present little risk for transmission of zoonotic disease to humans because these animals are kept in herds and thus good husbandry conditions usually exist. Q fever is a concern in certain research projects involving ungulate parturition products or materials contaminated by these products [43]. Other potential infections from this group of animals include Brucellosis, anthrax, melioidosis, *Yersinia* infection, Q fever, echinococcosis, coenuriasis, and, depending on the source of the animal (sheep) Rift Valley fever.

Nonhuman Primates

The two infectious agents that present major risks for transmission of zoonotic infection from nonhuman primates to humans are simian immunodeficiency virus (SIV) and herpes B virus [45-47]. The morbidity of human SIV infections has not been clearly defined [6]. The morbidity of herpes B virus is very clear. Although it causes minimal adverse effects in macaques, in humans it can cause rapidly progressive encephalomyelitis, with a fatality rate approaching 70%.

The best approach to either of these infections and other potential zoonoses transmitted by nonhuman primates is prevention of exposure via education about the risks of exposure. Animal handlers should receive instruction about protocols and procedures involved in handling nonhuman primates. They should be able to demonstrate steps to be taken in the event of a potential exposure. The use of restraint cages and chemical restraint should be encouraged whenever any interaction is planned with nonhuman primates. Protective equipment such as gloves, face shields, and arm protectors should be used [32]. This is especially important in handling macaques. When nonhuman primates have been experimentally inoculated with SIV or similar types of viruses, BSL 2 practices should be followed [45]. Other potential infections from this group of animals include histoplasmosis, *Mycobacteria* infection, *Entamoeba histolytica* infection, Monkeypox, rabies, rubeola, hepatitis A, *Shigella* infection and other more common human gastroenteritidies, Marburg virus infection, Ebola infection, and other hemorrhagic fevers, *Bertiella* infection, *Mesocstoides* infection, and other parasites.

CONTROL METHODS

It is generally accepted that engineering controls should be considered the best approach to reducing exposure risks. Using administrative or work practice controls is the next best approach. The least acceptable method is personal protective equipment. Animal care facilities are no exception to this approach to controlling hazards and exposures. Engineering controls generally are considered to be the best barriers to exposure to animals [27]. These barriers may consist singly or in combination of such items as fume hoods, biologic safety cabinets, special caging, and room ventilation. Administration and work practices consist of measures to reduce the number of employees exposed and reduce contacts with animals. For the protection of individual animal handlers, efforts are directed at reducing exposures by the percutaneous route, ingestion, and inhalation [27]. These measures should apply to handling, transporting, and restraining animals as well as to housekeeping, waste disposal, and cage cleaning. It is important also to address issues of personal hygiene to reduce the risk of exposure and provide facilities that make it easy to maintain a high standard of personal cleanliness [32]. Hand washing is very important in preventing the spread of infectious contaminants [43]. Eating, drinking, smoking, and applying cosmetics should not be permitted in laboratories or animal containment areas [27, 32, 43]. Personal protective equipment consists of equipment such as gloves, shoe covers, protective clothing, face shields, earplugs, and respirators. Animal handlers should be given the appropriate personal protective equipment based on potential exposure. [32]. The most important preventive strategy is education. Animal handlers must be trained in the use of control measures [27, 32, 43] and in proper handling of animals to avoid bites and scratches. It is also important to educate handlers on proper disposal methods for animal bedding and waste products and other contaminated body materials as well as on Universal Precautions and other good personal hygiene measures. The importance of immediately reporting accidents and adverse incidents is vital [27, 43] Training should be done at least annually and must be appropriate to animal handlers' education level, experience in the facility, and language skills [27, 32, 43].

TYPES OF MEDICAL EVALUATIONS

An important part of an animal handler's medical surveillance program is the medical evaluation. There are basically three types of medical evaluations: pre-placement, periodic, and episodic evaluations. These evaluations should be used to gather health information about the animal handler and for providing appropriate education to the animal handler. The encounter, for the most part, can be done by the use of questionnaires and focused interviews. A decision to conduct further evaluation should be based on information elicited during the history. The educational portion of the evaluation involves reiterating health exposure risks, reporting mechanisms for potential exposures and explaining how medical surveillance functions to protect the animal handler.

Preplacement Evaluation

The preplacement evaluation establishes a baseline of health information before an individual starts on the job and before experiencing any worksite exposures. The provider is expected to identify pre-existing conditions that may affect an individual's capacity to perform the essential functions of a position. This time also should be used to discuss medical conditions that might alter an individual's medical risk profile. Animal handlers should be informed about potential workplace risks, the proper use of personal protective equipment, and which medical symptoms should prompt an occupational health evaluation [27, 33, 48].

At the preplacement evaluation, the animal handler is given appropriate immunizations based on the animal contact he or she will have and in compliance with federal, state, and local regulations. The animal handler is started in a tuberculosis surveillance program. Rabies immunization and serologic monitoring should be offered to those considered at high risk of exposure to rabies. There should be serologic testing for toxoplasmosis for those at risk [49], namely, immunocompromised workers and any females with childbearing potential who will be exposed to cats or cat feces. If an animal handler in one of these categories lacks immunity to toxoplasmosis, the individual should be counseled about susceptibility and associated risk. The person's supervisor should be notified of the need for possible job reassignment of the worker. If there is a high risk of exposure to Q fever, counseling should be offered [49]. Animal handlers who will have direct involvement with *Coxiella burnetii* or handle products of parturition or other contaminated materials from sheep, goats, cattle, or cats are at risk. They should be advised of signs and symptoms and the importance of early treatment.

Additional services should be offered to those involved in work with nonhuman primates [49]. All animal handlers are enrolled in the TB surveillance program because TB has devastating consequences for nonhuman primates and may result in the loss of the whole colony. Rubeola screening is offered at preplacement. Rubeola is a common infection in nonhuman primate colonies. Hepatitis A and B vaccinations are offered if animal handlers will be working with experimentally infected nonhuman primates. Rabies immunization is offered to animal handlers who will be working with quarantined nonhuman primates. Additionally, animal handlers working with nonhuman primates are given instruction on appropriate measures to take in the event of potential exposure to herpes B virus from macaques and in the event of potential exposure to SIV from other monkeys and apes.

Periodic Evaluation

The periodic medical evaluation is the main component of a medical surveillance program and verifies the success of the occupational health and safety program in reducing exposure risk. Components of the evaluation focuses on the individual animal handler's risk of exposure. Inquiry should be made about the presence of symptoms that may be an early warning of disease. Physical examinations need not be a routine part of the periodic evaluation unless warranted by a change in health status or symptoms [27] It is imperative that the occupational health professional takes a careful history, based on knowledge of the animal handler's exposure risk. Periodic evaluations usually are given annually. An occupational history is conducted to detect early signs and symptoms of disease. Further medical evaluation is based on the findings of the history; at this time, tuberculin skin testing or other means of evaluating a worker's TB status is performed. Those working with nonhuman primates may need to have more frequent surveillance in the TB program. Immunization status is reviewed and updated as necessary. Those who received rabies immunization starting 2 years after the series was completed require serologic testing to determine their immune status.

Episodic Evaluation

Episodic health evaluations are evaluations of work-related injuries or medical follow-up of early warning symptoms of illness and persistent symptoms [27]. Animal handlers should be encouraged to report all suspected work-related injuries and ill-

nesses as soon as possible [49]. All accidental exposure incidents need to be evaluated to determine if they warrant medical evaluation. When confronted by a preexisting medical condition, an evaluation by the occupational health professional, with input from the employee's personal physician, will ensure proper medical surveillance and work assignment changes, thus helping to reduce the risk for the animal handler [43].

There should be a regular systematic review of these examinations by the animal care facility managers, the environmental health and safety professionals, and the occupational health professional. Changes in the program examinations should be based on changes in exposures of the animal handlers. The injury and illness experience and any new government regulation also will help determine if any changes are needed in the surveillance program.

SERUM BANKING

Serum banking allows for the ability to compare serum obtained after a worker's acute illness or exposure with prior samples from the same individual and is a standard component of animal handler surveillance programs. Guidelines from the late 1980s and early 1990s called for routine serum banking [27, 45, 46]. More recent guidelines recommend serum banking only in those cases in which serologic monitoring can follow the progression of a potential infection or disease. These guidelines also recommend testing of the serum specimen obtained along with its banking. In general, serum banking should be used only if there is a clear reason for obtaining the samples and there is a plan to analyze the data as part of a risk assessment strategy. Issues regarding chain of custody, confidentiality, identification of specimens, appropriate storage of specimens (to prevent deterioration), and security of specimens should be addressed in the serum banking policy. Employees should be afforded the opportunity to decline serum banking participation without punitive action by the employer.

IMMUNIZATIONS AND SEROLOGIC TESTING

Animal handlers should be offered immunizations known to be safe and effective. Recommendations for immunization vary according to risk and hazard assessments. This information will come from the institutional veterinarians and the occupational health and safety professionals.

- *Hepatitis B virus (HBV)*: Hepatitis B vaccination should be offered, based on the requirements of the OSHA Bloodborne Pathogen Standard (29 CFR 1910.1030).
- *Hepatitis A virus (HAV)*: Persons who work with HAV-infected primates or with HAV in a research laboratory setting should be HAV vaccinated. No other populations have been demonstrated to be at increased risk for HAV infection because of occupational exposure. Further details on the HAV vaccine are given below [49].
- *Tetatus/Diptheria*: All animal handlers should have current tetanus and diphtheria immunization status determination.
- *Rabies*: Rabies vaccine should be offered to animal handlers who work with animals potentially infected with rabies. It should be provided to those who capture or destroy wild animals on site. Those who inspect sites where rabies virus is also used should be considered for vaccination. Periodic serologic monitoring should be offered.
- *Toxoplasmosis*: Serologic testing for toxoplasmosis should be obtained for immunocompromised animal handlers or females capable of childbearing who anticipate exposure to cats or their feces. If titers are not interpreted as protective, then the animal handler should be counseled regarding potential health risks to themselves or the fetus. The supervisor needs to make the decision about providing job reassignments for these animal handlers [48].
- *Other vaccinations* offered might include those for yellow fever, rabies (see below), and polio.

GENERAL GUIDELINES AND SUMMARY FOR A PROGRAM

There must be a written policy statement about the medical surveillance program for animal handlers [27]. The purpose of an animal handlers' medical surveillance program needs to be stated. In essence, it is to protect the health of the worker. The clinical interactions are used to provide appropriate immunizations, to review good work practices, and to educate the animal handlers about risk assessment and exposure reduction. The program is available

not only to the animal handlers of the animal care facility [27, 32, 43, 49] but also to all who come in contact with animals on a routine basis. The animal handlers' surveillance program is divided into three categories:

1. Small animals, mainly rodents and rabbits
2. Large animals, mainly cats, dogs, and livestock
3. Nonhuman primates, namely, marmosets, monkeys, and apes

A medical surveillance plan for animal handlers should provide for the safety and good health of all those who work with animals. The program needs to focus on the specific needs of the animal handlers based on an adequate health risk assessment of the specific animal care facility. The occupational medicine service should be involved in policy and procedure issues that have an impact on the health of the animal handlers. The occupational health professional should have a good working knowledge of the facility and the hazards and risks involved. There should be regular interaction between the animal care facility managers, the environmental health and safety professionals, and the occupational health professional. There should be a computerized data-collection system that will augment the surveillance program; it should be used to review and aggregate information about the control methods and the surveillance program. The program should not add unnecessary items that eventually will dilute the services rendered to the animal handlers.

Medical Surveillance of Health Care workers with an Emphasis on Infectious Diseases

HEALTH CARE WORKERS

It is well recognized that health care workers are frequently exposed to a variety of infectious occupational insults that can result in serious acute or chronic adverse health effects [50]. Although occupational exposure to infectious disease is not a risk that solely affects health care workers, this group clearly has more intensity of such exposures and a far greater variety of exposures to potentially virulent infectious agents than most other occupational work groups. For these reasons alone, it is imperative that a well-organized surveillance program be in place in health care facilities. Those who run such facilities also must recognize that OSHA regulations mandate some infectious disease surveillance. However, the overriding incentive for infectious disease surveillance of health care workers should be that these programs benefit health care facility employees as well as the patient populations they serve, many of whom have compromised health. Surveillance programs for infectious diseases are already in place in most health care facilities. The remainder of this section details well-recognized infectious disease surveillance protocols and touches on other possible surveillance protocols that may be adapted depending on the potential for exposure that may exist in an individual facility. Surveillance programs always should coexist with primary and secondary prevention. Primary prevention of an infectious disease is action taken to prevent initiation of the disease process. These activities remove or reduce risk factors [48]. Such measures include Universal Precautions (e.g., for bloodborne pathogens), personal protective equipment (e.g., respirators, gowns, and gloves), engineering controls (e.g., ventilation and ultraviolet lighting), and preexposure vaccination. Secondary prevention of infectious disease involves intervention early in a disease process, when that process may be reversible or when the disease progression may be limited. For infectious diseases, secondary prevention may involve medical treatment such as medication, surgery, or postexposure vaccination [51].

Other chapters in this book cover specific infectious diseases, including surveillance for these diseases, in greater detail (see Chapters 24, 34, 35, and other chapters on specific infectious agents). The examples in this section cover the important elements that should be included in employee surveillance programs for most health care facilities.

SPECIFIC INFECTIOUS DISEASE SURVEILLANCE IN HEALTH CARE WORKERS
Hepatitis

Hepatitis B. Occupational exposure to HBV was a major impetus for OSHA's Bloodborne Pathogen Standard, which became effective March 6, 1992, and applies to all persons occupationally exposed to blood or other potentially infectious materials. According to the standard, exposure determination is based on the definition of occupational exposure without regard to personal protective clothing or equipment. Reviewing job classifications within the work environment and listing exposures into two groups are steps in making the exposure determination. The first group includes job classifications in which all the employees have occupational exposure, such as operating room scrub nurses. In such cases, it is not necessary to list specific work tasks. The second group includes job classifications in which some of the employees have occupational exposure, such as workers in a hospital laundry where some of the workers are assigned the task of handling contaminated laundry, whereas others are not.

Surveillance for HBV, either preplacement or postexposure, is based on blood tests for HBV antibodies and HBV antigen. These blood tests also help to determine whether or not an employee is a chronic carrier of the disease, carries the protective antibody, or needs to be vaccinated for the disease.

For those health care workers covered under OSHA's Bloodborne Pathogen Standard, a series of three HBV vaccines should be initiated at the time of the preplacement examination, provided that there is no previous history of HBV infection or previous administration of HB vaccine. If there is a history of previous disease or previous vaccine administration, then blood testing for the presence of HBV antibodies should be performed to determine whether immunity is present. Employers are not required to offer HBV vaccination (1) to employees who have previously completed the HBV vaccination series, (2) when immunity is confirmed by antibody testing, or (3) if the vaccine is contraindicated for medical reasons. Employee participation in a prescreening program is not required in order to obtain a HBV vaccination series. For prevaccination surveillance testing, when immunity or prior history of disease status is uncertain, one should consider performing blood testing for the HBV surface antigen (HBsAg) and the antibody to HBV surface antigen (anti-HBs). HBsAg is positive in chronic carriers. Anti-HBs indicates immunity following disease recovery or following a successful immunization series.

If necessary, postvaccination surveillance for immunity (anti-HBs) should be performed at least 1–6 months after completion of the vaccine series. If such results indicate a nonresponder, 15–25% achieve an adequate antibody response after one additional dose and 30–50% after three additional doses [52].

The HBV vaccine is a recombinant vaccine that carries no risk of bloodborne pathogen transmission. The standard schedule for immunization involves three injections in the deltoid muscle at 0, 1, and 6 months. The three-dose series confers a protective antibody response in more than 90% of healthy young adults. Response rates decline with age and may be as low as 50% in the elderly. Response is also lower in those with renal failure, diabetes mellitus, chronic hepatic disease, HIV infection, obesity, and smokers. The response rate is slightly better in women than in men [53].

Anti-HBs (hepatitis B surface antibody) is the major protective mechanism in individuals who have had an episode of HBV infection or have had the series of HBV vaccinations. Its presence usually indicates lifelong immunity [54].

The employer must make the HBV vaccine and the vaccination series available to all employees who experience an occupational exposure and must provide a postexposure evaluation and follow-up to all employees who experience an exposure incident. The vaccinations, and all medical evaluations and follow-up, must be made available by the employer at no cost to the employee.

For a health care employee who experiences an exposure to the blood or other body fluid from a patient potentially infected with HBV, the following procedural measures are recommended:

- The employee's hepatitis B history and vaccination status should be established and blood drawn for HBsAg and anti-HBs.
- If the patient is known to be HBsAg positive and is not known to be immune, the employee is immediately given HBV immune globulin (HBIG) at a dose of 0.06 mL/kg. Employees who received HBIG within the last 3 months do not need another injection.
- If the hepatitis B surface antigen (HBsAg) status of the patient is unknown, a blood sample is drawn from the patient and sent to the laboratory for HBsAg testing.
- After results of the preceding test are known, the following should be implemented:
  - If the health care employee's anti-HBs status is positive, indicating immunity, no further steps are taken.
  - If the patient's status is HBsAg negative and the health care employee's HBcoreAg and

anti-HBs are also negative, the employee is offered the HBV vaccine.
- If the patient's HBsAg status is positive, but the employee's HBcoreAg and anti-HBs are both negative, HBIG (0.06 mL/kg) is given along with the first dose of HBV vaccine. HBIG must be given within 7 days of exposure but preferably should be given within 24–48 hours. The vaccination series should be completed according to the recommended schedule (at 0, 1, and 6 months).

When noting preceding in an adult who has previously completed the HBV series, substantial evidence suggests that if an adult responded to HBV vaccination, that person is protected from chronic HBV infection for at least 20 years even if vaccinees lack detectable anti-HBs at the time of an exposure. For this reason, immunocompetent persons who have had postvaccination testing and are known to have responded to HBV vaccination with anti-HBs concentrations of 10 mIU/mL or more do not require additional passive or active immunization after an HBV exposure and do not need further periodic testing to assess anti-HBs concentrations [55].

Hepatitis A. HAV transmission in health-care institutions is rare. Outbreaks have been observed occasionally in neonatal intensive-care units because of infants acquiring the infection from transfused blood and subsequently transmitting hepatitis A to other infants and staff. Outbreaks of hepatitis A caused by transmission from adult patients to health care workers are typically associated with fecal incontinence, although the majority of hospitalized patients who have HAV infection are admitted after the onset of jaundice, when they are beyond the point of peak infectivity. Data from serologic surveys of health-care workers have not indicated an increased prevalence of HAV infection in these groups compared with that in control populations [49].

The risk for HAV infection related to occupational fecal contamination has been the subject of other studies. Data from serologic studies conducted outside the United States indicate that workers who had been exposed to sewage had a possible elevated risk for HAV infection; however, these analyses did not control for other risk factors (e.g., socioeconomic status). In published reports of three serologic surveys conducted among U.S. wastewater workers and appropriate comparison populations, no substantial or consistent increase in the prevalence of anti-HAV was identified among wastewater workers. No work-related instances of HAV transmission have been reported among wastewater workers in the United States [49].

When noting the preceding, the routine administration of HAV vaccine in health care personnel, is not recommended. Consequently, regular surveillance of health care workers for HAV infection is not standard procedure. Adherence to well-recognized precautions against transmission via the fecal-oral route is the best preventive measure. Administration of immune globulin within 2 weeks following a known hepatitis exposure is quite effective in preventing infection and may be advisable in outbreak situations.

If HAV vaccine is administered, two doses of the vaccine are needed for lasting protection. These doses should be given at least 6 months apart and may be given at the same time as other vaccines. Estimates of long-term protection for fully vaccinated people (i.e., that is the full two-dose series) suggest that protection from HAV infection could last for at least 25 years in adults.

Manufacturers have made available a combined HAV and HBV vaccine. Primary immunization consists of three doses, administered on a 0, 1, and 6 month schedule, the same schedule as that commonly used for single-antigen HBV vaccine. After three doses of the combination vaccine, antibody responses to both antigens are equivalent to responses seen after the single-HAV and HBV antigen vaccines are administered separately on standard schedules.

Hepatitis C. If the possibility of a health care worker's contracting HCV infection following a parenteral or mucous membrane exposure is of concern, the following procedural measures are recommended:

- The health care employee's HCV history should be established and blood drawn for anti-HCV antibodies.
- If the HCV status of the patient is unknown, then blood should be drawn from the patient and sent for testing of the antibody level to HCV (anti-HCV).

- If the source is found to be infected (anti-HCV positive) and the health care employee is anti-HCV negative, then the employee should be informed of the need for medical follow-up. Serologic monitoring for anti-HCV is repeated at 1 and at 6 months. Counseling should be made available to the employee.

There is no known effective immunoprophylaxis or chemoprophylaxis for hepatitis C. The CDC no longer considers the use of immune serum globulin an appropriate option.

Hepatitis D. Hepatitis D is caused by the hepatitis D virus (HDV), a defective virus that for pathogenesis needs the HBV HbsAg for its structural protein sheath. HDV is found in the blood of persons infected with the virus. HDV can be acquired either as a coinfection (occurs simultaneously) with HBV or as a superinfection in persons with existing chronic HBV infection.

Hepatitis E: Hepatitis E is a liver disease caused by the hepatitis E virus (HEV) transmitted in much the same way as HAV. Hepatitis E, however, rarely, if ever, occurs in the United States.

Tuberculosis

Health care workers, including home health nurses, staff in long-term care facilities, and emergency medical technicians should be included in a tuberculosis (TB) screening and prevention program [56, 57]. Such a program should include tuberculin skin testing for all health care workers upon employment and at intervals determined by their future risk of exposure in that facility.

Mantoux tuberculin skin testing is the standard method used for TB screening. This test is administered by intradermal injection of 0.1 mL of purified protein derivative (PPD) containing 5 tuberculin units (TU) into either the volar or dorsal surface of the forearm. A tuberculin syringe, with the needle bevel facing up produces a discrete, pale elevation of the skin (wheal), 6–10 mm in diameter.

Two-step TB skin testing is used to distinguish boosted reactions from those reactions owing to new infections. If the skin test reaction to an initial (first) test is read as negative, a second test should be done 1–3 weeks later. A positive reaction to this second test is most likely a boosted reaction indicating old infection with TB and not a new infection. Using the result of the second test in the two-step method, a person should be classified as either previously infected (but not a new converter) if the test is positive, or uninfected if the second test is negative. In the latter case (two-step negative), a positive reaction to any subsequent test is likely to represent a new infection with *Mycobaacterium tuberculosis* (new converter). Two-step TB skin testing is recommended for the initial (preplacement) testing of health care workers.

The tuberculin skin test should be interpreted within 48–72 hours of the injection. A positive reaction still may be read up to 1 week following the injection. However, if a patient who fails to return within 72 hours has a negative test, tuberculin testing should be repeated.

Measurement of the area of induration (palpable swelling) is the way a test is interpreted, not the erythema around the site of injection (Table 7-1). The appropriate cutoff measurement for a health care worker should be similar to the measurement limits used for persons not in health care occupations. The difference is that determination of what constitutes a positive tuberculin skin test for health care workers also depends on the prevalence of TB in the health care facility. In facilities with little if any exposure to TB, 15-mm induration may be an appropriate cutoff for persons with no other risk factors. On the other hand, for workers in facilities that regularly care for TB patients, 10-mm induration may be an appropriate cut-off. (See Chapter 9).

Varicella

Varicella vaccine was granted U.S. licensure in 1995. Vaccination is desirable for persons who lack a reliable history of varicella. Special efforts should be made to assess an individual health care worker's immunity to varicella by obtaining either a reliable history of disease or by measurement of serum antibody titers. Those who are susceptible—e.g., health care workers serving immunocompromised patients—should receive varicella vaccine. The oc-

currence of varicella in pregnant women is very rare because 90% of females of childbearing age are immune. However, a fetal varicella syndrome, characterized by multiple congenital malformations, has been described [58]. Therefore, it is advisable to weigh the risks and benefits of administering varicella vaccine to a nonimmune female health care worker of childbearing age.

Although historical information may be an important factor in predicting immunity, recent studies have shown that 2–5% of all health care workers are susceptible to varicella [59, 60]. Additionally, this study found that historical information was ineffective in predicting immune status for measles, rubella, mumps, and varicella.

Human Immunodeficiency Virus

Surveillance data suggest that most health care workers with acquired immunodeficiency syndrome (AIDS), acquired the human immunodeficiency virus (HIV) infection through a nonoccupational route [61]. However, as increasing numbers of patients with AIDS are hospitalized, the risk of exposure to HIV can be expected to increase further. Thus, preventing transmission of HIV to health care workers will require efforts to reduce the incidence and dosage of exposure to blood and body fluids through the use of Universal Precautions [62].

If, despite ongoing efforts to prevent HIV exposure, exposure takes place, in addition to appropriate medical treatment, surveillance of the exposed employee for the disease needs to begin immediately. Baseline testing of the health care worker to establish HIV antibody status at the time of exposure should be performed. If the source patient is seronegative and has no clinical evidence of AIDS or symptoms of HIV infection, further follow-up is usually not necessary. If the source person has recently engaged in behavior associated with contracting HIV infection, baseline and follow-up antibody titer measurements should be obtained at 6 weeks, 12 weeks, and 6 months postexposure

Table 7-1
Classification of Positive Tuberculin Skin tests in Health Care Workers

5-mm Induration	10-mm Induration	15-mm Induration
Known or suspected HIV	Medical conditions, excluding HIV	No known risk factors for TB
Close contacts of persons with infectious TB	IV drug users with known negative HIV	

[63]. It is unclear whether an extended follow-up period (e.g., 12 months) is indicated in certain cases. A recent study showed a mean seroconversion time frame of 46 days following exposure, with a median of 65 days [64]. (See Chapter 24).

Mumps

An effective vaccination program for those who are susceptible is the best approach to prevention of occupational transmission of mumps. Personnel should be considered immune if they have (1) documented physician-diagnosed mumps, (2) documentation of receipt of one dose of live mumps vaccine on or after their first birthday, or (3) serologic evidence of immunity. Persons born prior to 1957 may be considered immune from naturally acquired infection [65].

Rubella

Serologic screening of personnel for immunity to rubella need not be done before vaccinating against rubella, unless the medical facility considers it cost-effective or the person getting the vaccination requests it [27]. Rubella vaccination should be required for health care workers who work in a facility where exposure and consequent transmission to patients could have life-threatening consequences. This would include those who care for immunocompromised, pediatric, or obstetric patients. For the same reason, special consideration should be given to susceptible female health care workers of childbearing age who are at risk of exposure to rubella (such as those who work with pediatric patients). However, vaccination for rubella carries its own risk for this latter group, and women should be counseled to avoid pregnancy for a period of 30 days following the administration of vaccine.

Methicillin Resistant Staphyloccus Aureus (MRSA)

MRSA infection is caused by *Staphylococcus aureus* bacteria. Decades ago, a strain of *Staphylococcus* emerged in hospitals that was resistant to the broad-spectrum antibiotics commonly used to treat it. In the 1990s, a type of MRSA began showing up in the wider community. Today, that form of *Staphylococcus*, known as *community-associated MRSA* (CA-MRSA), is responsible for many serious skin and soft tissue infections and for a serious

form of pneumonia. MRSA infections that occur in otherwise healthy people who have not been hospitalized recently (within the past year) or had a medical procedure (such as dialysis, surgery, or catheters) are known as *community-associated MRSA* (CA-MRSA) infections. These infections are usually skin infections, such as abscesses, boils, and other pus-filled skin lesions [66].

MRSA has become a prevalent nosocomial pathogen in the United States. In hospitals, the most important reservoirs of MRSA are infected or colonized patients. Although hospital personnel can serve as reservoirs for MRSA and may harbor the organism for many months, they have been identified more commonly as a link for transmission between colonized or infected patients. The main mode of transmission of MRSA is via hands (especially health care workers' hands), which may become contaminated by contact with (1) colonized or infected patients, (2) colonized or infected body sites of the personnel themselves, or (3) devices, items, or environmental surfaces contaminated with body fluids containing MRSA. Standard precautions, as described in the *Guideline for Isolation Precautions: Preventing Transmission of Infectious Agents in Healthcare Settings 2007*, should control the spread of MRSA in most instances.

Routine surveillance for MRSA in asymptomatic health care workers is not recommended. However, the standard precautions to prevent potential transmission of MRSA include (1) hand washing after touching blood, body fluids, secretions, excretions, and contaminated items, whether or not gloves are worn (2) gloving (clean nonsterile gloves are adequate) when it can be reasonably anticipated that contact with blood or other potentially infectious materials, mucous membranes, nonintact skin, or potentially contaminated intact skin (e.g., of a patient incontinent of stool or urine) could occur (3) protection of the mucous membranes of the eyes, nose, and mouth during procedures and patient-care activities that are likely to generate splashes or sprays of blood, body fluids, secretions and excretions.(4) gowning appropriate to the task to protect skin and prevent soiling or contamination of clothing during procedures and patient care activities when contact with blood, body fluids, secretions, or excretions is anticipated (5) handle used patient care equipment soiled with blood, body fluids, secretions, and excretions in a manner that prevents skin and mucous membrane exposures, contamination of clothing, and transfer of microorganisms to other patients and the environment, and (6) handling, transporting, and processing used linen to avoid contamination of air, surfaces, and persons [67].

References

1. Fox J, Lipman N. Infections transmitted by large and small laboratory animals. *Infect Dis Clin North Am* 1991;5:131–59.

2. Colligan MJ, Sinclair RC. The training ethic and the ethics of training. *Occup Med State Art Rev* 1994; 9:127–34.

3. McCunney RJ, Anstadt G, Burton WN, et al. Advantage of a healthy work force. *J Occup Environ Med* 1997; 39:611–13.

4. Robinson ST. Role of industrial hygiene in medical surveillance. *Occup Med State Art Rev* 1990;5:469–78.

5. Burdorf A, Sorock GS, Herrick RF, et al. Advancing epidemiological studies of occupational injury—approaches and future directions. *Am J Ind Med* 1997;32:180–3.

6. Leigh JP, Miller TR. Job-related diseases and occupations within a large workers' compensation data set. *Am J Ind Med* 1998;33:197–211.

7. Maizlish N. Designing prevention-oriented software for workplace health and safety. *Am J Ind Med* 1997; 31:64–74.

8. Sorock GS, Smith GS, Reeve GR, et al. Three perspectives on work-related injury surveillance systems. *Am J Ind Med* 1997;32:116–28.

9. McCunney RJ. Preserving confidentially in occupational medical practice. *Am Fam Physician* 1996;53: 1751–6.

10. Rischitelli, DG. The confidentiality of medical information in the workplace. *J Occup Environ Med* 1995; 37:583–93.

11. Rothstein MA. A proposed revision of the ACOEM code of ethics. *J Occup Environ Med* 1997;39:616–22.

12. Rothstein MA. Legal and ethical aspects of medical screening. *Occup Med State Art Rev* 1996;11:31–9.

13. Tilton SH. Right to privacy and confidentiality of medical records. *Occup Med State Art Rev* 1996;11: 17–29.

14. American College of Occupational and Environmental Medicine. Position paper on the confidentiality of medical information in the workplace. *J Occup Environ Med* 1995;37:594–6.

15. Association of Occupational and Environmental Clinics. Patient bill of rights. 1987. Available at http://occ-env-med.mcduke.edu/oem/aoec.html .library.

16. Langer CS. Title I of the Americans with Disabilities Act. *Occup Med State Art Rev* 1996;11:5–16.

17. Stillman NG, Donmoyer KT. Occupational health issues under employment law. *Occup Med State Art Rev* 1996;11:41–55.

18. U.S. Department of Justice. Americans with Disabilities Act Home Page. Available at www.usdoj.gov/crt/ada/adahom1.html.

19. Baram M. Generic strategies for protecting worker health and safety. *Occup Med State Art Rev* 1996;11: 69–77.

20. Joseph AJ. Right-to-know training of workers with IQ less than 70: a pilot study. *Am J Ind Med* 1997;32: 417–20.

21. Manno M. Risk assessment. *Toxicol Lett* 1995;77: 45–7.

22. Bell JG, Bishop C, Gann M, et al. A systematic approach to health surveillance in the workplace. *Occup Med* 1995;45:305–10.

23. National Academy of Science. Risk assessment in the federal government: managing the process. Washington, DC: National Academy Press, 1983.

24. Jardine CG, Hrudey SE. Mixed messages in risk communication. *Risk Anal* 1997;17:489–98.

25. Matte TD, Fine L, Meinhardt TJ, et al. Guidelines for medical screening in the workplace. *Occup Med: State Art Rev* July–September 1990;5(3).

26. Agency for Toxic Substances and Disease Registry. *Taking an Exposure History. Case Studies in Environmental Medicine:* 26. Atlanta, GA: U.S. Department of Health and Human Services, 1992.

27. National Research Council. *Occupational health and safety in the care and use of research animals.* Washington, DC: National Academy Press, 1997.

28. Rom WH, Markowitz SB. Environmental and Occupational Medicine. 4th ed. Philadelphia: Lippincott Williams & Wilkins, 2006, Chap 26, p. 432.

29. Hunskaar S, Fosse R. Allergy to laboratory mice and rats: a review of its prevention, management and treatment. *Lab Anim* 1993;27:206–21.

30. National Institutes of Health. *Public Health Service Policy on Humane Care and Use of Laboratory Animals.* Rockville, MD: Department of Health and Human Services, 1996.

31. U.S. Department of Health and Human Services. *Biosafety in Microbiological and Biotechnical Laboratories.* Publication No. (CDC) 93-8395. Washington, DC: U.S. Government Printing Office, 1993.

32. National Research Council. *Guide for the Care and Use of Laboratory Animals.* Washington, DC: National Academy Press, 1996.

33. LaMontagne AD, Mangione TW, Christiani DC, et al. Medical surveillance for ethylene oxide exposure: practices and clinical findings in Massachusetts hospitals. *J Occup Environ Med* 1996;38:144–54.

34. Crook B. Review: methods of monitoring for process microorganisms in biotechnology. *Ann Occup Hyg* 1996;40:245–60.

35. Culver J. Preventing transmission of blood-borne pathogens: A compelling argument for effective device-selection strategies. *Am J Infect Control* 1997;25: 430–3.

36. Hathon L. Engineering controls for abating airborne biologic, chemical and physical contaminants in healthcare workplaces. *Occup Med State Art Rev* 1997;12:635–9.

37. Kacergis JB, Jones RB, Reeb CK. Air quality in an animal facility: particulates, ammonia, and volatile organic compounds. *Am Ind Hyg Assoc J* 1996;57:634–40.

38. Khuder SA, Arthur T, Bisesi MS, et al. Prevalence of infectious diseases and associated symptoms in wastewater treatment workers. *Am J Ind Med* 1998; 33:571–7.

39. LaMontagne AD, Rudd RE, Mangione TW, et al. Determinants of the provision of ethylene oxide medical surveillance in Massachusetts's hospitals. *J Occup Environ Med* 1996;38:155–68.

40. Plaut M, Zimmerman EM, Goldstein RA. Health hazards to humans associated with domestic pets. *Annu Rev Public Health* 1996;17:221–45.

41. Society for Healthcare Epidemiology of America position paper: Management of healthcare workers infected with hepatitis B virus, hepatitis C virus, human immunodeficiency virus, or other blood-borne pathogens. *Infect Control Hosp Epidemiol* 1997;18:349–63.

42. Stave GM. Control of biological hazards. *Occup Med State Art Rev* 1996;11:79–85.

43. National Institutes of Health. Health and Safety Manual/ Available at www.niehs.nih.gov/odhsb/manual/lftfrm.html.

44. Choice of Antibacterial Drugs. *Med Lett,* 2007: 5(57),44.

45. Centers for Disease Control and Prevention. Perspectives in disease prevention and health promotion guidelines to prevent simian immunodeficiency virus infection in laboratory workers and animal handlers. *MMWR* 1988;37:693–4, 699–704.

46. Holmes G, Chapman L, Stewart J, et al. Guidelines for the prevention and treatment of B-virus infections in exposed persons. *Clin Infect Dis* 1995; 20421–5.

47. National Institutes of Health. *Protection of NIH Personnel Who Work with Non-Human Primates.* Manual 3044-2. Washington, DC: NIH, 1993.

48. Prevention of Hepatitis A Through Active or Passive Immunization, Recommendations of the Advisory Committee on Immunization Practices (ACIP), *MMWR* 2006:55(RR07)1-23.

49. National Institutes of Health. Animal Exposure Surveillance Program. Available at http://oacu.od.nih .gov/exposure/aesp.html.

50. Rogers B. Health hazards in nursing and health care: an overview. *Am J Infect Control* 1997;25:248–61.

51. Pottinger JM, Herwaldt LA, Perl TM. Basics of surveillance—an overview. *Infect Control Hosp Epidemiol* 1997;18:513–27.

52. American Academy of Family Physicians. *Recommendations for Hepatitis B Pre-exposure Vaccination and Post-exposure Prophylaxis.* Reprint # 529. Kansas City, MO: AAFP, August 1992.

53. Reynolds EE, Baron RB, Perez-Stable EJ. *Who needs Hepatitis and Varicella vaccines? Fam Prac Recert* 1997;19(4):33–51.

54. Aach R, Hirschman SZ, Holland PV. The ABCs of viral hepatitis. *Patient Care* August 15, 1992.

55. A Comprehensive Immunization Strategy to Eliminate Transmission of Hepatitis B Virus Infection in the United States. Recommendations of the Advisry Committee on Immunization Practices (ACIP) Part II: Immunization of Adults. *MMWR* 2006; 55(RR16):1-25.

56. Centers for Disease Control. *Core Curriculum on Tuberculosis,* 3rd ed, Atlanta, GA: CDC, 1994.

57. Holmes SJ. Review of recommendations of the dvisory committee on immunization practices, Centers for Disease Control and Prevention, on varicella. *J Infect Dis* 1996;174(Suppl 3):S342–4.

58. Connan L, Ayoubi J, Icart J, et al. Intra-uterine fetal death following maternal varicella infection. *Eur J Obstet Gynecol Reprod Biol* 1996;68(1–2):205–7.

59. Sepkowitz K. Occupationally acquired infections in healthcare workers. *Ann Intern Med* 1996;125:826–34.

60. Oliveira J, da Cuhna S, Corte-Real R, et al. The prevalence of measles, rubella, mumps and chickenpox antibodies in a population of health care workers. *Acta Med Port* 1995;8(4):206–14.

61. Chamberland ME, Conley LJ, Bush TJ, et al. Healthcare workers with AIDS. National surveillance update. *JAMA* 1991;266(24):3459–62.

62. Lamphear BP. Trends and patterns in the transmission of bloodborne pathogens to health care workers. *Epidemiol Rev* 1994:16(2):437–50.

63. Centers for Disease Control and Prevention. Public Health Service guidelines for the management of health-care worker exposures to HIV and recommendations for postexposure prophylaxis. *MMWR* 1998;45:1–39.

64. Busch MP, Satten GA. Time course of viremia and antibody seroconversion following human immunodeficiency virus exposure. *Am J Med* 1997;102 (Suppl 5B): 117–24.

65. Bolyard EA, Tablan OC, Williams WW, et al. Guidelines for infection control in health care personnel. 1998. *Am J Infect Control* 1998;19:407–63.

66. MRSA Infection, MayoClinic.com. Available at www.mayoclinic.com/health/mrsa/DS00735.

67. Information About MRSA for Healthcare Personnel. October 10, 2007, Centers for Disease Control and Prevention. Available at www.cdc.gov/ncidod/dhap/ar_mrsa.html.

8

Employee Education and Training

William E. Wright

Background

Effective safety and health programs include employee education and training. Training targeted to specific infectious disease risks of a workplace can support primary prevention (preventing the occurrence of disease or injury) and secondary prevention (early detection of disease and early intervention). It can help employees to understand hazards and their control, improve morale, reduce workplace illness and injuries, and lower insurance premiums [1]. Effective training is essential for employees and good for business.

The need to prepare employees to respond to infectious disease risks has increased because of recent world events. U.S. postal workers and businesses faced intentional introduction of *Bacillus anthracis* into the mail-handling system in 2001. The New York World Trade Center and Pentagon bombings that year heightened awareness of a need for enhanced infection training for first responders and first receivers, as have more recent tidal waves and severe storms complicated by disrupted sanitation measures and mass casualties/fatalities. The world faces bioterrorism concerns, including variola virus (smallpox) and viral hemorrhagic fevers [2]. We face emerging issues of severe adult respiratory syndrome (SARS) related to a coronavirus, epidemics of avian influenza A (H5N1) in birds with outbreaks in humans [3], and potential pandemic influenza. International business travel and work assignments occur in areas of the world with high prevalences of tuberculosis, HIV, hepatitis B, malaria, and other serious endemic infections. Unlike the risks from machinery and familiar elements of the workplace, pathogens can be terrifying because they are an invisible threat that can seem mysterious. Training can demystify the threats, explain modes of transmission and risks, and communicate practical ways to control them.

Resources for Employee Training Programs on Infectious Diseases

Some employee training and education is mandated by the U.S. Occupational Safety and Health Administration (OSHA), parallel state plan standards, or other government regulations. OSHA has summarized training guidelines and training required in its standards [1] covering hundreds of situations in general industry in which training is needed. It is a useful resource for designing training programs. The Bloodborne Pathogens Standard (29 CFR 1910.1030) establishes minimum requirements for exposure control plans and training on proper handling of blood, other body fluids, and tissue. Most pathogens are not covered by their own standard or training mandate, but the need for employers to address them is covered by the general duty clause, Section 5(a)1 of the Occupational Safety and Health Act [4].

An example of hazard-related training is OSHA's Draft Model Training Program for Hazard Communication [5]. It focuses on chemical hazards but is applicable to training generally and hazards of pathogens. The World Health Organization (WHO) provides online training modules in occupational health, hygiene, and safety [6]. These are designed to provide education for professionals who are responsible for protecting the health of workers. Other useful resources cover general principles and approaches for training in industry that can be adapted for biohazard training [7–9].

The OSHA Standard on Hazardous Waste Operations and Emergency Response (HAZWOPER, 29 CFR 1910.120) is designed primarily for first responders at the primary release site of a chemical, biologic, or radiologic hazardous substance. The standard includes training requirements and reference to the Respiratory Protection Standard (29 CFR 1910.134) and its final rule [10]. Similar information for first receivers who are not at the primary release site but receive contaminated victims, their clothing, and their personal effects at hospitals (e.g., clinicians, hospital staff, and security) is available as a best practices document [11]. Training materials for respiratory protection are also available [12]. Guidance and training for other disaster site workers, such as those involved with utilities, demolition, debris removal, and heavy equipment operation, are available online and address pathogens and other hazards [13,14]. Further information related to training for emergency preparedness and response is available from the Centers for Disease Control and Prevention (CDC) [15].

Many of the chapters in this book contain sections on employee training and risks to employees or have other practical information that can be adapted for training programs. Chapter 3 covers many of the terms, principles, and infectious disease transmission considerations that are important foundation materials for training trainers and employees on infectious disease hazards. Chapter 27, on occupational travel, a new chapter for this edition, consolidates many general aspects of employee training for safe, healthy travel.

Some Key Elements of Training Programs

Employee training related to infectious diseases should be based on an exposure control plan that identifies workers who may be exposed to infectious diseases or organisms and specifies training and its delivery. The training should cover elements of the exposure control plan, including why individuals are considered to be at risk; ways infectious material can enter the body; signs and symptoms of infections that may result; infection control procedures; responses to spills or leaks; methods to clean, disinfect, or dispose of contaminated materials; procedures for investigating and documenting exposure incidents; procedures for investigation of infections; and available vaccines, medical evaluation protocols, and treatments.

The OSHA guidelines [1] cover how to tell whether a worksite problem can be solved by training. They address how to determine what training is needed and the role and utility of a job hazard analysis. The analysis identifies each step of a job and existing or potential hazards and determines the best way to perform the job to reduce or eliminate risks. The job hazard analysis helps guide the focus of training activities. Employee input and involvement are important to identify concerns about hazards, near-miss accidents, and risks so that this information can be incorporated into training. This can help training be job-specific and practical.

Training related to job hazards should be done at the time of initial assignment of the employee. New employees and those who are younger tend to have a higher incidence of work-related illness and injuries [1]. Training should occur during work hours at no cost to the employee. Programs should be designed to match the education level, literacy, and language diversity of the trainees. (Many of the standards and resource documents noted here are available in languages other than English.) Trainers should be knowledgeable about the workplace and its hazards and qualified to cover the subject matter based on their own training, certification, or experience. They should be committed to the importance of training for employee safety and health and able to communicate well. Training media should be selected that are simple, clear, and engaging for the target audience. Demonstrations, hands-on training, coverage of incidents or near-miss situations, and interactive sessions often help to get points across better than pedantic presentations or handing out pamphlets.

Training programs should have clear goals and objectives. After training, an evaluation should verify that employees understood the content and acquired the desired skills or knowledge. If the objectives are not achieved, then revised training or refresher training may be needed. Refresher training may be required by regulation [1]. Some other reasons for refresher training include observation that work is being done in an unsafe manner, occurrence of accidents or near-miss incidents, changes in assignments, change in the work processes or conditions of the workplace, presence of high-level risk for serious illness or injury, or development of new information about existing and potential hazards.

Records should be kept documenting the training content, when it occurred, the name of the trainer(s), who was trained, and measures of training effectiveness. Some standards for recordkeeping are covered in OSHA's guidance cited earlier. In some situations, training data can be integrated with measures such as absences, work-related illness or injury, disability, or occurrence of incidents and near misses to demonstrate the effectiveness of training.

Training is a broad and integrated business responsibility, not limited to formal, scheduled group sessions. Daily supervision and employee contacts with health and safety personnel can model safe behavior, reinforce training elements, and emphasize their importance. For example, at medical clinic visits, asking employees about work incidents, safety concerns, and use of personal protective equipment (PPE) can raise awareness of workplace safety.

Control of Infectious Hazards

Training is only one element of safety and health programs. It is not a substitute for reasonable control of hazards. Hazards are best addressed using the traditional hierarchy of control (i.e., substitu-

tion, engineering controls, administrative controls, and personal protective equipment). Substitution is usually not an option when dealing with microorganisms in work environments. Engineering and administrative measures, which are related to control and containment along the source and path of contaminants, work best in many situations. Good engineering and work process planning can reduce reliance on employee behavior and PPE for safety and lessen the need for training. When engineering and administrative controls are either not possible or incompletely control risks, work practices, including the use of PPE, are used to supplement these higher levels of control.

Work Practices and Infection Control

The exposure control plan and standing operating procedures for working with infectious materials should establish safe work practices and help to determine the training content. They should be available to supervisors and employees and used during the course of work. They should be updated at least annually.

People in the workplace are a source of infections. Some basic personal hygiene precautions can help to reduce the spread of pathogens and can be covered in training programs. These include minimizing hand contact to the eyes, nose, and mouth; covering sneezes and coughs effectively; and washing hands with soap and water (or alcohol-based wipes if no water is available) before eating; before, during, and after food preparation; before dressing a wound, taking or giving medication, or handling contact lenses; after covering sneezes and coughs or contact with other body fluids; after changing diapers or using a toilet; after working in other situations where hand contamination may occur; and when hands appear dirty. Hand washing should involve thorough coverage of the back of the hands, fingertips, and interdigital areas, as well as palmar surfaces, and be of adequate duration (at least 20 seconds, approximating the time it takes to completely sing "Happy birthday to you" twice; CDC "An Ounce of Prevention" campaign, 2007). Hand-washing trainers sometimes use an organic colorant that fluoresces under black light (e.g., GloGerm or others) as a surrogate marker for pathogens to assess the effectiveness of hand-washing technique

[16,17]. Training also should cover procedures for changing out of soiled or contaminated clothing and avoiding taking home work clothing that is significantly contaminated with pathogens. In some situations, ill workers may need to be assigned alternate duties, e.g., when work involves food handling or care of immunocompromised patients.

OSHA's Bloodborne Pathogens Standard and earlier citations related to first responders and first receivers contain detailed information on work practices and infection control. Exposure control plans, training, and recordkeeping are covered in the standard. Biosafety levels are used to stratify risk of pathogens and indicate control methods required. The standard addresses universal precautions (UPs), an approach to infection control consisting of treating blood and certain body fluids as if known to contain human immunodeficiency virus (HIV), hepatitis B, and other bloodborne pathogens (BBPs). The concept of UPs has evolved to combine the BBP practices with body substance isolation considerations and are now termed *standard precautions* (SPs) [18]. When SPs alone are not expected to completely interrupt routes of transmission, *transmission-based precautions* (TBPs—contact, droplet, and airborne) are used in addition to SPs. Use of PPE (e.g., gloves, masks, respirators, face shields, glasses or goggles for eye protection, boots, shoe coverings, coats, and gowns) is also covered. Requiring PPE creates a need for training related to their fit, proper use, effectiveness (e.g., protection factors), limitations (e.g., restricted vision and mobility), maintenance, and risks (e.g., latex allergy or heat injury). Proper cleaning of some equipment and decontamination procedures may result in use of materials that require training about their risks and safe use. Training also should include proper use of biosafety level equipment, how to tell if it is working properly, and what to do if defects or dysfunction are identified. Information on biosafety levels is covered in Chapter 3.

The need for training extends to administrative measures related to pathogens. It is important to ensure that employees know the meaning of posted warning signs and postings for no entry. Employees should be trained to know what to do if an alarm or emergency signal sounds and how to follow procedures for evacuation, quarantine, isolation, lockdowns, sheltering in place, and reentry.

Other Training Issues Related to Health Care

Work groups vary greatly in their sophistication regarding the use of medical services. It is often helpful to train employees on how and when to access medical care, why a delay in seeking care for some pathogen exposures can be detrimental, what to tell a treating health care provider about their work exposures and risks (e.g., importance of mentioning specific pathogens), and why it is important to take medication in the amount and duration prescribed. Training about some pathogens should include information on postexposure prophylactic regimens and availability, effectiveness, and risks of vaccines. Health care workers may need training and education regarding proper handling, storage, and refrigeration of vaccines to help ensure that viable supplies are maintained.

Training for International Travelers

Employees assigned to either travel or live overseas need training on infectious diseases, sanitation, food and water precautions, health care access, and procedures for emergencies and evacuations. If employees are to be accompanied overseas by their families, it is important to involve nonemployee adult family members in the training, especially if they will be caring for young children abroad. In addition to covering vaccinations and endemic and epidemic conditions related to the country of work, it is helpful to cover risks from food and drink, safe food selection and handling, how to make drinking water safe, and dealing with traveler's diarrhea; insect, arthropod, and animal vectors; sexually transmitted diseases; swimming precautions; and other issues specific to the location of work assignments. The CDC's "Yellow Book" is available online [19] and has sections that can be used to tailor training for employees and their families on these topics. Online updates for emerging infectious diseases in the United States and abroad are available from the CDC and from the WHO's Epidemic and Pandemic Alert and Response (ERP) website [20].

Conclusion

Infectious diseases are a growing global concern. Employee education and training about infectious diseases have become an integral and critical part of safety and health programs. Training can contribute to efficient work and reduction of risk and can be lifesaving. In a world of serious, unfamiliar, and mysterious-appearing pathogens, sound education and training can preempt some of the terrors of these hazards. Training can help organizations to meet their obligations to employees so that people are more confident in their daily lives and work and can respond safely and effectively to the challenges of workplace infections.

References

1. U.S. Department of Labor, Occupational Safety and Health Administration. Training Requirements in OSHA Standards and Training Guidelines. OSHA 2254. Washington: OSHA, 1998 (revised).
2. U.S. Department of Health and Human Services, Centers for Disease Control and Prevention. Emergency Preparedness and Response homepage. Available at www.bt.cdc.gov/.
3. World Health Organization (WHO). Cumulative Number of Confirmed Human Cases of Avian Influenza A (H5N1) Reported to WHO, Epidemic and Pandemic Alert and Response (EPR), November 2005. Available at www.who.int/csr/disease/avian_influenza/country/cases.
4. Occupational Safety and Health Act of 1970, 29 CFR 1910.
5. U.S. Department of Labor, Occupational Safety and Health Administration. Draft Model Training Program for Hazard Communication, October 17, 2003. Available at www.osha.gov/dsg/hazcom/mtp/101703.html.
6. World Health Organization. WHO Modules in Occupational Safety and Health, Hygiene and Safety, December 2005. Available at uic.edu/sph/glakes/who_modules/.
7. Zemke R and Kramlinger T. *Figuring Things Out: A Trainer's Guide to Needs and Task Analysis.* Reading, MA: Addison-Wesley, 1982.
8. Jacobs RL. *Structured On-the-Job Training: Unleashing Employee Expertise in the Workplace.* San Francisco: Berrett-Koehler, 2003.
9. Nadler L, Nadler Z. *Designing Training Programs: The Critical Events Model,* 2nd ed. Houston, TX: Gulf Publishing, 1994.
10. Respiratory protection: Final rules for Standards 1910 and 1926. *Fed Reg* 1998;63:1152–300.
11. U.S. Department of Health and Human Services. OSHA Best Practices for Hospital-Based First Receivers of Victims from Mass Casualty Incidents Involving the Release of Hazardous Substances. Washington: OSHA, 2005.
12. U.S. Department of Labor, Office of Training and Education, Occupational Safety and Health Administration. Outreach Training Materials for OSHA's Respirator Standard, 2007. Available at www.osha.gov/dcsp/ote/trng-materials/respiratorsrespirators.html.
13. U.S. Department of Labor, Office of Training and Education, Occupational Safety and Health Administration. OSHA Disaster Site Worker Outreach Training Program. Course no. 7600, 2008. Available at www.osha.gov/fso/ote/training/disaster/disaster.html.
14. U.S. Department of Labor, Office of Training and Education, Occupational Safety and Health Administration. Keeping Workers Safe During Clean Up and Recovery Operations Following Hurricanes, November 10, 2005. Available at www.osha.gov/OshDoc/hurricanesrecovery.html.
15. U.S. Department of Health and Human Services, Centers for Disease Control and Prevention. Emergency Preparedness and Response homepage. Available at www.bt.cdc.gov/ and www.bt.cdc.gov/training/.
16. Outbreaks of multiple drug-resistant *Shigella sonnei* gastoenteritis associated with day care centers183 Kansas, Kentucky, and Missouri, 2005. *MMWR* 2006;55:1068.
17. Olson SR, Gray GC. The Trojan Chicken Study, Minnesota. Centers for Disease Control and Prevention. *Emerg Infect Dis* 2006;12:795–9. Hospital Infection Control Practices Advisory Committee (HICPAC), Centers for Disease Control and Prevention. *Guidelines for Isolation Precautions in Hospitals.* Atlanta: CDC, 2007.
19. U.S. Department of Health and Human Services, Centers for Disease Control and Prevention. Health Information for International Travel, 2008. Available at www.cdc.gov/travel/.
20. World Health Organization, www.who.int/csr/outbreaknetwork.

Diseases

9

Occupational Tuberculosis

John D. Meyer and Douglas D'Andrea

Tuberculosis (TB), the "White Plague" of the nineteenth and early twentieth centuries, progressively declined with the introduction of public health measures at the turn of the century and then with the widespread use of antituberculous therapy in the 1940s and 1950s. This decline continued until the 1980s, when an upsurge in the incidence of TB in the United States coincided with the onset of the acquired immune deficiency syndrome (AIDS) epidemic. Relaxation of traditional public health measures aimed at the diagnosis and treatment of tuberculosis and alterations in social demographics—particularly increased immigration from endemic areas and a burgeoning homeless shelter and prison population—also contributed to the reversal of progress in TB control during this period. Coincident with the rise in tuberculosis incidence in the 1980s, the emergence of multidrug-resistant TB increased the risk of serious illness and death in those developing active tuberculosis. The number of new cases of tuberculosis continued to rise until the mid-1990s, when renewed commitment of resources to public health with improvements in recognition and treatment of TB in high-risk individuals combined to decrease the incidence of active and latent tuberculosis.

These trends increased the risk of tuberculosis among segments of the working population, particularly health care workers. The Occupational Safety and Health Administration (OSHA) estimated that over 5 million workers were exposed to TB in the course of their work [1], and while the incidence of tuberculosis continues to decline, health care workers remain at significant risk of exposure and possible infection. Health care has been the second fastest growing sector of the U.S. economy, employing over 12 million workers. The increase in workers with direct contact with infected individuals requires continued efforts to maintain effective measures to prevent tuberculosis, even as its overall incidence again declines in the United States. This chapter reviews the microbiology, pathogenesis, diagnosis, and epidemiology of tuberculosis, focusing on occupational exposure and surveillance measures to prevent tuberculosis infection among workers employed in health care and other high-risk jobs.

Pathogenesis and Transmission

Tuberculosis is caused by *Mycobacterium tuberculosis*, a member of a large and diverse genus of aerobic and nonmotile bacilli that differ in microbiology, biochemistry, and virulence. *M. tuberculosis* has a length of 1–4 μm and a thickness of 0.3–0.6 μm. Several characteristic biologic properties are clinically important. It is an obligate aerobe and grows best under conditions of high oxygen tension; as a result, infection typically involves the lungs in both animals and humans. Its cell wall has a high lipid content that resists both usual microbiologic stains and decolorization with alcohol. It also has a slow growth rate, with generation times between 12 and 18 hours, so laboratory isolation by culture typically may take weeks.

Almost all cases of tuberculosis are spread by person-to-person transmission through the respiratory route. Patients with active pulmonary or laryngeal tuberculosis shed infectious organisms into the ambient air through coughing, sneezing, or speaking. Larger droplets settle quickly onto nearby surfaces and generally are noninfectious despite containing large numbers of bacilli. In contrast, smaller droplets (1–5 μm in diameter), also called *droplet nuclei,* desiccate and remain suspended in the air for several hours, traveling substantial distances indoors. These particles, although containing only one to three active TB bacilli, are small enough to bypass upper respiratory defenses and impaction at the level of the bronchioles. They may be inhaled deep into the lungs, and once settling in the alveoli, tubercle bacilli may slowly multiply and initiate infection.

In response to infection, lymphocytes are stimulated and release cytokines that activate macrophages. Most of the bacteria are engulfed and killed, but some may survive and invade lymphatics and the bloodstream, draining to regional lymph nodes, and through hematogenous spread may infect virtually any organ. High blood flow and high local oxygen tension favor the development of infection when disseminated. Predictably, the most frequently infected parts of the body include the apices of the lungs, the renal cortex, the vertebrae, and the metaphyses of long bones. During the first 3 weeks, bacilli can multiply logarithmically; however, by the third week in the previously uninfected host, cell-mediated immune mechanisms have been initiated, and bacterial destruction by activated macrophages is increased. Granulomata form around and isolate foci of infection, encasing initial tuberculous lesions. These granulomatous tubercles characteristically have a necrotic or caseating center, a pathologic hallmark of TB.

M. tuberculosis does not produce enzymes or toxins, and in the immunocompetent host there is little tissue destruction or inflammation initially. Most patients remain asymptomatic after primary infection. In contrast, immunosuppressed individuals are particularly vulnerable to tubercle bacilli

and may develop symptomatic primary infection. Primary symptomatic tuberculosis historically was a pediatric disease, but with an increasing number of immunosuppressed adults, this is now observed more commonly among adults. It presents most commonly as an atypical pneumonia, but other common presentations include pleuritis with pleural effusions, pulmonary cavitations, and extrapulmonary tuberculosis. Primary extrapulmonary tuberculosis presented classically in children as cervical adenitis, miliary tuberculosis, or tuberculous meningitis. However, as with primary symptomatic infection, in general, primary extrapulmonary tuberculosis is now seen most commonly among persons infected with human immunodeficiency virus (HIV).

Although granuloma formation will contain the initial TB infection, viable bacteria can persist within granulomata. These can cause reactivation of infection when immunity wanes. Reactivation of latent tuberculous infection (LTBI), although more common soon after primary infection, may occur in an untreated person at any point in time, even decades after primary infection. Postprimary, or reactivation, pulmonary tuberculosis is the most common clinical form of tuberculosis. Reactivation typically occurs in the apical and posterior upper lobes of the lung, a reflection of the organism's affinity for regions of high oxygen tension. Reactivated TB may be manifested by pulmonary infiltrates, cavitations, empyema, fibrosis, and extrapulmonary tuberculosis with spread to other organs.

Although TB reactivation may occur at any time, the risk is greatest in the first years after primary infection. Approximately 5–15% of immunocompetent individuals develop active TB within 2 years of the initial infection. The incidence of reactivation of latent disease then declines to a low level for the remainder of an exposed individual's lifetime unless the immune mechanisms holding the infection in check are disrupted, often a consequence of aging or the development of chronic disease. The cumulative lifetime risk of tuberculosis reactivation has been estimated at 10%. This reflects both the high initial incidence of the infection and ongoing sporadic cases of reactivation among individuals with remotely acquired infection [2].

Reactivation of TB depends on many factors related to an individual's immune response to infection, which determines whether the infecting bacilli will be contained or will multiply and disseminate. Patient factors that appear to impair immunity and increase the risk of reactivation include older age, poor nutritional status, and concomitant illnesses such as HIV infection, AIDS, diabetes mellitus, renal insufficiency, hematologic malignancies, and silicosis. Chemotherapeutic agents and corticosteroids also impair the immune system and also may lead to reactivation of TB. The greatest incidence of reactivation occurs in individuals with HIV infection, up to 10% per year. Although overall prevalence of infection with *M. tuberculosis* is not increased in people with HIV infection, they do develop primary active TB at a higher rate and in a shorter period of time (as soon as 1 month after exposure) than do persons without HIV infection. Additionally, the clinical presentation of active tuberculosis in persons with HIV infection may differ, particularly once severe immunosuppression occurs, producing infections that are more widespread and severe.

Epidemiology of Occupational Tuberculosis

Since the 1950s, extraordinary progress has been made in the control and eradication of tuberculosis in the United States. Prior to the twentieth century, tuberculosis was the leading cause of death. With the advent of screening and public health programs beginning in the 1930s, followed by effective TB therapy in the 1940s and 1950s, the incidence of tuberculosis continued to decline every year from 1953 through 1985. The annual number of TB cases decreased by 74%, from 84,304 to 22,201 cases, and the case rate decreased by 82% from 53 to 9.3 cases per 100,000 population. In the early 1970s, many considered it no longer a public health problem, federal funding began to decrease, and TB public health services began to close. By the late 1980s, TB began to emerge again, and in 1986, a 2.6% increase in the number of TB cases marked the beginning of a resurgence of TB.

Several factors contributed to the resurgence: inadequate funding and dismantling of public health services providing screening and treatment of TB, the HIV and AIDS epidemic, the emergence of multidrug-resistant TB (MDRTB), and an increase in TB among the homeless, prison inmates, and other institutionalized persons. HIV infection is one of the greatest risk factors for active TB infection, and significant numbers of HIV-related TB outbreaks were reported among patients and health care workers and in correctional facilities and homeless shelters. There also was a proportionate increase among foreign-born persons. Excess cases of active TB infection (those that would not have been seen if previous trends had continued) in the period 1985–1992 were estimated at 52,100 [3].

The resurgence peaked in 1992 at 26,673 cases, or 10.5 cases per 100,000 persons. In response, renewed public health efforts, particularly targeted to well-defined risk groups and geographic locations, marked the beginning of a decrease in TB rates. Since 1993, rates of TB have once again declined, reaching an all-time low in 2004, with 2.6 cases per 100,000 persons. This represents a 61.9% decline in the incidence of tuberculosis since 1992 [4]. This trend has been attributed to the introduction of effective antiviral therapy for HIV infection, which has reduced the number of AIDS patients and their complications, including tuberculosis, combined with renewed public health efforts to identify and treat persons with both active and latent tuberculosis. During the same period, the incidence of MDRTB has declined by 76.5%. In 2003, about 1% of the 11,040 cases of TB were caused by MDRTB strains, a reduction owing primarily to public health efforts to ensure patients complete treatment for active or latent tuberculosis [4].

Despite the overall downward trend in rates of TB, not all groups have been affected equally. Rates among foreign-born residents of the United States, African-Americans, and Hispanics, although decreased, remain elevated in comparison with U.S.-born and white residents. Rates among foreign-born residents, although declining about 33% from the levels of the early 1990s, remain nearly 10 times higher than those of U.S.-born whites, at 22.5 cases per 100,000 persons. Worldwide, tuberculosis remains the second leading cause of infectious death after malaria, and it is estimated that 2 billion people, or one-third of the world's population, are infected. There are nearly 8 million new cases a year, with 3 million deaths, a figure that may be expected to increase because of the ongoing HIV epidemic in developing countries.

The recognition of TB as an occupational hazard, particularly among health care workers, lagged behind improvements in general public health measures aimed at its control. Standard texts from the 1920s and 1930s maintained that there was no danger from workers' breathing the expired air of consumptive patients or being coughed on by TB patients [5]. Pioneering studies by Heimbeck in Oslo in the 1920s demonstrated 95% tuberculin test conversion in nursing students by the time of graduation; furthermore, 22% of these initially negative nurses developed clinical tuberculosis compared with 1.5% of 200 initially tuberculin-positive nurses [5]. Despite similar compelling data from other studies, the recognition and control of TB as an occupational hazard were delayed decades after effective methods of diagnosis and therapy were available. With the advent of antituberculous therapy in the 1940s and 1950s, occupationally acquired TB became less frequent but, paradoxically, more conspicuous in light of the general trend toward reduced incidence of the disease.

One of the first comprehensive epidemiologic studies of the risk of tuberculosis among workers was a 1973–1974 survey of employees of the New York City Board of Education. This study found an overall 12% tuberculin reactivity in 61,000 employees; differences in prevalence within this cohort were related to ethnic group, socioeconomic status, age, and gender [6]. A second study by Berman and colleagues analyzed results of a 5-year (1971–1976) tuberculin-screening program in a Baltimore hospital [7]. The authors calculated an annual risk for TB infection of 1.4% among employees of the hospital, although the authors attributed the higher-than-expected conversion rate to a booster effect and to exposure in the community. Other studies among health care workers during this period found conversion rates of 0.11–4.5% depending on such factors as location and patient population. Despite evidence that tuberculin reactivity was prevalent in as much as one-fourth of some segments of the population, screening and treatment programs during the 1970s became underfunded, and previously successful public health measures atrophied, allowing for a substantial increase in incidence and prevalence of tuberculosis in the next decade.

An increase in TB, as a concomitant opportunistic infection in patients with HIV infection, paralleled the worldwide AIDS epidemic in the 1980s. Except for the period from 1979–1981, when an influx of refugees had slightly increased the incidence of tuberculosis, rates of tuberculosis in the United States had declined by about 6% a year since 1953. As noted earlier, between 1985 and 1992, the combination of the HIV and AIDS epidemic, homelessness, and an underfunded public health system led to an almost 20% increase in the rates of tuberculosis. As expected, risks to health care workers of TB infection became disproportionately skewed toward institutions that provided care to the homeless, indigent, and inner-city populations. Additionally, with the rise in cases of MDRTB, the perception of increased risk of severe illness and even death from TB became more widespread. Evidence for the increased risk to health care workers was drawn both from prevalence data on skin test conversions and from incidence data on new skin test conversions in outbreaks of TB in facilities. Postexposure rates of employee purified protein derivative (PPD) conversions have been noted to range from 4–77%, with most reported incidence rates from 15–30% [8]. Eight cases of active MDRTB developed in health care workers in New York and Miami hospitals in the period 1990–1991. Epidemiologic evidence linked these cases to nosocomial transmission from infected patients [9].

Routine exposure to patients in some hospitals has resulted in conversion rates of 5–10% per year [10]. In an attempt to quantify risk for a proposed standard, OSHA had calculated estimates of relative risk for TB skin test conversion ranging from 1.47–9.0, based on results from a 1994 Washington State hospital survey, a statewide survey in North Carolina, and data from 1989–1991 at Jackson Memorial Hospital in Miami [1]. Higher risks of PPD conversion (14.5% over 4 years) were found in employees who worked on wards where patients with culture-confirmed TB were cared for compared with 1.4% in those who did not work around these patients [11]. Furthermore, risk was not limited to those with direct patient contact; it also was increased in other workers, such as clerks, on the same wards. Health care tasks that increase the likelihood of contact with airborne bacilli also carry a particularly high risk. Pulmonary fellows converted at an 11% rate during their 2-year training period; this incidence compares with a 2.4% conversion rate in infectious disease fellows who would have cared for a similar patient population, indicating that respiratory aerosol generation by patients, particularly during instrumentation or procedures such as bronchoscopy, was an important determinant of infectivity [12].

Data on occupational risk outside hospital-based health care are sparse. Increased numbers of individuals with TB are isolated or cared for in settings such as prisons, homeless shelters, medical laboratories, hospices, and home health care services. Populations in correctional facilities, where high-risk individuals are overrepresented, have TB case rates that are estimated to be 3–11 times higher than in the general population. A 2-year employee screening program in New York State prisons found a PPD conversion rate of 1.9%. Relative risks for conversion were 1.64 in guards and 2.39 in medical employees in facilities with known TB cases [13]. Occupational exposure was estimated to account for 33% of new tuberculosis infections in this study. A recent multisite study of correctional health care workers found high prevalence rates of TB skin test reactivity (17.7%) and estimated an annual incidence rate of skin test conversion of 1.3%. Risks of a positive test were strongest, however, for those originating from outside the United States and those having a history of bacille Calmette-Guérin (BCG) administration, suggesting that demographic factors for skin test reactivity were more important than occupational risks [14].

Facilities for chronic and long-term care present another setting where workers may be exposed to infection. Facilities for the elderly continue to house a cohort of individuals for whom chemoprophylaxis of tuberculous infection had not yet been instituted and who thus present a risk for reactivation. Positive PPD rates among residents range from 10–40%. In addition, by virtue of age and illness, the uninfected may be particularly susceptible to primary infection from fellow residents. Large-scale screening studies of workers in these facilities do not exist; a smaller study from Canada [15] found a 15.7% rate of positive tuberculin testing in 286 staff members from a hospital and two chronic care facilities, paralleling a 14% rate among residents. A high rate of positive reactions (39.5%) was found among staff in elderly and mental health care services in a New Zealand hospital, implying that exposure may be much higher than had been suspected [16].

A fivefold risk for active TB in laboratory workers was noted in a large 1971 survey study in the United Kingdom [17]. Technicians in "morbid anatomy" departments (those working with tissue) were at the greatest risk for development of disease. Little current data exists on PPD conversion rates or transmission of TB in laboratories. Tuberculosis of the skin from primary inoculation, termed *prosector's wart,* is a well-known phenomenon in pathologists and related technical personnel [18]. Cutaneous inoculation of TB in laboratory personnel as a result of injuries by sharp instruments has been described [19].

The relationship of silicosis to the development of active tuberculosis infection has been well known for the last century and is the subject of an extensive literature. Active tuberculosis has been found to develop in as many as 25% of workers with silicosis; these workers have at least a threefold higher risk of death from TB infection. Work in silica-exposed occupations, such as quarrying, pottery, stone carving, and ship building and repair, is associated with a higher incidence of tuberculosis [20]. Because of the high rate of disease in these individuals, some authorities have suggested prolonged, even lifelong chemoprophylaxis for workers with silicosis who exhibit PPD conversion [21].

Diagnosis of Tuberculosis

Early diagnosis of both active TB and latent TB is key to the effective control and eradication of TB. A high index of suspicion is important to early identification and diagnosis of cases of TB, and no ideal single test is available for the diagnosis of either active or latent TB infection. Instead, diagnosis depends on the combination of clinical symptoms, chest radiography, microscopic examination and staining of appropriate specimens, microbiologic culture, and more recently, nucleic acid amplification assays.

Diagnosis of latent tuberculosis infection (LTBI) is based on the tuberculin PPD skin test, and until recently, the tuberculin skin test (TST) was the only reliable method of diagnosis of LTBI. The delayed-type hypersensitivity (DTH) reaction forms the basis for this common method of diagnosing TB infection. PPD of tuberculin, an extract of the bacterial cell wall prepared from the supernatant of cell cultures, stimulates a cell-mediated immune response when injected intradermally in subjects who have had tuberculous infection. The TST was designed originally for diagnosis of active infection, but its lack of sensitivity and specificity, and particularly its inability to distinguish between latent and active infection, make it unsuitable for the diagnosis of active TB. Both immunocompetent individuals with active TB infection and healthy subjects with LTBI but no evidence of active disease will react to this test. The inflammatory response produces an area of induration, the extent of which is used to assess the likelihood of infection and the need for preventive therapy. In individuals with primary TB infection, the PPD reaction becomes positive 4–12 weeks following exposure and initiation of infection. This time delay should be borne in mind when investigating TB outbreaks or exposure to active cases of TB.

Various TSTs have been available. The Mantoux test, using a single intradermal injection of an intermediate strength of PPD, is the most reliable method and has replaced multipuncture tests, such as the tine test. The preferred method for the test consists of intracutaneous injection of 0.1 mL of 5 tuberculin units (5 TU) of a standardized PPD preparation sufficient to result in a small wheal on the forearm or other injection site. The test is read 48 and 72 hours following injection and should be interpreted by personnel with adequate training and experience. A positive result is based on the extent of induration at the injection site; redness or erythema may be present in many individuals and may extend well beyond the injection site but should not be measured or considered positive.

Both false-negative and false-positive reactions can occur with the TST. Some persons with *M. tuberculosis* infection may not react to the TST. Persons with a weakened immune response from immunosuppressive drug therapy or HIV infection, children younger than 6 months of age, and persons acquiring a TB infection recently may not react to the skin test. The skin test also may be negative in cases of overwhelming infection, and negative skin testing should not be used to rule out active tuberculous infection. Expired PPD or an incorrectly administered skin test also can lead to false-negative results. The PPD must be administered intradermally; deeper subcutaneous injection can lead to a false-negative reaction. If the first test is administered incorrectly, another dose can be given immediately at another site. Table 9-1 summarizes how to administer and read the TST.

Table 9-1

Administering the Intradermal Mantoux Tuberculin Skin Test

1. The tuberculin skin test (TST) is performed by injecting 0.1 mL of tuberculin purified protein derivative (PPD) into the inner surface of the forearm. Select a smooth area on the forearm, and prepare it with alcohol.
2. The injection should be made intradermally with a tuberculin syringe, with the needle bevel facing upward. When placed correctly, the injection should produce a pale elevation of the skin, a wheal, 6–10 mm in diameter. Subcutaneous injection can result in a false-negative test. Another test dose can be given immediately at another site if the first test was administered improperly.
3. The skin test reaction should be read between 48 and 72 hours after administration. A patient who does not return within 72 hours will need to be rescheduled for another skin test.
4. Use a ballpoint pen or finger to measure the area of induration. Using a ballpoint pen, draw a line towards the area of induration. An increase in the resistence to movement of the pen will be noticed when the border of induration is reached. Repeat this step from the other side, and the overall width of the induration then can be measured with a ruler. (The diameter of the indurated area should be measured across the forearm, perpendicular to its long axis). When a pen is not available, the borders of induration can be identified with a finger.
5. The reaction should be measured and recorded in millimeters of induration. Do not measure erythema or redness. *The absence of induration should be recorded as "0 mm" induration and not "negative."*

False-positive results are also possible with the TST. Persons infected with nontuberculosis mycobacteria and those previously vaccinated with BCG can have false-positive reactions. Incorrect interpretation of the test also will lead to false-positive results. Only the area of induration in response to PPD should be measured and recorded. Erythema or redness at the site of injection occurs often but should not be included in the measurement; otherwise, the reaction may be incorrectly interpreted as positive.

The Centers for Disease Control and Prevention (CDC) have established guidelines for the interpretation of the test based on the likelihood of the degree of induration predicting the presence of infection and the risk of developing active TB. Since the predictive value of a positive test depends on the prevalence of a condition in the population, a higher positive threshold is set for use of the test in populations expected to have a low risk of exposure or development of infection and a lower positive threshold for populations at increased risk. For example, 5 mm of induration represents a positive reaction and is predictive of TB in persons with HIV infection or persons in close contact with patients known to have TB, whereas 15 mm of induration represents a positive reaction in persons with no identifiable risk factors. The CDC classification [22], shown in Table 9-2, outlines the criteria for a positive test in various population groups.

Screening for LTBI previously had been done by widespread tuberculin skin testing with limited consideration of the risk for TB in the population tested. The CDC now recommends TB testing be reserved for persons at high risk, and with the exception of initial testing of persons at low risk whose future work or other activities will place them at increased risk, screening of low-risk persons is no longer recommended. This strategy of targeted tuberculin testing, which should replace less discriminate screening, is a key strategic component of TB control. Targeted tuberculin testing identifies persons at high risk for developing active TB who would benefit from treatment of LTBI. Persons at increased risk include those who have had a recent infection and those with associated conditions that increase the risk of progression of LTBI to active TB. Infected persons at high risk should be offered treatment irrespective of age.

The tuberculin skin test in health care workers should be interpreted according to these same CDC guidelines. Two additional points, however, should be kept in mind in this interpretation. The first is that individual risk factors outside the work environment must be considered in the interpretation. For example, a worker who is receiving therapy that may be severely immunosuppressive or who has HIV infection will be considered to be in a higher-risk group for reactivation, and therefore, a skin test showing 5 mm of induration may represent a positive test. The second point is that in health care settings where TB is treated, close contact with infectious patients places workers at increased risk. In these workers, a skin test showing 10 mm of induration is probably sufficient to indicate a positive result, even in the absence of other risk factors. By contrast, if a facility presents a low or minimal risk for TB exposure, a cutoff point of 15 mm may be used to judge a result positive if the individual has no other risk factors. In general, in facilities that treat TB patients, an increase in skin test induration of 10 mm or more in a 2-year period indicates a skin test conversion; for facilities in which the risk of exposure is minimal, a cutoff point of 15 mm or more may be used. If a known exposure has occurred in a health care setting, an increase of 5 mm or more from a 0-mm baseline in a health care

Table 9-2
Criteria for Positive Tuberculin Reactivity

Size of Induration	Risk Group
Reaction ≥ 5 mm of induration	HIV-positive persons
	Recent contacts of TB case patients
	Fibrotic changes on chest radiograph consistent with prior TB
	Patients with organ transplants and other immunosuppressed patients (receiving the equivalent of ≥15 mg/d of prednisone for 1 month or more)
Reaction ≥10 mm of induration	Recent immigrants (i.e., within the last 5 years) from high-prevalence countries
	Injection drug users
	Residents and employees[a] of the following high-risk congregate settings: prisons and jails, nursing homes and other long-term facilities for the elderly, hospitals and other health care facilities, residential facilities for patients with AIDS, and homeless shelters
	Mycobacteriology laboratory personnel
	Persons with the following clinical conditions that place them at high risk: silicosis, diabetes mellitus, chronic renal failure, some hematologic disorders (e.g., leukemias and lymphomas), other specific malignancies (e.g., carcinoma of the head or neck and lung), weight loss of 10% or more of ideal body weight, gastrectomy, and jejunoileal bypass
	Children younger than 4 years of age or infants, children, and adolescents exposed to adults at high-risk
Reaction ≥ 15 mm of induration	Persons with no risk factors for TB

[a]For persons who are otherwise at low risk and are tested at the start of employment, a reaction of 15 mm or more of induration is considered positive.
Source: Adapted from Centers for Disease Control and Prevention. Targeted tuberculin testing and treatment of latent tuberculosis infection. *MMWR* 2000;49:24.

worker with close contact with the infected patient should be considered a positive result; however, if the employee's original baseline was more than 0 mm, a 10-mm increase remains the recommended cutoff for considering a test conversion [23].

Boosted reactions on TST can occur among hospital workers and other groups and may be mistaken for conversion. Reaction to tuberculin skin testing may wane gradually, and if many years have passed since initial TB infection or repeated antigenic challenge by skin testing, an individual beginning a screening program may have an initially negative skin test. However, after repeated testing, the reduction in cell-mediated hypersensitivity may be reversed, and the TST may become positive again, a phenomenon termed *boosting*. If not recognized in testing an individual, boosting can be misinterpreted as new PPD conversion, and the individual may be mistakenly diagnosed as a new case of TB. A two-step testing protocol has been recommended to avoid misinterpretation of the boosting phenomenon in subjects, including health care workers, who may need repeated testing [22]. An initially negative PPD test is followed by placement of a second 5-TU skin test 1–3 weeks later. If this second test is judged to be positive, any induration can be attributed to the booster phenomenon and considered to represent previous primary TB infection rather than a new conversion. If the second test remains negative, a subsequent test with a positive result indicates a newly converted case. In elderly populations, the booster phenomenon may not be present until three or more tests have been performed. All patients with positive TSTs, if not treated previously, should receive preventive therapy once active TB is excluded.

BCG vaccination also may complicate the diagnosis of TB infection because the PPD reaction that results cannot be distinguished from that produced by mycobacterial infection. BCG is used in many parts of the world to immunize individuals, primarily as a control measure in regions where TB incidence is high. The protection afforded by BCG vaccination is variable and may depend on host, environmental, and bacterial virulence factors. Reactivity to a TST develops soon after vaccination. Postvaccination skin test results may range from 3–19 mm of induration. The size of skin test reaction does not correlate with the degree of protec-

tion against TB that may be afforded by BCG [24]. Tuberculin reactivity owing to BCG vaccine wanes over time, however, and after 10 years may be minimal or absent. Previously, TSTs were interpreted differently in persons vaccinated with BCG. However, the CDC now recommends persons at high risk be tested irrespective of prior BCG administration and the results interpreted as if BCG vaccination had not occurred. For example, an adult health care worker who was immunized with BCG as a child in a country with a high TB prevalence would be considered to have a positive tuberculin skin test with a PPD reaction of 10 mm or greater. BCG vaccination should neither preclude participation in PPD screening nor lead the interpreter to conclude reflexively that BCG administration is the sole cause of an indurated skin test.

Subjects who, because of immunosuppressive illness, may be anergic previously were tested with other companion antigens at the time of PPD testing. Mumps, *Candida*, and tetanus toxoid antigens were administered in addition to PPD as an anergy panel; the absence of a response to these common antigens indicated a state of anergy, or inability to mount a delayed-type hypersensitivity reaction. The results of anergy panels were used to help interpret the results of PPD testing in individuals with impaired cell-mediated immunity, most notably HIV infection. A negative PPD test in the setting of a positive response to an anergy panel was considered a true negative and evidence of no infection. However, a negative PPD test in the setting of a negative response to an anergy panel was considered a false-negative result and did not exclude the possibility of TBI infection. However, because of such factors as selective loss of PPD reactivity and the booster phenomenon, anergy testing is unreliable and no longer routinely recommended in evaluating for tuberculous infection among patients with impaired cell-mediated immunity. Individuals with HIV infection should be assessed according to CDC guidelines, which describe reactions of 5 mm or greater as a positive result. Evaluation for preventive therapy in those who exhibit no response to skin testing should be made on the basis of additional clinical and epidemiologic information, such as evidence of exposure to another individual with active TB, and not the results of anergy testing.

Until 2001, the TST was the only test used to diagnose latent TB infection. Newer in vitro enzyme-linked immunosorbent assays (ELISAs) now have been approved for use in detection of LTBI by the U.S. Food and Drug Administration (FDA). This testing has been available since 2004 under the brand name QuantiFERON-TB Gold (QFT-G). The assay tests for interferon-gamma released from sensitized lymphocytes in whole blood incubated overnight with synthetic peptides simulating two proteins present in *M. tuberculosis:* early secretory antigenic target 6 (ESAT-6) and culture filtrate protein 10 (CFP-10). Compared with TST, QFT-G offers several advantages: It can be interpreted after a single patient visit, results are less subject to reader error, and the testing does not require that anamnestic immune responses be boosted for accurate interpretation. PPD contains hundreds of antigens, many shared by other mycobacteria common in the environment. The antigens used in QFT-G are more specific to *M. tuberculosis* and are absent from all BCG vaccine strains and many common nontuberculous mycobacteria, except *M. kansasii, M. szulgai,* and *M. marinum.* The CDC recommends use of QFT-G in all circumstances in which the TST is currently used, including contact investigations, evaluation of recent immigrants, and surveillance programs for infection control [25]. As with the tuberculin skin test, QFT-G testing should be targeted at diagnosing infected patients who will benefit from treatment. Before using QFT-G routinely, arrangements need to be made with a qualified laboratory to guarantee quality assurance and collection and transport of blood within 12 hours. Also QFT-G, like the TST, cannot differentiate between latent and active infection, a decision that must be made on other clinical grounds following a positive test.

For all individuals who exhibit a positive TST or QFT-G test, radiography is used to determine whether evidence of active or prior pulmonary tuberculosis infection is present. Additionally, any patient with symptoms suggestive of pulmonary TB infection should have radiography performed regardless of test results. A posteroanterior (PA) view is the standard radiographic procedure; additional views, such as apical lordotic views, may be needed. The classic, though infrequent, finding of healed initial TB infection is the *Ghon complex,* calcification of both a granuloma and its draining lymph node. Other diagnostic findings include multiple fibrotic or calcified pulmonary nodules; in many, if not most, subjects with LTBI, the chest radiograph is normal. A normal chest radiograph in an asymptomatic, healthy-appearing individual with a positive PPD test excludes the possibility of active pulmonary TB. Active pulmonary TB is characterized by patchy or nodular infiltrates in the apical or subapical upper lobes or the superior segments of the lower lobes, although radiographic abnormalities may occur throughout the lungs. In HIV-infected persons, particularly those with AIDS, pulmonary TB may present atypically, and infiltrates may be seen in any zone of the lungs, usually in conjunction with prominent hilar and mediastinal adenopathy. Cavitation, adenopathy, empyema, and pleural effusions also occur in active TB. Miliary spread of the disease appears as multiple nodular densities throughout the lung fields.

Microscopic examination and cultures of appropriate sputum specimens are still the cornerstones of diagnosis of active TB. To avoid mistakenly culturing saliva and nasal mucus, sputum specimens preferably should be obtained by individuals skilled in the appropriate techniques. Up to 30% of patients are unable to provide an expectorated sputum sample, but sputum production may be induced with saline aerosols. Failure to demonstrate acid-fast bacilli (AFB) on a smear does not exclude the diagnosis of TB; only 60% of patients with a positive culture have a positive AFB smear. Culture for mycobacteria is the diagnostic standard, with up to 93% sensitivity and 98% specificity. Culture with liquid media can provide results in as few as 2 weeks, in comparison with the 6–8 weeks required with solid media. A positive culture for *M. tuberculosis* makes the definitive diagnosis of TB. Since cultures may take up to 8 weeks to yield a positive identification, therapy may be instituted for a provisional diagnosis of active TB on the basis of clinical signs, symptoms, radiographic findings, and AFB smear results. Drug susceptibility testing is essential for all positive initial cultures, and the results should be used to guide modifications of antibacterial therapy. To assess effectiveness of, and response to, therapy, as well as to ascertain potential infectiousness of the patient, follow-up sputum examination and culture should be obtained at least monthly until cultures become negative.

Preventive Therapy

Isoniazid (INH) is the most widely used treatment for LTBI. It is bactericidal, relatively nontoxic, easily administered, and inexpensive. Treatment with INH has been demonstrated to reduce the risk of progression to active TB by as much as 90% in adults if a full course is completed. The recommended dose of INH for adults is 300 mg once daily. A minimum of 6 months of treatment with INH is essential. Nine months is often recommended, and there is a small but definite benefit to 12 months of therapy. The 2003 American Thoracic Society (ATS)/CDC/Infectious Diseases Society of America (IDSA) guidelines recommend a 9-month regimen of INH as the optimal regimen for almost all patients irrespective of HIV status or age [22,26]. Individuals with silicosis should receive a full 12-month course; more prolonged, even lifelong therapy in silicosis has been recommended by some [27].

INH should be dispensed only in monthly allotments to allow screening for symptoms of hepatotoxicity. From 10–20% of individuals taking INH develop asymptomatic transaminase elevations; many of these elevations resolve even if the drug is continued. Baseline laboratory is not routinely recommended at the start of treatment but is recommended in patients with a history of HIV infection or liver disease, in women who are pregnant or in the first 3 months of the postpartum period, and in patients whose history or physical examination suggests undiagnosed liver disease. Elevations of three to five times the upper limits of normal or symptomatic adverse reactions should lead the clinician to strongly consider halting therapy. Peripheral neuropathy also may develop as a side effect of INH therapy and generally can be prevented or ameliorated by concomitant pyridoxine (50 mg once daily) administration. Individuals with existing peripheral neuropathy or conditions such as diabetes that may predispose to its development should be evaluated and monitored carefully while undergoing prophylactic therapy.

Rifampin, once a day for 4 months, may be prescribed as an alternative to INH but should be reserved for individuals exposed to a patient with INH resistant but rifampin-sensitive *M. tuberculosis*. The CDC previously also had recommended a 2-month regimen of daily rifampin and pyrazinamide; data indicating high rates of hospitalization and death from liver injury associated with the use of rifampin and pyrazinamide prompted the CDC to issue a report recommending that this regimen generally should not be offered to persons with LTBI [28]. Rifampin and pyrazinamide should continue to be used as part of multidrug regimens to treat active TB.

Prevention and Control Strategies

ENGINEERING AND PROTECTIVE EQUIPMENT

Primary prevention strategies include rapid identification of patients with active TB and prompt isolation until they are determined to be noninfectious. The CDC recommends airborne infection isolation for all patients with pulmonary TB. Engineering controls, including negative-pressure isolation rooms, increased room ventilation, local exhaust ventilation, high-efficiency particulate air (HEPA) filtration, and ultraviolet (UV) radiation, are appropriate mechanisms for reducing the concentration of airborne droplet nuclei, limiting their dispersion throughout an institution and thus decreasing the potential for inhalation of pathogenic bacilli. The isolation area should receive at least 12 air changes per hour (ACH) for new construction as of 2001 and at least 6 ACH for construction before 2001 [29]. Increased ventilation to a patient or isolation room significantly reduces airborne particle concentration through dilution and will reduce the concentration of droplet nuclei by 99.75% under ideal conditions.

The room should be under negative pressure so that the direction of airflow is from the outside adjacent space into the room. Negative-pressure airflow, which results from maintenance of a pressure gradient between the interior of a hospital room and the surrounding work area, is an effective strategy for limiting the spread of airborne pathogens in hospitals and related facilities. Combined with appropriate ventilation controls, these systems reduce the risk of transmission to workers in adjacent areas. Negative-pressure mechanisms, however, are delicate and susceptible to a variety of disturbances, particularly in large facilities, where a number of influences can disrupt them. Reversal of normal pressure patterns can result from simply opening the door to the room, thus obviating the protective effect of airflow into the room. Maintenance and inspection of pressure systems must be frequent and systematic.

The air in the isolation room preferably is exhausted to the outside but may be recirculated, provided that the return air is filtered through a HEPA filter. HEPA filters designed to capture particles 0.3 μm in diameter with an efficiency of 99.97% will be effective in removing the 1- to 5-μm droplet nuclei that are infectious. HEPA filtration of a room or confined area generally is considered an adjunct to other ventilatory controls, particularly in situations in which ventilation is substandard or circulated air must, for engineering reasons, be reentrained back into the building. Disadvantages of HEPA filtration include the filters' resistance to entrainment of air through them, with consequent costs in energy and potential for leakage around the filter; the need for periodic maintenance and replacement, without which effectiveness is considerably reduced; and the failure of local or free-standing units to capture particulates in the vicinity. OSHA has recommended the use of HEPA filtration in cases in which air from isolation rooms cannot be exhausted away from employees, intake vents, and the public or must be recirculated within the building [1].

Ultraviolet germicidal irradiation (UVGI) has been suggested for use as a bactericide in several settings within hospitals, including isolation rooms, air-system ductwork, and recirculating room air cleaners. There remain differences of opinion regarding the efficacy of UVGI in reducing the airborne burden of *M. tuberculosis*. Claims have been made that irradiation results in reduction of viable organisms equivalent to over 20 ACH [30]. By contrast, other investigators have estimated the result of bacterial inactivation by UVGI at only 1.6 ACH and thus have not considered it an appropriate method of reducing bacterial aerosols in areas where they may be constantly generated [31]. The CDC recommends the use of UVGI as a supplemental air-cleaning mechanism in isolation, treatment, and waiting rooms; emergency facilities; and other areas where undiagnosed patients with active TB may be found [21]. It is not recommended as a stand-alone substitute for negative pressure in isolation rooms or for HEPA filtration of air that must be recirculated.

While these methods will reduce the number of infectious particles within an isolation room, the use of personal respiratory protection is also indicated for all persons entering airborne isolation rooms. Respiratory protection is also needed in procedure areas where the generation of aerosols with high infective potential is likely and in enclosed areas where engineering controls are not feasible, such as ambulances and other forms of transport. Respiratory protective devices must meet standards and performance guidelines developed by the National Institute of Occupational Safety and Health (NIOSH):

1. Filtration efficiency of 95% or greater for particles of 1 μm at flow rates of 50 L/min
2. Ability to be reliably quantitatively or qualitatively fitted such that fit testing results in leakage in no more than 10% of cases
3. Ability to fit faces differing in size and other characteristics
4. Ability to check for facepiece fit [32]

HEPA filter negative-pressure respirators, which filter particles of 0.3 μm with 99.97% efficiency, have been considered effective under these guidelines. The use of HEPA filter masks has been problematic because of evidence that particles leak around face seals in 10–20% of subjects, thereby reducing their protective effect. Cost and discomfort of the masks may hinder their widespread acceptance. Under more recent NIOSH criteria, N-95 respirators, which meet particle-removal efficiency standards of 95% for 0.3-μm particles, meet criteria for use in TB prevention guidelines.

Common surgical masks lack effective filtration for small particles and are of little use to the worker exposed to aerosols generated by a patient with TB. However, such a mask can be useful for temporary, short periods in patients who may present a risk within the facility, for example, those being transported for tests or procedures or those who have not yet been admitted to an isolation room. These masks will stop expulsion of most respiratory droplets and reduce the generation of droplet nuclei. Masks should be changed if wet with secretions or sputum because forceful coughing then may expel particles from the mask. Since surgical masks may be uncomfortable and stigmatizing for the patient, they should not be used as a prolonged substitute for effective isolation procedures.

In accordance with the OSHA respirator standard [33], individuals should undergo determination of medical fitness to wear a respiratory protective device. Although infrequent, some medical conditions may result in the inability to wear a respirator mask; individuals with such conditions should be kept from known or direct exposure to patients with active tuberculosis (e.g., direct patient contact or attendance at high-risk procedures). A related issue is the need for greater protection in performing procedures, such as bronchoscopy or chest physiotherapy, that result in the generation of large volumes of potentially infectious droplets. Positive-pressure or powered HEPA filter respirators may be more effective choices for individuals who perform these procedures regularly. Although data regarding the utility and efficacy of respiratory protection in the prevention of TB in institutions are sparse, the CDC recommendations for health care facilities are firm regarding the use of respirators, and individuals responsible for safety and health in these facilities must familiarize themselves with requirements for a respiratory protection program.

While engineering controls and personnel protective equipment are effective in reducing exposure and infection, overemphasis on ventilation and stationary engineering controls does little to reduce nosocomial spread from patients in whom active TB is not suspected [30]. A high index of suspicion, early isolation and institution of protective measures, and rapid diagnosis are essential to preventing the spread of TB throughout a health care facility.

SCREENING AND SURVEILLANCE

Secondary prevention or early diagnosis of LTBI before a person becomes symptomatic, and when treatment is effective, has been accomplished primarily through systematic screening of potentially exposed workers using tuberculin skin testing. The fundamental principles of tuberculin skin testing were outlined earlier; its application to workers exposed to TB is discussed in this section. Previously, tuberculin skin testing was the only test available for the diagnosis of LTBI. QFT-G is now available and may be substituted as an alternative to tuber-culin skin testing for surveillance; results are available after a single patient visit, are not subject to reader error, and are not confounded by a waning DTH skin reaction or the booster phenomenon.

Any facility that houses or cares for persons with suspected or confirmed TB, including hospitals, nursing homes, and homeless shelters, should develop an exposure control plan and complete a risk assessment that identifies the job tasks and individuals who potentially will be exposed to *M. tuberculosis*. This exposure assessment determines which workers should be included in a surveillance program and how frequently testing should be done. Every employee who potentially may be exposed to tuberculosis should participate in a medical surveillance program that systematically and periodically tests for LTBI. The exposure control plan also should include provisions for exposure incidents and should include appropriate medical evaluation and follow-up for all employees exposed to tuberculosis regardless of whether the employee had been participating in periodic screening and surveillance.

Health care facilities and other worksites should gather complete, reliable information on the baseline PPD skin test status of employees prior to initial assignment to jobs with occupational exposure to TB. An initial two-step protocol for PPD skin testing should be performed on hire or on initiation of a surveillance program for all employees not known to be previously positive or who cannot document a negative TST in the past 12 months. Individuals who exhibit the booster phenomenon (an initially negative test followed by a second positive PPD test), indicative of past TB infection with subsequent waning of the cell-mediated immune response, can be excluded from subsequent PPD skin testing. All individuals with a boosted reaction should be evaluated by a physician for treatment of LTBI. BCG vaccination should not be considered a contraindication to PPD testing; it is important to remember that these individuals also may exhibit a boosted reaction on two-step testing. The application and reading of skin tests (see Table 9-1) and interpretation of positive tests according to the CDC guidelines (see Table 9-2) should be performed by medical professionals trained in their interpretation. The employee should not, and should not be expected to, read and interpret his or her own test results.

Following the baseline PPD test, periodic retesting should be performed at least annually for employees at risk of exposure to TB. The CDC recommends that the frequency of PPD testing be based on a risk assessment of the health care facility, including the number of cases of infectious TB present and the potential for transmission to workers. The frequency of retesting will vary for different facilities; testing as frequently as every 3 months is suggested for workers in facilities with the highest risk, defined as areas with an elevated rate of skin test conversions, evidence of a cluster of conversions, or evidence of transmission between patients or from patients to workers [23, 25]. At the very least, employers should provide TB skin testing every 6 months for employees who routinely enter AFB isolation rooms, perform or are present during high-hazard procedures, transport suspected or confirmed infectious patients in enclosed vehicles, or work in intake areas of facilities where six or more confirmed cases of infectious TB have been encountered per year. These workers are considered to be exposed more intensely and frequently. In contrast, other workers with lower risks of exposure should be retested yearly.

Individuals in health care and other exposed work settings who have a positive PPD should have chest radiography performed to exclude the possibility of active tuberculosis. In the absence of radiographic evidence and clinical signs and symptoms of tuberculosis, treatment of latent tuberculosis with INH is indicated. When the source patient is known or strongly suspected to have MDRTB, a careful assessment of the exposed worker's health and immunologic status is mandated. Individuals at greater risk of developing active TB, particularly persons with HIV infection, immunosuppressed persons because of other medical conditions or therapies, the very young, and the elderly, should be considered for multiple-drug prophylactic therapy. This usually consists of the addition of rifampin to the prophylactic regimen but should be tailored to the known susceptibilities of the isolate or to the pattern of drug resistance in the facility. An infectious disease specialist with expertise in the treatment of MDRTB should be consulted.

A PPD conversion in the workplace may be a sentinel event, indicating that other workers or patients have had similar exposures. A history of contacts and possible exposures should be elicited from the individual with a newly converted skin test. If this history indicates that exposure took place within the facility, contacts of the suspected source should be identified and tested. A similar protocol should be followed in identifying contacts of a suspected or confirmed case of a worker with active TB within a facility; patients and coworkers must be identified and tested for evidence of TB infection [23]. If exposure is recent, sufficient time to convert to a positive skin test may not have elapsed, and any identified contacts that are skin test–negative should have repeat PPD testing in 3 months. If additional positive tests are found on follow-up, they are grounds for assessing current controls and preventive measures against the spread of TB within the facility.

Sometimes the probable source of infection cannot be readily identified within the facility at the time a PPD conversion is noted. The period within which the worker was likely to have become infected can be estimated based on previous negative skin test results and ranges from 10 weeks before the last negative PPD test to 2 weeks before skin test conversion. Hospital records during this time, including those from the laboratory and the infection control service, should be examined to determine possible sources of infection. Additional screening within the new converter's occupational group or among area coworkers may be necessary to determine the likelihood of transmission from a common source. If exposure occurred at work, the effectiveness of procedures and policies for TB control in the facility needs to be reviewed and evaluated. Since contact tracing and investigation require extensive work, it is essential to keep accurate and current records of the PPD status of all workers who may sustain TB exposures.

Workers who exhibit PPD conversion but have no symptoms or signs of active tuberculosis may continue work at their current job without restriction, whether or not they are taking INH. They should be advised to report any signs or symptoms of active TB. Prompt assessment for the possibility of active TB infection is indicated if symptoms develop in any skin test converter. Workers who cannot take INH or must have it discontinued before completing a full course should be made aware of the potential for development of active TB infection.

Workers with active pulmonary or laryngeal TB may transmit the infection to patients and coworkers. These workers should be excluded from the workplace until they have been demonstrated to be noninfectious through appropriate treatment. Adequate and continuing therapy, resolution of cough, and three consecutive negative AFB smears should be documented before an excluded individual is allowed to return to work. Special care must be taken to ensure that an infected individual continues with treatment, that treatment remains adequate (based on laboratory tests of sensitivity), and that sputum and other secretions remain negative for AFB. Patients who discontinue treatment before they are considered cured should be reevaluated immediately, and if evidence indicates that the employee may be infectious, he or she should be excluded from work immediately. Individuals with extrapulmonary TB are generally considered noninfectious with respect to the workplace and need not be excluded from work as long as concurrent pulmonary TB has been ruled out [22]. However, for individuals with cutaneous TB, appropriate precautions should be taken to ensure that exposure to actively infected lesions by direct contact does not occur.

The Future

Over the past decade, renewed public health funding and programs have been effective in reversing the resurgence of TB and renewing its progressive decline. Elimination of TB in the United States requires sustained efforts to identify and target populations at risk and requires adequate resources, a lesson brought home by the events of the 1980s. Major research programs are working to develop a safe and effective vaccine, pharmacologic trials are being conducted to study new drugs for the first-line treatment of TB, and molecular genotyping is becoming available as a tool to investigate outbreaks, to understand patterns of transmission, and to control TB.

Health care facilities and other employers whose workers may come into contact with infectious TB need to continue to define their population at risk, monitor employees' exposure status, institute appropriate and ongoing surveillance measures, and maintain effective controls and measures for the reduction of exposure among their personnel. Although evidence of the efficacy and cost-effectiveness of engineering controls and personal

protective equipment may not be complete [7], the failure to rapidly recognize and take adequate control measures for exposure appears to be the single most important factor in nosocomial transmission of TB infection.

Current guidelines provide a framework by which exposure reduction and surveillance can be instituted for the protection of exposed employees. From a public health perspective, reducing exposures also benefits those who may not fall under the immediate protection of health and safety standards but whose work may inadvertently put them at risk. Continued surveillance is needed to reduce the risk a new resurgence of TB may have on workers in health care, human services, and other high-risk jobs.

References

1. U.S. Department of Labor, Occupational Safety and Health Administration. Occupational exposure to tuberculosis: Proposed rule. *Fed Reg* 1997;62:54159–308.
2. Comstock GW. Frost revisited: The modern epidemiology of tuberculosis. *Am J Epidemiol* 1975; 101:363–82.
3. Schneider E, Moore M, Castro K. Epidemiology of tuberculosis in the United States. *Clin Chest Med* 2005;26:183–95.
4. Centers for Disease Control and Prevention. Trends in Tuberculosis—United States, 2004. *MMWR* 2005; 54:245–9.
5. Sepkowitz KA. Tuberculosis and the health care worker: A historical perspective. *Ann Intern Med* 1994;120:71–9.
6. Reichman LB, O'Day R. Tuberculous infection in a large urban population. *Am Rev Respir Dis* 1978;117: 705–12.
7. Berman J, Levin ML, Orr ST, et al. Tuberculosis risk for hospital employees: Analysis of a five-year tuberculin skin testing program. *Am J Public Health* 1981; 71:1217–22.
8. Bowden KM, McDiarmid MA. Occupationally acquired tuberculosis: What's known. *J Occup Med* 1994;36:320–5.
9. Centers for Disease Control and Prevention. Nosocomial transmission of multidrug-resistant tuberculosis among HIV infected persons—Florida and New York, 1988–1991. *MMWR* 1991;40:585–91.
10. Markowitz SB. Epidemiology of tuberculosis among health care workers. *Occup Med State Art Rev* 1994;9:589–608.
11. Boudreau AY, Baron SL, Steenland NK, et al. Occupational risk of *Mycobacterium tuberculosis* infection in hospital workers. *Am J Ind Med* 1997;32:528–34.
12. Malasky C, Jordan T, Potulski F, et al. Occupational

tuberculous infections among pulmonary physicians in training. *Am Rev Respir Dis* 1990;142:505–7.

13. Steenland K, Levine AJ, Seiber K, et al. Incidence of tuberculosis infection among New York State prison employees. *Am J Public Health* 1997;87:2012–7.

14. Mitchell CS, Gershon RR, Lears MK, et al. Risk of tuberculosis in correctional healthcare workers. *J Occup Environ Med* 2005;47:580–6.

15. Langille DB, Sweet LE. Tuberculin skin testing in a hospital and two chronic care facilities in Prince Edward Island. *Can J Infect Control* 1995;10:41–4.

16. Lawson J, Caygill J. Results from a Mantoux screening programme of staff in the care of elderly and mental health fields at Wakari Hospital, Dunedin. *NZ Med J* 1995;108:222–4.

17. Harrington JM, Shannon HS. Incidence of tuberculosis, hepatitis, brucellosis, and shigellosis in British medical laboratory workers. *Br Med J* 1976;1:759–62.

18. Goette DK, Jacobson KW, Doty RD. Primary inoculation tuberculosis of the skin: Prosector's paronychia. *Arch Dermatol* 1978;114:567–9.

19. Sharma VK, Kumar B, Radotra BD, et al. Cutaneous inoculation tuberculosis in laboratory personnel. *Int J Dermatol* 1990;29:293–4.

20. Rosenman KD, Hall N. Occupational risk factors for developing tuberculosis. *Am J Ind Med* 1996;30:148–54.

21. Morgan E. Silicosis and tuberculosis. *Chest* 1979;75:202–3.

22. Centers for Disease Control and Prevention. Targeted tuberculin testing and treatment of latent tuberculosis infection. *MMWR* 2000;49:1–51.

23. Centers for Disease Control and Prevention. Guidelines for preventing the transmission of *Mycobacterium tuberculosis* in health-care settings, 2005. *MMWR* 2005;54:46–52.

24. Snider DE. Bacille Calmette-Guérin vaccinations and tuberculin skin tests. *JAMA* 1985;253:3438–9.

25. Centers for Disease Control and Prevention. Guidelines for using the QuantiFERON-TB Gold test for diagnosing *Mycobacterium tuberculosis* infection—United States. *MMWR* 2005;54:49–55.

26. Blumberg HM, Burman WJ, Chaisson RE, et al. American Thoracic Society/Centers for Disease Control and Prevention/Infectious Diseases Society of America: Treatment of tuberculosis. *Am J Respir Crit Care Med* 2003;167:603.

27. Moulding, T. Preventive treatment of tuberculosis: A clinician's perspective. In Rossman MD, MacGregor RR (eds), *Tuberculosis: Clinical Management and New Challenges.* New York: McGraw-Hill, 1995, pp 89–105.

28. Centers for Disease Control and Prevention. Update: Adverse event data and revised American Thoracic Society/CDC recommendations against the use of rifampin and pyrazinamide for treatment of latent tuberculosis infection—United States, 2003. *MMWR* 2003;52:735–9.

29. Centers for Disease Control and Prevention. Guidelines for environmental infection control in healthcare facilities. Recommendations of CDC and the Healthcare Infection Control Practices Advisory Committee (HICPAC). *MMWR* 2003;52:1–42.

30. Nardell EA, Riley R L. Precautions to prevent transmission. In Rossman MD, MacGregor RR (eds), *Tuberculosis: Clinical Management and New Challenges.* New York: McGraw-Hill, 1995, pp 57–72.

31. Macher JM, Alevantis LE, Chang Y-L, et al. Effect of ultraviolet germicidal lamps on airborne microorganisms in an outpatient waiting room. *Appl Occup Environ Hyg* 1992;7:505–13.

32. Hodous TK, Coffey CC. The role of respiratory protective devices in the control of tuberculosis. *Occup Med State Art Rev* 1994;9:631–57.

33. 29 CFR 1910.134, Respiratory protection.

10 Occupational Legionellosis

William E. Wright

Legionellosis is an important water-borne environmental bacterial disease that can occur in outbreaks or in sporadic form. It is not recognized to be transmitted from person to person. Its importance in the occupational setting relates to its notoriety as a highly publicized lethal disease, its occurrence related to contaminated water in work settings, its relationship to travel, and its occurrence as a community-acquired pneumonia (CAP). When *Legionella* infection is reported in a member of a business organization, the occupational physician is often confronted with panicked managers and workers who need information and a well-ordered approach to address their concerns. Such an occurrence of *Legionella* raises the issue of potential contaminated water sources in the workplace, during travel, or in the general environment. Of particular concern are situations in which highly contaminated water sources occur in settings involving the elderly and infirm, particularly those with chronic respiratory disease and those who are immunosuppressed, treated with corticosteroids, and/or intubated, because these groups tend to have more severe disease.

The Organism

An outbreak of pneumonia at an American Legion Convention in Philadelphia in 1976 lead to the Centers for Disease Control and Prevention (CDC) publishing the details of this epidemic and the likely, previously unidentified bacterial pathogenic agent [1,2]. The disease was referred to as *legionnaires' disease* (sometimes termed *legionellosis*). The identified pathogen, an aerobic gram-negative, piliated, and pleomorphic-appearing bacillus, was later named *Legionella pneumophila*. It is now recognized to be one of a number of similar bacteria in a family now designated Legionellaceae. The family now consists of about 41 species, species members being assigned into about 64 serogroups (SGs). The species *L. pneumophila* currently has about 14 serogroups, SGs 1, 4, and 6 accounting for most *Legionella* infections and the most common pathogen in *Legionella*-related community-acquired pneumonia (CAP) being *L. pneumophila* SG 1. Further mention of SG 1 will refer to *L. pneumophia* species SG 1 unless otherwise specified. An international collaborative survey of culture-confirmed, sporadic, community-acquired legionellosis identified *L. pneumophila* in 91.5% of 508 isolates, SG 1 accounting for about 84% of these. SGs 2 to 13 accounted for 7.4% of *L. pneumophila* infections [3]. The main species and serogroups that are recognized to cause pneumonia in humans are listed in Table 10-1. The species designations and serogroup typing are important factors that help to determine whether a case or multiple cases are from a single source or are related.

The Legionellaceae are intracellular pathogens and are subject primarily to cell-mediated immunity for host defense mechanisms. The bacilli's attachment to host

Table 10-1
Legionnaires' Disease: Main Human Pathogens

Organism	Percentage of Cases*
Legionella pneumophila	91.5% (typically 80–90% of human infections in other series with SGs 1, 4, and 6 being the most common)
Legionella bozemanii	2.4%
Legionella longbeachae	3.9%; 30% of community-acquired *Legionella* isolates in Australia and New Zealand
Remaining species:	2.2%; these species include the following:
Legionella micdadei	(Pittsburgh pneumonia agent)
Legionella dumoffii	
Legionella feeleii	
Legionella wadsworthii	
Legionella anisa	

*Initial percentages shown are from an international collaborative survey [3]; local figures may vary from those shown.
Abbreviations: SG = serogroup.

cells, such as respiratory epithelial cells, is mediated by type IV pili and other outer-membrane proteins; they bind to complement CR1 and CR3 integrin receptors on the host cell surfaces using adsorbed C3bi ligands/adhesins [4]. The bacilli can attach to phagocytes, proliferate intracellularly, and be released when the cells rupture.

Legionella grow naturally in the environment in water. Colonization of natural and human-made water reservoirs is important in causing disease in humans. The organisms prefer warm water ($\geq 35°C$) and tend to grow on water surfaces, a behavior that facilitates contamination of aerosolized droplets and transmission to human respiratory tracts. However, *Legionella* organisms can live in refrigerated water for years, and some SGs have been cultured from soil. *Legionella* can invade and grow in ciliated protozoa living in water, which may account for some of its resistance to some water-treatment methods; these organisms, along with amebas, algae, water-dwelling bacteria, and sediment and scale, appear to promote *Legionella* proliferation in water. Although *L. pneumophila* has been found in ponds, lakes, and streams, it also can dwell in cooling-tower water, treated potable water sources, and other water sources.

Illnesses Caused by *Legionella* Organisms

The typical clinical illness resulting from *Legionella* infection is pneumonia. *Legionnaires' disease* is the

term used for pneumonia caused by species of Legionellaceae. There are no physical signs that distinguish it from other bacterial or viral pneumonias. The clinical course of legionnaires' disease tends to have more severe symptoms, a worse course, and poorer prognosis than atypical pneumonias owing to *Chlamydia, Mycoplasma,* and viruses. Early symptoms typically occur from 2–10 after exposure and most often include fever, cough, malaise, headache, and anorexia. Upper respiratory symptoms and coryza are rare. Body temperature may be over 40°C. Cough is typically nonproductive or productive of scant sputum. Pleuritic pain and hemoptysis may occur. Up to half of patients are reported to have watery diarrhea, and other gastrointestinal symptoms such as abdominal pain, nausea, or vomiting may occur. Myalgias and arthralgias may occur, and neurologic symptoms can include headache, photophobia, confusion, stupor, and encephalopathy. The illness can progress to respiratory failure and/or multisystem failure. In legionnaires' disease, hyponatremia (serum sodium < 131 meq/L) tends to occur more frequently than in other CAPs. Chest radiography typically shows patchy alveolar infiltrates or multilobular consolidation, but scattered discrete nodular densities can occur. Typical lung pathology findings include fibrinopurulent pneumonia with alveolitis and bronchiolitis. Less commonly, abscesses with central necrosis can occur.

Legionnaires' disease typically occurs with a low attack rate (up to 5%) when outbreaks occur. In hospitalized patients, the case-mortality rate can reach about 40%.

A less common form of *Legionella* illness is Pontiac fever, which was recognized as a distinct syndrome years prior to the 1976 outbreak that lead to the recognition of legionnaires' disease. Pontiac fever is an acute flulike illness with fever, chills, headache, malaise, and myalgias. Chest pain, mild cough, nausea, abdominal pain, and diarrhea can occur in fewer than half the patients. Onset of symptoms usually occurs 1–2 days after exposure (range 5–66 hours), and the illness typically resolves spontaneously in about 2–5 days without antibiotic treatment. Pontiac fever is thought to result from exposure to inhaled antigen and not bacterial invasion. Attack rates have been noted to be high (about 95%) in several outbreaks. The *Legionella* organism is virtually never isolated from the patient, and the case-fatality rate is essentially zero [5]. In some occupational settings, the symptom complex may raise questions about metal fume or polymer fume fever.

Respiratory tract illness without pneumonia owing to *L. pneumophila* and other *Legionella* species has been described. Its clinical presentation is not specific, and its incidence is not clear. Studies suggest that some people in the vicinity of an outbreak of legionnaires' disease seroconvert and may have mild or subclinical illness [6]. This is supported by seroprevalance studies in worksites with nosocomial outbreaks [7] and other studies [8,9]. This milder illness may resolve without antibiotic treatment.

Legionnella organisms have been implicated in other infections with signs and symptoms typical of the organs they infect. In cases of severe pneumonia, bacteremia can occur and result in myocarditis, pericarditis, and prosthetic valve endocarditis. Infection through a sternal wound has been reported, as has indwelling tube–related infections. In immunocompromised hosts, infections can include sinusitis, wound infections, septic arthritis, and abdominal infections such as peritonitis, pyelonephritis, and peritonitis [10].

Diagnosis

The most sensitive and specific methods of diagnosis of legionnaire's disease are culture of sputum, tracheal aspirates, or bronchoalveolar lavage fluid. Culture of appropriate samples of respiratory fluids can have a sensitivity of 80%. Microscopic examination of sputum samples tends to identify no or few organisms. The Gram stain in not particularly helpful for identifying legionnaires' disease because sputum samples during infection typically show many leukocytes but no organisms. Finding leukocytes (predominantly neutrophils) with no organisms or with some small gram-negative pleomorphic bacilli in sputum of a patient with pneumonia should result in consideration of legionnaires' disease. One species of Legionellaceae is weakly acid-fast on staining and can be mistaken for *Mycobacterium tuberculosis.* Culture of pleural fluid may detect a *Legionella* infection, and antibody testing of the fluid can increase the likelihood of positive results. Cultures tend to take 3–5 days to show visible growth, and

diagnosis can be complicated by overgrowth by other microflora. The Legionellaceae grow on buffered charcoal yeast extract (BCYE) but not on routine laboratory media. Sometimes antibiotics are added to the culture medium if competing flora from nonsterile sites are anticipated; the culture methods sometimes are not sensitive enough to make a diagnosis and need to be used in combination with serologic studies such as indirect fluorescent antibody tests [11] (see also Chapter 2). The serogroup-specific antigens can be identified with direct fluorescent antibody (DFA) testing. Polyclonal and monoclonal DFA tests are available, the latter having less cross-reactivity and more specificity (about 95%) for *L. pneumophila,* with variable sensitivity (25–75%) depending, in part, on the quality of the specimen [5]. DFA testing for SG 1 is available commercially and can be used with sputum, bronchoalveolar lavage cells, or lung tissue. The test sensitivity is generally about 70–75% and can be combined with culture and/or serologic evaluations for diagnosis.

Sometimes seroconversion in documented *L. pneumophila* illness does not occur or occurs as much as 4 weeks after the patient becomes ill; delayed seroconversion is more common with non-*pneumophila* species [11]. Seroconversion can last after inapparent illness or after nonpneumonia respiratory tract illness has resolved and can be present owing to exposure to antigen; therefore, a single antibody titer of any level is not diagnostic of legionellosis [5]. Some sources categorize a high single or static antibody titer against *L. pneumophila* (titer $\geq$ 1:1024) as supporting *L. pneumophila* as a possible cause of current pneumonia [12]. Paired sera (acute and convalescent) generally are done, with 4–6 weeks separating the two, with the longer period being favored owing to the potential for a delayed seroconversion response, particularly with non-*pneumophila* species.

Diagnosis sometimes can be made effectively by testing for *L. pneumophila* antigens in urine [13]. The rapid antigen test gives results in about 4 hours and has a 70% sensitivity and 99% specificity for SG 1 antigen [5,14]; it may crossreact with other serogroups. The antigen excretion is detectable about 3 days after the onset of clinical illness and may last for 6 weeks or longer. Some recommend that urine testing for SG 1 antigen be done in all patients with severe or rapidly progressing pneumonia depending on community patterns of disease [12]. The diagnosis of Pontiac fever usually is made by detecting seroconversion in antibody testing.

There are some polymerase chain reaction (PCR) tests available for detection of *L. pneumophila* DNA in material from nasopharyngeal swabbing. *L. pneumophila* is not known to colonize this area or be present there unless the organism is causing active pulmonary illness (pneumonia). These tests continue to be developed, but their clinical use is not yet clearly defined [12,15].

Diagnosis of either legionnaires' disease or Pontiac fever should result in expansion of the occupational, travel, and environmental history to determine whether likely exposure sources can be identified for further investigation.

Reporting of Cases

The CDC advises about methods of reporting cases of legionnaires' disease in addition to the applicable state and local reporting requirements and their reporting through the National Notifiable Diseases Surveillance System (NNDSS). Reporting methods include

1. Travel-associated cases should be reported to the CDC by e-mailing travellegionella@cdc.gov
2. Post a "call for cases" on Epi-X, the CDC's secure information-exchange network, which can help to identify clusters of cases related to outbreaks and travel-related cases.
3. For cruise ship–-related cases, in addition to using travellegionellaM@cdc.gov, inform the CDC Division of Global Migration and Quarantine and the CDC Vessel Sanitation Program by a single e-mail to VSP@cdc.gov and FMAO@cdc.gov.
4. Informing the cruise line is recommended.

The CDC Web site's legionnaires' disease homepage includes links for sample questionnaires that can be used for institutional outbreaks, travel-associated cases, and other situations. Also available is a sample letter to give to a hotel related to case identification.

The European Working Group for *Legionella* Infections (EWGLI) operates a surveillance system (EWGLINET) for legionnaires' disease among European travelers that can be accessed at www.ewgli.org.

Treatment

Recommendations for treatment of infection with *Legionella* species evolve over time. Current local patterns of antimicrobial resistance should be considered. Currently, the newer macrolides (e.g., azithromycin and clarithromycin) and respiratory tract quinolones (e.g., levofloxacin, ciprofloxicin, gemifloxacin, and moxifloxicin) are the drugs of choice and can be used as monotherapy. Tetracyclines (e.g., doxycycline), trimethoprim-sulfamethoxazole, and erythromycin are alternative drugs, but less preferred. Rifampin can be used in combination with a macrolide or a quinolone.

Current recommendations for initial therapy are for intravenous treatment until a clinical response is achieved (usually 3–5 days) and then oral therapy for 10–14 days for immunocompetent people, longer courses being required for immunosuppressed patients. *L. pneumophilia* is not susceptible to ß-lactam/ß-lactamase inhibitors, cephalosporins, or aminoglycosides. Pneumonia unresponsive to these agents should raise concern about legionnaires' disease and other resistant organisms [12,16]. Pontiac fever, a self-limited condition, requires no antibiotic therapy.

Other Epidemiologic and Occupational Considerations

Person-to-person transmission has not been documented. The Legionellacae are transmitted to people from water sources by airborne transmission. Aspiration of contaminated water also may be a route of transmission to the respiratory tract. Direct exposure of broken skin with contaminated water has been reported as a route of exposure for skin infection. In most studies of legionnaires' disease, the attack rates have been low (0.1–5%). The disease tends to occur more frequently in men than in women (ratio about 2.5:1.0), and reported cases occur most commonly in summer and autumn in the United States.

General risk factors for the occurrence of legionnaires' disease include advancing age, with most reported cases occurring after age 50, and cigarette smoking, chronic lung disease, diabetes mellitus, malignancy, chronic renal disease, inpatient surgery, and immunosuppression, including long-term treatment with corticosteroids and receipt of a transplanted organ. Occupational risk factors for legionnaires' disease relate to work with and around natural and human-made water sources that are contaminated with pathogenic Legionellaceae and offer opportunities for aerosolization of contaminated water.

A number of different contaminated water sources have been linked to outbreaks of legionnaire's disease. Water sources can be natural or human-made, indoors or outside, and can occur on ships as well as on land, in hospitals, in other health care facilities, and in non-health care-related buildings.

Historically, outbreaks have been identified from contamination in streams; ponds; decorative fountains; hot and cold tapwater; showers; cooling towers; dehumidifiers; hot tubs and whirlpool spas; evaporative coolers/condensers; standing water indoors from leaks, drips, seepage, and condensation; respiratory therapy equipment; and other water sources. The scope of the potential for contamination in industry is underscored by water being the most commonly used solvent.

In the few population studies that have been done, the seroprevalence of antibodies to *L. pneumophila* SG 1 range from about 1–20%. Few data are available on seroprevalence in occupational groups, although some studies carried out by the World Health Organization (WHO) identified an approximate 33% seroprevalence of antibodies in seafarers generally and 29% in cargo ship crews [17]. These workers may deal with a number of water sources in addition to the bodies of water on which they live and travel, including potable water systems; water in swimming pools and spas; water in heating tanks and condensed steam tanks; other nonpotable water systems; plumbing and wastewater systems; air-conditioning systems; and other condensate, bilge water, and transfers of water from land. A report cited below mentions an approximate 33% seroprevalence in hospital workers in a hospital with a contaminated water source and nosocomial infections [7]. Another relates a seroprevalence in professional drivers in cold climates of 4.6% and in warm climates (long-term frequent exposure to evaporative condensers/vehicle air conditioning) of 27.8% [18].

Some recent occupational and environmental settings in which cases or outbreaks of legionnaires' disease have been reported include a cruise ship whirlpool spa [19], a cruise ship water supply system [20], a Japanese spa [21], a hospital plumbing system causing nosocomial infections [22], groundwater supply, a hot-water tank, and potable water in a military hospital causing nosocomial infection [23]. Moreover, a university hospital's potable water system related to over 10 years of unrecognized nosocomial transmission of legionnaires' disease among transplant patients [24], another university hospital's water distribution network related to nosocomial infections [25], and a hospital cooling-tower pond and air-conditioning water system related to nosocomial infections and nearly one-third of the hospital staff having *Legionella* antibodies [7]. Other settings include travel-related hotels, camps, and cruise ships [26]; home and business water systems [27]; water supplies of hotels and camps [28]; cruise ship spa-bath filter stones [29]; cruise ships and other vessels, with illness said to occur more in passengers than in crew members [30]; an inadequate circulating and filtration system for commercial bath water in Japan [31]; a bathhouse with spa facilities in Japan [32]; a cooling tower [33]; aerosol generation through a cracked sight glass on a water flowmeter used for a plastics factory machine-cooling system (with an outdoor water supply tank) [34]; a cargo ship's cooling water circuit valve and water pumps (while under repair) [35]; spa baths/spa pools on display at a retail store in New Zealand [36]; an automotive plant finishing line [37]; a contaminated whirlpool filter and river water [38]; long-distance professional bus drivers using evaporative condensers/air conditioning in hot weather [18]; and a meat packing plant (retrospective serologic study of a 1957 outbreak of pneumonia in Minnesota) [39]. There is also a report of a case of fatal *L. pneumophila* pneumonia (SG 1, Olda and Camperdown subtypes, and SG 10) in a young calf of a dairy herd in Italy, said to be the first report of a naturally occurring *Legionella* pneumonia in an animal; the authors concluded that cattle probably act as an accidental host for Legionellacae [40].

Studies in Europe in 1998 estimated that travel-associated legionnaires' disease represents 16% of legionnaires' disease cases [26] (this reports defines travel as spending one or more nights away from home during the 10 days before becoming ill; European Surveillance Scheme for Travel-Associated Legionnaires' Disease). Other summary reports are based on the EWGLINET address travel-associated legionnaires' disease in Europe for 2002, 2004, and 2006 [41–44]. The CDC reports that about 21% of all legionnaires' disease reported to the CDC between 1980 and 1999 were travel-associated, the proportion rising as reporting of cases improved [45]. For assessment of travel-associated legionnaires' disease, the CDC recommends queries related to travel done in the 2 weeks prior to the onset of symptoms or activities 10–14 days prior to diagnosis (no standardized definition of travel is given) [45].

Community-Acquired Pneumonia (CAP) and *Legionella* Species

Historically, CAP was diagnosed as being primarily due to *Streptococcus pneumoniae* (up to 62% in the 1970s) [46]. Since then, in some studies, the proportion attributable to *S. pneumoniae* has decreased in hospital-based studies; in some studies, the causative agent of CAP could not be identified in at least 35% of patients (some estimates ranging from 50–75%) [46]. It was thought that *Chlamydia pneumoniae, L. pneumophila,* and *Mycoplasma pneumoniae* were common causes that were difficult to diagnose with accuracy. More recent data still list *S. pneumoniae* as the most common cause of CAP (about 30–50% of cases), with *Haemophilius influenza* and *Chlamydophila pneumoniae* (formerly *Chlamydia pneumoniae*) accounting for about 22% of cases. The estimates of the role of *L. pneumophila* in CAP vary, ranging from 3–15% or 2–7% [10,12]. Mixed flora aspiration pneumonia and *Mycoplasma pneumoniae* are estimated to account for about 10% and 5–10%, respectively. *Staphylococcus aureus* typically accounts for a smaller percentage of CAP in many hospital studies, but recent data at the time of this writing are of concern because of a rise in the occurrence of severe necrotizing CAP caused by methicillin-resistant *S. aureus,* some strains of which contain a gene for the production of a leukocidin, which is associated with severe disease (Panton-Valentine leukocidin [PVL]) [47,48]. Reports of community-acquired PVL in the United States, Canada, South America, Europe, and Asia indicate that it is a worldwide problem that is increasing. Influenza viral infection also should be considered as a factor in CAP, particularly during the typical flu season

and among travelers returning from areas in which influenza is likely to be present. Severe acute respiratory syndrome related to coronavirus (SARS-CoV), hantavirus, and other causes of viral pneumonia also should be considered.

The number of cases of CAP that occur in the United States is not entirely clear. It has been estimated that about 600,000 cases of CAP occur that require hospitalization each year [12]. If this figure is applied to the estimated proportions of *Legionella*'s contribution to CAP, then the number of people with *Legionella*-related CAP hospitalized annually would range from 12,000–42,000 (2–7%) or 18,000–90,000 (3–15%). If nonhospitalized cases of CAP were accounted for, the number of cases related to *Legionella* species likely would be much higher. The CDC estimates that from 8,000–18,000 people are hospitalized each year with legionnaires' disease [49]. Related to this estimate, the CDC also notes that many infections are not diagnosed or reported. This is consistent with other sources indicating that in a multihospital study, only about 3% of sporadic legionnaires' disease cases were thought to have been diagnosed correctly [10]. The CDC reported a total of 2,093 cases of legionellosis in the United States in 2004 [50] and 2,301 cases in 2005 [51].

Most cases of *Legionella*-associated CAP are related to infection with *L. pneumophila* SG 1. However, CAP has been reported owing to *L. pneumophila* SG 3 [52]; SG 6 [53]; SG 13 [38]; SGs 3, 5, 6, and 7 [54]; SGs 1–6 in a Brazilian study [55]; SGs 1, 3, 4, 6, and 8 [56]; *L. micdadei* and *L. longbeachea* SG 1 [56]; *L. longbeachae; L. anisa; L. bozemannii; Legionella*-like amoebal pathogens (LLAPs) [54]; and others (see Table 10-1). A number of species have been reported in nonpneumonia respiratory tract infections [9].

LLAPs are bacteria that grow only in amoebas and are closely related phylogenetically to *Legionella* species. These organisms include LLAPs 1–13, *Parachlamydia acanthamoeba* (BN9 and Hall's coccus), *Afipia felis, Simkania negevensis,* and others. These have been thought to play an infrequent role in CAP, sometimes as a copathogen and infrequently as a sole pathogen. *C. pneumoniae,* a well-recognized cause of CAP, is also known to infect amoebae, as are *Mycobacterium avium intracellulare, Listeria monocytogenes,* and some *Ehrlichia*-like species [57–59].

Treatment recommendations for CAP change. They may vary by geographic location, and they depend on the profile of local microorganisms, presence of outbreaks related to specific organisms, and patterns of antibiotic resistance. General recommendations for CAP treatment at the time of this writing are based on most cases being caused by *S. pneumoniae, C. pneumoniae, L. pneumophila,* and *M. pneumoniae.* Typically, ambulatory patients who are otherwise healthy are treated with an oral macrolide or doxycycline, fluoroquinolones being used in older patient with comorbid illness. In patients hospitalized with CAP a β-lactam (e.g., ceftriaxone or cefotaxime) plus a macrolide (e.g., erythromycin, azithromycin, or clarithromycin) or a fluoroquinolone to target *S. pneumoniae* (e.g., levofloxacin or moxifloxacin) are typical choices. The recommendations vary depending on specific organisms identified, local patterns of resistance, patient's history of previous antibiotic use, allergy history, etc. [60]. Summary tables of the 2007 guidelines on management of CAP give more details on treatment [12]. Many of these choices would cover *Legionella* species (see treatment section above).

Prevention and Control

When legionnaires' disease or Pontiac fever is diagnosed, there should be an expansion of the occupational, travel, and environmental history to determine whether likely exposure sources can be identified for further investigation. If a case or cases occur without a likely travel-related association, the weight of consideration falls on the general non-travel environment and work environment sources of exposure to contaminated water. Testing of water sources for *Legionella* species and subgroups may be done. If the species/subgroup in the suspected water source matches the organism identified in the legionellosis patient, this is usually taken to indicate a presumed connection. The occupational physician faced with a newly diagnosed case of legionnaires' disease in a work group should query the available medical data and local or state department of health information to see if other cases have occurred that may be related to the workplace. Reporting of cases, which is an important responsibility for health care providers and is essential to assist with identification of environmental and

workplace outbreaks, is covered in a previous section of this chapter.

Further prevention and control procedures are primarily in the area of engineering controls. Efforts involving substitution, administrative controls, work practices, and personal protective equipment have very limited roles in preventing *Legionella*-related diseases. Engineering controls include assessment for proper design and operation of the water sources/systems; proper maintenance or redesign to avoid leaks, seepage, condensation, unnecessary aerosolization, and stagnant areas (e.g., system reservoirs, dead-end pipes, etc.); removal of sludge, scale, and sediment (including removal of faucet aerators that can accumulate sediment in which *Legionella* can grow); treatment to remove and limit algae and biofilms in water; and water treatment to eliminate, prevent, or minimize contamination with *Legionella* species.

A number of water treatment options are available, including chlorination (which takes fairly high levels owing to the organism's tolerance to chlorine), ozonation, copper-silver ionization, ultraviolet light sterilization, thermal eradication, and instantaneous steam heating. Each of these approaches has pros and cons in terms of cost, effectiveness, risks, damage to water systems, and presence or absence of residual disinfectant effect [61]. The type and scope of a disinfection plan must be designed for water systems on a case-by-case basis, taking into account the amount of contamination, input water source, point sources of contamination (such as pumps, valves, and heat tanks), types of systems, and their design and peculiarities.

In some settings, particularly related to water systems recognized to be at high risk of contamination, hospitals in which *Legionella* contamination can result in serious nosocomial infections, settings frequented by immunosuppressed people or others at high risk for serious infection, and settings that have had previous contamination, environmental monitoring (biologic testing) is advisable. A hospital-based approach to prevention and control has been published [62]. Other resources are available online from the CDC and WHO.

The assessment of water systems is further addressed in Chapter 38. In addition, the American Society of Heating, Refrigeration, and Air-Conditioning Engineers (ASHRAE) has published guidelines for building water systems related to *Legionella* risks [63]. The WHO has published information on ship-related outbreaks of disease that includes water-borne diseases and legionnaires' disease [17], a drinking-water quality guide for ship sanitation [64], and other related resources. The CDC also has published a recent summary of cruise ship experience with legionnaires' disease [65].

A program of prevention and control includes employee education about legionnaires' disease and Pontiac fever, coverage of how these illness are transmitted, information on the types of workplaces and environmental factors that can be related to these illnesses, the importance of reporting illnesses that occur that resemble these conditions, and the approach taken to protect and ensure that water sources do not contain dangerous contamination.

References

1. Fraser DW, Tsai TR, Orenstein W, et al. Legionnaires' disease: Description of an epidemic of pneumonia. *N Engl J Med* 1977;297:1189–97.
2. McDade JE, Shepard CC, Fraser DW, et al. Legionnaires disease: isolation of a bacterium and demonstration of its role in other respiratory disease. *N Engl J Med* 1997;297:1197–1203.
3. Yu VL, Plouffe JF, Pastoris MC, et al. Distribution of *Legionella* species and serogroups isolated by culture in patients with sporadic community-acquired legionellosis: An international collaborative survey. *J Infect Dis* 2002;186:127–8.
4. Pier GB. Molecular mechanisms of microbial pathogenesis. In Kasper DL, Fauci AS, Longo DL, et al. (eds), *Harrison's Principles of Internal Medicine*, 16th ed. New York: McGraw-Hill, 2005, Chap 105, pp 700–1.
5. U.S. Centers for Disease Control and Prevention. Top 10 things every clinician needs to know about legionellosis. Legionellosis Resource Site (Legionnaires' Disease and Pontiac Fever), September 27, 2006. Available at *www.cdc.gov/legionella/top10.htm*.
6. Boshuizen HC, Neppelenbroek SE, van Vliet H, et al. Subclinical *Legionella* infection in workers near the source of a large outbreak of legionnaires' disease. *J Infect Dis* 2001;184:515–8.
7. O'Mahony MC, Stanwell-Smith RE, Tillett HE, et al. The Stafford outbreak of legionnaires' disease. *Epidemiol Infect* 1990;104:361–80.
8. Regan CM, McCann B, Syed Q, et al. Outbreak of legionnaires'disease on a cruise ship: Lessons for international surveillance and control. *Commun Dis Public Health* 2003;6:15206.
9. Lieberman D, Lieberman D, Korsonsky I, et al. *Legionella* species infection in adult febrile respiratory tract infections in the community. *Scand J Infect Dis* 2002;34:1–4.
10. Chang F-Y, Yu VL. *Legionella* infection. In Kasper DL, Fauci AS, Longo, et al. (eds), *Harrison's Principles of Internal Medicine*, 16th ed. New York: McGraw-Hill, 2005, Chap 132, pp 870–4.
11. Waterer GW, Baselski VS, Wunderick RG. *Legionella* and community-acquired pneumonia: A review of current diagnostic tests from a clinician's viewpoint. *Am J Med* 2000;110:41–8.
12. Marrie TJ. Community-acquired pneumonia. In Tan JS, File TM, Salata RA, et al. (eds), *Expert Guide to Infectious Diseases*, 2nd ed. Philadelphia: ACP Press, 2008, Chap 23, pp 450–79.
13. Kashuba ADM, Balows CH. *Legionella* urinary antigen testing: Potential impact on diagnosis and antibiotic therapy. *DMID* 1996;24:129–39.
14. Stout JE, Yu VL. Legionellosis. *N Engl J Med.* 1997; 337:682–7.
15. Ramirez JA, Ahkee S, Tolentino A, et al. Diagnosis of *Legionella pneumonphila, Mycoplasma pneumoniae,* or *Chlamydia pneumoniae* lower respiratory infection using the polymerase chain reaction on a single throat swab specimen. *Diagn Microbiol Infect Dis* 1996;24:7–14.
16. Treatment guidelines from The Medical Letter: Choice of antibiotics *Med Lett* 2007;544.
17. World Health Organization. *Sanitation on Ships: Compendium of Outbreaks of Foodborne and Waterborne Disease and Legionnaires' Disease Associated with Ships, 1970–2000.* Geneva: WHO, 2001 (available on Internet).
18. Polat Y, Ergin C, Kaleli I, et al. Investigation of *Legionella pneumophila* seropositivity in professional long-distance drivers as a risky occupation. *Mikrobiyol Bul* 2007;41:211–7.
19. Jernigan DB, Hoffman J, Cetron MS, et al. Outbreak of legionnaires' disease among cruise ship passengers exposed to a contaminated whirlpool spa. *Lancet* 1996;347:494–9.
20. Castellani Pastoris M, Lo Monaco R, Goldoni P, et al. Legionnaires' disease on a cruise ship linked to the water supply system: Clinical and public health implications. *Clin Infect Dis* 1999;28:33–8.
21. Nakadate T, Yamauchi K, Inoue H. An outbreak of legionnaires' disease associated with a Japanese spa. *Nihon Kokyuki Gakkai Zasshi* 1999;37:601–7.
22. Lepine LA, Jernigan DB, Butler JC, et al. A recurrent outbreak of nosocomial legionnaires' disease detected by urinary antigen testing: Evidence for long-term colonization of a hospital plumbing system. *Infect Control Hosp Epidemiol* 1998;19:905–10.
23. Blatt SP, Parkinson MD, Pace E, et al. Nosocomial legionnaires' disease: Aspiration as a primary mode of disease acquisition. *Am J Med* 1995;95:16–22.
24. Kool JL, Fiore AE, Kioski CM, et al. More than 10 years of unrecognized nosocomial transmission of legionnaires' disease among transplant patients. *Infect Control Hosp Epidemiol* 1998;19:898–904.

25. Boccia S, Laurenti P, Borella P, et al. Prospective 3-year surveillance for nosocomial and environmental *Legionella pneumophila:* Implications for infection control. *Infect Control Hosp Epidemiol* 2006;27:459–65.

26. Jarraud S, Reyrolle M, Riffard S, et al. Legionnaires' disease in travelers. *Bull Soc Pathol Exot* 1998;95:486–9.

27. Rota MC, Caporali MG, Massari M, et al. European guidelines for control and prevention of travel associated legionnaires' disease: The Italian experience. *Euro Surveill* 2004;9:10–1.

28. Decludt B, Campese C, Lacoste M, et al. Clusters of travel associated legionnaires' disease in France, September 2001–August 2003. *Euro Surveill* 2004;9:12–3.

29. Kura F, Amemura-Maekawa J, Yagita K, et al. Outbreak of legionnaires' disease on a cruise ship linked to spa-bath filter stones contaminated with *Legionella pneumophila* serogroup 5. *Epidemiol Infect* 2006;134:385–91.

30. Rowbotham TJ. Legionellosis associated with ships: 1977 to 1997. *Commun Dis Public Health* 1998;1:146–51.

31. Nakamura H, Yagyu H, Kishi K, et al. A large outbreak of legionnaires' disease due to an inadequate circulating and filtration system for bath water: Epidemiologic manifestations. *Intern Med* 2003;42:806–11.

32. Okada M, Kawano K, Kura F, et al. The largest outbreak of legionellosis in Japan associated with spa baths: Epidemic curve and environmental investigation. *Kansenshogaku Zasshi* 2005;79:365–74.

33. Isozumi R, Ito Y, Ito I, et al. An outbreak of *Legionella* pneumonia originating from a cooling tower. *Scand J Infect Dis* 2005;37:709–11.

34. Allen KW, Prempeh H, Osman MS. *Legionella* pneumonia from a novel industrial aerosol. *Commun Dis Public Health* 1999;2:294–6.

35. Cayla JA, Maldonado R, Gonzalez J, et al. A small outbreak of legionnaires' disease in a cargo ship under repair. *Eur Respir J* 2001;17:1322–7.

36. Ruscoe Q, Hill S, Blackmore T, et al. An outbreak of *Legionella pneumophila* suspected to be associated with spa pools on display at a retail store in New Zealand. *N Z Med J* 2006;119:U2253.

37. Outbreak of legionnaires' disease among automotive plant workers—Ohio, 2001. *MMWR* 2001;50:357–8.

38. Faris B, Faris C, Schousboe M, et al. Legionellosis from *Legionella pneumophia* serogroup 13. *Emerg Infect Dis* 2005;11:405-9.

39. Osterholm MT, Chin TD, Osborne DO, et al. A 1957 outbreak of legionnaires' disease associated with a meat packing plant. *Am J Epidemiol* 1983;117:60–7.

40. Fabbi M, Pastoris MC, Scanziani E, et al. Epidemiological and environmental investigations of *Legionella pneumophila* infection in cattle and case report of fatal pneumonia in a calf. *J Clin Microbiol* 1998;36:1942–7.

41. Ricketts K, Joseph C, European Working Group for *Legionella* Infections Health Protection Agency. Travel associated legionnaires' disease in Europe: 2002. *Euro Surveill* 2004;9:6–9.

42. Ricketts K, Joseph C, European Working Group for *Legionella* Infections. Legionnaires' disease in Europe, 2003–2004. *Euro Surveill* 2005;10:256–9.

43. Cano R, Prieto N, Martin C, et al. Legionnaires' disease clusters associated with travel to Spain during the period January 2001 to July 2003. *Euro Surveill* 2004;9:14–5.

44. Ricketts KD, McNaught B, Joseph CA, et al. Travel-associated legionnaires' disease in Europe: 2004. *Euro Surveill* 2006;11:107–10.

45. U.S. Centers for Disease Control and Prevention. Travel-associated legionnaires' disease: Common questions and answers for health departments. Legionellosis Resource Site (Legionnaires' Disease and Pontiac Fever), September 27, 2006. Available at www.cdc.gov/legionella/faq.htm.

46. Perkins BA, Relman D. Explaining the unexplained in clinical infectious diseases: Looking forward. *Emerg Infect Dis* 1998;4:395–7.

47. Francis JS, Doherty MC, Lopatin U, et al. Severe community-onset pneumonia in healthy adults caused by methicillin-resistant *Staphylococcus aureus* carrying the Panton-Valentine leukocidin genes. *Clin Infect Dis* 2005;40:100–7.

48. Roberts JC, Gulino SP, Peak KK, et al. Fatal necrotizing pneumonia due to Panton-Valentine leukocidin positive community-associated MRSA and influenza co-infection: A case report. *Ann Clin Microbiol Antibiocrob* 2008;7:5.

49. U.S. Centers for Disease Control and Prevention. Patient facts: Learn more about legionnaires' disease. Legionellosis Resource Site (Legoinnaires' Disease and Pontiac Fever), September 27, 2006. Available at *www.cdc.gov/legionella/patinet_facts.htm.*

50. Summary of notifiable diseases—United States, 2004. *MMWR* 2006;53:1–79.

51. Summary of notifiable diseases—United States, 2005. *MMWR* 2007;54:2–92.

52. Hespers BL, Bossink AW, Cohen-Stuart JW, et al. A patient with *Legionella pneumophila* sergroup 3 pneumonia detected by PCR. *Ned Tijdschr Geneeskd* 2005;149:2009–12.

53. Chen CY, Chen KY, Hsueh PR, et al. Severe community-acquired pneumonia due to *Legionella pneumophila* serogroup 6. *J Formos Med Assoc* 2006;105:256–62.

54. McNally C, Hackman B, Fields BS, et al. Potential importance of *Legionella* species as etiologies in community acquired pneumonia (CAP). *Diagn Microbiol Infect Dis* 2000;38:79–82.

55. Chedid MB, Ilha Dde O, Chedid MF, et al. Community-acquired pneumonia by *Legionella pneumophila* serogroups 1–6 in Brazil. *Respir Med* 2005;99:966–75.

56. Tang PW, Toma S. Broad-spectrum enzyme linked

immunosorbent assay for detection of *Legionella* soluble antigens. *J Clin Microbiol* 1986;24:556–8.

57. Marrie TJ, Raoult D, La Scola B, et al. *Legionella*-like and other amoebal pathogens as agents of community-acquired pneumonia. *Emerg Infect Dis* 2001;7:1026–9.

58. Greub G, Raoult D. Parachlamydiaceae: Potential emerging pathogens. *Emerg Infect Dis* 2002;8:625–30.

59. La Scola B, Boyadjiev I, Greub G, et al. Amoeba-resisting bacteria and ventilator-associated pneumonia. *Emerg Infect Dis* 2003;9:815–21.

60. Treatment guidelines from The Medical Letter: Choice of antibiotics. *Med Lett* 2007;5:35–8.

61. Stout JE, Yu VL. Experience of the first 16 hospitals using copper-silver ionization for *Legionella* control: Implications for evaluation of other disinfection modalities. *Infect Control Hosp Epidemiol* 2003;24:563–8.

62. Allegheny County Health Department. *Approaches to Prevention and Control of Legionella Infections in Allegheny County Health Care Facilities.* Pittsburgh: Allegheny County Health Department, 1997.

63. The American Society of Heating, Refrigeration, and Air Conditioning Engineers (ASHRAE). Minimizing the Risk of Legionellosis Associated with Building Water Systems, Guideline 12-2000. Available at www.ashrae.org.

64. World Health Organization. Rolling Revision of the WHO Guidelines for Drinking-Water Quality (draft): Guide to Ship Sanitation. Geneva: WHO, October 2004. Available at www.who.org.

65. Cruise ship-associated legionnaires' disease, November 2003–May 2004. *MMWR* 2005;54:1153–5

11A

Occupational Influenza: Recent Update

William E. Wright

This is a status report or synopsis of current and emerging issues regarding influenza and occupations. This update is presented because information on influenza is evolving rapidly, particularly related to avian influenza, pandemic flu preparedness, recent vaccines, vaccine development issues, and antiviral treatment.

The editor and publisher, not wanting to tamper with excellence, also have reprinted the original, comprehensive first-edition chapter entitled, "Occupational Influenza," by Dr. Daymon Evans, with that author's current second-edition revisions (Chapter 11B). That chapter provides a detailed background and history of influenza that is important for all occupational health practitioners to know. It also addresses virus nomenclature; characteristics of past pandemics and their viral strains; basic issues of influenza prevention, control, and education; and background on vaccines and treatment. It also sets the stage for what is added here regarding recent events and information related to influenza, recent and current vaccines, antiviral treatment considerations, concerns about H5N1 avian flu, and preparations for pandemic flu. Additional information on pandemic influenza can be found in Chapter 37.

2008 Update

As Dr. Evans noted in his first-edition chapter 8 years ago, concern about the next influenza pandemic is not *if* it will occur but *when*. Since the first edition of this book was published, there has been an increasing awareness that the stage may be set for another pandemic influenza. The current concern relates to the expanding presence of a particularly lethal A/H5N1 avian influenza virus [1–3]. Presence of this pathogen in chickens in Asia resulted in the killing of many millions of chickens in contaminated flocks in an attempt to limit its spread. Despite these efforts, and owing in part to humans living closely with chickens in parts of Asia, by 2005, outbreaks occurred in humans (in Thailand, Cambodia, Vietnam, Indonesia, and China). The mortality in these cases was about 50%. The population mortality rate may be lower depending on how well cases of mild or inapparent infection are identified. In early 2006, human cases were identified in Turkey, signifying a spread westward. In response to concern about worldwide spread of the virus through flyways by migratory birds such as ducks, in which the pathogen is not lethal, the Food and Agriculture Organization of the United Nations advised countries along migratory pathways to be on alert and noted concerns about the spread of avian flu through bird trafficking and commerce involving poultry products from endemic countries [4]. At the time of this writing, in February 2008, the World Health Organization

(WHO) has reported a total of 360 laboratory-confirmed human cases of avian influenza A(H5N1) that resulted in 226 deaths (62.8% mortality). About 64% of cases have occurred in Indonesia and Viet Nam, about 12% in Egypt, about 8% in China, 7% in Thailand, 3% in Turkey, 2% in Azerbaijan, 2% in Cambodia, and the remainder in Iraq, Lao People's Democratic Republic, Djibouti, Myanmar, Nigeria, and Pakistan [5].

Although this H5N1 avian influenza virus has high lethality, so far it appears to be inefficiently transmitted among humans. By early 2006, only two cases of human-to-human transmission had been identified in close-contact, high-exposure situations [6]. Later that year, in Indonesia, an initial case in a family was related to contact with infected poultry, and a total of eight family members were infected, with seven deaths occurring. Since then clusters of human cases have ranged from two to eight cases, nearly all among family members living in the same household [7]. Clustering of human cases in areas heavily populated by avian species makes it difficult to distinguish multiple-person sequential avian exposure from human-to-human transmission. Although the main route of exposure to H5N1 is respiratory and predominantly through poultry/birds, human family member transmission is likely through droplets or droplet nuclei, and two confirmed H5N1 cases were attributed to drinking uncooked blood of a duck. Although the clinical presentation is typically that of usual severe influenza, a confirmed H5N1 case in a child presented with a clinical picture of encephalitis with fever, headache, and diarrhea.

The evolutionary step that is anticipated with foreboding is that co-infection with seasonal human influenza virus and H5N1 avian influenza virus in humans or pigs (the two "mixing bowls" for human and other influenza viruses) will permit sufficient intermingling and recombinations of the genetic material of these viruses to generate a shift to a new pathogen that shares the avian H5N1's virulence and the traditional seasonal human influenza's high transmissibility. For the current H5N1 avian influenza virus of concern, this is the only step now lacking to achieve a pandemic. If this does not happen with this H5N1 form of avian influenza, other pathogenic avian influenza strains also have the potential to emerge in pandemic form (e.g., H7N2, H7N3, H7N7, and H9N2). More de-tails regarding avian influenza are covered in Chapter 37.

An indicator that the threat of pandemic influenza is being taken more seriously than previously in the United States is the recent Executive Order that added "influenza caused by novel or reemergent influenza viruses that are causing, or have the potential to cause, a pandemic" to the U.S. Centers for Disease Control and Prevention (CDC) list of quarantinable communicable diseases [8]. Influenza, a historic killer of huge dimensions, rightfully joins the ranks of other "classic" killers on the list, including cholera, diphtheria, infectious tuberculosis, plague, smallpox, yellow fever, and viral hemmorhagic fevers (all listed 1983) and severe acute respiratory syndrome (SARS, listed 2003).

Occupational Issues

Given the lethality and spread of the avian influenza virus H5N1, the CDC and other national and international agencies, including the WHO, are encouraging development of disaster plans to provide containment of point occurrences of lethal influenza and anticipate occupational and social disruptions in the event of more global spread [9–13]. Details of the U.S. Department of Health and Human Services (HHS) Pandemic Influenza Plan have been published [14]. The plan outlines strategies for businesses, governments, and other entities for pandemic influenza planning. It includes four tiers of priority for occupational and nonoccupational groups to receive antiviral treatment. The occupational groups, that is, essential health care workers, vaccine and antiviral manufacturers, key government leaders, and pandemic responders, are included in the first-priority tier, along with the highest-risk persons (based on age and underlying disease), pregnant women, and household contacts of the very young (<6 months old) and severely immunocompromised. The second tier of priority includes occupational groups (i.e., critical infrastructure and other pandemic responders), along with other high-risk persons. The third tier covers key government health decision makers and mortuary workers. The fourth tier is unrelated to occupation. It covers healthy people from ages 2–64 who are not in other, higher-priority groups.

Occupational physicians and other occupational health care providers need to be involved in the design and implementation of disaster plans for businesses, communities, and governments related to severe or pandemic influenza. Education and training of employee populations are very important. Activities also include encouraging and carrying out influenza vaccination programs, supporting personal and administrative practices that prevent transmission of influenza, using prophylactic and postexposure treatments optimally, and assisting in planning sustainable operations with a work force diminished by illness in a setting of potential breakdown of supply and distribution chains. Employers may need medical support and advice on reasonable and effective absence and return-to-work policies and leave policies for employees providing home care to ill relatives. Medical decision-making support related to plans for shifting some employees' work assignments to respond to a pandemic, shifting workloads to areas less affected by illness, and using telecommuting technology also may be needed.

The occupational physician also may be called on to help plan and implement cohorting of sick individuals (i.e., keeping influenza victims in the same, limited area of a health care facility), isolation procedures (i.e., separation and restriction of movements of people with specific infectious illness from healthy workers) and serve as liaisons to the CDC and state and local government plans for implementing orders for quarantine (i.e., separation and restriction of movements of people exposed to an infectious agent, not yet ill, who may become infectious). The current CDC recommendation for duration of quarantine for pandemic influenza is for one incubation period. The incubation period for seasonal influenza is generally up to 4 days, but the incubation period for a new pandemic influenza virus is not yet known.

Part of the occupational health role also involves communication and support to address the broader social issues that may occur with widespread severe or pandemic influenza. These include lack of well workers to provide basic services (e.g., health care, mortuary services, law enforcement services, transportation, and distribution of food, fuel, water, electricity, and other essential commodities and services); closure of schools, businesses, and borders; and the resulting chaos and social upheaval. Occupational health preparation

for a pandemic includes planning responses not only for sustainable business, social stability, and care of influenza victims but also for surges of people who fear they are infected but are not. The capacity of occupational and other health service facilities to handle the surge of ill and worried people may be one of the weakest links in preparedness for an influenza pandemic.

When a pandemic occurs, many employees may experience isolation, fear, anger, stress, grief, and exhaustion. The HHS Pandemic Influenza Plan includes a very useful section on psychosocial support of the work force related to a pandemic period. This supplement addresses psychosocial support for health care providers and other occupational groups (including disaster response workers and their families), implementation of work force resilience programs, and the importance of behavioral health responses and resources during pandemic and postpandemic periods [15].

Personal Protection and Practices

Extensive data on the efficacy of using respirators, face masks, and other personal protection for influenza and influenza pandemics are lacking. However, given the potential lethality of pandemic influenza, certain personal precautions are prudent, particularly in health care settings during pandemics. Based on information that influenza transmission occurs largely from exposure to respiratory large particles (droplets > 5 μm), the WHO has recommended recently that health care providers use surgical masks when working within 3 ft of patients who are considered potentially infected with pandemic influenza. Because studies cannot exclude the possibility that influenza can be transmitted through small-particle aerosols (droplet nuclei) at distances over 3 ft, the WHO recommends use of respirators (i.e., N-95 or a comparable alternative) when involved in medical procedures that may generate aerosols (e.g., endotracheal intubation, bronchoscopy, suctioning the upper respiratory track or airways, and nebulizer treatments). The recommendations also support discarding masks and respirators after leaving the patient or after seeing multiple influenza patients in one room. The WHO recommends hand washing with either soap and water or alcohol-based preparations after each encounter with a patient, before seeing a patient, and after discarding a respirator or mask [16].

HHS also has published new guidelines for personal protection in health care workplaces [17]. These guidelines for pandemic situations are evolving. They support use of respirators and masks (as noted by WHO). They also recommend single-use gloves for contact with body fluids and respiratory secretions, goggles or face shields if spray or splatter of infectious materials is likely, and single-use isolation gowns if soiling with body fluids or respiratory secretions is anticipated. The guidelines also mention potential for virus transmission by fomites or direct contact; warn against touching eyes, nose, or mouth with contaminated gloves or hands; support use of standard hospital environmental cleaning; and emphasize the importance of hand hygiene. Use of soap or antimicrobial soap and water is recommended if hands are visibly soiled with respiratory secretions. Soap and water or alcohol-based cleaners are recommended for hand washing in other situations.

The guidelines also recommend that during an influenza pandemic health care workplaces monitor the work force for illness and manage those who have symptoms or are ill. Management includes screening employees before they come on duty, sending employees home if they are ill or have symptoms, keeping ill employees off work until they are physically able to return to duty, offering administrative or alternate duties (away from influenza patient care areas) to those who are at high risk for complications of pandemic influenza (e.g., pregnant and immunocompromised employees), and prioritizing health care workers who have recovered from pandemic influenza for care of active pandemic influenza patients.

A recent study focused on attitudes about influenza prevention related to the 2003–2004 influenza season in the United States. Of those who sought medical attention for influenza-like illness (ILI) about 8% were asked to wear a mask at their health care provider's office. More than 80% said they would wear a mask while waiting at a doctor's office or hospital [18]. The efficacy of having ill or well people in workplaces and community settings wear masks to control the spread of pandemic influenza has not been established. The HHS guidelines recommend procedure or surgical masks for patients with respiratory symptoms entering health

care facilities. Masks are also suggested as a matter of personal choice for people with respiratory symptoms in community settings, as well as for well people, particularly those at high risk of influenza complications.

In non–health care occupational settings during influenza pandemics, it is recommended to keep those with respiratory illness away until well; encourage respiratory hygiene/cough etiquette (e.g., covering nose and mouth with tissues or sleeve at the elbow while coughing and sneezing); have easily accessible tissues, tissue disposal, and hand-washing materials; and use good hand hygiene.

In addition to the HHS guidelines, many organizations have developed pandemic preparedness programs. The overall goal is to not just address influenza, but to strengthen worldwide surveillance, public health systems, and planning and response capabilities that can be applied to epidemic and pandemic microbiologic threats. The WHO is a resource on pandemic preparedness worldwide, and the CDC Web site (*www.cdc.gov*) lists many evolving resources for pandemic flu and disaster preparedness and has a program to help developing countries with pandemic preparedness [9–13]. Many nations have organized programs to meet local needs and coordinate internationally.

Vaccine Update

Annual vaccination continues to be the most effective way to prevent infection and complications from influenza A and B. The efficacy of inactivated influenza vaccine in preventing influenza is about 80% but varies each year according to drifts and shifts in antigenicity of ambient strains and how well they match the strains selected for the annual vaccine. Despite media attention, some people still refrain from getting the vaccine.

The occupational physician has a role in educating employees about influenza vaccination, including benefits, limitations, and risks. Despite heightened awareness about influenza and a potential pandemic, studies of elderly people, a group at increased risk for hospitalization and death from influenza, have documented a reduction in the proportion vaccinated [19]. Some reasons given for not getting vaccinated include not knowing the vaccination was needed, concern that the vaccination might cause influenza or side effects, thinking it would not prevent influenza, thinking they were not at risk, and lack of available vaccine owing to shortages. These data were not representative of any work population but may reflect notions among the general public that could be targets for employee education and training.

The U.S. Food and Drug Administration (FDA) makes recommendations for influenza vaccine content for the U.S. influenza seasons. Composition of influenza vaccines in other countries may vary from these recommendations, particularly in the southern hemisphere. The viral contents of the influenza vaccines recommended for the United States since the first edition of this book are shown in Table 11A-1. For the recent influenza seasons in

Table 11A-1
Influenza Virus Vaccines: Recently Targeted Antigens for Influenza Vaccine Production in the United States

Season	Antigen Types in Vaccine*
2000–2001	A/New Caledonia/20/99(H1N1)-like A/Moscow/10/99(H3N2)-like B/Beijing/184/93-like
2001–2002	A/New Caledonia/20/99(H1N1)-like A/Moscow/10/99(H3N2)-like B/Sichuan/379/99-like
2002–2003	A/New Caledonia/20/99(H1N1)-like A/Moscow/10/99(H3N2)-like B/Hong Kong/330/2001-like
2003–2004	A/New Caledonia/20/99(H1N1)-like A/Moscow/10/99(H3N2)-like B/Hong Kong/330/2001-like
2004–2005	A/New Caledonia/20/99(H1N1) A/Wyoming/03/2003(H3N2) B/Shanghai/361/2002-like
2005–2006	A/New Caledonia/20/99(H1N1)-like A/California/7/2003(H3N2)-like B/Shanghai/361/2002-like
2006–2007	A/New Caledonia/20/99(H1N1)-like A/Wisconsin/67/2005-like(H3N2)-like B/Malaysia/2506/2004-like
2007–2008	A/Solomon Islands/3/2006(H1N1)-like A/Wisconsin/67/2005/H3N2-like B/Malaysia/2506/2004-like
2008–2009[†]	A/Brisbane/59/2007(H1N1)-like A/Brisbane/10/2007(H3N3)-like B/Florida/4/2006-like

*For nomenclature rules, see Chapter 11B.
[†]Recommended 02/21/08 by the U.S. FDA's Vaccines and Related Biological Products Advisory Committee (VRBPAC).
Note: Information in this table is derived from season lot release statements from the U.S. Food and Drug Administration, *www.fda.gov.* Southern hemisphere vaccine virus antigens may differ from those shown herein.

the United States, vaccines have included three inactivated split-virus vaccines (Fluarix by GlaxoSmithKline, Fluvirin by Novartis, and Fluzone by Sanofi-Pasteur) for intramuscular injection (0.5-mL dose in deltoid) and one live attenuated influenza virus (LAIV) vaccine (FluMist by MedImmune) for intranasal use (0.5-mL sprayer for giving 0.25 mL in each nostril) [20, 21]. The 2007–2008 vaccines included these as well as inactivated split-virus vaccines Afluria (CSL Biotherapies) and FluLaval (GlaxoSmithKline) [22].

FluMist, which was first approved for use in children, is now approved for use in healthy (not having an underlying medical condition that predisposes them to influenza complications), nonpregnant people in the 5- to 49-year-old range. The age range for FluMist covers part of the common occupational age range, but the approved range does not cover those individuals who are at greatest risk for complications of influenza. In 2007, the recommendation for use of LAIV also included healthy children aged 2–4 years without a history of asthma or recurrent wheezing [23]. FluMist is not recommended for people who are immunocompromised or people with chronic heart, lung, kidney, or metabolic diseases. The LAIV vaccine mimics a natural infection in the nasal passages and can result in rhinorrhea, headache, sore throat, and cough in adults. After vaccination, children can experience rhinorrhea, congestion, headache, fever, chills, muscle aches, sore throat, cough, wheezing, and exacerbation of asthma. Owing to a theoretical risk of transmitting the live attenuated virus, it is recommended that those who receive FluMist avoid contact with immunosuppressed people for 7 days after vaccination. The live and inactivated vaccines for influenza may contain traces of egg protein and have a potential to evoke a hypersensitivity reaction [20]. In clinical studies, transmission of vaccine virus to close contacts has occurred only rarely [24]. The CDC and FDA's Vaccine Adverse Event Reporting System (VAERS) can be reached at 1-800-822-7967 or www.vaers.hhs.gov. This reporting service does not included advice on treatment. The United States has created a federal program to help pay for care for those who are harmed by vaccines. The National Vaccine Injury Compensation Program can be contacted at 1-800-338-2382; the website is at www.hrsa.gov/vaccinecompensation.

Recently in the United States, there has been concern that the mercury from thimerosal in some of the vaccines may be related to autism. The current scientific information has not supported mercury from thimerosal-containing vaccine and immune globulins being causally related to deficits in neuropsychological functioning [22, 25]. Of the available influenza vaccines for the 2007–2008 season, the multidose vials have the highest mercury content per individual 0.5-mL dose (about 24.5–25 μg per dose), the prefilled individual-dose syringes have less than 1 μg per dose or none, and the available LAIV has none [22].

The influenza A strains for the 2005–2006 U.S. vaccines were based on a newly selected H3N2 virus (A/California/7/2004 or its antigenic equivalent) and an H1N1 virus (A/New Caledonia/20/99). The influenza B strain is B/Jiangsu/10/2003. The latter two were used in the 2004–2005 vaccine. The 2004–2005 vaccine contained the H3N2 strain A/Wyoming/3/2003, which is antigenically equivalent to a Fujian type of H3N2 that caused severe illness in children in the 2003–2004 season owing to antigenic drift from the H3N2 that was included in that season's vaccine [20,26]. The 2006–2007 vaccine retained the H1N1 New Caledonia strain and substituted a new H3N2 A/Wisconsin/67/2005-like and a new B/Malaysia/2506/2004-like viral strain [27]. The 2007–2008 vaccine changed the H1N1 antigen to A/Solomon Islands/3/2006-like [28].

In the United States, the 2007–2008 flu season started out with primarily H1N1 infections and then shifted to predominantly H3N2 infections that were not well covered by the seasonal vaccine. By mid-February 2008, 49 states had widespread influenza activity (Table 11A-2 lists activity level definitions), primarily influenza A (about 82%), with the influenza A viral isolates being predominantly H3 viruses (about 66%). Of the H3 isolates, only 16% matched the A/Wisconsin isolate in the seasonal vaccine, and 79% were A/Brisbane/10/2007-like (used in the 2008 southern hemisphere vaccine), which was an antigenic variant that evolved from the A/Wisconsin strain on which the U.S. vaccine was based [29]. This is a example of the natural drifting of the influenza viruses that can lead some vaccinees to think that the vaccine does not work. The 2008–2009 vaccine for the United States has been recommended to contain three new antigens to adjust to the shifting picture of in-

Table 11A-2
Geographic Levels of Spread of Influenza, United States

Activity levels and definitions:

No activity: No laboratory-confirmed cases and no reported increase in the number of ILI cases.

Sporadic: Small numbers of laboratory-confirmed cases or a single laboratory-confirmed outbreak of influenza, but no reported increase in cases of ILI.

Local: Outbreaks of influenza or increases in ILI cases and recent laboratory-confirmed influenza in a single region of the state.

Regional: Outbreaks of influenza or increases in ILI cases and recent laboratory-confirmed influenza in at least two but less than half the regions in a state.

Widespread: Outbreaks of influenza or increases in ILI cases and recent laboratory-confirmed influenza in at least half the regions in a state.

Source: U.S. Centers for Disease Prevention and Control. Seasonal Flu, Flu Activity and Surveillance, Reports and Surveillance Methods in the United States, Overview of Influenza Surveillance in the United States, February 29, 2008; available at www.cdc.gov/flu/weekly/fluactivity.htm.

fluenza activity: H1N1 A/Brisbane/59/2007-like, H3N2 A/Brisbane/10/2007-like, and B-Florida/4/2006-like [30]. Shortages of influenza vaccine occurred in the 2004–2005 season owing to temporary suspension of the license of one of the vaccine manufacturers. For the 2005–2006 season, a tiered approach for use of the inactivated influenza vaccine was recommended, taking into account potential shortages of vaccine [31,32]. Priority for adults includes health care workers, those at high risk of influenza complications (e.g., pregnant women in any trimester, people 65 years of age and older, and younger adults with chronic medical conditions), and household contacts or caregivers of infants. After reaching child and adult priority groups, the CDC recommended vaccination of everyone, particularly all adults aged 50 years or older. The occupational health physician should encourage pregnant employees to discuss influenza vaccination with their obstetricians [33]. The 2007 summation in *The Medical Letter* regarding their consultants' opinion is, "Everyone ≥ 6 months old without a contraindication should be vaccinated against influenza" [22].

There is no commercially available influenza vaccine for humans for avian influenza, but some lots of H5N1 influenza vaccine have been made for clinical trials and are included in the U.S. Strategic National Stockpile for use if the current H5N1 strain develops the capacity to be efficiently transmitted among humans. Provisionally, the dose schedule is two intramuscular injections a month apart. It is not known whether the N1 component of the H1N1 seasonal influenza vaccine will confer any protection against avian influenza, but some recent information suggests that some degree of protection may occur [34, 35] (see Chapter 37).

Antiviral Treatment Update

In the past, the adamantanes amantadine and rimantadine, inhibitors of the influenza virus's M2 ion channel, have been effective for treatment and prophylaxis of influenza A. They are not active against influenza B. Their record of success has included preventing influenza A illness in 70–90% of patients when started before exposure and continued for up to 6–8 weeks of the exposure period and shortening the duration of illness when taken within 48 hours of onset of illness [36].

In 2006, the CDC issued a health advisory recommending against the use of adamantanes for either treatment or prophylaxis of influenza during the 2005–2006 season [37]. This advice was based on the emergence of drug resistance related to point mutations in amino acids of the M2 protein that confer cross-resistance to amantadine and rimantadine. Adamantine resistance in the United States has reflected global trends. The U.S. prevalence of resistant influenza grew from 1.9% in 2004 to 14.5% during the 2004–2005 influenza season. In the 2005–2006 season, 91% of influenza A H3N2 virus isolates from 23 states in the United States were noted to be resistant to both drugs. At the time of this writing, for the 2007–2008 influenza season in the United States, the overall resistance of current-season influenza A isolates was 24%, with resistance among H3N2 strains being 98.9% and among H1N1 strains being 4.7%. Based on this, use of amantadine and rimantadine was not recommended for prevention or treatment of influenza [29].

When amantadine and rimantadine are appropriate for use in influenza A treatment or prophylaxis, the usual adult doses for each are 100 mg PO bid and 200 mg PO daily, respectively. The dose of amanadine should be reduced to 100 mg daily for people with reduced kidney function (CrCl < 50 mL/min) and in people 65 years of age and older. The dose of rimantadine should be reduced to this

level for people 65 years of age and older and for people with severe hepatic or renal failure [36].

The CDC 2006 advisory against the use of amantadine and rimantidine noted that all influenza viruses in the United States tested for resistance to adamantanes were susceptible to neuraminidase inhibitors. Therefore, the inhibitors of the influenza neuraminidase enzyme, namely, oseltamivir (Tamiflu, tablet, Roche) and zanamivir (Relenza, inhaled powder, GlaxoSmithKline), were recommended in situations in which antiviral prophylaxis and treatment were needed [37]. In Asia, viral resistance to oseltamivir has been reported in up to 18% of people being treated with it for H3N2 influenza A [38]. Further studies are needed to define whether the resistant virus is spread from person to person and whether it is still sensitive to zanamivir. Viral resistance to drug treatment may vary from region to region. Web sites at the CDC are updated as information on drug resistance evolves [39,40]. For the 2007–2008 influenza season, as of the date of this writing, the overall resistance of influenza virus isolates in the United States to neuraminidase inhibitors was 6.8%, the resistance being found in A(H1N1) viruses, 9.6% of which had a genetic mutation conferring resistance to oseltamivir. This type of resistance was seen sporadically in a number of surveillance areas but did not affect A(H3N2) or B influenza virus isolates. None of the isolates of influenza A or B were resistant to zanamivir. Based on these data, the CDC continued to recommend use of oseltamivir and zanimivir for prevention and treatment of influenza [29].

Similar to the past record of adamantanes, the neuraminidase inhibitors can prevent influenza in 60–90% of patients to whom they are given for preexposure and postexposure prophylaxis. They have the advantage over adamantanes of working against both influenza A and B. The neuraminidase inhibitors also can reduce the duration of influenza symptoms (by about 1–2 days), severity, and occurrence of complications if started within 48 hours of onset of the illness. As of early 2006, the FDA had approved zanamivir's role in influenza for treatment, not prophylaxis. Oseltamivir was approved for prophylaxis and treatment. The 2007–2008 recommendations include roles for treatment and prophylaxis with either zanamivir or oseltamivir. Utilization and dosage recommendations may change, so the reader should consult current prescribing information. At the time of this writing, the usual doses of oseltamivir for prophylaxis and treatment are 75 mg PO once daily and 75 mg PO bid, respectively. The doses need to be reduced to once every other day for prophylaxis and once daily for treatment when renal failure is present (CrCl = 10–30 mL/min). The dose for zanamivir is two 5-mg oral inhalations once daily [36], with no adjustment in dose for the presence of renal failure for a 5-day course [23]. An oral suspension form of oseltamivir is available; current recommendations should be checked for dosages of either of these medications for children. Employees who are pregnant should consult with their primary health care provider about the use of influenza antiviral drugs. All antiviral drugs mentioned here are classified as category C for use during pregnancy (see Chapter 33).

The most important way to prevent influenza occurrence is vaccination. The CDC recommends that people at high risk of complications from influenza be vaccinated even if an influenza outbreak has begun. If influenza virus is circulating, chemoprophylaxis can be given to people at high risk during the 2 weeks after vaccination, which is the typical period for adults to develop an adequate immune response to the vaccine. The same recommendation is made for people who care for or have frequent contact with those who are at high risk for complications of influenza. If influenza is being caused by a variant strain not likely to be covered by the vaccine, then these workers can be considered for chemoprophylaxis regardless of vaccination status. Chemoprophylaxis also should be considered for immunosuppressed people who are not likely to mount an adequate immune response to the vaccine and health care workers with direct care responsibilities who are unable to get vaccine [41]. The CDC does not recommend use of influenza antivirals for people in the community who are not at high risk when supplies of vaccine and antiviral drugs are insufficient to meet the demands for those at high risk.

Antiviral drugs are not recognized to interfere with the efficacy of inactivated influenza vaccines but can interfere with the efficacy of LAIV. Current recommendations are that antiviral drugs should not be given from 2 days prior to LAIV administration to at least 2 weeks or more after the vaccina-

tion [42]. Amantidine and rimantadine do not protect against most H5N1 viral strains, but neuraminidase inhibitors have been effective in animal studies, and some authorities consider them to be options for prophylaxis or early treatment of human H5N1 influenza. However, effective dosages are not known [42].

Diagnosing Influenza

Influenza-like illness (ILI) is common. Influenza shares symptoms and clinical presentation with a number of other respiratory pathogens. Influenza A and B cannot be distinguished from each other based on clinical presentation and symptoms. Most diagnoses of influenza are made clinically (based on abrupt onset of an illness consisting of some combination of fever, nonproductive cough, sore throat, aches, headache, rhinitis, and malaise), without testing, during periods of influenza activity in the community or region. Sensitivity and specificity of symptoms, such as fever and cough, for influenza vary depending on influenza activity in the community and the circulation of other respiratory pathogens. In studies of adults, the sensitivity and specificity of fever and cough symptoms compared with viral culture results for influenza have ranged from about 55–75% [43].

The laboratory standard for diagnosis of influenza is viral culture. Results of culture generally take 5–10 days, but some recently improved methods may take only 2 days. Acute and convalescent sera drawn 2–4 weeks apart can be useful in epidemiologic monitoring but are less useful for clinical decision making owing to the time to get results. Immunofluorescent tests and enzyme immunoassays are available in some laboratories and provide results regarding influenza A and B detection in several hours. A number of rapid diagnostic tests are available that give results in about 30 minutes. These have varying levels of sensitivity, specificity, and predictive value. Generally, sensitivity may be 70% or more and specificity 90% or more. Up to 30% of negative tests may be falsely negative. Results are more likely to be falsely negative if done on specimens that are inadequate or inappropriate. Specimens from nasopharyngeal aspirates, swabs, or washes tend to be favored over throat swabs. None of the rapid tests can identify the strain of influenza, but some can distinguish between influenza A and

B. The rapid tests are most useful when support for a decision regarding antiviral treatment needs to be made [44] (see also Chapter 2).

The CDC provides evolving guidance on influenza diagnostic testing and characteristics of rapid diagnostic tests [45]. Some can be used in an office setting with a certificate of waiver (CLIA-waived test) or laboratory certification. Many other rapid tests are complex enough to require specific laboratory certification.

Other Emerging Issues

As part of containment and disaster planning, emerging strategies include expanding and upgrading vaccine production technology (e.g., using recombinant technology) and improving vaccine technology to provide broader protection. The current one-egg, one-dose technology for vaccine production relies on a finite supply of eggs, can be subject to contamination, gives narrow protection, and involves a 9-month cycle just for production of seasonal influenza vaccine. Vaccine for a new pandemic strain likely would require significantly more antigen per dose that the 15 μg per strain in the seasonal vaccine. A multidose vaccination schedule may be needed to achieve protection from a pandemic influenza. Debate in the United States is ongoing about whether to forego production of a seasonal vaccine in order to produce large amounts of vaccine based on the avian H5N1 virus or other emerging pandemic strain for human use. The utility of this approach is unclear because no pandemic strain has yet been isolated, its characteristics for vaccine production are not known, and it is unknown whether a vaccine based on this avian strain would have clinical efficacy in a pandemic.

Other areas of investigation include assessing antibody response and clinical efficacy of intradermal administration of vaccine and reduction of the standard dose of antigen. These approaches may maintain or improve immunogenicity of vaccine while stretching the available supply [20]. Work has been done related to pharmacologic means of increasing concentrations of the prodrug oseltamivir's active metabolite Ro 64 0802 so that less oseltamivir can be used per dose. The metabolite is excreted by glomerular filtration and active tubular secretion. Probenecid can increase the systemic concentration

about 2.5-fold [46]. The clinical implications and efficacy of this finding are not yet clear.

Possibly more important than the technologies related to vaccines and drugs is how limited supplies of these materials are distributed globally. National and personal stockpiling of vaccines and antiviral drugs can lead to their maldistribution so that the materials are not available where they will have the greatest effect in pandemic situations. For instance, efforts are planned or ongoing to contain the H5N1 avian influenza virus at its source during early outbreaks of human illness in Asia and other regions, when feasible. This approach may be important for containing a pandemic influenza virus, but it requires prompt, sometimes large-scale responses with adequate supplies of antiviral materials.

Conclusion

Influenza continues to be a significant public health problem, resulting in morbidity and mortality that affect the general population, including the workplace. Approaches to the problem are evolving rapidly. When pandemic influenza occurs again, it likely will produce very challenging problems for the workplace and for society globally. The current global focus on pandemic influenza, with emphasis on prevention, containment, and planning, reflects awareness of the impact on population morbidity and mortality that influenza pandemics can bring. Many lives depend on the scale and effectiveness of this focus being sufficient in the workplace and society generally to avert or mitigate the threat. This update refers to a number of sources that can help occupational health practitioners prepare for seasonal influenza and pandemic influenza. Other resources are listed at the end of this update and in the revised and comprehensive first-edition chapter that follows.

References

1. Lewis DB. Avian flu to human influenza. *Annu Rev Med* 2006;57:139–54.
2. Wong SS, Yuen KY. Avian influenza virus infections in humans. *Chest* 2006;129:156–68.
3. Wu TZ, Huang LM. Avian influenza. *Chang Gung Med J* 2005;28:753–7.
4. Food and Agriculture Organization of the United Nations, Rome, Italy. Avian Influenza Control and Eradication. FAO's Proposal for a Global Pro-

gramme, January 2006; dDraft available at avian influenza sites at www.fao.org.

5. Cumulative Number of Confirmed Human Cases of Avain Influenza A/(H5N1) Reported to WHO, February 12, 2008; available at www.who.int/csr/disease/avian_influenza/country/cases_table_2008_02_12/en/.

6. Gellin B. Avian Influenza. Presentation at George Washington University Medical Center, January 18, 2006.

7. U.S. Centers for Disease Control and Prevention. Avian Influenza: Current H5N1 Situation, June 15, 2007; available at www.cdc.gov/flu/avian/outbreaks/current.htm.

8. Bush, G.W. Amendment to E.O. 13295 Relating to Certain Influenza Viruses and Quarantinable Communicable Diseases, The White House, April 1, 2005.

9. World Health Organization. Pandemic Preparedness. Epidemic and Pandemic Alert and Response (EPR), 2008; available at www.who.int/csr/disease/influenza/pandemic/; other WHO pandemic preparedness resources also are found at this site.

10. Genscheimer KF, Meltzer MI, Postema AS, et al. Influenza Pandemic Preparedness. Emerging Infectious Diseases (serial online) 2003;9(12); available at www.cdc.gov/ncidod/EID/vol9no12/03-0289.htm.

11. World Health Organization. WHO Global Influenza Preparedness Plan: The Role of WHO and Recommendations for National Measures Before and During Pandemics, March 2005; available at www.who.int/csr/resources/publications/influenza/WHO_CDS_CSR_GIP_2005_5/en/index.html.

12. Lokuge B, Drahos P, Neville W. Pandemics, antiviral stockpiles and biosecurity in Australia: What about the generic option? Med J Aust 2006;185:16–20.

13. Tam T, Sciberras J, Mullington B, et al. Fortune favours the prepared mind: A national perspective on pandemic preparedness. Can J Public Health 2005;96:406–8.

14. U.S. Department of Health and Human Services. HHS Pandemic Influenza Plan[JKM1]; available at www.hhs.gov/pandemicflu/plan.

15. U.S. Department of Health and Human Services. HHS Pandemic Influenza Plan, Supplement 11: Workforce Support: Psychosocial Considerations and Information Needs[JKM2]; available at www.hhs.gov/pandemicflu/plan.

16. World Health Organization. WHO Clarification: Use of Masks by Health-Care Workers in Pandemic Settings, November 2005; related to WHO Global Influenza Preparedness Plan: The Role of WHO and Recommendations for National Measures Before and During Pandemics, March 2005.

17. U.S. Department of Health and Human Services, Centers for Disease Control and Prevention. Professional Guidelines, Supplement 4: Infection Control, January 2006; available at www.hhs.gov/pandemicflu/plan/pdf/S04.pdf.

18. Experiences with influenza-like illness and attitudes regarding influenza prevention—United States, 2003–2004 Influenza Season. MMWR 2004;53:1156–8.

19. Influenza vaccination and self-reported reasons for not receiving influenza vaccination among Medicare beneficiaries aged 65 years—United States, 1991–2002. MMWR 2004;53:1012–5.

20. Influenza vaccine 2005–2006. Med Lett Drugs Ther 2005;47:85–7.

21. Influenza vaccine 2006–2007. Med Lett Drugs Ther 2006;48:81–3.

22. Influenza vaccine 2007–2008. Med Lett Drugs Ther 2007;49:81–3.

23. U.S. Centers for Disease Control and Prevention. Prevention and control of influenza: Recommendations of the Advisory Committee on Immunization Practices (ACIP), October 24, 2007. MMWR 2007;13:1–54.

24. U.S. Centers for Disease Control and Prevention. Seasonal Flu, Key Facts About Seasonal Flu Vaccine, October 19, 2007.

25. Thompson WW, Price C, Goodson B, et al. Early thimerosal exposure and neuropsychological outcomes at 7 and 10 years. N Engl J Med 2007;357:1281–92.

26. Influenza vaccine 2004–2005. Med Lett Drugs Ther 2004;46:83–4.

27. U.S. Food and Drug Administration. www.fda.gov/CBER/flu/flu2006.htm.

28. U.S. Food and Drug Administration. www.fda.gov/cber/flu/flu2007.htm

29. U.S. Centers for Disease Control and Prevention. 2007–2008 Influenza Season Week 8, Ending February 23, 2008. FluView; available at www.cdc.gov/flu/weekly/index.htm.

30. U.S. Food and Drug Administration. Influenza Virus Vaccine 2008–2009 Season: Vaccines and Related Biological Products Advisory Committee (VRBPAC), February 21, 2008; available at www.fda.gov/Cber/flu/flu2008.htm.

31. Update: Influenza vaccine supply and recommendations for prioritization during the 2005–2006 influenza season. MMWR 2005;54:850.

32. Tiered use of inactivated influenza vaccine in the event of a vaccine shortage. MMWR 2005;54:749.

33. Influenza vaccination in pregnancy: Practices among obstetrician-gynecologists— United States, 2003–2004 influenza season. MMWR 2005;54:1050–52.

34. Sandbulte MR, Jimenez GS, Boon ACM, et al. Cross-reactive neuraminidase antibodies afford partial protection against H5N1 in mice and are present in unexposed humans. PLoS Med 2007;4:e59.

35. Gillim-Ross L, Subbarao K. Can immunity induced by the human influenza virus N1 neuraminidase provide some protection from avian influenza H5N1 viruses? PLoS Med 2007;4:e91.

36. Antiviral drugs for prophylaxis and treatment of influenza. *Med Lett Drugs Ther* 2005;47:93–5.

37. Centers for Disease Control and Prevention. CDC Health Advisory, January 14, 2006.

38. Kiso M, Mitamura K, Sakai-Tagawa Y, et al. Resistant influenza A viruses in children treated with oseltamivir: Descriptive study. *Lancet* 2004;364:733–4.

39. Centers for Disease Control and Prevention. www.cdc.gov/flu/.

40. Centers for Disease Control and Prevention. www.cdc.gov/flu/protect/antiviral/index.htm.

41. Centers for Disease Control and Prevention. Influenza Antiviral Medications: 2005–2006 Interim Chemoprophylaxis and Treatment Guidelines (last modified January 14, 2006); available at www.cdc.gov/flu/professionals/treatment/0506antiviral-guide.html.

42. Antiviral durgs for prophylaxis and treatment of influenza. *Med Lett Drugs Ther* 2006;48:87–8.

43. Centers for Disease Control and Prevention. Influenza (Flu): Clinical Description and Diagnosis; available at www.cdc.gov/flu/professionals/diagnosis.

44. Centers for Disease Prevention and Control. Interim Guidance for Influenza Testing During the 2004–2005 Influenza Season[JKM3]; available at www.cdc.gov/flu/professionals/diagnosis/0405testingguide.html.

45. Centers for Disease Control and Prevention. Laboratory Procedures for Influenza[JKM4]; available at www.cdc.gov/flu/professionals/labdiagnosis.html.

46. Hill G, Cihlar T, Oo C, et al. The anti-influenza drug oseltamivir exhibits low potential to induce pharmacokinetic drug interactions via renal secretion: Correlation of in vivo and in vitro studies. *Drug Metab Dispos* 2002;30:13–9.

Other Resources

U.S. Centers for Disease Control and Prevention, contacts: 1-800-CDC-INFO (1-800-232-4636); cdcinfo@cdc.gov.

Barry J: *The Great Influenza: The Epic Story of the Deadliest Plague in History.* New York: Viking Press, 2004.

Davis M. *The Monster at Our Door.* New York: New Press, 2005.

Knobler SL, Mack A, Mahmoud A, et al. (eds). *The Threat of Pandemic Influenza: Are We Ready?* Workshop summary prepared for Forum on Microbial Threats, Board on Global Health, Institute of Medicine. Washington: National Academies Press, 2005.

11 B

Occupational Influenza

Daymon Evans

In common language, *the flu* has come to mean any generalized communicable illness of the upper respiratory or gastrointestinal systems. A wide discussion of all the possible pathogens and illnesses that could be mislabeled *the flu* is beyond the scope of this chapter. The discussion is limited to that relatively severe and highly communicable upper respiratory infection caused by the RNA orthomyxoviruses A, B, and C. Influenza should not be confused with *Haemophilus influenzae*, a bacteria that can cause upper respiratory infections. When first cultured from purulent sputum during outbreaks in 1892 by Pfeifer [1], it was presumed to be the pathogen responsible for clinical influenza [2]. Its etiology as the influenza pathogen was questioned after the 1918 pandemic, and its name was officially changed to *hemophilus influenza* in 1920 to recognize both its historical association with influenza and its dependence on blood components or the "blood loving" nature of the bacteria [3]. The virus responsible for human influenza was first isolated in 1933 [4]. *Haemophilus influenzae* B vaccine (HiB) is now part of the childhood immunization panel and should not be confused with influenza vaccines.

The size of this chapter is a reflection of the incidence of this disease in working populations, its dynamic epidemiologic characteristics, the challenges of surveillance, and the complexity of treatment and prevention options. Influenza and influenza-like illness (ILI) affect more workers annually than all diseases in this textbook combined and are responsible for spikes of absenteeism and financial costs to all employers. Since the writing of this chapter for the first edition, both the Occupational Safety and Health Administration (OSHA) and the Centers for Disease Control and Prevention (CDC) have published guidance documents for employers to prepare for pandemics.

OSHA. Guidance on Preparing Workplaces for an Influenza Pandemic. OSHA 3327-02N 2007; available at www.osha.gov/publications/influenza_pandemic .html, www.osha.gov/Publications/OSHA3327pandemic.pdf.

CDC. Business Pandemic Influenza Planning Checklist. Available at www.pandemicflu.gov/plan/businesschecklist.html.

"Occupational influenza" may be an administrative nonentity, in that influenza is rarely accepted as a compensable occupational disease. Influenza is considered a normal disease of life by most workers' compensation carriers and state statutes because there is no evidence that the risk, incidence, or prevalence varies among professions or worksites. Widening the definition of occupations to include students and military personnel will include a major population of influenza victims, include classic routes of transmission, and include the study groups for much of our scientific and observational knowledge of the disease.

Influenza is a disease of great consequence to employers because of the expense of absenteeism and medical care. The direct medical costs of influenza in mid-1990 dollars are estimated to be as much as $4.6 billion in an average year, but total and direct costs of a severe influenza season are at least $12 billion [5]. Much of this cost is absorbed by employers.

Especially vulnerable are hospitals and other acute health care facilities, with their simultaneous high patient workloads and high employee absenteeism [6–9]. Both may be attributable to influenza. Management is challenged to maintain adequate staffing of in-patient units during influenza epidemics and may have to resort to the expense of contracting workers from outside agencies. Well employees may be asked to work longer shifts or overtime, and the more dedicated caregivers may report to work despite their own illness and thus contribute to the nosocomial aspects of an epidemic [10–12].

However, the employer and the worksite can serve pivotal roles in community influenza prevention, education, and intervention. Employers offering influenza vaccine and/or prophylactic antiviral prescriptions will recover their costs in most years [13–19]. A case-control study by Campbell and Rumley [13] showed that a North Carolina textile plant saved $2.58 for each $1.00 invested in an employee vaccination program. A survey study by 3M showed that employees receiving sequential (annual) immunizations had reductions in absenteeism [19].

Practitioners of occupational and environmental medicine frequently will be asked to consult on and/or attend influenza prevention efforts. This is good public health and a wise business investment. Occupational medicine practitioners (OMPs) should enthusiastically accept these offers and maintain their up-to-date knowledge on influenza epidemiology, immunization, and other prevention strategies. They should be able to serve their client companies and patients as a year-round resource for influenza control and prevention planning. When influenza infects workers, it affects their health and productivity. Some occupations logically may seem more at risk than others, but there is little evidence that infection rates vary significantly among jobs or worksites. With most adults spending one-fourth of their life at or en route to or from work, there is little doubt that employment and the workplace are major factors in human-to-human influenza transmission. Society may not accept influenza as a compensable occupational disease but cannot deny its existence as an environmental disease. It remains one of the most studied, most fascinating, least understood, and prevalent human afflictions. The opportunity for implementation of adult influenza immunization and education at workplaces should not be missed.

Epidemiology

INCIDENCE AND PREVALENCE

Influenza is the world's leading respiratory infection and is a threat to all populations. Less than half of those hospitalized with acute respiratory disease during the influenza months are over age 65 or have a chronic medical condition [20] (the classic high-risk patient), and half of all patients hospitalized by complications of influenza are employed.

Influenza may seem to come in seasonal epidemics, but in reality, it is an endemic human disease continually encircling the Earth. A strain may take 1–2 years to circle the globe, and 20% of the Earth's human population will have at least one influenza infection in an average year [21]. A geographic area and its population have their season at any given point in time and likely serve as the reservoir for the disease, which seemingly disappears for much of the year. A *pandemic* is defined as "an epidemic occurring over a very wide area, crossing international boundaries and usually affecting a large number of people" [22].

History and Influenza

Only by understanding the history of human influenza can we afford this disease the respect it deserves. Its stealth motivates us to maintain our surveillance systems and to fund further research on surveillance, prevention, and treatment.

Pre-Twentieth-Century Outbreaks. A favorite exercise of medical historians is to diagnose the Great Plague of Athens, which occurred in 430 BC. Thucydides gave extensive descriptions of the clinical syndrome and spread of this epidemic [23], which killed a third of the Greek army and precipitated the downfall of the empire. Langmuir and colleagues have postulated that this plague was an especially virulent influenza strain with a high rate of secondary staphylococcal infection and toxic shock syndrome [24].

ILIs have been recorded throughout history [25] under many different names, such as "the grip." The English term comes from sixteenth-century Italians, who noted that the illness could "influence" others to have the illness and/or possibly that a winter constellation could "influence" the illness. Since the sixteenth century, at least 31 global pandemics of ILI have been recorded, averaging 4–5 per century [26].

The first publications on the quantitative impact of influenza can be attributed to Robert Graves [27]. He counted new graves in Dublin cemeteries starting in 1837. William Farr recorded details of the London epidemic of 1847 and first described the concept that death rates may vary by season [28]. We now call this *excess mortality*. Farr described peaks occurring in colder months, attributable to influenza complications. Both Graves and Farr were members of the London Epidemiological Society, one of the first professional organizations to formally study disease dynamics.

The 1918 Spanish Flu Pandemic. The great 1918 pandemic has been the most rapid and deadly communicable epidemic of the twentieth century. Five of every 1,000 Americans died, with a final U.S. death toll estimated at 675,000. This is more American deaths than those caused by all wars in that century. As an emergency measure, public gatherings were banned in many places, and there was an international shortage of caskets during the 1918 pandemic.

The illness would begin as a typical influenza case but could develop rapidly into severe pneumonia. Fever could reach 105°F and cause dementia and hallucinations. Mahogany-colored spots would appear over the cheekbones, and cyanosis and death could occur in a few hours. The case-fatality rate was about 10%. The mystery of why the disease targeted young adults was not solved for a generation.

It was called the *Spanish flu* because it was mistakenly believed to be the same virus responsible for an epidemic in Spain that spring. It spread along railroad lines and with the movement of troops. News of the epidemic was overshadowed by World War I. World War I caused 8.5 million deaths, but over 20 million people died in a few

weeks from this influenza, occurring near the end of the war.

In the Brevig Mission near Nome, Alaska, 90% of the residents died in a 5-day period in November 1918. The tribal and city councils allowed several of the 72 bodies buried in a mass permafrost grave to be studied. In 2005, nucleic acid viral mapping matched the formalin-fixed paraffin-imbedded tissue of the two 1918 soldier victims preserved by the Armed Forces Institute of Pathology [29]. The 1918 pandemic virus is now identified as GenBank entry 88776, or A/Brevig Mission/1/1918 (H1N1). It was likely due to a major change in the antigenic nature of an avian virus that adapted to humans and subsequently developed human-to-human contagion. This recent finding further vilifies the H5N1 ("bird flu") avian influenza currently emerging, which has not as yet developed effective human-to-human transmission.

Subsequent Pandemics. Other major changes in influenza antigens occurred with the 1957–1958 Asian flu A(H2N2), which was responsible for 70,000 deaths in the United States (Table 11B-1). The most recent pandemic was the Hong Kong flu A(H3N2), responsible for 34,000 deaths during 1968 and 1969. Gene segments for both the 1957 and 1968 subtypes were closely related to influenza viruses previously found in wild bird species. Pandemics "scares" have occurred with the swine flu in 1976, the Russian flu in 1977, and the current bird flu [30,31].

The Swine Flu. A deadly respiratory epizootic began in pigs in the midwestern United States in the early autumn of 1918. Swine veterinarian Dr. J. S. Koen believed this disease to be the same as the human Spanish influenza and named it *swine influenza* [32]. This influenza still occurs in pigs in the Midwest each autumn but is not as deadly as it was during the 1918 outbreak.

This swine virus was isolated by Shope in 1930 [33], three years before an influenza virus was isolated from a human [4]. Serologic surveys conducted by Shope in 1936 [34] showed that many humans over age 12 had antibodies to this swine virus isolate. This was confirmed by other studies and led to the assumption that the swine influenza isolate was closely related to the 1918 human pandemic strain and possibly identical.

This offered an explanation for why the 1918 disease was so deadly to young adults. Older

Table 11B-1
Pathogenic Human Influenza Viruses

Type	Subtype	Prototype	U.S. Mortality	Status
A	H1N1	A/New Jersey/8/76	500,000+ in 1918 Spanish Flu; 675,000 over ensuing several years	Swine reservoir?[a] Other H1N1s circulating
	H2N2	A/Japan/305/57	70,000+ in 1957 Asian Flu	Not in circulation at present
	H3N2	A/Hong Kong/1/68	34,000 in 1968 Hong Kong Flu; maybe 400,000 since 1968[b]	The most virulent in present circulation
	H5N1	Unnamed, first found in terns 1961	0 (but 6 in Hong Kong, 1997/8 "Bird Flu"?)[c]	Chickens slaughtered. Next global threat
B	None	B/Lee/40[d]	No data; but less than A subtypes	In circulation, but epidemics infrequent
C	None	C/Taylor/1233/47[e]	Believed to be minimal	In circulation, but clinically inapparent

[a]See discussion of swine influenza, page 11–4.
[b]See reference 64.
[c]See references 30, 31. All cases confined to Hong Kong area at present writing.
[d]First isolated by Francis in 1940. (Francis T Jr. A new type of virus from epidemic influenza. *Science* 1940;92:405–8.)
[e]First isolated by Taylor in 1947. (Taylor RM. Studies on survival of influenza virus between epidemics and antigenic variant of the virus. *Am J Public Health* 1949;39:171–8.)

persons had been exposed to a similar virus that had circulated in an 1890 pandemic, and they may have had some antibody cross-protection. Further comparative human birth cohort–swine serosurveys conducted by Davenport [35] and others in the 1950s confirmed that a virus very similar to the swine influenza virus circulated from 1918 until about 1928.

Laidlaw [36] postulated that swine influenza was the surviving form of the 1918 human virus. Shope proved that swine could be infected with influenza from humans under experimental conditions [37] and later by natural conditions [38]. He found older hogs on New Jersey farms with neutralizing antibodies to a human influenza virus; these antibodies were not found in younger hogs. In the Asian flu pandemic of 1957, it was again found that some hogs were infected with human influenza [39]. The 1968 pandemic strain also was found in pigs [40] in an area where humans and swine lived in close proximity on an island. However, these researchers did not believe that influenza could be spread from swine to humans, only that swine were the secondary victims of a human disease.

In the early 1960s, there were several unconfirmed reports of swine influenzas infecting humans behind the Iron Curtain. A collaborative team from the Illinois Department of Health and the University of Illinois Veterinary College studied human sera for swine virus in 1966 [41]. They found those with direct swine contact to have a rel-ative risk of 21 for having swine influenza antibodies. There may have been human-to-human spread because those who had contact with swine workers (but not swine) had a higher incidence of swine influenza antibodies than the general public (who were exposed to neither). They concluded that swine influenza was not a true occupational hazard because the infection was inapparent.

It was not until 1974 that swine influenza virus was isolated from a human, some 44 years after being isolated from hogs [42]. The victim was a 14-year-old immunosuppressed boy who did not have contact with swine until a few days before his death, when he came into contact with two pigs on a farm. Both pigs were seropositive for the strain, and both the boy's parents were negative. A year later, all members of a family of six who lived on a hog farm in Wisconsin were found to be positive, with the index case showing a positive paired sera [43]. Several more cases of illness owing to swine influenza were reported from Missouri, Wisconsin, and Minnesota, but it was the outbreak among recruits at Fort Dix, New Jersey, in 1976 that sparked international attention. No contact between soldiers and swine could be identified, so it was suspected that spread was human to human. The Fort Dix epidemic created a public health panic because

- The 230 infected recruits were young and healthy.
- Previous pandemics had begun in military units.

- There was evidence of human-to-human spread.
- The swine influenza endemic in New Jersey hogs had been found 40 years earlier and had a direct linkage to the 1918 pandemic.

Because of the fear of a return of the 1918 pathogen, a massive public health initiative resulted in one-fourth of the U.S. population receiving a monovalent swine influenza vaccine. An epidemic did not occur, but the rare and highly publicized vaccine complications of Guillain-Barré syndrome damaged public confidence in the influenza vaccine and the public health surveillance of influenza. Formal influenza control has yet to fully recover credibility, although a risk factor for Guillain-Barré syndrome has not been associated with subsequent vaccines [44,45].

Most recently, two workers became ill with an influenza-like illness after performing nasal swabs on pigs. The pigs were artificially infected with a swine influenza, A(H1N1), in experiments at the University of Wisconsin–Madison [46]. The two workers cultured the identical strain despite adhering to animal biosafety level 3 containment practices [47]. These workers were the eighth and ninth humans proved to have been infected with swine influenza directly from hogs [48–53]. Both survived, but the majority of patients in previously reported cases died.

Antigen Nomenclature and Clinical Correlation

An influenza virus was first isolated from chickens during a fowl plague in 1901 [32]; the pathogen is now known to be A(H7N7). Influenza B and C were isolated in 1940 and 1947, respectively. Influenza was found to grow in embryonated chicken eggs, and this led to many advances in culture technique, serologic testing, and eventually vaccine development. The influenza virus is a single-stranded RNA myxovirus that contains three sets of proteins. It is the nucleoprotein portion that distinguishes A, B, and C from one another.

Influenza C is the simplest in structure and contains only a single glycoprotein. It has been associated only with minor epidemics and less severe illness, and serosurveys confirm many inapparent infections and near 100% immunity for this type by age 5 [54]. Influenza C may be more endemic than epidemic. Influenza B, however, can cause epidemics, although much less often than the more prevalent influenza A. In addition, influenza B usually causes less severe illness than influenza A.

Influenzas A and B each have two types of projecting glycoproteins, the hemagglutinin (H) and the neuraminidase (N). These glycoproteins are responsible for the antigenic variations in the subtypes and are the sites of antibody attachment and inhibition.

A standard system of nomenclature was developed for influenza A and underwent revisions in 1971 [55] and 1980 [56]. It is as follows:

- Type (A, B, or C)
- Host of origin (influenza A), if and only if it is not human
- Geographic origin, a city or region where first found
- Isolation (strain) number, assigned sequentially
- Year of isolation
- If influenza A, then a description of antigenic specificity (subtype) of the surface antigens:
  - *H*: hemagglutinin (one of 12 types, 1, 2, 3, and 5 pathogenic to humans)
  - *N*: neuraminidase (one of 9 types, 1 and 2 pathogenic to humans)

Examples: B/Beijing/184/93: a human influenza B virus first isolated in Beijing in 1993.

A/Nanchang/933/95 (H3N2): a human influenza A (H3N2) virus first isolated in Nanchang in 1995.

A/duck/Ukraine/1/63 (H7N2): an avian influenza A (H7N2) virus first isolated from ducks in the Ukraine in 1963.

The World Health Organization (WHO) maintains reference isolates for both humans (WHO Collaborating Centres for Reference and Research on Influenza) and nonhumans (WHO Centres for the Study of Influenza Ecology in Animals). Reference matching is made on request.

An influenza A virus can undergo genetic recombinations and create newborn progeny subtypes. Genetic reassortment between two different influenza A viruses has been postulated to be the mechanism of the *antigenic shift* [57,58] when they simultaneously infect and replicate in the same victim cell. Shifts are believed to be changes of up to 50% of the nucleotide sequence and may be responsible for new pathogens and major epidemics or pandemics in a general population lacking immunity to this new subtype. The more minor changes are the *antigenic drift* (either influenza A or B) of less than 1% of the nucleotide sequence. Humans may have at least partial antibody protection from previously closely related infection.

Influenza A is known to be present both endemically and epidemically in many animal species (e.g., chickens, ducks, hogs, horses, mink, and seals) and theoretically could be the source for new human subtypes. Types B and C are primarily human viruses and are more antigenically stable than type A. H1N1 was the primary human subtype circulating until an antigenic "double" shift to H2N2 in 1957 created the Asian flu pandemic (see Table 11B-1). An antigenic shift to H3N2 in 1968 resulted in the Hong-Kong flu pandemic.

It was believed that only one subtype could circulate at a time until A(H1N1) reappeared in 1977 and subsequently cocirculated with A(H3N2). Some strains may "cycle" over a period of decades, possibly centuries. The antigenic shifts seen in the past century may not represent new human pathogens. There is some serologic evidence from birth cohorts that the strain that caused a severe epidemic in 1889 and 1890 was very similar to the influenza A (Hong Kong) strain (H3N2) of 1968 [59]. During the 1968 Hong Kong flu, persons over the age of 75 had lower morbidity and mortality than those ages 65–74 [60]. It also has been shown that 26% of persons born between 1857 and 1877 had antibodies to the A/Japan/305/7(H2N2) subtype, implying that an Asian-like flu may have circulated in the middle of the nineteenth century [61].

In December 1997, the entire chicken population of Hong Kong was slaughtered after 18 humans with chicken contact were infected with an A(H5N1) subtype [30,31]. There were 6 deaths including the 3-year-old boy who was the index case. At this writing, avian influenza has been reported in 14 nations of Asia, Africa, and the Middle East. Of 346 cases, 213 (62%) have been fatal.

Excess Mortality

Expanding on the principle first described by Graves and Pearl and Frost [62,63], the term *excess mortality* is used to describe the death toll from the 1918 pandemic. *Excess mortality* is defined as those

seasonal deaths that occur above the number predicted on the basis of a stable death rate. In the United States and other temperate areas, excess mortality occurs in the winter months and is essentially synonymous with influenza and its complications.

The excess mortality concept has undergone many statistical revisions, including the present P-I (pneumonia and influenza) index published weekly in *Morbidity and Mortality Weekly Reports*. Most of the 20,000 or so "excess" deaths in an average year in the United States are the elderly and chronically ill. Spikes occur with pandemics (Figure 11B-1). The most recent influenza A subtype (H3N2) continues to circulate and may have contributed to as many as 400,000 deaths in the United States since 1968 [64]. In the 20 flu seasons between 1972 and 1992, there were over 10,000 deaths in seven winters, over 20,000 deaths in nine winters, and over 40,000 deaths in four winters. These deaths may be only a fraction of the true deaths in which influenza was a precipitating factor.

Morbidity from influenza starts to rise at about age 40. Currently, at least 90% of influenza deaths occur in citizens over the age of 65 [65], up from 62% for the same age group in the 1970s [66]. Many fatalities occur in those with chronic cardiac, pulmonary, renal, or metabolic diseases; anemia; and/or immunosuppression. Even if those with chronic illnesses survive influenza and its complications, the illness may further weaken their conditions and contribute to shortened life spans. Mortality from influenza may continue to increase as life expectancy increases for all the high-risk populations, for example, organ-transplant recipients, premature neonates, persons with cystic fibrosis, congestive heart failure patients, and those living with acquired immunodeficiency syndrome (AIDS).

Seasonality

In North America, the influenza season runs from December through March, but surveillance is vigilant from October through April. Epidemics typically are concentrated in a 3-week period; the mode month is February [67]. In tropical areas, epidemics occur most often during the rainy season.

In localized outbreaks, epidemics can evolve rapidly, with little warning, and often end as suddenly as they start. There are also sporadic and

Figure 11B-1
Monthly mortality from influenza in Massachusetts from 1887–1921 and in 90 U.S. cities from 1922–1956. (From Collins SD, *Influenza in the United States,* 1887–1957. Public Health Monograph 48. Washington: Government Printing Office, 1957.)

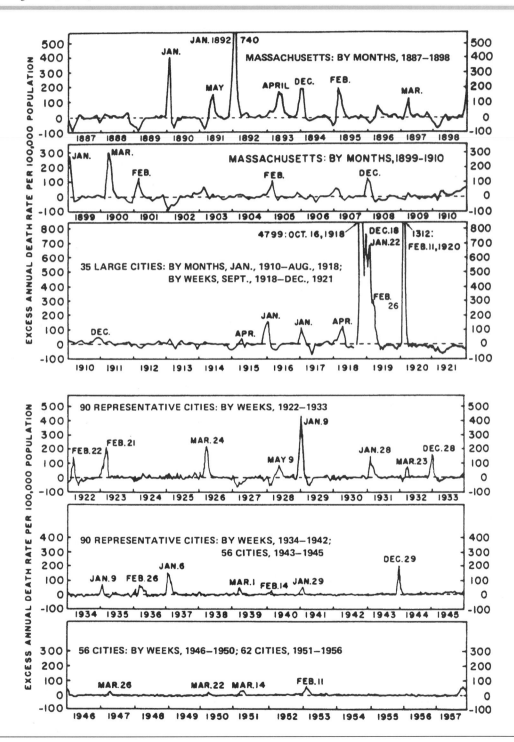

isolated cases, and serosurveys often confirm that subclinical, or asymptomatic, epidemics have occurred in the general population. Sporadic or isolated cases can occur anytime and anywhere, and in most cases, the origin is untraceable. With the speed of modern travel, an epidemic can jump oceans in a matter of hours.

TRANSMISSION RISK FACTORS=
Infectivity=

Influenza is spread by

1. Airborne respiratory droplets (see Chapter 3) from human to human
   With: respiratory or upper airway secretions
   From: the coughing and sneezing of those infected and infectious
   To: those susceptible and exposed
   By: air
2. Direct contact (see Chapter 3) from human to human
   With: respiratory secretions, possibly saliva
   From: those infected and infectious
   To: those susceptible and exposed
   By: mucous membrane to mucous membrane, directly or by fomites

The Centers for Disease Control and Prevention (CDC) and the Hospital Infection Control Practices Advisory Committee (HICPAC) jointly write the *Guideline for Isolation Precautions in Hospitals* [68]. Their recommended categories of isolation were changed in 1997 to "transmission-based precautions"; these are presented in detail in Chapter 3. The 2007 guidelines have added "respiratory hygiene/cough etiquette" to the standard precautions in response to information learned from the 2003 global severe adult respiratory syndrome (SARS) epidemic. Influenza is listed under "infections spread by droplet transmission" (along with adenovirus, rhinovirus, *Bordetella pertussis, Mycoplasma pneumoniae, Neisseria meningitides,* and SARS-associated coronavirus). Recommended droplet precautions are

1. Patient placement in a private room. If a private room is not available, then the patient should be put in a room with a patient infected with the same organism (*cohorting*).

2. Wearing of a mask (paper surgical) when working within 3 feet of the patient.
3. Limiting transporting of the patient from the hospital room (for essential purposes only).
4. The standard precautions, including handwashing, cough etiquette, and avoiding patient care when ill.

The expired infective influenza nuclei is believed to be about 1–5 μm in size [69] and is therefore inspirable into the deep lower lung, past the healthy body's physiologic and anatomic barriers. (This meets the CDC/HICPAC definition of *airborne transmission.*) An infective droplet nuclus (either an infected evaporated droplet or an infective dust particle vehicle) can remain suspended in the air for longer periods of time and be dispersed widely by air currents. Other airborne microorganisms include *Mycobacterium tuberculosis,* rubeola, and varicella.

As few as five particles may be an adequate infective dose for the lower lungs; approximately a hundredfold of that number is required for infection of the nasopharynx [69]. Deep inspiration of the influenza-contaminated expired air of another is the most efficient and infectious means of influenza transmission [69,70]. The infectivity and incubation period then depend on

1. The dose or number of infective viral particles inspired or direct contact with mucous membranes.
2. The site of inoculation. Deep pulmonary inoculation is more infectious and has a shorter incubation period than nasopharyngeal or oral inoculation.
3. The individual infectivity of the virus strain (which can have a great range) and its efficiency in invading and replicating in human respiratory tissues.
4. Host factors such as
   a. Preexisting full or partial immunity (which may be positively related to age).
   b. General ability of the body and immune system to fight infection, which may have a negative correlation with age in adults.
   c. Anatomic or structural susceptibility to infection, such as preexisting pulmonary disease or airway membrane damage.

The influenza virus is very stable in the cold and low humidity of winter and may be infective on fomites for hours. The virus can reproduce only in living cells and possibly only in the epithelial cells of the respiratory system. Transfusion or blood-borne spread has not been described.

Attack Rates

Attack rates can vary from 10–20% in the global community to 50% in more closed or crowded communities or schools. The highest attack rate recorded is 72% aboard an unventilated aircraft [71]. Population attack rates are also influenced by the four sets of factors mentioned earlier, plus a fifth factor, which is the virulence, or ability of an influenza strain to cause clinical disease. There is a range from predominantly inapparent infection (influenza C) to the 10% fatality rate of the 1918 pandemic. Socioeconomic class also appears to be a factor in community attack rates. Data from the comprehensive Houston observational studies have shown that small children in low-income families are at greater risk than preschool children of middle-income families [72,73]. Conversely, people in the higher socioeconomic group may have higher attack rates and more severe illness as adults. Those with a more hygienic and less crowded and exposed childhood will have less immunity as adults. This principle is operational in the attack rates of many other infections, such as hepatitis A, rubella, measles, varicella-zoster virus, mumps, cytomegalovirus (CMV), mononucleosis, and many other herpesviruses. This principle of immunity related to socioeconomic status also might be relevant to adults in their workplace job categories. Those working in crowded or high person-to-person contact positions may, over time, develop better influenza immunity than those working outdoors or in a more socially protected environment.

Incubation Period

The incubation period for influenza virus is 1–5 days. Studies have shown that nasal shedding begins one day before the onset of clinical illness [70]. This explains why isolating or cohorting the ill always has failed to prevent transmission. This relatively short incubation period accounts for both the rapid development and the rapid demise of epidemics when the susceptible pool is exhausted or was not exposed or infected.

Infective Period

The period of infectivity is usually up to 5 days [21] but may be as many as 7 days in coughing children [74]. Maximum infectivity occurs when viral concentrations are highest in nasal and respiratory secretions, and this is simultaneous with maximum symptoms [75]. Viral concentrations can be very high and infectivity prolonged in patients with influenza pneumonia [76].

Having all ill and infectious persons remain away from the public during the time of their illness may greatly reduce community and workplace spread. Blunting of the community epidemic curve can be seen when school Christmas vacations occur just after the start of an epidemic [77–79]. There is no evidence that infective periods are prolonged in immunocompromised individuals, nor is there evidence of chronic human carriers of the influenza virus.

Places of Transmission, the Workplace

Any settings where people "mix" in enclosed areas are conducive to the transmission of influenza, especially if ventilation or air exchange is inadequate. These settings include structures such as office buildings, schools, churches, theaters, and night-clubs, as well as commercial forms of transportation such as buses, aircraft, and ships and their gates, terminals, and docks. When persons from different geographic areas converge into crowded areas, a single index source can infect large numbers of people. This occurred, for example, aboard a commercial aircraft in Alaska in 1977 [71], when 72% of passengers were infected by a single coughing passenger after the plane was detained $4\frac{1}{2}$ hours. The ventilation system was off during this time. The epidemic was identified because passengers were diverted to an area where all cases were seen by one physician, who initiated an investigation. Outbreaks of influenza are also common on cruise ships [80] when the travel time is shorter than the incubation period. Many outbreaks in traveling military units have been reported. Influenza vaccines should be considered for any travel medicine itinerary.

Community Spread

The first signs of an influenza outbreak classically occur in primary schools and day-care centers. The association is with immature personal and respiratory hygiene and contamination of shared fomites. Influenza A(H3N2) viruses are generally more serious infections in children than influenza A(H1N1) or B [81]. The disease is then brought home to adults by the children. Longitudinal observation studies (in Seattle, Tecumseh, and Houston) have all shown higher attack rates in adults with school-age children in the home. In an 8-year study of Houston families [82], the highest age block for infection was ages 6–10, when 39.3% of the children had influenza illness and 47.7% of the children showed serologic evidence of influenza infection each year. The percentage of attack rates dropped with increasing age, but an average of 33% of adults in families with school-age children had an influenza infection each year.

Adults then transmit influenza to their workplace [79]. That is to say, transmission is "horizontal" among students at school, then "vertical" among generations at home, and then "horizontal" again among coworkers in the workplace in the latter part of an epidemic. Longini and colleagues have used data from the Seattle and Tecumseh studies to develop mathematical models to estimate the frequency of community-acquired infection and secondary attack rates [83,84].

Often, the elderly population and shut-ins are the last to be infected. Hospitalization rates rise relatively late in an epidemic season. When the P-I index curves are superimposed on influenza activity curves, they consistently show that pneumonia mortality peaks about 2 weeks after the peak of influenza morbidity.

Many communities have *action levels*, a preset percentage of absenteeism during which schools or nonessential businesses may close. The early closing of schools has been a controversial means of aborting an early influenza epidemic. The flattening of the epidemic curve seen with holiday breaks has been hard to reproduce on demand. (Often, it is the high absenteeism of faculty that necessitates school closures.) High absenteeism in primary schools portends heavy absenteeism in the workplace in a matter of a few days to a week or 10 days.

Susceptibility

Susceptibility to influenza is universal. There are no humans born who are immune to influenza infection, although some may have inapparent, subclinical infections. Infection confers immunity to the infecting influenza strain and closely related strains. When a new influenza subtype emerges (i.e., an antigenic shift occurs), people of all ages and locales are susceptible, and a pandemic is possible.

Cross-Species Transmission: The Reservoir

The origin of new human pathogenic strains has been one of the many mysteries of influenza. Influenza A has its reservoir in many wild birds and domestic farm animals and causes them both clinical and subclinical infections. There is little doubt that the major gene pool and reservoir for mammalian and avian influenza A is wild birds, but direct infection from bird to human is rare. Influenza A viruses become pathogenic to humans through a genetic intracellular mixing between strains. This may occur in birds or in humans but certainly occurs in the domestic pig [85]. The pig may be a genetic "mixing bowl" for new human influenza strains.

The duck ponds on farms in southern China are places where pigs, humans, and both wild and domestic birds share close contact. All three twentieth-century pandemics can be traced to origins in China or other parts of Asia. For this reason, the United States supports influenza research and new strain surveillance laboratories on the Chinese mainland. This surveillance monitors animals and the humans in close contact with them as an early warning system for the next pandemic [64]. Documented cases of transmission to or from humans remains mostly isolated and anecdotal, such as most avian influenza victims having direct contact with ill chickens. At this writing, there has not been a sustained human influenza epidemic that can be documented to have begun directly with animal-to-human transmission. Nor is there solid evidence that an animal species is serving as the reservoir for a recycling human influenza. It is very plausible, and even probable, that both occur, but this theory has so far escaped proof by the scientific method. It is interesting and fortunate to note that none of our more popular pet animals (i.e., cats, dogs, and parrots) have been found to carry influenza A. Nor has influenza B or C been found to be infectious to animals.

Much is written on the interspecies transmission of influenza and the potential threat of a new pandemic of animal origin. Please refer to any of the excellent reviews prepared by Webster and colleagues [86–88] for more information or the many links to the study of avian influenza (www.cdc.gov/flu).

OCCUPATIONAL RISK FACTORS
Exposure to Children

All observational and community studies show that the first signs of an influenza outbreak occur in schools and day-care centers. Children may have greater susceptibility and therefore higher attack rates than adults and also may have a longer period of infectivity. The immature personal hygiene and normal behavior of children may be contributory (e.g., not covering their face when coughing or sneezing, not washing their hands, and contaminating shared toys and other fomites with their saliva or respiratory secretions). Adult day-care workers, teachers, and pediatric clinic employees may be the earliest adults infected and should receive early vaccination for influenza each year.

Prolonged Face-to-Face Exposure

Prolonged one-on-one exposure to a single individual in a ventilation zone of 1 m or less can increase the chances of obtaining an infective viral dose. Occupations with such contact include dentists and dental hygienists, hairdressers and barbers, manicurists, massage and physical therapists, taxi drivers, and benefit agency workers. Unfortunately, none of these professions are included in the occupations recommended for annual immunization by the CDC [89]. The risk may be even higher if contact with an infected individual or individuals occurs in enclosed or poorly ventilated areas during cold weather.

High-Volume Population Exposure

Exposure also can be related to a high volume of brief encounters with the general public or in handling fomites such as money or tickets. Workers with this type of exposure include cafeteria cashiers and other food service workers, ticket takers, receptionists, tellers, sales and counter clerks, and even politicians on handshaking campaigns. These high-risk occupations should be considered in recommending influenza vaccine or anti-influenza medications for workers.

Enclosed Areas

Perhaps the greatest risk is associated with places where large numbers of persons from wide geographic areas gather in enclosed quarters for long periods of time. This type of exposure occurs in airline work, military barracks, college or boarding school dormitories, military ships or submarines, jails and detention centers, and tour buses. Temporary or episodic gatherings in offices or other sealed energy-efficient buildings also may increase exposure risk. These occur in cafeteria lines, time clock lines, or meetings. Designated smoking areas also may be transmission points, serving as nidi of higher-risk, coughing employees. A designated smoking area still may be preferred to a no-smoking policy, which often provokes workers to "meet and sneak" a smoke in poorly ventilated closets, toilet stalls, or other confined spaces.

Schools and Universities

Classroom students are particularly susceptible to all communicable respiratory or orally transmitted infections, including influenza, mycoplasma, mononucleosis, CMV, meningococcal meningitis, streptococcus, and other respiratory viruses. Student-related risk factors include

- Younger age and therefore less acquired immunity to influenza strains
- Crowding in classes, dorms, and lines for registrations or meals
- Frequent social gatherings or sporting events, either as participants or as spectators
- Dancing, kissing, or more intimate sexual contact
- Antigen "melting pot," as students from wide geographic areas converge after traveling in mass commercial transportation (buses, aircraft, and trains)

University students have been readily available subjects for study through campus student health services. Studies conducted on campus students have included analysis of individual risk factors, vaccine efficacy trails, antiviral drug efficacy [90], seroprevalence studies [91], age-related attack rates for Russian flu [92], and pulmonary function and influenza [90] and are the first studies to show that two antigenic variants can cocirculate in a given season [93]. Most notable have been the extensive studies conducted by the late Dr. Alfred S. Evans on students at Yale, the University of Wisconsin [94], and a university in the Philippines [95]. His studies show very little difference in campus epidemics among students in temperate climates versus those in tropical climates, but his study conducted in the Philippines did find that Philippine students very rarely have group A streptococcal, *Mycoplasma* pneumonia, adenovirus, or Epstein-Barr virus infections. The symptoms of ILIs are more specific for influenza if contracted in a tropical environment.

Influenza is a risk for all students, but that risk may decrease with each year on campus because one's immunity matures [94]. These serial serologic surveys show that as many as 4% of students have inapparent (subclinical) influenza infections. Taking one or more fall semester final examinations while ill is nearly a rite of passage for North American students.

The Military

Wars have been lost and empires have collapsed because of respiratory epidemics. Most military personnel, especially new recruits reporting for basic training, have the same risk factors listed earlier for students. Basic training is a risk epidemiologically equivalent to the freshman year. The dynamics of influenza epidemics often can be traced by troop movements [96] and often are the source of infection for civilian populations [97]. The onset of the 1986 influenza epidemic in the United States can be traced directly to a returning Navy squadron [96].

Troops have been the subject of influenza studies [98], influenza vaccine complication studies [99], and vaccine efficacy trials [100]. The Commission of Influenza of the Armed Forces Epidemiological Board (in the Department of Defense) monitored effectiveness of influenza vaccine and provided the most quoted statistic: "70–90% effective" for influenza vaccines [89]. The military is often one exception to influenza vaccinations being voluntary.

Animal Exposure

Only about a dozen cases of documented transmission of swine influenza to humans have been reported; several cases were fatal [48–53]. At least two cases occurred despite state-of-the-art precautions in a research facility. Nonetheless, it is known that much of the Earth's domestic swine population is endemically infected with influenza A subtypes H1N1 and, as of 1998, H3N2, closely resembling human subtypes. A study performed in Austria in 1994 showed that 24.5% of that country's fattening pigs, on 41% of Austrian farms, had antibodies to A(H1N1) [101]. A subsequent seroprevalence study of 137 veterinarians in Austria found that 8.8% were positive for this A(H1N1) [102]. A statistically significant number ($p \leq 0.01$) of these positive individuals were swine practitioners.

A complete review of all animal influenza studies is beyond the scope of this chapter. There are no practical or routine precautions recommended for influenza protection in livestock animal handlers other than receiving the yearly influenza vaccine and the general precautions of hand washing and avoiding direct mucous membrane contact with any animal respiratory fluids. A virulent human influenza pandemic originating from a pig, chicken, or other animal remains a theoretical day-to-day threat to the human population.

The Health Care Setting

Health care workers (HCWs) in health care institutions and health care students in training have risks similar to those listed earlier for classroom students. In addition, there is the direct hands-on contact that HCWs have with the sickest, hospitalized influenza sufferers. There are many reports of nosocomial epidemics of influenza [10, 11]; HCWs may be the index cases for these [12], especially in long-term or chronic-care facilities where the residents have limited exposure to others [9, 103–107].

HCWs are always a top priority for immunization programs [89]. Many advisory and accrediting agencies require or strongly recommend that employers offer influenza immunizations to their employees [108]. A randomized vaccine study of both HCWs and residents of long-term facilities in Scotland showed reduced patient mortality (odds ratio of 0.56) if over 60% of employees were immunized [109]. Immunizations of employees produced a better clinical outcome for the residents than for the workers themselves. There are many ongoing studies of influenza vaccines and neuramidase inhibitor efficacy in HCWs.

Nevertheless, HCWs probably do not have a higher overall rate of influenza infection than the general public. During an especially severe influenza season, this author conducted a nonscientific survey of ILI-associated absenteeism within a three-hospital network (Community Hospitals of Indianapolis). The survey covered a 30-day period from mid-December 1993 to mid-January 1994 and included absenteeism reports from 115 departments of nearly 5,000 employees. The overall ILI rate for direct caregivers in the hospital was 40.7%. The insurance office workers located off campus and with no patient contact had an 89.5% ILI rate. But 77.8% of the ill hospital caregivers used sick days compared with only 29.4% of the insurance office workers. Our county health department had requested that direct caregivers stay at home when symptomatic. These recommendations were publicized in employee newsletters, bulletin boards, and other highly visible places in the facilities. The higher percentage of ill clinical workers staying home may show some evidence of compliance.

Of particular interest were two urgent care centers serving similar populations and patient volumes. The North Clinic, a temporary modular building with poor ventilation, had 15 employees, all of whom lost work from illness in the 30-day period. None of the 10 employees in the newer and well-ventilated East Clinic were ill during that same period.

Immunosuppressed HCWs have dual indications for immunization and also should be considered for antiviral chemoprophylaxis by their primary care physicians. There has been no advantage achieved from giving two-dose immunizations to HIV-infected workers [110].

The Aerospace Environment

Very little has been published on respiratory infection in space travel, and there have been very few respiratory infections reported during space flight. Having an ILI disqualifies an astronaut from a mission, as was dramatically presented in the 1995 film *Apollo 13*.

Since the infective influenza virus is only a few microns in size, it is relatively unaffected by gravity.

A biophysical model in a paper by Knight and colleagues [69] speculates that influenza actually may be less infectious in zero gravity. But respiratory disease with larger infective particles (over 20 µm) may be more infective in zero gravity than in gravity because at zero gravity they are free-floating and have the potential for inoculation by inspiration.

Prevention and Control

ADMINISTRATIVE CONTROLS

The primary preventive measure for influenza continues to be immunization. Employers may not be able to control influenza as they might other occupational risks, but activities can be directed toward supporting employees' use of sick-time benefits. The following suggestions represent this author's own ideas developed from 30 years of on-site and institutional medical practice. Employers may take small steps to improve morale for the working ill and possibly reduce workplace transmission or absenteeism. These may include

- Providing boxes of tissues in widely available locations, with waste containers in very close proximity.
- Providing fresh drinking water or juices in widely available locations, with an ample supply of disposable drinking cups.
- Putting up signs reminding employees to cover their face while coughing or sneezing and to wash their hands after possible contamination with respiratory or oral secretions. Locations may include washrooms, dining areas, elevators, and multiple-user workstations.
- Offering temporary or brief periods of "amnesty" from termination for those calling in sick when they have no sick-time entitlement. Employees feeling forced to work even while ill could diminish workplace productivity and promote workplace infectivity.

Administrative actions to preserve productivity may include

- Allowing partial sick days or "sick hours" for those who need to leave because of illness.
- Relieving or reducing any procedural barriers for getting time off for doctor visits for workers or their dependent family members.

More long-range or proactive planning may include

- Having "action levels" of absenteeism at which certain nonessential departments or work areas will close.
- Considering temporary or contingency "work at home" options for employees in positions in which this may be possible.
- Providing on-site day care for ill children of employees (if practical and local regulations permit).

Actions for employers or agencies that maintain on-site occupational nursing or dispensaries may include

- Considering extended hours to cover shift workers.
- Being well stocked with medications to treat symptoms and printouts for the self-treatment of influenza or the common cold.
- Providing or arranging for discounts for antiviral medications prescribed by their own physician through benefits prescription plans or called into the dispensary (check local dispensing laws).

Ideally, employers should be able to record vacation or elective days off versus days off for illness or ILI. This is the only way to track true absenteeism owing to influenza or to conduct studies on the efficacy of immunization or other steps for prevention or intervention [19]. Employers also may insist that their health insurance vendors have prevention programs and have adequate availability of primary care physicians near the worksite(s). Employers also may insist that deductibles for after-hour or urgent-care clinics be financially reasonable.

When prevention fails, the best advice is for ill employees to remain at home during times of peak symptoms. Symptoms correlate positively with infectivity. This is especially important in health care or long-term care facilities, where ill employees are a risk to their vulnerable patients.

Once the influenza virus has invaded a worksite, influenza vaccine is not a practical solution. The immunizations may take 2 weeks to confer immunity, and stocks of vaccine may be exhausted by the time the epidemic begins. Antiviral medications are not a full substitute for immunization.

SAFE WORK PRACTICES AND ENGINEERING CONTROLS

Ventilation

Very few controlled scientific studies of the association between ventilation and human influenza activity have been conducted, but there have been enough episodic reports [70, 96, 97, 111, 112] of high infectivity rates in poorly ventilated areas to lend evidence to this logical and plausible assumption. The emergence of the SARS outbreak led to many recent studies of ventilation and airborne infection, and those studies were reviewed comprehensively by Li in 2006 [188]. Whenever possible, and when the task and facilities allow, workstations should be designed to allow 2–3 ft between the faces of workers and their coworkers, customers, or clients.

If the presumed 5-μm or less size of the infective influenza particle is correct, then influenza technically should fall under both "Airborne Precautions" and "Droplet Precautions" in the CDC/HICPAC recommendations [68]. This level of precaution calls for a private room with a negative pressure of 6–12 air exchanges per hour and vented either into a high-efficiency particulate air (HEPA) filter or outdoors. The tuberculosis isolation and controls (i.e., HEPA filtration, negative-pressure rooms, and N-95 respirators [113, 114]) could be the best "packaged process" when victims of a virulent strain receive medical care. This level of precautions also was found to contain human-to-human transmission of SARS. Research or laboratory workers who may be handling human respiratory secretions or other biologic hazards should do so only if wearing proper face protection or under a class II (or III) biological safety cabinet [115]. Those handling respiratory fluids from humans or other animals known to carry influenza or material that may have been in contact with the cloacae of potentially infected avian species are recommended to follow biosafety level 2 practices [47]. Note that these guidelines were published in 1993, before the swine-to-worker cases that were reported in 1997 despite biosafety level 3 precautions [46]. The best advice for those working with animals is, as for everyone, annual influenza immunizations and frequent hand washing after any biologic contamination.

Safe Work Practices

Appropriate safe work practices need to be specific for each workplace and its inherent tasks. For example, day-care workers should wash their hands frequently after potential contamination with children's respiratory or oral secretions. Some principles apply to all workplaces, however. These are

1. Good general housekeeping and clean, well-maintained hand-washing (and hand-drying) facilities in restrooms.
2. Trash containers should be readily available in all work areas and should be lined to minimize direct handling of trash by custodians.
3. Those who handle money or other potentially infected fomites (e.g., cashiers, ticket takers, and ushers) should wash their hands before and after work and before and after meals. They should avoid hand-to-mouth or other mucous-membrane contact in the interim between hand washings.

During influenza epidemics, employers may consider some methods to prevent close congregation of employees. For example, employers could schedule daily work times to avoid congestion at elevators, stairwells, and time clocks and schedule mealtimes to avoid cafeteria lines.

There are more formal recommendations for health care institutions to follow when dealing with their staff and with influenza patients [68, 108]. Specific infection control education is also mandated by various regulations and local statutes for health care facilities Recommendations also suggest restricting hospital visitors who have a febrile respiratory illness.

The only absolute protection is complete isolation from other humans from late fall to early spring yearly. The only practical protections remain vaccination, the observance of good personal hygiene by covering the face when coughing or sneezing, and politely encouraging the same behavior in symptomatic coworkers.

PERSONAL PROTECTIVE EQUIPMENT

> Obey the laws and wear the gauze. Protect your jaws from septic paws.
>
> —*Rhyme propagated by the San Francisco Board of Health during the 1918 Pandemic (Citizens could be jailed for not wearing their gauze masks.)*

Personal protective equipment is neither generally available nor practical for influenza control, although there is now increasing availability and training for N-95 or other paper particulate masks.

The plausible assumption is that influenza transmission may be interrupted by wearing a regular paper surgical mask within 3 ft.

If a health care institution chooses to apply "airborne" rather than "droplet" CDC/HICPAC precautions for influenza, National Institute of Occupational Safety and Health (NIOSH)–approved N-95 masks developed for tuberculosis protection theoretically could protect one from influenza. Demand for the N-95 masks peaked during the 2003 SARS global outbreak.

EMPLOYEE EDUCATION AND TRAINING

Education in good personal hygiene should include covering the mouth and nose when coughing or sneezing. Employees should wash their hands if there has been mucous contamination of the hands or if they have had contact with objects possibly contaminated by the respiratory or oral secretions of others.

Many non–health care employers are finding personal communicable disease prevention programs to be useful within their periodic training and development or health promotion programs. "Preventing Communicable Disease" is a common mandatory training in many workplaces now, along with timely topics on preventing workplace violence, preventing sexual harassment, and vigilance for terrorism. Commercial products such as Glo-Germ can aid training in hand-washing techniques.

Employees should be trained to seek early and adequate treatment when they first have symptoms of infection. This may shorten the time of illness, prevent organ damage or failure, and prevent secondary bacterial infection. Non–health care workers also should be encouraged to stay home when ill with symptoms of influenza, and such directives at times may be given from health departments. Employees also should be encouraged to "save" some sick days for when they are actually ill so that they will be less likely to report to work when ill but out of sick leave.

Most important are employee education about the value of the influenza vaccine and a concerted effort by employers to remove negative myths and misconceptions regarding influenza vaccines. This education should include the information that the vaccine is dead and does not and cannot cause nor spread influenza. The information should be in the language and writing style appropriate for the worker. Employers can share the "when's and where's" of local immunization efforts with their employees if unable to directly provide immunization on-site. An excellent public promotion resource for the Medicare population [65] is the U.S. Health and Human Services Centers for Medicare and Medicaid Services (Figure 11B-2). This Web address has uncopyrighted color posters available for downloading. An excellent multipage fact sheet on influenza for the consumer is available from the National Institute of Allergy and Infectious Disease at www.niaid.nih.gov/publications/. HCWs should be taught the importance of receiving immunizations as recommended by the CDC [68] and trained to answer questions on influenza vaccine asked by their patients. All workers in health care should be knowledgeable about influenza and be able to encourage vaccination and other precautions for their patients. It is unacceptable for physicians or other health care professionals to discourage patients from receiving influenza immunization based on their own ignorance or limited personal experience.

MEDICAL SURVEILLANCE
International Surveillance

It is only a question of when, not if, the next pandemic will occur. International surveillance has been coordinated by the World Health Organization since 1970 and is extensive, expensive, and truly global. An excellent source of information on influenza data should exist in the former Soviet Union, where all clinic visits were reported to a central computerized database. This same database was used to confirm excuses for work or school absence. Unfortunately, no studies analyzing these data have been published since 1977 [116].

A comparison of new antigenic variants of influenza found in laboratory experiments performed on sera from representative populations is one method used to predict population susceptibility and severity of epidemics. Information collected from influenza epidemics in various parts of the world is used in decisions about vaccine valency. The United States supports influenza research and new-strain surveillance laboratories on the Chinese mainland. This surveillance includes animals and humans in close contact with animals as an early warning system for possible epidemics [64].

U.S. Surveillance

Surveillance in the United States is coordinated by the Centers for Disease Control and Prevention National Center for Infectious Disease in Atlanta. Influenza is not a reportable illness in the United States and is not linked to the National Notifiable Disease System (NNDSS), but local and state health departments like to know of outbreaks or clustering of ILI, including reports from the workplace. In the United States, influenza surveillance has four levels:

1. *U.S./WHO Collaborating Laboratory Surveillance System.* Most of these 70 laboratories are within state or local health departments, and some are within universities or hospital networks. Each week of October through May, the collaborating laboratories report the total number of specimens received for respiratory virus testing and the number of influenza-positive isolates of A(H1N1), A(H3N2), A(nonspecific), and B. All donors are typed by age groups: 1, 1–4, 5–24, 25–44, 45–64, 65 or over, or unknown. Beginning in 1998, information has been submitted electronically to the CDC. Some representative isolates are submitted to the WHO Collaborating Center for Surveillance, Epidemiology, and Control of Influenza at the CDC for complete antigenic characterization and antiviral resistance testing.

Figure 11B-2
Example of a color poster available on the Internet: US "Fight Flu" Program [65].

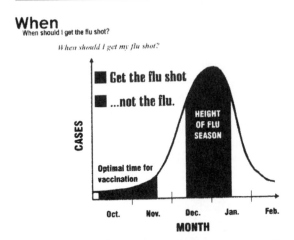

When
When should I get the flu shot?

2. *Sentinel Physician Surveillance Network.* Each week from October through May, approximately 140 preselected and representative primary care providers, called *sentinel physicians,* report the number of patient visits for the week and the number of those patients who were examined for ILI, according to the preceding age groups. Some of the physicians collect nasal and throat swabs for virus isolation in the collaborating laboratories. The data are reported to the CDC. Sentinel physicians also may participate in other community health surveillance projects, such as monitoring of lead levels.

3. *The 122 U.S. Cities Surveillance System.* Vital statistics from 122 major U.S. cities representing about half the U.S. population are reviewed weekly. Recorded are (a) the number of death certificates filed owing to all causes and (b) the number of deaths for which pneumonia was identified as the underlying cause of death and for which influenza was mentioned in any position on the certificate. This information is reported to the Epidemiology Program Office (EPO) of the CDC each week. A seasonal baseline is calculated using the proportion of pneumonia and influenza deaths observed since 1983 (the P-I index). If that number varies by a statistically significant amount, influenza deaths are said to be above epidemic threshold (excess mortality).

4. *State and Territorial Epidemiologists' Report.* In each week of October through May, epidemiologists from each state or territory report the estimated level of influenza activity in their area as

- No activity
- Sporadic activity, defined as sporadically occurring cases of ILI or culture-confirmed influenza with no outbreaks detected
- Regional activity, defined as outbreaks of ILI or culture-confirmed influenza occurring in counties representing less than or equal to 50% of that state or territory's population
- Widespread activity, defined as outbreaks of ILI or culture-confirmed influenza occurring in counties representing over 50% of that state or territory's population

These reports come to EPO-CDC via the National Electronic Telecommunications Systems for Surveillance (NETSS). Methods used to make the determination of influenza activity vary from state to state and may include local sentinel physician networks, reports on increased visits for respiratory illness to hospital emergency rooms or outpatient clinics, school or worksite absenteeism reporting, nursing home surveillance, and reports of laboratory-diagnosed influenza.

Other Surveillance Definitions

- *Expanded reporting period.* Influenza can occur at any time of the year. Information on isolates in the summer may provide valuable information on the strain coming in the usual season.
- *Expanded sources of surveillance.* State epidemiologists or local health officials may request that other institutions or facilities assist in data collection to accommodate special needs for information.

Published Sources of Surveillance Data

A report entitled, *Prevention and Control of Influenza: Recommendations of the Advisory Committee on Immunization Practices (ACIP)* [89], is published by the CDC each year in late April or early May as part of the *Morbidity and Mortality Weekly Report*'s "Recommendations and Reports" cosubscription. The report includes information on the trivalent vaccines being prepared for the upcoming season, updates on influenza epidemiology, recommendations for targeted groups, timing of vaccination, and the latest antiviral medication protocols for influenza. It is the best annual source for influenza information and is available over the Internet. A weekly "Influenza Update Summary, for the week ending mm/dd/yyyy" is posted by the CDC and can be viewed, download, or printed from the Internet at www.cdc.gov/flu/weekly/fluactivity.html. The report includes a map of the 50 states shaded by their influenza activity levels (Figure 11B-3).

Surveillance information is available through the CDC website at www.cdc.gov or by calling the CDC information line at 1-800-232-4636. These reports include percentages of upper respiratory illnesses that are cultured-positive for influenza, the prevalent strains, and age-related trends.

Individual cases of influenza are not investigated. Exceptions are the severe or fatal cases with rare complications (e.g., encephalitis, myocarditis, and rhabdomyolysis) that may suggest an especially

Figure 11B-3
Example of a Weekly Influenza Activity Report. (From National Centers for Infectious Disease, Centers for Disease Control and Prevention, available on the Internet at www.cdc.gov/ncidod/diseases/flu/weekly.html).

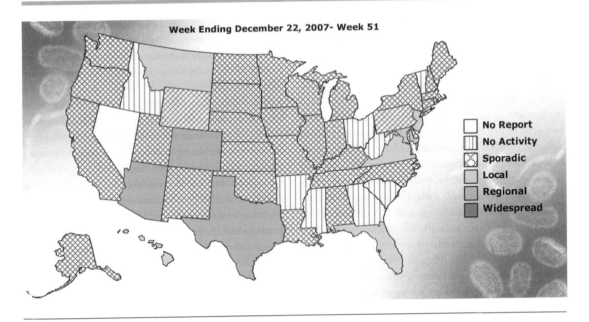

virulent strain with specific organ pathogenicity. Other exceptions include influenza suspected to be of animal origin. These influenza A viruses that cannot be subtyped by hemagglutination inhibition testing using the standard H1N1 antisera included in the influenza reagent kit distributed by the CDC should be sent to the CDC Influenza Branch immediately. In any of these situations, the state health department and the Influenza Branch of the CDC (404-639-3591) should be contacted immediately.

Excess Mortality and the P-I Death Index

Since 1918, excess mortality has been used systematically as an index for the recognition of influenza epidemics. The method of data collection was further refined by Collins and Lehmann [117]. Figure 11B-1 is from a monograph published in 1957 [118] and provides graphic evidence of influenza epidemics over a 70-year period in the state of Massachusetts and major U.S. cities. The graph is 1 year short of catching another pandemic.

The methodology of tracking excess mortality was refined by CDC biostatistician R. E. Serfling

[119] in 1963. He used a linear regression function to represent data in a smoother sine curve and to produce advanced warning of variation and excess deaths. Excess mortality is now called the *P-I deaths* (pneumonia- and influenza-attributable deaths) and is a method of reporting developed by Choi and Thacker in 1981 [120]. This is the statistic reported weekly in the *Morbidity and Mortality Weekly Report* from 122 U.S. cities of greater than 100,000 population and on the CDC website.

The defined *epidemic threshold* occurs when 7.2% of all deaths are attributable to pneumonia and influenza. This represents 1.645 standard deviations above the seasonal baseline. The expected seasonal baseline is projected using a robust regression procedure in which a periodic regression model is applied to observed percentages of deaths from pneumonia and influenza since 1983. Simonsen and colleagues have proposed adding a *severity index* to the equation for more accurately comparing the severity of individual epidemics [121].

Deaths "officially" or directly attributable to influenza may only be a fraction of the deaths in which influenza was a precipitating factor. Those with preexisting cardiac or pulmonary disease have a higher mortality from influenza, but this may not be reflected in their death certificates. Nosology protocols give a higher preference to the cardiac and pulmonary International Classification of Disease (ICD) codes. At present in the United States, at least 45,000 people die each year from combined influenza and pneumonia, ranking it as the sixth leading cause of death.

Family and Observational Studies

The most reliable morbidity data on influenza comes from longitudinal studies of defined and natural populations, or *observational studies*. These studies depend on the use of serosurveys to study patterns of infection and patterns of spread. It is from these studies that infectivity rates, community patterns of spread, and serosurvey data have been gathered. The largest studies have been conducted in Tecumseh, Cleveland, Seattle, and Houston. The Influenza Research Center in Houston has been the most prolific source of information on community-wide influenza.

Biologic Testing

Embryonated hen's eggs were the very first cultures used for diagnosing influenza and remain the standard culture technique. Various monkey kidney cultures are far superior but in recent years have become too expensive for routine use. Individual clinical influenza infection is proved by a fourfold increase in influenza-specific IgM antibody titer. Neither serologic testing nor viral culturing and typing are clinically useful in individual cases of influenza because results will be returned after the case outcome is determined. Such testing is done only within the formal surveillance systems described earlier or in various academic or research projects. The network of laboratories capable of conducting influenza studies is maintained by the WHO and the CDC. The major coordinating reference and "indexing" laboratories are maintained in Atlanta and London.

The sentinel physicians report the number of patients they see each week who have symptoms that meet the case definition of ILI. These symptoms are nearly 100% sensitive for finding cases of influenza but under 50% specific for lab-confirmed influenza. These same symptoms occurring in tropical settings may have a much higher specificity

for influenza [95]. A certain number of these patients are selected for laboratory studies. Blood is returned to reference laboratories and cultured and/or serotyped at public expense. It is from these local reports that national trends are reported in the influenza weekly reports in the *Morbidity and Mortality Weekly Report* and on the Internet. Employer-based medical clinics traditionally have not been a part of the sentinel system, and this is one reason why scientific knowledge on influenza in the workplace is less than adequate. An on-site occupational clinic is an epidemiologically ideal source for study, especially if the clinic is well staffed and efficient and cares for a stable work force population with little year-to-year change in demographic variables. A major corporation or occupational medical professional organization could be in an excellent position to initiate such observational studies or to conduct clinical trials of administrative, environmental, or behavioral control studies of influenza.

Pre- and Postexposure Influenza Vaccine

Influenza vaccine is the best method available for preventing the disease, even though it is one of the least efficacious of civilian vaccines, and its efficacy and use vary from year to year. Influenza vaccination is not considered a routine adult or childhood immunization, but it is recommended for specific populations. Antiviral medications are not a substitute for vaccination because they can only lessen the course of the disease and cannot prevent infection. Influenza vaccines are provided free to Medicare B recipients, members of most state Medicaid plans, and members of many health maintenance organizations (HMOs) and private insurance plans. Many health care plans restrict the availability of influenza vaccination—that is, they make it obtainable with restricted availability only through the designated primary care provider.

History of the Vaccine. Human influenza was first isolated in chicken embryos in the 1930s, and the first vaccines were developed from the allantoic fluid shortly thereafter [122]. The vaccinations frequently caused symptomatic reactions until the development of the zonal centrifuge [123] and improvements in attenuation techniques in the 1960s and 1970s. Only information on the adverse effects of influenza vaccines made available since the 1970s is applicable to modern vaccines [124].

Valency Selection Process ("the Committee"). Each year the Food and Drug Administration's Vaccine and Related Biological Products Advisory Committee (VRBPAC) recommends three strains to U.S. vaccine product makers. Decisions are based on antigenic analyses of recently isolated influenza viruses and the antibody responses of persons vaccinated in the previous season. The vaccination strains must be selected 9–10 months before the season, with no assurance that the selections are accurate or that antigenic drift may not occur by the time product is shipped. There are two major subtypes of influenza A in circulation: H1N1 and H3N2 (see Table 11B-1). The vaccine is updated annually to include the three strains most likely to circulate (a trivalent vaccine). Usually this is one of each circulating A subtype strain and one B strain. One or more will change from the previous year. Although the current influenza vaccine may contain one or more of the antigens administered in previous years, annual vaccination with the current vaccine is necessary because immunity declines in the year following a vaccination. Product remaining from the previous season should not be used. Annual changes made in the valency are reasons to retake the vaccine each year, and any similarity is not justification to avoid the vaccine. Repeated exposures to the same antigen can booster immunity [19].

Detailed information on the vaccine, the coming influenza season, and any changes in recommendations are published in the *Morbidity and Mortality Weekly Report*'s "Recommendations and Reports" in late April or early May and on the Internet at www.cdc.gov/epo/mmwr/mmwr_rr.html.

Influenza Vaccine Products Available in the United States. It takes months to produce, package, and distribute the vaccine each year, plus a month or more for nationwide administration. Now nearly 90 million doses are given in the United States each year. If a pandemic were to emerge, the manufacturing process could switch to a monovalent vaccine to maximize production, but there may not be time to produce enough vaccine to protect the entire population. The variability of the egg market and supply also may affect production during a crisis. (This is not affected by the price of tea in China but rather by the price of *eggs*.)

In 1996–1997, Parke-Davis voluntarily initiated a recall of some vaccine product because of decreased potency of one component antigen, namely, A/Nanchang/933/95(H3N2). The company discovered and reported the problem during its own postmanufacturing surveillance. This was not a product safety issue [125], but the company did drop out of the market for the following year. The vaccine is made from highly purified egg-grown viruses that have been made noninfectious (inactivated). The methods of production may vary among manufacturers and may include both proprietary purification methods and the use of antibiotics. All contain the mercury-based preservative thimerosal that is found in many other vaccines and which in rare cases can cause localized allergic reactions.

Mechanism of Action. All the influenza vaccines used in North America contain killed virus and work as a passive vaccine. All these products are "split virus," "subvirion," or "purified surface antigen." Whole-virus vaccines have a history of increased febrile reactions and side effects and are not recommended for children under the age of 13 [126].

Children who have not been exposed to influenza previously have a primary antibody response to the vaccine, and for children under age 9, it is recommended that they have a second dose to achieve an adequate antibody titer. The second dose should be given no sooner than 30 days after the first but still before December. Most revaccinated adults and children develop high postvaccination hemagglutination inhibition (HI) antibody titers in a booster-type immune response. These antibody titers are protective against illness caused by strains similar to those in the vaccine or the related variants that may emerge during outbreak periods [89]—that is, there may be an adequate booster reaction even if the two vaccine antigens are not exactly the same.

Elderly persons and persons with certain chronic diseases may develop lower postvaccination antibody titers than healthy young adults and may remain susceptible. If such persons develop ILI despite vaccination, the vaccine still can be effective in preventing lower respiratory tract involvement or other secondary complications. Vaccine reduces the risk of hospitalization and death.

Lasting antibodies to influenza are of the IgG class and are specifically reactive against the hemagglutinin and neuraminidase portions of the vaccine strain. Population data have shown that serum HI antibody titers correlate inversely with the occurrence of influenza virus infection [127]. Antibody titers peak at about 10–14 days after a vaccine booster and then decline over the coming months. This is the primary reason for the recommendation of annual revaccination.

The vaccine antigen stimulates production of antibodies only to the three strains. The vaccine will fail if infection is overwhelming or if the infecting strain is not closely related to the vaccine antigen and will not offer cross-protection from respiratory illness caused by other viruses or bacteria.

Timing: When to Immunize. Vaccine must be ordered months in advance, and supplies may be depleted before the epidemics actually start. Estimating the volume of vaccine to order should be based on past experience. Utilization may vary from year to year depending on the extent of the epidemic, severity of symptoms, and media coverage.

Epidemics occur from October to May in North America. Activity is usually low until December, with peaks usually occurring in late November to early March, although new subtypes may circulate a month or two earlier. An unusually early report of widespread activity may be taken as a sign of a highly vulnerable population and a severe epidemic. Vaccine products are usually available some time in September, and the ideal time for immunizing persons in the general population is mid-October to mid-November (see Figure 11B-2).

Health officials may issue recommendations for earlier immunization. Vaccine can be given later, however, especially if there is reason to believe that peak activity will occur later in the season, but no opportunities should be missed to offer vaccination to high-risk patients or to workers when they visit a health care provider's office or clinic.

Recently, there has been a pattern of offering discount influenza vaccines in "we are the first" marketing campaigns by supermarkets, pharmacies, and shopping malls. Public immunization dates may be moving to an earlier time each year, and "herd" immunization could be falling by the time of peak activity several months later. The vaccine should be offered up to as late as April in some years (if available). Clinics doing international travel preparation should consider having extra vaccine products available for the off-season.

Who Should Be Immunized. GENERAL GUIDELINES. Influenza vaccine is strongly recommended for anyone 6 months or older who, because of age or underlying medical condition, is at increased risk for complications of influenza. Health care workers and others (including household members) in close contact with persons in high-risk groups also should be vaccinated. Vaccine may be administered to any person who wishes to reduce the chance of becoming infected with influenza and missing work or school. The following groups are at increased risk for influenza-related complications and are strongly advised to be vaccinated [89]:

- Persons 65 years of age or older
- Residents of nursing homes or other facilities housing persons of any age with chronic medical conditions
- Adults and children with chronic disorders of the pulmonary or cardiovascular systems, including children with asthma
- Adults and children who have required regular medical follow-up or hospitalization during the preceding year because of chronic metabolic diseases, including diabetes mellitus, renal dysfunction, hemoglobinopathies, or immunosuppression, including that caused by medication
- Children and teenagers (6 months to 18 years of age) who are receiving long-term salicylate (aspirin) therapy and therefore may be at risk for developing Reye's syndrome after influenza infection
- Women who will be in the second or third trimester of pregnancy during the influenza season

PREGNANCY GUIDELINES. This sixth category was added during 1997 by the Advisory Committee on Immunization Practices (ACIP). Influenza-associated excess mortality among pregnant women was reported only during the 1918–1919 and 1957–1958 pandemics. Some case reports had suggested an increased risk for serious medical complications of influenza as a result of increases in heart rate, stroke volume, and oxygen consumptions; decreases in lung capacity; and changes in immunologic function.

An abstract [128] of the impact of influenza during 17 interpandemic influenza seasons documented that the relative risk of hospitalization for selected cardiorespiratory conditions among pregnant women increased from 1.4 during weeks 10–14 of gestation to 4.7 during weeks 37–42. The comparison (relative risk [RR] = 1.0) was to women who were 1–6 months' postpartum. Women in their third trimester of pregnancy were hospitalized at a rate comparable with that of non-pregnant women who have high-risk medical conditions, for whom influenza vaccine traditionally has been recommended. Using data from this study, it was estimated that an average of one to two hospitalizations among pregnant women could be prevented for every 1,000 pregnant women immunized.

However, pregnant women who have medical conditions that increase their risk for complications from influenza should be vaccinated before the influenza season regardless of the stage of pregnancy. Studies of influenza immunization of more than 2,000 pregnant women have demonstrated no adverse fetal effects associated with influenza vaccine [89]. Because influenza vaccine is not a live vaccine, major systemic reactions are rare. Many experts consider influenza vaccination safe during any stage of pregnancy, but because spontaneous abortion is common in the first trimester and unnecessary exposures traditionally have been avoided during this time, some experts and obstetricians prefer delaying influenza vaccination until the second trimester to avoid coincidental association of the vaccine with early pregnancy loss. There is no contraindication of vaccine during breast-feeding [89]. Recent issues of pregnancy and influenza are reviewed annually and published in the ACIP report [89].

GROUPS THAT CAN TRANSMIT INFLUENZA TO PERSONS AT HIGH RISK. Persons who are clinically or subclinically infected and who attend to and/or live with members of high-risk groups (e.g., the elderly, transplant recipients, or persons with AIDS) can and likely will transmit influenza virus to them. Efforts to protect these members of high-risk groups against influenza may be improved by reducing the chances of exposure to influenza from their care providers. Therefore, the following groups should be vaccinated [89]:

- Health care professionals
- Residents of nursing home or other chronic care facilities

- Children 6–59 months old
- All persons over age 50
- Children from 6 months to 18 years of age who are on chronic aspirin therapy and at risk of Reye's syndrome.
- Women who are or will be pregnant during influenza season
- Persons who have chronic pulmonary conditions, including asthma; cardiovascular disease (other than hypertension); and renal, hepatic, hematologic, or metabolic disorders, including diabetes.
- Persons who are immunosuppressed by medications or by diseases such as HIV infection
- Persons who have any condition that can compromise respiratory function or the handling or respiratory secretions or that can increase the risk of aspiration
- Healthy household contact and caregivers of children younger than age 5 and adults over age 50
- Healthy household contacts and caregivers of persons with medical conditions that put them at higher risk for severe complications from influenza

Those in these groups compromise 73% of the general population, but only about one-third were vaccinated in the 2006–2007 season [89].

VACCINATIONS OF OTHER OCCUPATIONAL GROUPS. Employers may want to consider offering vaccination to workers who provide essential community services, who reside in dormitory-type housing, or who have the occupational risks described previously, although these groups generally are not included in the recommended groups for vaccination.

VACCINATION OF INDIVIDUALS WITH HIV/AIDS. Vaccine is recommended for HIV-infected individuals [89]. The vaccine has produced protective antibody titers in HIV-infected persons who have minimal AIDS-related symptoms and high CD4+ T-lymphocyte cell counts. Those with lower counts have not had protective antibody levels develop [129], nor have they responded to boosters or second doses [110].

VACCINATION OF TRAVELERS. The influenza season is reversed to April to September in the southern hemisphere. Those traveling there during these times should receive the most recent vaccine. More up-to-date information can be obtained from travel services or the WHO Influenza Web site at *www.who.int/topics/influenza/en/.*

Contraindications. For those with contraindications to influenza vaccine, antiviral prophylaxis with the neuramidase inhibitors may be considered. Breast-feeding is not a contraindication to vaccination because it poses no safety risk to mother or infant. Breast-feeding does not adversely affect the immune response to vaccine [89]. Contraindications to influenza vaccine are

- People with known allergies to eggs or egg protein products (absolute) or to thimerosal preservative (relative) should *not* receive this vaccine until consulting with their physician. However, if the individual is at very high risk for influenza mortality, you may want to refer the person for allergy evaluation and desensitization protocols [130].
- Adults with acute febrile illnesses should not be vaccinated until symptoms have abated. However, minor upper respiratory tract infections or allergic rhinitis is not a contraindication to the vaccination of children.
- A past history of Guillain-Barré syndrome (of any etiology) within 6 weeks of an influenza vaccine is a precaution.
- First-trimester pregnancy. Women who have medical conditions that increase their risk for complications from influenza should be vaccinated before the influenza season regardless of the stage of pregnancy.

Dosage. For all adults, the dosage of all U.S. products is 0.5 mL intramuscular, with the deltoid as the muscle of choice. All studies are based on intramuscular injections. Infants and young children should be immunized in the anterolateral aspect of the thigh. Manufacturers' recommendations should be followed for storage of vaccine products; generally, they need to be refrigerated and protected from light.

Local Reactions. The most common side effect is a mild local reaction (at the vaccination site), which occurs in 10–15% of people. The reaction is usually mild, generally lasts less than 24 hours, and does not inhibit daily activities.

Systemic Reactions. Low-grade fever, malaise, myalgia, and headache may occur following vacci-

nation. These symptoms, if they occur, usually begin 6–12 hours after injection and can persist for up to 2 days. Systemic reactions occur in only 10–15% of children who have not been exposed to influenza virus in the past and in only about 1–2% of adults who are receiving yearly vaccines.

IMMEDIATE SENSITIVITY REACTIONS. Immediate sensitivity (allergic) reactions (e.g., hives, angioedema, allergic asthma, and systemic anaphylaxis) occur rarely after influenza vaccination. These are most likely due to the traces of egg protein that remain in the product. Any individual with a history of similar reaction to dietary egg products should avoid influenza shots.

DELAYED SENSITIVITY. Delayed hypersensitivity reactions to the thimerosal used as a preservative in all influenza and many other vaccines have been reported. However, thimerosal sensitivity is not an absolute contraindication because these reactions are confined to local reactions [131]. A past history of recurrent and significant local reactions with other immunization or purified protein derivative (PPD) tuberculin injection sites may be related to thimerosal sensitivity. A true positive PPD reaction, with induration, should not be confused with thimerosal allergy by the patient or providers.

Drug Interactions. There has been one study [132] showing decreased theophylline clearance (increased half-life of 122%) after influenza immunization, but this finding has been refuted by others [133–137]. Likewise, one study [138] showed an effect of influenza vaccine on warfarin efficacy, but this finding was refuted by another study [139]. Most manufacturers of vaccine do not include warnings of theophylline or warfarin interactions.

Great Britain has reported several small series in which there has been a high incidence of exacerbation of asthma after influenza vaccine [140,141]. This finding has been refuted by other studies, including the United Kingdom Committee on Safety of Medicines, which had only five reports of alleged asthma or bronchospasm exacerbations in 40 million doses administered between 1963 and 1991 [142]. This controversy was reviewed by Watson in 1997 [143]. At present, no manufacturer or agency states that asthma is a contraindication to influenza immunization.

Late Complications. The most publicized and significant complication of influenza vaccination has been the Guillain-Barré syndrome (GBS) associated with the 1976–1977 monovalent influenza (swine flu) vaccine. The Nationwide Influenza Immunization Project was halted abruptly on December 16, 1976, after clusters of this complication were reported. A rapid nationwide study showed a relative risk of four to eight times (compared with the unvaccinated) for the incidence of GBS. The excess risk for GBS was about 1 in every 100,000 immunizations [144]—2–3 cases per 100,000—compared with a rate of about 1–2 cases per 100,000 in the general population. Analysis of the 1976–1977 cases showed associations with ages 18–64, with most cases of GBS starting the second week after vaccination. There also was an association with having had a past history of GBS.

Surveillance of the influenza vaccinations since that time has not shown an increased relative risk for GBS associated with influenza vaccine [44,45]. Many manufacturers still list GBS as a possible complication, and most providers still list GBS on the informed consent form for influenza vaccine. A past history of GBS is no longer considered an absolute contraindication to inactivated vaccine, however. The postulated mechanism for the inactivated influenza antigens causing GBS is molecular mimicking of myelin by viral protein in the vaccine, which triggers an autoimmune response. Theories of a persistent influenza virus gene in neural cells as a cause of chronic degenerative diseases of the central nervous system are unproved [145].

False-positive HIV and hepatitis C screening tests (ELISA) in blood donors who had received influenza vaccine with 1991 products was first reported in 1992 by blood banks in the Great Lakes area. Immunization with the 1991 product had an odds ratio of 81 for false-positive test results, which is significant at $p \leq 0.01$ [146]. Donors reverted to HIV-negative status on HIV screening tests in an average of 75 days, but false-positive results on hepatitis C screening may persist longer. Donors with false-positive test results were accepted as future donors after proof of false-positive status. If an influenza vaccine is suspected of being responsible for any transient false-positive test, it should be reported to Vaccine Adverse Event Reporting System (VAERS; 1-800-822-7967) [147].

Efficacy. When vaccine and epidemic strains of virus are well matched, achieving high vaccination rates among persons living in close proximity (e.g., nursing homes and other chronic care facilities) can reduce the risk for outbreaks by inducing "herd" immunity. The Commission on Influenza of the Armed Forces Epidemiological Board, U.S. Department of Defense, oversaw and measured the effectiveness of the influenza vaccine for many years. It reported an effectiveness of 70–90% for those under age 65 [35,89], and this remains the best single source of long-range efficacy.

All 17- to 21-year-old recruits at Lowry Air Force in Denver were vaccinated for a period of 30 years (3,000–5,000 per year), which resulted in vaccine efficacy of 72–95% in 70% of the years [100]. Only the antigenic shift of 1968 and the major drift of 1972 reduced efficacy below 60%. This study also included immunizations for adenovirus, which essentially made that disease extinct at the Air Force base; the only maker of the adenovirus vaccine discontinued the product in 1996 despite its high efficacy [148]. The military still considers an adenovirus vaccine a high priority.

One study of healthy working adults has shown that those who receive the vaccine have 25% fewer respiratory infections, 43% fewer sick days, and 44% fewer physician visits for respiratory illness [14]. Vaccination reduced direct medical costs by $5.99 and indirect costs by $40.86 per person vaccinated. In the elderly and those with chronic medical conditions, the efficacy may be less. Vaccine reduces hospitalization by 70% and deaths by about 85% for the elderly not in nursing homes [149]. Among elderly nursing home residents, the vaccine can reduce the risk of hospitalization and pneumonia by about 50–60% and the risk of death by 75–80% [89].

If antigenic drift results in the circulating virus becoming different from the vaccine virus strain, the overall efficacy of the vaccine may be reduced to near zero in preventing illness in a single season [18]. However, the vaccine is still likely to lessen the severity of the illness and prevent influenza complications and death.

Concomitant Administration of Other Vaccines. The target groups for influenza and pneumococcal vaccines have great overlap, such as those aged 65 or older and those with increased susceptibility to infection (e.g., patients with HIV infection, splenectomy, sickle cell disease, diabetes mellitus, chronic disorders of the lungs or heart, and cirrhosis). Influenza and pneumococcal vaccines may be administered together, at different sites, without an increase in side effects. Pneumococcal vaccine is covered by Medicare when ordered by a physician. It may be given at any time of the year and is a once-in-a-lifetime vaccination for most people.

Live Influenza Vaccine. More than 30 years' usage of "cold adapted" live influenza vaccines in Russia and the former Soviet Union [150] did lead to development of the live attenuated influenza vaccine (FluMist) by intranasal administration. It is well described in the ACIP report [89] and has been reformulated for 2007.

Antiviral Chemotherapy and Prophylaxis for Influenza A

Two drugs with indications for the treatment of influenza A viruses, amantadine and the closely related drug rimantadine hydrochloride, are no longer recommended [151]. A significant degree of drug resistant was reported and efficacy became questioned. Nevertheless, they may have utility in a global pandemic if other means of treatment or prevention are unavailable. Neither was indicated for B, C, or parainfluenza viruses. Because these drugs do not interfere with the immunogenicity or efficacy of influenza vaccines, vaccine and antiviral medication can be given together, although these medications should never be substituted for vaccination.

History and Usage. The initial indication for amantadine chloride was for Parkinsonism and other extrapyramidal diseases. In 1976, it was approved for use against type A influenza virus for both the treatment and prophylaxis of adults and children over the age of 12 months. Rimantadine was approved in 1993 for influenza A treatment.

Mechanism of Action. The mechanisms of action of these two drugs are unknown, but they appear to prevent the release of infectious viral nucleic acid into the host cells by interfering with the function of the transmembrane domain of some viral proteins. They also may prevent virus assembly during virus replication.

Therefore "prophylaxis" with these drugs is not true prophylaxis. They cannot prevent infection but rather only can significantly inhibit viral replication to the point of preventing clinical illness if the person is taking adequate doses of the drug at the time of infection. Thus "treatment" is started after apparent infection has begun, whereas "prophylaxis" is treatment at the time of infection.

When these drugs were used to arrest an influenza A epidemic in progress, the goal was to reduce the viral load and shedding from those infected, thus protecting susceptible persons. Fortunately, these drugs do not seem to block or reduce antibody response or future immunity to the infecting strain. Because of the removal of indications for these drugs owing to drug resistance, they will not be discussed further in this chapter. Detailed information can be found in the ACIP annual recommendations prior to 2005 at *www.cdc.gov/mmwr.*

Recent Advances. Research on the use of neuraminidase inhibitors has recently produced two new Food and Drug Administration (FDA)–approved type A and B anti-influenza drugs—Glaxo's inhaled powder, zanamivir (Relenza), and Roche's oral capsule, oseltamivir phosphate (Tamiflu). Both medications must be taken within 2 days of symptom onset, zanamivir as two inhalations (10 mg total) twice daily at 2-hour intervals on the first day and then two inhalations twice daily at 12-hour intervals for 5 days and oseltamivir as a 75-mg capsule twice daily for 5 days. These drugs can reduce the duration of illness by 1–3 days but are indicated only for type A and B influenza in adults. Possible side effects include nausea and/or vomiting, bronchitis, insomnia, and vertigo. Detail descriptions of the drugs and their annual recommendations are available in the ACIP annual recommendations [89].

Compliance with Recommendations

Although efforts to protect the general public from exposure to influenza usually prove unsuccessful, efforts aimed at high-risk groups can be effective. Special efforts have been made to target individuals over the age of 65 because of their higher mortality from influenza, and compliance with recommendations has improved greatly. Medicare initiated reimbursement for influenza vaccine in 1993 [152], although the paperwork involved generally was not cost-effective for many private influenza campaigns or employers. However, reimbursement was doubled in 2002 by the Centers for Medicare and Medicaid Services (CMS).

Many older people remember vaccines from the 1940s to mid-1960s that were less pure and had more side effects owing to impurities. Since these vaccine side effects of fever, headache, muscle aches, and fatigue were essentially the same as those of influenza, many mistakenly assumed that the vaccine infected them with influenza. Although no influenza vaccine ever used in the United States could have been capable of transmitting influenza infection, this misconception persists and has continued to have a negative effect on use of the influenza vaccine.

Even with the massive public health campaigns for immunization with the 1976 swine flu, only about 25% of the U.S. population was immunized. National health objectives for the year 2010 include vaccination of 90% of those at risk for severe influenza-related illness. The public expects modern vaccines to be highly efficacious, and they remain relatively disappointed with influenza products. But vaccine does fail when there is circulation of an influenza virus that is dissimilar from that used in the vaccine and offers little, if any, protection. And it has been shown that individuals can get more than one influenza A subtype infection in a single season [153]. The Japanese have vaccinated nearly 100% of their children, but epidemics persist.

Until very recently, few studies had been done on the use of influenza vaccines in health care workers. Doebbeling and colleagues [154] studied factors associated with use of influenza vaccines by hospital workers over two seasons. Among the professional nursing staff, they found positive associations with age, salary, and employment time and negative associations with absenteeism. Nonprofessional support staff showed positive associations with age, female gender, salary, and length of employment. Nonprofessional staff had an association only with age. An assumption can be made that the more one knows about influenza and the more experience one has with its complications, the more likely one is to elect annual immunization.

If employers cannot offer the vaccine to employees on-site, they should provide information on immunizations through their benefit plans or community services. Employers also should be cooperative in allowing health care providers to publicize times and places of influenza vaccinations, especially those convenient to the workplace. Table 11B-2 summarizes factors that may increase use of the influenza vaccine. The left column denotes minimal effort, service, or employer cost, whereas the right column moves the spectrum toward increased effort, convenience, and cost.

Metrics to Assess Adequacy of Preventive Measures

The best incentive for taking measures to prevent influenza is the dollar. Many articles have been published on the efficacy and cost-benefit analysis of influenza vaccine, although most studies have concentrated on immunization for the elderly [14, 155–158] and Medicare [159, 160], HMO, HIV-infected [161], and chronic lung disease [162] populations rather than for workers per se [13, 14, 163]. All studies show a positive benefit from immunization, and influenza vaccine is often used as an example of cost-benefit efficacy in methodology papers [164, 165].

Direct costs of influenza illness include physician and office fees, cost of laboratory tests, cost of prescription and nonprescription drugs, hospital charges for acute and/or extended care, and cost of supplies. But these costs may represent only 20–30% of the total cost. Indirect costs are those of absenteeism to industry, schools, and government and the economic costs of years of life lost (e.g., life insurance, burial, and dependent support) for individuals who die from influenza. Costs of prevention are those of vaccine and antiviral medications, the staff and facilities to immunize or examine, medical treatment for adverse effects of vaccinations and antiviral medications, and the loss of employees' productive time going to and from the provider's facility or the pharmacy.

In light of these direct and indirect costs, why do so many individuals choose not to take the vaccine? An "individual" decision-analysis model was con-

Table 11B-2
Spectrum of Factors That Impact Employees' Utilization of Influenza Vaccine

Factor	Positive Impact	Negative Impact
Education	Provided	Not provided
Educator	Knowledgeable provider	Less knowledgeable
Place	At worksite	Off worksite
Time	Organized availability	Make own arrangements
	During work time	Outside work time
	All shifts	Limited shifts
	Multiple dates	Limited dates
Ends	When vaccine gone	When scheduled times for immunization end
How	Walk-in	Appointment
	No waiting	Waiting lines
Cost	Free to employees	Employee pay/co-pay
Who	Employee and family	Employee only

structed by Dr. Stephen C. Schoenbaum of the Harvard Pilgrim Health Plan of New England in 1987 [166]. He presented two decision equations applicable to the individual, one during the preseason and one during an influenza epidemic. They are summarized in Tables 11B-3 and 11B-4. Table 11B-5 presents a model for estimating work loss for the individual worker.

Those at high risk for morbidity or mortality from influenza have higher relative costs associated with illness than those with higher incomes. Schoenbaum's model fails to consider the occupational or social variables that may affect the individual's chances of being infected (attack rates). Employers and their contracted providers can best influence the individual equations by offering convenient low-cost vaccination (see Table 11B-2).

Symptoms and Signs

CLINICAL EPIDEMIOLOGY

For the purpose of epidemiologic surveillance, the classic case definition for an *influenza-like illness* (ILI) is a fever over 100°F (37.8°C) and either a sore throat or cough [167]. This definition is highly sensitive for the diagnosis of clinically apparent influenza but has poor specificity. Onset of symptoms can be as soon as 24 hours after exposure and viral invasion but is usually 48–96 hours postexposure. The communicable (infective) period may precede symptoms by a few hours and peaks with the peak illness and symptoms of fever, cough, and/or nasal discharge. Communicability and viral shedding ends 2–3 days after peak symptoms but may persist for up to 7 days in children and those with primary influenza pneumonia.

Table 11B-3
General Benefit-Cost Model of Preseason Influenza Immunization from an Individual's Perspective

Expected benefits = cost of having influenza
  × average annual probability of an epidemic (0.33)
  × average attack rate if an epidemic year (0.2–0.3)
  × vaccine efficacy rate if taken (0.6–0.7)
    = 0.33 × 0.2 × 0.6 = 4% of the cost of having influenza *or*
    0.33 × 0.3 × 0.7 = 7% of the cost of having influenza
Expected costs = cost of receiving the vaccine + cost of having a significant reaction

Source: Reprinted from Schoenbaum SC. Economic impact of influenza. The individual's perspective. *Am J Med* 1987;82:26–30. © 1987 with permission from Excerpta Medica Inc.

Table 11B-4
Benefit-Cost Model for Protection of an Individual Against Influenza During an Epidemic

Expected benefit = preseason expected benefits (from Table 11-3)
  × 1/preseason probability of an epidemic
  × anticipated residual occurrence rate
    = preseason expected benefits × 1/0.33 × approx 1.0[a]
    = 3 × (preseason expected benefits)
    = 12 – 20% of the cost of having a case of influenza
Expected costs = cost of receiving vaccine
  + cost of having a reaction
  + cost of receiving antiviral medication for 2 weeks
  + cost of reaction to antiviral medication

[a]Early in an epidemic, the residual occurrence rate is almost as high as the originally anticipated occurrence rate
Source: Reprinted from Schoenbaum SC. Economic impact of influenza. The individual's perspective. *Am J Med* 1987;82:26–30. © 1987 with permission from Excerpta Medica Inc.

Table 11B-5
Annual Work-Loss Benefit Model of Influenza Vaccine, Individual Perspective

Severe epidemic year, not vaccinated:	
Chance of illness (40% attack rate)[a]	0.40
Chance will have work absenteeism (50%)[b]	0.50
Days absent (average 4)	4.00
Average number of days absent (multiply all three above)	0.80
Mild epidemic year, not vaccinated:	
Chance of illness (20% attack rate)[a]	0.20
Chance will have work absenteeism (30%)[b]	0.30
Days absent (average 3)	3.00
Average number of days absent (multiply all three above)	0.18
Severe epidemic year, vaccinated:	
Chance of illness (40% attack rate)[a]	0.40
Divided by vaccine efficacy (40%, 60% failure)[c]	0.24
Chance will have work absenteeism (50%)[b]	0.50
Days absent (average 4)	4.00
Average number of days absent (multiply all above)	0.48
Mild epidemic year, vaccinated:	
Chance of illness (20% attack rate)[a]	0.20
Divided by vaccine efficacy (80% success, 20% failure)[c]	0.04
Chance will have work absenteeism (30%)[b]	0.30
Days absent (average 3)	3.00
Average numbers of days absent (multiply all above)	0.04

[a]Assumes that severe epidemic years have an influenza attack rate of 40%, and mild epidemic years 20%.
[b]Assumes that in severe epidemic years, there is more severe illness, with 50% of workers becoming ill and losing an average of four days, and in milder epidemic years, there is milder illness, with 30% of workers becoming ill and losing an average of three days.
[c]Assumes that vaccine is one half as effective in severe epidemic years, compared with mild epidemic years—40% versus 80%—due to antigenic drift and/or mismatching.

The attack rate in the general public is 10–20% annually but can reach over 70% in closed or less ventilated environments, including the workplace [21, 71]. The observational influenza studies performed in Cleveland [168], Seattle [169], Houston [170], and Tecumseh [171] consistently showed higher attack rates (20–50%) in adults living in households with infected children. Houston HMO studies of 1981–1983 showed that the rate of physician visits for acute respiratory disease during the 10-week peak influenza season was about 12% for employed persons and their adult family members [172]. A U.S. study showed that vaccinated workers averaged 0.31 physician visits for ILI compared with 0.55 for unvaccinated workers [14]. Scandinavian studies showed an average work absence owing to influenza of 4.9 days [163].

PREVALENCE OF SYMPTOMS

Of all healthy people infected by influenza, about 20% have inapparent illness, and 30% have some respiratory symptoms without fever. However, 50% have a full-blown illness, that is, respiratory symptoms, chills and fever, sore throat, myalgia, headaches, malaise, and persistent cough [74, 153, 173–177]. Severity of symptoms varies from strain to strain and year to year depending on host-related factors such as age and previous immunity.

CLINICAL COURSE

Onset of influenza symptoms is usually abrupt. The first symptoms are usually fever, sore throat, and myalgia, followed closely by cough (usually nonproductive), coryza, headache, and fatigue. Easy fatigability may last a week or more, and a dry cough may be protracted, lasting 2 weeks or more. Temperatures can range from 100–103°F (37.8–39.4°C) and possibly higher in children. Gastrointestinal symptoms are less prevalent in adults than in children but may include loss of appetite or tussive vomiting. Constipation from decongestants, antihistamines, or antitussive medication; abdominal pain or vomiting from nonsteroidal anti-inflammatory medications; and diarrhea secondary to antibiotic prescriptions are often mistakenly blamed on the primary illness. Predominant primary gastrointestinal symptoms generally are not attributable to influenza viruses. *Stomach flu* and *intestinal influenza* are misnomers used to describe illnesses caused by other organisms.

COMPLICATIONS

Influenza is usually a self-limited illness; healthy American adults who contract it usually lose about 4 calendar days from work. About 5% of adults who become ill develop significant lower respiratory tract conditions such as tracheobronchitis or pneumonitis. The pneumonitis can be either primary influenza or a secondary bacterial pathogen. Common bacteria influenza-associated pneumonias include those caused by *Streptococcal pneumoniae, Staphylococcus aureus,* and *Haemophilus influenzae.* If death occurs from secondary bacterial pneumonia, it usually happens within 1–2 weeks of the onset of pneumonia symptoms. Secondary infections of the sinus or middle ear are common after influenza.

Most influenza-related deaths occur in those with preexisting heart or lung disease who are over age 65. Rates of hospitalization of the elderly may increase two- to fivefold [89] during a major influenza epidemic. Those with weakened immune systems or heart or lung disease are more prone to succumb to pneumonia and/or pulmonary edema with hypoxia. Some have theorized that influenza can precipitate myocardial infarction owing to primary myocardial invasion [177, 178], but no association between myocardial infarction and viral antibodies has been found [179]. Myocarditis and rhabdomyolysis in association with some strains of influenza A [180] have been documented, however [180].

Most adults hospitalized with acute respiratory infections clinically or epidemiologically related to influenza are not in a high-risk group recommended for influenza vaccination [20]. Most are employed.

Reye's syndrome is a rare complication of influenza [181]. Hallmarks of the syndrome are encephalopathy and fatty microvesiculation of the liver associated with the use of salicylate by individuals with influenza B (more than A), especially children and young adults. The syndrome has a mortality rate of up to 40% and also may complicate primary varicella infection. The use of salicylates is contraindicated for all children and young adults with any ILIs.

Some of the more rarely reported cases of organ failure—cardiac, liver, and renal failure—have been associated with specific influenza strains, particularly new or pandemic strains. One report suggested that influenza virus may infect peripheral lymphocytes [182]. A toxic shock–like syndrome as a complication of influenza infection also has been reported.

The Asian influenza of 1957–1958 was suspected of causing viremia and contributing to a higher incidence of schizophrenia in children born of mothers infected in midpregnancy [183, 184]. An association between influenza and schizophrenia would support the hypothesis of schizophrenia as a neurodevelopmental disorder. Reviews have been published by Hayase and Tobita [145] and McGrath and Castle [184]. A nested case-control study of a 1959–1966 birth cohort with a 30- to 38-year follow-up showed a sevenfold increased risk of schizophrenia in offspring exposed to influenza in the first trimester [185]. This same article reviews earlier studies.

PATHOPHYSIOLOGY

Infection may result from as few as 5 influenza-infected droplet nuclei inspired into the deep lung or approximately 100 or more droplet nuclei coming into contact with the nasopharyngeal mucosa [69]. The degree and depth of tissue reaction may be positively correlated with both the infectivity and the severity of symptoms and illness associated with the specific influenza strain.

The columnar epithelium is destroyed by the replicating intracellular influenza virus, possibly stripping it down to the bare basement membrane [186]. The dead and infected epithelium is then sloughed off, and lymphocytic infiltrates can develop in the lung, causing fibrosis or pulmonary edema. The slow regeneration of the columnar epithelium may be responsible for the prolonged dry throat and cough that are characteristic of influenza. Repair of the mucosal surfaces is necessary to restore the mucociliary escalator clearance systems, which protect the lower respiratory tree and help to clear damaged tissue. Influenza injury of the lung also may impair the function of pulmonary macrophages. It may be this impairment that increases the infected individual's vulnerability to other pulmonary pathogens and thus increases the chance of bacterial pneumonia.

There is no evidence to support the belief that the mammalian influenza virus can replicate anywhere other than in respiratory system cells [187]. The neuraminidase portion of the influenza virion may be the part responsible for invasion of the very susceptible lower respiratory mucous membranes, but there are several case reports of the culturing of influenza from other body organs, including skeletal muscles, cardiac muscle, and lymphocytes. The actual pathogenesis of influenza complications such as encephalitis, myositis, myalgia, and Reye's syndrome is unknown.

IgA- or mucous membrane–mediated immunity to specific influenza viruses may offer partial protection from closely related strains, but it is IgG immunity that seems to provide the most lasting natural immunity.

Differential Diagnosis

Because of the nature of this text, this discussion of differential diagnosis pertains only to adults. As mentioned previously, the definition of *influenza-like illness* (ILI) is any febrile illness with either a sore throat or a cough regardless of the season in which the illness occurs. Synonyms for self-limited upper (above the epiglottis) respiratory infection are *upper respiratory infections* (URIs), *acute viral rhinitis,* the *common cold* (or ICD-9 460, ICD-10 J00), *pharyngitis,* and *laryngitis.*

Since influenza (ICD-9 487 and ICD-10 J10,11) is not a reportable disease, clinical epidemiologic information is not collected. A definitive diagnosis can be made only by confirmatory laboratory studies. Dozens of microorganisms with hundreds of serotypes can cause ILI. Many more serious infections can begin with ILI symptoms, including many viral and some bacterial meningitides (see Chapter 23), *Legionella* (see Chapter 10), other upper respiratory tract infections (see Chapter 14), and chlamydial infections (see Chapter 12).

BACTERIA
Mycoplasma Pneumonia

Also known as *primary atypical pneumonia, Mycoplasma* pneumonia shares many characteristics with influenza, including fever, headache, malaise, and persistent paroxysmal coughing. Like influenza, *Mycoplasma* pneumonia also may occur in epidemics in military units or institutions and has a higher frequency in older children and young adults. However, with *Mycoplasma* pneumonia, there is a much flatter epidemic curve owing to its longer incubation of 6–32 days and its communicable period of several weeks. Also, it is more likely to occur in late summer or early fall, unlike influenza, which occurs from late fall through early spring.

Streptococcus (Group A Beta-Hemolytic)

Streptococcal infection shares with influenza the symptoms of fever and sore throat but is less likely to cause significant cough. An individual with streptococcal sore throat usually presents with more physical findings, such as cervical lymphadenopathy, tonsillitis, and edema, redness, or petechiae of the throat or palate. Rapid tests for streptococcus may aid in the diagnosis.

Other Viral Infections

If it were practical to perform viral cultures on all adults with upper respiratory cold symptoms, not all would be positive. Overall, influenza viruses would represent about 10–15% of positive cultures, but during a midwinter outbreak of upper respiratory illness, these viruses could account for over 50%. Coronaviruses would represent another 10–15%, but the largest class represented would be the over 100 serotypes of rhinoviruses (20–40%), and this would be even higher in the fall [21]. The clinical course for all the viruses is essentially the same, as are their short incubation periods. But many other viruses can cause ILI if there is associated viremia. Even the initial seroconverting viremia of HIV most often described as an "influenza-like illness."

Significant fever is almost always present with influenza, whereas it is less characteristic of other respiratory viruses (Figure 11B-4 and Table 11B-6). Cervical adenopathy, productive cough, pleuritic pain, and visible lesions of the oropharynx are more characteristic of other viruses (such as mononucleosis, coxsackievirus, CMV, or other herpesviruses) and bacterial pharyngitis. Influenza is most accurately diagnosed "epidemiologically" by the prevalence of similar illness in the community or worker cohorts. Health care practitioners should not hesitate to access up-to-date surveillance information to aid in diagnosis (at www.cdc.gov/flu).

Diagnostic Evaluation

White blood cell counts are usually normal (5,000–10,000/mm^3) in persons with influenza, but there is a relative lymphocytosis. Leukopenia may be present in up to 50% of patients during the acute phase of the illness. White counts over 15,000/mm^3 suggest bacterial or secondary infection. Diagnostic laboratory tests should focus on secondary infection in the seriously ill, especially if there is preexisting cardiac or pulmonary disease. Other diagnostic testing should be performed on the basis of symptoms, for example, chest radiography or arterial blood gas measurement for individuals with respiratory crisis and electrocardiography or heart monitoring for persons with cardiovascular complications.

Performing specific virology studies for most patients is not clinically practical because test results will not be available until after the illness has run its clinical course. Some surveillance using the sentinel physician system is done for epidemiologic and planning purposes, and more intensive studies may be indicated when an epidemic is suspected of having an animal origin and/or there is the threat of a major antigenic shift [30,31]. Bedside rapid diagnostic aids are increasing in availability and utility and are described by Dr Wright in Chapter 11A.

Influenza cannot be distinguished from other respiratory illnesses by clinical examination of the patient. Definitive diagnosis requires specific influenza testing by one of several methods. These include the following:

VIRUS ISOLATION

Virus isolation methods have the advantage of producing virus of sufficient quantity for full antigenic characterization, which is needed for matching with vaccines. The disadvantage is that results are not available for several days and thus are of little use to the clinician. Rapid culture assays detect viral antigens in cell culture and are available in a shorter time period. State health departments should be contacted for information on local laboratory support for influenza surveillance.

ANTIGEN-DETECTION ASSAYS

There are several methods for the diagnosis of influenza infection directly from clinical material. Cells from the clinical specimen can be stained using immunofluorescent antibody to detect the presence of viral antigen. Nasal washes, nasopharyngeal aspirates, nasal throat swabs, gargling fluid, transtracheal aspirates, and bronchoalveolar lavage specimens are suitable.

Figure 11B-4
Example of an educational poster available on the Internet. (From the National Institute of Allergy and Infectious Disease at www.niaid.nih.gov/.)

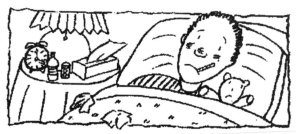

Is It a Cold or the Flu?

Symptoms	Cold	Flu
Fever	Rare	Characteristic, high (102-104°F); lasts 3-4 days
Headache	Rare	Prominent
General Aches, Pains	Slight	Usual; often severe
Fatigue, Weakness	Quite mild	Can last up to 2-3 weeks
Extreme Exhaustion	Never	Early and prominent
Stuffy Nose	Common	Sometimes
Sneezing	Usual	Sometimes
Sore Throat	Common	Sometimes
Chest Discomfort, Cough	Mild to moderate; hacking cough	Common; can become severe
Complications	Sinus congestion or earache	Bronchitis, pneumonia; can be life-threatening
Prevention	None	Annual vaccination; amantadine or rimantadine (antiviral drugs)
Treatment	Only temporary relief of symptoms	Amantadine or rimantadine within 24-48 hours after onset of symptoms

Other methods include immunostaining, visualization of viral antigens by electron microscopy, detection of viral RNA by molecular hybridization, and reverse transcriptase polymerase chain reaction (PCR). When direct antigen-detection methods are used for the diagnoses of influenza, it is important to save an aliquot of the clinical sample for further testing, if necessary. These samples may be used for culture confirmation of direct test results and virus isolation for subtyping of influenza A isolates by a public health laboratory. Full antigenic characterization of the virus may be performed by the U.S. World Health Organization (WHO Collaborating Center for Surveillance, Epidemiology, and Control of Influenza, Influenza Branch, CDC). This characterization is necessary for the detection and tracking of antigenic variants, an essential part of the selection of optimal influenza vaccine components.

SEROLOGIC TESTING: SERODIAGNOSIS

Because most human sera contain antibodies to influenza, the diagnosis of influenza cannot be made from a single serum sample. Paired serum

Table 11B-6
Characteristics of Adult Upper Respiratory Infections: Acute and Early Symptoms

Characteristic	Influenza	Other Virus	Bacteria
Symptoms			
High fever	+++	+	++
Acute onset	+++	++	+
Swollen cervical lymph nodes	+	++	++
Oral or pharyngeal lesions	0	++	++
Productive cough	+	++	+++
Shortness of breath	0	+	++
Copious nasal discharge	++	+++	+
Conjunctivitis	+	++	++
Pleuritic chest pain	+	++	+++
Complications			
Rapid recovery	+++	+	++
Secondary sinusitis	+	++	+++
Secondary bronchitis	+	+	++
Secondary pneumonitis	++	+	++
Epidemiology			
Short incubations	++	+	−
Mid-winter epidemic	+++	++	+
Children ill first	+++	++	+
Quick epidemic curve	+++	+	0
Excess mortality	+++	0	+

specimens are required for serologic diagnosis of influenza infection. The presence of a fourfold increase in specific monoclonal IgG or IgM during the disease course confirms recent infection: IgM peaks at 2 weeks and IgG at 4–7 weeks following infection. A finding of high IgG early in the course of the illness or a stable IgG after a second serologic test indicates immunity that preexists the illness. A complement fixation or hemagglutinin test showing a fourfold increase of IgG or IgM in sera compared with the level during the acute phase and convalescence a few weeks later confirms recent influenza infection.

The acute specimen should be collected within a few days of the onset of illness, and the convalescent sample should be collected approximately 2–3 weeks later for IgM or 4 weeks later for IgG. A positive result is a fourfold or greater rise in titer between the acute and convalescent samples to one subtype of virus. For example, starting with an initial serum dilution of 1:10, a twofold (doubling) serum dilution would result in a concentration of 1:20. A fourfold or higher increase in titer between the acute and convalescent phase sera—that is, an increase from 1:20 to 1:80 or higher—would be considered positive. A twofold increase between the two sera is within the margin of error for the test and should not be considered a positive finding. To ensure that a rise in titer is due to infection rather than to recent influenza vaccination, the vaccination history of the patient also must be taken into account.

Treatment and Rehabilitation

The 1918 pandemic occurred many years before vaccines, antiviral medications, or antibiotics were available, yet 90% of infected persons survived and acquired lifelong partial protection from A(H1N1) influenza. Influenza is usually a self-limited illness, but the severity of the illness and an individual's risk for complications may well correlate with whether and to what degree the illness is self-limited.

Rest is the best treatment, and the profound fatigue of early illness may be nature's best defense mechanism. Hydration is essential to replace body fluids lost because of fever and to assist repair of respiratory tissues damaged by viral invasion. Frequent sips and swallows of fluids may help to relieve coughing stimulated by the damaged respiratory epithelium. Hydration is needed for the proper operation of the mucociliary escalator functions and for coughing to clear infected sections.

The use of prescription cough suppressive medication in influenza is controversial. Salt water or analgesic gargles may relieve coughing, and smokers should abstain from smoking. A cool-mist humidifier in the bedroom may assist rest, but the water should be changed every 8 hours to prevent *Pseudomonas* contamination. Although appetite may be suppressed, the patient should eat regular meals of nonspicy but nutritious foods. The complex carbohydrates of fruits and vegetables may help to provide energy and reduce fatigue.

Over-the-counter analgesics, decongestants, and antihistamines may afford some symptomatic relief. Acetaminophen, not aspirin, should be used for fever in children and adolescents. Amantadine or rimantadine may lessen the severity and course of influenza A if started within 48 hours of onset of symptoms, although they are no longer recommended because of resistance. The same dose is used as that for prophylaxis (200 mg daily for healthy adults, 100 mg daily for those over age 65 and those known to have renal impairment). Oseltamivir (Tamiflu) orally or zanamivir (Ralenza) intranasally may reduce symptoms and the duration of illness if given within 36 hours of onset of illness. Antibiotics should be used only for confirmed or strongly suspected secondary bacterial infection, evidenced by a positive chest radiogram, purulent or bloody sputum, pleuritic pain, positive Gram's stain, or a positive rapid antigen test.

Some have claimed that influenza may cause permanent impairment of pulmonary function [90], but recovery is usually complete, and permanent sequelae from influenza or its treatment are very rare.

Occupational Considerations

Companies and other organizations should have business and operating contingency plans for periods of high employee absenteeism owing to influenza. Every few years this could be as high as 50% over a period of a few days. Companies should remove as many administrative, financial, and time barriers as possible for their workers to receive in-

fluenza immunizations and/or treatment (see Table 11B-2) in an effort to maximize use of vaccination. If an employer is unable to provide on-site administration of influenza vaccine by its own or contracted nurses, then benefits managers should pressure the health plan vendors to cover prevention services such as influenza vaccine and anti-influenza chemoprophylaxis. An organization's plans should include access to health care providers near the workplace and reasonable copayments for outpatient visits for vaccination and ILI treatment. Formal employee-sponsored health-promotion or wellness programs should include credits and incentives for use of annual influenza immunizations. Other recommendations for administrative support are discussed on pages 235–238. Publications and protocols for employer preparations for pandemic influenza have been published since the first edition of this chapter [188–190]. The U.S. Army also has published nonvaccine recommendations to reduce acute respiratory infections in close-quarter living [191].

There has been a tendency since the 1990s for human resources and benefits departments to combine previous categories of days off into a single bank of paid time off to simplify their recordkeeping. This impairs the ability to study workers' illnesses in detail [19]; thus questions such as the efficacy of influenza vaccines or other prevention programs will remain unanswered ("No data in, no data out").

Occupational health providers should be aware of the factors that put an individual at high risk for influenza and of recommendations for immunization, and they should make a year-round effort to identify workers for education about and offering of vaccination. Providers also should be familiar with the epidemiology of influenza and the community and occupational risk factors for the disease. All occupational health practitioners should be able to provide information on the disease and its prevention and how to implement and promote influenza prevention programs.

References

1. Pfeifer R. Vorlaufige mitt heilunger uber die erreger der influenzae. Dtsch Med Wochenschr 1892;18:28–34.
2. Pfeifer R. Die aetiologie der influenza. *Z Hyg Infektioskr* 1893;13:357–86.

3. Winslow CE, Broadhurst J, Buchanan RE, et al. The families and genera of the bacteria: Final report of the Committee of the Society of American Bacteriologists on Characterization and Classification of Bacterial Types. *J Bacteriol* 1920;5:191–229.

4. Smith W, Andrewes CH, Laidlaw PP. A virus obtained from influenza patients. *Lancet* 1933;2:66–8.

5. *Influenza Factsheets.* Bethesda, MD: National Coalition for Adult Immunizations, June 1997.

6. Pachucki CT, Walsh Pappas SA, Fuller GF, et al. Influenza A among hospital personnel and patients: Implications for recognition, prevention, and control. *Arch Intern Med* 1990;149:77–80.

7. Hammond GW, Cheang M. Absenteeism among hospital staff during an influenza epidemic: Implications for immunoprophylaxis. *Can Med Assoc J* 1984;131:449–52.

8. Williams WW, Preblud SR, Reichedlderfer PS, et al. Vaccines of importance in the hospital setting. *Infect Dis Clin North Am* 1989;76:501–4.

9. Mast EE, Harmon MW, Gravenstein S, et al. Emergency and possible transmission of amantadine-resistant viruses during nursing home outbreaks of influenza (AH3N2). *Am J Epidemiol* 1991;134:986–97.

10. Balkovic ES, Goodman, A, Rose FB, et al. Nosocomial influenza A(H1N1) infection. *Am J Med Technol* 1980;46:318–20.

11. Van Voris LP, Belshe RB, Shaffer JL. Nosocomial influenza B virus infection in the elderly. *Ann Intern Med* 1982;96:153–8.

12. Centers for Disease Control and Prevention. Suspected nosocomial influenza cases in an intensive care unit. *MMWR* 1988;37:3.

13. Campbell DS, Rumley MH. Cost-effectiveness of the influenza vaccine in a healthy, working-age population. *J Occup Environ Med* 1997;39:408–14.

14. Nichol KL, Lind A, Margolis KL, et al. The effectiveness of vaccination against influenza in healthy working adults. *N Engl J Med* 1995;333:889–93.

15. Smith JWG, Pollard R. Vaccination against influenza: A five-year study of the post office. *J Hyg (Lond)* 1979;83:157–70.

16. Greene CC, Beaver GT. A study of mass influenza inoculation in a large industry. *J Occup Med* 1960;2:263–70.

17. Philipp R, Harvey K, Fletcher G, et al. Sickness absence from work and influenza immunization. *J Soc Occup Med* 1987;37:128–9.

18. Wiengarten S, Staniloff H, Ault M, et al. Do hospital employees benefit from the influenza vaccine? A placebo-controlled clinical trail. *J Gen Intern Med* 1988;3:32–7.

19. Olsen GW, Burris JM, Burlew MM, et al. Absenteeism among employees who participated in a workplace influenza immunization program. *J Occup Environ Med* 1998;40:311–6.

20. Glezen WP, Decker M, Perrotta DM. Survey of underlying conditions of persons ospitalized with acute respiratory disease during influenza epidemics in Houston, 1978–1981. *Am Rev Respir Dis* 1987;136:550–5.

21. Benenson AS (ed). *Control of Communicable Diseases Manual,* 16th ed. Washington: American Public Health Association, 1995, pp 245–51.

22. Last JM (ed). *A Dictionary of Epidemiology,* 3rd ed. New York: Oxford University Press, 1995, p 121.

23. Jones HS. *Thucydidis Historiae.* Exfor, England: Clarendon Press, 1942.

24. Langmuir AD, Worthen TD, Solomon J, et al. Thucydides syndrome: A new hypothesis for the cause of the plague of Athens. *N Engl J Med* 1985;313:1027–30.

25. Townsend JF. History of influenza epidemics. *Ann Med History* 1933;5:533–47.

26. Douglas RG. Influenza. In Goldman L, Bennett JC (eds), *Cecil Textbook of Medicine,* 19th ed. Philadelphia: Saunders, 1992, Chap 36, p 1815.

27. Graves RJ. Influenza. In Graves RJ, Gerhard WW (eds), *System of Clinical Medicine.* Philadelphia: Barrington and Hasvwell, 1848, p 462.

28. Farr W. *Tenth Annual Report of the Registrar General.* London: HMSO, 1847.

29. 1918 Killer flu virus sequence in GenBank. *NCBI News* 2006;14:2; available at www.ncbi.nlm.nih.gov/Web/NewsltrV15N1/1918.html.

30. Centers for Disease Control and Prevention. Update: Isolation of an avian influenza A (H5N1) viruses from humans—Hong Kong, 1997–1998. *MMWR* 1998;46,52,53:1245–7.

31. World Health Organization. *Emerging and Other Communicable Diseases,* Fact Sheet no 188: *Influenza A(H5N1),* January 9, 1998; available at www.who.ch/programmes/emc/flu/h5n1.htm.

32. Centanni E, Savonuzzi O (cited by Stubbs EL). Fowl plague. In Bister HE, Schwarte OH (eds), *Diseases of Poultry,* 4th ed. Ames, IA: Iowa State University Press, 1965.

33. Shope RE. Swine influenza (a series of papers). *J Exp Med* 1931;54:349–85.

34. Shope RE. The incidence of neutralizing antibodies for swine influenza virus in the sera of human beings of different ages. *J Exp Med* 1936;63:669–84.

35. Davenport FM, Hennessy AB, Francis T. Epidemiologic and immunologic significance of age distribution of antibody to antigenic variants of influenza virus. *J Exp Med* 1953;98:641–56.

36. Laidlaw PP. Epidemic influenza: A virus disease. *Lancet* 1935;1:1118.

37. Shope RE, Francis T. The susceptibility of swine to the virus of human influenza. *J Exp Med* 1936;64:791.

38. Shope RE. Serological evidence for the occurrence of infection with human influenza virus in swine. *J Exp Med* 1938;67:739–48.

39. Kaplan MM, Payne AM. Serological survey in animals for type A influenza in relation to the 1957 pandemic. *Bull WHO* 1959;20:465–88.

40. Kundin WD. Hong Kong influenza virus infection among swine during a human epidemic in Taiwan. *Nature (London)* 1970;228:857.

41. Schnurrenberger PR, Woods GT, Marti RJ. Serologic evidence of human infection with swine virus. *Am Rev Respir Dis* 1970;102:356–61.

42. Smith TF, Burgert EO, Dowdle WR, et al. Isolation of swine influenza virus from autopsy lung tissue of man. *N Engl J Med* 1976;294:708–10.

43. O'Brien RJ, Noble GR, Easterday BC, et al. Swine-like influenza virus infection in a Wisconsin farm family. *J Infect Dis* 1977;136:S390–6.

44. Hurwitz E, Schonberger LB, Nelson DB, et al. Guillain-Barré syndrome and 1978–1979 influenza vaccine. *N Engl J Med* 1981;304:1557.

45. Kaplan JE, Katona P, Hurwitz ES, et al. Guillain-Barré syndrome in the United States, 1979–1980 and 1980–1981: Lack of association with influenza vaccination. *JAMA* 1982;248:698–700.

46. Wentworth DE, McGregor MW, Macklin MD, et al. Transmission of swine influenza virus to humans after exposure to experimentally infected pigs. *J Infect Dis* 1997;175:7–14.

47. Department of Health and Human Services. *Biosafety in Microbiological and Biomedical Laboratories,* 3rd ed. Publication no (CDC) 93-8395. Washington: US Government Printing Office, 1993, pp 44–67; available at www.cdc.gov/od/ohs/biosfty/.

48. Top FH, Russell PK. Swine influenza at Fort Dix: IV. Summary and speculation. *J Infect Dis* 1977;135:S376–80.

49. Hinshaw VS, Bean WJ Jr, Webster RB, et al. The prevalence of influenza viruses in swine and the antigenic and genetic relatedness of influenza viruses from man and swine. *Virology* 1978;84:51–62.

50. Dasco CC, Couch RB, Six HR, et al. Sporadic occurrence of zoonotic swine influenza virus infections. *J Clin Microbiol* 1984;20:833–5.

51. Patriarca PA, Kendal AP, Xakowski PC, et al. Lack of significant person-to-person spread of swine influenza-like virus following fatal infection of an immunocompromised child. *Am J Epidemiol* 1984;119:152–8.

52. Rota PA, Rocha EP, Harmon MW, et al. Laboratory characterization of a swine influenza virus isolated from a fatal case of human influenza. *J Clin Microbiol* 1989;27:1413–6.

53. Wentworth D, Xian X, Cooley AJ, et al. An influenza A(H1N1) virus closely related to swine influenza responsible for a fatal case of human influenza. *J Virol* 1994;68:2051–8.

54. Dykes AC, Cherry JD, Nolan DE. A clinical, epidemiologic, serologic, and virologic study of influenza C virus infection. *Arch Intern Med* 1980;140:1295–8.

55. A revision of the system of nomenclature for influenza virus. *Bull WHO* 1971;45:119–124.

56. A revision of the system of nomenclature for influenza viruses: A WHO memorandum (meeting February, 1980). *Bull WHO* 1980;58:585–91.

57. Laver WG, Webster RG. Studies on the origin of pandemic influenza: III. Evidence implicating duck and equine influenza viruses as possible progenitors of the Hong Kong strain of human influenza. *Virology* 1973;51:383–91.

58. Scholtissek C. Influenza virus genetics. *Adv Genet* 1979;20:1–36.

59. Schoenbaum SC, Coleman MT, Dowdle WR, et al. Epidemiology of influenza in the elderly: Evidence of virus recycling. *Am J Epidemiol* 1976;103:166–73.

60. Houseworth WJ, Spoon MM. The age distribution of excess mortality during A2 Hong Kong influenza epidemics compared with earlier A2 outbreaks. *Am J Epidemiol* 1974;94:348–50.

61. Masurel N, Marine WM. Recycling of Asian and Hong Kong influenza A virus hemagglutinins in man. *Am J Epidemiol* 1973;97:44–9.

62. Pearl R. Influenza studies: On certain general statistical aspects of the 1918 epidemic in American cities. *Public Health Rep* 1919;34:1743–83.

63. Frost WH. The epidemiology of influenza. *Public Health Rep* 1919;34:1823–6.

64. Gross PA. Preparing for the next influenza pandemic: A reemerging infection. *Ann Intern Med* 1996;124:682–5.

65. US Health and Human Services, Centers for Medicare and Medicaid Services. Available at cms.hhs.gov.

66. Glezen WP, Payne AA, Snyder DN, et al. Mortality and influenza. *J Infect Dis* 1982;146:313–21.

67. Couch RB, Kasel JA, Glezen WP, et al. Influenza: Its control in persons and populations (Houston Surveillance Program). *J Infect Dis* 1986;153:431–40.

68. Siegel JD, Rhinehart E, Jackson M, Chiarello L, and the Healthcare Infection Control Practices Advisory Committee. 2007 Guideline for Isolation Precautions: Preventing Transmission of Infectious Agents in Healthcare Settings, June 2007; available at www.cdc.gov/ncidod/dhqp/pdf/isolation2007.pdf.

69. Knight V, Couch RB, Landahl HD. The effect of the lack of gravity on airborne infection during space flight. *JAMA* 1970;214:513–8.

70. Couch RB. Epidemiology of influenza: Summary of influenza, Workshop IV. *J Infect Dis* 1973;128:361–86.

71. Moser MR, Bender TR, Marelolis NS, et al. An outbreak of influenza aboard a commercial airliner. *Am J Epidemiol* 1979;110:1–7.

72. Glezen WP, Frank AL, Taber LH, et al. Influenza in childhood. *Pediatr Res* 1983;17:1029–32.

73. Glezen WP, Paredes A, Taber LH. Influenza in children: Relationship to other respiratory agents. *JAMA* 1980;243:1345–9.

74. Frank AL, Taber LH, Wells JM, et al. Patterns of shedding of myxoviruses and paramyxoviruses in children. *J Infect Dis* 1981;144:433–41.

75. Couch RB, Douglas RG Jr, Feson DS, et al. Correlated studies of a recombinant influenza virus vaccine: III. Protection against experimental influenza in man. *J Infect Dis* 1971;124:473–80.

76. Lefrak EA, Stevens PM, Pitha J, et al. Extracorporeal membrane oxygenation for fulminant influenza pneumonia. *Chest* 1974;66:385–8.

77. Glezen WP. Consideration of the risk of influenza in children and indications for prophylaxis. *Rev Infect Dis* 1980;2:408–20.

78. Glezen WP, Couch RB, Taber LH, et al. Epidemiological observations of influenza B virus infections in Houston, Texas, 1976–1977. *Am J Epidemiol* 1980; 111:13–22.

79. Glezen WP, Couch RB. Interpandemic influenza in the Houston area, 1974–1976. *N Engl J Med* 1978; 298:587–92.

80. Acute respiratory illness among cruise-ship passengers—Asia. *MMWR* 1988;37:63–6.

81. Frank AL, Taber LH, Wells JM. Comparison of infection rates and severity of illness for influenza A subtypes H1N1 and H3N2 (Houston). *J Infect Dis* 1985;151:73–80.

82. Glezen WP, Couch RB. Influenza viruses. In Evans AS, Kaslow RA (eds), *Viral Infections of Humans, Epidemiology and Control*, 4th ed. New York: Plenum Press, 1997, p 482.

83. Longini IM Jr, Kiipman JS. Household and community transmission parameters from final distribution of infections in households. *Biometrics* 1982;38:115–26.

84. Longini IM Jr, Koopman JS, Montao AS, et al. Estimating household and community transmission parameters for influenza. *Am J Epidemiol* 1982;115: 736–48.

85. Webster RG, Bean WJ, Gorman OT, et al. Evaluation and ecology of influenza A viruses. *Mirobiol Rev* 1992;56:152–79.

86. Webster RG. Influenza virus: Transmission between species and relevance to emergency of the next human pandemic. *Arch Virol* 1997;13:S105–13.

87. Webster RG, Shortridge KF, Kawaoka Y. Influenza: Interspecies transmission and emergency of new pandemics. *FEMS Immunol Med Microbiol* 1997;18: 275–9.

88. Webster RG, Sharp GB, Claas ED. Interspecies transmission of influenza viruses. *Am J Respir Crit Care Med* 1995;152:S25–30.

89. Centers for Disease Control and Prevention. Prevention and control of influenza: Recommendations of the Advisory Committee on Immunization Practices. *MMWR* 2007;56:1–54.

90. Little JW, Hall WJ, Douglas RG Jr, et al. Airway hyperactivity and peripheral airway dysfunction in influenza A infection. *Am Rev Respir Dis* 1978;118: 295–303.

91. Evans AS, Niederman JC, Sawyer RN, et al. Prospective studies of a group of Yale University freshmen: II. Occurrence of acute respiratory infections and rubella. *J Infect Dis* 1971;123:271–8.

92. Layd PM, Engelberg AL, Dobbs HI, et al. Outbreak of influenza A/USSR/77 at Marquette University. *J Infect Dis* 1980;142:347–52.

93. Kendal AP, Schieble J, Cooney MK, et al. Cocirculation of two influenza A(H3N2) antigenic variants detected by virus surveillance in individual communities (Berkeley and Seattle). *Am J Epidemiol* 1978; 108:308–11.

94. Evans AS, Dick EC, Nystuden K. Influenza in University of Wisconsin students. *Arch Environ Health* 1963;6:62–9.

95. Evans AS, Espiritu-Campos L. Acute respiratory diseases in students at the University of the Philippines, 1964–69. *Bull WHO* 1971;45:103–12.

96. Klontz KC, Hynes NA, Gunn RA, et al. An outbreak of influenza A/Taiwan/1/86 H1N1 infections at a naval base and its association with airplane travel. *Am J Epidemiol* 1980;129:341–8.

97. Lebiush M, Rannon L, Kark JD. An outbreak of A/USSR/90/77 H1N1 influenza in army recruits: Clinical and laboratory observations. *Mil Med* 1982; 147:43–8.

98. Evans AS. Serologic studies of acute respiratory infection in military personnel. *Yale J Biol Med* 1975; 48:201–9.

99. Roscelli JD, Bass JW, Pang L. Guillain-Barré syndrome and influenza vaccination in the U.S. Army, 1980–1988. *Am J Epidemiol* 1991;133:952–5.

100. Meikejohn G. Viral respiratory disease at Lowry Air Force Base in Denver, 1952–1982. *J Infect Dis* 1983; 148:775–84.

101. Nowotny N, Mostl K, Maderbacher R, et al. Serological studies in Austrian fattening pigs with respiratory disorders. *Acta Vet Hung* 1994;42:377–9.

102. Nowotny N, Armin D, Klemens F, et al. Prevalence of swine influenza and other viral, bacterial, and parasitic zoonoses in veterinarians. *J Infect Dis* 1997; 76:1414–5.

103. Horman JT, Stetler HC, Israel E, et al. An outbreak of influenza A in a nursing home. *Am J Public Health* 1986;124:114–9.

104. Patriarca PA, Weber JA, Parker RA, et al. Risk factors for outbreaks of influenza in nursing homes: A case-control study. *Am J Epidemiol* 1986;76:501–4.

105. Centers for Disease Control and Prevention. Outbreak of influenza A in a nursing home—New York, December 1991 to January 1992. *MMWR* 1992;41: 129–31.

106. Gross PA, Rodstein M, LaMontagne JR, et al. Epidemiology of acute respiratory illness during an influenza outbreak in a nursing home. *Arch Intern Med* 1988;148:559–61.

107. Catter ML, Renzullo PO, Helgerson SD, et al. Influenza outbreaks in nursing homes: How effective is influenza vaccine in the institutionalized elderly? *Infect Control Hosp Epidemiol* 1990;11:473–8.

108. Centers for Disease Control and Prevention. Guidelines for infection control in health care personnel, 1998 (Sec 22, Respiratory Viral Infections); available at www.cdc.gov/ncidod/dhqp/gl_hcpersonnel.html.

109. Potter J, Stott DJ, Roberts MA. Influenza vaccination of health care workers in long-term-care hospitals reduces the mortality of elderly patients. *J Infect Dis* 1997;175:1–6.

110. Miotti PG, Nelson KE, Dallabetta GA, et al. The influence of HIV infection on antibody responses to a two-dose regimen of influenza vaccine. *JAMA* 1989;262:779–83.

111. Cheson F, Hewitt D. Spread of influenza in a factory. *Br J South Med* 1952;6:68–75.

112. Ksaizek TG, Olson JG, Irving GS, et al. An influenza outbreak due to A/USSR/77-like (H1N1) virus aboard a U.S. Navy ship. *Am J Epidemiol* 1980;112:487–94.

113. Centers for Disease Control and Prevention. Guidelines for preventing the transmission of *Mycobacterium* tuberculosis in health-care facilities. *MMWR* 1994;43:69–88.

114. Department of Health and Human Services and Centers for Disease Control and Prevention. Guidelines for preventing the transmission of *Mycobacterium* tuberculosis in health-care facilities, Notice (Supplement no 3, Engineering Controls). *Fed Reg* 1994;59:54276–88.

115. Occupational Health and Safety Administration. *Technical Manual, Sec V: Hospital Investigations, Health and Hazards.* Washington: OSHA, 1988.

116. Baroyan OV, Rvachev LA, Ivannikow YG. *Modeling and Forecasting of Influenza Epidemics for the Territory of the USSR.* Moscow: Gameleya Institute of Epidemiology and Microbiology, 1977.

117. Collins SD, Lehmann J. Trends and epidemics of influenza and pneumonia, 1918–1951. *Public Health Rep* 1951;6:1487–505.

118. Collins SD. *Influenza in the United States, 1887–1957.* Public Health Monograph no 48. Washington: US Government Printing Office, 1957.

119. Serfling RE. Methods for current statistical analysis of excess pneumonia-influenza deaths. *Public Health Rep* 1963;78:494–506.

120. Choi K, Thacker SB. An evaluation of influenza mortality surveillance, 1962–1979: 1. Time-series forecasts of expected pneumonia and influenza deaths. *Am J Epidemiol* 1981;113:215–22.

121. Simonsen L, Clarke MJ, Williamson GD, et al. The impact of influenza epidemics on mortality: Introducing a severity index. *Am J Public Health* 1997;87:1944–50.

122. Salk JE. Reactions to concentrated influenza virus vaccines. *J Immunol* 1948;58:369–95.

123. Baker RS, van Frank RM. Purification of large quantities of influenza virus by density gradient centrifugation. *J Virol* 1967;1:1207–16.

124. Tyrrell DAJ, Schild GC, Dowdle WR, et al. Development and use of influenza vaccines. *Bull WHO* 1981;59:165–73.

125. Poland GA. Lessons from the influenza vaccine recall of 1996–1997. *JAMA* 1997;278:1022–3.

126. *Physicians' Desk Reference,* 52 nd ed. Montavale, NJ: Medical Economics Company, 1998.

127. Hobson D, Curry RL, Beare AS, et al. The role of serum hemagglutination-inhibiting antibody in protection against challenge infection with influenza A and B viruses. *J Hyg (Lond)* 1972;70:767–77.

128. Neuzil KM, Reed GW, Mitchel EF, et al. Influenza morbidity increases in late pregnancy. In *Abstracts of the IDSA,* 34th Annual Meeting, 1996, p 48.

129. Safrin S, Rush JD, Mills J. Influenza in patients with human immunodeficiency virus infection. *Chest* 1990;98:33–7.

130. Murphy KR, Strunk RC. Safe administration of influenza vaccine in asthmatic children hypersensitive to egg proteins. *J Pediatr* 1985;106:931–3.

131. Aberer W. Vaccination despite thimerosal sensitivity. *Contact Dermatitis* 1991;24:6–10.

132. Renton K. Decreased elimination of theophylline after influenza vaccination. *Can Med Assoc J* 1980;123:288.

133. Goldstein RS. Decreased elimination of theophylline after influenza vaccination. *Can Med Assoc J* 1982;126:470.

134. Britton L, Ruben FL. Serum and theophylline levels after influenza vaccination. *Can Med Assoc J* 1982;126:1375.

135. Fischer RG. Influence of trivalent influenza vaccine on serum theophylline levels. *Can Med Assoc J* 1982;124:1312.

136. San Joaquin VH, Reyes S, Marks MI. Influenza vaccination in asthmatic children on maintenance theophylline therapy. *Clin Pediatr* 1982;21:724–6.

137. Stults B, Hasisaki P. Influenza vaccination and theophylline pharmacokinetics in patients with chronic obstructive lung disease. *West J Med* 1983;139:651–4.

138. Kramer P. Effect of influenza vaccine on warfarin anticoagulation. *Clin Pharmacol Ther* 1984;35:416.

139. Lipsky GA. Influenza vaccination and warfarin anticoagulation. *Ann Intern Med* 1984;100:835–7.

140. Hassan WU, Henderson AF, Keaney NP. Influenza vaccination in asthma. *Lancet* 1992;339:194.

141. Daggett P. Influenza and asthma. *Lancet* 1992;339:367.

142. Palache AM, van der Velden JW. Influenza vaccination in asthma. *Lancet* 1992;339:741.

143. Watson JM, Cordier JF. Nicholson KG. Does influenza immunization cause exacerbations of chronic airflow obstruction or asthma? *Thorax* 199752:190–4.

144. Schonberger L, Bregman DJ, Sullivan-Bolyai JZ, et al. Guillain-Barré syndrome following vaccination in the national immunization programs, United States 1976–1977. *Am J Epidemiol* 1979;110:105–23.

145. Hayase Y, Tobita K. Influenza virus and neurological diseases. *Psychiatr Clin Neurosci* 1997;51:181–4.

146. Mac Kenzie WR, Davis JP, Peterson DE, et al. Multiple-false positive serologic tests for HIV, HTLV-1, and hepatitis C following influenza vaccination. *JAMA* 1992;268:1015–7.

147. Vaccine Adverse Event Reporting System, P.O. Box

1100, Rockville, MD 20849-1100. Toll-free phone: 1-800-822-7967.

148. Howell MR, Nang RN, Gaydos CA, et al. Prevention of adenoviral acute respiratory disease in army recruits: Cost-effectiveness of a military vaccination policy. *Am J Prev Med* 1998;14:168–75.

149. Centers for Disease Control and Prevention. *Influenza Vaccine, 1998.* Factsheet. Atlanta: CDC, 1998; available at www.cdc.gov/ncidod/diseases/flu/fluvac.htm.

150. Kendal AP. Cold-adapted live attenuated influenza vaccines developed in Russia: Can they contribute to meeting the needs for influenza control in other countries? *Eur J Epidemiol* 1997;13:591–609.

151. Centers for Disease Control and Prevention. Health Alert: CDC Recommends Against the Use of Amantadine and Rimantadine for the Treatment or Prophylaxis of Influenza in the United States During the 2005–06 Influenza Season; available at www.cdc.gov/flu/han011406.htm.

152. Centers for Disease Control and Prevention. Implementation of the Medicare influenza benefit program. *MMWR* 1994;43:771–3.

153. Frank AL, Taber LH, Wells JM. Individuals infected with two subtypes of influenza A virus in the same season. *J Infect Dis* 1983;147:120–4.

154. Doebbeling BN, Edmond MD, Davis CS, et al. Influenza vaccination of health care workers: Evaluation of factors that are important in acceptance. *Prev Med* 1997;26:68–77.

155. Mullooly JP, Bennett MD, Hornbrook MC, et al. Influenza vaccination programs for elderly persons: Cost-effectiveness in a health maintenance organization. *Ann Intern Med* 1994;121:947–52.

156. Fedson DS. Influenza and pneumococcal vaccination of the elderly: Newer vaccines and prospects for clinical benefits at the margin. *Prev Med* 1994;23:751–5.

157. Gross PA, Hermogenes AW, Sacks HS, et al. The efficacy of influenza vaccine in the elderly person: A meta-analysis and review of the literature. *Ann Intern Med* 1995;123:518–27.

158. Hampson AW, Irving LB. Influenza vaccination: Cost-effective health care of the older adults? *J Qual Clin Prac* 1997;17:3–11.

159. Centers for Disease Control and Prevention. Medicare influenza vaccine demonstration—Selected states, 1988–1992. *JAMA* 1992;267:1734–5.

160. Final results: Medicare influenza vaccine demonstration—Selected states, 1988–1992. *MMWR* 1993;42:601–4.

161. Rose DN, Schechter CB, Sacks HS. Influenza and pneumococcal vaccination of HIV-infected patients: A policy analysis. *Am J Med* 1993;94:160–8.

162. Gorse GJ, Otto EE, Daughaday CC, et al. Influenza vaccination of patients with chronic lung disease. *Chest* 1997;112:1221–33.

163. Kumpulainen V, Makela M. Influenza vaccination among healthy employees: A cost-benefit analysis. *Scand J Infect Dis* 1997;29:181–5.

164. Jefferson T, Mugford M, Gray A, et al. An exercise on the feasibility of carrying out secondary economic analysis. *Health Econ* 1996;5:155–65.

165. Kent DL. The basics of decision analysis. *J Dent Educ* 1992;56:791–9.

166. Schoenbaum SC. Economic impact of influenza: The individual's perspective. *Am J Med* 1987;82:26–30.

167. Wharton M, Chorba TL, Vogt RL, et al. Case definitions for public health surveillance. *MMWR* 1990;39:1–45.

168. Jordan WS Jr, Badger GF, Dingle JA. A study of illness in a group of Cleveland families: XVI. The epidemiology of influenza, 1948–1953. *Am J Hyg* 1958;68:169–89.

169. Fox JP, Hall CE, Cooney MK, et al. Influenza virus: Infection in Seattle families, 1975–1979. *Am J Epidemiol* 1982;116:212–27.

170. Taber LH, Paredes A, Glezen WP, et al. Infection with influenza A/Victoria virus in Houston families, 1976. *J Hyg (Camb)* 1981;86:303–13.

171. Monto AS, Davenport FM, Napier JA, et al. Effect of vaccination of a school-age population upon the course of an A2/Hong Kong influenza epidemic. *Bull WHO* 1969;41:537–42.

172. Glezen WP, Decker M, Joseph SW, et al. Acute respiratory disease associated with influenza epidemics in Houston, 1981–1983. *J Infect Dis* 1987;155:1119–26.

173. Frank AL, Taber LH. Variation in frequency in natural reinfection with influenza A viruses. *J Med Virol* 1983;12:17–23.

174. Frank AL, Taber LS, Glezen WP, et al. Influenza B virus infections in the community and the family: The epidemics of 1976–1977 and 1979–1980 in Houston, TX. *Am J Epidemiol* 1983;118:313–25.

175. Frank AL, Taber LH, Glezen WP, et al. Reinfection with influenza A (H3N2) virus in young children and their families. *J Infect Dis* 1979;140:829–35.

176. Frank AL, Taber LH, Porter CM. Influenza B virus reinfection. *Am J Epidemiol* 1987;125:576–86.

177. Bainton D, Jones GR, Hole D. Influenza and ischemic heart disease: A possible trigger for acute myocardial infarction. *Int J Epidemiol* 1978;7:231–9.

178. Pönka A, Jalanko H, Pönka T, et al. Viral and mycoplasmal antibodies in patients with myocardial infarction. *Ann Clin Res* 1981;13:429–32.

179. Finland M, Parker F, Barnes M. Acute myocarditis in influenza A infection. *Am J Med Sci* 1945;207:455–68.

180. Leebeek FW, Baggen MG, Mulder LJ, et al. Rhabdomyolysis associated with influenza A virus infection. *Netherlands J Med* 1995;46:189–92.

181. Corey L, Rubin RJ, Hattiwick MA, et al. A nationwide outbreak of Reye's syndrome. *Am J Med* 1976;61:615–25.

182. Wilson B, Planterose DN, Naginton J, et al. Influenza A antigens on human lymphocytes in vitro and probably in vivo. *Nature* 1976;259:582–4.

183. O'Callaghan E, Sham P, Takei N. Schizophrenia after

prenatal exposure to 1957 A2 "(H2N2)" influenza epidemic. *Lancet* 1991;25:1248–50.

184. McGrath J, Castle D. Does influenza cause schizophrenia? A five-year review. *Aust NZ J Psychiatry* 1995;29:23–31.

185. Brown AS, Begg MD, Gravenstein S, et al. Serologic evidence of prenatal influenza in the etiology of schizophrenia. *Arch Gen Psychiatry* 2004 61;774–80.

186. Schiff LJ. Studies on the mechanisms of influenza virus infection in hamster trachea organ culture. *Arch Ges Virus Forsch* 1974;44:195–204.

187. Larson EW, Dominik JW, Rowberg AH, et al. Influenza virus population dynamics in the respiratory tract of experimentally infected mice. *Infect Immunol* 1976;13:438–47.

188. Li Y, Leung, GM, Tang, JW, et al. Role of ventilation in airborne transmission of infectious agents in the built environment: A multidisciplinary systematic review. *Indoor Air* 2007;17:2–18

189. Guidance on Preparing Workplaces for an Influenza Pandemic. OSHA 3327-02N. 2007; available at www.osha.gov/publications/influenza_pandemic.html, /www.osha.gov/Publications/OSHA3327pandemic.pdf.

190. Business Pandemic Influenza Planning Checklist. Available at www.pandemicflu.gov/plan/business-checklist.html.

191. U.S. Army Center for Health Promotion and Preventive Medicine. Non-vaccine recommendations to prevent acute infectious respiratory disease among U.S. Army personnel living in close quarters. USACHPPM Technical Guide 314. May 2007.

12 Occupational Chlamydial and Rickettsial Respiratory Infections

Daniel J. Martin

Chlamydial and rickettsial agents have been found to be important pathogens in the workplace. They are nonmotile, gram-negative, obligate intracellular organisms. *Chlamydia* species have a biphasic life cycle [1], and while they are prokaryotic, they are distinct from the eubacteria. *Chlamydia* have a sporelike extracellular elementary body (EB) that attaches to the host cell, enters via endocytosis [2], and reorganizes via growth and replication into the reticulate body (RB). Eventually, these form more elementary bodies, which are then released via cell lysis, initiating further infection. The family Chlamydiaceae has been the subject of some taxonomic controversy, with the general consensus being to establish two genera, *Chlamydia*, which includes *C. trachomatis*, and a new genus, *Chlamydophila*, which now includes *C. pneumonia* and *C. psittaci* [3]. Both names are still used commonly to refer to these organisms, however. Nine species of Chlamydiaceae are felt to exist, with three being human pathogens—*Chlamydophila psittaci*, *Chlamydophila pneumoniae*, and *Chlamydia trachomatis*. Infection with these organisms may result in a wide variety of clinical presentations, most importantly respiratory infection. Clinical features and serologic findings may be similar for these species, providing the physician with some diagnostic difficulty.

The family Rickettsiaceae includes two groups of the genus *Rickettsia*—the typhus group and the spotted fever group. *Rickettsia* are members of the alpha group of purple bacteria, members of the order Rickettsiales and the family Rickettsiaceae. They may be related to the primitive bacteria that evolved into the mitochondrial organelle of the eukaryotic cell [4].

Rickettsia use a cycle of mammalian reservoirs and arthropod vectors. Primarily zoonotic diseases, they tend to be fastidious and may produce endotoxin [5]. Their clinical manifestations reflect the proliferation of the organism in the endothelium of small blood vessels, resulting in characteristic rashes and vasculitic complications.

Coxiella burnetii, the agent of Q fever, and *Bartonella* are two species related to *Rickettsia*. *C. burnetii* is unique among this group in that it is quite a hardy organism and has the potential of causing severe economic damage when outbreaks occur among livestock. *Bartonella* species include *B. quintana*, *B. henselae*, and *B. elizabethae*. These organisms cause bacteremic illness and should be considered in the differential diagnosis of cases of culture-negative endocarditis.

Orientia tsutsugamushi was formerly considered a member of the *Rickettsia* genus. In its endemic area, it is a relatively common arthropod-borne zoonosis that causes infection in a considerable percentage of those exposed.

This chapter focuses primarily on *Chlamydophila psittaci,* the agent of psittacosis; *Chlamydophila pneumoniae,* the TWAR agent, and *C. burnetii,* the agent of Q fever. Mention is also made of *Chlamydia trachomatis, Rickettsia prowazekii, R. typhi, R. rickettsia, O. tsutsugamushi,* and *B. quintana* (see Table 12-1).

Pathogens

CHLAMYDIA/CHLAMYDOPHILA

In 1879, Dr. J. Ritter described seven patients who became ill after exposure to his brother's parrots in Uster, Switzerland. He termed their illness *pneumotyphus* [6]. In 1892, Morange observed similar events related to parrots and coined the term *psittacosis* (*psittakos,* Greek for "parrot") [7]. In 1907, Halberstaedter and von Prowazek examined the "mantled" intracytoplasmic organisms in tissue from patients with trachoma. They classified these organisms as Chlamydozoaceae (*chlamys,* Greek for "mantle") [8]. Laboratory isolation and microscopic examination of the etiologic agent involved in a human outbreak of psittacosis were performed in 1930 [9]. Similar identifications were taking place in British, U.S., and German laboratories [10]. Subsequent reports showed that transmission could be achieved via nonpsittacine birds, such as chickens, turkeys [11], petrels [12], pigeons [13], and ducks [14]. Initially felt to be viral agents, these organisms were correctly classified as bacteria in 1966 [15], and the agents of trachoma, psittacosis, and lymphogranuloma venereum (LGV) were grouped together under the genus *Chlamydia.* It is now apparent that virtually any bird species may act as a reservoir for *C. psittaci,* and the terms *psittacosis,* or *ornithosis,* for human infection and *avian chlamydiosis* (AC) for bird infection are more properly used [16–18].

C. trachomatis is the cause of ocular trachoma (serotypes A–C), genitourinary tract infections (serotypes D–K), and lymphogranuloma venereum (serotypes L1–3) [19]. Recognized in antiquity, treatments for trachoma were first described in China in the twenty-seventh century BC and Egypt in the nineteenth century BC [20]. The characteristic cytoplasmic inclusions were first noted in tissue from an infant with trachoma in 1909 [21] and

later were found in the cervical and urethral cells of an infected child's parents [22] and in the urethrae of men with nongonococcal urethritis [23]. Currently, *C. trachomatis* is recognized as a common sexually transmitted pathogen worldwide, making it an important public health issue.

A third chlamydial species, *Chlamydophila pneumoniae* (TWAR), was first isolated from the conjunctiva of a child in Taiwan in 1965 and termed *TW 183* (for "Taiwan"). The same agent later was isolated in Seattle in 1983 and was referred to as *AR 39* (for "acute respiratory") [24]. A retrospective analysis of sera stored from a 1978 springtime epidemic among young adult Finns revealed positive complement fixation (CF) titers in 78% of these pneumonias. This indicated that the organism also could cause epidemic outbreaks of respiratory disease [25]. In 1986, Grayston isolated the organism [26] and confirmed its etiologic role via use of the microimmunofluorescent antibody (MIF) test in a group of Washington University students with pneumonias and bronchitis. Combining the *TW* and *AR* prefixes, he referred to it as the *TWAR agent.* Originally considered a strain of *C. psittaci,* the organism ultimately was recognized as a new species and given the name *C. pneumoniae* because of its most frequently recognized manifestation [27]. Subsequent reports have illuminated the role of this organism in close-population and barracks outbreaks [28–33]. *C. pneumoniae* also may cause bronchitis, sinusitis, and other milder forms of respiratory disease [34].

RICKETTSIA AND RELATED PATHOGENS

In 1935, an Australian medical officer named E. H. Derrick described a febrile illness that afflicted 20 employees of a Brisbane, Queensland, meat-processing plant. The puzzling disease was named *Q* (for "query") *fever* [35]. Burnett and Freeman showed that a rickettsial organism could be isolated from the blood and urine of Derrick's patients [36], and the organism was soon recovered from the Rocky Mountain wood tick in Montana by Davis and Cox [37]. The agent thus came to be known as *Coxiella burnetii. C. burnetii,* an important occupational pathogen, now has been found in 51 nations on five continents [38], and both acute and chronic forms of infection have been described. *C. burnetii* is a pleomorphic gram-negative coccobacillus, an intracellular parasite that is highly infectious to

Table 12-1
Chlamydial and Rickettsial Infections and Their Epidemiology and Clinical Features

Disease	Organism	Vector/Reservoir	Geographic Distribution	Clinical Aspects	Diagnosis	Therapy
Psittacosis	*Chlamydophila psittaci*	Birds	Worldwide	Fever, headache, tracheobronchitis or atypical pneumonia	Culture, MIF, CF titers, PCR	Tetracycline Doxycycline, 10–14 days
Trachoma	*Chlamydia trachomatis*	Humans	Worldwide	Ocular/urethritic/pneumonitic presentations; female sterility	Culture with FA, ELISA, MIF, DFA, PCR	Azithromycin 1 gm single-dose Doxycycline, ofloxacin, erythromycin for 7 days
TWAR pneumonia	*Chlamydophila pneumoniae*	Humans	Worldwide/favors tropics	Upper and lower respiratory infection	IgG and IgM MIF, CF, Cell culture of throat swab	Tetracycline, erythromycin, azithromycin, clarithromycin for 10–14 days
Q fever	*Coxiella burnetii*	Domestic ungulates	Worldwide (except New Zealand)	Acute form with flu-like onset, then atypical pneumonia; chronic forms include endocarditis	IFA, CF, MIF, ELISA, blood culture	Tetracycline, doxycycline, erythromycin for 2–4 weeks for acute; doxycycline, quinolone combinations for chronic, for 2–3 years or more
Epidemic typhus	*Rickettsia prowazekii*	*Pediculus humanus-corporis*/humans	Worldwide	Headache, fever, chills, truncal rash with facial and palmar sparing	ELISA, MIF, tissue staining	Single-dose doxycycline, 100 mg, for epidemic; longer courses of doxycycline, chloramphenicol, or tetracycline for Brill-Zinsser disease
Murine typhus	*Rickettsia typhi*	*Xenopsylla cheopsis/Rattus* spp.	Worldwide; parallels rodent populations	Milder than *Rickettsia prowazekii*; headache, fever, truncal rash	IFA, LA, Dip-S-Ticks	Doxycycline, chloramphenicol, tetracycline, quinolones effective
Rocky Mountain spotted fever	*Rickettsia rickettsii*	*Dermacentor andersonii*	Worldwide (various spotted fevers)	Fever, headache, wrist and ankle rash that spreads centripetally	IF Staining of rash biopsy, IFA, CF, LA, ELISA	Tetracycline, chloramphenicol, doxycycline for 7 days
Scrub typhus	*Orientia tsutsugamushi*	Chiggers (larval *Leptotrombidium* spp.)/rodents	Eastern Asia, Western Pacific	Eschar, local adenopathy, fever, headache, spreading truncal rash	IFA, IIP, ELISA (Dip-S-Ticks)	Tetracycline (7 days) or doxycycline (3 day course) Erthromycin, doxycycline,
Trench fever	*Bartonella quintana*	*Pediculus humanus*	Worldwide	Variable duration of fever, bacteremia, shin pain	IFA, blood "subculture," EIA, PCR	tetracycline (optimum regimen)

CF = complement fixation; DFA = direct immunofluorescent antibody; ELISA/EIA = enzyme-linked immunosorbent assay; FA = fluorescent antibody; IFA = immunofluorescent antibody; IIP = indirect immunoperoxidase; LA = latex agglutination; MIF = microimmunofluorescence; PCR = polymerase chain reaction.

humans. It exhibits phase variation, with transformation between a phase I "virulent" and phase II "avirulent" form [39]. Within cells, it multiplies within acidic phagolysosomes, making it difficult to eradicate. While animal infection is usually subclinical, human infection can result in a variety of febrile illnesses, including pneumonitis.

Rickettsial diseases are infections by a group of organisms that have developed a small genome via reductive evolution and thus depend on the host cell for many functions. They tend to disrupt the adherens junctions of the endothelial cells they infect, resulting in increased microvascular permeability and characteristic rashes [40]. Louse-borne typhus (also known as *jail fever*) is an ancient disease that continues to command our attention. Epidemics were first noted in the 1400s, and 3 million deaths in Europe and the Soviet Union were attributed to typhus between 1918 and 1922 [41]. The causative organism, *R. prowazekii*, is transmitted from person to person by the human body louse, *Pediculus humanus corporis.* Transmission is aided by crowded, unsanitary conditions such as those that occur during wars or following natural disasters [42]. Recrudescence of epidemic typhus may occur years later and is called *Brill-Zinsser disease.* Murine typhus is caused by *R. typhi* and parallels the worldwide distribution of *Rattus* rats, its primary reservoir. Originally differentiated from the clinically similar typhus-like illnesses in 1926, it was isolated eventually from rats and its main vector, the flea, *Xenopsylla cheopis* [43]. Transmission occurs when infected flea feces is rubbed into a pruritic bite. *R. rickettsii* is a tick-borne organism that causes a characteristic vasculitic rash on the trunk and extremities, a disease known as *Rocky Mountain spotted fever* (RMSF). The first descriptions of the disease came from the Native American tribes of Montana [44]. The role of ticks in transmission was demonstrated when the disease was contracted by volunteers bitten by ticks removed from a patient with RMSF [44]. Similar illness is produced by other members of the spotted fever group. Organisms such as *R. conorii, R. australis,* and *R. akari* are also transmitted from mammals and marsupials to humans through an arthropod vector, resulting in characteristic rashes and clinical syndromes. These illnesses appear to occur within certain geographic areas, an important epidemiologic clue to their identity. RMSF

was investigated by Howard Taylor Ricketts in the Bitterroot Valley of Montana in the early 1900s, and the organism subsequently was named in recognition of his work [4, 45]. The main vectors of spotted fevers are several species of ticks, and the main reservoirs of disease are mammalian vertebrates such as rodents and dogs. The Rocky Mountain wood tick, *Dermacentor andersonii,* appears to be the most important vector in cases of RMSF.

Scrub typhus is also due to an obligate intracellular organism. Formerly classified as a rickettsial infection, it is now considered to represent a distinct genus, *Orientia tsutsugamushi* [46]. The prototype strains were termed *Gilliam, Karp,* and *Kato.* The organism can be grouped into serotype clusters, which include Gilliam, Karp, Kato, Kuroki, Saitama, and Kawasaki [47]. It is now apparent that there is great heterogeneity within the species, investigators having identified more than 40 strains in Japan alone [48]. Subsequent analysis has shown that there is an impressive degree of genotypic and immunotypic variation even between strains recovered within a given country [49]. Scrub typhus is an illness that results when humans are infected as accidental hosts. It derives its name from the vegetation that most frequently harbors its vector, the larval stage (chigger) of trombiculid mites [50]. This illness is seen mostly in eastern Asia and the western Pacific, including Australia. Field troops in Vietnam were noted to be at risk [51], and other occupations are at risk as well [52, 53].

Bartonella species are members of the α₂ subgroup of the proteobacteria. Many of the species cause disease in humans, most important of which are *B. quintana, B. henselae,* and *B. bacilliformis. B. quintana* (named for its supposed 5-day fever) was first described as a cause of febrile outbreaks in World War I troops and thus was termed *trench fever* [54]. Affecting up to 1 million troops in Europe in World War I, the organism made an epidemic reappearance in World War II. *B. quintana* is likely spread via the body louse or fleas, with rodents and bats as a reservoir. Transmission and epidemics are related to conditions of poor sanitation and hygiene [55]. In England, control of the organism was achieved to a large degree by the issuance of new clothing to returning trench warfare soldiers [56]. *B. henselae* was isolated in 1986 [57]. Transmitted by cats or their fleas, *B. henselae* poses a special danger to immunocompromised individuals, especially those infected with the human immunodeficiency virus (HIV).

Epidemiology

INCIDENCE AND PREVALENCE
Chlamydophila psittaci

C. psittaci is commonly found in birds, including companion (pet) birds and poultry. Cases occur both sporadically and in outbreaks. The latter are often associated with a commercial source, such as an abattoir (slaughterhouse). Seroprevalence studies suggest that the disease occurs much more commonly than is reported [58]. It is likely that any bird species can be host to this organism, although psittacine birds (e.g., parrots, parakeets, and cockatoos) are infected most often. Outbreaks in ducks and turkeys are especially important for economic reasons. In 1978, a single infected flock of turkeys resulted in a cost of $19,000 for a Nebraska poultry-processing plant [59].

Vertical transmission has been seen and is believed most likely to be the result of exposure to the organism in the urogenital tract or, in some cases, as a result of postnatal exposure. Intrauterine infection occurs in some species, such as chickens [60], and not in other species [61]. The usual route of transmission among animals is most likely inhalation of infectious aerosols, but fecal ingestion is also a potential route [62]. Sexual transmission has been noted in sheep [63]. Infected birds may be either asymptomatic or acutely, subacutely, or chronically infected. The disease tends to be systemic, with multiple organs showing involvement. There is a 5–15% carriage rate among asymptomatic birds, which may increase to 100% when birds are subjected to the stresses of overcrowding and breeding [10, 64–66]. Selected avian populations have surprisingly high rates of prevalence. Belgian commercial turkeys were antibody-positive in 50–75% [67], and testing of German turkey flocks revealed positive results on enzyme-linked immunosorbent assay (ELISA) in 20–70% of apparently healthy birds [68]. Approximately 18% of pigeons from a public park in Spain had *Chlamydia* isolated from their feces, and approximately 30% had positive antibody tests [69]. Up to 13% of free-living raptors in the Munich area had positive cloa-

cal swabs by the ELISA method [70]. Asymptomatic captive birds at the Ninoy Wildlife Rescue Center in the Philippines were ELISA-positive at a rate of 25% [71]. Birds also may develop an acute version of the illness after years of latent infection [72, 73].

Many other species of animals have been noted to be susceptible to infection with *C. psittaci*, including horses [74, 75], crocodiles [76], sheep [77], cows [78], goats [79], swine [80], bears [81], dogs [82], cats [83], and koalas [84]. Transmission from these reservoirs to humans also has been noted to occur [85,86]. Orthozoonotic infection (between species) has been documented [87].

The incidence of human infection with *C. psittaci* (psittacosis) is difficult to determine with certainty. Problems in diagnosis, serologic cross-reactivity with other *Chlamydia* species, and low rates of reporting contribute to what is likely a considerable underestimate of the true incidence and prevalence of the disease. Only 100–200 cases of *C. psittaci* are reported to the Centers for Disease Control and Prevention (CDC) and the British CDSC each year [88], although seroprevalence studies suggest that a much higher rate of infection is actually occurring. Most of the reported cases involve adults 15–44 years of age [88]. Children appear to be infected at a higher rate than would be expected in view of a presumed low rate of exposure. A Japanese study of 223 infants and children with pneumonia found that 2.2% were IgM-positive for *C. psittaci* antibodies.

Infectivity is likely high among exposed humans: 44% of veterinary surgeons developed ornithosis after visiting a duck processing plant [89], and 49% of new employees in a duck processing plant showed evidence of recent infection within 90 days of employment, although only 28% of them were clinically ill [90]. Genotypes A or E/B were detected in 14.9% of workers at 39 psittacine breeding facilities [91]. An Israeli study found that 81% of individuals exposed to diseased birds showed serologic evidence of acute infection. In a population with no recent outbreaks or avian illnesses, serology was positive in 43% of farm workers [92]. Screening of employees at an Australian duck processing plant in the wake of a *C. psittaci* outbreak revealed that over 76% had serologic evidence of infection, but only 12% had evidence of recent infection. Infection was usually acquired during the first year of employment [93].

Chlamydophila pneumoniae

C. pneumoniae exhibits a basic endemic rate and also shows periodic epidemicity. In contrast to *Mycoplasma pneumoniae*, it appears somewhat less likely to infect the young and more prone to infect the elderly [24]. In both adults and children, tropical regions have a higher prevalence of *C. pneumoniae* than northern regions [24, 94]. Seroprevalence studies show that more than 50% of U.S. residents have IgG to *C. pneumoniae*, indicating past infection. Overall, it is responsible for approximately 10% of pneumonias, making it the third to fourth most common etiologic agent. In studies involving children, only 1% of children hospitalized with pneumonia (average age 3.7 years) had evidence of acute *C. pneumoniae* infection [95], and in another study, only 5% of Japanese infants and children with pneumonia were IgM-positive for *C. pneumoniae* on microimmunofluorescence (MIF) testing [94]. After infancy, incidence rates rise rapidly. In one study, an annual attack rate of 6–9% was found in the 5- to 14-year-old age group [96]. Many of these converters experienced minimal, if any, symptoms. Attack rates level off after the teenage years, and eventually, 70% of older adults exhibit evidence of previous infection [97].

There is an unexplained gender difference, with males having positive serology at higher rates than females [96]. Experts feel that infection is likely universal, with the presence of negative antibodies indicating clearance after infection, and that reinfection is common [98]. Most likely owing to its preferential infection of the elderly, in 11.4% of all hospitalized pneumonia patients, the cause is probably *C. pneumoniae*. Other respiratory infections are also quite commonly caused by the organism. Up to 20% of acute bronchitis is due to *C. pneumoniae* [99], and the organism is also responsible for approximately 4% of exacerbations of chronic obstructive pulmonary disease (COPD) [100]. The relationship between chronic bronchitis and infection with *C. pneumoniae* deserves attention because 72% of COPD patients exhibit evidence of past infection [101]. Interestingly, infection with the pathogen causes ciliary stasis early on, which is believed to be responsible for frequent co-infec-

tions. These findings have led some to speculate that *C. pneumoniae* has a pathogenetic role in chronic bronchitis [99, 102].

Chlamydia trachomatis

C. trachomatis appears to be an exclusively human pathogen. It is the most common bacterial sexually transmitted disease (STD) in developed countries [103] and also has a high prevalence in developing nations. There is an incidence of approximately 4 million new cases in the United States each year [104]. High rates of prevalence are sustained by the fact that asymptomatic individuals may remain infectious for months, thereby infecting others without their knowledge [104].

Certain populations have extremely high rates of infection. For instance, 95% of commercial street sex workers in Jamaica were MIF-positive, indicating past or present infection, as opposed to 53% of blood donors, and active infection was found in 25% of these workers [105]. Sex workers in Istanbul had a much lower rate (12.9%) of seropositivity by direct fluorescent antibody (DFA) for unexplained reasons [106]. Female sex workers in Dakar had positive polymerase chain reaction (PCR) assays of endocervical specimens, 47.6% of which were genotype E [107].

The high rates of infection that are sometimes seen in sex workers are felt to be due primarily to infection contracted while employed. High exposure rates in this population were illustrated by the finding that approximately 5% of seminal fluid samples recovered from a Copenhagen massage parlor demonstrated the presence of *C. trachomatis* [108]. The overall prevalence of infection among sexually active asymptomatic men is approximately 10% [109]. Sexually active women have approximately a 15% prevalence rate [110]. Prevalence is highest among adolescent females and is also high among African-Americans, inner-city residents, and the poor [104].

C. trachomatis is also known to cause pneumonia. A Japanese study found 22% of children hospitalized with pneumonia to have IgM to *C. trachomatis* [94]. This pathogen is also the cause of ocular trachoma and lymphogranuloma venereum (LGV). Ocular trachoma is a frequent cause of blindness, accounting for up to 9 million new cases per year and afflicting 500 million individuals worldwide [111]. LGV is caused by a distinct strain of *C. trachomatis* that exhibits high endemicity in South America, Africa, and Southeast Asia.

Coxiella burnetii

C. burnetii is the agent of Q fever, existing in animal reservoirs such as sheep, goats, and cattle. It is maintained in ticks as its main reservoir and vector. The organism is prevalent throughout the world, with the exception of New Zealand, which remains free of *Coxiella* infection [112]. The term *coxiellosis* has been applied to animal infection, which is usually asymptomatic. Abortion may result from infection with the organism in domestic animals. *C. burnetii* is also found in fish, arthropods, birds, rodents, cats, and other livestock [113]. The organism can be found in the milk, urine, feces, and placentae of infected animals. The amniotic fluid and placenta can be the site of a tremendously high concentration of organisms [114], and not surprisingly, transmission appears to be highly correlated with parturition. It is believed that physiologic stress and the immunosuppression of pregnancy may encourage multiplication of the organism. Infected animals may continue to shed the organism for weeks [39]. Prevalence rates among livestock are often quite high. Sheep (24%) and goats (57%) were frequently seropositive in one California study [115], and commercial and noncommercial animals showed the same prevalence rates. Another study found that 82% of California dairy cows are antibody-positive [116]. In cattle herds, serologic evidence of infection may be seen in 80% of animals [117].

Humans become infected via inhalation of infected aerosols, with the organism typically infecting monocytic cells. Males have a higher incidence than females, likely as a result of exposure differences [118]. In the Spanish southwest, the male:female ratio of infection was 4:1 [119]. In Nova Scotia, 12% of blood donors exhibited antibody to *C. burnetii* [120], as did 49% of veterinarians and 35% of abattoir workers [121]. In Toronto, a more urban environment, only 0.6% of blood donors were positive, whereas 18% of staff at a Toronto animal research facility were infected, including 68% of the animal handlers. Of the 60 research laboratory workers in the Toronto study who had positive serology results, there were 12 cases of clinical illness, and 2 required hospital admission [122]. A study of the general population in California revealed positive serology results in 6% [115].

The incidence of the organism varies geographically; it is reported most frequently in regions where medical authorities are most vigilant. In countries without appropriate testing facilities, the reported incidence is quite low [123]. Owing to the nonspecific nature of the illness and the fact that it is usually self-limited, many cases likely go undiagnosed. Highly endemic areas include parts of southern France, where the prevalence is felt to be 50 per 100,000 and where 15% of cases of endocarditis are due to *C. burnetii*. Spain, Switzerland, and Nova Scotia also have high prevalence rates. In other areas, such as California and Great Britain, the rates have declined tremendously over the last 40–50 years [124]. A large survey of rural Welsh residents found only 21 individuals with positive serology, with a higher frequency among farmers [125]. In Carpathia, prevalence decreased from approximately 10% in the wake of a mid-1970s' outbreak to a 2–3% rate after 20 years [126]. Only 228 cases were reported in the United States between 1978 and 1986, half in California [127]. In regions where the main reservoir is sheep, such as the Basque region, a defined lambing period likely provides a seasonal variation to the incidence of acute Q fever, with the highest incidence in the spring and early summer [128]. The chronic forms of Q fever infection probably develop in only 1–10% of acute cases [129, 130].

Rickettsia prowazekii

R. prowazekii, the agent of epidemic typhus, is unusual in that humans are the primary reservoir, with body lice (*Pediculus humanus corporis*) transmitting the organism from a rickettsemic individual to a new host. In the United States, the southern flying squirrel (*Glaucomys volans*) is also a reservoir [131]. Vertical transmission among animals also has been reported [132]. The infection is prominent in areas and settings that predispose humans to lice infestation, including the rural highlands of South and Central America, as well as northeastern and central Africa [133, 134]. Periods of societal strife are also known to promote epidemics of infection. In wartime Bosnia and Herzegovina, for example, 4.3% of the general population was found to have antibodies to *R. prowazekii* [135]. Napoleon's Grand Army also suffered from typhus, and 3 of 35 soldiers' remains in a mass grave at Vilnius contained the DNA of *R. prowazekii* [136]. The potentially epidemic nature of the disease caused by this agent was illustrated by an outbreak of typhus in a jail in Burundi, followed by more extensive spread into refugee camps in Rwanda, Burundi, and Zaire [137]. The last U.S. typhus epidemic occurred in 1922, and since then, only rare, sporadic cases have been seen. Very few cases of epidemic typhus have been diagnosed in the United States; in fact, by 1996, only 28 had been reported [41]. Among European immigrants after World War II, *R. prowazekii* infection, almost always Brill-Zinsser disease, was seen with some frequency.

Rickettsia typhi

R. typhi has a worldwide distribution, especially in the warmer coastal areas, where its reservoir (*Rattus* rats) and vector (the flea, *Xenopsylla cheopis*) abound. Both sporadic cases and epidemics of murine typhus occur. During the 1940s, approximately 5,000 new U.S. cases were reported annually. By 1989, aggressive control measures had decreased this number to less than 100 [138]. U.S. prevalence is highest in California and Texas and varies seasonally, increasing during the warmer months. In most of the world, infection is usually related to the indoor presence of rats and their infected fleas. Other factors that increase endemicity are those that promote increases in the rodent population. War, poor sanitation, and crowding appear to be problematic. In 1995, 61% of individuals in northeastern Bosnia and Herzegovina were found to have antibody to *R. typhi* [135]. Other areas of high endemicity exist. For example, 28% of pregnant Tanzanian women were immunofluorescence assay (IFA)–positive for *R. typhi* [135]. In Malang, Indonesia, 36% of peridomestic rodents were seropositive for *R. typhi,* and 35% of civilians also had antibodies [139]. Other areas of Africa (e.g., Morocco) show much lower rates. A 1995 study found that only 1.7–4% of Moroccans were IFA-positive for *R. typhi* [140]. On the Greek island of Evia, 91% of *Rattus norvegicus* were antibody-positive, as were 2.6% of *Xenopsylla cheopis* [141]. Transmission in suburban areas also may be higher than generally expected. In suburban Bangkok, 8% of individuals showed evidence of recent *R. typhi* infection [142]. In the southeastern United States, it is felt that a shift to a peridomestic cycle of trans-

mission is occurring, with free-roaming dogs and cats, opossums, and their fleas now the predominant reservoirs and vectors [143].

Rickettsia rickettsii

R. rickettsii [Rocky Mountain spotted fever (RMSF)] is transmitted via tick bite. RMSF is closely related to a number of other spotted fever illnesses, some of which occur in Asia, Australia, Brazil [144], and Europe [145]. RMSF is the second most common tick-borne disease in the United States. It is reported in every state except Vermont, Maine, and Hawaii and can be contracted during any season [44]. The incidence of RMSF rose to a peak of 1,100 cases per year between 1977 and 1983. This increase was believed to be related to increased awareness of the disease as well as a population shift to more geographically remote areas [44]. The incidence declined thereafter, with only 590 annual cases reported in 1995 [146], but rose again to an annual incidence of over 1,000 as of 2002 [147]. The true incidence of RMSF and murine typhus is probably underestimated by a factor of 4 or more [148]. The average annual U.S. incidence has been estimated at 2.2 cases per million [149]. The reported incidence within the United States varies regionally: 0.53 cases per 100,000 population in the West and South Central states and 0.83 per 100,000 in the South Atlantic states [145]. For unknown reasons, more cases are now being seen in the Southeast. In 1994, 37% of all U.S. cases occurred in Georgia and the Carolinas. Between 1997 and 2002, 56% of all U.S. cases were from the Carolinas, Tennessee, Oklahoma, and Arizona [149]. Most cases occur during the warmer months, likely reflecting levels of outdoor activity as well as seasonal variation in tick populations. Among the general population under age 65, infection rates appear to be similar in all age groups [146], although a tendency for higher rates in the 40- to 64-year-old age group may be explained by a greater likelihood of clinically evident disease and thus reporting [149]. Children are likely frequently infected, with milder and thus undetected infection. Men are infected more frequently, probably because of increased exposure via recreation and occupation. Infection rates during periods of intense exposure may be quite high. In a 2-week training exercise in Arkansas, 38% of U.S. Army soldiers deployed in the field became infected

[150]. RMSF is also seen in Argentina, Brazil, Columbia, Costa Rica, Mexico, and Panama [149].

Orientia tsutsugamushi

Scrub typhus is a disease of the Far East caused by the organism *O. tsutsugamushi*. It is prominent in eastern Asia and the western Pacific. It is also seen as far west as Afghanistan and Pakistan. One case report suggests that Africa may be a source as well [151], but most cases seen outside the typical region of distribution are in travelers from endemic areas. The disease is transmitted by the bite of the larval stage of Trombiculidae mites, including *Leptotrombidium pallidum* and *L. scutellare*, which parasitize rodents. Humans are accidental hosts [152]. These vectors are prominent in scrublike vegetation but also can be found in tall grass and other ecological niches [153]. It appears that the vector population itself is heavily infected. A Korean study of six different localities showed an overall chigger parasitization rate of 69%, with a wide geographic variation in prevalence and mite identity [152]. The incidence and prevalence of scrub typhus infection in humans can vary markedly according to geography, socioeconomic development, and age. Earlier studies showing sex differences likely reflect occupationally related exposure differences. In Thailand, as many as 59–77% of rural residents exhibit antibodies to *O. tsutsugamushi*, indicating previous infection [154, 155]. In metropolitan Bangkok, 21% of blood donors showed evidence of recent infection [156]. Evidence of antibody was found in approximately 20% of all civilian residents of the Pescadores Islands of Taiwan in the mid-1970s, with no sex difference. Infection before age 10 occurred in only 1%, but 41% had antibodies by age 50. Only 16% of urban dwellers had been infected versus 38% of rural dwellers [52]. In Palau, IgG positivity went from 5–47% in 8 years as a consequence of an outbreak [157]. Among all Thai Army conscripts, the baseline seroprevalence rate varied between 6% and 18% but was higher in the Thai Rangers, who routinely perform patrol missions [158]. Febrile U.S. soldiers in Viet Nam were screened routinely for *O. tsutsugamushi*, and 7% of a total of 1,650 were positive in one study [51]. The overall annual attack rate was calculated at 59 per 100,000, with 86% of cases occurring in certain heavily exposed combat units, which themselves accounted for less than 20% of the total military population. All documented exposures were noted to occur on the geographic "fringes" of the centers of population [51].

Bartonella

B. quintana and *B. henselae* are found worldwide. *B. quintana* is probably transmitted by the body louse, *Pediculus humanus* [159], although scabies are potential vectors as well [160]. It is believed that the louse sheds the organism in its feces when it bites, which then inoculates the human host when the bite is scratched [161]. Interestingly, however, many of the victims do not have body lice, and efforts to isolate the organism from fleas have been unsuccessful [162]. *B. quintana* has been isolated from lice found on infected patients [163]. *B. henselae* is associated with cats and possibly with feline fleas [164, 165]. *Bartonella* cases appear to be mostly sporadic; outbreaks are associated with conditions of poor sanitation and hygiene. Seroprevalence is very difficult to determine owing to a lack of data; however, a serologic study performed in Seattle after a 1993 outbreak among the homeless found that 20% of homeless individuals had positive MIF titers for *B. quintana* versus 2% of random blood donors [166]. *B. elizabethae* was isolated from 46% intravenous drug users in Central and East Harlem in New York [167]. Among veterinary professionals, seroprevalence for *Bartonella* infection is approximately 7% [168]. Although other species of *Bartonella* have been isolated from mice, rats, cats, and dogs, the reservoirs for *B. quintana* are not known. It has been proposed that humans may serve as a reservoir [169].

TRANSMISSION RISK FACTORS
Chlamydia psittaci

Transmission of *C. psittaci* between birds is heightened by stress, such as overcrowding, chilling, and malnutrition. Transmission to nestlings also occurs, along with potentially protective maternal antibodies [170]. The birds' clinical syndromes involve shedding of potentially infective material in copious ocular or nasal discharge, urate excretion, or diarrhea [18]. Direct contact by humans with these secretions or their aerosols results in infection in a high proportion of cases. These secretions and their aerosols are highly infectious and remain so for several months because the organism in the form of the elementary body (EB) is highly resistant to acid, alkali, and drying. Close contact, such as petting birds, is risky, although relatively trivial exposure (e.g., aviary visits) is also a risk factor. The organism also may be transferred by bird bites and by handling the feathers of infected birds. Preexisting skin injuries heighten susceptibility to transmission [59]. Among reported human cases, 70% of identified sources involved caged birds, and employment in situations where exposure was likely also was a risk [18]. In an outbreak among veterinary surgeons, handling of infected duck feathers was found to be a risk factor for transmission [124]. Handling the products of gestation of infected birds appears to be quite risky as well [171, 172]. Interestingly, 25% of cases have no discernible avian exposure history [74, 173], with infection likely owing to an unnoticed transient exposure to infected droppings. Six of the eight known serovars (A–F) have been isolated from birds [174], with differing degrees of virulence. Serovar D, for instance, was found to be highly pathogenic when inoculated into turkeys and less so in other species [175]. The more virulent strains are believed to have larger and more numerous inclusions and to replicate more freely in the host cell's cytoplasm [175]. Certain orders of birds appear to be more susceptible to infection with a given serovar [176]. Psittacine and turkey strains are the most virulent for humans, resulting in more severe clinical symptomology [73]. Psittacosis also can be transmitted between humans, including nosocomially [177], and results in more clinically severe infection in these cases.

Chlamydophila pneumoniae

Transmission of C. pneumoniae is believed to be exclusively human to human, with respiratory secretions the likely method of infection. The organism does remain viable on environmental surfaces, including countertops, but is less viable and infectious in these cases and survives only 10 minutes on human hands [178]. Closed populations, including families, appear to be at risk for outbreaks. Students have higher seropositivity rates, also likely owing to closer living and working arrangements [179]. It appears that some asymptomatic individuals are capable of spreading the disease and some actively infected individuals are not [24]. Epidemic outbreaks occur in closed populations and may persist for 6 months at a time [24]. Patients with HIV infection appear to be more prone to infection with C. pneumoniae, as evidenced by their higher seroprevalence rate, and the pathogen has been isolated from the bronchoalveolar lavage (BAL) fluid of 10% of HIV-positive patients with pneumonia [180].

Chlamydia trachomatis

Genital infection with C. trachomatis is transmitted more easily from men to women [181]. Sex with a symptomatic partner poses a higher risk of transmission than with an asymptomatic one [182]. Pregnancy also appears to be a risk factor [183]. Concomitant infection with Neisseria gonorrhoeae increases the risk of transmission [184]. Higher frequency of sexual intercourse is correlated with increased rates of infection [185], and use of nonbarrier methods of contraception is a known risk factor [186]. Use of latex condoms decreases the risk of transmission and also protects against viral pathogens such as HIV [187]. Condom breakage and slippage occur in a small percentage of encounters, resulting in potential pathogen exposure.

Vertical transmission is common, occurring in 60% of babies born to infected females. Infection in these cases causes inclusion conjunctivitis in 18% and pneumonia in 16% [188]. Pneumonia owing to C. trachomatis is seen most frequently in infants and is also prominent in immunocompromised patients [189].

Coxiella burnetii

C. burnetii is transmitted to humans by inhalation of aerosols. C. burnetii may remain in a sporelike state for months, resistant to drying and temperature extremes, and may remain viable in the soil for 5 months. Air samples may remain positive for 2 weeks after the local parturition of an infected animal [190]. Historically important sources of infection include domestic ungulates such as cattle, sheep, and goats. Cats, dogs, and deer are also potential sources [191]. In northern climates, parturient cats in particular have been noted to initiate outbreaks [192]. Infection typically occurs in proximity to a stationary source; however, more obscure sources have been seen. There have been reports of a high incidence in individuals living by roadsides over which infected animals and their products were transported [193, 194]. These reports illustrate the high infectivity of the organism, which can, in fact, be transmitted by inoculation with a single organism [195]. Disease also may be transmitted via transfusion, gastrointestinal ingestion, drinking raw milk, skin trauma, sexual contact [196], vertically [197], and possibly ticks [124]. Person-to-person transmission occurs rarely [198]. There is one case of a physician who was infected after delivering the child of an infected patient [199]. Articles of clothing can become contaminated and thus infectious to those who do laundry or are otherwise exposed to clothing [200, 201]. Only a handful of person-to-person instances of transmission have been reported [202, 203]. High attack rates, short incubations, and more severe clinical syndromes are associated with exposure to the high inoculum involved in cleaning up the products of conception of infected parturient cats [204]. Patients who are immunocompromised owing to HIV infection, neoplasia, or corticosteroid use are more susceptible to developing the chronic forms of the disease. Patients with preexisting valvulopathy are more likely to develop Q fever endocarditis. Q fever also can be reactivated by the induction of immunosuppression [205].

Rickettsia

R. prowazekii is transmitted in conditions that favor lice infestation. Poor sanitation, crowding, infrequent washing, and infrequent changing of clothing are risk factors [42]. Periods of war, famine, and migration frequently foster these conditions. Epidemics of typhus were seen in Europe in the aftermath of World War I and in the concentration camps of World War II. *R. typhi* transmission is increased in regions and situations in which the rat population is high. As with *R. prowazekii,* war and periods of societal strife lead to conditions that favor outbreaks. One case of transmission owing to a laboratory accident has been reported [169]. *R. rickettsii* transmission is higher in those with tick exposure [206] and is also possible in those who crush infected ticks between their fingers [145]. Pet ownership was not found to be a statistical risk factor, although the dog tick, *Dermacentor variabilis,* is the main vector in the eastern and Pacific coastal areas [149]. Person-to-person infection probably does not occur, except in cases of direct percutaneous inoculation [44].

Orientia tsutsugamushi

Scrub typhus infection occurs in humans with environmental exposure to the chiggers (larval forms) of specific mites that infest rodents. Humans become infected as accidental hosts. Exposure occurs in proximity to the scrublike vegetation that harbors populations of rodents, with both mice and rats potentially infected. Transmission occurs via the bite of a chigger. Infection rates rise during the early rainy season owing to a corresponding increase in arthropod population density. Soldiers who are deployed under simulated battlefield conditions are markedly susceptible to infection [158]. Outdoor activities such as hiking and mountain climbing also put humans at risk for scrub typhus [207]. Sitting or lying on the ground in endemic areas places an individual at particular risk [208]. In addition to arthropod-to-human transmission, human-to-human transmission may occur. Scrub typhus infection can be spread vertically [209] and via needlestick [210]. It appears that there are variations in strain virulence among *O. tsutsugamushi* that probably affect the likelihood of disease transmission. These differences were actively exploited by the Japanese in the 1930s, who infected volunteers with the less virulent strains of the Pescadores, protecting them from the more virulent strains of Japan [211].

Bartonella

B. quintana outbreaks also appear to be related to conditions that promote body louse infestation. The homeless, alcoholics, and HIV-infected people seem most vulnerable. The risk for transmission of *B. henselae* is believed to be increased by exposure to cats and their fleas. Ownership of kittens, cat bites, and cat scratches are risk factors [165].

OCCUPATIONAL RISK FACTORS
Psittacosis

Occupations associated with increased risk for acquiring psittacosis include veterinarians, veterinary technicians [212], poultry industry workers [213], farmers, zoo and aviary employees, laboratory workers [214], abattoir workers, wildlife rehabilitators [215], and pet shop employees. Pigeon fanciers and other pet owners are particularly at risk, accounting for over 40% of all cases [18]. Although humans who have the most intimate contact with the animals or their products are at highest risk, microbial aerosols have been documented to infect employees who have had no direct animal contact [216]. Within a turkey processing plant, workers from the evisceration area or the "live hang" room were 5.6 and 3.4 times, respectively, as likely to be-come infected in the course of an outbreak than were individuals who worked in other areas of the plant, exhibiting 34% and 21% seropositivity rates, respectively. Mink room workers and deboning line workers also had high attack rates, and the clean-up crews in the deboning room had even higher rates of infection than the deboning line workers [217]. It also was noted that workers at a "further pro-cessing" plant became infected, proving that even a presumably trivial exposure to defeathered, eviscer-ated, chilled carcasses is potentially infectious [217].

Chlamydophila pneumoniae

C. pneumoniae presents a risk to closed populations such as families and those in military garrisons and schools [99]. The attack rates among military gar-risons during documented outbreaks ranges from 6–8% [25]. Outbreaks also have been reported among family groups and in schools, nursing homes, long-term health care facilities, and hospi-tals [31]. Physicians who care for these patients are also at risk for infection as well as reinfection.

Chlamydia trachomatis

C. trachomatis is an occupational hazard for com-mercial sex workers. Obviously, their clients are at risk as well. An interesting finding arose from a study of commercial sex workers in Copenhagen. It was found that owing to a high rate of condom use by prostitutes when involved with paying cus-tomers, the rate of infection with *C. trachomatis* ac-tually was lower than that from encounters with nonpaying individuals, presumably spouses and lovers [108].

Q Fever

C. burnetii presents potential risks for veterinari-ans, farmers, abattoir workers, wool processors [218], textile workers [214], laundry workers, and laboratory personnel. Outbreaks have occurred in meat-packing plants, dairies, and stockyards [117]. The outbreaks at research facilities are likely related to the use of goats and gravid sheep in experimen-tal studies. Personnel who have direct contact with the animals or their products have the highest rates of infection. It is now known that any personnel with exposure to infected aerosols (including visi-tors) are also at relatively high risk for infection [218–221]. In the past, Q fever was studied by the U.S. military as a proposed agent for biologic war-

fare [222], and its potential to infect troops or even metropolitan areas with some impact has been ex-plored [223]. Owing to the organism's resistance to drying and inactivation, as well as its high infectiv-ity, *C. burnetti* remains a major source of concern as a potential agent of bioterrorism [224].

Rickettsial Infections

R. prowazekii may be transmitted to individuals, such as prison guards, who work in close proximity to lice-infested individuals. *R. typhi* transmission to laboratory personnel has been reported [225]. The rate of *R. rickettsii* infection is believed to be higher in outdoor workers with heavy exposure to ticks. Soldiers also may contract the disease from expo-sure during field exercises [150]. Travelers to en-demic areas are at risk for any of the rickettsioses [226].

Scrub Typhus

Those at risk for scrub typhus, *O. tsutsugamushi* in-fection, include individuals who have exposure to the mites *Leptotrombidium leptobromidium* and *L. scutellare* in endemic areas. Historically, this has in-cluded military personnel, outdoorsmen, un-schooled children (who presumably spend a high proportion of time outdoors), and farmers [52].

Bartonella Infections

Individuals at risk for *B. quintana* include soldiers, who may be exposed to prolonged conditions of poor sanitation and crowding. Cat owners and vet-erinarians are at risk for *B. henselaea*. A random serologic survey of attendees at a veterinary confer-ence revealed that 7% had antibodies to *B. hense-laea* or *B. quintana,* suggesting a considerable incidence of occupational transmission [168].

Prevention and Control

ADMINISTRATIVE CONTROLS
Chlamydophila psittaci

Importation of birds is tightly regulated by the Vet-erinary Services of the Animal and Plant Health In-spection Service (APHIS), U.S. Department of Agriculture (USDA). Birds and poultry (e.g., chick-ens, ducks, geese, guinea fowl, and turkeys) are both subject to a separate set of stringent importation requirements, as detailed in the *Code of Federal Reg-ulations* (CFR) [227]. Canadian imports and re-turning U.S. pet and performing birds are subject to a slightly modified set of regulations, also detailed in the CFR. For standard bird and poultry importation, prior to shipping, the importer requires an import permit from the USDA and a health certificate from a veterinarian of the exporting nation [227]. Permits are available from APHIS, Veterinary Services, National Center for Import-Export, 4700 River Road Unit 38, Riverdale, MD 20737-1231. The USDA may prohibit or restrict importation from areas that are known to harbor highly dangerous communicable disease, such as Newcastle disease or certain strains of Avian flu. The USDA inspects all imports at the port of entry and enforces a minimum 30-day quarantine to ensure freedom from infection. The specific ports of entry for birds and poultry and sites of quarantine are also specified in the CFR [227]. Ideally, birds are quarantined in the country of origin for 45 days prior to transport [227]. During U.S. quarantine, birds are fed a medicated feed containing not less than 1% chlortetracycline (CTC) and not more than 0.7% calcium to treat potential *C. psittaci* infection. An additional 15 days of this dietary therapy are strongly recommended to ensure adequate therapy. Birds with documented infection or known exposure to *C. psittaci* should be placed in isolation. Treatment should be provided for all confirmed cases and possibly for all suspected ones. Isolation of the birds should be continued until all cases involving potential exposure are resolved, thus preventing reinfection of a treated bird. Other procedures are as follows:

- Overcrowding and malnutrition should be avoided, especially during transport.
- All parties involved in bird transactions should keep accurate records in order to allow retrospective identification of potential contacts and facilitate their treatment. This helps to prevent propagation of an outbreak.
- Quarantine of all potentially infected birds from a site where infection has been known to occur should be implemented by the state's public health or animal authorities [228].
- At the discretion of public authorities, epidemiologic investigation may be undertaken to determine the source of infection and to alert all potentially exposed individuals. In cases involving newly acquired birds, elucidating the identity of the primary source of infection is vital.

Important considerations in such investigations include the number and types of birds involved, human exposures and illnesses, condition of storage and transportation facilities, ventilation factors, and the treatments initiated, if any.

- Physicians should report cases of *C. psittaci* infection to the appropriate health authorities. Suspected cases in birds should be referred to a veterinarian.
- Suspected outbreaks should be reported to the CDC's Childhood and Respiratory Diseases Branch, Division of Bacterial and Mycotic Diseases, National Center for Infectious Diseases, (404) 639-2215 [18].
- Industrial processing of birds is generally overseen by state agencies and USDA meat inspectors. Ill-appearing birds should trigger serologic investigation for *C. psittaci*, followed by treatment or sacrifice of the infected specimens [217]. Since infected birds may be asymptomatic and still remain infectious, routine screening of flocks prior to their processing using a rapid and reliable test is optimal.

Chlamydophila pneumoniae

Isolation of cases is not generally felt to be necessary. The prolonged nature of outbreaks indicates a long incubation period, and asymptomatic carriage further complicates the issue of infection control. Prompt therapy of any suspected case, especially among health care workers, is recommended.

Chlamydia trachomatis

Cases of *C. trachomatis* infection should be reported to the appropriate public health authorities. A high degree of coordination among health care professionals, educators, and outreach workers is required. Health departments must ensure that all sexual partners of known cases are identified and notified and that adequate therapy and follow-up have been arranged. The CDC recommends that all states have laws that facilitate the collection of information regarding chlamydial cases. The CDC stresses primary and secondary prevention strategies:

- *Primary prevention* includes changes in behavior to include lower numbers of sexual partners, judicious partner selection, and the use of barrier methods of contraception.

- *Secondary prevention* includes (1) screening of women to identify and treat those at high risk for the sequelae of infection and (2) prompt and accurate recognition of chlamydial syndromes and timely, appropriate testing of those potentially infected.

Coxiella burnetii

Cases of *C. burnetii* should be reported to the appropriate public health authorities so that an epidemiologic investigation may be initiated. Research facilities should be constructed with prevention of transmission in mind. Airtight segregation of potentially infectious laboratory specimens is imperative. Other procedures include the following:

- All laboratory animals ideally should be evaluated for *C. burnetii* prior to transfer to research laboratories.
- In flocks of animals with significant prevalence (>20%), culling and chemoprophylaxis should be strongly considered [113].
- Access to the animal research facility should be limited, and visitation should be considered a risky practice.
- Accurate records of all animal transactions should be kept. Q fever is reportable in approximately 24 states [229].

The Australian government, using a whole-cell vaccine, instituted a National Q Fever Management Program that ran from 2000–2006. This vaccine had proven efficacy, decreasing the rate of infection among meat industry workers from 4–0.08% over a 5-year period [115a]. Despite institution of the program, 106 occupational cases were confirmed, with 71% of those not having been vaccinated. [230].

Chlamydia trachomatis

C. trachomatis is reportable in all 50 states. Notification of partners can be performed by the appropriate public health authorities if partner referral fails [231]. Counseling and education can be provided to infected individuals and their contacts at that time. Cases also can be reported on the national level to the CDC National Electronic Disease Surveillance System (NEDSS) [123].

Rickettsia typhi

Control of *R. typhi* can be achieved by eradication of rats and rat fleas. Insecticide dusting campaigns are of some use in bringing epidemics under control [41]. Proper sanitation and waste disposal help to prevent the conditions that encourage rat infestations [226]. Assessment of rodent populations and serologic testing in areas of outbreaks are likely to be helpful [232].

Rickettsia rickettsii

During the 1970s, a South Carolina program that attempted to test all submitted ticks for RMSF proved unsuccessful in decreasing the incidence of infection. However, the program was believed to have been some benefit insofar as it raised the public's and the medical profession's awareness of the importance of the disease [45].

SAFE WORK PRACTICES AND ENGINEERING CONTROLS

Chlamydophila psittaci

In any facility that accepts birds for boarding, sale, or consignment and thus houses populations of birds, the cages should be positioned so that material such as food and feathers cannot contaminate nearby cages. The sides of the cages should be solid, not mesh, and stacking of the cages is unwise. The bottoms of the cages should be made of wire mesh, and litter that will not produce dust, such as newspapers, should be placed underneath the mesh [215]. Cages and bowls should be cleaned daily (washed with soap and water), rinsed, disinfected, and rinsed again. The cage itself should be thoroughly disinfected between occupants, and exhaust ventilation should be adequate to prevent aerosol accumulation.

Newly acquired birds should be quarantined for 14–30 days before being added to a group. They should be treated prophylactically for *C. psittaci* unless they have previously tested negative. Only birds who test negative for *C. psittaci* should be accepted for boarding or consignment, and boarders should be maintained in an area with separate air-handling equipment.

In the case of an infected specimen, thorough cleaning of the cage that held the bird should be performed while the bird is held in isolation. The cage itself should be scrubbed with detergent, rinsed, disinfected, and rinsed again.

Effective disinfectants include a 1:1,000 solution of quarternary ammonium compounds [alkyl-dimethylbenzylammonium chloride (Roccal,

Zephiran)], 70% isopropyl alcohol, a 1:100 dilution of household bleach (2.5 tbsp/gal), chlorophenols, or 1% lysol. The disinfectant should be allowed to have a minimum of 5 minutes' contact with the material being cleansed.

The cage itself should have a wire-mesh bottom, and litter that does not produce dust should be used. The litter should be moistened prior to removal and should be burned or double-bagged.

The room that houses the cage also should be cleaned and disinfected. Material not amenable to disinfection, such as litter and wooden perches, should be discarded. The floor should be mopped with disinfectant or an oil-impregnated sweeping compound.

The ventilation system also should be disinfected because it may harbor the organism. During the cleaning of rooms and cages, ventilation and air currents should be minimized to prevent contamination of other areas. To prevent aerosolization of the organism, standard vacuum cleaners should not be used, and the floor itself should be disinfected or at least mopped with water.

The caretaker should observe the birds daily, weighing them every 3–7 days. Birds undergoing treatment should be segregated by sex. The recommended antibiotic treatment protocol must be followed (see below). Necropsy rooms in veterinary establishments should include a laminar flow hood to decrease the possibility of transmission [227].

During importation quarantine, the facility is required to have TV monitoring, leakproof waste-bags, and 24-hour security monitoring, either on-site or electronically. All walls, floors, and ceilings must be impervious and able to withstand cleaning and disinfection. There must be a separate necropsy area and separate equipment cleansing areas [227]. Quarantine workers should wear appropriate protective clothing and footwear. They should shower when entering and leaving the work area. They should work exclusively with one lot of birds until the quarantine period is over. Public visitation of the facility is forbidden [227].

Chlamydophila pneumoniae

Good respiratory hygiene to minimize droplet transmission during infection is recommended. Strict respiratory isolation is not specifically recommended [31]; however, the cryptic etiology of many respiratory outbreaks is likely to lead to the institution of measures known to reduce short- and long-range transmission of disease via droplet nuclei. These include negative-pressure ventilation as well as the use of personal protective equipment such as masks [32].

Chlamydia trachomatis

Transmission of C. trachomatis during sexual intercourse can be reduced by the use of latex condoms. The male variety is preferred, although the female condom may provide some protection [233].

Coxiella burnetii

C. burnetii presents a challenge to workplace prevention:

- Proper air handling to minimize exposure to infected aerosols must be achieved.
- Avoidance of infected animals is the key to prevention.
- Laboratories that culture C. burnetii should do so under strict environmental control. This includes using sealed hoods, proper ventilation, and safe culturing techniques [234].
- Disinfection of the facility must be performed regularly.
- Excessive transport of specimens within the facility should be avoided [232].

The CDC also recommends [235] the following:

- Educate the public on sources of infection.
- Appropriately dispose of placenta, birth products, fetal membranes, and aborted fetuses at facilities housing sheep and goats.
- Use only pasteurized milk and milk products.
- Use appropriate procedures for bagging, autoclaving, and washing of laboratory clothing.
- Vaccinate (where possible) individuals engaged in research with pregnant sheep or live C. burnetii.
- Quarantine imported animals.
- Ensure that holding facilities for sheep are located away from populated areas. Animals should be tested routinely for antibodies to C. burnetii, and measures should be implemented to prevent airflow to other occupied areas.
- Counsel persons at highest risk for developing chronic Q fever, especially persons with preexisting cardiac valvular disease or individuals with vascular grafts.

Rickettsia prowazekii

Outbreaks of *R. prowazekii* in jail populations have been controlled by shaving and dusting all prisoners with 0.5% permethrin, changing mattresses and clothes, and cleaning the infected facility with cyfluthrin, for example. Treating all personnel simultaneously with a single dose of doxycycline should minimize the potential for spread of the organism [236].

Rickettsia rickettsii

Strategies aiming at decreasing disease incidence via targeting resident populations of ticks have been successful in some cases. These include the use of acaricides and eliminating tick habitats (e.g., uncut grass and brush). Novel methods of tick control include application of the acaricides to the host mammals via baited tubes, boxes, and feeding stations [147].

Orientia tsutsugamushi

Control of the mite and rodent populations can be effective. On Pingtan Island in China, preventive strategies directed against these elements resulted in no clinical cases being detected in 2003–2004 [237].

PERSONAL PROTECTIVE EQUIPMENT AND PREVENTIVE MEASURES
Chlamydophila psittaci

Personnel who handle potentially infected birds should wear gloves, protective clothing and footwear, paper surgical hats, and a respirator with at least an N-95 rating (a dust-mist mask may be substituted if the respirator is not available) [18]. Surgical masks may not be effective in transmission prevention.

Necropsies on potentially infected birds should be performed under a hood equipped with an exhaust fan. The carcass should be wetted with detergent and water to prevent aerosolization of infectious particles.

Any individual at risk who develops an influenza-like illness after even trivial bird exposure should seek immediate medical evaluation [215].

Chlamydophila pneumoniae

Protective equipment such as masks can be considered when exposure is to active cases with presum-

ably active droplet generation. It is not clear if, as with *C. psittaci*, N-95 respirators are effective.

Coxiella burnetii

The use of protective equipment to reduce transmission is vitally important. Because clothing also may be contaminated when working with infected animals or their products, proper handling of potentially contaminated clothing is essential.

Vaccination of animals used in research would greatly diminish the possibility of zoonotic infection. Careful laboratory technique can minimize the possibility of infection. Avoidance of mouth pipetting and spills and prompt disposal of needles and syringes are important [238].

The CDC recommends biosafety level 2 (BSL-2) practices and facilities for individuals performing nonpropagative laboratory procedures such as serology. BSL-2 includes the following:

- Open bench work is permissible if personnel wear appropriate protective clothing or gear.
- Techniques that may produce splatter or aerosols of infectious materials should be done inside a biological safety cabinet (BSC) or other containment device.
- Waste materials need to be segregated into chemical, radioactive, biohazardous, and general waste streams. Infectious waste should be decontaminated (by treating with chemical disinfectants or by steam autoclaving).
- All the microbiologic practices and procedures delineated for the lower levels are carried forward to the next higher level (e.g., BSL-3).
- Attention should be given to wearing gloves, using mechanical pipetting devices, and handling sharps carefully.
- Only limited access is allowed to the BSL-2 laboratory.
- A leakproof box, preferably equipped with a gasket-seal lid, should be used for transport of infectious materials.
- Other special practices include decontaminating work surfaces after completing the work with the infectious materials, keeping nonresearch animals out of the laboratory, and reporting all spills and accidents. An incident log book is a useful means for recording events that have gone wrong; it is important to document these events, not for punitive action, but to be able to better

understand what happened with an eye to preventing similar events in the future.

- The supervisor of a BSL-2 laboratory should be a competent scientist who has a technical understanding of the risks associated with the microbiologic agents in use.

BSL-3 is recommended for individuals working with infected tissues or embryonated eggs or cell cultures and includes double-door access and sealed penetrations [232, 239].

- Secondary barriers are needed at BSL-3.
- Double-door entry is required.
- Venting is needed to ensure that air moves from areas of lesser contamination to areas of higher contamination and is also single-pass. Thus exhaust air is not recirculated. Exhaust air does not have to be HEPA filtered unless local conditions are such that reentrainment into building air supply systems is possible.
- Wall, ceiling, and floor penetrations are sealed to keep in all aerosols and gaseous decontaminants. The floor is monolithic, and there are continuous cove moldings that extend at least 4 in up the wall. Ceilings should be waterproof for ease of cleaning.
- Vacuum lines in the BSCs are protected with HEPA filters so that maintenance personnel are not exposed to infectious aerosols.
- Standard microbiologic practices are the same as for BSL-2 laboratories.
- Additional personnel protective devices may be worn, such as respirators, and laboratory workers must have appropriate medical evaluations and be trained in proper fit testing and care of their respirators [239].

Rickettsial Infections

Outbreaks of *R. prowazekii* can be controlled by delousing programs. Infected individuals require delousing to effect cure. DDT, lindane powder, malathion, or carbaryl may be used [42] on the body, and permethrin may be used on articles of clothing. Prophylactic doxycycline may help to prevent infection and interrupt the spread of an outbreak [41]. Correcting the conditions that promote lice infestation is quite important. Washing regularly, laundering, and use of insecticides are helpful.

R. typhi infection rates can be decreased through aggressive rat and flea control.

R. rickettsii infection can be prevented by the use of insect repellents and the wearing of protective clothing. DEET-containing products can be applied to the skin and clothing. Permethrin applied to clothing also helps to prevent *R. rickettsii* infection. Avoidance of highly endemic areas is wise. A hair and skin survey after a possible exposure is important, and pets should be inspected as well. Forceps removal of arthropods will help to prevent transmission of tick-borne disease because 6 hours of attachment is likely necessary for transmission. Proper technique requires anterior grasping of the ticks, with complete removal of all body parts, followed by washing the area with soap and water [45].

BSL-2 practices and facilities are recommended for nonpropagative laboratory procedures. BSL-3 practices and facilities are recommended for laboratories using known or potentially infectious materials, those handling experimentally infected animals, and those involved in growing the organism in cell culture [232].

Orientia tsutsugamushi

Some measures for preventing scrub typhus include avoiding exposure to the tall grass and scrub vegetation that harbors the chiggers. Visitors to endemic areas should wear clothing that covers the arms and legs. Use of insect repellents such as DEET, including application to the tops of boots and socks [240], should be encouraged. Using cots instead of placing sleeping bags on the ground also reduces exposure. Use of pesticides to control the population of mites may be considered if deployment and exposure are unavoidable [241]. Chemoprophylactic treatment with doxycycline appears to be effective. A study of 1,125 military personnel exposed to a hyperendemic area of Taiwan showed that 200 mg orally each week resulted in a fivefold decrease in disease incidence [242]. Weekly doses of doxycycline (200 mg orally) also were found to be protective against experimental inoculation [243]. Chloramphenicol (4 g orally each week, continued for 4 weeks after exposure) also was successful [244]. Doxycycline has a favorable half-life and is likely to be better tolerated than chloramphenicol. Doxycycline prophyaxis should be continued for up to 6 weeks after exposure.

EMPLOYEE EDUCATION AND TRAINING
Chlamydophila psittaci

Employees need to be well versed in the preventative measures outlined earlier. They also should be educated as to the highly infectious nature of *C. psittaci* and should be made aware of the routes of infection and the methods used to reduce risk. They should report any illnesses observed in birds to the appropriate veterinary authority immediately and should report any human illnesses promptly as well. Personnel involved in the sale of birds should be instructed never to sell an ill-appearing bird or other animal. Physicians caring for infected patients should be alerted to the patient's exposure history and should have a low threshold to begin treatment. Patients with respiratory illnesses who have a known exposure to *C. psittaci* probably should be started on empirical therapy while awaiting test results.

Chlamydia trachomatis

Commercial sex workers should be made aware of the benefit of using latex condoms. They should become well skilled in the technical aspects of their use so that breakage and slippage rates are decreased [245]. Proper use involves using a new condom before each act, using water-based lubricants only, and using correct methods for applying and removing condoms [231]. Female condoms can be used if male condom use is not possible [231]. The general population should be made aware of the intricacies of *C. trachomatis* infection. Schools are a possible venue for the provision of information. The availability of confidential testing and treatment will enhance control efforts, especially among adolescents.

Coxiella burnetii

Individuals who handle animals or specimens potentially infected with *C. burnetii* should become well versed in the various manifestations of the disease and should understand the potential modes of transmission and methods used for prevention. In addition, they should be well acquainted with the proper procedures for ventilation, transport, and waste removal [122]. Laboratory workers also need to be properly fitted with appropriate respiratory protective gear [239].

MEDICAL SURVEILLANCE
Chlamydophila psittaci

Screening and prophylactic therapy for *C. psittaci* take place at the portal of entry in the instance of importation of birds and poultry. Testing birds prior to boarding or consignment is also recommended [215]. Epidemiologic evaluation in response to confirmed and suspected cases and outbreaks is performed by authorities at the state and local levels. These outbreaks, especially if multistate, should be reported to the CDC Respiratory Disease Branch at 404-639-2215 [215].

Chlamydia trachomatis

Screening for *C. trachomatis* in highly endemic areas may be of benefit, especially if the seroprevalence rate is greater than 5% [183]. The CDC recommends screening in a multitude of situations listed in the next section.

Coxiella burnetii

Skin testing for *C. burnetii* allows identification of individuals who are presumably at risk for acute Q fever infection [115]. Identification of those at risk allows for the administration of vaccine in certain circumstances that may be protective. Individuals with valvulopathy or immunosuppressive conditions are poor candidates for occupations likely to result in *C. burnetti* exposure. Serologic testing of groups with high rates of seroprevalence can identify groups and individuals at risk and determine the efficacy of interventions such as vaccination [230].

Bartonella quintana/Rickettsia prowazekii

Screening individuals for lice on a periodic basis, which may be performed in schools or as a public health measure during periods of societal strife, can be effective in detecting and eliminating lice infestation, thus eliminating the vectors of *B. quintana* and *R. prowazekii*.

BIOLOGIC TESTING
Chlamydophila psittaci

Testing of birds for AC should be performed in cases of illness consistent with *C. psittaci* and, when possible, exposure to AC has occurred. Testing prior to boarding or consignment is also recommended [215].

Chlamydia trachomatis

The CDC recommendations of 2006 for screening for *C. trachomatis* include [246]

- Sexually active females age 25 years or younger
- Females age 25 years and older at high risk
- Pregnant women (at initial visit in all and prior to the third trimester if under age 25 and if at high risk)

The initial CDC recommendations of 1993 also included [104]

- Women undergoing induced abortion
- Women attending clinics for sexually transmitted diseases
- Women in detention facilities
- Women with mucopurulent cervicitis

The U.S. Department of Preventive Health Services issued a set of guidelines in 2007 [247]:

- Screening of sexually active females age 24 and younger
- Screening of females age 25 and older at increased risk
- Screening of pregnant females age 24 and younger
- Screening of pregnant females age 25 and older at increased risk
- No routine screening for females over age 25 who are not at risk
- No evidence to support screening of males

High-risk females include those with new or multiple partners, a previous history of an STD, nonbarrier contraception, low socioeconomic status, and active symptoms. Sex workers have a particularly high prevalence of disease, and routine screening and treatment may be of benefit. In the United States, legalized brothels in Nevada have their workers tested for chlamydia and treated, if necessary, prior to employment and every week thereafter. Males at high risk (e.g., in STD clinics or correctional facilities and adolescents) also can be considered for screening. Frequency of testing remains unspecified. Yearly testing in high-risk groups may be advisable, although 6-month intervals may be considered in some groups such as adolescents.

Coxiella burnetti

Testing and quarantine of animals prior to importation and testing prior to transfer to research facilities are advised [235].

Rickettsial Infections

Monitoring the size and serology of rodent populations can be employed as part of an effective rodent depopulation program [248]. In Hawaii in 2002, in response to an outbreak of *R. typhi*, the Hawaii Department of Health (HDH) applied rodenticide ($ZnPO_4$ oat bait) to areas where rodent populations were high. The HDH also conducted rodent trapping, environmental assessments, and resident education with emphasis on rodent-proofing domiciles. Physicians and other officials used mass media to educate the public about the clinical aspects of disease, mode of transmission, and pest control. A dramatic decrease in the rodent populations followed [248]. The CDC also issues guidelines on protecting human dwellings from infestation. These measures include sealing up all holes with steel sool and caulk or using metal sheet and cement for larger holes. Trapping the rodents and storing food items and trash in rodent-proof containers are also important. Cleaning up the droppings and urine of rodents should be done with a mixture of water and bleach, with care taken to avoid aerosolization [249].

IMMUNIZATION AND PROPHYLACTIC MEASURES

Pre- and Postexposure Measures

Chlamydophila psittaci. Electron microscopy is being used to investigate potential targets of vaccine against *C. psittaci*, with antigens on the elementary body of particular interest [250]. A lyophilized vaccine using the temperature-sensitive 1B strain of *C. psittaci* has been used successfully in ewes to prevent abortion [251]. Genetic immunization involving the plasmid DNA expressing the major outer membrane protein (MOMP) of a serovar strain did produce IgG antibodies and T-cell memory priming in vaccinated turkeys [252].

Further studies in which turkeys received plasmid DNA with MOMP from a D serovar showed significant protection against *C. psittaci* challenge, with even higher antibody levels seen with adjuvant administration of 1α,25-dihydroxy vitamin D_3 [253]. Vaccines for cats are also under study [254].

No vaccine is currently available commercially for birds. Previous *C. psittaci* infection does not confer immunity. Empirical antibiotic therapy in influenza-like illnesses in workers with AC exposure can be considered.

Chlamydophila pneumoniae. No human vaccine is currently available commercially against *C. pneumoniae*. Researchers have developed a vaccine based on a surface protein that was effective in eliminating infection in mice [255].

Chlamydia trachomatis. Commercial sex workers in Turkey frequently use prophylactic antibiotics [100] effective against *C. trachomatis*. One survey found that approximately 65% followed this practice. When infection is found in any individual, it is imperative that his or her sex partners be treated. Pregnant females who test positive can be treated with erythromycin, 250–500 mg orally four times daily for 7 days, which reduces the chance of maternal-fetal transmission to 10% [183]. Perinatal application of erythromycin or tetracycline to prevent ocular trachoma is not effective [256], but the infected neonate can be treated effectively with systemic erythromycin, as well as topical tetracycline if conjunctivitis is present [183]. Outreach programs targeting condom use in China also have resulted in decreased rates of infection [246]. A study in the Philippines found that one round of presumptive therapy for *Chlamydia* and *N. gonorrhoeae,* coupled with improved preventative practices, was helpful. These interventions resulted in a decrease in *N. gonorrhoeae* and/or *C. trachomatis* seroprevalence from a baseline of 52% and 41% for brothel workers and street sex workers, respectively, down to 23% and 28% at 7 months [257].

Currently, no effective vaccines against *C. trachomatis* are available. Research is focusing on identification of the protective antigens and on novel plasmid or viral delivery systems, as well as on immunomodulatory adjuvants [258].

Coxiella burnetii. Vaccine against *C. burnetii* (Q-Vax) is available commercially in Australia and eastern Europe. It is being given to Australian abattoir workers and Russian laboratory personnel [259]. Q-Vax proved to be nearly 100% protective over a 5-year period when given to 2,555 Australian abattoir workers [260]. As noted earlier, an Australian program of widespread immunization met with mixed success, with the target population being essentially undervaccinated, possibly owing

to administrative problems or possibly difficulties arising from prevailing attitudes among those to be vaccinated [227, 261]. U.S. efforts aimed at vaccine development continue [262]. A chloroform: methanol residue vaccine (CMR) appears efficacious and should be unlikely to result in sterile abscesses and granulomas [263]. Provision of vaccine to those likely to be exposed may become more widespread. Individuals with known valvulopathy, diabetes mellitus, cancer, or other immunocompromised states may benefit most from the development and provision of an efficacious vaccine. A skin test to determine previous infection status will help to avoid severe local reactions and should be performed prior to vaccination. Those who test positive should not be vaccinated [122]. Immunization of animals is also being investigated. The prospect of decreasing the reservoir of disease via vaccination is appealing, and studies using pregnant goats, for example, showed at least partial protection from an inactivated phase I vaccine [264].

Rickettsial Infections. Vaccine against *R. prowazekii* is available. It is recommended for individuals who travel to endemic areas and live in close proximity to the indigenous populations (e.g., missionaries, anthropologists, and construction workers), medical personnel in endemic areas, and *R. prowazekii* laboratory workers [265]. The available vaccines use crude rickettsial antigen or attenuated strains and may produce some toxicities [266]. Development of new vaccines directed against DNA sequences involved in important bacterial activities hold promise [267]. Prophylactic doxycycline, 200 mg in a single-dose regimen once a week during travel to endemic areas, has been recommended by some [268].

While no effective vaccine is available for *R. typhi*, previous infection results in long-lasting natural immunity. Vaccine against *R. rickettsii* is also not available, but research in this area continues [269].

Orientia tsutsugamushi. Prophylaxis with doxycycline is highly effective, as noted earlier. Despite extensive research [270], effective vaccines against scrub typhus are not available mostly because of the antigenic diversity among the various serotypes.

Metrics to Assess Adequacy of Preventive Measures

Coxiella burnetii. Air sampling to detect the Q fever pathogen is possible. Dust from air treatment ducts also can be tested for the presence of the organism. Serologic testing of animals and workers can determine the efficacy of prevention programs such as vaccination, quarantine, and engineering controls [230].

Chlamydia trachomatis. Screening of sex workers for *C. trachomatis* infection is facilitated by the availability of nucleic acid amplification tests (NAATs) of endocervical specimens or, even more simply, urine specimens. These tests can detect the seroprevalence of infection and assess the adequacy of intervention with a high degree of accuracy [246].

Rickettsial Infections. Serologic surveys of domestic animals such as cats may provide useful information about the adequacy of measures designed to control *R. typhi* and *R. prowazekii* [267]. IFA and PCR can be used to detect the prevalence of infection in fleas and rats [271], as well as ticks [272]. Ticks also may be tested for the presence of *R. rickettsii*, although the usefulness of such testing is in doubt [44].

SYMPTOMS AND SIGNS
Chlamydophila psittaci

C. psittaci in birds (avian chlamydiosis) presents differently depending on the virulence of the infecting strain and the species infected. Upper respiratory findings—mainly cough, dyspnea, sinusitis, poor flying performance, and nasal, conjunctival, and ocular discharge—are most frequent [273]. Ruffled feathers, lethargy, anorexia, yellow-green urate excretion, weight loss, and diarrhea also may occur. Neurologic symptoms such as seizure and tremor are seen in many species [274]. Autopsy findings include elements of serofibrinous polyserositis, such as airsacculitis, pericarditis and peritonitis [275], rhinitis, pneumonia, and hepatosplenomegaly [276]. Some species, such as chickens, are somewhat resistant to infection, and other species, such as pigeons and gulls [177], are often infected subclinically [17]. Ducks and geese may have unusual neurologic presentations such as disequilibrium [277]. Abortion is seen in sheep, cattle, goats, and horses. Conjunctivitis is noted in cats, cattle, sheep, hamsters, and guinea pigs, whereas enteritis has been reported in hares, cattle, and pigs. Arthritis may be a manifestation of infection in pigs, cattle, sheep, and horses [17].

The incubation period of *C. psittaci* is 6–20 days

in humans [89]. Rarely, the inoculum may infect the pulmonary parenchyma directly, resulting in an abbreviated 1- to 3-day incubation period [58]. Normally, the bacteria infect the epithelial cells of the lower respiratory tract and then produce a two-stage bacteremia, which initially affects the reticuloendothelial cells of the liver and spleen and then involves the lungs [58]. Infection in humans may be asymptomatic or result in severe systemic infection with pneumonia [278]. The typical clinical scenario involves tracheobronchitis or atypical pneumonia manifested by the abrupt development of fever, chills, myalgia, headache, and dry cough. The headache may be severe. A "typical" pneumonia resembling that associated with community-acquired bacterial pathogens may occur [279]. Relative bradycardia and an unimpressive pulmonary examination (belying an impressive degree of pulmonary infiltrates) are often noted. Crackles may be heard in the lower lung fields [58]. Other presentations include a mononucleosis-like syndrome manifested by fever, pharyngitis, and lymphadenopathy [278, 280] and a typhoid-like syndrome manifested by fever, malaise, and splenomegaly [14]. Rash, neurologic symptoms, and gastrointestinal symptoms such as diarrhea also have been reported. Headache and photophobia may mimic meningitis, and lumbar puncture is performed frequently [281]. Chest radiography shows pulmonary infiltrates in more than half of patients. Horder's spots, a pink maculopapular eruption, is seen in less than 50%. Unusual presentations are common, making for an extensive list of differential diagnoses. Unusual presentations include myopericarditis [282], endocarditis [283], hemorrhagic macular choroidopathy [284], psychiatric symptoms [285], hearing loss [286], intracranial hypertension [287], acute interstitial nephritis [288], acute glomerulonephritis [289], acute renal failure [290], transverse myelitis [291], cerebellar dysfunction [19], bilateral fourth nerve palsies [292], and elevated hepatic enzymes. These entities often occur in conjunction with the respiratory symptoms, confirming the systemic nature of the illness. In some cases, progression to severe hypoxemia, requiring mechanical ventilation, and ultimately death may occur [293]. In the pre-antibiotic era, mortality was likely 30–40% of patients with psittacosis [14]. Presently, overall mortality is estimated at 0.7% [173]. Gestational psittacosis appears to be particularly virulent. Transmitted from birds or sheep, it may present as a fulminant illness with pneumonia, disseminated intravascular coagulation (DIC), elevated transaminases, and abnormal renal function [172]. In pregnant patients, placental insufficiency may result in miscarriage [294]. Chest radiography typically shows a unilobar infiltrate (90%), although migratory [295], multilobar, reticular [296], ground-glass [297], and miliary patterns have been reported. Hilar adenopathy is common [58].

Chlamydophila pneumoniae

C. pneumoniae has a variety of presentations. In some cases, infection is asymptomatic, in others, flulike [99]. C. pneumoniae most frequently causes bronchitis or pneumonia, which is usually symptomatic of reinfection. The severity of the clinical syndrome that emerges is heavily influenced by the presence of comorbid illnesses and the patient's overall condition. In the elderly, pneumonitis occurs more commonly and is more likely to require hospitalization. In HIV-infected patients, a severe and ultimately fatal pneumonitis may ensue [298]. In some individuals, a prolonged syndrome characterized by bronchitic symptoms persisting for weeks may occur. Chronic infection that persists despite antibiotic therapy is seen in a small percentage of cases [299]. Pharyngitis, otitis, and sinusitis are frequent accompaniments to the respiratory tract symptoms [300]. Rarely, pharyngitis may be the sole manifestation of infection [34]. Reinfection is usually clinically milder, with less fever and a lower rate of hospitalization [33, 301]. A typical clinical scenario for patients with C. pneumoniae infection is one of biphasic disease. First, pharyngitis and laryngitis occur, followed by cough after several days. Fever occurs early, especially in primary infection. The disease then enters a second phase involving lower respiratory tract symptoms, with rales and possibly wheezing [33]. Sinusitis, with sinus tenderness, may be seen. The onset of asthma may occur in the wake of a C. pneumoniae infection, and there may be a pathogenetic role for the organism in this disease [302]. Other studies have shown that appropriate antibiotic treatment of asthmatics who are culture-positive for C. pneumoniae results in improvement of their reactive airway disease [303] and that infected steroid-dependent asthmatics can be weaned

off oral steroids successfully [304]. Rarely, neurologic syndromes, including Guillain-Barré syndrome, meningitis, and cerebellar syndrome occur in patients with C. pneumoniae infection [305]. Other associated findings may include erythema nodosum, fibromyalgia [306], arthritis [307], myocarditis, pericarditis, and endocarditis [24]. C. pneumoniae has been serologically linked to atherosclerotic heart disease and myocardial infarction [308] and has been isolated from atheromatous plaques [309]. One study found 90% of patients with acute myocardial infarction to be MIF-positive for C. pneumoniae IgG [310]. While some believe that the organism's presence itself promotes atherogenesis, the significance of these findings is being debated. C. pneumoniae also has been detected by PCR in 49% of aortic valves that required replacement [311], and 45% of stroke/TIA patients were found to have antibody to C. pneumoniae versus 19.4% of controls [312]. Future investigations into the role of C. pneumoniae in atherosclerotic and valvular heart disease offer the possibility that screening and treatment eventually may have an important role in the prevention of these diseases and their considerable morbidity and mortality. Some feel that C. pneumoniae may contribute to vascular disease by infecting the vascular wall directly or by initiating a local chronic low-grade inflammation. However, trials have failed to show that antibiotic treatment of C. pneumoniae can reduce the incidence of new cardiovascular events in patients with known disease [313].

Chlamydia trachomatis

Genital C. trachomatis also has a variable presentation depending on the strain involved, the age and sex of the infected individual, and the mode of transmission. The greatest danger posed by this pathogen is that it causes minimal, if any, symptoms in most of those it infects, whether men or women, and therefore may go undetected. Up to 70% of females who have endocervical infection exhibit minimal symptoms, typically experiencing various degrees of dysuria, vaginal discharge, or bleeding [314]. Examination at this point reveals cervical erythema and mucopurulent discharge [315]. Other manifestations in women include acute urethral syndrome and pelvic inflammatory disease (PID). Salpingitis develops in approximately 8% [316], which, if untreated, can lead to female sterility [317]. In pregnant females, chorio-amnionitis and premature delivery are possible [183]. In males, *C. trachomatis* infection is usually asymptomatic. Some males develop urethritis after a 7- to 14-day incubation. Dysuria and scant penile discharge may be noted. Males also may develop epididymitis and prostatitis [325], proctocolitis (in homosexuals) [319], reactive arthritis [320], and conjunctivitis (presumably owing to self-inoculation from genital infection) [321]. Other possible manifestations include neonatal inclusion conjunctivitis, pneumonia (seen in infants and immunocompromised patients) [322,323], and meningoencephalitis [324]. Lymphogranuloma venereum (LGV) is due to a strain of *C. trachomatis* that rarely occurs in the United States. LGV typically causes a genital ulcer at the site of inoculation and later leads to inguinal and femoral adenopathy or perirectal disease [231].

Rickettsia Infections

R. prowazekii infection is heralded by 1–3 days of malaise, followed by severe headache, fever, chills, and prostration. A truncal rash typically appears in the region of the axillary folds and spreads centrifugally. Eventually only the palms, soles, and face are spared. The rash may be petechial or maculopapular [41]. Meningismus, delirium, and coma have been seen. Symptoms may last for 2 weeks or more, and convalescence may be prolonged [42]. Mortality occurs at a variable frequency. Antibiotics shorten the febrile phase to 72 hours or less. Digital gangrene and cerebral thrombosis are potential adverse outcomes [41]. Thrombocytopenia and elevated transaminases may be seen. Brill-Zinsser disease is a recrudescence of epidemic typhus. It manifests up to 30 years after the original infection, often in the elderly and immunocompromised. It is characterized by a 10- to 14-day course of fever, intense headache, and mental status change. A scant, milder form of the rash typically occurs on days 4–6. Mortality is rare [325].

R. typhi causes fever in almost all victims. Headache, rash, gastrointestinal symptoms, cough, and myalgia are seen in less than half of patients at presentation. The rash is truncal in 88%, when present. Anemia is seen in almost 65% of patients [138]. Rarely, the disease manifests as meningitis [326] or retinitis [327]. The elderly and those with comorbid conditions tend to have more severe symptoms, although murine typhus is generally milder than louse-borne typhus.

R. rickettsii causes fever, headache, and rash in 80–90% of those it infects. Onset may be nonspecific, with fever, chills and myalgiae. Anorexia, nausea, and vomiting are often seen, as well as abdominal pain. This is followed in 2–4 days by rash, originally small, blanching, pink macules on the ankles or wrists. In approximately half of patients, the rash evolves into a petechial exanthem over the next several days. The rash spreads centripetally, usually sparing the face [147]. The organisms infect the endothelial cells and thus injure the microcirculation, leading to the petechiae and possibly gangrene. Meningismus and other neurologic abnormalities have been reported, and pulmonary manifestations such as pneumonia and pleural effusion are also seen [328]. Nausea and vomiting are noted frequently, and hepatosplenomegaly occurs in the more severe cases [44]. Conjunctivitis is seen in 30% or more, and periorbital edema may indicate severe infection in children [44].

Coxiella burnetii

Coxiellosis is the term used to describe *C. burnetii* infection in animals. Infection in animals is usually asymptomatic, although abortion outbreaks have been noted. *C. burnetii* produces symptoms in up to 50% of infected humans [117]. The presentation in humans appears to vary geographically for unknown reasons. For example, Q fever pneumonia is rare in Australia but is seen in up to 50% of cases in the United States and Great Britain [118]. In France, hepatitis is the most common presentation [329].

The typical incubation period for Q fever after exposure is 2–4 weeks. The inoculum size affects the duration of incubation inversely [330]. Symptoms typically begin with a flulike syndrome. Fever ranges up to 104°F, and the patient may experience chills, rigors, malaise, anorexia, myalgia, and headache. The fever may persist for 3 weeks. Relative bradycardia is often noted, and a severe retroorbital headache [330] may be the most prominent symptom. A macular or purpuric exanthem is seen in 20% of patients with acute infection [329]. A vasculitic rash appearing later in the course of the disease occurs in fewer than 10%.

Up to half of patients have pneumonia [331]. A

dry cough is seen in up to 28% of the patients who have abnormal chest radiographs [332]. Dry crackles on lung auscultation are more typical than signs of consolidation [117]. Pleuritic chest pain occurs in up to 34% of infected individuals [195]. Pneumonia is usually mild but may progress to respiratory failure [39]. Radiographic films of the chest typically show patchy or rounded opacities in the lower lung fields. In one series, the lower lobes were involved in 100% of patients with pneumonia [333]. Multiple round lesions, effusions, air bronchograms, reticular infiltrates, hilar adenopathy, pseudotumor, and atelectasis also have been reported [37]. Clearing of the lungs may take more than 70 days [117]. Nausea, vomiting, and diarrhea are seen in a minority of patients. Hepatomegaly was seen in half the patients in one series [118] but was absent in all patients in another study [334]. Splenomegaly also occurs in a small percentage of infected individuals [334].

Untreated, patients may develop a typhoidal state characterized by delirium and stupor. In the pre-antibiotic era, recovery took several weeks or even months.

Acute Q fever also may present as an isolated fever, pneumonia, meningitis, hepatitis, myocarditis, or pericarditis [258]. Other manifestations of acute Q fever include optic neuritis, choroidal neovascularization [335], rhabdomyolysis [336], thyroiditis, pancreatitis, syndrome of inappropriate antidiuretic hormone (SIADH), deep vein thrombosis, epididymitis, orchitis, abortion, and erythema nodosum [334]. The presentation of Q fever tends to vary geographically, perhaps reflecting differences in strain.

Chronic Q fever by involves symptoms beyond 6 months. It is seen in less than 5% of those infected. It appears to develop more slowly and may have an insidious onset. Chronic Q fever is more prominent in the elderly, the immunocompromised, and individuals with valvulopathy. Manifestations of chronic infection include endocarditis, osteomyelitis, abortion, and pseudotumor [258]. Endocarditis, which is usually indolent, is seen almost exclusively in those with preexisting valvulopathy or prosthetic valves [337] and accounts for approximately 65% of chronic cases of Q fever [234]. Large vegetations and major embolic events have been noted, and fever with congestive heart failure is a frequent presentation [338]. Since routine

blood cultures do not detect *C. burnetii*, a high index of suspicion is required to make the diagnosis. Associated clues to the diagnosis include clubbing (seen in 37% of patients) [130], as well as indicators of an underlying inflammatory state, such as an elevated erythrocyte sedimentation rate, rashes, and splenomegaly [234].

Orientia tsutsugamushi

O. tsutsugamushi infection also has a variable clinical presentation. There appear to be considerable differences in virulence between different strains, with some causing a typically mild flulike illness and others leading to an overwhelming infection resulting in death. Virulence factors are segregated geographically, so the result of infection varies dramatically with the area of endemicity. Host factors, specifically the issue of primary infection versus reinfection, are also important [339].

Infection with the agent of scrub typhus begins with inoculation of the host by the bite of the chigger. Within 2 days, a papule appears; it develops into a bulla and eventually ulcerates. Local multiplication of the organism often results in the formation of an eschar, a black crust surrounded by raised, erythematous borders [51]. Asian patients appear less likely to have eschars, possibly owing to a partial immunity derived from previous infection [340]. Lymphadenopathy begins regionally and becomes generalized in most patients. Only the nodes in close proximity to the inoculation site tend to be tender, however [51]. After an average of 16 days' incubation, symptoms begin in a characteristic flulike manner. Fever of 104°F or more may be seen, along with myalgia, anorexia, and headache Dizziness is common [208].

In one study, fever and headache occurred in 100% of patients, chills in 80%, and cough in 45%. Adenopathy was noted in 85%, whereas an eschar was seen in only 46% [51]. When present, the eschar was on the leg or scrotum approximately 66% of the time [51]. In some patients, a generalized vasculitis ensues [341]. Other cutaneous manifestations include a macular or papular rash, which begins on the trunk, spreads to the extremities, and involves the palms and soles [208]. This rash also may reappear during clinical relapse, providing an important clue to therapeutic failure. The organism also may involve the central nervous system, causing mononuclear meningitis [342]. Many other clinical syndromes have been described: ocular problems such as conjunctival injection and subconjunctival hemorrhage [341], granulomatous hepatitis [343], "acute abdomen" [344], and interstitial pneumonitis [345]. Other pulmonary manifestations include interstitial edema and hemorrhage caused by vasculitis [346]. Pleural and pericardial effusion [208], meningoencephalitis, and acute respiratory distress syndrome also have been reported [347]. Untreated, the illness lasts approximately 2 weeks, with a mortality that varies from 0–30%. Antimicrobial therapy shortens the clinical course of the infection and decreases mortality to essentially zero [348].

Bartonella quintana and *Bartonella henselaea*

As with virtually all the organisms discussed in this chapter, *B. quintana* has an impressive variety of clinical presentations. *B. quintana* causes trench fever, a bacteremic illness in which victims classically develop a single 5-day fever. However, infected individuals also may remain afebrile, have recurrent episodes of 5-day fever, or develop persistent fever [349]. Associated symptoms and signs, including myalgia, headache, bone pain, splenomegaly, and an evanescent maculopapular rash [350], are common. Shin pain may be a distinctive finding. *B. henselaea* presentation also may involve recurrent fever depending on the host's immune status. Disseminated infection by either species may cause bacillary angiomatosis, peliosis, or other inflammatory conditions [351]. *B. henselaea* is also implicated as a cause of cat-scratch disease. Endocarditis has been reported with both species, as well as with *B. elizabethae* [352]. Optic disc edema, retinal lesions, and optic nerve head inflammatory masses have been seen with *B. henselaea* [353, 354]. While 50% of patients with *Bartonella* infections have self-limited disease, the remainder suffer relapses or develop more chronic forms of infection [161].

Differential Diagnosis

PSITTACOSIS

The differential diagnosis of psittacosis includes virtually any organism that can produce the clinical picture of atypical pneumonia. These would include *C. burnetii*, *M. pneumoniae*, *C. pneumoniae*, *Legionella*, *Francisella tularensis*, influenza, and other viruses. The protean manifestations of the disease may mimic meningitis, endocarditis, and extrapulmonary diseases such as gastroenteritis and hepatitis. Epidemiologic clues are vital and are often obtained by thorough history taking. Patients with potential psittacosis always should be questioned regarding exposure to animals, specifically birds. Q fever is suggested by a history of exposure to cats, goats, or other farm animals. Clinical clues are relatively nonspecific, being common to many of the illnesses just listed. With *C. psittaci* infection, severe headache and dry cough are prominent. Photophobia, epistaxis, and Horder's spots, if present, are helpful diagnostically. Confirmation of *C. psittaci* infection may not be available until serologic testing is complete; testing for complement fixation (CF) titers or microimmunofluorescence (MIF) is particularly useful [215, 355].

Like psittacosis, *M. pneumoniae* infection also produces atypical pneumonia, with dry cough, malaise, and sore throat. Positive cold agglutinins are suggestive [356], and CF or immunoelectroprecipitation (IEP) of serum will detect antibody to *M. pneumoniae* [355]. ELISA, which detects IgG or IgM to *M. pneumoniae*, is also available and appears to be quite useful [357]. Legionnaire's disease also may present with atypical pneumonia, mental status changes, relative bradycardia, and high fever. Chills and rigors are less frequent symptoms in legionnaire's disease than in psittacosis, and pharyngitis is quite rare, in contrast to Q fever and *M. pneumoniae* infection [39]. Specialized culture, DFA of sputum, or urine antigen detection can be used to diagnose *Legionella* [358, 359].

Chlamydophila pneumoniae

C. pneumoniae tends to be less virulent than psittacosis [360]. Specialized serology is necessary to distinguish this infection from psittacosis owing to crossreactivity among *Chlamydia* species. *Francisella tularensis* causes tularemia, which presents as pneumonia 7–20% of the time [361]. The diagnosis is suggested by a history of tick or deerfly bite, contact with wild rabbits, ulceroglandular lesions, or hilar adenopathy [362]. Diagnosis of tularemia may be accomplished serologically using agglutination assay or ELISA [363]. Influenza and other viruses also may present with pneumonitis. Differentiation may be impossible on clinical grounds. Prominent upper respiratory symptoms and a typical seasonal attack pattern favor a diagnosis of viral infection, but ultimately, culture and serology may be required [364]. Psittacosis also may present as culture-negative endocarditis, mimicking organisms of the HACEK (*Haemophilus parainfluenza, H. aphrophilus, Actinobacillus, Cardiobacterium, Eikenella,* and *Kingella*) group or other fasitidious bacteria [58]. Gestational psittacosis may present with DIC, elevated transaminases, and abnormal renal function. These cases mimic some of the aspects of thrombotic thrombocytopenic purpura (TTP), hemolytic-uremic syndrome, and the hemolysis, elevated liver function tests, and low platelets (HELLP) syndrome [172].

C. pneumoniae typically presents as a mild respiratory illness. When pneumonia occurs, it may easily be confused with other causes of atypical pneumonia, as mentioned earlier. The age of the patient may be a helpful clue because *M. pneumoniae* is more likely in younger patients, as opposed to *C. pneumoniae,* which is somewhat more prevalent in the elderly [87]. Prominent sore throat with laryngitis is, as noted, more common in patients with *C. pneumoniae* infection than in those with *M. pneumoniae* [26]. Viral causes of pharyngitis and bronchitis also must be considered. Respiratory viruses such as influenza, respiratory syncytial virus (RSV), and adenovirus may present similarly. Atypical presentations may mimic meningitis and other reactive arthritides.

Chlamydia trachomatis

Genital infection with *C. trachomatis,* when symptomatic, can be differentiated from *Neisseria gonorrhoeae* by a longer incubation with less copious and purulent discharge [365]. Nongonococcal urethritis (NGU) also can be due to *Ureaplasma urealyticum* [366] or *Trichomonas vaginalis* [367]. PID also can be due to *N. gonorrhoeae* or anaerobic bacteria. *C. trachomatis* should be included in the differential diagnosis of patients with suspected meningoencephalitis [292].

Coxiella burnetii

The differential diagnosis of Q fever depends on presentation. When pneumonia is present, agents that cause atypical pneumonia should be consid-

ered, as detailed earlier. Differentiation between *C. burnetii, M. pneumoniae,* and *L. pneumophila* can be quite difficult. When flulike symptoms predominate, influenza must be considered, especially during the brief winter flu season. Influenza typically exhibits a high attack rate in a given community for only a brief 2-week period each year. A history of exposure to domestic animals raises the possibility of brucellosis or leptospirosis [229]. When elevated transaminases are the presenting sign, confusion with viral hepatitis may occur. Chronic *C. burnetii* infection may present as culture-negative endocarditis, raising the possibility of infection with fungus, *C. psittaci, Legionella,* or HACEK organisms. Other chronic vascular infections may be confused with chronic Q fever, and endocarditis with hepatomegaly may be confused with Q fever endocarditis.

Rickettsia prowazekii/Rickettsia typhi

The differential diagnosis of typhus includes many exanthematous diseases. The rash of typhus typically begins in the axillary folds and progresses centrifugally, distinguishing it from the centripetal rash of RMSF, which classically begins on the wrists and ankles. Meningococcemia, measles, secondary syphylis, Kawasaki's disease, and rubella are other exanthematous diseases that should be considered in the differential diagnosis of typhus [42]. Epidemiologic clues are often helpful, especially if the appearance of the rash is delayed.

R. typhi has a nonspecific clinical appearance, making it difficult to differentiate from other febrile illnesses, even when rash is present. A central maculopapular rash develops in 70% of those infected with *R. typhi* [226]. Epidemiologic evidence may be lacking because the bite of the flea may not be recalled [145]. The differential diagnosis is similar to that for *R. prowazekii* and includes RMSF, secondary syphilis, ehrlichiosis, and Kawasaki's disease. Other rickettsioses, stroke, pneumonia, and gastroenteritis also should be considered [145]. The cutaneous signs of measles, rubella, or roseola may be mistaken for those of *R. typhi* [226]. The differential diagnosis for *R. rickettsii* includes the other spotted fevers, typhoid fever, measles (especially if the rash is atypical), mononucleosis, and meningococcemia [145]. A rash on the palms and soles is not pathognomonic because it may mimic drug reactions, infective endocarditis, and other agents, such as *Treponema pallidum, Erlichia chaffeensis,* and enteroviruses [147]. Immune thrombocytopenic purpura (ITP) and thrombotic thrombocytopenic purpura (TTP) enter the differential if thrombocytopenia develops. A presentation of fever and headache in the absence of rash poses great diagnostic difficulty, even during the expected seasonal period. The presence of pulmonary infiltrate may suggest other atypical pneumonia pathogens. The various spotted fevers may be distinguished from each other according to geographic clues. Influenza also can presents with fever, chills, and myalgiae. The abdominal pain may suggest acute appendicitis.

Orientia tsutsugamushi

The presentation of tsutsugamushi's disease may be clinically nonspecific. Infectious mononucleosis is a frequent misdiagnosis because both illnesses may present with malaise, fever, and adenopathy. Diagnostic serologic tests, including the monospot test, are widely available and reliable [368]. The distinctive eschar is a useful diagnostic finding in patients with scrub typhus but is seen in fewer than half of patients [51]. Other diagnostic considerations include typhus, typhoid, brucellosis, leptospirosis, toxoplasmosis, and flavivirus [42]. Typhus can be distinguished by the lack of an eschar and a centrifugally spreading rash that emerges in the setting of lice infestation. Serologic testing, including ELISA and PCR, are helpful [369, 370]. Typhoid fever is due to *Salmonella typhi* and may be indistinguishable clinically from typhus and scrub typhus. In patients with typhoid fever, cultures of blood, stool, and bone marrow, as well as duodenal string culture, should be performed. This will result in a diagnostic sensitivity of 90% [371], which is helpful because serologic testing for typhoid is felt to be unreliable [372]. *Brucella* causes brucellosis, another zoonosis with nonspecific symptomology. A history of exposure to cows, camels, or unpasteurized milk and an occupational history of abattoir or veterinary work are helpful clues [373]. Diagnosis of brucellosis is usually achieved via isolation of the organism from blood or bone marrow [374]; serology also may be helpful [375]. Leptospirosis also may present in a flulike fashion, with nonspecific findings. Con-

junctival injection and hemorrhage, if present, are distinctive [376]. A history of exposure to dogs, rodents [384], or livestock, either recreationally or occupationally, is an important clue [377, 378]. Isolation of *Leptospira* from blood, cerebrospinal fluid (CSF), and urine is possible. Serologic tests for *Leptospira* are available and useful diagnostically [379, 380]. Toxoplasmosis may present with lymphadenopathy and mimic mononucleosis. A history of exposure to cat feces or ingestion of undercooked meat may be present [381], and isolation of the organism in body fluids may be successful early in the course of the disease. A number of serologic tests are also available for toxoplasmosis, including PCR [382, 383]. The flaviviruses also may present with fever, relative bradycardia, and myalgia [384]. CF, ELISA, and PCR testing are useful diagnostically.

Bartonella Quintana/Bartonella henselaea

B. quintana and *B. henselaea* must be differentiated from other causes of recurrent fever, including the diverse causes of endocarditis. Other arthropod-borne infections should be considered when infestation or bites are evident. In patients with HIV infection, the possibility of infection with fungal or mycobacterial organisms should be considered. Infection after a cat scratch may be due to *Pasteurella multocida* or other organisms. When endocarditis is present, the wide differential diagnosis of culture-negative endocarditis must be employed; this involves ruling out anaerobes, fungi, and fastidious organisms [385].

Diagnostic Evaluation

CHLAMYDIA PSITTACI
Avian Chlamydiosis

According to the CDC's 1997 guidelines, avian chlamydiosis (AC) cases are classified by the CDC as suspected, probable, or confirmed [386].

- A *suspected* case involves
  1. Clinical illness consistent with AC, with an epidemiologic link to another case of AC
  2. Asymptomatic birds with equivocal serologic evidence of infection
  3. Clinical illness with a positive, nonstandardized laboratory test result

4. A clinical illness consistent with AC that responds well to antibiotic therapy
- A *probable* case of AC involves an illness compatible with AC and either
  1. A high serologic titer obtained after symptom onset
  2. Fecal, cloacal, or respiratory/ocular exudate that is ELISA- or fluorescent antibody (FA)–positive for *C. psittaci*
- A *confirmed* case of AC requires either
  1. Isolation of *C. psittaci* from a clinical specimen
  2. ELISA- or FA-positive *C. psittaci* antigen in the bird's tissue
  3. A serologic titer that increases more than fourfold in two specimens obtained at least 2 weeks apart
  4. Giminez stain– or Machiavello stain–positive AC organisms in the bird's tissues

Methods of diagnosing AC include isolation of the organism from the bird's organs or secretions. While pharyngeal samples are the most likely to be positive, to increase sensitivity, sampling of multiple sites should be considered, especially if only a single animal is being investigated [387]. The sample is used to inoculate cell cultures, and staining subsequently reveals the organism's presence in the cellular inclusions. This can be accomplished by staining the tissue with chromatic or immunologic stains. Impression smears of actively infected tissues using Giemsa, Giminez, or Macchiavello stain are also useful [275]. For technical reasons and because of safety concerns, few laboratories culture the organism. When sending specimens to these laboratories, pooling 3–5 days of specimens and transporting the specimens packed in ice are recommended. Culture of the organism is still considered the reference standard for detection [17]. Antigen can be detected using ELISA [388], although the reliability of this test has been questioned. Other antigen-detection methods historically include cytologic staining [389], electron microscopy [390], PCR [391], elementary body agglutination (EBA), immunoperoxidase [392], peroxidase-antiperoxidase [393], and microimmunofluorescence (MIF). In some studies, PCR assay was found to be more sensitive than culture and ELISA [394, 395].

Serologic testing to detect antibodies to *C. psittaci* has several limitations. Chief among these is the fact that false-negative results are common early in the clinical course owing to low serum levels of antibody. Later, false-positive results are seen because of the persistence of antibodies (CF detects both IgM and IgG) despite adequate therapy. It is also difficult for laboratories to differentiate *Chlamydia* from *Chlamydophila* species. Some authorities feel that serologic testing is most useful in epidemiologic studies and less useful in the clinical setting [17]. Serologic tests most commonly used to detect antibody to *C. psittaci* include CF assay, which is sensitive but may remain elevated after treatment, and ELISA. Latex agglutination (LA) is also available; this test detects IgM to identify acute *C. psittaci* infection but fails to identify the more chronic forms of infection [67]. EBA is available but is performed in only one laboratory. Furthermore, EBA test results may remain positive despite therapy. In the absence of positive culture results, the most reliable diagnosis would be if a bird suspected to be a source of infection tests positive for both antibody and antigen. A fourfold increase in titer or a positive titer with antigen detection is generally considered significant.

Psittacosis

The CDC defines a *probable* case of psittacosis as

1. Clinical findings consistent with psittacosis, with an epidemiologic link to a known case
2. MIF or CF titer of 1:32 after symptom onset

A *confirmed* case of psittacosis requires

1. Positive *C. pstittaci* culture
2. Clinical findings consistent with psittacosis: either a greater than fourfold increase in CF or MIF titer over 2 weeks or more or an MIF assay positive (>1:32) for IgM

Psittacosis is human infection with *C. psittaci*. The disease presents the clinician with a diagnostic challenge. Rapid diagnosis is desirable because delays may result in poor outcomes. One study found that because an average of 8 days elapsed prior to diagnosis in five of eight patients with respiratory failure, they eventually died [396]. The diagnostician can be aided by epidemiologic clues, especially occupational or recreational exposures to birds. Such exposures are noted in 85% of patients with *C. psittaci* infection and may prompt effective empirical antibiotic therapy [293].

Chest radiography is minimally useful owing to its nonspecificity. While culture of the organism is possible, it is performed infrequently, mostly because of logistic and safety considerations. Specimens contaminated with *C. psittaci* are quite infectious and therefore hazardous to laboratory personnel [58]. The usual diagnostic method for psittacosis involves finding a greater than fourfold rise in CF titer over more than a 2-week period, although a single titer of 1:32 or greater is good presumptive evidence of infection, especially when the clinical findings are consistent with psittacosis. MIF assays are available and can distinguish between infection with the various chlamydial species. A fourfold rise in antibody or a titer of greater than 1:16 appears diagnostic. MIF also appears to be more sensitive than the standard CF titer (61% versus 46%), but false-negative results may occur [397]. DFA using monoclonal antibodies against the antigens of *C. psittaci* is available and allows more rapid diagnosis [398]. DFA can be performed on sputum, for example, providing a means of rapid and accurate diagnosis. A false-positive result owing to the presence of *C. pneumonia* or *C. trachomatis* infection is possible, and in such cases, the more species-specific MIF can be used. If results are equivocal because of a sluggish antibody response owing to therapy, a third sample may be checked later in the clinical course of the infection. In cases of suspected endocarditis, culture of the organism may be performed using the patient's serum; staining and immunofluorescence of the involved heart valve constitute another method for detecting the pathogen [399]. PCR testing is now available commercially. PCR has great promise in that it may be able to safely provide rapid diagnosis without the need to wait for convalescent sera. PCR can be performed on respiratory samples and has been performed experimentally as well on blood and urine [400]. One study found high degrees of sensitivity and specificity in detecting *C. psittaci* DNA in human sputum, throat swabs, and BAL fluid [401]. The use of PCR remains somewhat limited at present. Other methods of detection reported include analysis of BAL fluid, which also may yield the organism [402]. Lung biopsy tissue examined by di-rect immunofluorescence also may be positive [403].

Chlamydia trachomatis

Diagnosis of *C. trachomatis* requires a high index of suspicion because most cases are subclinical. Historically, specimens were best obtained from the endocervix in women and the urethra in men, with simultaneous urethral sampling in women increasing sensitivity [404]. The reference standard to measure the accuracy of diagnostic methods involved growing the organism in cell culture, followed by staining for the fluoroscein-conjugated monoclonal antibody directed against the major outer membrane protein (MOMP) of *C. trachomatis* [104]. Lung tissue also can be cultured in cases of suspected *C. trachomatis* pneumonia. However, these culture techniques are difficult to standardize and perform, as well as being expensive. Newer techniques that have proven to be highly sensitive and specific include nucleic acid amplification tests (NAAT) such as PCR. Nonculture tests also include DFA, ELISA, DNA probes, and MIF. DFA testing will detect chlamydial antigen in clinical specimens, although a DFA test with a *C. trachomatis*–specific anti-MOMP monoclonal antibody is highly specific. EIA testing that uses an enzyme linked to a monoclonal antibody is helpful, although use of chlamydial lipopolysaccharide (LPS) as an antigen may render an ELISA assay non-species-specific, resulting in false-positive results. PCR is quite sensitive and specific. Point-of-care testing is available commercially. It is rapid (<30 minutes) and may be performed in office settings. These tests rely on the LPS antigen, however, and are non-species-specific [405]. Specimens for testing also can be obtained from the rectum, conjunctiva, urine, and serum [104]. Serologic testing for *C. trachomatis* is available in some locations but is not recommended for routine screening. An IgM MIF of 1:32 or greater for *C. trachomatis* is presumptive evidence of infection [231]. A presumptive diagnosis of *C. trachomatis* should be made in patients with NGU, with PID, with epididymitis (if the patient is less than age 35), with sexual partners of known cases, and with gonorrhea. In all cases, the treatment regimens should include antibiotics effective against *C. trachomatis* infection. Despite a presumptive diagnosis, testing still should be performed for epidemiologic reasons as well as to determine appropriate care and follow-up [104].

Chlamydophila pneumoniae

C. pneumoniae infection is usually a mild respiratory illness. Leukocytosis rarely occurs in patients with *C. pneumoniae* infection, although an elevated erythrocyte sedimentation rate (ESR) is common. A single subsegmental infiltrate on chest radiogram is seen most commonly [406], although a diffuse interstitial pattern has been noted in HIV-infected patients [298]. Pleural effusion secondary to *C. pneumoniae* sometimes occurs, and the organism has been isolated from pleural fluid. However, the organism is best isolated using nasopharyngeal swabs to inoculate a cell culture. Fluorescent-antibody staining of the culture may be performed after several days of incubation; a positive result confirms the presence of *Chlamydia* species. Culture techniques are somewhat cumbersome, require several days of incubation, and are only 65% sensitive. These considerations have led to the development of several serologic diagnostic modalities. CF may be performed; the result is considered positive if there is a fourfold rise in titer or if a single titer is 1:64 or greater. Unfortunately, CF appears to be less sensitive than MIF and is genus-specific. Thus a positive CF result does not distinguish between pneumonia owing to *C. pneumoniae, C. psittaci,* or *C. trachomatis* [24]. Using IgM- and IgG-specific MIF appears to be the most sensitive and specific method and can distinguish acute from previous infection [24]. Unfortunately, IgM is often absent in patients with reinfection as well as in younger patients. IgA-specific MIF may help in cases of reinfection, however, because one study showed all individuals with reinfection to have MIF IgA titers of 1:64 or greater [33]. MIF may be considered positive if there is a fourfold rise in titer, if the IgM titer is 1:16 or greater, or if IgG is 1:512 or greater [24]. A new microimmunofluorescence test (MRL) appears to be somewhat more sensitive than the standard MIF test [407]. PCR appears to be quite useful, allowing a rapid diagnosis not available with culture techniques. Sensitivities and specificities as high as 100% and 98%, respectively, have been reported on BAL fluid specimens [408]. PCR may be performed on throat swabs, sputum, or BAL fluid specimens [409,410]. Unfortunately, real-time PCR may detect the presence of *C. pneumonia* DNA but cannot reliably distinguish among active infection, persistent infection, and asymptomatic carriage, thus severely limiting PCR's clinical usefulness [411].

Coxiella burnetii

Q fever has a mild, nonspecific presentation and thus can be difficult to diagnose. While a cluster of cases related to the same source may be seen, sporadic cases occur frequently. A history of occupational exposure and headache is an important clue for the physician. The clinical presentation and laboratory findings are quite variable. *C. burnetii* infection may present as pneumonitis, with interstitial or nodular infiltrates present in the lower lobes [214]. The white blood cell count is abnormal in approximately 30% of patients with this infection [39], thrombocytopenia is seen in 25% [117], and thrombocytosis owing to platelet counts as high as 1,000,000 may be seen [334]. Elevated transaminases (two to three times normal) are seen in approximately 50% of patients, whereas jaundice is rare [334]. Hemolytic anemia has been noted [118], and the ESR may be elevated. Hypoxemia parallels the radiographic extent of disease. In one study, 26% of patients had Pa_{O_2} of less than 60 mmHg [334]. CSF pleocytosis and elevated protein also have been seen in patients with *C. burnetii* infection [119].

Since infection with *C. burnetti* is often clinically nonspecific, serologic tests such as IFA classically have been used to diagnose infection. IFA is the reference method for diagnosis. A single IFA titer of 1:256 or greater is felt to be diagnostic [234]. *C. burnetti* exists in two antigenic phases, phase I and II. Interestingly, testing for antibodies to phase II antigens is used to detect acute infection, whereas testing for phase I antigens is useful in the detection of chronic infection [117]. Positive titers for IgM indicate likely acute infection, although they may persist for 1 year [234]. Positive IgA and IgG (≥1:800) to *C. burnetii* phase I antigens indicate chronic infection with a high sensitivity and specificity and may be associated with endocarditis [234]. Antibody titers may wane slowly over time, remaining positive for years in some patients [117]. Combined detection of IgM and IgA in addition to IgG improves the specificity of the assays and provides better accuracy in diagnosis. In acute cases of Q fever, patients will be test positive for IgG antibodies to phase II antigens and IgM antibodies to phase I and II antigens. Infection can be confirmed by culture of the organism or, more commonly, by serologic methods. The organism can be grown in cell culture, chicken embryo, and animals [234]. Owing to the significant hazard to laboratory personnel, culture requires a BSL-3 laboratory. It is now possible to culture the organism more safely using, for example, the shell-vial cell culture technique. This method of culture may be performed on tissue biopsies and buffy coat samples; it requires only 6 days of incubation [234]. Culture techniques still may be useful for patients in whom early diagnosis is required because if *C. burnetii* infection is present, the culture result is likely to be positive before serologic conversion (7–15 days) occurs [412]. PCR is being investigated in the hope that it will lead to earlier diagnosis and treatment. One study using LightCycler nested PCR found that 24% of patients were PCR-positive in the first 2 weeks after symptom onset versus 14% positive for IFA [413]. A Japanese study found that nested PCR was 10 times more sensitive than their regular PCR assay and was able to detect as few as 10 organisms. Technical problems with cross-contamination were felt likely to be an issue, however [414]. Much more promising was a South Australian study of 27 patients during an outbreak. Using two PCRs in concert, one using the 27-kDa outer membrane protein and the other using the insertion sequence, the mean time to PCR-based diagnosis was 4 days versus 17 days with serology [415]. IFA also may be performed on valvular tissue or the supernatant of cell cultures but is currently less convenient than serology. *C. burnetii* also can be detected directly using immunologic staining methods in tissues such as heart valves. When Q fever hepatitis is present, autoantibodies to smooth muscle, a positive antinuclear antibody (ANA) test, or a positive Coombs' test may be seen [234]. Q fever endocarditis may be diagnosed by using the criteria of the Duke Endocarditis Service [416]. Analysis has shown that the sensitivity of this method is increased when a positive *C. burnetii* blood culture or a high phase I titer of 1:800 or greater for IgG is considered the major diagnostic criterion [417].

Rickettsia prowazekii/Rickettsia typhi

Prompt diagnosis of rickettsial diseases is important to decrease morbidity and mortality. Unfortu-

nately, serologic diagnosis may not be timely, and serologic testing may be misleading in the early stages of infection. Epidemiologic clues, a high index of suspicion, and empirical therapy are important tools for the clinician. Skin biopsy offers a chance for early diagnosis of rickettsial infection, provided that rash is present. The organism may be demonstrated using Giemsa or Giminez staining. *R. prowazekii* may be diagnosed by culture, serologically, or by PCR [418]. EIA testing for *R. prowazekii* is available [369], as is MIF and IFA [137]. Immunohistochemical staining of tissues is possible and may be useful in acute cases [358]. Real-time PCR appears promising for early diagnosis, with positive serologic identification of *R. prowazekii* at day 3 in infected mice [419].

R. typhi can be diagnosed serologically by IFA or by latex agglutination (LA). Immunohistologic identification of *R. typhi* in tissue [420] and PCR [421] are also available. Rapid diagnosis also was shown to be possible through the use of the Dip-S-Ticks, which have 88% sensitivity and 87% specificity for *R. typhi* in testing IFA-positive sera [422].

R. rickettsii is potentially lethal, so early diagnosis is important. Up to 20% of untreated cases and 5% of treated cases are fatal [147]. *R. rickettsii* may cause nonspecific laboratory abnormalities such as anemia, thrombocytopenia, and hyponatremia [44]. The organism may be cultured from blood, although some feel that this poses a biohazard to laboratory personnel. The organism is classified as a BSL-3 agent. Serology is often confirmatory because serologic positivity may not develop for 7–10 days. IFA remains the most widely used serologic test for the diagnosis of RMSF [370]. IFA demonstrating titers of 1:128 or greater or demonstration of a fourfold increase to 1:64 or greater is considered positive [138], although results are not species-specific. LA (≥1:64), CF, and indirect hemoagglutination (≥1:128) are also felt to be serologically diagnostic of RMSF [145]. ELISA is also becoming more widely available. PCR has somewhat limited sensitivity when used on sera owing to low levels of rickettsemia. PCR techniques are more likely to be useful when testing skin biopsy specimens [147, 148, 423].

The pathology of the rash in RMSF is characteristic, revealing lymphohistiocytic capillaritis and venulitis, with extravasation of erythrocytes [424]. Timely diagnosis may be achieved by immunofluorescent staining of a punch biopsy of the rash. This technique appears to be 70% sensitive and almost 100% specific. Immunoperoxidase staining is less timely because it is performed on a processed specimen, but it exhibits the same sensitivity and specificity as immunofluorescent staining [425].

Orientia tsutsugamushi

Historically, scrub typhus has been exquisitely responsive to appropriate antimicrobial therapy, so much so that a prompt response was felt to be diagnostic and a poor response to cast doubt on the diagnosis. The emergence of drug-resistant strains has made the availability of serologic diagnosis more essential [426]. Routine laboratory testing is of little help in diagnosing scrub typhus. Frequent findings include elevated ESR, serum lymphocytosis (>50% lymphs in 70% of cases), and increased transaminases [208]. Several serodiagnostic tests are available for diagnosing scrub typhus. IFA is now the mainstay of serologic diagnosis. Lack of standardization among available assays has led to the recommendation that diagnosis should be based on a fourfold increase in titer between the paired sera, although an isolated high titer is suggestive of disease [427]. An ELISA test, known commercially as Dip-S-Ticks, proved to be 94% sensitive and 98% specific at a cutoff of one or more positive dots. PCR may be useful in that it may be positive when specific antibody tests are unrevealing [428, 429]. Nested PCR of eschar lesions had a sensitivity of 86% and a specificity of 100% in one study, and PCR of the buffy coat layer was positive in 19 of the 22 patients who were still IgM-negative [430, 431]. Real-time PCR also appears promising [432]. The classic slide agglutination Weil-Felix reaction (crossreactive antibodies to the *Proteus* X strain) was found to lack sensitivity and is not considered useful [433].

Bartonella quintana/Bartonella henselaea

B. quintana and *B. henselaea* are difficult to culture. Sensitivity of culture is highly variable, with various techniques and specimen sources yielding sensitivities of 28–98% in one study [434]. Bone, skin, and valvular and blood specimens may yield the organism. In endocarditis patients, previous administration of antibiotics typically will render the specimen culture-negative. A direct IFA test has been available for *Bartonella* infection since 1992

[385], with IFA titers of 1:64 or greater originally being considered positive. IFA has some limitations clinically, with relatively low sensitivity, non–species specificity, and a confusing degree of seroprevalence in noninfected individuals [435]. The sensitivity and specificity of IFA for *Bartonella* infection were felt to be 83% and 98% in one study, [436], although crossreactivity with *C. pneumoniae* appeared to occur [360]. EIA also may detect infection but is not available commercially. Studies have shown EIA to have lower sensitivity than IFA, however, limiting its usefulness [437]. PCR is now available and is likely to become a useful tool for detection of *Bartonella* infection [438,439]. The sensitivity and specificity of PCR have been measured at 61% and 100%, respectively [379].

Treatment and Rehabilitation

CHLAMYDOPHILA PSITTACI

Treatment of avian chlamydiosis includes several established options. Effective treatments include medicated feed impregnated with chlortetracycline (CTC), ideally maintaining a serum concentrations of 1 µg/mL [440]. Mash diets and pellets with greater than 1% CTC can be bought or mixed. White millet seed with CTC is available (e.g., Keet Life) and can be used to treat parakeets, canaries, finches, and budgerigars [67]. Larger psittacines and lovebirds require treatment with 1% CTC either via medicated pellets (e.g., Psittacin or Psittavit) or as a cooked mash or nectar diet to which CTC powder (e.g., Cyanamid or Mix 66) has been added [67]. CTC can be added to hen feed to medicate pigeons [67]. Oral doxycycline, 25–50 mg/kg once a day, is another option for most psittacines. Doxycycline probably should be given at a dosage of 25–30 mg/kg each day for cockatoos and macaws and 25 mg/kg each day for African gray parrots, Goffin's cockatoos, and blue, gold, and green-winged macaws. A dose of 40–50 mg/kg each day is needed for cockatiels, Senegal parrots, and blue-fronted and orange-winged Amazon parrots. All these treatments should be continued for 45 days.

Adequate antibiotics cannot be provided via drinking water because the psittacines have very low water requirements [67]. Turkeys require treatment with pelleted feed with CTC at a concentration of 400 g/ton, which should be continued for 2 weeks or more; the turkey should be held for at least 2 days prior to slaughter [67, 277]. Intramuscular doxycycline is available in Europe and Canada. A dose of 75–100 mg/kg is injected into the pectoral muscle each day for 4 weeks and then every 5 days. Birds who are too ill to eat can be tried on injectable oxytetracycline; 75 mg/kg every 3–4 days has been successful in some species. Tissue necrosis is a problem with intramuscular CTC and oxytetracycline [440]. Quinolones and macrolides may be beneficial, but proof is lacking at present. Enofloxacin is available for use and can be considered if other therapies have proved ineffective [441]. Supportive therapy with fluids, heat, and vitamins also may be helpful [442], and a diet low in calcium (<0.7%) will allow for sufficient tetracycline absorption from the gastrointestinal tract.

Treatment of infected humans is more straightforward. Untreated psittacosis may result in a persistent fever for 3–4 weeks, often resulting in death [14]. Isolation of *C. psittaci* patients has not been traditional owing to a perceived low rate of infectivity, although transmission from patient to doctor or nurse has been described [14]. The CDC does not officially recommend patient isolation or prophylactic therapy of contacts [18]. Possible human-to-human transfer [177] suggests that respiratory isolation or at least extreme care in handling the secretions and biologic specimens of these patients is prudent. Tetracyclines are the drugs of choice for the treatment of psittacosis. Doxycycline, 100 mg orally twice daily, and tetracycline, 500 mg orally twice daily, can be used. Treatment should be continued for at least 10–14 days after resolution of fever. Intravenous tetracycline at a dosage of 10–15 mg/kg per day or intravenous doxycycline at 4.4 mg/kg per day in two divided doses can be used in severely ill patients. The macrolides may be effective, but there are several reported cases in which the patient died despite erythromycin therapy [293, 443]. Macrolides may be considered for pregnant women and children under age 9. Quinolones such as ofloxacin [444, 445] also may be useful [446], whereas sulfonamides are usually not. Appropriate therapy should result in clinical improvement within 48–72 hours. Although unusual, reinfection with *C. psittaci* can occur [92].

CHLAMYDOPHILA PNEUMONIAE

C. pneumoniae is sensitive to tetracyclines, erythromycin, clarithromycin, and azithromycin [444]. Doxycycline 100 mg PO bid for 10–14 days should be adequate therapy in most cases. The organism is not sensitive to sulfonamides and is less sensitive to quinolones [447]. Despite adequate therapy, relapse may occur, necessitating retreatment. Antibiotic resistance may develop in patients who are treated with azithromycin therapy [448], as well as in those treated with doxycycline [449]. Some authorities have recommended 2 g/day of erythromycin or tetracycline given in divided doses [214]. Animal studies suggest that short-term courses of antibiotics may become acceptable [450]. Patients with elevated IgA and IgG titers are considered to have chronic *C. pneumoniae* infection and have been treated in one study with 4 months of doxycycline therapy without effect [451]. Optimal therapy for such patients remains to be determined, but benefit appears to be lacking. Newer agents such as tigecyclin, a glycylcycline, may hold promise in view of increasing tetracycline TCN resistance [452].

CHLAMYDIA TRACHOMATIS

C. trachomatis can be treated with doxycycline, 100 mg orally twice daily for 7 days. The treatment of choice in uncomplicated cases is azithromycin, 1 g orally, which allows one-dose therapy. Alternatives to these two regimens for uncomplicated *C. trachomatis* include ofloxacin (not for adolescent or pregnant patients), 300 mg orally twice daily for 7 days, erythromycin base, 500 mg orally four times daily for 7 days (recommended in pregnant patients), erythromycin succinate, 800 mg orally four times daily for 7 days [231], and levofloxacin 500 mg orally each day for 7 days [104, 246]. Pregnant patients can be treated with amoxicillin, 500 mg orally twice daily for 7 days, or azithromycin 1 g PO in a single dose, with erythromycin base as an alternate regimen [231]. All strains of *C. trachoma* exhibit susceptibility to sulfonamides. Rare cases of tetracycline resistance have been reported [453]. Treatment failure rates of up to 8% have been reported and likely are related to a high chlamydial load as opposed to true resistance [454]. Therapy for PID should include the doxycycline regimen noted earlier in order to cover infection and co-infection with *C. trachomatis*. LGV requires doxycycline or erythromycin for 21 days. Bubo aspiration may be necessary [231]. Treatment of mucopurulent cervicitis should await test results unless the patient is unlikely to return for follow-up [231]. The patient should be advised to observe sexual abstinence for 7 days and until all partners have completed a full course of antibiotics. Testing for cure can be considered after 3 weeks. Testing for cure is recommended for pregnant women and when treatment failure is suspected. Ophthalmia neonatorum and infant pneumonia caused by *C. trachomatis* can be treated with erythromycin, 50 mg/kg per day in four doses for 10–14 days. Mothers of newborns with *C. trachomatis* pneumonia also should be screened and treated if necessary [231].

COXIELLA BURNETTI

Although acute Q fever, including Q fever pneumonitis, is usually self-limited, treatment should be provided to reduce the risk of chronic Q fever infection. Treatment of *C. burnetii* is difficult owing to the vacuolar location of the organism. Antibiotic sensitivities are somewhat heterogeneous; variable susceptibilities to quinolones, tetracyclines, rifampin, and erythromycin have been reported. Doxycycline is now the treatment of choice owing to its being efficacious and well tolerated. A dosage of 100 mg orally twice daily for 2–3 weeks can be used in adults [117]. Tetracycline antibiotics are also quite effective for acute Q fever, decreasing the duration of fever by 50% if started in the first 72 hours [455]. A dose of 25 mg/kg per day in four doses for a total of 2–4 weeks can be given to adults and children over age 8 with pneumonitis. Erythromycin, 500 mg orally four times daily for 10 days, also appears effective, although there are concerns regarding safety [456, 457]. Some experts have recommended combining doxycycline or macrolide therapy with rifampin [39]. Using a macrolide with rifampin has the advantage of coverage for other atypical pathogens such as *Legionella* while awaiting serologic results [334]. Quinolones penetrate the CSF well and should be considered for patients with Q fever meningoencephalitis [234].

Chronic forms of Q fever such as endocarditis theoretically should be treated with a bactericidal agent. Traditionally, these entities were treated with tetracyclines, sometimes in combination with other antibiotics. Current recommended therapies include two potentially useful regimens, doxycycline with a quinolone for at least 4 years and doxycycline in combination with hydroxychloroquine for

1.5–3 years. The second therapy appears to lead to fewer relapses [456], but mortality in both regimens was only 5%. Adding hydroxychloroquine to doxycycline increases the pH within the phagolysosome and may allow for regimens as short as 18 months [258, 458]. Late relapses are frequent and may result in a high mortality [419]. Monitoring serum doxycycline minimum inhibitory concentration (MIC) ratios may prove to be beneficial [459], as may maintaining a serum doxycycline level of at least 5 µg/mL [460]. Some practitioners consider cure to have been achieved once phase I IgA and IgG are negative, with titers of 1:200 or less [234]. Monitoring serology seems the best approach to determining the length of therapy, with continuation of antibiotics if the patient remains positive [337]. Lifetime therapy may be necessary for some patients. Valve replacement has been used by some physicians in an attempt to cure Q fever endocarditis, and it probably should be considered in the case of hemodynamic compromise or recurrent embolization [337, 234]. In cases of prosthetic valve endocarditis, valve replacement after several weeks of antibiotic therapy is often required for cure [461], although some successes are reported [462].

RICKETTSIA PROWAZEKII/RICKETTSIA TYPHI

Louse-borne typhus from *R. prowazekii* can be cured with a single dose of doxycycline, 100 mg orally [463], and 200-mg doses also have been seen to be highly effective [464]. More prolonged courses of therapy are advocated by some [268] and are likely to be used extensively in the critically ill. Endogenously acquired *R. prowazekii* (Brill-Zinsser disease) and *R. typhi* should be treated with doxycycline, 100 mg orally twice daily, chloramphenicol, 50 mg/kg per day in four divided doses, or tetracycline, 25 mg/kg per day in four divided doses [42]. *R. typhi* may also be treated with quinolones, although clinical data are limited. Time to defervescence was 2.9 days for doxycycline versus 4 or more days for chloramphenicol and ciprofloxacin [465].

R. rickettsii can be treated with doxycycline, 100 mg orally twice daily, TCN, 25–50 mg/kg per day, or chloramphenicol, 50–75 mg/kg per day [145]. Doxycycline is the drug of choice in adults as well as children. The pediatric dose is 2.2 mg/kg twice daily (orally or intravenously) for children under

100 lb. Intravenous therapy is recommended for hospitalized patients. Treatment should be continued for at least 3 days after the fever subsides and until there is improvement clinically. Therapy usually is needed for 5–7 days, although the critically ill may require longer courses of treatment [147]. Tetracycline likely can be used safely in children because the risk of dental discoloration is minimal with limited use [437]. Chloramphenicol appears to be less effective than doxycycline and is no longer available in the oral form in the United States. Chloramphenicol typically had been the preferred treatment for *R. rickettsii* during pregnancy [147].

ORIENTIA TSUTSUGAMUSHI

Death from scrub typhus in the pre-antibiotic era was approximately 50% but is now near zero when appropriate antibiotic therapy is instituted [426]. Doxycycline is the mainstay of treatment for scrub typhus. Treatment with appropriate antimicrobials (e.g., doxycycline, 100 mg orally twice daily for 7 days, or TCN, 500 mg orally four times daily) historically has been quite successful, leading to rapid defervescence, which is sufficiently characteristic to allow empirical diagnosis. In 60 U.S. servicemen who acquired scrub typhus in Vietnam, the fever resolved within 28 hours [466]. No relapses were seen with 10 days of TCN therapy [51]. Virulent strains that are resistant to doxycycline and chloramphenicol have been found in northern Thailand [426]. Rifampin [467] may be useful in these cases. Shorter courses of therapy, especially for mild disease, may suffice. A Korean study found a 94% cure rate with 3 days of doxycycline versus 100% with 7 days of tetracycline ($p \geq 0.05$) [468]. Single-dose azithromycin proved equally effective as 7 days of doxycycline [469]. Azithromycin proved successful against a resistant strain in vitro and may come to be important in the treatment of children and pregnant women [470]. Intravenous minocycline has been used in severe cases [347]. The occurrence of relapse after therapy initially was thought to be related to the initiation of therapy quite early in the course of the disease [244]. However, risk of relapse is now felt to be more likely owing to the virulence of the infecting strain [468]. Some authorities have recommended 14 days of antibiotic therapy to reduce this risk [50]. Reinfection with scrub typhus also may occur, necessitating retreatment [468].

BARTONELLA QUINTANA/BARTONELLA HENSELAEA

B. quintana and *B. henselaea* seem highly susceptible to antibiotics in vitro; however, only the aminoglycosides have proved to be bactericidal for these organisms [471]. Experts have recommended azithromycin 500 mg once daily for 3 months (replacing erythromycin 500 mg four times daily, the former drug of choice). Immunocompromised patients with serious infection should receive intravenous azithromycin or erythromycin plus oral rifampin 300 mg PO bid. *B. quintana* bacteremia should receive doxycycline 100 mg PO twice daily for 4 weeks plus gentamycin 3 mg/kg intravenously each day for the first 2 weeks [472]. For *B. quintana* endocarditis, the American Heart Association recommends ceftriaxone 2 g intravenously each day for 6 weeks, along with gentamycin 1 mg/kg intravenously three times a day for the first 2 weeks. Doxycycline may be added to the preceding for the 6-week course [473].

References

1. Moulder JW. Looking at *Chlamydiae* without looking at their hosts. *Am Soc Microbiol News* 1984; 50:353–62.
2. Moulder JW. Interaction of *Chlamydiae* and host cells in vitro. *Microbiol Rev* 1991;55:143–90.
3. Everett KD, Bush RM, Andersen AA. Emended description of the order Chlamydiales, proposal of Parachlamydiaceae fam. Nov. and Simkaniaceae fam. nov. *Int J Syst Bacteriol* 1999;49:415–440.
4. Sagan L. On the origin of mitosing cells. *Journal of Theoretical Biology* 1967;14(3):225–274.
5. Saah AJ. Rickettsiosis. In: Mandel GL, Bennett JE, Dolin R (eds). *Principles and Practice of Infectious Diseases*, 4th Ed. New York: Churchill Livingstone, 1995. Pp 1719–20.
6. Harris RL, Williams TL. Contribution to the question of pneumotyphus: a discussion of the original article by J. Ritter in 1880. *Rev Infect Dis* 1985;7: 119–22.
7. Morange A. *De la psittacose, ou infection speciale determinee par les perruches*. PhD thesis, Academie de Paris, Paris, 1895.
8. Halberstaedter L, von Prowazek S. Zur aetiologie des trachoma. *Dtsch Med Wochensch* 1907;33:1285–7.
9. Coles AC. Micro-organisms in psittacosis. *Lancet* 1930;1:1011–2.
10. Macfarlane JT, Macrae AD. Psittacosis. *Med Bull* 1983;39:163–7.
11. Meyer KF, Eddie B. Characteristics of a psittacosis viral agent isolated from a turkey. *Proc Soc Exp Biol Med* 1932;83:99–101.

12. Haagen E, Mauer G. Dir psittacose in Deutschland. *Zentralb Bakteriol* 1938;143:81–2.

13. Pinkerton H, Swank RL. Recovery of virus morphologically identical with psittacosis from thiamin-deficient pigeons. *Proc Soc Exp Biol Med* 1940;45:704–6.

14. Wolins W. Ornithosis (psittacosis), a review with a report of eight cases resulting from contact with the domestic Pekin duck. *Am J Med Sci* 1948;216:551–64.

15. Moulder JW. The relation of the psittacosis group (chlamydia) to bacteria and viruses. *Ann Rev Micro* 1966;20:107–30.

16. Schlossberg D. *Chlamydia psittaci* (psittacosis). In: Mandel GL, Bennett JE, Dolin R (eds), *Principles and Practice of Infectious Diseases*, 4th Ed. New York: Churchill Livingstone, 1995. Pp 1693–6.

17. Vanrompay D, Ducatelle R, Haesebrouck F. *Chlamydia psittaci* infections: a review with emphasis on avian chlamydiosis. *Vet Micro* 1995;45:93–119.

18. Compendium of psittacosis (chlamydiosis) control, 1997. *MMWR* 1997 (suppl);46(RR-13):1–13.

19. Korman TM, Turnidge JD, Grayson ML. Neurological complications of chlamydial diseases: case report and review. *Clin Inf Dis* 1997;25(4):847–51.

20. Schacter J, Dawson CR. *Human Chlamydial Infections.* Littleton, MA: PSG Publishing, 1978. Pp 63–96.

21. Halberstaedter L, von Prowazek S. Ueber chlamydozoenbefunde bei blenorrhea neonatorum non gonorrhoica. *Klin Wochenschr* 1909;46:1839–40.

22. Heymann B. Ueber die fundorte der Prowazek'schen korperchen. *Berl Klin Wochenschr* 1910;47:663–6.

23. Lidner K. Zur atiologie der gonokokkenfrein urethritis. *Wien Klin Wochenschr* 1910;23:283–4.

24. Grayston JT. Infections caused by *Chlamydia pneumoniae* strain TWAR. *Clin Infect Dis* 1992; 15:757–63.

25. Saikku P, Wang SP, Kleemola M, et al. An epidemic of mild pneumonia due to an unusual strain of *Chlamydia psittaci. J Infect Dis* 1985;151:832–9.

26. Grayston JT, Kuo C-C, Wang S-P, et al. A new *Chlamydia psittaci* strain, TWAR, isolated in acute respiratory tract infections. *N Engl J Med* 1986;315:161–8.

27. Grayston JT, Kuo C-C, Campbell LA, Wang S-P. *Chlamydia pneumoniae* sp. nov. for *Chlamydia* sp. strain TWAR. *Int J Syst Bacteriol* 1989;39:88–90.

28. Mordhorst CH, Wang SP, Grayston JT. Epidemic 'ornithosis' and TWAR infection, Denmark 1976–85. In: Oriel D, Ridgway G, Schacter J, et al. (eds), *Chlamydial Infections.* Cambridge, Engl.: Cambridge University Press, 1986. Pp 325–8.

29. Eng J, Flottorp A. Pra-ornithose; en epidemi av akutt luftveisinfeksjon med positiv Lygranum-KBR. *Tidsskr Nor Laegeforen* 1957;77:51–6.

30. Fraser PK, Hatch LA, Shell GN, et al. Minor respiratory illnesses caused by an agent of the psittacosis/lymphogranuloma-venereum group. *Lancet* 1964;2:306–8.

31. Miyashita N, Ouchi K et al. Outbreak of Chlamydophila pneumonia infection in long-term care facilities and an affiliated hospital. *J Med Microbiol* 2005;54:1243–7.

32. Tang JW, Eames I et al. Factors involved in the aerosol transmission of infection and control of ventilation in healthcare premises *J Hosp Infection* 2006;64:100–114.

33. Ekman M-R, Graystn JT, Visakorpi R, et al. An epidemic of infections due to *Chlamydia pneumoniae* in military conscripts. *Clin Infect Dis* 1993;17:420–5.

34. Grayston JT, Aldous MB, Easton A, et al. Evidence that *Chlamydia pneumoniae* causes pneumonia and bronchitis. *J Infect Dis* 1993;168:1231–5.

35. Derrick EH. "Q" fever, a new fever entity: clinical features, diagnosis and laboratory investigation. *Med J Aust* 1937;2:281–99.

36. Burnett FM, Freeman M. Experimental studies on the virus of "Q" fever. *Med J Aust* 1937;2:299–305.

37. Davis GE, Cox HR. A filter-passing infectious agent isolated from ticks: I. Isolation from *Dermacentor andersoni*, reactions in animals, and filtration experiments. *Public Health Rep* 1939;53:2259–67.

38. Leedom JM. Q fever; an update. In: Remington JS, Schwartz MN (eds), *Current Clinical Topics in Infectious Diseases.* New York: McGraw-Hill, 1980. Pp 304–31.

39. Marrie TJ. *Coxiella burnetii* (Q fever) pneumonia. *Clin Infect Dis* 1995;21(suppl 3):S253–64.

40. Walker DH, Rickettsiae and rickettsial infections: the current state of knowledge. *Clin Infect Dis* 2007; 45 Suppl 1:S39–44.

41. Baxter JD. The typhus group. *Clin Dermatol* 1996; 14(3):271–8.

42. Saah, AJ. *Rickettsia prowazekii.* In: Mandel GL, Bennett JE, Dolin R (eds), *Principles and Practice of Infectious Diseases.* 4th Ed. New York: Churchill Livingstone, 1995. Pp 1735–7.

43. Azad AF. Epidemiology of murine typhus. *Ann Rev Entomol* 1990;35:553–69.

44. Silber JL. Rocky Mountain spotted fever. *Clin Derm* 1996;14:245–58.

45. Harden VA. Koch's postulates and the etiology of rickettsial diseases. *J Hist Med Allied Sci* 1987;42(3):277–95.

46. Tamura A, Ohashi N, Urakami H, et al. Classification of *Rickettsia tsutsugamushi* in a new genus, *Orientia* gen. nov., as *Orientia tsutsugamushi* comb. nov. *Int J Systematic Bacteriol* 1995;45(3):589–91.

47. Fournier PE, Siritantikorn S et al. Detection of new genotypes of Orientia tsutsugamushi infecting humans in Thailand. *Clin Microbiol Infect* 2008;14(2):168–73.

48. Ohashi N, Kayama Y, Urakami N, et al. Demonstration of antigenic and genotypic variation in *Orientia tsutsugamushi* which were isolated in Japan, and their classification into type and subtype. *Microbiol Immunol* 1996;40(9):627–38.

49. Tamura A, Ohashi N, Koyama Y, et al. Characterization of *Orientia tsutsugamushi* isolated in Taiwan by immunofluorescence and restriction fragment length polymorphism analyses. *FEMS Microbiol Lett* 1997; 150(2):225–31.

50. Saah AJ. *Rickettsia tsutsugamushi* (scrub typhus). In: Mandel GL, Bennett JE, Dolin R (eds), *Principles and Practice of Infectious Diseases,* 4th Ed. New York: Churchill Livingstone, 1995. Pp 1740–1.

51. Berman SJ, Kundin WD. Scrub typhus in South Vietnam, a study of 87 cases. *Ann Intern Med* 1973; 79:26–30.

52. Olson JG, Bourgeois AL. Changing risk of scrub typhus in relation to socio-economic development in the Pescadores Islands of Taiwan. *Am J Epidemiol* 1979;109:236–43.

53. Brown GW, Robinson DM, Huxsoll DL, et al. Scrub typhus: a common cause of illness in indigenous populations. *Trans R Soc Trop Med Hyg* 1976;70: 444–8.

54. McNee JW, Renshaw A. "Trench fever": a relapsing fever occurring with the British troops in France. *Br Med J* 1916;1:225–34.

55. Tappero JW, Moele-Boetani J, Koehler J, et al. The epidemiology of bacterial angiomatosis and bacillary peliosis. *JAMA* 1993;269(6):770–5.

56. Daly JS. *Bartonella* species. In: Gorbach SL, Bartlett JG, Blacklow NR (eds), *Infectious Diseases.* Philadelphia: W.B. Saunders, 1998. Pp 1961–7.

57. Slater LN, Welch DF, Hensel D, et al. A newly recognized fastidious gram-negative pathogen as a cause of fever and bacteremia. *N Engl J Med* 1990;323: 1587–89.

58. Gregory DW, Schaffner W. Psittacosis. *Sem Respir Med* 1997;12(1):7–11.

59. Anderson DC, Stoesz PA, Kaufmann AF. Psittacosis outbreak in employees of a turkey-processing plant. *Am J Epidemiol* 1978;107(2):140–8.

60. Wittenbrink MM, Mrozek M, Bisping W. Isolation of *Chlamydia psittaci* from a chicken egg: evidence of egg transmission. *Zentralblatt Fur Veterinarmedizin—Reihe B* 1993;40(6):451–2.

61. Williams AF, Beck NF, Williams SP. The production of EAE-free lambs from infected rams using multiple ovulation and embryo transfer. *Vet J* 1998; 155(1):79–84.

62. Page LA. Experimental ornithosis in turkeys. *Avian Dis* 1959;3:51–66.

63. Papp JR, Shewen PE. Pregnancy failure following vaginal infection of sheep with *Chlamydia psittaci* prior to breeding. *Infect Immunol* 1996;64(4):1116–25.

64. Centers for Disease Control. *Psittacosis Surveillance, 1975–84.* Atlanta: CDC, June 1984.

65. Janeczek F, Gebermann H. Comparison of the cell culture method and ELISA for detection of *Chlamydia psittaci. Proc Symp Avian Dis, Munich* 1988:296–306.

66. Dorrestein GM, Wiegman LJJM. Inventaris onderzoek naar de uitscheiding van *Chlamydia psittaci* door parkieten in de omgeving van Utrecht door middel van ELISA. *Tijdschr Diergeneeskd* 1989;114: 1227–32.

67. Vanrompay D, Butaye P, Van Nerom A, et al. The prevalence of *Chlamydia psittaci* infections in Belgian commercial turkey poults. *Vet Microbiol* 1997; 54(1):85–93.

68. Ryll M, Hinz KH, Neumann U, et al. Pilot study of the occurrence of *Chlamydia psittaci* infections in commercial Turkey flocks in Niedersachsen. *Deutsche Tierarztliche Wochenschrift* 1994;101(4): 163–5.

69. Salibnas J, Caro MR, Cuello F. Antibody prevalence and isolation of *Chlamydia psittaci* from pigeons (*Columba livia*). *Avian Dis* 1993;37(2):523–7.

70. Gerbermann H, Korbel R. The occurrence of *Chlamydia psittaci* infections in raptors from wildlife preserves. *Tierartliche Praxis* 1993;21(3): 217–24.

71. Maluping RP, Oronan RB, Toledo SU. Detection of Chlamydophila psittaci antibodies from captive birds at the Ninoy Aquino Parks and Wildlife Nature Center, Quezon City, Philippines. *Ann Agric Environ Med* 2007;14(1):191–3.

72. Psittacosis (editorial). *Br Med J* 1972;1:1–2.

73. Compendium of psittacosis (chlamydiosis) control. *MMWR* (suppl) 1997;46(RR-13):1–13.

74. Mair TS, Wills JM. *Chlamydia psittaci* infection in horses: results of a prevalence survey and experimental challenge. *Vet Record* 1992;130(19):417–9.

75. Miyamoto C, Takashima I, Karaiwa H, et al. Seroepidemiological survey of chlamydial infections in light horses from Japan. *J Vet Med Sci* 1993; 55(2): 333–5.

76. Huchzermeyer FW, Gerdes GH, Foggin CM, et al. Hepatitis in farm hatchling Nile crocodiles (*Crocodylus niloticus*) due to chlamydial infection. *Tidjskr S Afr Vet Ver* 1994;65(1):20–2.

77. Papp JR, Shewen PE. Pregnancy failure following vaginal infection of sheep with *Chlamydia psittaci* prior to breeding. *Infect Immunol* 1996;64(4):1116–25.

78. Wittenbrink MM, Kirpal G, Thiele D, et al. Detection of *Chlamydia psittaci* in vaginal discharge of cows: a necessary enlargement of bacteriologic diagnosis for the etiologic clarification of fertility disorders in the female cow. *Zentralblatt Fur Veterinarmedizin—Reihe B* 1994;41(7–8):492–503.

79. Liao K, Chain CY, Lu YS, et al. Epizootic of *Chlamydia psittaci* infection in goats in Taiwan. *J Basic Microbiol* 1997;37(5): 327–33.

80. Thoma R, Guscetti F, Schiller I, et al. *Chlamydiae* in porcine abortion. *Vet Pathol* 1997;34(5):467–9.

81. Madic J, Huber D, Lugovic B. Serologic survey for selected viral and rickettsial agents of brown bears (*Ursus arctos*) in Croatia. *J Wildlife Dis* 1993; 29(4): 572–6.

82. Gresham AC, Dixon CE, Bevan BJ. Domiciliary out-

break of psittacosis in dogs: potential for zoonotic infection. *Vet Record* 1996;138(25):622–3.

83. Kik MJ, van der Hage MH, Greydanus–van der Putten SW. Chlamydiosis in a fishing cat (*Felis viverrina*). *J Zoo Wildlife Med* 1997;28(2):212–4.

84. Martin JL, Cross GF. Comparison of the omp I gene of *Chlamydia psittaci* between isolates in Victorian koalas and other animal species. *Aust Vet J* 1997; 75(8):579–82.

85. Villemonteiz P, Agius G, Decroz B et al. Pregnancy complicated by severe *Chlamydia psittaci* infection acquired from a goat flock: A case report. *Eur J Obstet Gynecol Reprod Biol* 1990;37:91–4.

86. Barnes MG, Brainerd H. Pneumonitis with alveolar-capillary block in a cattle rancher exposed to epizootic bovine abortion. *N Engl J Med* 1964;271: 981–5.

87. Lipman NS, Yan LL, Murphy JC. Probable transmission of *Chlamydia psittaci* from a macaw to a cat. *J Am Vet Med Assoc* 1994;204(9):1479–80.

88. Wreghitt T. Chlamydial infection of the respiratory tract. *Comm Dis Rep* 1993;3(9):R119–24.

89. Palmer SR. A common-source outbreak of ornithosis in veterinary surgeons. *Lancet* 1981;2:798–9.

90. Newman CP, Palmer SR, Kirby FD, et al. A prolonged outbreak of ornithosis in duck processors. *Epidemiol Infect* 1992;108(1):203–10.

91. Vanrompay D, Harkinezhad T, et al. Chlamydophila psittaci transmission form pet birds to humans. *Emerg Infect Dis* 2007;13(7):1108–10.

92. Huminer D, Pitlik S, Kitayin D. Prevalence of *Chlamydia psittaci* infection among persons who work with birds. *Isr J Med Sci* 1992;28:739–41.

93. Hinton DG, Shipley A, Galvin JW, et al. Chlamydiosis in workers at a duck farm and processing plant. *Aust Vet J* 1993;70(5):174–6.

94. Numazaki K, Chiba S, Umetsu M. Detection of IgM antibodies to *Chlamydia trachomatis, Chlamydia pneumoniae,* and *Chlamydia psittaci* from Japanese infants and children with pneumonia. *In Vivo* 1992; 6(6):601–4.

95. Jantos CA, Wienpahl B, Schiefer HG, et al. Infection with *Chlamydia pneumoniae* in infants and children with acute lower respiratory tract disease. *Pediatr Infect Dis J* 1995;14:117–22.

96. Aldous MB, Grayston JT, Wang S-P, et al. Seroepidemiology of *Chlamydia pneumoniae* in Seattle families, 1966–79. *J Infect Dis* 1992;166:646–9.

97. Thom DH, Wang SP, Grayston JT, et al. *Chlamydia pneumoniae* strain TWAR and angiographically demonstrated coronary artery disease. *Arterio Throm* 1991;11:547–51.

98. Thom DH, Grayston JT, Campbell LA, et al. Respiratory infection with *Chlamydia pneumoniae* in middle-aged and adult outpatients. *Eur J Clin Microbiol Infect Dis* 1994;13(10):785–92.

99. Cosentini R, Blasi F. New pathogens for respiratory infections. *Curr Opin Pulmon Med* 1996;2(3):174–80.

100. Blasi F, Legnani D, Lombardo VM, et al. *Chlamydia pneumoniae* infections in acute exacerbations of COPD. *Eur Respir J* 1993;6:19–22.

101. Verkooyen NA, van Lent NA, Mousavi Joulandan SA, et al. Diagnosis of *Chlamydia pneumoniae* infection in patients with chronic obstructive pulmonary disease by micro-immunofluorescence and ELISA. *J Med Microbiol* 1997;46:959–64.

102. Maaertens G, Lewis SJ, de Goveia C, et al. Atypical bacteria are common cause of community-acquired pneumonia in hospitalized adults. *S Afr Med J* 1994;84:678–82.

103. Ronsmans C, Bulut A, Yolsal N, et al. Clinical algorithms for the screening of *Chlamydia trachomatis* in Turkish women. *Genitourin Med* 1996;72:182–6.

104. Recommendations for the prevention and management of *Chlamydia trachomatis* infections, 1993. *MMWR* 1993;42:1–39.

105. Dowe G, King SD, Brathwaite AR, et al. Genital *Chlamydia trachomatis* (serotypes D-K) infection in Jamaican commercial street sex workers. *Genitourin Med* 1997;73:362–4.

106. Agacfidan A, Chow JM, Pashazade H, et al. Screening of sex workers in Turkey for *Chlamydia trachomatis*. *Sex Trans Dis* 1997;10:573–5.

107. Sturm-Ramirez K, Brumblay H et al. Molecular epidemiology of genital *Chlamydia trachomatis* infection in high-risk women in Senegal, West Africa. *J Clin Micro* 2000;38 (1):138–45

108. Worm AM, Lauritzen E, Jensen IP, et al. Markers of sexually transmitted disease in seminal fluid of male clients of female sex workers. *Genitourin Med* 1997;73:284–7.

109. Karam GH, Martin DH, Flotte R, et al. Asymptomatic *Chlamydia trachomatis* infections among sexually active men. *J Infect Dis* 1986;154:900–3.

110. Cates W, Wasserheit JN. Genital chlamydial infections: epidemiology and reproductive sequellae. *Am J Obstet Gynecol* 1991;164:1771–81.

111. Thylefors B. Development of trachoma control programs and the involvement of national resources. *Rev Infect Dis* 1985;7:774–6.

112. Hilbink F, Penrose M, Kovacova E, et al. Q fever is absent from New Zealand. *Int J Epidemiol* 1993; 22:945–9.

113. Baca OG, Paretsky D. Q fever and *Coxiella burnetti*: a model for host-parasite interaction. *Microbiol Rev* 1983;47:127–49.

114. Babudieri B. Q fever: a zoonosis. *Adv Vet Sci Comp Med* 1959;5:82–182.

115. Ruppanner R, Brooks D, Morrish D, et al. Q fever hazards from sheep and goats used in research. *Arch Environ Health* 1982;37(2):103–10.

116. Biberstein EL, Behymer DE, Bushnell R, et al. A survey of Q fever (*Coxiella burnetti*) in California dairy cows. *Am J Vet Res* 1974;35:1577–82.

117. Antony SJ, Schaffner W. Q fever pneumonia. *Sem Respir Infect* 1997;12(1):2–6.

118. Spelman DW. Q fever: a study of 111 consecutive cases. *Med J Aust* 1982;1:547–53.

119. Munoz-Sanz A, Vera A, and Rodriguez Vidigal FF. Q Fever in Extremadura: an emerging infection. *Enferm Infecc Micro Clin* 2007;25(4):230–4.

120. Marrie TJ, Van Buren J, Faulkner RS, et al. Seroepidemiology of Q fever in Nova Scotia and Prince Edward Island. *Can J Microbiol* 1984;30:129–34.

121. Marrie TJ, Fraser J. Prevalence of antibodies to *Coxiella burnetti* among veterinarians and slaughterhouse workers in Nova Scotia. *Can Vet J Res* 1985;26: 181–4.

122. Simor AE, Brunton JL, Salit IE, et al. Q fever: hazard form sheep used in research. *Can Med Assoc J* 1984;130:1013–6.

123. National Electronic Disease Surveillance System working group. National Electronic Disease Surveillance System(NEDSS): a standards-based approach to connect public health and clinical medicine. *J Public Health Manag Pract* 2001:7:43–50.

124. Palmer SR, Young SE. Q-fever endocarditis in England and Wales. *Lancet* 1982;2:1448–9.

125. Davies TR, Edwards Y, Margan A, et al. Prevalence of Q fever in a rural practice. *J Public Health Med* 1997;19(3):324–7.

126. Klymchuk MD, Kushnir ZH, Kiriiak OP, et al. The characteristics of the spread of *Coxiella burnetii* in the Carpathian region. *Mikrobiolohichnyi Zhurnal* 1997;59(5):46–52.

127. Sawyer LA, Fishbein DB, McDade JE. Q fever: current concepts. *Rev Infect Dis* 1987;9:935–46.

128. Pascual F, Carrascosa M. The epidemiology of Q fever (letter). *Eur Heart J* 1997;18:1190.

129. Brouqui PB, Dupont HT, Drancourt M, et al. Chronic Q fever. *Arch Intern Med* 1993;153(5): 642–8.

130. Stein A, Raoult D. Q fever endocarditis. *Eur Heart J* 1995;16(suppl B):19–23.

131. Bozeman FM, Masiello SA, Williams MS, et al. Epidemic typhus rickettsiae isolated from flying squirrels. *Nature* 1975;255:545–7.

132. Kurganova II, Klimchuk ND. Transplacental transmission of the causative agent in experimental rickettsial infection. *Mikrobiolohichnyi Zhurnal* 1996; 58(4): 80–5.

133. Perine RL, Chandler BP, Krause DK, et al. A clinicoepidemiological study of epidemic typhus in Africa. *Clin Infect Dis* 1992;14(5):1149–58.

134. Saah AJ. *Rickettsia prowazekii* (Epidemic or louseborn typhus). In: Mandel GL, Bennett JE, Dolin R (eds), *Principles and Practice of Infectious Diseases*, 4th Ed. New York: Churchill Livingstone, 1995. Pp 1735–7.

135. Punda-Polic V, Leko-Brbic J, Radulovic S. Prevalence of antibodies to rickettsiae in the north-western part of Bosnia and Herzegovina. *Eur J Epidemiol* 1995; 11(6):697–9.

136. Raoult D, Dutour O et al. Evidence for louse-transmitted diseases in soldiers of Napoleon's Grand Army in Vilnius. *J Infect Dis.* 2005;193(1):112–20.

137. Raoult D, Roux V, Ndihokubwayo JB, et al. Jail fever (epidemic typhus) outbreak in Burundi. *Emerging Infect Dis* 1997;3(3):357–60.

138. Dumler JS, Walker DH. Murine typhus. In: Mandel GL, Bennett JE, Dolin R (eds), *Principles and Practice of Infectious Diseases*, 4th Ed. New York: Churchill Livingstone, 1995. Pp 1737–9.

139. Richards AL, Soeatmadji DW, Widodo MA, et al. Seroepidemiologic evidence for murine and scrub typhus in Malang, Indonesia. *Am J Trop Med Hyg* 1997;57(1):91–5.

140. Meskini M, Beati L, Benslimane A, et al. Sero-epidemiology of rickettsial infections in Morocco. *Eur J Epidemiol* 1995;11(6):655–60.

141. Chaniotis B, Psarulaki A, Chaliotis G, et al. Transmission cycle of murine typhus in Greece. *Ann Trop Med Parasitol* 1994;88(6):645–7.

142. Strickman D, Tanksul P, Eamsila C, et al. Prevalence of antibodies to Rickettsiae in the human population of suburban Bangkok. *Am J Trop Med Hyg* 1994; 51(2):149–53.

143. Azad AF, Radulovic S, Higgins JA, et al. Flea-borne rickettsioses: ecologic considerations. *Emerging Infect Dis* 1997;3(3):319–27.

144. deLemos ER, Machado RD, Coura JR. Rocky Mountain spotted fever in an endemic area in Minas Gerais, Brazil. *Memorias do Instituto Oswaldo Cruz* 1994; 89(4):497–501.

145. Walker DH, Raoult D. *Rickettsia rickettsii* and other spotted fever group Rickettsiae (Rocky Mountain spotted fever and other spotted fevers). In: Mandel GL, Bennett JE, Dolin R (eds), *Principles and Practice of Infectious Diseases*, 4th Ed. New York: Churchill Livingstone, 1995. Pp 1721–7.

146. Summary of notifiable diseases, United States, 1995. *MMWR* 1996;44:1.

147. www.cdc.gov/ncidod/dvrd/rmsf/index.htm, last reviewed May 20, 2005.

148. Walker DH, Dumler JS. Emerging and reemerging rickettsial diseases (editorial). *N Engl J Med* 1994; 331(24):1651–2.

149. Diagnosis and management of tickborne and Rickettsial diseases: Rocky Mountain Spotted Fever, Ehrlichioses, and Anaplasmosis—United States. Chapman AS. *MMWR* 2006;55(RR04):1–27

150. Sanchez JL, Candler WH, Fishbein DB, et al. A cluster of tick-borne infections: association with military training and asymptomatic infections due to *Rickettsia rickettsii*. *Trans R Soc Trop Med Hyg* 1992; 86:321–5.

151. Ghorbani RP, Ghorbani AJ, Jain MK, et al. A case of scrub typhus probably acquired in Africa. *Clin Infect Dis* 1997;25(6):1473–4.

152. Song HJ, Kim KH, Kim SC, et al. Population density of chigger mites, the vector of tsutsugamushi disease in Chollanam-do, Korea. *Korean J Parasitol* 1996; 34(1):27–33.

153. Traub R, Wisseman CL Jr. The ecology of chigger-borne rickettsiosis (scrub typhus). *J Med Entomol* 1974;11:237.
154. Takada N, Khamboonruang C, Yamaguchi T, et al. Scrub typhus and chiggers in northern Thailand. *Southeast Asian J Trop Med Public Health* 1984;15:402–6.
155. Johnson DE, Crumm JW, Hanchalay S, et al. Sero-epidemiological survey of *Rickettsia tsutsugamushi* infection in a rural Thai village. *Trans R Soc Trop Med Hyg* 1982;76:1–3.
156. Strickman D, Tanskul P, Eamsila C, et al. Prevalence of antibodies to rickettsiae in the human population of suburban Bangkok. *Am J Trop Med Hyg* 1994;1(2):149–53.
157. Demma LJ, McQuistan JH et al. Scrub typhus, Republic of Palau. *Emerg Infect Dis.* 2006;12(2):290–5.
158. Eamsila C, Singsawat P, Duangvaraporn A, et al. Antibodies to *Orientia tsutsugamushi* in Thai soldiers. *Am J Trop Med Hyg* 1996;55(5):556–9.
159. Vinson JW, Fuller HS. Studies on trench fever. I. Propagation of rickettsia-like organisms from a patient's blood. *Pathol Microbiol* 1961;24 (suppl):152–5.
160. Spach DO, Candor AS, Dougherty MJ, et al. *Bartonella (Rochalimaea) quintana* bacteremia in inner-city patients with chronic alcoholism. *N Engl J Med* 1995;332:424–8.
161. Gluckman SJ. Q fever and trench fever. *Clin Dermatol* 1996;14(3):283–7.
162. Maurin M, Raoult D. *Bartonella (Rochalimea) quintana* infections. *Clin Microbiol Rev* 1996;9(3):273–92.
163. Brouqui P, Lascola B, Roux V and Raoult D. Chronic *Bartonella quintana* bacteremia in homeless patients. *NEJM.* 1999;340(3):184–9.
164. Koehler JE, Glaser CA, Tappero JW. *Rochalimea henselaea* infection: a new zoonosis with the domestic cat as a reservoir. *JAMA* 1994;16:553–4.
165. Zangwill KM, Hamilton DH, Perkins BA, et al. Cat-scratch disease in Connecticut. *N Engl J Med* 1993;329:8–13.
166. Jackson LA, Spach DH, Kippen DA, et al. Seroprevalence to *Bartonella quintana* among patients at a community clinic in downtown Seattle. *J Infect Dis* 1996;173(4):1023–6.
167. Comer JA, Diaz T et al. Evidence of rodent-associated *Bartonella* and *Rickettsia* infections among intravenous drug users from Central and East Harlem, New York City. *Am J Trop Hyg* 2001;65(6):855–60.
168. Noah DL, Kramer CM, Verbsky MP, et al. Survey of veterinary professionals and other veterinary conference attendees for antibodies to *Bartonella henselaea* and *B quintana*. *J Am Vet Assoc* 1997;210(3):342–4.
169. Rolain JM, Foucault C et al. *Bartonella quintana* in human erythrocytes. *Lancet* 2002;360(9328):226–8.
170. Kocianova E, Rehacek J, Lisak V. Transmission of antibodies to *Chlamydia psittaci* and *Coxiella burnetti* through eggs and "crop milk" in pigeons. *Eur J Epidemiol* 1993;9(2):209–12.
171. Bano Aracil M, Gonzalez Moran F, Bertomeu Blanch F, et al. Familial outbreak of pneumonia by psittacosis. *Medicina Clinica* 1992;99(7):258–60.
172. Hyde SR, Benirschke K. Gestational psittacosis: case report and literature review. *Modern Pathology* 1997;10(6):602–7.
173. Centers for Disease Control. *Psittacosis surveillance. Annual summary 1975–84.* Atlanta: CDC, June 1987.
174. Andersen AA. The stereotyping of *Chlamydia psittaci* isolates using serovar-specific monoclonal antibodies with the micro-immunofluoroscence test. *J Clin Microbiol* 1991;29:707–11.
175. Vanrompay D. Avian *Chlamydia psittaci* phyla and their pathogenic significance for turkeys. *Verhandelingen—Koninklijke Academie voor Geneeskunde van Belgie* 1996;58(6):701–9.
176. Vanrompay D, Andersenn AA, Ducatelle R, et al. Serotyping of European isolates of *Chlamydia psittaci* from poultry and other birds. *J Clin Microbiol* 1993;31(1):134–7.
177. Hughes C, Maharg P, Rosario P, et al. Possible nosocomial transmission of psittacosis. *Infect Cont Hosp Epidemiol* 1997;18(3):165–8.
178. Falsey R, Walsh EE. Transmission of Chlamydia pneumonia, *J Infect Dis* 1993;168(2):493–6.
179. Ferrari M, Poli A et al. Seroprevalence of Chlamydia pneumonia antibodies in a young adult population sample living in Verona. *Infection* 2000;28(1):38–41.
180. Augenbraun MH, Robin MR, Chirwing K, et al. Isolation of *Chlamydia pneumoniae* from lungs of patients infected with the human immunodeficiency virus. *J Clin Microbiol* 1991;29:401–2.
181. Katz BP, Caine VA, Jones RB. Estimation of transmission probabilities for chlamydial infection. In: Bowie WR, Calswell HD, Jones RP, et al. (eds), *Chlamydial Infections.* Cambridge, Engl: Cambridge University Press, 1990. Pp 567–70.
182. Ramstedt K, Forssman L, Giesecke J, et al. Epidemiologic characteristics of two different populations of women with *Chlamydia trachomatis* infection and their male partners. *Sex Transm Dis* 1991;18:205–10.
183. Smith JR, Taylor-Robinson D. Infections due to *Chlamydia trachomatis* in pregnancy and the newborn. *Baillieres Clin Obstet Gynecol* 1993;7(1):237–55.
184. Batteiger BE, Fraiz J, Newhall WJ, et al. Association of recurrent chlamydial infection with gonorrhea. *J Infect Dis* 1989;159:661–9.
185. Blythe MJ, Katz BP, Orr DP, et al. Historical and clinical factors associated with *Chlamydia trachomatis* genitourinary infection in female adolescents. *J Pediatr* 1988;112:1000–4.
186. Mardh PA, Paavonen J, Puolakkainen M. *Chlamydia.* New York: Plenum Press, 1989.
187. From the Centers for Disease Control and Prevention. Update: barrier protection against HIV

infection and other sexually transmitted diseases. *JAMA* Aug 25;270(8):933–4.

188. Schachter J, Grossman M, Sweet RL, et al. Prospective study of perinatal transmission of *Chlamydia trachomatis*. *JAMA* 1986;255:3374–7.

189. Meyers JD, Hackman RC, Stamm WE. *Chlamydia trachomatis* infection as a cause of pneumonia after human bone marrow transplantation. *Transplantation* 1983;36(2):130–4.

190. Lennette EH, Welsh HH. Q fever in California. Recovery of *Coxiella burnetti* from the air of premises harboring infected goats. *Am J Hyg* 1951;54:44–9.

191. Marrie TJ. Epidemiology of Q fever. In: Marrie TJ (ed), *Q fever: The Disease*. Vol 1. Boca Raton, FL: CRC Press, 1990. Pp 49–70.

192. Marrie TJ, Haldane EV, Faulkner RS, et al. The importance of *C burnetii* as a cause of pneumonia in Nova Scotia. *Can J Public Health* 1985;76:233–6.

193. Q fever outbreak—Switzerland. *MMWR* 1984; 33:355–61.

194. Salmon MM, Howells B, Glencross EJF, et al. Q fever in an urban area. *Lancet* 1982;1:1002–4.

195. Sawyer LA, Fishbein DB, McDade JE. Q fever: current concepts. *Rev Infect Dis* 1987;9:935–46.

196. Kruszewska D, Tylewska-Wierzbanowska SK. *Coxiella burnetii* penetration into the reproductive system of male mice, promoting sexual transmission of infection. *Infect Immunol* 1993;61:1448–95.

197. Raoult D, Stein A. Q fever during pregnancy—a risk for women, fetuses and obstetricians (letter). *N Engl J Med* 1994;330:371.

198. Deutsch DL, Petersen ET. Q fever: transmission form one human being to another. *JAMA* 1950; 1943:348–50.

199. Laughlin T, Waag D, Williams J, et al. Q fever: from deer to dog to man (letter). *Lancet* 1991;337:676–7.

200. Marrie TJ, Langille D, Papukna V, et al. Truckin' pneumonia—an outbreak of Q fever in a truck repair plant probably due to aerosols from clothing contaminated by contact with newborn kittens. *Epidemiol Infect* 1989;102:119–27.

201. Mann JS, Douglas JG, Inglis JM, et al. Q fever: person-to-person transmission within a family. *Thorax* 1986;41:974–5.

202. Deutsch DL, Peterson ET. Q fever: transmission from one human being to others. *JAMA* 1950;143: 348–50.

203. Marrie TJ, Durant H, Williams JC, et al. Exposure to parturient cats: a risk factor for acquisition of Q fever in maritime Canada. *J Infect Dis* 1988;158: 101–8.

204. Sidwell RW, Thorpe BD, Gebhardt LP. Studies of latent Q fever infections. II. Effects of multiple cortisone infections. *Am J Hyg* 1964;79:320–7.

205. Norazah A, Mazlah A, Cheong YM, et al. Laboratory-acquired murine typhus—a case report. *Med J Malaysia* 1995;50(2):177–9.

206. Wilfert CM, McCormack JN, Kleeman K, et al. Epidemiology of Rocky Mountain spotted fever as determined by active surveillance. *J Infect Dis* 1984;150:469–79.

207. Kitahama S, Suzuki J, Kawakami Y. A case of tsutsugamushi disease infected by mountain climbing in the Republic of Korea. *Kansenshogaku Zasshi (J Jap Assoc Infect Dis)* 1996;70(5):516–9.

208. Marschang A, Nothdurft HD, Kumlien S, von Sonnenburg F. Imported rickettsioses in German travellers. *Infection* 1995;23(2):94–7.

209. Suntharassaj T, Janjindamai W, Krisanapan S. Pregnancy with scrub typhus and vertical transmission: a case report. *J Obstet Gynecol Res* 1997;23(1):75–8.

210. Jee HG, Chung MH, Lee SG, et al. Transmission of scrub typhus by needlestick from a patient receiving perfloxacin. *Scand J Infect Dis* 1996;28(4):411–2.

211. Kawamura R, Kasahara S, Toyama T, et al. On the prevention of tsutsugamushi disease (2nd report). Results of preventive inoculations for people in the endemic regions and laboratory tests with the Pescadores strain. *Tokyo Iji Shinshi* 1938;3115: 3323–6.

212. Filstein MR, Ley AB, Vernon MS. Epidemic of psittacosis in a college of veterinary medicine. *J Am Vet Med Assoc* 1981;179(6):569–72.

213. Durfee PT, Pullen MM, Currier RW, et al. Human psittacosis associated with commercial processing of turkeys. *J Am Vet Assoc* 1975;167(9):804–8.

214. Esposito AL. Pulmonary infections acquired in the workplace. *Clin Chest Med* 1992;13(2):355–65.

215. Smith KA, Bradley K et al. Compendium of measures to control Chlamydophila psittaci (formerly Chlamydia psittaci) infection among humans (psittacosis) and pet birds, *J Am Vet Med Assoc* 2005:226: 532–9.

216. Buchanan TM, Hendricks SL, Patton CM, et al. Brucellosis in the United States, 1960–72: an abattoir-associated disease. *Medicine* 1974;53(6):427–39.

217. Hedberg K. An outbreak of psittacosis in Minnesota turkey industry workers: implications for modes of transmission and control. *Am J Epidemiol* 1989;130: 569–77.

218. Sigel MM, McNair Scott TF, Henle W. Q fever in a wool and hair processing plant. *Am J Public Health* 1950;40:524–32.

219. Hall CJ, Richmond SJ, Caul EO, et al. Laboratory outbreak of Q fever acquired from sheep. *Lancet* 1982;1:1004–6.

220. Meiklejohn G, Reimer LG, Graves PS, et al. Cryptic epidemic of Q fever in a medical school. *J Infect Dis* 1981;144(2);107–13.

221. Dupuis G, Petite J, Peter O, et al. An important outbreak of human Q fever in a Swiss Alpine valley. *Int J Epidemiol* 1987;16:282–7.

222. Vol. II, Feb 24, 1977. Unclassified document; *U.S. Army Activity on the U.S. Biological Warfare Programs*. L–3,4,5,6.

223. Franz DR, Jahrling PB, Friedlander AM, et al. Clinical recognition and management of patients exposed to biological warfare agents. *JAMA* 1997; 278(5):399–411.

224. Raoult D, Marrie T, Mege L. Natural history and pathophysiology of Q fever. *Lancet* 2005;5(4): 219–26.
225. Centers for Disease Control. Laboratory-acquired endemic typhus. *MMWR* 1978;27(26):215–216.
226. McDonald JC, MacLean JD, McDade JE. Imported rickettsial disease: clinical and epidemiologic features. *Am J Med* 1988;85:799–805.
227. U.S. Dept of Agriculture, Animal and Plant Health Inspection Service. *Importation of Certain Animals, Birds, and Poultry and Certain Animal, Bird and Poultry Products: Requirements for Means of Conveyance and Shipping Containers.* CFR Title 9, Part 93. 101–7, Jan 1, 2007.
228. U.S. Dept of Agriculture, Animal and Plant Health Inspection Service. *Importation of Certain Animals, Birds, and Poultry and Certain Animal, Bird and Poultry Products: Requirements for Means of Conveyance and Shipping Containers.* CFR Title 9, Part 92. 101–7, Jan 1, 1997.
229. Q fever among slaughterhouse workers—California. *MMWR* 1986;35(14):223–4.
230. Palmer C, McCall B et al. "The dust hasn't settled yet": The National Q fever Management Program, missed opportunities for vaccination and community exposures. *Aust N Z J Public Health* 2007;31(4): 330–2.
231. 1998 guidelines for treatment of sexually transmitted diseases. *MMWR* 1998;47(RR-1):1–116.
232. www.cdc.gov/OD/OHS/biosfty/bmbl/sect7d.htm, Accessed March 21, 2008. Last reviewed January 2, 1997.
233. Update on barrier protection against HIV infection and other sexually transmitted diseases. *MMWR* 1993;42(30):589–91.
234 Raoult D, Marrie T. Q fever. *Clin Infect Dis* 1995;20: 489–96.
235. www.cdc.gov/ncidod/, accessed March 21, 2008– Last reviewed February 13, 2003.
236. Bise G, Coninx R. Epidemic typhus in a prison in Burundi. *Trans R Soc Trop Med Hyg* 1997;91(2): 133–4.
237. Hengbin G, Min C, Kaihua T and Jiaqi T. The foci of scrub typhus and strategies of prevention in the Spring in Pingtan Island, Fujina Province. *Ann NY Acad Sci.* 2006;1078:188–96.
238. Pike RM. Past and present hazards of working with infectious agents. *Arch Path Lab Med* 1978;102:333–6.
239. Richmond, JY and RW McKinney, *1993: Biosafety in Microbiological and Biomedical Laboratories.* US Department of Health and Human Services, CDC/NIH, 3rd Ed. Washington, DC: US Government Printing Office.
240. Mehr ZA, Rutledge LC, Echano NM, et al. U.S. Army soldiers' perceptions of arthropod pests and their effects on military missions. *Milit Med* 1997;162(12): 804–7.
241. Ho TM, Fauziah MK, Saleh I. Laboratory evaluation of five pesticides for control of *Leptobromidium*
242. *fletcheri* (Acari: Trombiculidae). *Southeast J Trop Med Public Health* 1992;23(1):125–7.
242. Olson JG, Bourgeois AL et al. Prevention of scrub typhus. Prophylactic administration of doxycycline in a randomized double-blind trial. *Am J Trop Med Hyg* 1980;29(5):989–97.
243. Twartz JC, Shirai A, Selvaraju G, et al. Doxycycline prophylaxis for human scrub typhus. *J Infect Dis* 1982;146:811–8.
244. Smadel JE, Traub R, Frick L, et al. Chloramphenicol (chloromycetin) in the chemoprophylaxis of scrub typhus (tsutsugamushi disease). III. Suppression of overt disease by prophylactic regimens of four-week duration. *Am J Hyg* 1950;51:216–28.
245. deGraaf R, Vanwesenbeeck I, van Zessen G, et al. The effectiveness of condom use in heterosexual prostitution in the Netherlands. *AIDS* 1993;7:265–9.
246. Workowski KA, Berman SM. Sexually transmitted diseases treatment guidelines. *MMWR* 2006; 55(RR11):1–94.
247. *Screening for Chlamydial Infection,* Topic Page. June 2007. Rockville, MD: U.S. Preventive Services Task Force. Agency for Healthcare Research and Quality. www.ahrq.gov/clinic/uspstf/uspschlm.htm.
248. Murine Typhus—Hawaii 2002. *MMWR.* 2003; 52(50):1224–6.
249. Prevent rodent infestations. In www.cdc.gov/ rodents/prevent_rodents/index.htm. Updated May 26, 2006.
250. Burstein GR, Gaydos CA et al. Incident *Chlamydia trachomatis* infection among inner-city adolescent females. JAMA 1998;280:521.
251. Chalmers WS, Simpson J, Lee SJ, et al. Use of a live chlamydial vaccine to prevent ovine enzootic abortion. *Vet Record* 1997;141(3):63–7.
252. Vanrompay D, Vanloock M, et al. Genetic immunization for Chlamydia psittaci. *Vehr K Acad Geneeskd Belg* 2001;63(2):177–88.
253. Protection of turkeys against Chlamydophila psittaci challenge by DNA and rMOMP vaccination and evaluation of the immunomodulating effect of 1 alpha,25-dihydroxyvitamin D(3). *Vaccine* 2005; 23(36):4509–16.
254. Sturgess CP, Gruffydd-Jones TJ, Harbour DA, et al. Studies on the safety of *Chlamydia psittaci* vaccination in cats. *Vet Record* 1995;137(26):668–9.
255. Thorpe C, Edwards L et al. Discovery of a vaccine antigen that protects mice from Chlamydia pneumonia infection. *Vaccine* 2007;25(12):2252–60.
256. Hammerschlag MR, Cummings C, Roblin PM, et al. Efficacy of neonatal ocular prophylaxis for the prevention of chlamydial and gonococcal conjunctivitis. *N Engl J Med* 1989;320:769–72.
257. Wi T, Ramos Er et al. STI declines among sex workers and clients following outreach, one time presumptive treatment and regular screening of sex workers in the Philippines. *Sex Trans Infect* 2006; 82(5):386–91.
258. Igetsieme J, Eko F et al. Delivery of Chlamydial vaccines. *Exp Opin Drug Deliv* 2005;2(3):549–62.

259. Raoult D. Q fever: still a query after all these years (edit). *J Med Microbiol* 1996;44(2):77–8.

260. Acklund JR, Worswick DA, Marmion BP. Vaccine prophylaxis of Q fever. *Med J Aust* 1994;160:704–8.

261. Milazzo A, Featherstone KB, Hall RG. Q fever vaccine uptake in South Australian meat processors prior to the introduction of the National Q Fever Management Program. *Commun dis Intell.* 2005; 29(4):400–6.

262. Marmion BP, Ormsbee RA, Krykor M. Vaccine prophylaxis of abattoir-associated Q fever. *Epidemiol Infect* 1990;104:275–87.

263. Waag DM, England MJ, Pitt ML. Comparative efficacy of a *Coxiella burnetii* chloroform: methanol residue (CMR) vaccine and a licensed cellular vaccine (Q-Vax) in rodents challenged by aerosol. *Vaccine* 1997;15(16):1779–83.

264. Arricau-Bouvery N, Souriau A et al. Effect of vaccination with phase I and phase II *Coxiella burnetti* vaccines in pregnant goats. *Vaccine* 2005;23(35): 4392–402.

265. Typhus vaccine. *MMWR* 1978;27:189.

266. Raoult D, Woodward T, and Dumler JS. The history of epidemic typhus. *Infect Dis Clin North Amer.* 2004;18(11):127–40.

267. Matthewman L, Kelly P, Hayter D, et al. Domestic cats as indicators of the presence of spotted fever and typhus group Rickettsiae. *Eur J Epidemiol* 1997; 13(1):109–11.

268. Sexton DJ and Dasch GA. Rickettsial and Erlichial Infections. *In:* Roos, KL (ed). *Principles of Neurologic Infectious Diseases.* New York: McGraw-Hill Professional, 2005. Pp 328–342.

269. Dumler JS, Wisseman CL Jr, Fiset P, et al. Cell-mediated immune responses of adults to vaccination, challenge with *Rickettsia rickettsii*, or both. *Am J Trop Med Hyg* 1992;46(2):105–15.

270. Yu Y, Wen B et al. Induction of protective immunity against scrub typhus with a 56-kilodalton recombinant antigen fused with a 47-kilodalton antigen of *Orientia tsutsugamushi* Karp. *Am J Trop Med.* 2005; 72(4):458–64.

271. Tselentis Y, Psaroulaki A, Maniatis J, et al. Genotypic identification of murine typhus *Rickettsia* in rats and their fleas in an endemic area of Greece by the polymerase chain reaction and restriction fragment length polymorphism. *Am J Trop Med Hyg* 1996; 54(4):413–7.

272. Gage KL, Gilmore RD, Karstens RH, et al. Detection of *Rickettsia rickettsii* in saliva, hemolymph and triturated tissues of infected *Dermacentor andersoni* ticks by polymerase chain reaction. *Mol Cell Probes* 1992;6(4):333–41.

273. Harrison GJ. A practitioner's view of the problem of avian chlamydiosis. *J Am Vet Assoc* 1989;195:1525–8.

274. Wages DP. Diseases of pigeons. *Vet Clin North Am* 1987;37:1089–107.

275. Avian Chlamydiosis. In: Kahn, Cynthia M (ed), *Merck Veterinary Manual* 9th Ed. Whitehouse Station, NJ: Merck & Co. Inc., 2006.

276. Vanrompay D, Ducatelle R, Haesebrouck F, et al. Primary pathogenicity of a European isolate of *Chlamydia psittaci* from turkey poults. *Vet Microbiol* 1993;38(1–2):103–13.

277. Grimes JE, Wyrick PB. Chlamydiosis (ornithosis). In: Calnek BW (ed), *Diseases of Poultry.* 9th Ed. Iowa State University Press, 1991. Pp 311–25.

278. Schaffner W, Drutz DJ, Duncan GW, et al. The clinical spectrum of endemic psittacosis. *Arch Intern Med* 1967;119:433–43.

279. Monsieur I, Maysman M, Vincken W, et al. Severe community-acquired pneumonia caused by atypical organisms. *Acta Clinica Belgia* 1997;52(2):112–5.

280. Byrom NP, Walls J, Mair HJ. Fulminant psittacosis. *Lancet* 1979;1:353–6.

281. Yung AP, Grayson ML. Psittacosis: A review of 135 cases. *Med J Aust* 1988;148:228.

282. Diaz F, Collazos J. Myopericarditis due to *Chlamydia psittaci*: the role of autoimmunity. *Scand J Infect Dis* 1997;29(1):93–4.

283. Lamaury J, Sotto A, Le Quellec A, et al. *Chlamydia psittaci* as a cause of lethal bacterial endocarditis. *Clin Infect Dis* 1993;17(4):821–2.

284. Duprat F, Akoum N, Le Hoang P. Hemorrhagic macular choroidopathy in young adults. *J Francais d' Opthal* 1995;18(3):226–9.

285. Hain C, Demisch S, Langer B. Organically-induced delusional syndrome in psittacosis. *Psychiatrische Praxis* 1997;24(4):198–9.

286. Brewis C, McFerran DJ. "Farmer's ear": sudden sensorineural hearing loss due to *Chlamydia psittaci* infection. *J Laryngol Otol* 1997;111(9):855–7.

287. Prevett M, Harding AE. Intracranial hypertension following psittacosis (letter). *J Neurol Neurosurg Psychol* 1993;56(4):425–6.

288. Branley P, Speed B. Acute interstitial nephritis due to *Chlamydia psittaci* (letter). *Aust NZ J Med* 1995; 25(4):365.

289. Jeffrey RF, More IA, Carington D, et al. Acute glomerulonephritis following infection with *Chlamydia psittaci*. *Am J Kidney Dis* 1992;20(1): 94–6.

290. Mason AB, Jenkins P. Acute renal failure in fulminant psittacosis. *Respir Med* 1994;88(3):239–40.

291. Crook T, Bannister B. Acute transverse myelitis associated with *Chlamydia psittaci* infection. *J Infection* 1996;32(2):151–2.

292. Newton P, Lalvani A, Conlon CP. Psittacosis associated with bilateral 4th cranial nerve palsies. *J Infection* 1996;32(1):63–5.

293. Verweij P, Meis JF, Eijk R, et al. Severe human psittacosis requiring artificial ventilation: case report and review. *Clin Infect Dis* 1995;20(2):440–2.

294. Jorgensen DM. Gestational psittacosis in a Montana sheep rancher. *Emerging Infect Dis* 1997;3(2):191–4.

295. Yamato H, Segawa K, Tsuda T, et al. A case of psittacosis with migratory infiltrates. *Japan J Thorac Dis* 1992;30(1):100–5.

296. Taniguchi H, Mukae N, Ihibashi H, et al. A case of fulminant psittacosis necessitating mechanical ven-

tilation diagnosed by chlamydial isolation from BALF. *J Japan Assoc Infect Dis* 1995;69(12):1396–401.

297. Miyashita Y, Nakamori Y. A family outbreak of *Chlamydia psittaci* infection. *J Japan Assoc Infect Dis* 1996;70(4):377–81.

298. Comandini UV, Maggi P, Santopadre P, et al. *Chlamydia pneumoniae* respiratory infections among patients infected with the human immunodeficiency virus. *Eur J Clin Microbiol Infect Dis* 1997; 16(10):720–6.

299. Hammerschlag MR, Chirgwin K, Roblin PM. Persistent infection with *Chlamydia pneumoniae* following acute respiratory illness. *Clin Infect Dis* 1992; 14(1):178–82.

300. Ekman MR, Grayston JT, Visakorpi R. An epidemic of infections due to *Chlamydia pneumoniae* in military conscripts. *Clin Infect Dis* 1993;17:420–5.

301. Thom D, Grayston JT, Campbell LA, et al. Respiratory infection with *Chlamydia pneumoniae* in middle-aged and older adult patients. *Eur J Clin Microbiol Infect Dis* 1994;13:785–92.

302. Hahn DL, Dodge RW, Galugjatnikov R. Association of *Chlamydia pneumoniae* (strain TWAR) infection with wheezing, asthmatic bronchitis, and adult-onset asthma. *JAMA* 1991;266:225–30.

303. Emre U, Roblin PM, Gelling M, et al. The association of *Chlamydia pneumoniae* infection and reactive airways disease in children. *Arch Pediatr Adoles Med* 1994;148(7):341–2.

304. Hahn DL, Bukstein D, Luskin A, et al. Evidence for *Chlamydia pneumoniae* infection in steroid-dependent asthma. *Ann Allergy Asthma Immunol* 1998; 80(1): 45–9.

305. Korman TM, Turnidge JD, Grayson ML. Neurological complications of chlamydial infections: case report and review. *Clin Infect Dis* 1997;25:847–51.

306. Machtey I. *Chlamydia pneumoniae* antibodies in myalgia of unknown cause (including fibromyalgia) (letter). *Br J Rheumatol* 1996;36(10):1189–90.

307. Moling O, Pegoretti S, Rielli M, et al. *Chlamydia pneumoniae*-reactive arthritis and persistent infection. *Br J Rheumatol* 1996;35(11):1189–90.

308. Naidu BR, Ngeow YF, Kannan P, et al. Evidence of *Chlamydia pneumoniae* infection obtained by the polymerase chain reaction in patients with acute myocardial infarction and coronary heart disease. *J Infect* 1997;35:199–203.

309. Shor A, Kuo C-C, Patton DL. Detection of *Chlamydia pneumoniae* in coronary artery fatty streaks and atheromatous plaques. *S Afr Med J* 1992;82:158–61.

310. Mazzoli S, Tofani N, Fantini A. *Chlamydia pneumoniae* antibody response in patients with acute myocardial infarction and their follow-up. *Am Heart J* 1998;135:15–20.

311. Nystrom-Rosander C, Thelin S, Hjelm E, et al. High incidence of *Chlamydia pneumoniae* in sclerotic heart valves of patients undergoing aortic valve replacement. *Scand J Infect Dis* 1997;29(4):361–5.

312. Cook PJ, Honeybourne D, Lip GY, et al. *Chlamydia*

pneumoniae antibody titers are significantly associated with acute stroke and transient cerebral ischemia: the West Birmingham Stroke Project. *Stroke* 1998;29(2):404–10.

313. Visseren FL, Spiering W, Hoepelman IM. Infection induced vascular disease—little evidence according to the Koch's postulates. Ned Tijdschr Geneeskd. 2007;151(52):2883–7.

314. Cates W, Wasserheit JN. Genital chlamydial infections: epidemiology and reproductive sequelae. *Am J Obstet Gynecol* 1991;164:1771–81.

315. Brunham RC, Paavonen J, Stevens CE, et al. Mucopurulent cervicitis: the ignored counterpart in women of urethritis in men. *N Eng J Med* 1984;311: 1–6.

316. Westrom L, Svensson L, Wolner-Hanssen P, et al. Chlamydial and gonococcal infections in a defined population of women. *Scand J Infect Dis* 1982; 32(suppl):157–62.

317. Paavonen J. Genital *Chlamydia trachomatis* infections in the female. *J Infect Dis* 1992;25(suppl 1):39–45.

318. Berger RE, Alexander ER, Harnisch JP, et al. Etiology, manifestations and therapy of acute epididymitis: prospective study of 50 cases. *J Urol* 1979;121: 750–4.

319. Quinn TC, Goodell SE, Mkrtichian E, et al. *Chlamydia trachomatis* proctitis. *N Engl J Med* 1981;305: 195–200.

320. Keat A. Extra-genital *Chlamydia trachomatis* infection as sexually-acquired reactive arthritis. *J Infect* 1992;25(suppl 1):47–9.

321. Stenberg K, Mardh P-A. Genital infection with *Chlamydia trachomatis* in patients with chlamydial conjunctivitis: unexplained results. *Sex Transm Dis* 1991;18:1–4.

322. Schacter J, Grossman M, Sweet RL, et al. Prospective study of perinatal transmission of *Chlamydia trachomatis*. *JAMA* 1986;255:3374–7.

323. Ito JI, Comess KA, Alexander ER, et al. Pneumonia due to *Chlamydia trachomatis* in an immunocompromised adult. *N Engl J Med* 1982;307:95–8.

324. Goldman JM, McIntosh CS, Calver GP, et al. Meningoencephalitis associated with *Chlamydia trachomatis* infection. *Br Med J* 1983;286:517–8.

325. Reilly PJ and Kalinske RW. Brill-Zinsser disease in North America. *West J Med.* 1950; 1333(4):338–48.

326. Toumi A, Loussaief C et al. Meningitis revealing *Rickettsia typhi* infection. *Rev Med Interne.* 2007; 28(2):131–3.

327. Hudson HL, Thach AB and Lopez PF. Retinal manifestations of acute murine typhus. *Int Opthalmol.* 1997;21(3):121–6.

328. Helmick CG, Bernard KW, D'Angelo LJ. Rocky Mountain spotted fever: clinical, laboratory, and epidemiologic features of 262 cases. *J Infect Dis* 1984;150:480–6.

329. Tissot Dupont H, Raoult D, Brouqui P, et al. Epidemiologic features and clinical presentations of

acute Q fever in hospitalized patients. *Am J Med* 1992;93:427–34.

330. Tiggert WD, Benenson AS. Studies of Q fever in man. *Trans Assoc Am Physicians* 1956;69:98–104.

331. Dupont HT, Raoult D, Broqui P. Epidemiological features and clinical presentations of acute Q fever in hospitalized patients: 323 French patients. *Am J Med* 1992;93:427–34.

332. Feinstein M, Yesner R, Marks JL. Epidemic of Q fever among troops returning from Italy in the spring of 1945: clinical aspects of the epidemic at Fort Patrick Henry, Virginia. *Am J Hyg* 1946; 44:72–87.

333. Sobradillo V, Ansola P, Baranda F, Corral C. Q fever pneumonia: a review of 164 community-acquired cases in the Basque country. *Eur Respir J* 1989;2: 263–6.

334. Marrie TJ. Q fever pneumonia. *Semin Respir Infect* 1989;4(1):47–55.

335. Ruiz-Moreno JM. Choroidal neovascularization in the course of Q fever. *Retina, J Ret Vitr Dis* 1997; 17(6):553–5.

336. Carrascosa M, Pascual F, Borobia MV, et al. Rhabdomyolysis associated with acute Q fever. *Clin Infect Dis* 1997;25:1243–4.

337. Siegman-Igra Y, Kaufman O, Keysary A, et al. Q fever endocarditis in Israel and a worldwide review. *Scand J Infect Dis* 1997;29:41–9.

338. Tunkel AR, Kaye D. Endocarditis with negative blood cultures (letter). *N Engl J Med* 1992;326(18): 1215–6.

339. Shiga K, Ogawa M, Ono T, et al. Analysis of clinical severity of tsutsugamushi disease according to the serotype of pathogenic rickettsia. *Kansenshogaku Zasshi—J Japan Assoc Infect Dis* 1997;71(4):299–306.

340. Smadel JE, Traub R, Ley HL, et al. Chloramphenicol (chloromycetin) in the chemoprophylaxis of scrub typhus (tsutsugamushi disease). II. Results with volunteers exposed in hyperendemic areas of scrub typhus. *Am J Hyg* 1949;50:75–91.

341. Kato T, Watanabe K, Katori M, et al. Conjunctival injection, episcleral vessel dilation, and subconjunctival hemorrhage in patients with new tsutsugamushi disease. *Japan J Opthal* 1997;41(3):196–9.

342. Pai H, Sohn S, Seong Y, et al. Central nervous system involvement in patients with scrub typhus. *Clin Infect Dis* 1997;24(3):436–40.

343. Chien RN, Liu NJ, Lin PY, et al. Granulomatous hepatitis associated with scrub typhus. *J Gastro Hepat* 1995;10(4):484–7.

344. Yang CH, Young TG, Peng MY, et al. Unusual presentation of acute abdomen in scrub typhus: a report of two cases. *Chin Med J* 1995;55(5):401–4.

345. Chan CH, Lai F, Daly B, et al. Scrub typhus pneumonitis with delayed resolution. *J Trop Med Hyg* 1995;98(2):114–6.

346. Jeong YJ, KimS et al. Scrub typhus: clinical, pathologic, and imaging findings. *Radiographics* 2007; 27(1):161–72.

347. Fang CT, Ferng WF, Hwang JJ, et al. Life-threatening scrub typhus with meningoencephalitis and acute respiratory distress syndrome. *J Formosan Med Assoc* 1997;96(5):390.

348. Saah AJ. *Rickettsia tsutsugamushi* (scrub typhus). In: Mandel GL, Bennett JE, Dolin R (eds), *Principles and Practice of Infectious Diseases,* 4th Ed. New York: Churchill Livingstone, 1995. Pp 1740–1.

349. Liu WT. Trench fever: a resume of literature and a note on some obscure phases of the disease. *Chin Med J* 1984;97:179–90.

350. Relman DA. Has trench fever returned? *N Engl J Med* 1995;332(7):463–4.

351. Slater LN, Welch DF. *Rochalimaea* species (recently renamed *Bartonella*). In: Mandel GL, Bennett JE, Dolin R (eds), *Principles and Practice of Infectious Diseases,* 4th Ed. New York: Churchill Livingstone, 1995. Pp 1741–7.

352. Drancourt M, Mainardi JL, Brouqui P, et al. *Bartonella (Rochalimaea) quintana* endocarditis in three homeless men. *N Engl J Med* 1995;332:419–23.

353. Bafna S, Lee AG. Bilateral optic disc edema and multifocal retinal lesions without loss of vision in cat-scratch disease (letter). *Arch Ophthal* 1996;114(8): 1016–7.

354. Cunningham ET Jr, McDonald HR, Schatz H, et al. Inflammatory mass of the optic nerve head associated with systemic *Bartonella henselaea* infection. *Arch Ophthal* 1997;115(12):1596–7.

355. Peter O, Dupuis G, Burgdorfer W, et al. Evaluation of the complement fixation and indirect immunofluorescence tests in the early diagnosis of primary Q fever. *Eur J Clin Microbiol* 1985;4:394–6.

356. Leo A, Enders G, Roelcke D. Increase of post-infection cold agglutinins after infection with *Mycoplasma pneumoniae,* varicella-zoster and rubella virus. *Beitrage Zur Infusionstherapie und Transfusionsmedizin* 1994;32:197–9.

357. Uldum SJ, Jensen JS, Sondergard-Andersen J, et al. Enzyme immunoassay for detection of immunoglobulin M (IgM) and IgG antibodies to *Mycoplasma pneumoniae. J Clin Microbiol* 1992;30: 1198.

358. Kashuba AD, Ballow CH. Legionella urinary antigen testing: potential impact on diagnosis and antibiotic therapy. *Diag Microbiol Infect Dis* 1996;24(3):129–39.

359. Kazandjian D, Chiew R, Gilbert GL. Rapid diagnosis of *Legionella pneumophila* serogroup 1 infection with the Binax enzyme immunoassay urinary antigen test. *J Clin Microbiol* 1997;35(4):954–6.

360. Chirgwin K, Roblin PM, Gelling M, et al. Infection with *Chlamydia pneumonia* in Brooklyn. *J Infect Dis* 1991;163:757–61.

361. Cox SK, Everett ED. Tularemia. An analysis of 25 cases. *Missouri Med* 1981;78:70–4.

362. Gill V, Cunha BA. Tularemia pneumonia. *Semin Respir Infect* 1997;12(1):61–7.

363. Snyder MJ. Immune responses to *Francisella tularensis.* In: Rose NR, Friedman H, Fahey JL (eds),

Manual of Clinical Laboratory Immunology. Washington, DC: American Society of Microbiology, 1986. Pp 377–8.

364. George RB, Ziskind MM, Rasch JR, et al. Mycoplasma and adenovirus pneumonias: comparison with other atypical pneumonias in a military population. *Ann Intern Med* 1966;65:931–42.

365. Stamm WE, Koutsky LA, Benedetti JK, et al. *Chlamydia trachomatis* urethral infections in men. Prevalence, risk factors, and clinical manifestations. *Ann Intern Med* 1984;100:47–51.

366. Bowie WR, Wang SP, Alexander ER, et al. Etiology of nongonococcal urethritis. Evidence for *Chlamydia trachomatis* and *Ureaplasma urealyticum. J Clin Invest* 1977;59:735–42.

367. Krieger JN, Verdon M, Siegel N, et al. Risk assessment and laboratory diagnosis of trichomoniasis in men. *J Infect Dis* 1992;166:1362–6.

368. Sevic S. Serologic diagnosis of acute infectious mononucleosis. *Medicin Pregled* 1997;50(9–10):403–8.

369. Bise G, Coninx R. Epidemic typhus in a prison in Burundi. *Trans R Soc Trop Med Hyg* 1997; 1(2):133–4.

370. Kostman JR. Laboratory diagnosis of rickettsial diseases. *Clin Dermatol* 1996;14(3):301–6.

371. Gilman RH, Terminel M, Levine MM, et al. Relative efficacy of blood, urine, rectal swab, bone-marrow and rose-spot cultures for recovery of *Salmonella typhi* in typhoid fever. *Lancet* 1975;1:1211–3.

372. Wicks ACB, Cruickshank JG, Musewe N. Observations of the diagnosis of typhoid fever in an endemic area. *S Afr Med J* 1974;48:1368–70.

373. Applebaum GD, Mathisen G. Spinal brucellosis in a southern California resident. *West J Med* 1997;166(1):61–5.

374. Gotuzzo E, Carrillo C, Guerra J, et al. An evaluation of diagnostic methods for brucellosis: the value of bone marrow cultures. *J Infect Dis* 1986;153:122–5.

375. Young EJ. Serologic diagnosis of human brucellosis: analysis of 214 cases by agglutination tests and review of the literature. *Rev Infect Dis* 1991;13:359–72.

376. Saltoglu N, Aksu HZ, Tasova Y, et al. Leptospirosis: twelve Turkish patients with the Weil syndrome. *Acta Medica Okayama* 1997;51(6):339–42.

377. Vinetz JM, Glass GE, Flexner CE, et al. Sporadic urban leptospirosis. *Ann Intern Med* 1996;125(10):794–8.

378. Katz AR, Sasaki DM, Mumm AH, et al. Leptospirosis on Oahu: an outbreak among military personnel associated with recreational exposure. *Milit Med* 1997;162(2):101–4.

379. Petchclai B, Hiranras S, Potha U. Gold immunoblot analysis of IgM-specific antibody in the diagnosis of human leptospirosis. *Am J Trop Med Hyg* 1991;45:672–5.

380. Gussenhoven GC, van der Hoorn MA, Goris MG, et al. LEPTO dipstick, a dipstick assay for detection of *Leptospira*-specific immunoglobulin M antibodies in human sera. *J Clin Microbiol* 1997;35(1):92–7.

381. Wallace GD. The role of the cat in the natural history of *Toxoplasma gondii. Am J Trop Med Hyg* 1973;22:313–22.

382. Szenasi Z, Nagy E, Ozsvar Z, et al. Serodiagnosis of toxoplasmosis. *Orvosi Hetilap* 1997;138(51):3241–7.

383. Bretagne S, Costa JM, Kuentz M, et al. Late toxoplasmosis evidenced by PCR in a marrow transplant recipient. *Bone Marrow Trans* 1995;15(5):809–11.

384. Zaki AM. Isolation of a flavivirus related to the tick-borne encephalitis complex from human cases in Saudi Arabia. *Trans R Soc Trop Med Hyg* 1997;91(2):179–81.

385. Case records of the Massachusetts General Hospital. Weekly clinicopathological exercises. Case 2-1997. A 38-year-old man with digital clubbing, low-grade fever, and a murmur. *N Engl J Med* 1997;336(3):205–10.

386. Case definitions for infectious conditions under public health surveillance. *MMWR* 1997;46(No. RR-10):27.

387. Andersen AA. Comparison of pharyngeal, fecal, and cloacal samples for the isolation of *Chlamydia psittaci* from experimentally infected cockatiels and turkeys. *J Vet Diag Invest* 1996;8(4):448–50.

388. Fudge AM, Connely F. Diagnosis of avian chlamydiosis infections using enzyme immunoassay methods. *Proc Assoc Avian Vet* 1990;263–9.

389. Stamp JT, McEwen AG, Watt JAA, et al. Enzootic abortion in ewes. *Vet Rec* 1950;62:251–4.

390. Grimes JE, Daft BE, Grumbles LC, et al. *A Manual of Methods for Laboratory Diagnosis of Avian Chlamydiosis.* Kennet Square, PA: American Association of Avian Pathology, 1987.

391. Hewinson RG, Griffiths PC, Bevan BJ, et al. Detection of *Chlamydia psittaci* from avian field samples using the PCR. *Vet Rec* 1991;199:129–30.

392. Tappe JP, Andersen AA, Cheville NF. Respiratory and pericardial lesions in turkeys infected with avian or mammalian strains of *Chlamydia psittaci. Vet Pathol* 1989;26:386–95.

393. Moore FM, McMillan MC, Margaret L, et al. Comparison of culture, peroxidase-antiperoxidase reaction and serum latex agglutination methods for the diagnosis of chlamydiosis in pet birds. *J Am Vet Med Assoc* 1991;199:71–73.

394. Messmer TO, Skelton SK, Moroney JF, et al. Application of a nested, multiplex PCR to psittacosis outbreaks. *J Clin Microbiol* 1997;35(8):2043–6.

395. Hewinson RG, Griffiths PC, Bevan BJ, et al. Detection of *Chlamydia psittaci* DNA in avian clinical samples by polymerase chain reaction. *Vet Microbiol* 1997;54(2):155–66.

396. Verweij P, Meis JF, Eijk R, et al. Severe human psittacosis requiring artificial ventilation: case report and review. *Clin Infect Dis* 1995;20(2):440–2.

397. Wong KH, Skelton SK, Daugharty H. Utility of complement fixation and microimmunofluorescence assays for detecting serologic responses in patients with clinically diagnosed psittacosis. *J Clin Microbiol* 1994;32(10):2417–21.

398. Oldach DW, Gaydos CA, Mundy LM, et al. Rapid diagnosis of *Chlamydia psittaci* pneumonia. *Clin Infect Dis* 1993;17(3):338–43.

399. Shapiro DS, Kenney SC, Johnson M, et al. Brief report: *Chlamydia psittaci* endocarditis diagnosed by blood culture. *N Engl J Med* 1992;326(18):1192–5.

400. Branley JM, Roy B et al. Real time PCR detection and quantitation of *Chlamydophila psittaci* in human and avian specimens from a veterinary cluster. *Eur J Clin Micro Infect Dis* 2008;27(4)269–73.

401. *Heddema ER, Beld MG et al.* Development of an internally controlled real-time PCR assay for detection of *Chlamydophila psittaci* in the LightCycler 2.0 system *Clin Micro Infect* 2006;12:571–75.

402. Taniguchi H, Mukae H, Ihiboshi H, et al. A case of fulminant psittacosis necessitating mechanical ventilation diagnosed by chlamydial isolation from BALF. *J Japan Assoc Infect Dis* 1995;69(12):1396–401.

403. Essig A, Zucs P, Susa M, et al. Diagnosis of ornithosis by cell culture and polymerase chain reaction in a patient with chronic pneumonia. *Clin Infect Dis* 1995;21(6):1495–7.

404. Jones RB, Katz BP, Van Der Pol B, et al. Effect of blind passage and multiple sampling on recovery of *Chlamydia trachomatis* from urogenital specimens. *J Clin Microbiol* 1986;24:1029–33.

405. Johnson RE, Newhall WJ et al. Screening tests to detect *Chlamydia trachoma* and *Neisseria gonorrhoeae* infections—2002. *MMWR* 2002;51(RR15):1–27.

406. Cook PJ, Honeybourne D. *Chlamydia pneumoniae*. *J Antimicrob Chemother* 1994;34:859–73.

407. Freidank HM, Vogele H, Eckert K. Evaluation of a new commercial microimmunofluorescence test for detection of antibodies to *Chlamydia pneumoniae*, *Chlamydia trachomatis*, and *Chlamydia psittaci*. *Eur J Clin Microbiol Infect Dis* 1997;16(9):685–8.

408. Ginerva C, Barranger C et al. Development and evaluation of Chlaylege, a new commercial test allowing simultaneous detection and identification of Leginella, Chlamydophila pneumonia, and Mycoplasma pneumonia in clinical respiratory specimens by multiplex PCR. *J Clin Microbiol* 2005;43(7):3247–54.

409. Tong CYW, Sillis M. Detection of *Chlamydia pneumoniae* and *Chlamydia psittaci* in sputum samples by PCR. *J Clin Pathol* 1993;46:313–7.

410. Maass M, Dalhoff K. Comparison of sample preparation methods for detection of *Chlamydia pneumoniae* in bronchoalveolar lavage fluid by PCR. *J Clin Microbiol* 1994;32:2616–9.

411. Miyashita N, Fukuda M et al. Evaluation of the diagnostic usefulness of real-time PCR for detection of *Chlamydophila pneumonia* in acute respiratory infections. *J Infect Chemother* 2007;13(3):183–7.

412. Kostman JR. Laboratory diagnosis of rickettsial diseases. *Clin Dermatol* 1996;14(3):301–6.

413. Fournier PE, Raoult D. Comparison of PCR and serology assays for early diagnosis of acute Q fever. *J Clin Micro* 2003;41(11):a5094–8.

414. Ogawa M, Setiyono A et al. Evaluation of nested PCR and nested PCR assays currently used for detection of *Coxiella burnetti* in Japan. *Southeast Asian J Trop Med Public Health* 2004;34(4):852–5.

415. Turra M, Chang G et al. Diagnosis of acute Q fever by PCR on sera during a recent outbreak in rural South Australia. *Ann NY Acad Sci.* 2006;1078:566–9.

416. Durack DT, Lukes AS, Bright DK. New criteria for diagnosis of infective endocarditis: utilization of specific echocardiographic findings. *Am J Med* 1994;96:200–9.

417. Fournier PE, Casalta JP, Habib G, et al. Modification of the diagnostic criteria proposed by the Duke Endocarditis Service to permit improved diagnosis of Q fever endocarditis. *Am J Med* 1996;100:629–33.

418. Aniskovich LP, Motin VL, Lichoded LJ, et al. Identification of *Rickettsia prowazekii* using the polymerase chain reaction. *Eur J Epidemiol* 1993;9(6):645–9.

419. Svraka S, Rolain JM et al. *Rickettsia prowazekii* and real-time polymerase chain reaction. *Emerg Infect Dis.* 2006;12(3):428–32.

420. Walker DH, Parks FM, Betz TB, et al. Histopathology and immunohistologic demonstration of the distribution of *Rickettsia typhi* in fatal murine typhus. *Am J Clin Pathol* 1989;91:720–4.

421. Carl M, Tibbs CW, Dobson ME, et al. Diagnosis of acute typhus infection using the polymerase chain reaction. *J Infect Dis* 1990;161:791–3.

422. Kelly DJ, Chan CT, Paxton H, et al. Comparative evaluation of a commercial enzyme immunossay for the detection of human antibody to *Rickettsia typhi*. *Clin Diag Lab Immunol* 1995;2(3):356–60.

423. Sexton DJ, Kanj SS, Wilson K, et al. The use of a polymerase chain reaction as a diagnostic test for Rocky Mountain spotted fever. *Am J Trop Med Hyg* 1994;50(1):59–63.

424. Kao GF, Evancho CD, Ioffe O, et al. Cutaneous histopathology of Rocky Mountain spotted fever. *J Cutan Pathol* 1997;24(10):604–10.

425. Procop GW, Burchette JL Jr, Howell DN, Sexton DJ. Immunoperoxidase and immunofluorescent staining of *Rickettsia rickettsii* in skin biopsies. A comparative study. *Arch Pathol Lab Med* 1997;121(8):894–9.

426. Watt G, Chouriyagune C, Ruangweerayud R, et al. Scrub typhus poorly responsive to antibiotics in northern Thailand. *Lancet* 1996;348(9020):86–9.

427. Blacksell SD, Bryant NJ et al. Scrub typhus serologic testing with the indirect immunofluoresence method as a diagnostic gold standard: a lack of consensus leads to a lot of confusion. *Clin Infect Dis.* 2007;44(3):391–401.

428. Shieh GJ, Chen HL, Chen HY, et al. Detection of *Rickettsia tsutsugamushi*–specific DNA from the lymphocyte of patients by polymerase chain reaction. *Proc Natl Sci Counc Repub China B, Life Sciences* 1995; 19(1):43–6.

429. Furuya Y, Katayama T, Hara M, et al. The patients

without specific antibodies were diagnosed by PCR as tsutsugamushi disease. *J Japan Assoc Infect Dis* 1997;71(5):474–6.

430. Kim DM, Kim HL et al. Clinical usefulness of eschar rolymerase chain reaction for the diagnosis of scrub typhus: a prospective study. *Clin Infect Dis* 2006: 43(10):1296–1300.

431. Kim DM, Yun NR et al. Usefulness of nested PCR for the diagnosis of scrub typhus in clinical practice: A prospective study. *Am J Trop Hyg* 2006;75(3): 542–5.

432. Pars DH, Blacksell SD et al. Real-time multiplex PCR assay for detection and differentiation of rickettsiae and orientiae. *Trans R Soc Trop Med Hyg* 2008;102(2):186–93.

433. Pradutkanchana J, Silpapojakul K, Paxton H, et al. Comparative evaluation of four serodiagnostic tests for scrub typhus in Thailand. *Trans R Soc Trop Med Hyg* 1997;91(4):425–8.

434. LaScola B and Raoult D. Culture of *Bartonella quintana* and *Bartonella henselae* from human samples: a 5 year experience (1993 to 1998). *J Clin Microbiol* 1999;37(6):1899–905.

435. Maurin M, Rolain JM and Raoult D. Comparison of in-house and commercial slides for detection by immunofluorescence of immunoglobulins G and M against Bartonella henselae and Bartonella Quintana. *Clin Diagn Lab Immunol* 2002;9(5):1004–9.

436. Szelc-Kelly CM, Goral S, Perez-Perez GI, et al. Serologic responses to *Bartonella* and *Afipia* antigens in patients with cat scratch disease. *J Pediatr* 1995; 127:23–6.

437. Lochary ME, Lockhart PB and Williams WT. Doxycycline and staining of permanent teeth. *Pediatr Infec Dis J* 1998;17:429–31.

438. Rodriguez-Barradas MC, Hamill RJ, Houston ED, et al. Genomic fingerprinting of *Bartonella* species by repetitive element PCR for distinguishing species and isolates. *J Clin Microbiol* 1995;33:1089–93.

439. Breathnach AS, Hoare JM, Eykyn SJ. Culture-negative endocarditis: contribution of *Bartonella* infections. *Heart* 1997;77(5):474–6.

440. Flammer K. Treatment of avian chlamydiosis in exotic birds in the United States. *J Am Vet Med Assoc* 1989;195:569–72.

441. Lindensruth H. Feldversuch zur Wirksamkeits-und Vertraglichkeitsprufung von Baytril bei importierten Psittaciden im Rahmen der Staatlichen Psitta-koseprophylaxe und therapie. *Vet Med Diss, Giessen*, 1992.

442. Harrison GJ. A practitioner's view of the problem of avian chlamydiosis. *J Am Vet Med Assoc* 1989; 195:1525–8.

443. van Berkel M, Dik H, van der Meer JW, et al. Acute respiratory insufficiency from psittacosis. *Br Med J* 1985;290:1503–4.

444. Leroy Q, Bouscart C et al. Treatment of pneumonia caused by Legionella, Mycoplasma, Chlamydiae and Rickettsiae using ofloxacin. *Pathol Biol* 1989; 37: 1137.

445. Miyashita N, Niki Y, Kishimoto T, et al. In vitro and in vivo antichlamydial activities of HSR-903, a new fluoroquinolone antibiotic. *Antimicrob Agents Chemother* 1997;41(4):857–9.

446. Roblin PM, Montalban G, Hammerschlag MR. Susceptibilities to clarithromycin and erythromycin of isolates of *Chlamydia pneumoniae* from children with pneumonia. *Antimicrob Agents Chemother* 1994; 38(7):1588–9.

447. Roblin PM, Kutlin A, Hammerschlag MR. In vitro activity of trovafloxacin against *Chlamydia pneumoniae*. *Antimicrob Agents Chemother* 1997;41(9): 2033–4.

448. Roblin PM, Hammerschlag MR. Microbiologic efficacy of azithromycin and susceptibilities to azithromycin of isolates of *Chlamydia pneumoniae* from adults and children with community-acquired pneumonia. *Antimicrob Agents Chemother* 1998; 42(1):194–6.

449. Nystrom-Rosander C, Hulten K, Gustavsson I, et al. Susceptibility of *Chlamydia pneumoniae* to azithromycin and doxycycline: methodological aspects in the determination of minimal inhibitory and minimal bactericidal concentrations. *Scand J Infect Dis* 1997; 29(5):513–6.

450. Malinveerni R, Kuo C-C, Campbell LA, et al. Effects of two antibiotic regimens on course and persistence of experimental *Chlamydia pneumoniae* TWAR pneumonitis. *Antimicrob Agents Chemother* 1995;39(1):45–9.

451. Sinisalo J, Mattila K, Nieminen MS, et al. The effect of prolonged doxycycline therapy on *Chlamydia pneumoniae* serological markers, coronary heart disease risk factors and forearm basal nitric oxide production. *J Antimicrob Chemother* 1998;41(1): 85–92.

452. Felmingham D. Tigecyclin—the first glycylcycline to undergo clinical development: an overview of in vitro activity compared to tetracycline. *J Chemother* 2005:17 Suppl 1:5–11.

453. Lefevre JC, Lepargneur JP, Guion D, et al. Tetracycline-resistant *Chlamydia trachomatis* in Toulouse, France. *Pathol Biol* 1997;45(5):376–8.

454. Horner P. The case for further treatment studies of uncomplicated *Chlamydial trachomatis* infection. *Sexually Transmitted Infections*. 2006;82:340–343.

455. Powell OW, Kennedy KP, McIver M, et al. Tetracycline in the treatment of Q fever. *Aust Ann Med* 1962;11:184–8.

456. Ray WA, Murray KT et al. Oral erythromycin and the risk of sudden death from cardiac causes. *NEJM* 2004;351(11):1089–96.

457. Sobradillo V, Zalacain R, Capelastegui A, et al. Antibiotic treatment in pneumonia due to fever. *Thorax* 1992;47:276–8.

458. Maurin M, Benoliel AM, Bongrand P, et al. Phagolysosomal alkalinization and the bactericidal effects of antibiotics: the *Coxiella burnetii* paradigm. *J Infect Dis* 1992;66:1097–102.

459. Rolain JM, Boulos A et al. Correlation between ratio

of serum doxycycline concentration to MIC and rapid decline of antibody levels during treatment of Q fever endocarditis. *Antimicrob Agents Chemother.* 2005; 49(7): 2673–6.

460. Rolain JM, Mallet MN, and Raoult D. Correlation between serum doxycycline concentrations and serologic evolution in patients with *Coxiella burnetti* endocarditis. *J Infect Dis.* 2003;188:1322–5.

461. Berbari EF, Cockerill FR, Steckelberg JM. Infective endocarditis due to unusual or fastidious organisms. *Mayo Clin Proc* 1997;72:532–42.

462. Calza L, Attard L et al. Doxycycline and chloroquine as treatment for chronic Q fever endocarditis. *J Infect* 2002;45(2):127–9.

463. Perine PL, Krause DW, Awoke A, et al. Single-dose doxycycline treatment of louse-born relapsing fever and epidemic typhus. *Lancet* 1974;2:742–4.

464. Huys J, Kayhigi J, Freyens P and Berghe GV. Single-dose treatment of epidemic typhus with doxycyline. *Chemotherapy* 1973; 18:314–7.

465. Gikas A, Doukakis S et al. Comparison of the effectiveness of five different antibiotic regimens on infection with *Rickettsia typhi*: Therapeutic data from 87 cases. *Am J Trop Med Hyg* 2004;70(5):576–9.

466. Sheehy TW, Hazlett D, Turk RE. Scrub typhus: a comparison of chloramphenicol and doxycycline in its treatment. *Arch Intern Med* 1973;132:77–80.

467. Watt G, Kantipong P et al. Doxycycline and rifampicin for mild scrub-typhus infections in northern Thailand: a randomized trial. *Lancet* 2000; 356(9235):1057–61.

468. Song JH, Lee C, Chang WH, et al. Short-course doxycycline treatment versus conventional tetracycline therapy for scrub typhus: a multicenter randomized trial. *Clin Infect Dis* 1995;21(3):506–10.

469. Kim YS, Yun HJ et al. A comparative trial of a single dose of azithromycin versus doxycycline for the treatment of mild scrub typhus. *Clin Infect Dis* 2004;39(9):1329–35.

470. Strickman D, Sheer T, Salata K, et al. In vitro effectiveness of azithromycin against doxycycline-resistant and susceptible strains of *Rickettsia tsutsugamushi*, etiologic agent of scrub typhus. *Antimicrob Agents Chemother* 1995;39(11):2406–10.

471. Maurin M, Raoult D. In vitro susceptibilities of spotted fever group *Rickettsiae* and *Coxiella burnetii* to clarithromycin. *Antimicrob Agents Chemother* 1993;37(12):2633–7.

472. Rolain M, Brouqui P et al. Recommendations for treatment of human infections caused by *Bartonella* species. *Antimicrob agents Chemother* 2004;48(6): 1921–33.

473. Baddour LM, Wilson WR et al. Infective endocarditis: diagnosis, antimicrobial therapy, and management of complications: a statement for healthcare professionals from the committee on Rheumatic Fever, Endocarditis, and Kawasaki Disease, Council on Cardiovascular Disease in the Young, and the Councils on Clinical Cardiology, Stroke, and Cardiovascular Surgery and Anesthesia, American Heart Association—executive summary: endorsed by the Infectious Diseases Society of America. *Circulation* 2005;111(23):3167–84.

13 Fungal Pneumonias in the Occupational Setting

Mary Anne Morgan and David R. Trawick

Background

Although human contact with fungal species is universal, the development and expression of fungal pneumonia depend on a number of variables. In the occupational setting the burden of the inoculum, rather than the pathogenicity of the organism itself, may be of primary importance. Many outbreaks of fungal pneumonias have occurred when the ambient spore count is increased by such work-related activities as construction or renovations or through contamination of duct systems. Inhalation, the primary route of exposure, occurs because many fungal spores are optimally sized (2–10 μm in diameter) for deposition in the upper and lower respiratory tracts [1, 2]. Aerosolization of the fungus at the worksite occurs through a variety of mechanisms, including human activity in contaminated areas and dispersal from heating, ventilation, and air-conditioning (HVAC) systems [1]. However, inhalation of fungal spores alone is often insufficient to trigger infection. In many instances, factors such as preexisting cardiopulmonary disease and host immunity play important roles in disrupting the complex balance between coexistence and disease.

In general, fungal lung disease (FLD) can be infectious, noninfectious, or both. The range of disease presentations caused by interaction with *Aspergillus fumigatus*, a ubiquitous organism found in the soil, exemplifies how a single organism can exert diverse effects ranging from invasive pneumonia in the immune-compromised host, to asthma or allergic bronchopulmonary aspergillosis (ABPA) in the atopic individual [3, 4], to the formation of fungus balls (mycetomas) in those with underlying structural lung disease. In the occupational setting, workers exposed to high concentrations of fungi, such as those working with tobacco plants (*Aspergillus* species), moldy hay (*Thermophilic actinomycetes*), or grapes during wine production (*Botrytis cincrea*) can develop an acute hypersensitivity pneumonitis [5].

The focus of this chapter will be on the *infectious* illnesses caused by exposure to fungi in the workplace (fungal pneumonias). With our increasingly diverse workforce, including individuals with human immunodeficiency virus (HIV) infection, those taking chronic steroids or other immunosuppressants, and those having returned to work following organ transplantation, the spectrum of workplace-related fungal illness has broadened. However, for the purposes of this chapter, we will concentrate on fungal pneumonias affecting the immunocompetent worker.

Host Immunity

Fungal pneumonias are relatively uncommon, are generally self-limiting, and are often mistaken for other, more common infectious illnesses such as the flu. Fungal causes of invasive pulmonary disease may be classified as *T-cell opportunists, phagocyte opportunists,* or entities causing *overlap disease.*

The T-cell opportunists include the endemic mycoses *Histoplasma, Blastomyces, Coccidioidomyces, Paracoccidioidomyces,* and less commonly, *Cryptococcus* [6]. These organisms are not killed by neutrophils; they are ultimately controlled by T cells. Normal hosts usually recover from infection unless overwhelmed by a large inoculum. In the face of T-cell deficiency, however, progressive disease can occur.

The phagocyte opportunists include *Aspergillus,* the zygomytes causing mucormycosis, and *Candida* [6]. Humans regularly inhale the spores of the first two, and the spores of all three are vulnerable to neutrophilic killing. Even in the presence of immune deficiencies such as acquired immunedeficiency syndrome (AIDS), the risk of invasive disease is small. However, when phagocyte number is compromised (such as owing to prolonged neutropenia following chemotherapy), or when phagocyte function is impaired (as in chronic granulomatous disease), invasive infection can occur. Because of the fact that they typically affect severely immunosuppressed individuals and are therefore relatively rare as a workplace complication, the phagocyte opportunists will not be discussed further in this chapter.

Candidiasis is also included in the category of overlap disease [6]. It differs from the other fungal infections in that it is not a soil organism but is instead part of the endogenous flora colonizing the skin, mucous membranes, and gastrointestinal tract. Transmigration across the bowel and invasion from the skin are the usual means of infection rather than inhalation. As a result, although candidal pneumonias do exist, they are rarely the primary focus of infection and are not seen commonly outside the health care setting.

In the workplace, the fungi most commonly linked to pulmonary disease include *Histoplasma capsalatum, Blastomyces dermatiditis,* and *Coccidioides immitis.* The remainder of this chapter will be devoted to exploring the nature of these T-cell opportunists in further detail, specifically in regard to occupational acquisition.

Occupational Fungal Pneumonia

HISTOPLASMOSIS
Epidemiology

H. capsulatum is a dimorphic soil fungus found throughout the world. In the United States, it is most prevalent in central and northeastern states, especially along the Ohio and Mississippi River valleys. The organism grows as hyphae in nitrogenous soil enriched by bird or bat excrement, which enhances growth by accelerating sporulation. The infective particles are spores, and there are two sizes: microconidia, ranging from 2–6 μm, and macroconidia, which are 6–14 μm in diameter [7]. Most infections follow inhalation of microconidia, which are smaller and more numerous and therefore are more likely to be deposited in the lung. There are rare cases of transmission via fomites, direct inoculation, infection following solid organ transplant, and infection after sexual contact, but inhalation remains the most common route of transmission. Unlike birds, which do not themselves acquire the infection owing to their higher body temperature, bats may harbor the fungus in their intestinal tract and spread the disease via fresh droppings [8, 9].

Pathogenesis

Following inhalation, *H. capsulatum* spores germinate and convert to yeast forms at human body temperature. The yeast forms then are phagocytosed by macrophages. The organism multiplies within the macrophages and spreads to draining lymph nodes and, subsequently, throughout the body via the bloodstream and lymphatics [7, 10]. Specific cellular immunity typically develops within 2 weeks of exposure, after immune thymus-derived lymphocytes activate macrophages to assume fungicidal properties. Interleukin-12 (IL-12), tumor necrosis factor alpha (TNF-α), and interferon-gamma (IFN-γ) are thought to be key mediators of this defense [11]. This primarily cell-mediated defense generally prevents the development of severe, progressive disease in immunocompetent adults [12]. In those with impaired immune defense or at the extremes of age, progressive disseminated disease can ensue, marked by granulomas and necrosis both in the lung and at distant sites. Even after mild infections, calcified lesions may be found in the liver and spleen [7, 10].

Clinical Presentation

Following inhalation of *H. capsulatum* spores, the spectrum of disease is largely determined by the magnitude of exposure and the fortitude of the host immune system. *Histoplasma* infection following low-level exposure is largely asymptomatic, but a minority of individuals (5%) present with nonspecific flulike symptoms, including fever, chills, myalgias, headache, anorexia, and a nonproductive cough [13].

Inhalation of a higher concentration of organisms can result in more persistent or severe pulmonary manifestations, such as dyspnea, pleurisy, severe pneumonitis, or even the acute respiratory distress syndrome (ARDS). In acute pulmonary histoplasmosis, chest radiographs often show enlarged mediastinal and hilar lymph nodes, as well as patchy or nodular parenchymal opacities, with overt cavitation being rare. Histology may reveal acinar or lobular bronchopneumonia, with neutrophilic inflammation initially followed by formation of granulomata. Resolution of radiographic and pathologic changes may take months [14].

Following heavy exposure, some patients may progress to a systemic or disseminated disease, marked by weight loss, pericarditis, mediastinitis, arthritis, gastrointestinal symptoms, lymphadenopathy, and hepatosplenomegaly. In most cases, these symptoms begin 1–4 weeks after exposure and last anywhere from a few days to 3 weeks and then resolve. Although most immunocompetent individuals recover from even heavy exposure without treatment, fatigue and dyspnea can persist for months [7, 12, 14, 15].

Patients with underlying chronic lung disease are susceptible to chronic pulmonary histoplasmosis. They will continue to experience productive cough, dyspnea, chest pain, fevers, and fatigue, with chest imaging demonstrating apical fibrosis and even cavitation. Bronchopleural fistulas, broncholithiasis, and new/enlarging cavity formation can occur [14]. Importantly, immunosuppression is not itself a risk factor for chronic pulmonary histoplasmosis. Pathologically, the degree of inflammation is disproportionate to the fungal burden, suggesting that it is hypersensitivity to the fungal antigen, in conjunction with underlying or pre-existing pulmonary disease, rather than the number of infecting organisms themselves, that leads to the development of chronic pulmonary histoplasmosis [16]. Of note, coexisting infection with mycobacteria, including *M. tuberculosis,* as well as the atypical mycobacteria, can occur and often must be considered [16, 17].

Although histoplasmosis spreads hematogenously during acute illness before cellular immunity develops, progressive or disseminated illness is unusual except at extremes of age or in the immunodeficient host. Severity of disease depends on the degree of immunosuppression and extent of exposure. In many cases of progressive or disseminated disease, untreated histoplasmosis is fatal. Death usually occurs by overwhelming infection and attendant complications of shock, respiratory distress, multi–organ system failure, and coagulopathy. Disseminated disease also can cause adrenal crisis, which, if unrecognized, may contribute to high mortality even in the face of adequate antifungal therapy. Importantly, while dissemination occurs most commonly during primary illness, it also may occur during reinfection or reactivation, resulting from a further decrement of immunocompetence [14]. HIV infection is a major risk factor for disseminated histoplasmosis, but other immune-deficiency states, such as that wrought by anti-TNF therapy or methotrexate, also may predispose to disseminated disease [11].

As indicated earlier, both reinfection and reactivation of latent histoplasmosis can occur, even decades after the initial infection [18, 19]. This is thought to be due to the ability of small numbers of yeast to lie dormant but viable in granulomas, but the pathophysiology is poorly understood. The current hypothesis is that reactivation occurs coincident with a "blow" to the immune system [20, 21], as is seen in experimental models of CD4/CD8 cell depletion. However, the hypothesis of reactivated histoplasmosis has been difficult to prove and remains controversial.

Diagnosis

The vast majority of cases of histoplasmosis remain undiagnosed owing either to the typical self-limited nature of the illness or to the failure of health practitioners to consider the disease when confronting the appropriate clinical scenario. Cultures, fungal stains, serologic tests for antibodies, and methods of antigen detection are all available and relatively specific, but all have significant shortcomings. The role of each test in establishing the diagnosis depends on the severity/manifestation of disease, as well as host factors.

Isolation of the organism by culture is the "gold standard" for detection, but the test is marred by a very high rate of false negativity and by the organism's sluggish growth. Even in patients with disseminated disease, 20% of cultures can be negative; in patients with chronic pulmonary histoplasmosis, half of all cultures will fail to reveal the culprit [22]. In the relatively rare case of active cavitation, the yield is higher [17]. Cultures need to be held for 4 weeks to rule out the disease. Histopathologic diagnosis is more rapid yet often requires an invasive procedure and carries a sensitivity of less than 50% [22].

Anti-*Histoplasma* antibodies may be detected in the serum of up to 90% of patients with histoplasmosis [22]. However, the 2–6 weeks needed for antibody formation, the lack of a powerful antibody response in patients with impaired immune defense, and the inability to differentiate between active infection and prior exposure all impair the usefulness of serologic testing as a sole means for diagnosis. Baseline seropositivity in endemic regions has been estimated to range from 0.5% by immunodiffusion to 4% by complement fixation [12]. Currently available serologic testing techniques include immunodiffusion (ID), which identifies H and M precipitin bands to *H. capsulatum,* and complement fixation (CF). CF is preferred over ID for its enhanced sensitivity, and it is felt that higher antibody titers are more diagnostic of active disease. However, up to one-third of patients with histoplasmosis have low titers (1:8 or 1:16), and ID may be more specific [12]. In addition, antibody crossreactions commonly occur in patients with other fungal infections (up to 40% in blastomycosis, paracoccidiomycosis, and aspergillosis, less in coccidiomycosis or candidiasis) and therefore, when present, may not specifically indicate active *Histoplasma* infection. Lastly, although antibodies typically clear following recovery from disease, they can persist in chronic infection or prolonged exposure or in the presence of continued low-level exposure. The significance of enduring antibody titers is unknown.

Antigen detection has the advantage of providing a tool for rapid diagnosis, well before organism growth in culture or development of antibodies in serum. In addition, antigen detection is more helpful in monitoring therapy and detecting relapse. Sensitivity is highest in patients with disseminated or acute pulmonary disease and is significantly greater in urine than in serum. Antigen was detected in the urine of 92% of patients with severe/disseminated histoplasmosis and in 75% of patients with acute pulmonary histoplasmosis, and this is enhanced in patients with AIDS or other immunodeficient states. Sensitivity is significantly less in patients with chronic pulmonary histoplasmosis (10–15%) and in patients with subacute disease (34%) [22]. Although a negative urine assay cannot rule out disease, severe illness and a negative test should prompt consideration of other diagnoses.

Less is known about the sensitivity of antigen testing of bronchoalveolar lavage fluid, but studies in AIDS patients with acute pulmonary histoplasmosis are promising. Recently, a "second generation" antigen assay was studied in non-AIDS patients with pulmonary histoplasmosis and demonstrated both sensitivity and specificity profiles greater than 90% [23].

Finally, antigen detection is useful both in following the effect of anti-*Histoplasma* therapy and in determining relapse. However, in patients with a high degree of exposure, more than a year may pass before antigen levels are undetectable. Maintenance of high antigen levels suggests treatment failure or nonadherence. Of note, false positivity can occur either owing to crossreactions with other endemic mycoses (e.g., blastomycosis or paracoccidiomycosis) or, rarely, owing to the presence of rheumatoid factor or other underlying conditions such as collagen diseases, malignancy, and cirrhosis.

Other diagnostic approaches include polymerase chain reaction (PCR) and DNA probe, neither of which has been validated at this point. There is no longer a commercially available histoplasmin skin test, although it continues to be used to define outbreaks and patterns of endemicity.

Treatment

Treatment is generally only required for acute life-threatening conditions (such as hypoxemia or meningitis), prolonged infection (>1 month), or in patients with progressive disseminated disease [12, 15, 24]. Amphotericin B is the drug of choice in these situations, generally followed by a prolonged course of itraconazole. The use of concurrent steroids, at least in early treatment, remains controversial [24]. For mild or self-limited pulmonary disease, either no treatment or, if symptoms persist for more than 1 month, a 6- to 12-week course of itraconazole is recommended. Mild, disseminated infection requires prolonged courses of itraconazole. In patients with HIV infection and disseminated disease, lifelong suppressive therapy is recommended following an initial course of amphotericin B [12, 15]. Itraconazole is also often effective for chronic cavitary disease.

Occupational Hazards

Immunocompetent individuals who develop active, symptomatic infections often have experienced intense point-source exposure after such activities as cleaning an area where bird and bat excrement is likely to accrue (such as a chicken house or an attic), working in building demolition, or transporting wood or dead trees. A classic example involves the case of a farmer and his two sons, aged 5 and 21, all of whom became acutely ill 3 weeks after cleaning a silo. All developed bilateral nonsegmental, patchy areas of consolidation on chest radiographs, the resolution of which took months. All had diffuse calcifications on repeat radiographs done years later. The father was the most ill, growing *H. capsulatum* from both his sputum and bone marrow [25]. Other cases have developed in individuals employed in the inspection or maintenance of bridges; chimney cleaning; building construction, restoration, or demolition work; installation of heating or air-conditioning systems; agricultural processing plants; and microbiology laboratories [18]. One famous outbreak occurred after Earth Day in 1970 after a small group of middle school students swept a 20-year accumulation of debris from the school courtyard. Nearly 400 people, including some who had been absent on the day of the cleaning, subsequently developed histoplasmosis, likely owing to contamination of the school's forced-air ventilation system [26]. There was a similar outbreak in 2001 after a 10- by 45-ft area of a school playground was rototilled [27]. In some cases, epidemics of histoplasmosis

can last for years, particularly in cases of ongoing construction and sporadic, low-level exposure. In one example, 29 cases of histoplasmosis occurred among employees of a medical school over a 7-year period. All cases began during periods of building renovation and were thought to be acquired inside. The school was located in a wooded area and was adjacent to a bird sanctuary [28]. In many cases, occupational outbreaks of histoplasmosis occurred following the disruption of contaminated soil or accumulations of bird or bat manure. Risk for disease acquisition in individuals who lack competent immune systems is clearly higher.

Prevention

The most recent National Institute for Occupational Safety and Health (NIOSH) report on workplace-acquired histoplasmosis was published in 2004 [18]. Its preventative recommendations included barring birds or bats from buildings, in order to prevent the accumulation of manure, using such techniques as ultrasonic devices, installing lights in a bat roosting area, and sealing entry/exit points. If exclusion is not successful, the committee recommended posting health risk warnings. Removing or disinfecting contaminated materials should occur under conditions that minimize the risk of aerosolization, such as spraying water on dusty or dry material before collecting it in heavy-duty, secure containers. Alternatively, a truck or trailer-mounted vacuum system can be used to minimize dust exposure. Waste should be disposed of immediately. There are currently no Environmental Protection Agency (EPA)–registered fungicidal soil disinfectants.

During such activities as construction, excavation, or demolition, water sprays and other dust-suppressing techniques should be used to minimize the risk of aerosolization, which are considerable. The three largest *Histoplasma* outbreaks in Indiana all involved demolition or construction, infecting several hundred thousand individuals and causing multiple deaths [12, 29–31]. In addition, such activities should be avoided during particularly windy periods. All construction vehicles should be outfitted with air conditioning to protect the drivers. In some situations, such as when manure is plentiful, removal may be necessary before proceeding with demolition.

The use of personal protective equipment such as respirator masks to reduce exposure to *H. capsulatum* is recommended during activities such as cleaning enclosed areas or working in poultry houses. Importantly, cases of histoplasmosis have been described in workers despite wearing either a respirator or a mask, although the higher-level protection systems (such as pressure-controlled self-contained breathing apparatus) are thought to be protective. Considerations of level of exposure, need for mobility, cost, and comfort also guide the choice of an appropriate air-purifying respirator [18]. For example, a disposable half-facepiece air-purifying respirator (protection factor of 10) may be adequate for low-risk activities such as monitoring bird roosts, whereas higher-risk activities, such as working in a dusty, enclosed area, would mandate higher protection, such as a powered air-purifying, full-facepiece respiratory (protection factor of 50).

Finally, disposable clothing, hoods, and shoe coverings should be worn whenever *H. capsulatum*–containing dust may be present. These should be disposed of in sealed heavy-duty plastic bags.

In workers known to be immunosuppressed, such as those infected with HIV, the U.S. Public Health Service and Infectious Disease Society of America (IDSA) have jointly published guidelines recommending that such individuals "avoid activities known to be associated with increased risk," such as working with surface soil or other dusty endeavors; cleaning chicken coops or other locations with bird droppings; cleaning, remodeling, or demolishing old buildings; or exploring caves [32].

BLASTOMYCOSIS
Epidemiology

B. dermatiditis, like *H. capsulatum*, is a dimorphic soil fungus that exists as a mycelial form in nature but converts to a yeast form in body tissue. Branched hyphae are 2–3 μm in diameter and possess oval or round conidia, which are 2–10 μm. Like *Histoplasma*, *B. dermatiditis* is endemic within the great river valleys, but its range extends to the southeast along the coastal areas of the Carolinas and further to the northwest through northern Wisconsin and Minnesota toward Canada [10, 33]. Accurate mapping has been hindered by the difficulty in isolating the organism from the soil and by the lack of an accurate skin test [33]. Clinical illness

is estimated to occur only one-tenth as often as histoplasmosis [10], with approximately 4 cases per 100,000 people living in endemic areas [34]. In epidemics, isolation of the fungus has been associated with the proximity of soil containing decaying vegetation to bodies of water. However, whether humidity or the presence of water itself is the primary factor in promoting growth of the organism and therefore spread of disease or is simply an explanation for greater exposure related to recreational or occupational activities is unknown [35].

Pathogenesis

Infection begins with inhalation of the spores, followed by clearing of the organism by bronchopulmonary phagocytes. Fungi that escape phagocyte defense undergo transition to the larger and more phagocyte-resistant yeast phase, with increasing virulence. The encapsulated organism then may spread hematogenously to other organs. Unlike histoplasmosis, *B. dermatiditis* may spread to skin and bone at any stage of the infection and with any type of pulmonary involvement [10, 33]. As immunity evolves, distinctive, noncaseating granulomas develop [10, 33]. Ultimately, immunity is conferred through antigen-specific T-lymphocytes and lymphokine-activated macrophages. Although pneumonia may resolve spontaneously, reactivation also may occur in both pulmonary and extrapulmonary sites with or without previous therapy [36].

Clinical Presentation

Blastomycosis exhibits a male predominance, with a reported male:female ratio of 4:1–5:1 in the nonepidemic setting [33]. The typical patient is a young man aged 25–50 who works outside or who engages in outdoor recreation [33]. In an outbreak, women and children are as likely to be infected. Otherwise, diagnoses in children are rare [37]. Exposure to contaminated soil seems to be the common link between sporadic cases and true epidemics.

Symptoms of infection are relatively nonspecific and include malaise, weight loss, and fever. The acute pneumonia of blastomycosis mimics that of bacterial pneumonia, with fever, chills, and a productive cough. The radiographic manifestations of pulmonary blastomycosis range from an asymptomatic infiltrate, to acute pneumonia, to chronic fibrocavitary pneumonia resembling tuberculosis, and occasionally, to indolent masslike entities resembling bronchogenic carcinoma [38]. Multiple extrapulmonary manifestations are possible and are likewise nonspecific. They include, in order of frequency, cutaneous (frequently verrucous or cavitary lesions), osseous (osteomyelitis), genitourinary (such as prostatitis), and less commonly, meningeal involvement [33].

Most patients with blastomycosis are immunocompetent. However, there appears to be an increasing prevalence among the immunosuppressed population, including diabetics, patients on systemic corticosteroids, and those with HIV infection or a history of solid or hematologic transplantation [39]. The incidence of severe complications, such as ARDS or central nervous system or other multiorgan involvement, is also higher, as is the rate of relapse. Early recognition and treatment therefore are essential.

Diagnosis

In contrast to histoplasmosis, pulmonary blastomycosis produces gross purulent sputum that often contains the characteristic yeast forms and is therefore easier to diagnose, once suspected. The organisms can be viewed in 10% potassium hydroxide–digested preparations of sputum, as well as in cytology specimens prepared with Papanicolaou's stain [40]. Cultures of sputum and infected tissue also have a high yield but may take several weeks [33]. Skin testing is neither sensitive nor specific and is generally not available clinically [33]. Serologic testing, including immunodiffusion tests, complement fixation, and enzyme immunoassays, all have undergone evaluation, but none has yet proven to have the diagnostic utility of the antigen testing described for *H. capsulatum* [41].

Treatment

The decision to treat is premised on the severity of the disease, the immune competence of the individual, and the toxicity of the antifungal agent employed [42]. Reports of self-limiting disease during epidemics exist [36, 43]. Thus, in some cases of acute pulmonary blastomycosis, the physician may elect to withhold therapy and carefully observe the patient [42]. Antifungal therapy is mandatory, however, in immunocompromised individuals and in patients with chronic pulmonary and extrapulmonary blastomycosis [42]. If treatment does

occur, itraconazole, 400 mg/day for 6 months, is very effective for mild to moderate cases but should not be used in patients with central nervous system involvement. Severely ill patients require amphotericin B. Exact dosing regimens and duration of therapy are unclear, but relapse rates are less than 5% in immunocompetent patients [33]. Patients who have AIDS, are transplant recipients, or are on chronic systemic corticosteroids also should receive initial therapy with amphotericin B, followed by long-term suppressive azole therapy [42].

Occupational Hazards

Delayed diagnosis, difficulty isolating *B. dermatiditis* in nature, and absence of a sensitive and specific test to assess exposure make outbreaks of this disease difficult to study [44]. Yet, in 1998, two cases of pulmonary blastomycosis were reported in young immunocompetent males who had worked together on a prairie dog relocation project in Colorado [45]. Work practices included using a gasoline-powered auger and hand trowels to excavate abandoned prairie dog burrows that were used by many animal species. The workers had spent the majority of several days digging and creating large amounts of dust and did not use protective clothing or masks. Rain was frequent during the project. Only the two ill workers had abnormalities on chest radiographs. The presence of highly nitrogenous, acidic, and moist soil likely fostered the growth of the fungus, contributing to the development of fungal pneumonia in these workers [45–47]. Other reports of work-related blastomycosis have occurred in individuals employed in forestry, hunting, or mycobiology laboratory.

Prevention

There are no formal recommendations for preventing exposure to *B. dermatiditis* in the workplace. The disease is unusual and sporadic, and no epidemiologic evidence exists to suggest that personal protective gear significantly alters the occurrence of disease. Extrapolating from the broader experience with other endemic mycoses (i.e., histoplasmosis and coccidiomycosis), similar measures recommended for protecting workers in these settings likely would be protective against soil contaminated by *B. dermatiditis*. These measures include wearing a NIOSH-approved respirator mask, donning protective clothing, and implementing an educational program for workers [45].

COCCIDIOIDOMYCOSIS
Epidemiology

C. immitis is a fungus endemic in the southwestern United States of the lower Sonoran Desert. It also inhabits adjacent areas of northern Mexico and desert areas of Central and South America. Areas of highest concentration are the southern San Joaquin Valley of California and in southern Arizona [48, 49]. In young adults moving to these areas for the first time, asymptomatic skin conversion rates are reported to be 2.5–3.5% per year [50]. *C. immitis* thrives in the mycelial form in desert soil in a semi-arid climate in which the summers are hot and dry, the winters mild, and the rainfall moderate [10]. Spore formation occurs along hyphae, which disarticulate from the mycelium and are carried and spread by wind. Infection occurs by inhalation of the spores (anthroconidia) [48]. Outbreaks of coccidioidomycosis have occurred during archeological digs, construction, and oil exploration in areas where anthroconidia density within the soil is high [51]. Outbreaks also occur after dust storms or, in at least one case in southern California, after an earthquake [52]. In the United States, inhalation of anthroconidia is thought to cause 100,000 *Coccidioides* infections annually [53].

Pathogenesis

The inhalation of arthroconidia into the alveoli initiates a predominately neutrophilic inflammatory response. However, the neutrophils cannot phagocytose the spores, which grow into spherules of 30–80 μm in diameter [10]. Each spherule reproduces by progressive cleavage of the cytoplasm, forming endospores (endosporulation). Eventually, the spherule ruptures, releasing endospores into the tissue. Each endospore possesses the potential to become another spherule.

Specific cell-mediated immunity is the main mechanism by which the body resists infection, and this generally occurs within 2 weeks [51]. Therefore, individuals with reduced function or numbers of T cells are at risk for progressive disease [51].

Clinical Presentation

Coccidioidomycosis may present as primary pulmonary infection, progressive pulmonary disease, or disseminated disease [51, 53]. Sixty percent of those individuals with the primary pulmonary disease have no symptoms or have an illness indistinguishable from an upper respiratory infection [48, 54]. Exposure in such patients is documented by a positive skin test. The remaining 40% will develop influenza-like symptoms, with onset typically 1–3 weeks after exposure. Approximately one-fourth of the symptomatic individuals exhibit more severe manifestations, including pleuritic chest pain [51]. Erythema nodosum and erythema multiforme may occur in primary disease but do not portend a better outcome, as thought previously. A symmetric arthritis, predominantly in the ankles but potentially involving several joints, may evolve during the primary infection as an immune-complex phenomenon. This "desert rheumatism" is generally self-limited [48, 51].

The chest radiograph usually exhibits an alveolar infiltrate or nodular density. The infiltrate often is subpleural and may abut the fissure. Other findings include hilar adenopathy or a pleural effusion. Five percent of patients will develop chronic changes such as nodules or thin-walled cavities [38].

Chronic progressive coccidioidal pneumonia resembles cavitary tuberculosis and is rare [38]. Although it may evolve from the primary infection, it often occurs subsequent to apparent healing of the primary infection and progresses in an indolent fashion. Those afflicted include diabetics and individuals with compromised immune systems. Empyemas and bronchopleural fistulas can result and are difficult to treat [53]. The frequency of symptomatic extrapulmonary complications of *C. immitis* ranges from as low as 0.5% of infections for persons of Caucasian ancestry to several-fold higher for persons of African or Filipino ancestry. In individuals with significant immunosuppression, such as those with AIDS, those with malignancy, those on chronic corticosteroids or anti-TNF therapies, and those who have undergone solid-organ transplantation, estimates of extrapulmonary disease run as high as 30–50% of infections. Pregnant women are also more vulnerable to dissemination. Although the manifestation of disseminated disease can be quite varied, the most frequent extrapulmonary organs involved include the skin, the bones, and the meninges. Meningitis accounts for the majority of deaths from disseminated disease [49, 53–56].

Diagnosis

A positive skin test will develop in most individuals within 2 weeks of infection. Unfortunately, this may simply reflect a legacy of a prior infection, especially if the individual lives in an endemic area. In the case of disseminated coccidiomycosis, anergy may develop. As in histoplasmosis, dermal hypersensitivity testing is therefore not clinically useful but may be helpful in defining *Coccidioides* epidemics. Direct examination of sputum smears after 10% KOH digestion or Papanicolaou staining may be diagnostic, but these tests are not very sensitive. Histologic examination of infected tissues may demonstrate organisms when special stains are employed. Culture results are more sensitive than direct histopathologic examination, with growth usually occurring within the first week. However, the mycelial growth form is highly infective; therefore, laboratory workers should be forewarned so that appropriate safety measures can be undertaken. Fortunately, serologic diagnostic methods for coccidioidomycosis are more advanced than for other pathogenic mycoses [57]. Positive IgM titers are consistent with acute infection and can be detected in 75% of people with acute infection. Complement-fixing (IgG) antibodies occur later in the course in most patients. Although highly specific when the results are positive, false-negative results may occur early in the course of an illness [57].

Treatment

Treatment is generally not required for mild to moderate primary pulmonary coccidioidomycosis. However, it should be considered for patients who are at risk for disseminated disease, including the immunosuppressed, diabetics, and pregnant women [49]. Treatment is also recommended in severe primary infections or in persistent and progressive disease. Disseminated disease always requires urgent therapy. Fluconazole, 400 mg/day for 6–12 months, is used in high-risk patients. Shorter courses of fluconazole have been used in lower-risk patients, as has itraconazole. Amphotericin B may be used in severe primary and disseminated disease [49].

Occupational Hazards

A coccidioidomycosis outbreak from a common point source confirmed by soil cultures occurred during the summer of 1970 among 103 archeology students excavating Indian ruins near Chico, California [58]. The outbreak involved at least 61 of 103 students and faculty members participating in a 5-week summer course in archeology sponsored by Queens College of the City University of New York and Chico State College. Most had never been in areas known to be endemic for coccidioidomycosis. The work involved sifting shovels of dry dirt through screens to filter out artifacts. Dust clouds often obscured vision or provoked coughing spells. No precautions were taken, and no masks were used. The conditions were hot and dry, with temperatures often reaching 43°C. The first illness with laboratory confirmation occurred 13 days after the first exposure to soil. One particularly ill woman presented with fever, shaking chills, headache, malaise, and a generalized maculopapular, pruritic rash. A chest radiograph revealed extensive bilateral pneumonia with hilar adenopathy.

This report emphasized dust control to reduce the degree of exposure of archeological workers. It also served as a basis for providing such workers with "informed consent" regarding the hazards of the work. Finally, it encouraged skin testing all workers without previous positive reactions and close observation of individuals more predisposed to serious infections (see above). A similar outbreak occurred in workers at an archaeological site in 2001 in Dinosaur National Monument in Utah, an area not commonly thought to be affected by *Coccidioides*. Again, work involved sifting dust, laying stone steps, and building a retaining wall. Workers did not wear protective masks. In all, 10 of 18 individuals developed acute, serology-positive coccidioidomycosis, with illness directly correlated with degree of exposure to dust. Later that summer, four workers wearing N-95 approved respirators finished building the retaining wall; one developed symptoms and laboratory evidence consistent with acute infection [59].

Prevention

Current recommendations include the use of NIOSH-approved N-95 respirators, activities to minimize soil disturbance (such as spraying soil), and avoiding work during highly windy days [60].

Prevention and Control

Hurricane Katrina made landfall in Louisiana on August 29, 2005, causing massive flooding in New

320

Table 13-1

Population-Specific Recommendations for Protection from Exposure to Mold in Buildings after Hurricanes and Major Floods,* by Specific Activity† and Risk Factor

Risk Factor	Observing from outside the demolition area (disturbs no dust)	Inspecting or assessing damage (disturbs little dust or mold)	Recovering moldy personal belongings (disturbs some dust or mold)	Sweeping, light cleaning, removing mold (disturbs much dust or mold)	Using power tools, cleaning, demolishing (disturbs all dust and mold)
None	No special precautions needed	No special precautions needed	Respiratory protection (RP)§ and gloves and dermal protection (GDP)	RP, GDP, and occlusive eye protection (OEP)¶	RP, GDP, and OEP
Persons at high risk for infection or colonization					
Profound immunosuppression**	Avoid exposure	Avoid exposure	Avoid exposure	Avoid exposure	Avoid exposure
Immunosuppression††	RP	RP, GDP, and OEP	Avoid exposure	Avoid exposure	Avoid exposure
Obstructive or cavitary lung disease§§	RP	RP	RP and GDP	RP, GDP, and OEP	Avoid exposure
Persons who have diseases with immune sensitization¶¶					
Allergic rhinoconjunctivitis (exacerbated by moldy materials)	RP	RP	RP, GDP, and OEP	RP, GDP, and OEP	Avoid exposure
Asthma (exacerbated by moldy materials)	RP	RP	RP, GDP, and OEP	Avoid exposure	Avoid exposure
Hypersensitivity pneumonitis caused by moldy materials	RP	RP	RP, GDP, and OEP	Avoid exposure	Avoid exposure
Persons with unknown risk* *					
Aged <12 years†††	Consult health-care provider	Consult health-care provider	Consult health-care provider	Consult health-care provider	Consult health-care provider
Pregnant	RP	RP	RP, GDP, and OEP	Avoid exposure	Avoid exposure
Aged >65 years	RP	RP	RP, GDP, and OEP	Avoid exposure	Avoid exposure

*Extensive mold contamination is assumed if the building's interior was saturated with water for >48 hours, extensive water damage is present, extensive mold growth is visible, or "mildew" odors are clearly stronger than before hurricanes.

†A visible dust cloud suggests high potential for exposure. However, activities can be associated with high fungal exposure even without visible dust. Consider more protective interventions for activities of longer duration or greater frequency.

§Recommended respiratory protection for residents is a respirator at least as protective as an N-95 filtering face piece. Respirator protection for workers in isolated areas of mold contamination (≤100 square feet) or small isolated areas of heating, ventilation, and air conditioning (HVAC) systems (≤10 square feet) where mold is disturbed is a respirator at least as protective as an N-95 filtering face piece. For working in areas of extensive contamination (>100 contiguous square feet) or HVAC systems with large areas of contamination (>10 square feet) and substantial mold-containing dust, full face-piece respirators with N100, R100, P100 particulate filters (or for powered air-purifying respirators, HEPA filters) are recommended.

¶Occlusive eye protection includes safety goggles, not regular eyeglasses.

**Transplant recipients, including organ or hematopoietic stem cell recipients within 6 months of transplant or during periods of substantial immunosuppression; neutropenia (neutrophil count <500/µL) associated with any cause (including neoplasm, cancer chemotherapy); CD4+ lymphopenia (lymphocyte count <200/µL) associated with any cause, including HIV infection. Affected persons should consult with their physicians before entering the affected area.

††Includes immunosuppressant drug therapy (e.g., cancer chemotherapy, corticosteroid, or other immunosuppressive drug therapy), and diseases impairing host defense such as leukemia or lymphoma. Affected persons should consult with their physicians before entering the affected area. Duration and frequency of exposures should be minimal.

§§Such diseases include chronic obstructive pulmonary disease, asthma not exacerbated by mold, cystic fibrosis, and cavitary tuberculosis. Risk for airway colonization and subsequent diseases following mold exposure is unknown. Recommendations are based on best professional judgment.

¶¶The optimal treatment for allergic rhinitis, allergic asthma, or hypersensitivity pneumonitis is avoidance of the sensitizing agent. If symptoms occur despite the recommended preventive measures, avoidance of exposure is indicated. In many cases, allergic etiology of rhinitis or asthma needs to be inferred from clinical information, since the available diagnostic reagents for documenting IgE-sensitization to fungi are mostly unstandardized. Similarly, the precise antigenic agent causing hypersensitivity pneumonitis is often unclear.

***The level of risk associated with exposure activities and the potential benefit of recommended personal protective equipment are unknown for these vulnerable populations.

†††Exposure-reducing behavior and respiratory protection can be difficult to achieve in children aged <12 years. Infants should avoid exposure at all activity levels.

Orleans and its surrounding parishes. The extent and duration of flooding and the number of structures exposed to and saturated with water rendered mold contamination inevitable. Heavy mold growth affected 40,000 homes, with an additional 100,000 manifesting significant growth. Reconstruction has resulted in higher degrees of mold exposure for both workers and the general public, with uncertain health consequences. Given the prediction that we may now be entering a 10-year cycle of enhanced hurricane activity, lessons from Katrina will be important in minimizing both fungal respiratory infections and adverse health effects in general.

Key principles in achieving these goals have been outlined by the Centers for Disease Control and Prevention and include both recommendations for avoidance of exposure and symptom-specific interventions for heavy mold contamination [1]. Table 13-1 refers to population-specific recommendations for those working in potentially contaminated areas [1].

Conclusions

- The development of fungal pneumonia depends on a number of factors, including the burden of inoculum, the pathogenicity of the organism, and the immune status of the individual.
- The most common organisms leading to occupational fungal pneumonia in the immunocompetent worker include *H. capsulatum*, *B. dermatiditis*, and *C. immitis*.
- Most occupational fungal pneumonia has a self-limited course; however, in cases of immunodeficiency or overwhelming exposure, specific treatment may be warranted.
- As our workforce evolves to include more individuals of impaired immunity, and as the environmental fungal burden swells, increased surveillance for fungal infection is imperative.

References

1. Brandt M, Brown C, Burkhart J, et al. Mold prevention strategies and possible health effects in the aftermath of hurricanes and major floods. *MMWR* 2006;55:1–27.
2. Dismukes WE, Pappas PG, Sobel JD. *Clinical Mycology.* New York: Oxford University Press, 2003.
3. Kauffman H, Tomee J, van der Werf T, et al. Review of fungus-induced asthmatic reactions. *Am J Respir Crit Care Med* 1995;151:2109–16.
4. Fraser RS. Pulmonary aspergillosis: Pathologic and pathogenetic features. *Pathol Annu* 1993;28:231–77.
5. Greenberger PA. Mold-induced hypersensitivity pneumonitis. *Allergy Asthma Proc* 2004;25:219–23.
6. Mandell GL, Simberkoff M. *Pleuropulmonary and Bronchial Infections.* New York: Churchill Livingstone, 1996.
7. Gurney JW, Conces DJ. Pulmonary histoplasmosis. *Radiology* 1996;199:297–306.
8. Greer DL, McMurray DN. Pathogenesis of experimental histoplasmosis in the bat, *Artibeus lituratus*. *Am J Trop Med Hyg* 1981;30:653–9.
9. Hasenclever HF, Shacklette MH, Young RV, Gelderman GA. The natural occurrence of *Histoplasma capsulatum* in a cave: I. Epidemiologic aspects. *Am J Epidemiol* 1967;86:238–45.
10. *Pulmonary and Critical Care Medicine* St Louis: Mosby-Year Book, 1997.
11. Deepe GS Jr. Modulation of infection with *Histoplasma capsulatum* by inhibition of tumor necrosis factor-alpha activity. *Clin Infect Dis* 2005;41:S204–7.
12. Wheat J. Histoplasmosis: Experience during outbreaks in Indianapolis and review of the literature. *Medicine* 1997;76:339–54.
13. Wheat LJ. Diagnosis and management of histoplasmosis. *Eur J Clin Microbiol Infect Dis* 1989;8:480–90.
14. Wheat LJ, Kauffman CA. Histoplasmosis. *Infect Dis Clin North Am* 2003;17:1–19.
15. Adderson E. Histoplasmosis. *Pediatr Infect Dis J* 2006;25:73–4.
16. Goodwin RA Jr, Owens FT, Snell JD, et al. Chronic pulmonary histoplasmosis. *Medicine* 1976;55:413–52.
17. Wheat LJ, Wass J, Norton J, et al. Cavitary histoplasmosis occurring during two large urban outbreaks: Analysis of clinical, epidemiologic, roentgenographic, and laboratory features. *Medicine* 1984;63:201–9.
18. Lenhart SW, National Institute for Occupational Safety and Health, National Center for Infectious Diseases (U.S.). *Histoplasmosis: Protecting Workers at Risk,* rev ed. Cincinnatti: US Department of Health and Human Services, Public Health Service, Centers for Disease Control and Prevention, National Center for Infectious Diseases, 2004.
19. Murray PR, Baron EJ, American Society for Microbiology. *Manual of Clinical Microbiology,* 8th ed. Washington: ASM Press, 2003.
20. Durkin M, Kohler S, Schnizlein-Bick C, et al. Chronic infection and reactivation in a pulmonary challenge model of histoplasmosis. *J Infect Dis* 2001;183:1822–4.
21. McKinsey DS, Spiegel RA, Hutwagner L, et al. Prospective study of histoplasmosis in patients infected with human immunodeficiency virus: Incidence, risk factors, and pathophysiology. *Clin Infect Dis* 1997;24:1195–203.
22. Wheat J. Current diagnosis of histoplasmosis. *Trends Microbiol* 2003;11:488–94.
23. Hage CA, Davis TE, Egan L, et al. Diagnosis of pulmonary histoplasmosis and blastomycosis by detection of antigen in bronchoalveolar lavage fluid

using an improved second-generation enzyme-linked immunoassay. *Respir Med* 2007;101:43–7.

24. Wheat J, Sarosi G, McKinsey D, et al. Practice guidelines for the management of patients with histoplasmosis. Infectious Diseases Society of America. *Clin Infect Dis* 2000;30:688–95.

25. Procknow JJ. Pulmonary histoplasmosis in a farm family: Fifteen years later. *Am Rev Respir Dis* 1967;95:171–88.

26. Brodsky AL, Gregg MB, Loewenstein MS, et al. Outbreak of histoplasmosis associated with the 1970 Earth Day activities. *Am J Med* 1973;54:333–42.

27. Chamany S, Mirza SA, Fleming JW, et al. A large histoplasmosis outbreak among high school students in Indiana, 2001. *Pediatr Infect Dis J* 2004;23:909–14.

28. Luby JP, Southern PM Jr, Haley CE, et al. Recurrent exposure to *Histoplasma capsulatum* in modern air-conditioned buildings.[erratum appears in *Clin Infect Dis* 2005;41:769]. *Clin Infect Dis* 2005;41:170–6.

29. Wheat LJ. Histoplasmosis in Indianapolis. *Clin Infect Dis* 1992;14:S91–9.

30. Schlech WF 3rd, Wheat LJ, Ho JL, et al. Recurrent urban histoplasmosis, Indianapolis, Indiana, 1980–1981. *Am J Epidemiol* 1983;118:301–12.

31. Wheat LJ, Slama TG, Norton JA, et al. Risk factors for disseminated or fatal histoplasmosis: Analysis of a large urban outbreak. *Ann Intern Med* 1982;96:159–63.

32. US Public Health Service, Infectious Diseases Society of America, Centers for Disease Control and Prevention (US). 2001 USPHS/IDSA Guidelines for the Prevention of Opportunistic Infections in Persons Infected with Human Immunodeficiency Virus. Atlanta, GA: US Department of Health and Human Services, Centers for Disease Control and Prevention, 2001.

33. Bradsher RW, Chapman SW, Pappas PG. Blastomycosis. *Infect Dis Clin North Am* 2003;17:21–40.

34. Dworkin MS, Duckro AN, Proia L, et al. The epidemiology of blastomycosis in Illinois and factors associated with death. *Clin Infect Dis* 2005;41:e107–11.

35. Bradsher RW. Water and blastomycosis: Don't blame beaver. *Am Rev Respir Dis* 1987;136:1324–6.

36. Recht LD, Philips JR, Eckman MR, Sarosi GA. Self-limited blastomycosis: A report of thirteen cases. *Am Rev Respir Dis* 1979;120:1109–12.

37. Steele RW, Abernathy RS. Systemic blastomycosis in children. *Pediatr Infect Dis* 1983;2:304–7.

38. McAdams HP, Rosado-de-Christenson ML, Lesar M, et al. Thoracic mycoses from endemic fungi: Radiologic-pathologic correlation. *Radiographics* 1995;15:255–70.

39. Pappas PG, Threlkeld MG, Bedsole GD, et al. Blastomycosis in immunocompromised patients. *Medicine* 1993;72:311–25.

40. Sutliff WD, Cruthirds TP. *Blastomyces dermatitidis* in cytologic preparations. *Am Rev Respir Dis* 1973;108:149–51.

41. Wheat LJ, Kohler RB, Tewari RP. Diagnosis of disseminated histoplasmosis by detection of *Histoplasma capsulatum* antigen in serum and urine specimens. N Engl J Med 1986;314:83–8.

42. Chapman SW, Bradsher RW Jr, Campbell GD Jr, et al. Practice guidelines for the management of patients with blastomycosis. Infectious Diseases Society of America. *Clin Infect Dis* 2000;30:679–83.

43. Sarosi GA, Davies SF, Phillips JR. Self-limited blastomycosis: A report of 39 cases. *Semin Respir Infect* 1986;1:40–4.

44. MacDonald PD, Langley RL, Gerkin SR, et al. Human and canine pulmonary blastomycosis, North Carolina, 2001–2002. *Emerg Infect Dis* 2006;12:1242–4.

45. Centers for Disease and Prevention. Blastomycosis acquired occupationally during prairie dog relocation-Colorado, 1998. *MMWR* 1999;48:98–100.

46. Klein BS, Vergeront JM, Weeks RJ, et al. Isolation of *Blastomyces dermatitidis* in soil associated with a large outbreak of blastomycosis in Wisconsin. N Engl J Med 1986;314:529–34.

47. Davies SF, Sarosi GA. Epidemiological and clinical features of pulmonary blastomycosis. *Semin Respir Infect* 1997;12:206–18.

48. Anstead GM, Graybill JR. Coccidioidomycosis. *Infect Dis Clin North Am* 2006;20:621–43.

49. Galgiani JN, Ampel NM, Blair JE, et al. Coccidioidomycosis. *Clin Infect Dis* 2005;41:1217–23.

50. Kerrick SS, Lundergan LL, Galgiani JN. Coccidioidomycosis at a university health service. *Am Rev Respir Dis* 1985;131:100–2.

51. Einstein HE, Johnson RH. Coccidioidomycosis: New aspects of epidemiology and therapy (see comment). *Clin Infect Dis* 1993;16:349–54.

52. Schneider E, Hajjeh RA, Spiegel RA, et al. A coccidioidomycosis outbreak following the Northridge, Calif., earthquake. *JAMA* 1997;277:904–8.

53. Stevens DA. Coccidioidomycosis. N Engl J Med 1995;332:1077–82.

54. Drutz DJ, Catanzaro A. Coccidioidomycosis, part I. *Am Rev Respir Dis* 1978;117:559–85.

55. Chiller TM, Galgiani JN, Stevens DA. Coccidioidomycosis. *Infect Dis Clin North Am* 2003;17:41–57.

56. Drutz DJ, Catanzaro A. Coccidioidomycosis, part II. *Am Rev Respir Dis* 1978;117:727–71.

57. Galgiani JN. Coccidioidomycosis: A regional disease of national importance. Rethinking approaches for control. *Ann Intern Med* 1999;130:293–300.

58. Werner SB, Pappagianis D, Heindl I, Mickel A. An epidemic of coccidioidomycosis among archeology students in northern California. N Engl J Med 1972;286:507–12.

59. Centers for Disease Control and Prevention. Coccidioidomycosis in workers at an archeologic site-Dinosaur National Monument, Utah, June–July 2001. *MMWR* 2001;50:1005–8.

60. Fisher F, Bultman M, Pappagianis D. Operation Guidelines (version 1.0) for Geological Fieldwork in Areas Endemic for Coccidioidomycosis (Valley Fever) 2000.

14

Occupational Upper Respiratory Tract Infections

Paul C. Levy and Paul S. Graman

Infections of the upper respiratory tract include a broad variety of illnesses caused by a large number of different viruses and bacteria. Often referred to as the *common cold* by health care professionals, as well as by members of society at large, symptoms include varying degrees of nasal stuffiness, rhinorrhea, sore or scratchy throat, cough, and chest congestion [1]. Despite having similar clinical symptoms and signs, a large number of specific agents have been identified as causing this illness (Table 14-1). Most of these infections are caused by viruses from the rhinovirus, coronavirus, and parainfluenza and respiratory syncytial virus groups [1, 2]. Importantly, bacterial respiratory infections, such as those caused by group A beta-hemolytic streptococci, can be indistinguishable on clinical grounds from viral causes of colds. In about a third of patients, no identifiable infectious agent can be identified. Fortunately, the majority of upper respiratory tract infections (URIs) are self-limited and rarely lead to significant morbidity or mortality. Nevertheless, URIs are one of the most common causes for absenteeism and reduced worker productivity. Estimates of the economic costs of the common cold run in the billions of dollars, largely the result of lost worker productivity, visits to health care providers, and treatment costs [3].

This chapter reviews the most common causes of URIs and their associated clinical syndromes. It discusses their role in occupation-related illness as well as measures targeted at their prevention, control, and treatment. The spectrum and occupational issues related to influenza virus infection are discussed in Chapter 11.

Epidemiology

Infections of the upper respiratory tract occur in all age groups. In general, children average six to eight colds per year, whereas the rate for adults is roughly half that observed in children. There is a clear seasonal variation in attack rates throughout the world, with most infections occurring during the months of September through April [2], the colder months in the United States. However, attack rates are similar in warmer regions. It is a common misunderstanding that exposure to cold predisposes to infection. Studies have failed to demonstrate increased rates of infections in otherwise healthy individuals after controlled exposure to cold temperatures. Occupationally acquired URIs have not been well studied. Reports of outbreaks caused by specific agents are largely confined to military recruits and health care facilities [4].

Table 14-1
Infectious Agents Associated with Upper Respiratory
Tract Infections

Viruses	Nonviral Pathogens
Rhinovirus	*Mycoplasma pneumoniae*
Coronavirus	Group A beta-hemolytic
Parainfluenza virus	streptococci
Respiratory syncytial virus	*Moraxella catarrhalis*
Influenza virus	
Adenovirus	

Organisms Associated with Upper Respiratory Tract Infections

VIRAL PATHOGENS
RNA Viruses

Rhinoviruses. Rhinoviruses are the most common cause of the common cold, accounting for upwards of 50% of infections in adults [1,2]. These viruses are composed of single-stranded RNA and are members of the Picornaviridae family. There are approximately 100 antigenic serotypes, all of which are capable of causing disease in humans. The prevalence of rhinovirus-neutralizing antibody first appears in childhood and tends to peak in young adults. In older adults, the prevalence declines somewhat, probably as a result of reduced exposure. Although rhinoviruses cause infections of the upper respiratory tract throughout the year, there are usually peaks in the fall and spring in the United States. In the tropics, infection tends to occur during the rainy season. The reasons for seasonal and geographic variation in the prevalence of rhinovirus infections are not entirely clear, although changes in living conditions (e.g., indoor crowding) may play a role [2].

It appears that close contact is required for rhinovirus to spread. Infected nasal secretions containing the virus are typically spread by direct contact (e.g., from hand to hand), followed by self-inoculation of mucosal surfaces such as the nose and conjunctiva. Inhalation of infected aerosols also will result in transmission of infection, but this mechanism is felt to be a less important means of spread than direct contact. The slightly lower temperature of the nasal passages (33–34°C) provides a more favorable temperature to support growth than that found in the lower respiratory tract. In fact, core body temperatures of 37°C or higher actually may inhibit viral replication. Recent data have shown that rhinoviruses infect mucosal cells by first attaching to a specific surface protein, intercellular adhesion molecule 1 (ICAM-1). Methods to inhibit cellular attachment of the virus are currently under study and may provide a novel way to prevent infection in the future.

A typical rhinovirus infection lasts 7 days, although 25% of individuals may have symptoms for up to 2 weeks. In general, symptoms of rhinorrhea, sore or scratchy throat, and nasal stuffiness are most common. Complications include bacterial sinusitis and otitis media. Individuals with underlying asthma and chronic obstructive pulmonary disease (COPD) are at an increased risk of an acute exacerbation of lower respiratory symptoms during rhinovirus infection. The recent detection of rhinovirus RNA in lower airway cells of infected individuals may be part of the explanation for exacerbations in this setting [5].

Parainfluenza Virus. Human parainfluenza virus infections are found worldwide [6]. In addition to causing URIs, parainfluenza virus infections are a primary cause of lower respiratory tract diseases in the very young, the elderly, and individuals with compromised immune systems. Parainfluenza virus infections are responsible for approximately one-third of lower respiratory tract infections in children under 5 years of age.

Parainfluenza virus is an enveloped, single-stranded RNA virus. The viral envelope is embedded with two different proteins. These envelope proteins possess neuraminidase and hemagglutinin activity similar to that of influenza virus and have been used in serotyping. The distinct serotypes have antigens in common with several other members of the Paramyxoviridae family and have been linked with specific patterns of respiratory tract disease [6].

The clinical symptoms of parainfluenza virus infections include those often associated with the common cold, such as rhinitis, pharyngitis, and conjunctivitis. In addition, symptoms associated with infection of the lower respiratory tract, such as cough, wheeze, and sputum production, also may appear. The clinical spectrum of parainfluenza virus infections tends to bear a closer similarity to infections caused by respiratory syncytial virus (RSV) than to those usually associated with rhinoviruses. Parainfluenza viral infections in immunocompromised individuals (e.g., organ transplant recipients) can cause severe disease associated with significant risk of mortality [6].

Coronaviruses. Coronaviruses account for approximately 10–15% of upper respiratory tract infections but also have been associated with diarrheal illnesses. Similar to rhinoviruses, coronaviruses are also single-stranded RNA viruses but are much more difficult to culture. Only four antigenic types have been associated with human disease. The seasonal prevalence of coronavirus is different from that of rhinoviruses; it is observed most commonly in late fall, winter, and early spring. Recently, a severe acute respiratory syndrome (SARS) has been described and is caused by the coronavirus SARS-CoV. An up-to-date discussion of SARS is beyond the scope of this chapter, but further information can be found in Chapters 28 and 37 and on the website of the Centers for Disease Control and Prevention [7].

Respiratory Syncytial Virus. Respiratory syncytial virus (RSV) is an enveloped, single-negative-stranded RNA virus from the Paramyxoviridae family that derives its name from the characteristic syncytia observed in pathologic specimens [8]. Replication of the virus within host cells results in fusion of neighboring cells into large multinucleate syncytia. A lipid envelope bearing two important glycoproteins surrounds the viral genome. These proteins, G and F, facilitate attachment and fusion, respectively, of the virus to the host cell. The clinical significance of the two distinct antigenic groups and different subtypes is not yet known.

RSV is a major cause of respiratory tract disease in infants and young children, with the highest infection rates observed in babies during the first 6 months of life. Annual epidemics can last more than 5 months and occur worldwide. In the United States, infections may develop as early as November or December but not uncommonly may be delayed until spring. When outbreaks occur in day-care centers, attack rates are very high, with nearly 100% of susceptible infants being infected. Lower respiratory tract disease develops in more than 40% of infants infected with RSV, leading to clinical pneumonia, bronchiolitis, or tracheobronchitis. Repeated infections are common throughout all age groups, with attack rates of over 50% reported in studies of second exposures.

Recent epidemiologic studies have shown that RSV is also a significant cause of respiratory disease in adults [9]. The illness is usually milder than that observed in children, with symptoms similar to those associated with the common cold. However, data in the elderly suggest that RSV causes a similar number of respiratory-related illnesses as nonpandemic influenza A. Severe lower respiratory tract disease may develop in adults, especially individuals with significant comorbid health problems and transplant patients receiving immunosuppressive therapy. Complications of severe bronchitis, prolonged cough, and pneumonia are not uncommon. A significant number of hospitalizations for pneumonia, COPD, heart failure, and asthma are associated with adult RSV infections.

DNA Viruses

Adenovirus. Adenoviruses are best known clinically for their ability to cause infection in both the upper respiratory tract and the conjunctiva [10]. In contrast to most viruses associated with URIs, adenoviruses are composed of double-stranded DNA. The outer protein coat is made up of 252 capsomere subunits. These viruses belong to the genus *Mastadenovirus,* and at least 47 distinct serotypes have been identified. Human adenoviruses have been further classified into six subgenera (A–F). Adenoviruses interact with human cells in three distinct ways. When human epithelial cells are infected, the virus goes through a replicative cycle producing a large number of viral progeny. In addition, a latent or chronic infection that produces very few infectious particles has been described in lymphoid cells. Last, adenovirus has been shown to integrate itself into certain host cell DNA. This integration is termed *oncogenic transformation,* in which viral DNA is replicated with host cell division, but no infectious particles are produced.

Adenoviruses are found worldwide. Infection usually occurs from fall to spring, but sporadic cases may occur throughout the year. Over half of adenovirus infections do not lead to clinical symptoms. Approximately 2% of acute respiratory tract infections in adults and 5% in children are caused by adenoviruses. The high prevalence of serum antibodies to multiple serotypes in adults suggests frequent exposure throughout an individual's life span. The different serotypes are associated with age-specific infections [10]. For example, types 1, 2, 5, and 6 are often found in young children, whereas types 3, 4, and 7 are observed more often in young adults. Certain serotypes have been linked with outbreaks in military recruits.

Adenoviruses cause a wide spectrum of illnesses. The symptoms of clinically apparent respiratory tract infections are very similar to those observed with influenza and RSV, including rhinorrhea, fever, sore throat, and cough. Typically, these symptoms subside within 7 days. Lower respiratory tract involvement is more likely to occur in infants and children, but this is much less common than with RSV. A whooping cough–like syndrome has been described in patients with adenovirus infection, although a direct causal link has not been firmly established.

A great number of additional clinical infections are caused by adenoviruses [2, 10]. Pharyngoconjunctival fever occurs in small outbreaks and is associated with conjunctivitis and adenopathy in addition to the URI symptoms described earlier. Environmental sources such as contaminated swimming pools and ponds have been associated with outbreaks of adenovirus infection. Epidemic keratoconjunctivitis is caused by several serotypes of adenovirus and has been described in shipyard workers as well as outbreaks linked to contaminated ophthalmic solutions and a roller towel used for face and hand drying [10, 11].

NONVIRAL PATHOGENS
Moraxella catarrhalis

M. catarrhalis is a gram-negative diplococcal organism that has been recognized only in recent decades as an important cause of upper and lower respiratory tract disease in humans [12]. Originally classified as a species of the genus *Neisseria* and later *Branhamella,* it has been reclassified several times based on studies of its fatty acids and DNA.

Approximately 5% or more of healthy adults are colonized by *M. catarrhalis* in the upper respiratory tract. Colonization is more common, however, in children, the elderly, and individuals with underlying medical conditions. Similar to other upper respiratory tract infections, *Moraxella* infections are observed more commonly in the winter months. Recent studies have demonstrated that colonization is a dynamic process, with frequent elimination and recolonization cycles occurring spontaneously among carriers.

In general, *Moraxella* has been implicated in

causing disease in both the upper and lower respiratory tracts. Upper tract disease is more common in children, among whom *Moraxella* has been frequently linked with sinusitis and otitis media. Conditions of the lower respiratory tract that are observed most commonly are exacerbations of COPD, pneumonia in the elderly, and nosocomial pneumonia [12].

The generally accepted criteria for implicating *M. catarrhalis* as causing an exacerbation of COPD rely on securing sputum smears showing a predominance of intracellular gram-negative diplococci and/or sputum cultures. Even when these criteria are fulfilled, however, it is often unclear whether the organism is a colonizer or a true pathogen. The frequency with which *Moraxella* infections are associated with bronchitis and worsening COPD has been estimated to run as high as 30% of patients. *Moraxella* also may be responsible for upward of 10% of cases of pneumonia in the elderly. Generally, these patients have associated medical conditions such as COPD, heart failure, or diabetes. On clinical grounds alone, it is not possible to differentiate pneumonia caused by *Moraxella* from other causes of pneumonia. Diagnosis requires culture of the organism from sputum, blood, or pleural fluid (if present).

Mycoplasma pneumoniae

M. pneumoniae is one of 14 different mycoplasmal species found in humans [13]. Additional species infect plants and animals. Species of *Mycoplasma* are the smallest known free-living organisms. The small size of the *Mycoplasma* genome, which limits biosynthetic capabilities, explains the complex nutritional requirements of these organisms. They must first attach themselves to host cells for colonization or disease to occur. While the majority of mycoplasmas remain attached to the cell surface, intracellular translocation has been described and may protect the organism from the host's immune response.

Children and young adults are especially prone to disease caused by *M. pneumoniae.* Approximately 10–20% of pneumonias that originate in the community setting are attributable to *Mycoplasma* infections. The incubation period is long (2–4 weeks) prior to the development of fever, chills, headache, and sore throat. Cough is usually moderate to severe, especially worse at night, and generally nonproductive. Cough symptoms often can dominate the clinical picture and may persist for 3–4 weeks. While most patients develop only tracheobronchitis, about 3% of individuals have findings of pneumonia on chest radiographs. A number of extrapulmonary complications have been reported, including aseptic meningitis, meningoencephalitis, hemolytic anemia, arthritis, myopericarditis, and heart failure, among others. Mucocutaneous lesions can be observed in 25% or more of infected individuals.

A diagnosis of infection with *Mycoplasma* is usually made on clinical grounds because serologic markers may not develop until the second or third week of the illness. Cold agglutinin titers of 1:64 or greater are supportive of a diagnosis but are observed in fewer than 50% of patients and thus are nonspecific. Paired specimens, obtained 2–4 weeks apart, that demonstrate significant titers of IgM and/or IgG antibodies are diagnostic. Unfortunately, the clinical utility of serologic testing for early detection is limited. Therapy is usually empirical because there are no readily available and reliable diagnostic tests that will detect infection with *Mycoplasma* early in the illness [13, 14]. Treatment guidelines are discussed below.

Streptococcus pyogenes (Group A Streptococci)

Although *S. pyogenes* is the only species in the Lancefield group A streptococci, this organism is responsible for a wide variety of diseases in humans [15]. The more common clinical infections are streptococcal pharyngitis, impetigo, pneumonia, and empyema. Recently, it has been recognized that exotoxin-producing strains of group A streptococci can trigger a toxic shock–like syndrome with clinical characteristics very similar to the better-known staphylococcal toxic shock syndrome. In addition, the postinfectious syndromes of acute rheumatic fever and poststreptococcal glomerular nephritis can follow infection by *S. pyogenes*. With respect to URIs, this chapter focuses on pharyngitis caused by *S. pyogenes*. The reader is referred elsewhere for a more thorough discussion of the entire spectrum of disease caused by group A streptococci [15, 16].

Group A streptococcal pharyngitis, which is spread by contact with an infected individual, is one of the most common bacterial infections in childhood. Although infection also can develop after contact with an asymptomatic carrier, this is

thought to occur much less commonly. Outbreaks described in military barracks have been well characterized, showing that the likelihood of developing an infection is linked directly to the distance between one's bunk and the nearest carrier. Surveillance cultures have shown that about 15% of the population are asymptomatic carriers of group A streptococci. The incubation period is brief, with only 1–4 days between significant exposure and development of symptoms. The posterior pharynx usually appears reddened and swollen, and the tonsils often display a mottled grayish-white exudate. Tender lymph nodes are frequently found at the angle of the jaw and along the anterior cervical chain.

A number of investigators have tried to develop clinical criteria, such as exudative pharyngitis, tender adenopathy, and fever, to predict whether or not a patient's symptoms are due to infection by group A streptococci. Unfortunately, the sensitivity and specificity of these criteria have ranged between 50% and 75%. The recently available rapid diagnostic testing kits tend to be highly specific (about 90–95%) but less sensitive (50–90%). Sensitivity of the rapid detection kits hinges on the quality of the specimen obtained and the experience of the individual performing the rapid test. Thus it is reasonable to initiate treatment on the basis of a positive rapid test, but the Infectious Disease Society of America (ISDA) recommends that children with a negative test still should be evaluated with a properly obtained throat culture [17].

Prevention and Infection Control

Prevention of transmission of the broad group of infections just discussed is a major challenge. Although many of these agents have predictable seasonal attack rates, they all are ubiquitous in the general population. Simple measures in areas providing clinical care to patients are effective at reducing the risk of transmission. Unfortunately, these strategies generally require a large amount of time and effort, making them impractical in industry, schools, day-care centers, or other areas outside of patient care settings. In addition, there are few well-designed studies on the prevention and control of URIs outside health care settings. The recommendations detailed in Table 14-2 and discussed below have been best studied in hospital settings and have been developed by the Hospital Infection Control Practices Advisory Committee (HICPAC) and the Centers for Disease Control and Prevention (CDC) [18]. Especially in the non–health care setting, such as industry or schools, a strategy to keep infected individuals at home and out of the workplace needs to be seriously considered because this is usually the most effective means of controlling the spread of highly contagious URIs.

The backbone of infection control in hospitals is education and periodic monitoring of employee compliance with precautions, because employee knowledge and adherence to infection control recommendations are essential. HICPAC/CDC recently recommended a two-tiered approach to infection control. The first tier, termed *standard precautions*, details precautions that should be implemented in all clinical areas regardless of a patient's symptoms or diagnosis. Standard precautions include hand washing both before and after patient contact. Also, wearing gloves when touching blood, body fluids, secretions, and contaminated items cannot be overemphasized. Employees should perform hand hygiene before and after patient contact regardless of the patient's diagnosis or presumed infectious status and regardless of whether gloves are worn [18]. Health care facilities are also strongly encouraging patient visitors to abide by these recommendations as well.

While hand hygiene has been shown to reduce transmission from direct contact and autoinoculation, individuals with URIs also can spread infection through the generation of infectious aerosols (i.e., usually particle sizes of more than 5 μm in diameter) when coughing, sneezing, or talking. Transmission to health care workers or patient visitors can occur when infectious droplets come in contact with mucous membranes. Thus the second tier of infection control is *transmission-based precautions*, which are used in the care of patients with known or suspected specific pathogens [18]. Transmission-based precautions include three categories: airborne, contact, and droplet precautions. These more intensive preventive measures are important in minimizing the risk of acquiring infection from an ill patient as well as reducing the possible spread of infection from a clinical provider. Since most of the agents that cause URIs are spread by contact and/or droplet formation, *droplet precautions* are recommended in addition to standard precautions for the care of patients with URIs. However, in infants and young children who may have RSV, HICPAC/CDC recommends both contact and droplet precautions be implemented until a diagnosis is established [18].

Droplet precautions for hospitalized patients with URIs include placement in a private room (when available) or a room with another patient who has active infection with the same organism. Masks also should be worn by health care workers when working within 3 ft of these patients. Surgical masks are acceptable for droplet precautions. From a logistical standpoint, however, masks should be in place on entering a patient's room. Masks and eye protection (i.e., goggles or face shields), as well as clean, nonsterile gowns, should be used during encounters or procedures that may expose providers to splashes or sprays of body fluids or secretions. Proper and careful donning and removal of protective attire are essential to prevent accidental autoinoculation with pathogens. Currently recommended precautions for the individual infectious agents discussed in this chapter are outlined in Table 14-2.

The most recent HICPAC/CDC guidelines added new elements to standard precautions based on experiences gained in several workplace outbreaks of respiratory tract infections. This was an especially important lesson learned from the 2003 SARS outbreak, where infected patients placed concerned family members and health care providers at significant risk. The new strategy has been termed *respiratory hygiene/cough etiquette* (Table 14-3) and incorporates broad education efforts directed at health care providers, visitors, and patients with the use of language-appropriate signage in key areas (e.g., examination and waiting rooms). Individuals with symptoms of URIs are encouraged to wear a surgical mask (if tolerated) and cover their mouths and noses with a tissue when coughing. Hand hygiene by the infected individual, his or her accompanying family and/or friends, and examining providers is essential in reducing the risk of spread. Although difficult to sustain, implementation of hand hygiene in non–health care settings has been shown to be effective in reducing the frequency of respiratory illnesses [19, 20].

Table 14-2
Isolation Precautions to Reduce Transmission of Infections to Health Care Employees

Organism	Isolation Precautions	Duration of Precautions
Rhinovirus	Standard	None specified
Adenovirus[a]	Standard + droplet + contact	Duration of illness
Parainfluenza	Standard + contact	Duration of illness
Respiratory syncytial virus	Standard + contact	Duration of illness
Mycoplasma pneumoniae	Standard + droplet	Duration of illness
Branhamella catarrhalis	Standard	None specified
Streptococcus pyogenes[b]	Standard + droplet	24 hours after effective therapy initiated

[a]It is also important to eliminate potential environmental reservoirs such as solutions and/or equipment in eye clinics.
[b]In the event that a nosocomial case of group A streptococcal disease is identified, culture specimens of pharyngeal, rectal, vaginal, and/or skin lesions should be obtained, as appropriate, from employees who are potential sources.

Table 14-3
Elements of Respiratory Hygiene/Cough Etiquette

Education of staff, patients, and visitors
Language-appropriate signage in waiting room areas
Source control measures:
  Cover mouth/nose with tissue while coughing and prompt disposal of used tissues
  Surgical masks on the coughing person (if tolerated)
  Hand hygiene after contact with respiratory secretions
  Spatial separation if possible (>3 ft for persons with URI symptoms)

Source: Siegel JD, Rhinehart E, Jackson M, Chiarello L, and the Healthcare Infection Control Practices Advisory Committee. 2007 Guideline for isolation precautions: Preventing transmission of infectious agents in healthcare settings. June 2007; available at www.cdc.gov/ncidod/dhqp/pdf/isolation2007.pdf.

PREVENTION OF SPECIFIC INFECTIONS IN THE WORKPLACE
Respiratory Syncytial Virus

During seasonal community-wide RSV infections, health care workers are at increased risk of acquiring the infection themselves. Several studies have shown that a large number of clinical staff become infected in community outbreaks of RSV [8]. In general, implementation of infection control procedures such as hand washing, use of eye/nose goggles, patient isolation, and use of gowns and gloves reduces nosocomial spread. In one small prospective study, when use of eye/nose goggles in combination with standard precautions was compared with use of standard precautions alone, the infection rate of clinical staff was markedly reduced in the former group [21]. Only 8% of staff became infected with RSV, as determined by viral isolation and/or serology, compared with 34% of staff when eye/nose goggles were not used routinely. Implementation of respiratory hygiene/cough etiquette measures by patients, visitors, and staff in patient care areas is recommended. Additional outbreaks have been reported in long-term care facilities, bone marrow transplant centers, and intensive care units.

The incubation period for RSV ranges from 2–8 days, and viral shedding can last as long as 3–4 weeks. Compliance with *contact precautions* markedly reduces nosocomial spread. Most hospitals have found it impractical to restrict the work activity of health care employees with symptomatic viral upper respiratory tract infections. HICPAC suggests, however, that in the setting of a community outbreak of RSV or influenza, providers with symptoms of URI should be assigned to duties other than the care of high-risk patients until acute symptoms resolve [18].

Adenovirus

Infections caused by adenovirus may be especially difficult to control. Adenoviral keratoconjunctivitis is highly contagious, with outbreaks reported in ophthalmology clinics [11], as well as in hospitals and long-term care facilities [18]. In ophthalmology clinic outbreaks, attack rates were highest in persons evaluated for eye problems (21% of those at risk) and was especially high for those who underwent procedures that resulted in manipulation of the eyelids, tonometry (74%), or minor surgery (38%). Respiratory symptoms of URI are common but do not always accompany eye symptoms. The incubation period ranges from 5–12 days, and shedding of infectious virus may continue for 2 weeks after the onset of symptoms. Although

HICPAC recommends that an infected health care worker be relieved of his or her job responsibilities for as long as the worker remains symptomatic, the long period of viral shedding suggests that it may be reasonable to minimize high-risk patient contact for a more extended period. To minimize risk of transmission to care providers, standard precautions as well as contact precautions should be observed in the care of patients with adenovirus. Perhaps even more important, though, symptomatic patients should be educated to practice respiratory hygiene/cough etiquette while in health care facilities (see Table 14-3).

Group A Streptococcus

Patients with group A streptococcal infections can transmit infection to care providers by contact and/or through aerosols, although the latter mechanism is thought to be less common. Care providers who become infected may develop a wide variety of manifestations of group A streptococcal disease, including pharyngitis, cellulitis, and the group A toxic shock–like syndrome. Rarely have asymptomatic carriers been linked to nosocomial outbreaks of infection, although asymptomatic hospital personnel have been found to carry the organism in the pharynx, skin, rectum, and female genital tract [22].

The incubation period for group A streptococcal pharyngitis is 2–5 days. Other illnesses caused by group A streptococci have different incubation periods. Culture surveys of hospital personnel are not recommended unless an outbreak triggers the need for epidemiologic investigation. If an employee is identified as a carrier through culture surveys, the individual's activities should be restricted until 24 hours after starting appropriate therapy. Workers who are discovered to be carriers in the absence of a hospital outbreak are generally not treated, nor is there any need to restrict their patient care activities [14, 16].

Treatment

Employees with uncomplicated URI caused by the respiratory viruses discussed earlier generally need only supportive care [1, 2, 23, 24]. First-generation antihistamines are usually effective in reducing rhinorrhea and sneezing, perhaps related to the associated anticholinergic effects of these drugs. Topical as well as systemic decongestants may provide symptomatic relief of nasal obstruction but should be used with caution in patients with hypertension. If topical decongestants are used consistently for more than 3–4 days, symptoms may rebound when they are discontinued (rhinitis medicamentosa). Topical use of anticholinergic medications (e.g., ipratropium bromide) has been shown to reduce symptoms of rhinitis and nasal congestion owing to URIs [25].

Supportive care is largely all that is needed, with a few important exceptions pertaining to individuals with impaired immune function. Workers who have received bone marrow transplantation and those who are immunosuppressed because of solid-organ transplantation or immunosuppressive therapy are at a particularly high risk for developing lower respiratory tract disease. The associated risk for severe disease in workers infected with human immunodeficiency virus 1 (HIV1) appears to be less than that of organ transplant patients. Although there are no specific guidelines regarding these populations of workers, common sense dictates that individuals with these associated health problems should make strong efforts to avoid situations in which they would need to provide care for patients potentially infected with influenza and RSV. There are currently no definitive recommendations as to whether prophylactic ribavirin should be given to high-risk individuals in the event of significant exposure [8].

A number of additional treatments for the common cold have been studied, but their potential benefits are likely minimal or insignificant. Unproven therapies include inhalation of steam, large doses of vitamin C (e.g., greater than 1 g/day), zinc supplements, and nonsteroidal anti-inflammatory medications. Data on these treatments are mixed [23, 24].

Antibiotics are not indicated in the treatment of an uncomplicated URI. Despite this well-known fact, overuse of antibiotics runs rampant in many primary care office settings. It has been estimated that over 20% of antibiotic prescriptions in the United States are for "treatment" of upper respiratory tract infections. Ideally, antibiotic use should be reserved for treatment of specific complications such as bacterial sinusitis and pneumonia. More liberal use of antibiotics has been recommended in patients with underlying obstructive airways disease, especially if patients experience increased dyspnea and a change in sputum color or volume [26].

Antibiotic regimens recommended for individuals with *M. pneumoniae* infection include the use of doxycycline or macrolide antibiotics (e.g., erythromycin, clarithromycin, or azithromycin). An extended course of 2–3 weeks has been recommended to minimize the risk of relapse. A fluoroquinolone medication can be used as an alternative [13, 14].

M. catarrhalis susceptibility to antibiotics has evolved over the past 25 years. Beta-lactam antibiotics were highly effective until the development of resistance. Currently, nearly all isolates from both the United States and Europe produce beta-lactamase. Antibiotic susceptibility testing suggests that *M. catarrhalis* can be treated with oral cephalosporins (e.g., cefixime, cefaclor, or cefuroxime), trimethoprim-sulfamethoxazole, or ampicillin-clavulanate. Macrolides (e.g., azithromycin or clarithromycin) or fluoroquinolones also can be used [13].

The drug of choice for treatment of group A streptococcal pharyngitis remains penicillin, given its long track record of efficacy and safety [17]. Erythromycin or other macrolide antibiotics are recommended for individuals who are allergic to penicillin. It is worth emphasizing that treatment with penicillin reduces the incidence of acute rheumatic fever and suppurative complications of group A streptococcal infection, such as peritonsillar abscess, lymphadenitis, and mastoiditis, but constitutional symptoms such as fever and malaise may well resolve spontaneously in 3-4 days even in the absence of treatment. The ISDA guidelines offer advice for the management of individuals who have persistent carriage of group A streptococcus despite treatment with penicillin. Most authorities do not recommend retreatment of asymptomatic carriers because they are not thought to be at risk for postinfection sequela, nor are they thought to be a significant potential source of infection to others.

References

1. Heikkinen T, Jarvinen A. The common cold. *Lancet* 2003;361:51–9.
2. Gwaltney JM Jr. The common cold. In Mandell GL, Bennett JE, Dolin R (eds), *Principles and Practice of Infectious Diseases*, 6th ed. Philadelphia: Churchill Livingstone, 2005, pp 747–52.
3. Fendrick AM, Monto AS, Nightengale B, et al. The economic burden of non-influenza-related viral respiratory tract infection in the United States. *Arch Intern Med* 2003;163:487–94.
4. Wald TG, Shult P, Krause P, et al. A rhinovirus outbreak among residents of a long-term care facility. *Ann Intern Med* 1995;123:588–93.
5. Detection of rhinovirus RNA in lower airway cells during experimentally induced infection. *Am J Respir Crit Care Med* 1997;155:1159–61.
6. Wright PF. Parainfluenza viruses. In Mandell GL, Bennett JE, Dolin R (eds), *Principles and Practice of Infectious Diseases*, 6th ed. Philadelphia: Churchill Livingstone, 2005, pp 1998–2003.
7. Centers for Disease Control and Prevention. Severe Acute Respiratory Syndrome (SARS). Altanta: CDC, 2008 available at www.cdc.gov/ncidod/sars/index .htm.
8. Hall CB, McCarthy CA. Respiratory syncytial virus. In Mandell GL, Bennett JE, Dolin R (eds), *Principles and Practice of Infectious Diseases*, 6th ed. Philadelphia: Churchill Livingstone, 2005, pp 2008–26.
9. Falsey AR, Hennessey PA, Formica MA, et al. Respiratory syncytial virus infection in elderly and high-risk adults. *N Engl J Med* 2005;352:1749–59.
10. Baum SG. Adenovirus. In Mandell GL, Bennett JE, Dolin R (eds), *Principles and Practice of Infectious Diseases*, 6th ed. Philadelphia: Churchill Livingstone, 2005, pp 1835–41.
11. Dawson C, Darrell R. Infections due to adenovirus type 8 in the United States: I. An outbreak of epidemic keratoconjunctivitis originating in a physician's office. *N Engl J Med* 1963;268:1031–7.
12. Murphy TF. Lung infections: 2. *Branhamella catarrhalis:* Epidemiological and clinical aspects of a human respiratory tract pathogen. *Thorax* 1998;53:124–8.
13. Baum SG. *Mycoplasma pneumoniae* and atypical pneumonia. In Mandell GL, Bennett JE, Dolin R (eds), *Principles and Practice of Infectious Diseases*, 6th ed. Philadelphia: Churchill Livingstone, 2005, pp 2271–80.
14. Mandell LA, Wunderink RG, Anzueto A, et al. Infectious Diseases Society of America/American Thoracic Society consensus guidelines on the management of community-acquired pneumonia in adults. *Clin Infect Dis* 2007;44:S27–72.
15. Wessels MR. Streptococcal and enterococcal infections. In: Fauci AS, Braunwald E, Isselbacher KJ, et al (eds), *Principles of Internal Medicine*, 14th ed. New York: McGraw-Hill, 1998, pp 885–92.
16. Bisno AL, Stevens DL. Streptococcus pyogenes. In: Mandell GL, Bennett JE, Dolin R (eds), *Principles and Practice of Infectious Diseases*, 6th ed. Philadelphia: Churchill Livingstone, 2005, pp 2362–79.
17. Bisno AL, Gerber MA, Gwaltney JM, et al. Practice guidelines for the diagnosis and management of group a streptococcal pharyngitis. *Clin Infect Dis* 2002;35:113–25.

18. Siegel JD, Rhinehart E, Jackson M, Chiarello L, and the Healthcare Infection Control Practices Advisory Committee. 2007 Guideline for isolation precautions: Preventing transmission of infectious agents in healthcare settings. June 2007; available at www.cdc.gov/ncidod/dhqp/pdf/isolation2007.pdf.

19. Ryan MA, Christian RS, Wohlrabe J. Handwashing and respiratory illness among young adults in military training. *Am J Prevent Med* 2001;21:79–83.

20. White C, Kolble R, Carlson R, et al. The effect of hand hygiene on illness rate among students in university residence halls. *Am J Infect Control* 2003;31: 36470.

21. Gala CL, Hall CB, Schnabel KC, et al. The use of eye-nose goggles to control nosocomial respiratory syncytial virus infection. *JAMA* 1986;256:2706–8.

22. Nosocomial Group A streptococcal infections associated with asymptomatic health-care workers—Maryland and California, 1997. *MMWR* 1999;48: 163–6.

23. Spector SL. The common cold: Current therapy and natural history. *J Allergy Clin Immunol* 1995;95: 1133–8.

24. Mossad SB. Clinical review: Fortnightly review—treatment of the common cold. *Br Med J* 1998;317: 33–6.

25. Hayden FG, Diamond L, Wood PB, et al. Effectiveness and safety of intranasal ipratropium bromide in common colds. *Ann Intern Med* 1996;125:89–97.

26. The COPD Guidelines Group of the Standards of Care Committee of the BTS. British Thoracic Society guidelines for the management of chronic obstructive pulmonary disease. *Thorax* 19;52:S1–28.

15 Occupational Plague

Shadaba Asad and Andrew W. Artenstein

Historical Background

Throughout history, plague has occupied an important role in shaping the course of human events. It has been the cause of pandemic disease and innumerable deaths, it has altered the geopolitical and military balance among civilizations [1, 2], and it may have led to genetic selection within Europeans, thus possibly affecting the course of future epidemic diseases such as human immunodeficiency virus (HIV) infection [3]. Three distinct plague pandemics have been recorded to date [4].

THE FIRST PANDEMIC

The plague epidemics that occurred between AD 541 and 750 are referred to as the *first*, or *Justinian*, *pandemic*. The first of these epidemics began in Ethiopia and spread quickly from Pelusium and Egypt, through the Middle East to the Mediterranean basin, and to a limited extent, to Mediterranean Europe. The second through eleventh epidemics (AD 558–654) occurred in 8- to 12-year cycles and affected all the "known world" at the time, that is, North Africa, Europe, central and southern Asia, and Arabia. Mortality rates of 15–40% were recorded, and it has been estimated that 50–60% of the population perished between AD 541 and 700. A number of economic, social, and political consequences, including the weakening of Byzantine Europe, have been attributed in part to this first pandemic [5].

THE SECOND PANDEMIC

Plague in Asia spread westward from AD 1330–1346 along the trade routes, arriving in Sicily in 1347 and heralding the beginning of the *second pandemic* [5]. The first epidemic wave (AD 1347–1351), which later came to be known as "the Black Death," was one of the worst natural disasters in history. It was estimated to have killed one-fourth of the population of Europe and to have changed the course of history [1]. Epidemics continued to occur in 2- to 5-year cycles from AD 1361–1480 and well into the seventeenth century.

THE THIRD PANDEMIC

The *third*, and *current*, *pandemic* is believed to have begun in the nineteenth century near the China-Tibet border, reaching the ports of Hong Kong in 1894 and Bombay in 1898 [6,7]. Over the next two decades, the pandemic expanded globally because infected rats disembarked from ships in the ports of Africa, Australia, Europe, Asia, the Middle East, South America, and the United States. A major epidemic occurred in the San Francisco area during the first part of the twentieth century. In the 1960s and 1970s, Vietnam reported thousands of cases annually; more than 10,000 cases of plague were reported during the U.S. military involvement there [7].

Microbiology

Alexandre Yersin isolated *Yersinia pestis,* the causative agent of plague, during the Hong Kong epidemic of 1894 [7]. *Y. pestis* belongs to the genus *Yersinia* within the family Enterobacteriacae and is a gram-negative, nonmotile, nonsporulating coccobacillus measuring 1–3 μm in length [8]. It exhibits bipolar staining on Giemsa, Wayson, or Wright's staining, thus explaining its characteristic "safety pin" appearance in stained smears of clinical specimens [4]. It grows aerobically, albeit slowly, on most culture media, including blood and MacConkey agar; small colonies are visible on the latter after 24–48 hours at 35°C. *Y. pestis* does not ferment lactose and is citrate-, urease-, and indole-negative [9].

Three biotypes of *Y. pestis* have been identified based on their ability to ferment glycerol and reduce nitrate: Antiqua, Orientalis and Medievalis. They do not appear to differ in their pathology or virulence. The Orientalis biotype is the etiologic agent of the third pandemic in Southeast Asia, Africa, and the western hemisphere. The Antiqua biotype occurs in parts of Africa, southeastern Russia, and central Asia. The Medievalis biotype, thought to have been responsible for the Black Death, occurs in natural foci around the Caspian Sea [10]. The organism harbors a number of virulence and transmission factors that enable its survival and transmission in the mammalian host and flea vector: pesticin sensitivity factor, associated with reduced siderophore-binding capability, thus affecting iron uptake; a plasminogen-activating protease that endows the organism with fibrinolytic activity and affects dissemination, especially in the pneumonic form of disease [11]; *Yersinia* outer protein, which may interfere with host responses such as phagocytosis and thrombin-platelet aggregation; murine toxin, a requirement for survival in fleas; F1 capsular antigen, serving an antiphagocytic function; serum resistance factor, conferring resistance to complement-mediated lysis; pH 6 antigen, mediating entry into naive macrophages; and endotoxin (lipopolysacchride),

which is responsible for the major pathogenic effects of plague, including sepsis and multi–organ system failure with its associated adult respiratory distress syndrome (ARDS) and disseminated intravascular coagulation (DIC) [12]. The entire genome of *Y. pestis* has been decoded recently; the genetic sequence suggests possible evolution from *Y. pseudotuberculosis* within the last 20,000 years [13].

Epidemiology

INCIDENCE AND PREVALENCE

Plague continues to evoke fear and panic in disproportion to the relatively low number of annually reported cases. Human plague occurs worldwide; most cases are reported from rural areas and developing countries. In the 15-year period from 1989–2003, 25 countries reported a total of 38,310 cases, with 2,845 plague-associated deaths, an overall mortality rate of 7.5% [14]. During this time, cases of human plague were reported nearly every year from eight countries: Democratic Republic of the Congo, Madagascar, and the United Republic of Tanzania in Africa; Peru and the United States in the Americas; and China, Mongolia, and Vietnam in Asia. However, 80.3% of plague cases and 84.5% of deaths were reported from Africa during the 1990s [14].

Since the early 1990s, an increased incidence of human plague has been observed, and this is particularly apparent in Africa. Such a trend may be due to both an actual increase in plague activity in its natural foci and an improvement in notification to the World Health Organization (WHO) by member countries. Additionally, recent modeling research points to the phenomenon of climate change as a possible potentiator of plague activity in animal reservoirs; an increase in spring temperatures of 1°C is predicted to have a major amplifying effect on the prevalence of *Y. pestis* in its natural hosts [15]. Over the past decade, at least three geographic areas experienced resurgent outbreaks of human plague after silent periods of more than 30 years: India in 1994 and 2002, Indonesia in 1997, and Algeria in 2003 [14]. Plague also has reemerged recently in sub-Saharan Africa, specifically East Africa and Madagascar [16]. The most recent outbreak occurred in the Democratic Republic of Congo, Zobia, Bas Uele district, Oriental Province, involving 130 suspected cases of pneumonic plague and 57 deaths [17].

Unlike the situation in other parts of the world, nearly all the diagnosed cases of human plague in the United States are reported to public health authorities. The occurrence of plague in the United States is sporadic and seasonal, with the highest incidence of cases during the spring and summer months, when people spend more time outdoors and are more likely to come into contact with the vector. During the 50-year period from 1947–1996, 390 cases of human plague were reported in the United States, with 60 deaths (15%) [18]. All these cases occurred in the following 10 states, listed in rank order by prevalence: New Mexico, California, Arizona, Colorado, Utah, Oregon, Idaho, Nevada, Wyoming, and Texas [7]. Over the 26-year period from 1970–1995, an average of 13 cases per year were reported to the Centers for Disease Control and Prevention (CDC); nearly 90% of these occurred in New Mexico, Arizona, Colorado, and California [19]. In November 2002, two human bubonic plague cases were diagnosed in New York City, yet acquired in New Mexico [20]. Because the two patients became ill in a nonendemic region, especially coming on the heels of the anthrax attacks of 2001, these cases raised the specter, subsequently ruled out, of bioterrorism using plague.

LIFE CYCLE, TRANSMISSION, AND PATHOGENESIS

Plague is primarily a zoonotic disease; humans are incidental hosts. Rodents serve as the primary host for plague and are the major sources of human exposure. Natural animal reservoirs include dozens of wild and domestic mammal species, most notably wild urban and sylvatic rodents and larger predators/carnivores [21]. Throughout the world, rats are the most important urban reservoir of plague, although other important sylvatic reservoirs include ground squirrels [22], rock squirrels [7], prairie dogs [23, 24], mice, bobcats, rabbits, voles, and chipmunks [7]. Domestic cats have become an increasingly recognized source of human infection [25–27]. Plague is transmitted among its animal reservoirs by the bite of infected fleas or, less commonly, by ingestion of contaminated animal tissues by the host. Fleas are the only arthropod vectors known to transmit *Y. pestis* in nature, and more than 30 species of fleas can perform this task, al-

though the Oriental rat flea, *Xenopsylla cheopsis,* may be the most important [28]. The human body louse also has been shown to be a potential vector of *Y. pestis* transmission in an experimental rabbit model [29].

Transmission usually occurs once the bacteria have multiplied in the proventriculus of the flea to such an extent during repetitive blood meals that the flea gut becomes obstructed by the bacilli, and infected blood is regurgitated into the wound of the host [7]. The coagulase enzyme of *Y. pestis* contributes to this "blocking" of the flea gut by causing ingested blood to clot [7]. The flea continues to feed, and the cycle of regurgitation continues, increasing the vector's efficiency of transmission. Other potential mechanisms of flea-borne transmission include penetration of infected flea feces into abraded skin, either directly or through inoculation by scratching, or mechanical transmission via contaminated flea mouthparts [7].

Human infection with plague occurs when infected fleas leave their small mammal hosts and infest humans. The greatest risk, historically, exists when epizootics cause high mortality in rodent populations (i.e., "ratfall") because fleas will leave a dead rat on cooling of its body temperature and tend to seek alternative hosts in close proximity. This explains the increased incidence of human urban plague during times of war, social upheaval, and natural disaster, all settings that lead to crowding and unsanitary conditions. In the United States, most human cases are acquired in or around the patient's residence through the bite of an infected flea either from a sylvatic source [7] or a domestic cat or dog [7, 25, 26]. Because domestic cats may develop clinical plague and die of overwhelming infection, they may represent an additional human risk factor during epizootics; in fact, primary plague pneumonia has been reported to be transmitted directly from cats to humans [27].

Human cases of plague in the southwestern United States are therefore most closely associated with activities that result in contact with infected fleas or their hosts, such as camping, hunting, or working in enzootic areas. Additional risk factors associated with acquiring plague in endemic areas include the presence of harborage (e.g., debris) and food sources (e.g., garbage) for wild rodents in close proximity to the home and, possibly, failure to control fleas on domestic pets [7]. Native American peoples, especially the Navajo, account for a dispro-portionate share of the reported cases probably be-cause of socioeconomic and cultural factors that place them in close contact with infected animals [7, 30]. Human plague also may occur as a result of direct inoculation with body fluids or tissues of in-fected animals, events that may supervene during the skinning or consuming of dead squirrels or rab-bits [7, 30]. Entry appears to be mediated through breaches in the skin or mucosa of the susceptible host. Finally, human-to-human transmission of plague pneumonia is theoretically possible but has not been reported from the United States since the Los Angeles outbreak of 1924 [31], although the 1994 epidemic in India heightens concern about this mode of transmission and spread [32]. *Y. pestis* has the potential to be used as a biological weapon and is considered to be a category A threat agent owing to the high mortality rate of pneumonic plague, the potential for secondary spread of cases during an epidemic, and the proven potential for mass production in aerosol form [33].

OCCUPATIONAL RISK FACTORS

Aside from the obvious occupational risks for hunters, taxidermists, archeologists, veterinarians, and other animal handlers, there have been rare re-ports of laboratory-acquired infection in humans. The first report, in 1901, was of a medical student working to prepare plague antiserum using samples from the San Francisco outbreak [34]. Burmeister and colleagues reviewed the existing literature in 1962 and presented four additional cases of labora-tory-acquired pneumonic plague and a secondary case in one of the contacts [35]. The likely portal of entry was inhalation, and the resulting illness was similar to the naturally occurring disease. The po-tential for laboratory-acquired plague probably has increased, in large part resulting from an expansion of funded research investigation under the auspices of biodefense.

Prevention and Control

PREVENTIVE MEASURES (NONBIOLOGIC)

Attempts to eliminate fleas and rodents from their natural environment in endemic areas is impracti-cal; therefore, preventive measures should be di-rected to home, work, and recreational settings where the risk of acquiring plague is high. A com-bined approach using environmental sanitation, public education on exposure avoidance, and pre-ventive antibiotics for suspected exposures is the recommended approach to prevent human plague [36]. Effective environmental sanitation reduces the risk of persons being bitten by infectious fleas of rodents and other animals in places where peo-ple live, work, and recreate. Removal of rodent food sources and harborage around human habitats and rodent-proofing homes, buildings, warehouses, and feed sheds are fundamental approaches to re-ducing the risk of plague exposure and can be im-plemented by the lay public. The application of chemical insecticides and rodenticides by trained professionals may be necessary under select cir-cumstances. Similarly, trained professionals can in-spect and fumigate shipping cargoes to control the importation of plague-infected rat populations.

In areas where plague is enzootic among wild rodents, such as the western United States, public health education for both the general public and the medical community is critical to limiting human plague cases. Such messages are intended to foster avoidance of exposure to disease-bearing an-imals and their fleas and must include recommen-dations regarding environmental sanitation (see above), reporting of sick or dead animals to the local health department, the use of gloves if han-dling potentially infected animals is unavoidable, and the regular flea-control treatment of pet dogs and cats.

Health authorities advise that antibiotics be given for a brief period to people who have been exposed to the bites of potentially infected rodent fleas (e.g., during a plague outbreak) or who have handled an animal known to be infected with the plague bacillus [36]. Prophylactic antimicrobials should be given to someone who has had close ex-posure to a person or an animal (e.g., domestic cat) with suspected plague pneumonia and to health care workers who have had close exposure to a pa-tient with suspected or proven pneumonic plague [19]. Close exposure, generally defined as within 2 m (~6.5 ft) of the patient, uniformly applies to household contacts; thus prophylaxis recommen-dations extend to these groups as well [7, 19]. The current recommendations for postexposure pro-phylaxis are discussed in detail below.

Veterinary workers and others known to be at high risk of contact with infected animals should be educated on ways to minimize exposure to infection and should wear gloves and eye protection when handling animals [19]. Droplet respiratory precautions, including the use of masks, should be adopted when treating severely ill domestic cats in enzootic areas [19].

INFECTION CONTROL

All suspected cases of plague should be reported promptly to the state health authorities for confirmation of diagnosis and epidemiologic investigation. Patients diagnosed with bubonic plague without pulmonary involvement warrant standard infection control precautions only. Individuals suspected of having plague pneumonia should be placed in isolation and managed under strict respiratory droplet precautions [37, 38] for at least 48 hours after the institution of appropriate antimicrobial therapy. Droplet precautions necessitate the use of disposable surgical masks, gloves, gowns, and eye protection. Those with confirmed plague pneumonia should be kept in respiratory isolation until their sputum cultures are negative [9].

Microbiology personnel should be alerted when a diagnosis of plague is suspected. Routine clinical specimens are managed in the laboratory under Biosafety Level 2 (BSL-2) precautions; however, manipulation of cultures, such as centrifuging, grinding, and vigorous shaking, and animal studies should be performed in a negative-pressure biosafety cabinet using BSL-3 precautions [9].

Bodies of patients who have died of plague should be handled with strict standard precautions by trained personal only. Precautions for transporting corpses for burial should be similar to those that apply to transporting sick patients. Aerosol-generating procedures such as bone sawing during surgery or postmortem examination would be associated with special risk and are not recommended. If such procedures are necessary, high-efficiency particulate air-filtered masks and negative-pressure rooms should be used, as is done in cases of tuberculosis [33].

As mentioned earlier, close contacts of plague patients should be offered postexposure prophylaxis. If this is refused, they should be observed carefully for the next 7 days; the development of signs and symptoms of plague warrants immediate treatment. In addition to beginning antibiotic prophylaxis, people in close contact with pneumonic plague patients should follow droplet precautions and use a surgical mask for 48 hours following initiation of antibiotic prophylaxis. *Y. pestis* is very sensitive to sunlight and heating and does not survive for long outside the host; hence there is no need for environmental decontamination of an area exposed to an aerosol of plague [33].

MEDICAL SURVEILLANCE

Because of the high case-fatality rate and the potential for epidemic disease, plague has been designated a class I notifiable disease and is therefore subject to regulations that require mandatory reporting of suspected cases to state health departments [19]. These authorities are required to investigate cases and subsequently report to the CDC, under whose authority further investigation is carried out. Laboratory-confirmed cases are subsequently reported to the WHO in Geneva, Switzerland. Once sporadic cases in humans have been confirmed, epidemiologic surveillance must be undertaken to identify potential geographic areas of risk and to assess the potential for additional cases. Such surveillance measures may include detailed risk and exposure histories from patients and contacts, assessment of the environment in which a case has occurred, and evaluation of the geographic vicinity for evidence of epizootic disease, such as obtaining information about rodent die-offs, performing autopsies of dead rodents and other potential hosts, and trapping live animals for serologic testing, as well as flea assessments [7]. Environmental control measures should be carried out in concert with surveillance. Education of those at risk, maintenance of strict hygienic standards, vector control by insecticide use, rodent control by rodenticides and trapping, rat-proofing of houses, and vaccination of high-risk individuals are all strategies believed to be effective in the control of plague [7]. The CDC and the WHO also have continued to reassess and enhance international surveillance systems for the detection and control of epidemic plague [7, 39], most recently in the contexts of the 1994 epidemic in India [32] and ongoing bioterrorism planning.

IMMUNIZATION

There is currently no licensed vaccine in routine use to prevent plague. A formalin-killed vaccine, Plague Vaccine USP, was available previously for use by persons at high risk of exposure, such as laboratory personnel. Its manufacture in the United States was discontinued in 1999, and at present, it is only produced by one source worldwide (Commonwealth Serum Laboratories, Ltd., Parkville, Australia). The killed vaccine does not protect against pneumonic plague and has limited utility compared with modern sanitation and prophylactic antibiotics in combating epidemic disease [19].

Research to produce improved vaccines that may protect against pneumonic plague is underway. Recombinant subunit vaccines that express both the F1 and V antigens of *Y. pestis* appear to elicit robust protection against subcutaneous or aerosolized challenge in mice [40, 41]. A phase I trial of such a combination vaccine in 24 healthy adults demonstrated immunogenicity at each dose level, although no clear dose response was noted [42]. In addition to the parenteral route, plague vaccine formulations are being developed for delivery via the inhaled, oral, and transcutaneous routes [43–45].

Clinical Manifestations

Plague generally presents in either the bubonic, septicemic, or pneumonic form. Occasionally, less common presentations predominate. Bubonic plague is the most common form of the disease, accounting for more than 80% of cases in the United States [4], although in a review of 27 cases of plague that occurred over a 25-year period at the Gallup Indian Medical Center in New Mexico, only 37% presented with classic bubonic symptoms and signs [46]. During an incubation period that averages 2–8 days following the bite of an infected flea, bacteria proliferate in regional lymph nodes. The patient subsequently develops an abrupt onset of fevers, rigors, malaise, prostration, and headache, sometimes with prominent gastrointestinal symptoms, followed within 24 hours by a bubo, a 1- to 10-cm, exquisitely tender, firm mass of lymph nodes in the area draining the site of infection [47]. Buboes most commonly occur in the groin; femoral nodes are affected more frequently than inguinal nodes; axillary or cervical lymph nodes are involved less commonly [30]. Involvement of intraabdominal nodes may mimic a surgical abdomen. Skin lesions are uncommon in bubonic plague, and the typical absence of a lesion at the site

of the flea bites, as well as the absence of an ascending lymphangitis, may distinguish this form of plague from other bacterial infections [9]. Occasionally, vasculitic lesions of the distal extremities occur as a result of the sepsis syndrome that may accompany bubonic plague. The bubonic presentation of plague may result in a fulminant clinical course progressing rapidly to death in 50–60% of untreated patients [19], but because of its distinctive clinical presentation in endemic areas, most patients are treated appropriately and early, with more than an 85% survival rate [9].

Septicemia in plague infection can occur during the course of bubonic disease or, less frequently, without detectable lymphadenopathy. Primary septicemic plague presents as a nonspecific febrile illness and tends to progress to septic shock and death in approximately 50% of cases owing in large part to delays in diagnosis and treatment [46]. If not treated expeditiously, septicemic plague with its attendant endotoxemia can progress to a systemic inflammatory response causing DIC, hemorrhage, multi–organ system failure, and irreversible shock [9].

Primary pneumonic plague is acquired via the inhalation route from a patient or domestic animal (e.g., cat) with pneumonic plague or by exposure to aerosols of plague cultures in a laboratory. This form of plague is rare and is associated with an exceedingly high mortality. Secondary pneumonic plague accounted for more than 90% of the 36 reported cases of pneumonic plague in the United States between 1950 and 1983 [48]. Secondary pneumonic plague results from hematogenous dissemination of bacteria from a bubo and presents in the setting of fever and lymphadenopathy with cough and/or hemoptysis, pleuritic chest pain, radiographic findings of patchy bronchopneumonia, cavities or confluent consolidation, and purulent sputum containing plague bacilli [9]. Pneumonic plague is highly contagious by the droplet route.

Plague meningitis is a rare complication of inadequately treated bubonic plague and presents with symptoms and signs similar to those of other forms of bacterial meningitis. This form of plague is seen most commonly in children and is associated with a high mortality rate. Plague also can present as a pharyngitis or tonsillitis and is thought to occur rarely in these forms following inhalation or ingestion of bacilli [7]. Nearly 20% of the cases in a recent series presented in this fashion, and mortality was high, largely owing to diagnostic delays [46].

Differential Diagnosis

The finding of a bubo, especially of the groin, in concert with constitutional symptoms and potential exposure history in an endemic area is highly suggestive of plague and certainly warrants empirical treatment for this diagnosis. Other potential causes of inguinal lymphadenitis in areas known to be endemic for plague include secondary syphilis, lymphogranuloma venereum, granuloma inguinale, chancroid, primary genital herpes, cat scratch disease, loiasis, onchocerciasis, and glandular tularemia [49]. The latter infection shares many characteristics of plague, including exposure history and systemic signs, but it usually presents as an ulceroglandular syndrome with an ulcer or pustule at the site of vector inoculation and typically affects the axillary or epitrochlear chains more commonly than the groin [7]. The differential diagnosis of bubonic plague involving the axillary or cervical lymph nodes includes acute pyogenic infections caused by streptococci and staphylococci; scrofula, owing to either tuberculosis or nontuberculous mycobacteria [50]; cat scratch disease; tularemia; deep mycotic infections; toxoplasmosis; and typical or atypical forms of viral mononucleosis [49].

The clinical presentation of patients with pneumonic plague is similar to that of other severe, typical and atypical forms of community-acquired pneumonia, as well as pneumonia owing to tularemia, psittacosis, Q fever, and influenza. This has been reviewed elsewhere recently [51]. When pneumonia occurs following dissemination from a bubo, the diagnosis is generally apparent. Patients with primary septicemic plague present similarly to those with sepsis from other causes. A history of potential exposure in an endemic area should raise the possibility of both plague and septicemic tularemia. Additional diagnoses that should be considered in the differential diagnosis of septicemic plague include meningococcemia, viral hemorrhagic fevers, acute leukemia, and Rocky Mountain spotted fever [51]. In patients who present with a predominance of gastrointestinal symptoms and signs, an intraabdominal source of sepsis, such as appendicitis, cholecystitis, or bowel obstruction,

should be considered. Plague pharyngitis typically presents as a bacterial pharyngitis, tonsillitis, or sinusitis, and therefore, the symptoms are frequently attributed to streptococcal disease. In the series of Crook and colleagues, all the patients who presented with pharyngitis were treated initially with penicillin, thus resulting in a therapeutic delay and, subsequently, a higher mortality rate [46].

Diagnostic Evaluation

The diagnosis of plague should be considered in patients presenting with an acute febrile illness, lymphadenitis, or fulminant pneumonia who have a history of potential exposure to rodents or other small mammals in known plague-enzootic regions or who have traveled recently to such areas. Additional clinical vigilance should be exercised regarding the possibility of bioterrorism. Once a clinical diagnosis is suspected, blood, respiratory, and tissues specimens should be collected, the laboratory notified of the clinical suspicion, and consideration given to empirical treatment. Routine laboratory data generally are consistent with those of a systemic infection but are otherwise nondiagnostic [46]. The radiographic appearance of pneumonic plague is also not diagnostic.

Blood cultures should be obtained before administration of antibiotics. Blood cultures, using standard bacteriologic media, were noted to be positive for *Y. pestis* in 96% of patients in a recent series of mixed clinical presentations [46], but in the early stages of bubonic plague, only 27% of blood cultures were found to be positive in previous reports [7]. A bacteriologic diagnosis may be accomplished in more than 75% of patients through smear and culture of a bubo aspirate or sputum (the latter in patients with pneumonic disease) [7, 46]. Because buboes are not typically fluctuant, aspirates may require an initial injection of a small amount of saline. Aspirated sanguineous material should undergo Gram and Wayson staining. The Gram stain reveals polymorphonuclear leukocytes and plump gram-negative coccobacilli; on Wayson stain, *Y. pestis* appear as light blue bacilli with dark blue polar bodies, giving the organism a "closed safety pin" appearance that is characteristic but not pathognomonic. A direct immunofluorescence test also can be applied to clinical specimens [9].

Serologic diagnosis via a passive hemagglutination test using fraction I of *Y. pestis* can be performed on acute- and convalescent-phase serum [9]. Serologic testing may be used to diagnose plague in those with negative cultures; a fourfold or greater increase in titer or a single titer of 1:16 or greater is presumptive evidence of infection. A single titer of 1:128 may be considered diagnostic. Most patients seroconvert 1–2 weeks after the onset of symptoms, although early antibiotic treatment may delay seroconversion by several weeks. Positive titers diminish gradually over months to years. A rapid antigen-detection dipstick test using monoclonal antibodies to *Yersinia* F1 antigens has been developed and deployed recently in endemic areas of Madagascar; the concordance between field testing and reference laboratory testing is nearly 90% [52]. The rapid test detects 42% more positive clinical specimens than culture and 31% more than the enzyme-linked immunosorbent assay (ELISA) with overall positive and negative predictive values of 90.6% and 86.7%, respectively [52]. Polymerase chain reaction (PCR) also can be used for the presumptive identification of *Y. pestis*, although this is not available in most clinical settings [53].

Treatment

Case fatality owing to plague depends on a number of factors, including time to initiation of antibiotics, access to advanced supportive care, and dose of inhaled bacteria. To avoid excess mortality, early administration of antimicrobial therapy that is effective against *Y. pestis* is essential [46]. Parenteral streptomycin has been the drug of choice for plague for more than 50 years and has reduced the mortality in bubonic plague to less than 5% [9]. It is not readily available in the United States owing to the absence of manufacturers. However, gentamicin is readily available and has shown efficacy in the treatment of plague. Both in vitro antimicrobial susceptibility studies of *Y. pestis* and animal studies suggest noninferiority of gentamicin compared with streptomycin [54, 55]. Additionally, one retrospective review of 75 human plague cases in the United States during the period 1985–1999 noted no significant clinical or survival differences between those treated with gentamicin versus streptomycin [56]. In this study, bubonic disease

accounted for the majority (84%) of cases; no cases of primary pneumonic plague were included. Thus the efficacy of gentamicin in pulmonary disease was not shown.

A single prospective, randomized clinical trial compared gentamicin with doxycycline for the treatment of bubonic plague in children and adults in Tanzania [57]; both therapies were found to be effective, with low rates of adverse events. For patients with contraindications to the use of aminoglycosides, alternatives include not only doxycycline but also fluoroquinolones or chloramphenicol [32]. Chloramphenicol has been recommended for plague meningitis because of its penetration across the blood-brain barrier. The clinical efficacy of fluoroquinolones cannot be ascertained with certainty from the literature, although in vitro data suggest efficient bacterial killing with less resistance selection using levofloxacin than with streptomycin [58]. While most patients show rapid clinical improvement and become afebrile within 3 days, a 10-day course should be completed because buboes may continue to harbor viable bacteria despite clinical improvement [7]. For children, aminoglycosides are preferred; alternatives include doxycycline, chloramphenicol, and fluoroquinolones [32]. Gentamicin is the therapy of choice in pregnancy [32]. Doxycycline or a fluoroquinolone may be used for postexposure prophylaxis in the setting of a mass-casualty (e.g., bioterrorism) event [33].

Multidrug resistance has been reported in a strain of *Y. pestis* isolated from a 16-year-old boy with bubonic plague in Madagascar [59, 60]. Outbreaks of multidrug-resistant plague have not as yet been documented but are of concerning because resistance is plasmid-mediated. It has been theorized that horizontal genetic transfer of plasmids may occur in the flea midgut, resulting in the potential for the spread of drug-resistant *Y. pestis* [61]. Of additional public health concern is the finding of mobile resistance elements, similar in structure to the backbone of the multidrug-resistant *Y. pestis* plasmid, in chicken, pork, and beef samples from various regions in the United States, suggesting a possible agricultural reservoir to mediate drug resistance in plague [62]. Therefore, surveillance of resistance patterns, as well as modification of treatment regimens based on susceptibility patterns, is important.

Occupational Considerations

As discussed earlier, plague is an uncommon occupational disease of hunters, taxidermists, veterinarians, animal handlers, and others whose livelihood or avocations place them in potential contact with the bacteria's hosts or vectors in endemic areas. There are also rare reports of plague as a laboratory-acquired infection [35]. The major risk factors in the laboratory setting include direct contact with cultures or infectious materials from humans or small mammal hosts, infectious aerosols generated during manipulation of cultures or infected animal tissues, and percutaneous injuries from contaminated laboratory equipment [63]. The appropriate prevention and control measures were discussed earlier. Plague also may be viewed as an occupational disease risk of health care providers, especially in the case of pneumonic disease, in which the disease may be spread by droplets. Droplet precautions plus eye protection should be used for patients with suspected plague until pneumonia has been excluded or until the patient has received 72 hours of therapy and clinical improvement occurs. Similar precautions should be taken while aspirating buboes. Close contacts (i.e., contact with a patient at 2 m of distance) of patients with pneumonic plague should receive postexposure prophylaxis, as outlined earlier [64]. Individuals who have died of plague should be handled with standard precautions [33]. Contact with remains should be limited to trained personnel, and the safety precautions for transporting corpses for burial should be the same as those for transporting ill patients. Aerosol-generating procedures, such as bone sawing associated with surgery or postmortem examinations, are associated with heightened risks of transmission and are not recommended [33]. If such aerosol-generating procedures are necessary, high-efficiency particulate air-filtered masks (N-95 or greater) and negative-pressure respiratory isolation should be used [33].

References

1. Cantor NF. *In the Wake of the Plague: The Black Death and the World It Made.* New York: Simon & Schuster, 2002.
2. Trevisanato SI. Did an epidemic of tularemia in Ancient Egypt affect the course of world history? *Med Hypoth* 2004;63:905–10.
3. Galvani AP, Slatkin M. Evaluating plague and smallpox as historical selective pressures for the CCR5-delta 32 HIV- resistance allele. *Proc Natl Acad Sci USA* 2003;100:15276–9.
4. Perry RD, Fetherston JD. *Yersinia pestis:* Etiologic agent of plague. *Clin Microbiol Rev* 1997;10:35–66.
5. Drancourt M, Raoult D. Molecular insights into the history of plague. *Microbes Infect* 2002;4:105–9.
6. Barnes AM, Quan TJ. Plague. In Gorbach SL, Bartlett JG, Blacklow NR (eds), *Infectious Diseases.* Philadelphia: Saunders, 1992, pp 1285–91.
7. Butler T. Plague and Other Yersinia Infections. In Greenough WB, Merigan TC (eds), *Current Topics in Infectious Diseases.* New York: Plenum Press, 1983.
8. Farmer JJ, Kelly MT. Enterobacteriaceae. In Balows A, Hausler W, Herrmann K, et al (eds), *Manual of Clinical Microbiology.* Washington: American Society of Microbiology, 1991, p 381.
9. Butler T. *Yersinia* species (including plague). In Mandell GL, Bennett JE, Dolin R (eds), *Principles and Practice of Infectious Diseases,* 6th ed. New York: Elsevier Churchill Livingstone, 2005, pp 2691–700.
10. Guiyoule A, Grimont F, Iteman I, et al. Plague pandemics investigated by ribotyping of *Yersinia pestis* strains. *J Clin Microbiol* 1994;32:634–41.
11. Lathem WW, Price PA, Miller VL, et al. A plasminogen-activating protease specifically controls and development of primary pneumonic plague. *Science* 2007;315:509–13.
12. Dennis DT, Gage KL. Plague. In Cohen J, Powderly W (eds), *Infectious Diseases,* 2d ed. New York: Elsevier, 2004, pp 1641–48.
13. Zhou D, Han Y, Song Y, et al. Comparative and evolutionary genomics of *Yersinia pestis. Microbes Infect* 2004;6:1226–34.
14. World Health Organization. *Weekly Epidemiological Report,* August 13, 2004; 79(33):301–308; available at *www.who.int/wer.*
15. Stenseth NC, Samia NI, Viljugrein H, et al. Plague dynamics are driven by climate variation. *Proc Natl Acad Sci USA* 2006;103:13110–5.
16. Chanteau S, Ratsifasoamanana L, Rasoamanana B, et al. Plague a reemerging disease in Madagascar. *Emerg Infect Dis* 1998;4:101–4.
17. World Health Organization. Communicable Diseases Surveillance and Response (CSR), March 15, 2005.
18. Centers for Disease Control and Prevention. Fatal human plague—Arizona and Colorado, 1996. *MMWR* 1997;46:617–20.
19. Centers for Disease Control and Prevention. Prevention of plague: Recommendations of the Advisory Committee on Immunization Practices (ACIP). *MMWR* 1996;45:1–15.
20. Imported plague—New York City, 2002. *MMWR* 2003;52:725–28.
21. Madon MB, Hitchcock JC, Davis RM, et al. An overview of plague in the United States and a report of investigations of two human cases in Kern County, California, 1995. *J Vector Ecol* 1997;22:77–82.

22. Craven RB, Maupin GO, Beard ML, et al. Reported cases of human plague infections in the United States, 1970–1991. *J Med Entomol* 1993;30:758–61.

23. Anderson SH, Williams ES. Plague in a complex of white-tailed prairie dogs and associated small mammals in Wyoming. *J Wildl Dis* 1997;33:720–32.

24. Cully JF Jr, Barnes AM, Quan TJ, et al. Dynamics of plague in a Gunnison's prairie dog colony complex from New Mexico. *J Wildl Dis* 1997;33:06–19.

25. Kaufmann AF, Mann JM, Gardiner TM, et al. Public health implications of plague in domestic cats. *J Am Vet Med Assoc* 1981;179:875–8.

26. Eidson M, Tierney LA, Rollag OJ, et al. Feline plague in New Mexico: Risk factors and transmission to humans. *Am J Public Health* 1988;78:1333–5.

27. Werner SB, Weidmer CE, Nelson BC, et al. Primary plague pneumonia contracted from a domestic cat at South Lake Tahoe, CA. *JAMA* 1984;251:929–3.

28. Wilson ME. The power of plague. *Epidemiology* 1995;6:458–60.

29. Houhamdi L, Lepidi H, Drancourt M, et al. Experimental model to evaluate the human body louse as a vector plague. *J Invest Dermatol* 2006;194:1589–96.

30. Cleri DJ, Vernaleo JR, Lombardi LJ, et al. Plague pneumonia disease caused by *Yersinia pestis*. *Semin Respir Infect* 1997;12:12–23.

31. Centers for Disease Control and Prevention. Human plague—United States, 1981. *MMWR* 1982;31:74–6.

32. Centers for Disease Control and Prevention. Human plague—India, 1994. *MMWR* 1994;43:689–91.

33. Inglesby TV, Dennis DT, Henderson DA, et al. Plague as a biological weapon: Medical and public health management. *JAMA* 2000;283:2281–90.

34. Link VB. *A History of Plague in the United States of America.* Washington: US Department of Health, Education and Welfare, US Government Print Office, 1955.

35. Burmeister RW, Tigertt WD, Overholt EL. Laboratory-acquired pneumonic plague: Report of a case and review of previous cases. *Ann Intern Med* 1962;56:789–800.

36. CDC Plague Home Page. Available at www.cdc.gov/ncidod/dvbid/plague/index.htm.

37. Benson AS. Plague. In *Control of Communicable Diseases Manual.* Washington: American Public Health Association, 1995, pp 335–8.

38. Garner JS. Guideline for isolation precautions in hospitals. The Hospital Infection Control Practices Advisory Committee. *Infect Control Hosp Epidemiol* 1996;17:53–80.

39. Fritz CL, Dennis DT, Tipple MA, et al. Surveillance for pneumonic plague in the United States during an international emergency: A model for control of imported emerging diseases. *Emerg Infect Dis* 1996;2:30–6.

40. Glynn A, Freytag L, Clements J. Effect of homologous and heterologous prime boost on the immune response to recombinant plague antigens. *Vaccine* 2005;23:1957–65.

41. Reed DS, Martinex MJ. Respiratory immunity is an important component of protection elicited by subunit vaccination against pneumonic plague. *Vaccine* 2006;24:2283–89.

42. Williamson E, Flick-Smith H, LeButt C, et al. Human immune response to plague vaccine comprising recombinant F1 and V antigens. *Infect Immun* 2005;73:3598–608.

43. Eyles JE, Williamson ED, Speirs ID, et al. Protection studies following bronchopulmonary and intramuscular immunization with *Yersinia pestis* F1 and V subunit vaccines coencapsulated in biodegradable microspheres: A comparison of efficacy. *Vaccine* 2000;18:3266–71.

44. Eyles JE, Elvin SJ, Westwood A, et al. Immunization against plague by transcutaneous and intradermal application of subunit antigens. *Vaccine* 2004;22:4365–73.

45. Balada-Llasat JM, Panilaitis B, Kaplan D, et al. Oral inoculation with type III secretion mutants of *Yersinia pseudotuberculosis* provides protection from oral, intraperitoneal, or intranasal challenge with virulent *Yersinia. Vaccine* 2007;25:1526–33.

46. Crook L, Tempest B. Plague: A clinical review of 27 cases. *Arch Intern Med* 1992;152:1253–6.

47. Butler T. *Yersinia* infections: Centennial of the discovery of the plague bacillus. *Clin Infect Dis* 1994;19:655–61.

48. Barnes AM, Poland JD. Plague in the United States—1983. *MMWR* 1984;33:15–21SS.

49. Swartz MN. Lymphadenitis and lymphangitis. In Mandell G, Bennett J, Dolin R (eds), *Principles and Practice of Infectious Diseases,* 4th ed. New York: Churchill Livingstone, 1995, pp 936–44.

50. Artenstein AW, Kim JH, Williams WJ, et al. Isolated peripheral tuberculous lymphadenitis in adults: Current clinical and diagnostic issues. *Clin Infect Dis* 1995;20:876–82.

51. Artenstein AW. Bioterrorism and biodefense. In Cohen J, Powderly WG (eds), *Infectious Diseases,* 2d ed. St Louis: Mosby, 2003, pp 99–107.

52. Chanteau S, Rahalison L, Ralafiarisoa L, et al. Development and testing of a rapid diagnostic test for bubonic and pneumonic plague. *Lancet* 2003;361:211–6.

53. Loeiz C, Herwegh S, Wallet F, et al. Detection of *Yersinia pestis* in sputum by real time PCR. *J Clin Microbiol* 2003;41:4873–5.

54. Wong JD, Barash JR, Sandfort RF, et al. Susceptibilities of *Yersinia pestis* strains to 12 antimicrobial agents. *Antimicrob Agents Chemother* 2000;44:1995–6.

55. Frean JA, Arntzen L, Capper T, et al. In vitro activities of 14 antibiotics against 100 human isolates of *Yersinia pestis* from a Southern African plague focus. *Antimicrob Agents Chemother* 1996;40:2646–7.

56. Boulanger LL, Ettestad P, Fogarty JD, et al. Gentamicin and tetracyclines for the treatment of human plague: Review of 75 cases in New Mexico, 1985–1999. *Clin Infect Dis* 2004;38:663–9.

57. Mwengee W, Bulter T, Mgema S, et al. Treatment of

plague with gentamicin or doxycycline in a random-ized clinical trial in Tanzania. *Clin Infect Dis* 2006; 42:614–21.

58. Louie A, Deziel MR, Liu W, et al. Impact of resis-tance selection and mutant growth fitness on the relative efficacies of streptomycin and levofloxacin. *Antimicrob Agents Chemother* 2007;51:2661–7.

59. Galimand M, Guiyoule A, Gerbaud G, et al. Mul-tidrug resistance in *Yersinia pestis* mediated by a transferable plasmid. *N Engl J Med* 1997;337:677–80.

60. Dennis DT, Hughes JM. Multidrug resistance in plague. *N Engl J Med* 1997;337:702–4.

61. Galimand M, Carniel E, Courvalin P. Resistance of *Yersinia pestis* to antimicrobial agents. *Antimicrob Agents Chemother* 2006;50:3233–6.

62. Welch TJ, Fricke WF, McDermott PF, et al. Multiple antimicrobial resistance in plague: An emerging public health risk. *PLoS One* 2007;3:1–6.

63. Richmond JY, McKinney RW (eds). *Biosafety in Mi-crobiological and Biomedical Laboratories,* 3rd ed. Washington: US Department of Health and Human Services, 1993.

64. Prentice MB, Rahalison L. Plague. *Lancet* 2007;369: 1196–207.

16 Occupational Hantavirus Pulmonary Syndrome

Randall L. Updegrove

Viruses classified into the *Hantavirus* genus [1] of the family Bunyaviridae were first isolated in Korea in 1978. However, sporadic epidemics have been attributed to these viruses since the 1930s and, possibly, earlier. The hantaviruses are trisegmented, single-stranded RNA viruses that are lipid-enveloped. During the Korean conflict in the 1950s, some 3,000 members of the United Nations forces developed an illness characterized by fever, hemorrhage, and acute renal failure. This illness complex became known by several names, including *Songo fever, hemorrhagic nephrosonephritis, Korean hemorrhagic fever, Manchurian fever,* and *epidemic hemorrhagic fever.* Since then, the illness has been classified as *hemorrhagic fever with renal syndrome* (HFRS). In 1993, intense multiagency collaborative efforts led to the identification and characterization of a second illness, first seen in the southwestern United States, caused by a different hantaviral type, known as *hantavirus with pulmonary symptoms* (HPS). Information as to the nature of these illnesses, as well as the causative viruses, continues to be refined and expanded, and ongoing research identifies new viral hosts and viral serotypes of this genus.

Hantavirus Pulmonary Syndrome

HPS was first identified in May of 1993, after an outbreak of a fatal respiratory illness in the southwestern United States. The first cases were reported in New Mexico, when two Native American residents of the same house died within 5 days of each other. Over the next months, several other states throughout the southwest, including Arizona, Colorado, and Utah, reported similar cases. Using nucleotide sequence analysis and polymerase chain reaction (PCR) on extracted RNA from autopsy specimens, as well as the identification of antibodies crossreactive to hantaviruses—rodent-borne viruses responsible for HFRS in Eurasia [1]—suspicion grew surrounding a probable association of this disease with HFRS. The patterns of crossreactivity in human convalescent and rodent serum specimens, the fact that the clinical syndrome was dissimilar to HFRS, and the pattern of immunohistochemical reactivity associated with this disease led to the identification of a previously unrecognized hantavirus. Shortly thereafter, the clinical and pathologic features of this syndrome were clarified, risk factors for infection were identified, and the primary rodent host was found [2–5]. The virus was named the *Four Corners virus* and, later, the *Sin Nombre virus* or *Muerto Canyon virus,* and molecular diagnostic assays, as well as serologic testing, were quickly developed.

EPIDEMIOLOGY

Although HPS was first identified in 1993, retrospective serologic testing showed evidence of a case as early as 1959 [6], with another case identified retroactively from 1978. Up to 1996, the Centers for Disease Control and Prevention (CDC) confirmed 131 U.S. cases of HPS, with an overall case-fatality rate 49.6%. Of confirmed cases, the mean age of patients is 35 years, with a range of 11–69 years. Gender analysis shows no predilection for either sex, with approximately 50% of patients male and 50% female. Cases have occurred in Caucasians as well as in African Americans, with any racial or age variations in infection rates most likely attributable to differences in activities that facilitate exposure to the rodent reservoir for the hantavirus, usually in rural settings.

Although the initial cases occurred in the Southwest in Native Americans, 24 additional states have reported cases since 1993. Although most of these cases are west of the Mississippi River, cases have been reported in Rhode Island, New York, Florida, and Louisiana. Outside the United States, HPS has been identified in Argentina, Canada, Brazil, and Paraguay [7].

TRANSMISSION RISK FACTORS

HPS appears to be caused by multiple agents that together form a distinctive evolutionary clade [8]. Three hantavirus serotypes have been identified that cause HPS: Sin Nombre virus (SNV), Black Creek Canal virus (BCCV), and Bayou virus (BV). SNV has been associated with a case-fatality rate that is 10 times that of the other hantaviruses. SNV acts as the prototypical HPS and was the first virus isolated from HPS patients in the spring and summer of 1993 [9]. BCCV has been associated with HPS in Florida [10]. Antigens and viral sequencing of patients with HPS in Texas and Louisiana have identified the presence of BV in that area. In 1993, nucleotide sequence analysis of amplified DNA products from three PCR-positive humans and six PCR-positive rodents of the species *Peromycus maniculatus* (deer mouse) showed a closely related, direct genetic link between the hantavirus sequences in the rodents and the human cases. The deer mouse is found throughout the United States, except the Southeast. It acts as the principal reservoir for the hantavirus responsible for HPS, carrying SNV.

Rodent infection parallels that found with the hantaviruses associated with HFRS, with the virus shed in saliva, urine, and feces. Human infection occurs in a similar manner as that of the HFRS viruses as well, primarily occurring via aerosolized virus inhaled from rodent excreta that inoculates arid materials. In addition, transmission can occur when dried materials contaminated with rodent saliva are disturbed and introduced into disrupted skin, the conjunctivae, or water or food. Human-to-human transmission has not been seen. The deer mouse is the primary reservoir for the virus in the southwestern United States and Canada [4]. The white-footed mouse (*Peromyscus leucopus*) acts as the main host for an SNV-like virus in the eastern United States [11]. In Florida (southern Florida), the cotton rat (*Sigmodon hispidus*) is the reservoir for BCCV, and the rice rat (*Oryzomys palustris*) is the reservoir for BV [12]. In addition, hantavirus antibodies have been found in the pinon mouse (*P. truei*), the chipmunk (*Eutamias dorsalis*), the brush mouse (*P. boylii*), and the western chipmunk (*Tamias* species).

Similar to HFRS virus, outbreaks of HPS appear to be geographically and seasonally influenced and parallel rodent migrations and eradication efforts. Although little is known about activities that lead to a high risk of infection, studies indicate that entering buildings or areas that are infrequently opened or disturbed contributes to increasing risk [2]. The number of rodents in a house or building also obviously contributes to this risk, with rodent-infested structures found to be associated with several cases [13]. Geographic distribution of HPS cases in the United States is strongly tied to the relatively more frequent close proximity of humans and certain rodent species habitats. For example, the deer mouse and white-footed deer mouse often live near residents and domestic settings. Therefore, the density of their populations can be high in areas frequently visited by humans. Additionally, the rodents tend to migrate indoors, particularly during colder months, and to farms during the fall and spring. Seeking cooler areas, rodents may move to forested areas in the warmer summer months.

OCCUPATIONS AT RISK

Occupations found to be at risk for HPS viral infection, therefore, are logically those that tend to place workers in the proximity of the higher rodent populations during the higher-risk seasons, with clustering of cases common. Fortunately, cases of occupationally related HPS virus infection are infrequent [14, 15]. Occupations at or potentially at risk include grain farmers, farm workers, laborers, repairmen, construction workers, animal pest control workers, livestock specialists, field biologists, forestry workers, park rangers, mill workers, utility workers, feedlot workers, various technicians, hikers, and service industry workers, as well as others (Table 16-1). In 1994, a study showed the presence of antibody to SNV in 6 of 528 mammalogists and rodent workers with varying degrees of rodent exposures in the United States [15]. Although person-to-person transmission, particularly among hospital employees and patients, has not occurred, infection has occurred in laboratory workers handling rodents. Some of these cases may have involved transmission of the virus via rodent bite.

Table 16-1A
HPS: Occupations at Risk

Laboratory workers	Farm workers
Service repairmen	Technicians
Ranch workers	Service industry workers
Shepherds	Longshoremen
Pest control workers	Immunologists
Maintenance workers	Plumbers
Animal handlers	Granary workers
Construction workers	Mammologists
Field biologists	Park rangers
Mill workers	Utility employees
Laborers	

Table 16-1B
CDC: Situations Associated with Hantavirus Infection

- Increasing number of host rodents in human dwellings
- Occupying or cleaning previously vacant cabins or other dwellings that are actively infested with rodents
- Barn and other outbuilding cleanings
- Disturbing excreta or rodent nests around the home or workplace
- Residing in or visiting areas where substantial increases have occurred in numbers of host rodents or numbers of hantavirus-infected host rodents
- Handling mice without gloves
- Keeping captive wild rodents as pets or research subjects
- Handling equipment or machinery that has been in storage
- Disturbing excreta in rodent-infested areas while hiking or camping
- Sleeping on the ground
- Hand plowing or planting

PREVENTION AND CONTROL
Administrative Controls

Recommendations to decrease hantavirus exposure risk include precautions for individuals or groups working in occupations associated with rodent, rodent excreta, or contaminated dust exposure [16]. In addition, state health departments and the CDC have formed the *HPS Registry,* through which the effectiveness and usefulness of recommended risk-reduction efforts are assessed. Reporting of new cases by health care providers to this registry remains paramount for the ongoing identification of additional pathogenic hantaviruses, rodent hosts, and risk factors for infection.

Prevention and effective treatment of HPS, as well as HFRS, are based on three goals: minimization of rodent population clusters in the workplace, avoidance of exposure to contaminated materials or aerosolized excreta, and awareness of the early signs of disease to allow for rapid treatment and medical support. Prevention begins with public awareness, particularly among occupational groups at risk for exposure, routinely engaging in certain relatively higher-risk activities. Some of these activities include inhabitation of previously vacant buildings, field crop harvesting or planting, barn cleaning, disturbing rodent-infested areas while in woods or fields, or residing or working in areas with an increasing or relatively high rodent population (including laboratories). Eradication of the rodent reservoirs, however, is infeasible. Risk reduction can occur through proper environmental hygiene activities that deter rodents from colonizing the work area. The CDC has issued recommendations for eliminating rodent infestations by rodent-proofing urban and suburban buildings and reducing the rodent populations via modification of the rodent habitat and sanitation [17, 18] (Table 16-2).

Additionally, the CDC has issued general precautions for residents of affected areas, including ways that the rodent population of a residence (or workplace) can be reduced, affecting primary prevention strategies for hantavirus risk reduction (Table 16-3).

The clean-up of rodent-contaminated areas also involves adherence to recommended procedural steps (Table 16-4).

When working with vacant dwellings with large amounts of rodents or in areas previously occupied by an individual with a confirmed hantavirus

Table 16-2
CDC Recommendations for Elimination of Rodent Infestation

- Before rodent elimination work is begun, ventilate closed buildings or areas inside buildings by opening doors and windows for at least 30 minutes. Use an exhaust fan or cross-ventilation, if possible. Leave the area until the airing-out period is finished. This airing may help to remove any aerosolized virus inside the closed-in structure.
- Seal, screen, or otherwise cover all openings into the home that have a diameter of more than $\frac{1}{4}$ inch. Then set rodent traps inside the building, using peanut butter as bait. Use only spring-loaded traps that kill rodents.
- Treat the interior of the structure with an insecticide labeled for flea control; follow specific label instructions. Insecticide sprays or powders can be used in place of aerosols if they are appropriately labeled for flea control. Rodenticides also may be used while the interior is being treated, as outlined below.
- Remove captured rodents from the traps. Wear rubber or plastic gloves while handling rodents. Place the carcasses in a plastic bag containing a sufficient amount of a general-purpose household disinfectant to thoroughly wet the carcasses. Seal the bag, and then dispose of it by burying in a 2- to 3-ft-deep hole or by burning. If burying or burning are not feasible, contact the local or state health department about other appropriate disposal methods. Rebait and reset all sprung traps.
- Before removing the gloves, wash gloved hands in a general household disinfectant and then in soap and water. A hypochlorite solution (prepared by mixing 3 tablespoons of household bleach in 1 gallon of water) may be used in lieu of a commercial disinfectant. When using the chlorine solution, avoid spilling the mixture on clothing or other items that may be damaged. Thoroughly wash hands with soap and water after removing the gloves.
- Leave several baited spring-loaded traps inside the house at all times as a further precaution against rodent reinfestation. Examine the traps regularly. Disinfect traps no longer in use by washing in a general household disinfectant or the hypochlorite solution. Disinfect and wash gloves as described above, and wash hands thoroughly with soap and water before beginning other activities.

Table 16-3
CDC Recommendations for Reducing Rodent Populations

- Keep all food and water covered and stored in rodent-proof containers with tight-fitting lids.
- Store all garbage inside the building or in outbuildings in rodent-proof metal or thick plastic containers with tight-fitting lids.
- Wash dishes and cooking utensils immediately after use, and remove all spilled food.
- Dispose of trash and clutter.
- Use spring-loaded rodent traps continuously.
- For an adjunct to traps, use rodenticide with bait under a plywood or plastic shelter (covered bait station) on an ongoing basis inside the house.
- Keep rodents from entering the building:
  - Use steel wool or cement to seal, screen, or otherwise cover all openings into the home that have a diameter of $\frac{1}{4}$ in or more.
  - Place metal roof flashing as a rodent barrier around the base of wooden, earthen, or adobe dwelling up to a height of 12 in and buried in the soil to a depth of 6 in.
  - Place 3 inches of gravel under the base of homes or under mobile homes to discourage rodent burrowing.
- Within 100 ft of the building, reduce food and shelter sources for rodents:
  - Used raised cement foundations in new construction of sheds, barns, outbuildings, or woodpiles.
  - When possible, place woodpiles 100 ft or more from the house, and elevate wood at least 12 in from the ground.
  - Store grains and animal feed in rodent-proof containers.
- Near buildings, remove food sources that might attract rodents, or store food and water in rodent-proof containers.
- Store hay on pallets, and use traps or rodenticide continuously to keep hay free of rodents.
- Do not leave pet food in feeding dishes.
- Dispose of garbage and trash in rodent-proof containers that are elevated at least 12 in off the ground.
- Haul away trash, abandoned vehicles, discarded tires, and other items that may serve as rodent nesting sites.
- Cut grass, brush, and dense shrubbery within 100 ft of the home.
- Place spring-loaded rodent traps at likely spots for rodent shelter within 100 ft around the building, and use continuously.
- Use and EPA-registered rodenticide approved for outside use in covered bait stations at places likely to shelter rodents within 100 ft of the building.

Table 16-4A
CDC Recommendations for Clean-Up of Contaminated Areas

- Persons involved in the clean-up should wear rubber or plastic gloves.
- Spray dead rodents, nests, droppings, foods, or other items that have been tainted by rodents with a general-purpose household disinfectant or chlorine solution. Soak the material thoroughly, and place in a plastic bag. When clean-up is complete, or when the bag is full, seal the bag. Then place the sealed bag into a second plastic bag, and seal it. Dispose of the bagged material by burying in a 2- to 3-ft-deep hole or by burning. If these alternatives are not feasible, contact the local or state health department concerning other appropriate disposal methods.
- After the preceding items have been removed, mop floors with a solution of water, detergent, and disinfectant or chlorine solution [such as $1\frac{1}{2}$ cups household bleach diluted in 1 gallon of water (1:10 solution)]. Spray dirt floors with a disinfectant solution. A second mopping or spraying of floors with a general-purpose household disinfectant is optional. Carpets can be effectively disinfected with household disinfectants or by commercial-grade steam cleaning or shampooing. To avoid generating potentially infectious aerosols, do not vacuum or sweep dry surfaces before mopping. Spray dirt floors with a disinfectant or chlorine solution.
- Disinfect countertops, cabinets, drawers, and other durable surfaces by washing them with a solution of detergent, water, and disinfectant, followed by an optional wiping-down with a general-purpose household disinfectant.
- Rugs and upholstered furniture should be steam cleaned or shampooed. If rodents have nested inside furniture and the nests are not accessible for decontamination, the furniture should be removed and burned.
- Launder potentially contaminated bedding and clothing with hot water and detergent, handling the dirty laundry with rubber, latex, nitrile, or vinyl gloves and then washing or disinfecting the gloves. After removing the clean gloves, thoroughly wash bare hands with soap and warm water. Machine-dry laundry of a high setting, or hang out to air dry in the sun.

Table 16-4B
CDC Recommendations for Clean-Up of Dead Rodents and Rodent Nests

- Wear rubber, latex, vinyl, or nitrile gloves.
- In the western United States, use insect repellent (containing DEET) on clothing, shoes, and hands to reduce the risk of fleabites that might transmit plague.
- Spray dead rodents and rodent nests with a disinfectant or a chlorine solution, soaking them thoroughly.
- Place the dead rodent or nest in a plastic bag or remove the dead rodent from the trap and place it in a plastic bag.
- When cleanup is complete, seal the bag, place it into a second plastic bag, and seal the second bag. Dispose of the material in the double bag by (1) burying it in a 2- to 3-ft-deep hole, (2) burning it, or (3) discarding it in a covered trash can that is regularly emptied. Contact local or state health department concerning other appropriate disposal methods.

Table 16-5
CDC Recommendations for Work in Contaminated Areas

- A baseline serum sample, preferably drawn at the time these activities are initiated, should be available for all persons conducting the clean-up of homes or building with heavy rodent infestation. The serum sample should be stored at −20°C.
- Persons involved in the clean-up should wear coveralls (disposable, if possible), rubber boots or disposable shoe covers, rubber or plastic gloves, protective goggles, and an appropriate respiratory protection device [half-mask air-purifying (or negative-pressure) respirator with a high-efficiency particulate air (HEPA) filter or a powered air-purifying respirator (PAPR) with HEPA filters]. Respirators (even positive-pressure types) are not considered protective if facial hair interferes with the facial seal because proper fit cannot be assured. Respirator practices should follow a comprehensive user program and be supervised by a knowledgeable person [21, art. 9].
- Personal protective equipment (PPE) should be decontaminated on removal at the end of the day. If the coveralls are not disposable, they should be laundered on site. If no laundry facilities are available, the coveralls should be immersed in liquid disinfectant until they can be washed.
- All potentially infective waste material (including respirator filters) from clean-up operations that cannot be burned or deep buried on site should be double bagged in appropriate plastic bags. The bagged material then should be labeled as infectious (if it is to be transported) and disposed of in accordance with local requirements for infectious waste.
- Workers who develop a febrile or respiratory illness with 45 days of the last potential exposure should seek medical attention immediately and inform the attending physician of the potential occupational risk of hantavirus infection. The physician should contact local health authorities promptly if hantavirus-associated illness is suspected. A blood sample should be obtained and forwarded with the baseline serum through the state health department to the CDC for hantavirus antibody testing [Art. 9].

infection, the precautions listed in Table 16-5 should be followed, according to the CDC.

MEDICAL SURVEILLANCE

Individuals who work in areas where rodents are likely to congregate, work with rodents directly (particularly those identified as frequent harbingers of the hantavirus), or are involved in clean-up operations or in any other capacity associated with a high risk of hantavirus exposure (see above) should undergo medical surveillance for early signs of infection. Medical surveillance is based on a combination of worker education and early detection, as shown in Table 16-6.

Laboratory workers handling rodents should obey additional precautions. Certain high-risk techniques, such as intubation of laboratory animals or other activities that tend to generate aerosols, should be completed in biologic safety cabinets with proper exhaust ventilation and filter systems [19]. Laboratory work that may result in propagation of hantaviruses should be conducted in a Biosafety Level 3 (BSL-3) facility [20], with BSL-2 practices recommended for handling clinical specimens and BSL-3 practices recommended for handling infected tissue and viral cell cultures [21]. In general, however, laboratory workers practicing

universal precautions while processing routing clinical specimens (e.g., blood, urine, or respiratory secretions) are not considered to be at increased risk of hantavirus infection.

BIOLOGIC TESTING

All individuals whose occupations place them in a high-risk group for hantavirus exposure should consider obtaining a baseline serum sample to be stored at −20°C. Should the individual become infected, this sample can be tested (along with acute sera) for presence of the hantavirus antigen and antibodies. In addition, convalescent serum is obtained from infected individuals. Analysis with an enzyme-linked immunoglobulin capture immunosorbent assay (ELISA) can be used to detect the presence of immunoglobulin M (IgM) and/or rising titers of immunoglobulin G (IgG) antibodies (to indicate acute infection). In laboratories, frequent serologic testing of laboratory rats and replacement of infected rodents with seronegative animals are recommended [19]. Serologic surveillance of laboratory personnel is also useful to identify early hantavirus infection. It should be noted that studies have demonstrated evidence of hantavirus antibody (to SNV and Hantaan virus, which is the prototypical HFRS virus) in asymptomatic

Table 16-6
CDC Recommendations for Medical Surveillance of Workers in High-Risk Areas

- Obtain a baseline serum sample (at time of hire) and store at −20°C.
- Educational program(s) should be organized and provided to all workers to be involved in potentially high-risk jobs. This program should include, at a minimum, details regarding the types of work associated with the virus, the CDC recommendations for disease prevention as well as clean-up of high-risk sites, and signs and symptoms associated with the disease (both HFRS and HPS).
- Employers should provide a comprehensive medical screening and surveillance program to workers, including medical clearance for respirator use, baseline evaluation, and periodic examination as indicated. The physician responsible for the program should be familiar with methods used for screening and early detection of infection in high-risk populations, as well as with the physical demands of the job and the medical requirements for use of personal protective equipment. On-call medical services should be provided, and workers should be able to contact these services for 45 days after the last potential exposure.
- If a high-risk worker develops a febrile or respiratory illness within 45 days of the last potential exposure, he or she should be instructed to seek immediate medical attention and inform the treating health care provider of the possible risk of hantavirus infection. If the provider then suspects hantavirus infection, he or she should alert local health authorities. A serum sample should be obtained and sent to the state health department for forwarding to the CDC for antibody testing for hantavirus.
- Employers should mandate the wearing of a half-face, tight-seal, negative-pressure respirator or a (positive pressure) PAPR (powered air-purifying respirator) equipped with N-100 or P-100 filters (formerly designated high-efficiency particulate air, or HEPA, filters) when removing rodents from traps or handling rodents in the affected area(s). The use of respirators should be in conjunction with a full respirator protection program at the workplace. Therefore, any hantavirus surveillance program also should include a concurrent respirator medical clearance evaluation based on the anticipated environmental conditions of use and the respirator types to be worn.
- Workers should wear rubber, latex, vinyl, or nitrile gloves when handling rodents or handling traps containing rodents. Before removing the gloves, wash gloved hands in a disinfectant or chlorine solution and then wash bare hands in soap and water.
- Mammalogists, wildlife biologists, or public health personnel who handle wild rodents for research or management purposes should refer to published safety guidelines and the CDC Web site "All About Hantaviruses."

laboratory workers and mammologists with varying degrees of rodent exposure.

IMMUNIZATION

At present, there is no immunization available for the different serotypes of hantavirus.

CASE STUDY: HPS

Two days prior to hospital admission, a 30-year-old plumber sought care at an emergency room complaining of a 2-day history of fever, chills, headache, myalgia, nausea with vomiting, and dry, nonproductive cough. Shortly prior to the onset of symptoms, he recalled working in an old basement, where he noticed several piles of rodent droppings adjacent to the pipes. Admission oral temperature was 103°F (39°C), with a pulse rate of 118 beats/min. Complete blood count indicated a white blood cell count of 6600/mm^3 (normal 4500–11,000/mm^3) and a decreased platelet count of 117,000/mm^3 (normal 130,000–400,000/mm^3). Chest x-ray was normal. The patient was diagnosed as having an acute febrile illness, treated symptomatically, and released to outpatient follow-up.

Two days later, the patient again presented to the emergency room, this time with a persistent fever of 101–104°F, tachycardia (heart rate of 140 beats/min), and hypotension, with a blood pressure of 70/50 mmHg. On repeat laboratory testing, his white blood cell count had risen mildly to 12,000/mm^3, with a cell differential including 18% neutrophils, 55% bands, 18% lymphocytes, and 2% immature granulocytes. His platelet count had dropped to 35,000/mm^3. Additional laboratory testing showed a blood urea nitrogen (BUN) concentration of 38 mg/dL (consistent with mild azotemia), a creatinine concentration of 2.0 mg/dL (mild elevation), and elevated serum liver enzyme levels [LDH 2,487 units/L (normal 297–628 units/L), AST 226 units/L (normal 14–50 units/L), and ALT 152 units/L (normal 7–56 units/L)]. Hypoalbunemia was present, with a serum albumin level of 2.0 g/dL. Serum lipase and amylase levels also were elevated, at 771 and 226 units/L, respectively, although the patient did not complain of abdominal pain and had a normal abdominal physical examination. Admission chest x-ray showed perihilar interstitial infiltrates. The patient was hypoxic, with an O$_2$ saturation (room air) of 80%. Over the next 3 days, he became progressively hypoxemic and developed pulmonary edema and oliguria. With supportive care, including careful fluid monitoring, his symptoms resolved, and he was released.

SYMPTOMS AND SIGNS

The spectrum of disease, including severity and clinical presentation, is distinctly different in HPS than in HFRS. No defined set of signs and symptoms dependably identifies HPS, at the time of presentation, from other types of noncardiogenic pulmonary edema or adult respiratory distress syndrome (ARDS). In HPS, patients commonly present with a prodromal illness consisting of *myalgias, fever, cough,* and *headache* (similar to that of HFRS). Although gastrointestinal symptoms (e.g., abdominal pain, nausea, and vomiting) can be seen, their occurrence is atypical. The initial symptoms usually persist for up to 5 days prior to hospitalization. Evidence of *respiratory distress,* including tachypnea and tachycardia, develop quite abruptly, with laboratory findings of leukocytosis, vascular volume contraction with hemoconcentration (76% of patients), hypoalbuminemia, and thrombocytopenia (71% of patients). In addition, a moderate increase in serum creatinine (>2.5 mg/dL) can be seen but is present in only 10% of all fatal cases. Rhabdomyolysis can occur, as can lactic acidosis. Although hemorrhagic signs may be evident, they are not usually as significant as with HFRS. Chest x-ray findings may be lacking initially (during the prodromal phase) but later typically provide a picture of evolving pulmonary edema, with extensive bibasilar or perihilar airspace disease found in 70% of patients and pleural effusions in 60% [22].

The two major life-threatening pathophysiologic changes in HPS are increased permeability pulmonary edema and an atypical form of septic shock caused by myocardial depression and hypovolemia [23]. Hypoxia is progressive and can be rapid (as can the development of pulmonary edema), not infrequently occurring within the first 24 hours of admission. Survival is linked to the development of hypotension and hypoxia, with death more likely if both develop. Hypotension is not necessarily a direct consequence of hypoxia because patients can maintain adequate oxygenation while developing progressive hypotension [24, 25]. Patients develop severe pulmonary capillary leak syndrome with abnormal gas exchange. Although this sometimes can be reversed by mechanical ventilation, patients frequently die as a result of cardiovascular collapse [26]. Myocardial involvement in the infection is suggested by the onset of death, often secondary to diminished cardiac output and terminal electromechanical dissociation, with dysrhythmias preterminally [27]. The mortality rate of HPS is approximately 50%. In those who survive, however, recovery is usually complete.

Pulmonary histology of patients with HPS shows alveoli engorged with proteinaceous fluid with few inflammatory cells. Heart and kidney tissue, however, show no evidence of necrosis or inflammation [28].

In addition to clinical diagnosis, serologic tests (detection of Four Corners virus–specific antibodies in serum by Western blot assays) in combination with reverse transcriptase polymerase chain reaction (RT-PCR) (to identify Four Corners virus RNA in peripheral blood mononuclear cells) and detection of hantavirus antigen by immunohistochemistry (IHC) should be used to confirm the clinical diagnosis of acute infection. Detection of hantavirus IgM antibodies in serum or a fourfold or greater rise in serum IgG antibodies to hantavirus confirms the diagnosis.

The CDC, in an attempt to alert clinicians to the usual presentation of this initially nondescript illness, has identified clinical features that help to identify patients (Table 16-7).

TREATMENT

There is no current definitive treatment for HPS. The foundations of treatment include early recognition and rapid provision of full supportive measures. Rapid recognition of the probability of hantavirus infection and immediate institution of full supportive measures in an intensive care unit setting have been associated with better patient outcome. Prolonged periods of hypoxia or hypotension prior to stabilization portend a higher risk of death [24]. Mechanical ventilation or supplemental oxygen is needed frequently. To maintain adequate cardiac output, inotropic and pressor agents are used often, with judicious use of fluid administration and central pressure and cardiac monitoring. Ribavirin, an antiviral agent, has been used with mixed results in vivo but has been found to be active against hantavirus in vitro. However, to date, ribavirin has not been shown to improve mortality from HPS, although it may have some use in treatment in the future. Adverse effects seen from the use of ribavirin have necessitated blood transfusions in several patients [26, 29].

DIFFERENTIAL DIAGNOSIS

Particularly in the early stages of disease, hantavirus is very easily misdiagnosed owing to its nonspecific symptomatology. The hantavirus prodrome very closely resembles the symptoms of influenza, with fever, myalgias, headache, and chills.

Table 16-7
Screening Criteria for Hantavirus Pulmonary Syndrome in Persons with Unexplained Respiratory Illness

Potential case-patients must have one of the following:

- A febrile illness [>101°F (38.3°C)] occurring in a previously healthy person characterized by unexplained ARDS *or* bilateral interstitial pulmonary infiltrates developing within 1 week of hospitalization with respiratory compromise requiring supplemental oxygen,

  or

- An unexplained respiratory illness resulting in death in conjunction with an autopsy examination demonstrating noncardiogenic pulmonary edema without an identifiable specific cause of death.

Potential case-patients are to be *excluded* if they have any of the following:

- A predisposing underlying medical condition (e.g., severe underlying pulmonary disease, solid tumors, or hematologic malignancies), congenital or acquired immunodeficiency disorders, or medical conditions (e.g., rheumatoid arthritis or organ transplant recipients) requiring immunosuppressive drug therapy (e.g., steroids or cytotoxic chemotherapy).

- An acute illness that provides a likely explanation for the respiratory illness (e.g., recent major trauma, burn, or surgery), recent seizures or history of aspiration, bacterial sepsis, and another respiratory disorder such as respiratory syncytial virus in young children, influenza, or *Legionella* pneumonia.

Confirmed case-patients must have the following:

- At least one specimen (e.g., serum and/or tissue) available for laboratory testing for evidence of hantavirus infection.

  and

- In a patient with a compatible clinical illness, either serology (presence of hantavirus-specific IgM or rising titers of IgG), polymerase chain reaction for hantavirus ribonucleic acid, or immunohistochemistry for hantavirus antigen is positive.

However, influenza patients are more likely to present with sore throat and cough [30]. The presence of, at times, marked abdominal pain can lead to the diagnosis of an acute abdomen, with the occasional hantavirus patient admitted to a surgical ward. Aseptic meningitis can present similarly; however, the absence of sore throat, coryza, and meningismus acts as a distinguishing factor. Pneumococcal pneumonia usually can be distinguished from HPS by the more likely presence of lobar infiltrates on chest x-ray in pneumococcal pneumonia than in HPS [30]. In one study, multivariate discriminate analysis revealed that three clinical characteristics at admission (i.e., nausea and/or vomiting, lack of cough, and dizziness), along with three initial laboratory abnormalities (i.e., decreased platelet count and serum bicarbonate level and increased hematocrit level), acted to identify all patients with HPS and to exclude HPS in at least 80% of patients with unexplained ARDS [30]. The classic hantavirus pulmonary virus infection is marked by a nonspecific prodrome, followed by *abrupt* deterioration of pulmonary function and develop of ARDS and hypotension. This pattern of infection, along with characteristic laboratory findings (noted earlier) and confirmation of hantavirus antibodies, along with strong clinical suspicion and a recent history consistent with probable rodent excreta exposure, allows astute clinicians to distinguish HPS from several other infectious agents (Table 16-8).

Hemorrhagic Fever with Renal Syndrome

EPIDEMIOLOGY

The hantaviruses associated with HFRS generally cause an acute interstitial nephropathy with fever, hemorrhage of variable severity, and renal insufficiency, not infrequently leading to hypotension and shock [31–33]. Historically, hantaviruses were rec-

Table 16-8
Differential Diagnosis: HPS

Influenza	Aseptic meningitis
Unexplained ARDS	Pneumonic plague
Pneumococcal bacteremia	Psittacosis
Histoplasmosis	Severe *Mycoplasma* pneumonia
Tularemia (pulmonary)	Legionellosis
Meningococcemia	Leptospirosis
Disseminated fungal infection	Rickettsial infection

ognized as falling into four types: Hantaan (the prototypical hantavirus), Seoul, Puumula, and Prospect Hill. Five additional serotypes (Dobrava/Belgrade, Leakey, Thailand, and Thottapayalam) have been identified as additional serotypes [4, 33–36]. A fairly unique feature of the hantaviruses (among the other members of the Bunyaviridae family) is their high specificity for rodent species. The hantaviruses are rarely transmitted by arthropod vectors [37]. The viruses thus are endemic to regions that harbor the rodent populations that are associated with specific hantavirus types. The first hantavirus was discovered in 1976, although hantavirus-induced disease has been identified since the 1930s [37, 38].

Study of the epizootology of the hantavirus types responsible for HFRS unveils a large distribution throughout the world. Hantaan virus (HV) is found most often in rodents in Asia. Puumula virus (PV), on the other hand, is found in Scandinavia and eastern Europe, including eastern Russia, again in rodent hosts [39]. Prospect Hill virus (PHV) was first isolated in Maryland [39, 41]. Seoul virus (SV) is found in the common rat, explaining its largest geographic distribution of all the hantaviruses, thanks largely to worldwide shipping [37]. Phylogenetically, HV and SV are most closely related, and PV and PHV are the closest linked [42].

The primary reservoir for the hantaviruses are rodents [37]. Exposure to nesting materials heavily contaminated with infectious secretions and excretions, grooming behavior, and intraspecies wounding by biting are significant factors in the continuation of the enzootic cycle [40, 49]. Rats weighing in excess of 300 g, reproductively mature, and displaying aggressive behavior appear to have a higher seroprevalence of infection [43–46].

The individual viral serotypes are rodent-specific and infect the rodents with no or little manifestation of apparent disease [47]. The virus appears to persist in the reservoir animals and is shed very slowly. Once rodent infection occurs, viremia ensues for a short period of time, with the production of host antibodies to the virus and viral dissemination to the lung, salivary glands, and kidney. Although the antibodies probably are present throughout the remainder of the host's life (and protect the host from acquiring disease), viral shedding persists. Human infection usually occurs after the disruption of reservoir rodent populations.

Infection occurs primarily via inhalation of aerosolized infected rodent excreta, although rodent saliva also contains virus, making bites another means of transmission. In addition, direct contamination of food or household items with infected rodent excreta can lead to human transmission.

The severity of infection varies significantly depending on the causative virus involved. For example, although antibodies for the Prospect Hill virus (PHV) have been identified frequently in individuals' sera, no manifestations of illness have been associated with the virus to date. Prior to the identification of HPS, PHV was the only indigenous North American hantavirus. Of the four major serotypes, Hantaan, Puumala, and Seoul are known human pathogens. PV is associated with a mild form of disease (without shock and hemorrhage) known as *nephropathia epidemica* [3, 4]. Although usually associated with mild disease, infection by SV occasionally can lead to severe illness and death. HFRS attributed to HV usually begins with an abrupt onset and progresses through five stages before resolution. DV has been identified mostly in the Balkans, where it can also be associated with severe HFRS [50].

Person-to-person transmission of any of the hantaviruses has not been reported. Health care workers therefore do not appear to be vulnerable to infection via treatment of infected patients [1]. Laboratory workers handling infected laboratory rodents, however, have been found to be at risk [43, 48–51].

Although no confirmed cases of HFRS have been identified in North America, the illness is well known to various other regions of the world. In China, cases of HFRS during the period of 1931–1942 have been identified retrospectively as occurring in Japanese soldiers and known as *atypical scarlet fever, acute nephritis, hemorrhagic typhus,* and others [52]. From 1950–1990, 904,995 people residing in China became infected with the disease, with an average morbidity of 2.69 per 100,000 persons, with 38,965 deaths (case-fatality rate of 4.31%) [52]. Currently, outbreaks of HFRS continue to occur in approximately 30 Chinese areas.

In addition to being region-specific in its distribution, hantavirus infection is also seasonal. A periodicity of infection and epidemics exists, related to host ecology, human control efforts, and human and (host) animal natural immunity [53]. Generally, epidemic peaks occur in winter (rural regions), summer (forest regions), and spring (urban regions). The reason for this lies in the host ecology. In the spring and fall (less harsh months), rodents preferentially reside in fields. In the summer months, the forests provide a cool respite from the hot sun's rays. In the winter months, however, many rodents seek warmer, more pleasant shelter indoors. This migration of the host provides the foundation for the relatively increased incidence in human infection in the spring and fall months in farm workers, in park rangers and hikers in the summer, and in indoor workers in the winter months. Eradication efforts aimed at minimizing the rodent population have been successful at lowering the incidence of disease, whereas large rodent populations in areas with no or poor population-reduction efforts have been attributed to an increased incidence of infection.

HV-induced HFRS is found in eastern Russia, Korea, and China. The distribution parallels the range of the striped field mouse [38,39]. HV-infected mice in Korea display a seasonal movement pattern that mirrors the HV disease rates in that country. The mice are reproductively active in the fall and spring, producing large numbers of gravid mice. Gravid mice excrete more urine than nongravid mice, leading to higher amounts of aerosolized virus in the air during these seasons. Fall and spring also happen to be the planting and harvesting times [28]. The combination of increased aerosolized virus in the fields and increased work time spent in the fields by field workers (during planting and harvesting) leads to greater potential viral exposure and infection risk. In Sweden, PV is found in the bank vole, and disease incidence has been correlated with the size of the vole population for a given year [39]. In HFRS-endemic areas in eastern Europe, Asia, and Scandinavia, well-demarcated microfoci of disease are found, making this a "place disease" [54]

Lee and Lee first isolated HV from the lung tissue of striped field mice from a region of Korea endemic for HFRS in 1976. Following this discovery, serologic diagnosis of HV infection allowed for the identification of several genera of rodents in varied geographic areas that harbor the virus [32] (Table 16-9). The principal reservoirs of hantaviruses are rodents of the superfamily Muroidea and the family

Muridae (genera: *Apodemus, Mus,* and *Rattus*) and the family Arvicolidae (genera: *Microtus* and *Clethrionomys*). *R. norvegicus* (Norway rats), as well as some species of *Clethrionomys* and *Microtus,* are found in Scandinavia and the Americas. The prototypical rodent HV reservoir, (mouse) genus *Apodemus,* are not found in the Americas. However, serologic evidence of a relative of HV, the Prospect Hill virus (PHV), has been isolated from the meadow vole (*Microtus pennsylvanicus*), particularly those weighing more than 50 g [55, 56]. Also, the Seoul virus (SV) has been isolated from Norway rats found in the United States, in Philadelphia, Houston, New Orleans, and Baltimore [58–61]. Although no verified cases of HFRS have occurred in the United States to date, hantaviruses found in members of the *Rattus* genus were identical to hantaviruses in Japan and Korea responsible for causing disease [1, 50, 51]. Hantavirus-infected rats also have been identified in other areas of the United States, including Columbus, Ohio, New York City, Honolulu, and San Francisco. Leakey, Texas, is the home of the Leakey virus (LV), identified in a mouse frequently found in homes, *Mus musculus,* and antigenically dissimilar to the previously recognized hantavirus serotypes [50]. PHV-like hantavirus antibodies also have been found in other species, including *Clethrionomys rutilus, Peromyscus difficilis, P. truei, Neotoma mexicana, N. cinerea, P. maniculatus, P. californicus, C. gapperi, Microtus californicus,* and *P. leucopus* in Virginia, West Virginia, California, Minnesota, Colorado, Alaska, Maryland, and New Mexico [44–46, 55–57, 61].

Beside rodents, other animals have been associated with hantavirus and HFRS. In Maryland, for example, cats (*Felis catus*) have shown antibodies to hantavirus, whereas in China, musk shrews (*Suncus murinus*) have been implicated in the spread of disease [62]. Other small mammals (the short-tailed shrew, *Blarina brevicauda,* and the long-tailed weasel, *Mustela frenata*) [45, 46, 56], as well as bats [63], may harbor hantavirus related viruses (see Table 16-9).

CLINICAL MANIFESTATIONS

Each of the hantavirus types infects a single rodent species and produces lifelong asymptomatic infection. The virus is transmitted horizontally among rodents, and infected rodents shed virus in saliva,

urine, and feces for several weeks after infection. The incubation period for human infections ranges from 4 days to 6 weeks (average 12–16 days).

Hantaan Virus and Dobrava Virus

The most severe form of HFRS occurs with infection by HV, with fatality rates from 5–15%. This virus occurs in Asia and acts as the prototypical model of HFRS. HFRS caused by HV is usually abrupt in onset. Five distinct clinical phases have been described as infection progresses in an infected individual: *febrile, hypotensive, oliguric, diuretic,* and *convalescent.* The delineation of these phases may be less evident in milder infections. Similar severe infection usually occurs with DV. The first, or febrile, phase usually spans over 3–5 days and is marked by the onset of headache, widespread petechiae, facial flushing, and lumbar and abdominal pain. This is followed by the hypotensive phase, marked by the onset of shock, with low cardiac output and increased systemic vascular resistance. The cause of shock is unknown; however, involvement of several mediators, including kinin activation, has been studied [22]. During this phase, thrombocytopenia, hemoconcentration, and leukocytosis are seen. The oliguric phase follows, with associated hypertension. If careful fluid monitoring does not occur, pulmonary edema and respiratory distress can occur owing to volume overload. Hemorrhagic complications and DIC can occur during this phase, as they can during the preceding two stages. If the patient survives the first three stages, the diuretic phase ensues, marked by possible electrolyte abnormalities. Hyposthenuria marks the beginning of the final, convalescent phase, often persisting for weeks. Full recovery is common.

Seoul and Puumula Viruses

Infection with SV or PV usually leads to a milder form of HFRS than that with HV, with fatality rates of less than 1%. SV is distributed worldwide, although no reported cases of infection have been reported in the United States. PV, identified in Scandinavia and several European countries, is associated with a form of HFRS known as *nephropathia epidemica* [63–65]. This infection is characterized by fever, abdominal pain, back pain, and renal impairment. Nephropathia epidemica usually

Table 16-9
U.S. Hantavirus infection: Rodent and Mammal Hosts

Region	Species	Region	Species
Northeast		**Southwest**	
New York City	*R. norvegicus*	Los Angeles	*R. norvegicus*
Philadelphia	*R. norvegicus*	New Mexico	*P. maniculatus*
Pennsylvania	*M. pennsylvanicus*		*M. californicus*
Mid-Atlantic			*P. truei*
Baltimore	*R. norvegicus*		*P. boylii*
	M. pennsylvanicus		*P. crinitus*
	P. leucopus		*N. cinerea*
	M. musculus		*P. difficilis*
	Tamias striatus		*N. Mexicana*
	B. brevicauda	**West**	
	Sciurus carolinensis	San Francisco	*R. norvegicus*
		Denver	*R. norvegicus*
Fairfax, VA		Seattle	*R. norvegicus*
Frederick, MD	*M. pennsylvanicus*	Tacoma, WA	*R. norvegicus*
	M. leucopus	Portland, OR	*R. norvegicus*
	Tamiasciurus hudsonicus	Sacramento, CA	*R. norvegicus*
	B. brevicauda	Oakland, CA	*R. norvegicus*
	Pitymys pinetorum	Monterey, CA	*M. californicus*
West Virginia	*M. pennsylvanicus*	San Mateo, CA	*M. californicus*
	P. maniculatus	California (general),	*P. maniculatus*
	M. chrotorrhinus	Colorado (general),	*N. mexicana*
	P. leucopus	and New Mexico (general)	*N. cinerea*
	C. gapperi		*P. californicus*
			P. truei
Pocahontus, Wv	*C. gapperi*		*P. difficilis*
Southeast			*M. californicus*
New Orleans	*R. norvegicus*		*P. crinitus*
Miami	*R. norvegicus*		*P. boylii*
South		Snow Canyon, UT	*P. boylii*
Houston, TX	*R. norvegicus*		*P. eremicus*
Galveston, TX	*R. norvegicus*		*P. crinitus*
Arkansas	*R. norvegicus*		*Onychomys torridus*
			Dipodomys merriami
Del Rio And Leakey, TX	*P. flavus*		*Neotoma lepida*
	P. hispidus	**Far West**	
	M. musculus	Alaska	*C. rutilus*
	S. hispidus		*M. pennsylvanicus*
		Hawaii (Hilo, Oahu, Maui)	*R. norvegicus*

carries a favorable prognosis, but permanent renal effects may occur. PHV, indigenous to North America, is currently not associated with disease, but serologic evidence of infection has been identified in individuals. Mild cases of HFRS may have occurred in the United States but may have been easily overlooked or attributed to other causes. Additionally, several other strains of hantavirus, such as the Girard Point virus (isolated from *R. norvegicus* in Philadelphia and Houston [59]) and the Baltimore isolate [58] have been identified, although their contribution to disease is unclear.

As noted earlier, in HFRS, as in HPS, the reservoirs for the viruses are rodents. In addition, the modes of transmission from rodent to human are identical. Therefore, recommended methods of disease control, safe work practices, preventive and medical treatment measures, as well as occupational groups at risk, are similar for both diseases. Additionally, treatment measures are the same, based on early recognition and intensive supportive measures. The reader is therefore referred to the preceding discussion regarding these topics (see "Hantavirus Pulmonary Syndrome" above) for further review.

References

1. Schmaljohn CS, Hasty SE, Dalrymple JM, et al. Antigenic and genetic properties of viruses linked to hemorrhagic fever with renal syndrome. *Science* 1985;227:1041–4.

2. Zeitz PS, Butler JC, Cheek JE, et al. A case-control study of hantavirus pulmonary syndrome during an outbreak in the southwestern United States. *J Infect Dis* 1995:171:864–70.

3. Duchin JS, Koster FT, Peters CJ, et al. Hantavirus pulmonary syndrome: A clinical description of 17 patients with a newly recognized disease. *N Engl J Med* 1994;14:949–1005.

4. Childs JE, Ksiazek TG, Spiropoulou CF, et al. Serologic and genetic identification of *Peromyscus maniculatus* as the primary rodent reservoir for a new hantavirus in the southwestern United States. *J Infect Dis* 1994;169:1271–80.

5. Zaki SR, Greer PW, Coffield LM, et al. Hantavirus pulmonary syndrome: Pathogenesis of an emerging infectious disease. *Am J Pathol* 1995;146:552–79.

6. Frampton JW, Lanser S, Nichols CR, et al. Sin Nombre virus infection in 1959. *Lancet* 1995;346:781–2.

7. Laboratory Centre for Disease Control. First reported cases of hantavirus pulmonary syndrome in Canada. *Can Commun Dis Rep* 1994;20:121–8.

8. Hjelle B, Krolikowske J, Torrez-Martinez N, et al. Phylogenetically distinct hantavirus implicated in a case of hantavirus pulmonary syndrome in the northeastern United States. *J Med Virol* 1995;46:21–7.

9. Elliott LH, Ksiazek TG, Rollin PE, et al. Isolation of the causative agent of hantavirus pulmonary syndrome. *Am J Trop Med Hyg* 1994;51:102–8.

10. Khan AS, Spiropoulou CF, Morzunov S, et al. Fatal illness associated with a new hantavirus in Louisiana. *J Med Virol* 1995;46:281–6.

11. Song JW, Lack LJ, Gajdusek DC, et al. Isolation of pathogenic hantavirus from white-footed mouse (*Peromyscus leucopus*). *Lancet* 1994;344:1637.

12. Torrez-Martinez N, Hjelle B. Enzootic of Bayou hantavirus in rice rats (*Oryzomys palustris*) in 1983. *Lancet* 1994;344:1637.

13. Armstrong LR, Zaki SR, Goldoft MW, et al. Hantavirus pulmonary syndrome associated with entering or cleaning rarely used, rodent-infested structures. *J Infect Dis* 1995;172:1166.

14. Zeitz PS, Graber JM, Voorhees RA, et al. Assessment of occupational risk for hantavirus infection in mammalogists and rodent workers (abstract H57). In *Abstracts of the 35th Interscience Conference on Antimicrobial Agents and Chemotherapy.* Washington: American Society for Microbiology, 1995, p 190.

15. Armstrong LR, Khabbaz RF, Childs JE, et al. Occupational exposure to hantavirus in mammalogists and rodent workers (abstract). *Am J Trop Med Hyg* 1994;51:94.

16. Centers for Disease Control and Prevention. Hantavirus infection—Southwestern United States: Interim recommendations for risk reduction. *MMWR* 1993;42:ii-13.

17. Pratt HD, Brown RZ. *Biological Factors in Domestic Rodent Control.* DHEW publication no (CDC) 79-8144. Washington: US Government Printing Office, 1979.

18. Scott HG, Borom MR. *Rodent-Borne Disease Control Through Rodent Stoppage.* DHEW publication no (CDC) 77-8343. Washington: US Government Printing Office, 1977.

19. Wong TW, Chan YC, Yap EH, et al. Serological evidence of hantavirus infection in laboratory rats and personnel. *Int J Epidemiol* 1988;17:887–90.

20. Centers for Disease Control and Prevention/National Institutes of Health. *Biosafety in Microbiological and Biomedical Laboratories,* 2d ed. DHHS publication no (CDC) 88-8395. Atlanta: US Department of Health and Human Services, CDC, 1988.

21. Sewell DL. Laboratory-associated infections and biosafety. *Clin Microbiol Rev* 1995;8:389–405.

22. Butler JC, Peters CJ. Hantaviruses and hantavirus pulmonary syndrome. *Clin Infect Dis* 1994;19:387–95.

23. Hallin GW, Simpson SQ, Crowell RE, et al. Cardiopulmonary manifestations of hantavirus pulmonary syndrome. *Crit Care Med* 1996;24:252–8.

24. Centers for Disease Control and Prevention. Update: Hantavirus pulmonary syndrome—United States, 1993. *MMWR* 1993;42:816–20.

25. Duchin JS, Koster FT, Peters CJ, et al. Hantavirus pulmonary syndrome: A clinical description of 17 patients with a newly recognized disease. *N Engl J Med* 1994;330:949–55.

26. Levy H. Clinical course, management and pathology of hantavirus pulmonary syndrome (abstract from Session 67). Presented at the American Society for Microbiology's 34th Interscience Conference on Antimicrobial Agents and Chemotherapy, Orlando, FL, October 4–7, 1994.

27. Jenison S, Hjelle B, Simpson S, et al. Hantavirus pulmonary syndrome: Clinical, diagnostic, and virologic aspects. *Semin Respir Infect* 1995;10:259–69.

28. Morrison YY, Rathbun RC. Hantavirus pulmonary syndrome: The Four Corners disease. *Ann Pharmacol* 1995;29:57–63.

29. Chapman LE, Mertz G, Khan AS, et al. Open label intravenous ribavirin for hantavirus pulmonary syndrome (abstract H111). Presented at the American Society for Microbiology's 34th Interscience Conference on Antimicrobial Agents and Chemotherapy, Orlando, FL, October 4–7, 1994.

30. Moolenaar RL, Dalton C, Lipman HB, et al. Clinical features that differentiate hantavirus pulmonary syndrome from three other acute respiratory illnesses. *Clin Infect Dis* 1995;21:643–9.

31. Lahdevirta J. Nephropathia epidemica in Finland: A clinical, histological and epidemiological study. *Ann Clin Res* 1971;3:1–154.

32. Yanagihara R, Gajdusek DC. Hemorrhagic fever with renal syndrome: A historical perspective and

review of recent advances. In Gear JHS (ed), *CRC Handbook of Viral and Rickettsial Hemorrhagic Fevers.* Boca Raton, FL: CRC Press, 1988, pp 151–88.

33. Xiao SY, LeDuc JW, Chu YK, et al. Phylogenetic analyses of virus isolates in the genus *Hantavirus,* family Bunyaviridae. *Virology* 1994;198:205–17.

34. Avsic-Zupanc T, Xiao SY, Stojanovic R, et al. Characterization of Dobrava virus: A hantavirus from Slovenia, Yugoslavia. *J Infect Dis* 1992;38:132–7.

35. Gligic A, Dimkovic N, Xiao SY, et al. Belgrade virus: A new hantavirus causing severe hemorrhagic fever with renal syndrome in Yugoslavia. *J Infect Dis* 1992;166:113–20.

36. Chu YK, Rossi C, LeDuc JW, et al. Serological relationships among viruses in the *Hantavirus* genus, family Buvyaviridae. *Virology* 1994;198:196–204.

37. LeDuc JW, Childs JE, Glass GE. The hantaviruses, etiologic agents of hemorrhagic fever with renal syndrome: A possible cause of hypertension and chronic renal disease in the United States. *Ann Rev Public Health* 1992;13:79–98.

38. Lee HW, Lee PW, Johnson KM. Isolation of the etiologic agent of Korean hemorrhagic fever. *J Infect Dis* 1978;137:298–308.

39. LeDuc JW. Epidemiology of Hantaan and related viruses. *Lab Anim Sci* 1987;37:413–8.

40. Lee HW, Lee PW. Korean hemorrhagic fever: II. Isolation of etiologic agent. *Korean J Virol* 1977;7:19–29.

41. Lee PW, Amyx HL, Gajdusek DC, et al. New hemorrhagic fever with renal syndrome-related virus in indigenous wild rodents in United States (letter). *Lancet* 1982;2:1405.

42. Nichol ST, Spiropoulou CF, Morzunov S, et al. Genetic identification of a hantavirus associated with an outbreak of acute respiratory illness. *Science* 1993;262:914–7.

43. Childs JE, Korch GW, Smith GA, et al. Geographical distribution and age-related prevalence of Hantaan-like virus in rat populations of Baltimore, Maryland, USA. *Am J Trop Med Hyg* 1985;34:385–7.

44. Korch GW, Childs JE, Glass GE, et al. Serological evidence of hantaviral infections within small mammal communities of Baltimore, Maryland: Spatial and temporal patterns and host range. *Am J Trop Med Hyg* 1989;41:230–40.

45. Childs JE, Glass GE, Korch GW, et al. Prospective seroepidemiology of hantaviruses and population dynamics of small mammal communities of Baltimore, Maryland. *Am J Trop Med Hyg* 1987;37:648–52.

46. Childs JE, Glass GE, Korch GW, et al. The ecology and epizootiology of hantaviral infections in small mammal communities of Baltimore, Maryland: A review and synthesis. *Bull Soc Vector Ecol* 1988;13:113–22.

47. Lee HW, Baek LJ, Johnson KM. Isolation of Hantaan virus, the etiologic agent of Korean hemorrhagic fever, from wild urban rats. *J Infect Dis* 1982;146:638–44.

48. Lee PW, Gibbs CJ Jr, Gajdusek DC, et al. Serotypic classification of hantaviruses by indirect immunofluorescent antibody and plaque reduction neutralization tests. *J Clin Microbiol* 1985;22:940–4.

49. Baek LJ, Yanagihara R, Gibbs CJ Jr, et al. Leakey virus: A new hantavirus isolated from *Mus musculus* in the United States. *J Gen Virol* 1988;69:3129–32.

50. Dantas JR Jr, Okuno Y, Tanishita O, et al. Viruses of hemorrhagic fever with renal syndrome (HFRS) grouped by immunoprecipitation and hemagglutination inhibition. *Intervirology* 1987;27:161–5.

51. Sugiyama K, Matsuura Y, Morita C, et al. Determination of immune adherence HA of the antigenic relationship between *Rattus-* and *Apodemus-*borne viruses causing hemorrhagic fever with renal syndrome. *J Infect Dis* 1984;149:472.

52. Chen, HX, Qiu FX. Epidemiological survey: Epidemiologic surveillance on the hemorrhagic fever with renal syndrome in China. *Chin Med J* 1993;106:857–63.

53. Chen HX, Qiu FX, Dong BJ, et al. Epidemiological studies on hemorrhagic fever with renal syndrome in China. *J Infect Dis* 1986;154:394.

54. Smadel JE. Epidemic hemorrhagic fever. *Am J Public Health* 1953;43:1327–30.

55. Lee PW, Amyx HL, Gajdusek DC, et al. New hemorrhagic fever with renal syndrome-related virus in indigenous wild rodents in United States. *Lancet* 1982;2:1405.

56. Lee PW, Amyx HL, Yanagihara, R, et al. Partial characterization of Prospect Hill virus isolated from meadow voles in the United States. *J Infect Dis* 1985;152:826–9.

57. Tsai TF, Bauer SP, Sasso DR, et al. Epizootiologic and epidemiologic investigations of Hantaan virus-related infections in the United States. In Bender TR, Diwan AR, Raymond JS (eds), *Hemorrhagic Fever with Renal Syndrome.* Honolulu: School of Public Health, University of Hawaii, 1985, pp 18–22.

58. Childs JE, Korch GW, Glass GE, et al. Epizootiology of hantavirus infections in Baltimore: Isolation of a virus from Norway rats and characteristics of infected rat populations. *Am J Epidemiol* 1987;126:55–68.

59. LeDuc JW, Smith GA, Johnson KM. Hantaan-like viruses from domestic rats captured in the United States. *Am J Trop Med Hyg* 1984;33:992–8.

60. LeDuc JW, Smith GA, Johnson KM, et al. Urban rats as hosts of Hantaan-like viruses in the Americas. In Bender TR, Diwan AR, Raymond JS (eds), *Hemorrhagic Fever with Renal Syndrome.* Honolulu: School of Public Health, University of Hawaii, 1985, pp 15–7.

61. Lee PW, Yanagihara R, Franko MC, et al. Preliminary evidence that Hantaan or a closely related virus is enzootic in domestic rodents. *N Engl J Med* 1982;307:624–5.

62. Tang YW, Xu ZY, Zhu ZY, et al. Isolation of a haemorrhagic fever with renal (HFRS) virus from *Suncus murinus,* an insectivore. *Lancet* 1985;1:513–4.

63. Kim GR, Lee YT, Park CH. A new natural reservoir of hantavirus: Isolation of hantaviruses from lung tissues of bats. *Arch Virol* 1994;134:85–95.

64. Gajdusek DC. Virus hemorrhagic fevers: Special reference to hemorrhagic fever with renal syndrome (epidemic hemorrhagic fever). *J Pediatr* 1962;60: 841–57.

65. Lee HW, Lee PW, Baek LJ, et al. Geographical distribution of hemorrhagic fever with renal syndrome and hantaviruses. *Arch Virol* 1990;1:5–18.

66. Settergren B. Nephropathia epidemica (hemorrhagic fever with renal syndrome) in Scandinavia. *Rev Infect Dis* 1991;13:736–44.

17

Occupational Hepatitis

Daniel A. Nackley and Ralph L. McLaury

*H*epatitis is a general term that indicates hepatic inflammation. *Viral hepatitis* is reserved for diseases characterized by inflammation of the liver owing to several infectious viruses [1].

Hepatitis may be inapparent, with a subclinical presentation, or may cause a period of self-limited incapacitation. Depending on the etiology, the disease may become chronic. In rare instances, it progresses to fulminant hepatic inflammation [2].

Infectious hepatitis is not unique to any one population or group, but it was the emergence of the acquired immune deficiency syndrome (AIDS) epidemic in the early 1980s that drew renewed attention to the significant risks of hepatitis and other infectious diseases in health care workers. Increasing attention was focused on the use of universal precautions (which now have been replaced with standard precautions), as well as immunizing health care workers against hepatitis B. Several landmark pieces of legislation and recommendations were promulgated by the National Institutes of Occupational Health and Safety (NIOSH) and by Congress. These included the Guidelines for Protecting the Safety and Health of Health Care Workers (NIOSH); Public Law 100-607; the Health Omnibus Programs Extension Act of 1988, Title II, Programs with Respect to Acquired Immune Deficiency Syndrome; and Guidelines for Prevention of Transmission of Human Immunodeficiency Virus and Hepatitis B Virus to Health-Care and Public Safety Workers: A Response to Public Law 100-607, the Health Omnibus Programs Extension Act of 1988.

These pieces of legislation and agency recommendations culminated in the Occupational Safety and Health Administration's (OSHA's) blood-borne pathogens standard. Today, countless numbers of workers benefit from this landmark legislation. However, there is a constant influx of new information that emanates from the isolation of new bacteria and viruses, as well as from improved understanding of the pathogen, host, and transmission/vector relationships. There exist new means of preventing and treating diseases, with new vaccines, immunobiologics, and medications. In addition, populations and groups other than health care workers—daycare workers, law enforcement officers, firefighters, and penal corrections employees—are affected. Thus occupational medicine physicians are challenged by the increasing array of work settings and types of jobs that put workers at risk for contracting hepatitis. This challenge expands the scope of traditional occupational medicine practice further into the arena of infectious disease, infection control, and public health.

In addition to the clinical and laboratory features of occupationally acquired infectious hepatitis, this chapter reviews the historical aspects, epidemiology, prevention, and treatment of viral hepatitis, as well as other infectious viral and nonviral sources of hepatic inflammation. There is also an in-depth discussion of special populations with unique risks for contracting hepatitis (with which the authors have had extensive experience). These are the populations that have the greatest risk of contracting work-related viral hepatitis. The chapter also briefly discusses work accommodations for employees who have hepatitis and current recommendations for the work management of infected individuals who perform invasive procedures. The chapter closes with a review of the prevention of occupational infectious hepatitis.

General Principles

Viral hepatitis is caused by a pathogenic virus that invades hepatocytes. Viruses responsible for viral hepatitis are hepatitis A, B, C, D, and E. Other viruses that may cause hepatic inflammation, one characteristic of the disease process, are Epstein-Barr virus, cytomegalovirus, herpes simplex virus, yellow fever virus, and rubella virus.

Pathologically and histologically, the typical lesion consists of necrosis of the hepatocyte, with a mononuclear lymphocytic inflammatory response. However, these features are not specific for any one particular infective agent, or cause, of hepatic inflammation [2].

Clinical and Laboratory Manifestations

Symptoms of acute viral hepatitis are nonspecific and predominantly constitutional and gastrointestinal. Prodromal symptoms include malaise, fatigue, anorexia, nausea, vomiting, and arthralgias. Following the prodromal symptoms, there is an icteric phase characterized by hepatic inflammation, abdominal pain, and jaundice. Symptoms often lessen during the icteral phase, particularly in children.

Physical manifestations may include mild fever, hepatomegaly, splenomegaly, jaundice, and pruritus. Spider nevi and telangiectasia may be present in chronic cases as a result of hepatic insufficiency that results in an estrogenic effect.

The hallmark of laboratory studies is significant elevation of serum aminotransferases. The alanine aminotransferase (ALT) elevation often exceeds that of the aspartate aminotransferase (AST). Other laboratory manifestations include elevations of serum bilirubin, alkaline phosphatase, and pro-

thrombin time. There may be a decrease in the serum albumin, resulting in hyperglobulinemia. Hemolysis may occur, and urinalysis often reveals the presence of bilirubin.

Among the possible complications of viral hepatitis are massive hepatic necrosis, cholestatic hepatitis, aplastic anemia, vasculitis, and pancreatitis. In cases of hepatitis B, C, and D, the process may evolve to chronic hepatitis [2].

Epidemiologic studies have linked the occurrence of hepatic cell carcinoma (HCC) with the hepatitis B virus. The lifetime risk of developing HCC is estimated to be 10–25 times greater in carriers of HBV compared with noninfected populations. Hepatitis C virus (HCV) also has been identified as a cause of HCC, although the epidemiology is less established at this time [3]. The incidence of HCC secondary to HCV is expected to rise as a result of an aging population [4]. Hepatitis D is associated with a threefold increase in HCC, although the confounding factor of concomitant HBV infection cannot be underestimated.

Historical Aspects

Awareness of hepatitis dates back many centuries. References to disorders characterized by jaundice appear in the literature of the ancient Greeks, Babylonians, and Chinese [5].

It was not until 1963 that the Australian antigen of hepatitis B was characterized by Blumberg [6]. Since then, testing methodologies have expanded to include specific serologic tests of the host antibody response, the characterization of seven different viral hepatitides, and the development of polymerase chain reaction technology in characterizing various strains of a given virus.

Hepatitis A

BACKGROUND AND EPIDEMIOLOGY

Hepatitis A (HAV) is a 27-nm RNA *Hepatovirus,* a member of the family Picornaviridae. While HAV occurs worldwide, it tends to occur in sporadic and epidemic proportions in developed portions of the world. It is historically a disease associated with poor public sanitation or poor hygiene. In developing countries, adults are typically immune, and the disease occurs as part of the endemic illnesses. Humans and nonhuman primates are the reservoirs for the virus. The typical modes of transmission are person to person (via the fecal-oral route), common source (through food or water), sexual, and blood/intravenous [7–9].

In developed parts of the world, where good sanitation and public health practices are common, most adults do not contract HAV infection. As a result, when an outbreak does occur, it tends to be proportionally more epidemic. Transmission rates are high in day-care centers, long-term residential facilities, and other settings where there is high risk of fecal-oral transmission [7]. In the United States, epidemic cycles appeared to have ended by the 1980s. Since 1983, however, HAV rates have increased, with one of the most recent epidemics occurring in 1997 owing to contaminated strawberries from Mexico [7, 8]. In the United States, other outbreaks have been attributed to common-source exposures, that is, food or water contamination.

The incubation period averages 28–30 days but may range from 15–50 days. The period of communicability begins in the latter half of the incubation period and continues into the first few days of the onset of jaundice [7].

WORK ISSUES

If HAV infection is detected during the incubation period, the infected individual should be placed on enteric precautions during the first 2 weeks of illness but for no more than 1 week after the onset of jaundice. Quarantine is not required. After the period of communicability, accommodation may be required. Individuals with resolving infection may need to be placed on light duty, with frequent rest breaks or an abbreviated work day or work week. Typically, recovery is complete after HAV infection [7].

ACTIVE AND PASSIVE IMMUNIZATION

There are three variants of hepatitis A vaccine licensed for use in the United States: Havrix, Twinrix (HAV-HBV combination), and Vaqta. Each is highly effective in individuals over 18 years of age when administered according to the manufacturer's direction. The high immunogenicity of the two vaccines makes postvaccination serologic testing unnecessary. In addition, standard commercially available assays may not detect neutralizing antibodies to HAV in actively immunized individuals because the HAV vaccine induces an antibody

response much weaker than that owing to natural infection [9].

The vaccine's long-term effectiveness has not been fully characterized, but it appears that protective levels of anti-HAV are sustained for 20 years or more. Typically, most HAV vaccine recipients are immune within 2 weeks of the first immunization; 100% of recipients are immune within 4 weeks of the first vaccination. Current recommendations are for vaccination 4 weeks prior to anticipated exposure (e.g., travel to an endemic area). The full vaccination series consists of two vaccines over 6 months.

Before HAV vaccine was available, passive immunization with serum immune globulin (IG) was the method of protecting individuals, both before and after exposure. If an individual plans to travel to an endemic area within 4 weeks after active immunization with HAV vaccine, current recommendations are that he or she receive 0.02 mL/kg of IG, which will provide up to 3 months of protection. HAV vaccine may be administered concurrently with IG, but different injection sites should be used. While concurrent administration may reduce the immunogenicity of HAV vaccine, the effect is not considered to be clinically significant.

POSTEXPOSURE PROPHYLAXIS

When exposure to HAV is likely or anticipated, such as when traveling to an endemic area, active immunization with HAV vaccine is preferable. When nonimmune individuals are exposed to HAV, a single dose of intramuscular IG is recommended because of its high level of efficacy in preventing disease. The standard dose of IG is 0.02 mL/kg. Current guidelines recommend the use of IG for postexposure prophylaxis as soon as possible. It may be administered up to 2 weeks after HAV exposure. Efficacy more than 2 weeks after exposure is not known [9].

IG is prepared by the pooling of human plasma that has been screened for HBV surface antigen, HIV, and anti-HCV. There has been no documented transmission of any bloodborne infectious disease with IG for intramuscular injection (IGIM). In 1994, however, the Centers for Disease Control and Prevention (CDC) reported outbreaks of HCV infection among individuals who had received certain lots of intravenous immune globulin (IGIV) for primary immunodeficiency disorder.

After this outbreak, the contaminated lots of IGIV were removed from the medical marketplace [10]. Since that time, there has been a market shortage of IGIM [11].

IGIM, however, has an excellent track record, with no documented cases of transmission of bloodborne infection. There are currently two sources of IGIM in the United States: FFF Enterprises (1-800-843-7477) and Talecris (www.Talecris.com, 1-800-243-4153). Currently, IGIM should be reserved for postexposure prophylaxis. Now that there is a safe and effective vaccine against HAV, preexposure prophylaxis with the vaccine is preferable to using IGIM. Using HAV vaccine in cases of potential exposure ensures that the current supplies of IGIM will be adequate when it is needed for postexposure prophylaxis. Table 17-1 details the recommended doses of IG for HAV pre- and postexposure prophylaxis [11].

Hepatitis B

BACKGROUND AND EPIDEMIOLOGY

It is now known that there are at least two viruses responsible for bloodborne hepatitis: hepatitis B virus and hepatitis C virus. Hepatitis B virus (HBV) was formerly referred to as *serum hepatitis*. It is a 42-nm DNA virus in the family Hepadnaviridae. HBV may be transmitted via the bloodborne (e.g., percutaneous or intravenous), perinatal, or sexual route [7]. Humans are the natural reservoir for the virus. Worldwide, HBV is a major cause of acute and chronic hepatitis, cirrhosis, and primary hepatocellular carcinoma. Five percent of the adult U.S. population is positive for the anti-HB core antigen

Table 17-1
Recommended Doses of Immune Globulin (IG) for Hepatitis A Pre- and Postexposure Prophylaxis[a]

Setting	Duration of Coverage	IG Dose[b]
Preexposure	Short term (1–2 mos)	0.02 mL/kg
	Long term (3–5 mos)	0.06 mL/kg[c]
Postexposure	—	0.02 mL/kg

[a]Infants and pregnant women should receive a preparation that does not include thimerosal.
[b]IG should be administered by intramuscular injection into either the deltoid or gluteal muscle. For children younger than 24 months of age, IG can be administered in the anterolateral thigh muscle.
[c]Repeat every 5 months if continued exposure to HAV occurs.
Source: From prevention of hepatitis A through active or passive immunization: Recommendations of the Advisory Committee on Immunization Practices (ACIP). *MMWR* 2006;55:1–23.

and 0.5% is positive for the HB surface antigen (HBsAg; infectious).

Infectious HBV virions have been found in nearly all human bodily fluids; however, only blood, blood products, semen, saliva, and vaginal fluids are considered to be infectious. The incubation of HBV ranges from 45–180 days, with an average of 60–90 days [7]. Infectious individuals can infect others for many weeks before the onset of symptoms and throughout the clinical phase. Unlike HAV infection, which has a fairly typical disease course followed by complete resolution, HBV infection has a variety of clinical outcomes. Approximately 95% of healthy adults with acute HBV infection recover completely, but 5–10% remain HBsAg-positive after resolution of symptoms and are at risk for developing chronic hepatitis.

All seronegative individuals are susceptible to HBV infection. The risk of contracting infection after a bloodborne exposure ranges from 2–40%, depending on the absence or presence of HBV antigen in the infectious source. Overall, the attack rate is 30% [7, 12].

Individuals with serologic resolution of previous infection have lifelong immunity. Immunity is characterized serologically by the following findings on blood studies: anti-HBs positive, HBsAg negative, and anti-HBcore positive. Typically, the anti-HBs and anti-HBcore serologic findings are lifelong.

PREVENTION

Individuals who have received the complete series of one of the four commercially available vaccines and who demonstrate serologic evidence of immunity are protected (i.e., anti-HBs positive). The four vaccines for hepatitis B that have been used in the United States are Heptavax (made from pooled sera of HBV carriers; no longer available in the United States), Engerix HB, Recombivax, and Twinrix (a combination of HAV and HBV antigens). It is not certain how long protection lasts, but it is anticipated to be indefinite in individuals who are known responders.

HBV vaccine–induced antibodies to HBV are known to wane gradually, and many individuals (60% or more) of the initial responders lose detectable antibodies within 12 years. However, among adults who responded to the initial series, even with declining or undetectable levels of antibody, booster doses are considered to be unnecessary and are not recommended by some clinicians. However, previously published recommendations by the CDC have suggested that individuals be tested for anti-HBs unless an adequate level has been demonstrated within the past 24 months. If the anti-HBs is considered to be inadequate, a booster dose of HBV vaccine should be administered [13–15].

Some individuals who have been documented responders to HBV immunization nonetheless have developed asymptomatic HBV infection, demonstrated by the presence of anti-HBcore with no subsequent development of HBsAg. These individuals with mild, asymptomatic infection have not demonstrated any of the sequelae associated with either acute or chronic HBV infection [15, 16].

HBV vaccine typically is administered to adults in three doses. After the initial dose, subsequent doses are administered at 1 and 6 months. Postvaccination testing is not mandatory; however, in populations in which there is a high rate of HBV carriage or where the risk of exposure is significant (e.g., health care workers), postvaccination testing should be considered.

TREATMENT OF NONRESPONDERS TO THE PRIMARY VACCINE SERIES

Serologic response rates are highest in individuals who receive the vaccination in the first and second decades of life. More than 90% of healthy adults and 95% of infants, children, and adolescents develop protective antibody responses from the primary series [13]. However, with each successive decade of life, the response rate lessens. Only 80–85% of the vaccine recipients who receive the primary series at the ages of 40–45 years develop protective antibodies. Smoking and obesity also lessen the immunologic response to the primary series.

Between 15% and 20% of individuals who are nonresponders to the primary vaccine series develop adequate antibody response after one additional dose of HBV vaccine (one booster, lifetime total of four HBV vaccines) and between 30% and 50% after three additional doses (three boosters, lifetime total of six HBV vaccines) [15]. If an individual sustains an exposure and is a known nonresponder, serologic testing for HBsAg should be performed to determine if the individual is a

chronic carrier. In a study of nonresponders, Jarroson found that 75% of nonresponders in his series did demonstrate HBV-specific cellular immune responses [17].

In addition, because of the possible waning of immunity with time in those who have been vaccinated previously with HBV vaccine, some clinicians perform periodic serologic testing of previously vaccinated responders to ensure that they are immune when a significant exposure occurs. Current CDC recommendations, however, do not mandate such an approach in previously vaccinated known responders because follow-up studies have revealed no clinical HBV illness in this population. With a continuing focus on cost-effective medicine, follow-up testing in previously known responders (even with exposure to an HBsAg source) appears to be unnecessary.

The CDC has published updated guidelines for postexposure prophylaxis for percutaneous or mucosal exposure to HBV (Table 17-2) [22].

PASSIVE IMMUNIZATION WITH HBIG

HBV immune globulin (HBIG) should be used in individuals who have not been vaccinated or who are nonresponders to the HBV vaccine. HBIG provides an instant method of protection that lasts approximately 3 months. Current recommendations for the use of HBIG as postexposure prophylaxis are that it be administered at a dose of 0.06 mL/kg intramuscularly as soon as possible after exposure. It is recommended that the total HBIG dose be split into two equally divided doses and then injected in each gluteal muscle. HBV vaccine series should be initiated concurrently. If HBV vaccine is not initiated, then HBIG should be repeated in 1 month [14]. HBIG is available from Bayer Pharmaceuticals as of 2005 in 2- and 10-mL vials.

HBIG should be administered no later than 7 days after exposure because there are no data as to its efficacy after 7 days [14]. In addition, there are uncertainties as to the maximum recommended doses of HBIG. Previous recommendations have cited a maximum dose of 5 mL in adults [16]. However, at a dose of 0.06 mL/kg, individuals over 80 kg (176 lb) would require larger doses. Thus, for large or obese adults, some physicians may exceed the 5-mL maximum dose.

As part of counseling after an exposure, the treating physician should thoroughly inform the

Table 17-2

Recommended Postexposure Prophylaxis for Exposure to Hepatitis B Virus

Vaccination and Antibody Response Status of Exposed Workers[a]	Treatment		
	Source HBsAg-Positive[b]	Source HBsAg-Negative[b]	Source Unknown or Not Available for Testing
Unvaccinated	HBIG[c] ×1 and initiate HB vaccine series[d]	Initiate HB vaccine series	Initiate HB vaccine series
Previously vaccinated			
Known responder[e]	No treatment	No treatment	No treatment
Known nonresponder[f]	HBIG × 1 and initiate revaccination or HBIG × 2[g]	No treatment	If known high-risk source, treat as if source were HBsAg-positive
Antibody response unknown	Test exposed person for anti-HBs[h]	No treatment	Test exposed person for anti-HBs[h]
	1. If adequate,[e] no treatment is necessary		1. If adequate,[d] no treatment is necessary
	2. If inadequate,[f] administer HBIG x 1 and vaccine booster		2. If inadequate,[d] administer vaccine booster and recheck titer in 1–2 months

[a]Persons who have previously been infected with HBV are immune to reinfection and do not require postexposure prophylaxis.
[b]Hepatitis B surface antigen.
[c]Hepatitis B immune globulin; dose is 0.06 mL/kg intramuscularly.
[d]Hepatitis B vaccine.
[e]A responder is a person with adequate levels of serum antibody to HBsAg (i.e., anti-HBs >10 mIU/mL).
[f]A nonresponder is a person with inadequate response to vaccination (i.e., serum anti-HBs < 10 mIU/mL).
[g]The option of giving one dose of HBIG and reinitiating the vaccine series is preferred for nonresponders who have not completed a second three-dose vaccine series. For persons who previously completed a second vaccine series but failed to respond, two doses of HBIG are preferred.
[h]Antibody to HBsAg.
Source: From Updated US Public Health Service guidelines for the management of occupational exposures to HBV, HCV, and HIV and recommendations for postexposure prophylaxis. *MMWR* 2001;50:1–23.

exposed worker about the risks of contracting disease or infection, a follow-up plan, and precautions. The precautions relevant to HBV, HCV, HDV, and HIV include avoiding childbearing for up to 1 year after exposure and refraining from donations of blood, from breast-feeding, and from sharing of razor blades or toothbrushes. In addition, the physician should counsel exposed individuals to use a latex condom (in a monogamous relationship) or refrain from sexual intercourse and high-risk sexual practices (if not in a monogamous relationship). Often, the spouse or sexual partner may have questions that need to be answered by the physician.

Hepatitis C

BACKGROUND AND EPIDEMIOLOGY

Hepatitis C (HCV) historically has been called *non-A, non-B hepatitis* (NANB). Prior to 1989, the etiologic agent was unknown, and there were no serologic markers. The infectious agent, HCV, was later identified using sera of chimpanzees who carried NANB hepatitis [1,2] and has been characterized as an RNA virus with a genome similar to that of *Flavivirus* and *Pestivirus,* each a genus in the Flaviridae family [2], and has been classified recently as a *Hepacivirus* in the Flavivridae family [23].

HCV has six genotypes, with subtypes within each genotype. As a result, there are several perplexing issues regarding the diagnosis, presentation, and treatment of HCV infection [1]:

1. The difficulty in identifying infection by serologic tests—even with the resulting development of second- and third-generation tests, which attempt to increase the sensitivity and specificity.

2. Naturally acquired infection with HCV apparently does not lead to immunity against reinfection secondary to the genomic variability.

3. As a result of the genomic variability of HCV, it has been difficult to develop a vaccine to prevent infection.

HCV infections remain persistently present in more than 70% of adult-onset infections [24]. As such, it is thought to be a major cause of chronic liver disease with cirrhosis.

ROUTES OF TRANSMISSION

HCV can be found in serum, saliva, semen, urine, stool, and vaginal secretions. Typically, transmission is via large-volume inoculation, such as that which occurs with blood transfusion. However, HCV can be spread via perinatal or sexual contact.

HCV is commonly transmitted by way of intravenous drug abuse, renal dialysis, and administration of untreated clotting factor concentrates. Approximately 0.5% of blood donors in the United States are positive for HCV antibodies. It has been found that about 40% of acute sporadic cases of HCV are not associated with any risk factors. Thus, while interpersonal spread may occur, the mechanism has not been determined.

The incubation period for HCV may range from 2 weeks to 6 months but commonly is 6–9 weeks. The attack rate is considered to be 3%, with a range of 1.2–10.05% for percutaneous exposure [12]. Infected individuals may be contagious prior to the development of ALT elevation, and infectiousness may persist indefinitely. HCV titers appear to be low, and ALT activity correlates with peaks in virus concentration [2, 7].

Occupational exposure to HCV is of equal concern as with HBV. At least 85% of persons with HCV infection develop chronic infection, and of these, approximately 70% develop chronic liver disease and enzyme elevation [25].

Individuals with chronic HCV infection are at increased risk for cirrhosis of the liver. In addition, chronic HCV infection appears to be associated with hepatocellular carcinoma [26].

Currently, there is no pre- or postexposure prophylaxis for those with chronic HCV infection. At the present time, clearance of the HCV from the blood has been accomplished in many patients with treatment using interferon and ribavirin [27]. The means of transmission are not well defined in sexual or household contacts; thus it is somewhat difficult to recommend specific guidelines to pre-

vent secondary transmission (other than avoidance of sharing toothbrushes or razor blades).

Prevention of exposure in susceptible individuals is the current preventive approach. Health care workers and workers in long-term residential facilities or correctional systems should adhere to standard precautions. Current postexposure guidelines are as follows [12, 25]:

1. Source testing for antibody to anti-HCV and ALT should be performed.
2. Individuals exposed to an anti-HCV-positive source should have baseline testing for anti-HCV and ALT.
3. Confirmation of anti-HCV-positive results should be obtained by supplemental assay.
4. IG has not been shown to be efficacious in postexposure prophylaxis against HCV.
5. Some authorities advocate the use of interferon-a in early cases of HCV infection. It has been proposed that using polymerase chain reaction (PCR) testing for HCV RNA will detect infections earlier, thus leading to early treatment with interferon. However, PCR is currently not a licensed assay, and there is a high degree of variability in the results. Early treatment of acute HCV hepatitis with interferon has shown a 30–40% reduction in progression to chronic HCV in meta-analyses. The data are insufficient to draw firm conclusions as to which patients to treat, when to begin, and optimal dosage of medication [47].
6. Follow-up surveillance testing should be performed for 6–9 months following exposure.

A vaccine for HCV is not available; however, recent discovery of natural immunity and vaccine efficacy in chimpanzees has encouraged optimism that an effective vaccine can be developed. Also, in up to 50% of acute human infections, spontaneous clearance of the virus takes place [28].

Hepatitis D

BACKGROUND AND EPIDEMIOLOGY

Hepatitis D virus (HDV) is also known as the *delta hepatitis agent* [1]. It is a defective RNA virus that uses HBsAg for its structural protein sheath. HDV requires coinfection in an individual who is HBsAg-positive, either acutely or chronically [26].

HDV can occur as one of two entities: (1) acute coinfection of HDV simultaneous with acute HBV or (2) acute HDV superinfection concomitant with chronic HBV.

Acute Simultaneous HDV Coinfection

Patients with acute simultaneous coinfection of HDV with acute HBV typically have a better prognosis. Fewer than 5% of cases of acute HDV infection result in chronic delta hepatitis. Coinfection typically is characterized by a low-level titer of anti-HDV and is short-lived. Thus anti-HDV tests typically may not detect HBV/HDV coinfection secondary to low titers.

Acute HDV Superinfection Concomitant with Chronic HBV

This entity runs a more virulent course than simultaneous HDV coinfection: 70% of all HDV superinfections result in chronic hepatitis. HDV superinfection with chronic HBV is more easily detected than acute simultaneous HDV confection because there are higher levels of anti-HDV.

HDV infection (whether coinfection or superinfection) runs a more severe course than isolated HBV or HCV infection. Acute infection with HDV has a mortality of 2–20%. In chronic HDV hepatitis, 60–70% of patients develop cirrhosis within 15–20 years.

EPIDEMIOLOGY

HDV infection occurs worldwide. Humans are the natural reservoir. Experimentally, HDV can be transmitted in chimpanzees infected with HBV. HDV also can be modeled experimentally in the woodchuck infected with woodchuck hepatitis virus. Although there is evidence of intrafamilial spread and sexual infection, HDV is spread more commonly and more easily by parenteral exposure. The incubation period is 2–8 weeks.

The primary means of preventing HDV infection is the prevention of HBV through HBV vaccination. In individuals who already have HBV infection, whether acute or chronic, avoidance of risks for HDV exposures is the only effective means of preventing the disease [7].

In southern Europe, at least, the prevalence of HDV has declined from a level of 23% in 1987 to 8% in 2005. This decreased incidence is attributed to improvement in hygiene, economic conditions, and HBV vaccination campaigns [29].

Hepatitis E

BACKGROUND AND EPIDEMIOLOGY

Hepatitis E virus (HEV) is a 32-nm RNA virus that is structurally similar to calicivirus [26] and similar epidemiologically to HAV. HEV has been referred to as *enterically transmitted non-A, non-B hepatitis* (ETNANB). The infection was first documented in New Delhi, India, during a 1955 epidemic. It is transmitted by the fecal-oral route; contaminated drinking water is the typical vehicle for outbreaks [18, 26].

Usually, the incubation period is 2–9 weeks, with a mean of 45 days. During epidemics, however, the incubation period is 15–64 days, with a mean of 26–42 days. The actual period of communicability is not well defined, but HEV has been detected in stool samples for up to 14 days after the onset of jaundice. The reservoir is unknown, but it is known that HEV is transmissible to chimpanzees, cynomolgus macaques, tamarins, and pigs [7].

The attack rate is highest in the 15- to 40-year-old population. There is a 15–20% case-fatality rate among pregnant women; the greatest risk is during the third trimester [1, 7, 18]. HEV does not progress to a chronic liver condition, with full recovery expected in most population groups except as noted earlier [30].

Prevention of HEV is best achieved via strict adherence to the hygienic and dietary principles one follows to avoid infectious diarrhea—avoidance of local water in endemic areas (unless boiled or carbonated), avoidance of uncooked foods, and avoidance of fruits that one does not peel. In the United States, the use of IG is unlikely to prevent HEV secondary to the country's low endemic rate [18]. A vaccine is not available.

Hepatitis G

Hepatitis G (HGV) is a bloodborne virus that appears to have transmission characteristics in common with HCV. The virus and its epidemiology have been defined recently. It has a serologic occurrence rate of 15 per 1,000 blood donors (1.5%). The HGV and GB virus types have been found to be isolates of the same virus and are closely related to the HCV. They are commonly found, frequently persist in humans, but have not been associated with any known disease state [31]. Whether they continue to be known as hepatits G is uncertain because many workers in the field feel that this is misleading and incorrect [31].

SEN, TT Viruses

These two viruses have been found in many posttransfusion patients. As with the HGV, the relation to hepatic disease is still under investigation because, to date, clear evidence linking them to hepatitis has not been found [32, 33].

Other Sources of Infectious Hepatic Inflammation

Various viral and nonviral infectious diseases can cause hepatic inflammation. These diseases should be included, along with noninfectious etiologies (e.g., drug, chemical, and autoimmune), in the differential diagnosis of workers with elevated liver enzymes [1]. For purposes of discussion of infectious hepatitis, the classification can be considered as (1) acute hepatitis owing to other viruses and (2) hepatitis owing to nonviral infectious agents [26].

ACUTE HEPATITIS OWING TO OTHER VIRUSES

The liver may be affected by several viral agents. One of the most common causes of hepatic inflammation is Epstein-Barr virus (EBV), the etiologic agent associated with heterophile-positive infectious mononucleosis. Other viruses that can cause hepatic inflammation are cytomegalovirus (heterophile-negative mononucleosis syndrome), rubella, rubeola, mumps, and coxsackie B virus.

Typically, in these cases of viral infection, the hepatic inflammation is mild, with liver enzymes ranging from two to five times normal and little, if any, jaundice. With EBV-associated hepatitis, an acute icteric syndrome can occur, although this is relatively uncommon. In the immunocompromised host with a systemic viral infection, however, hepatic inflammation can be severe, resulting in hepatic necrosis and possibly death from hepatic failure. This scenario has been associated with herpes simplex virus, cytomegalovirus, and varicellazoster virus [26]. Yellow fever, a zoonosis transmitted by several variants of mosquito [7], also can cause severe hepatitis, resulting in significant elevations in the liver enzymes and mortality approaching 20–50%. While yellow fever is not endemic in the United States, it is endemic in Central America, South America, and Central Africa.

HEPATITIS OWING TO NONVIRAL INFECTIOUS AGENTS

Liver inflammation and dysfunction can result from bacteria, mycobacteria, rickettsiae, fungi, brucellosis, tularemia, plague, bacterial sepsis, and legionnaires' disease. There are three nonviral infectious agents that can produce an acute hepatitis syndrome: syphilis, leptospirosis, and Q fever [26].

Syphilis

Primary and early secondary syphilis can cause ALT and AST elevations of four to eight times normal. The diagnosis of syphilis-related hepatitis is made on the basis of the history, physical examination, and serologic tests for syphilis.

Leptospirosis

Leptospirosis is a febrile illness caused by the spirochete *Leptospira,* which occurs worldwide. *Leptospira* infection has protean manifestations, including sudden and severe onset of fever, headache, chills, rash, and severe myalgia, and may affect the hepatic and pulmonary systems. Leptospirosis has a relatively low case-fatality rate, but in affected individuals with hepatic and renal involvement, the rate is over 20%.

Leptospirosis is contracted by exposure to water contaminated with the urine of infected animals, typically infected rats. It is an occupational hazard for sewage workers, farmers, veterinarians, and those with potential exposure to infected waters. It is an unusual cause of jaundice in the United States [7].

Q Fever

Q fever is a rickettsial disease caused by *Coxiella burnetii.* The natural reservoirs are infected farm animals, some wild animals, and ticks. The infection is transmitted by the airborne route, with contaminated airborne dust or other particles containing the rickettsiae. It also can be transmitted by ingestion of contaminated raw milk.

Direct transmission by blood or bone marrow transfusion has been reported [8]. The hepatic manifestations of Q fever range from subclinical hepatic involvement and inflammation (the typical course) to overt jaundice. It is transmitted by infected farm animals.

Special Populations with Unique Risk for Exposure

SEWAGE WORKERS

The health of sewage workers has been of concern for centuries. Bernardino Ramazzini, the "father of occupational medicine," described the plight of sewage workers in *Diseases of Workers* (*De Morbis Artficium*). In particular, he described the maladies of those who clean privies and cesspits [20]. There have been several illnesses described in sewage workers. These descriptions range from "sewage worker's syndrome" [21] to various bacterial, parasitic, and enteric infections contracted through exposure to sewage [34, 35].

Several authorities have suggested an epidemiologic link between HAV seroprevalence and exposure to sewage at work. Skinhoj and colleagues described an increased prevalence of anti-HAV antibodies in sewage workers compared with gardeners and municipal clerks [36], and several investigators have recommended immunization of sewage workers with HAV vaccine [37–40]. Formal recommendations by the CDC and the Advisory Committee on Immunization Practices (ACIP) have not been publicly promulgated, however. It is reasonable to consider vaccination of sewage workers with HAV vaccine, considering the low endemic rate in the U.S. population and relatively low cost of the vaccine compared with the health care costs associated with hepatitis A illness. This view is not universally accepted, however, and several authors do not support vaccination of sewage workers against HAV [41–33,47]. Another hepatic risk for sewage workers is leptospirosis, but the hepatic inflammation associated with it is often subclinical and usually is not the focal aspect of the disease.

HEALTH CARE WORKERS

HBV infection is a major threat to health care workers (along with HIV and HCV infection). In 1993, there were an estimated 1,450 cases of occupationally acquired HBV infection in health care workers (HCWs). This represents a 90% decrease from the estimated number of HBV infections in HCWs in 1985 [14]. The decrease in incidence is attributable to wide-scale voluntary immunization of HCWs with the HBV vaccine.

In 1991, the OSHA bloodborne pathogens standard became law, and health care institutions were required to provide active HBV immunization to susceptible employees with potential exposure to blood or other potentially infectious bodily fluids. This mandatory provision for the protection of HCWs has greatly contributed to the significant decline in occupationally acquired HBV infection in HCWs.

LAW ENFORCEMENT AND CORRECTIONAL DEPARTMENT PERSONNEL

HBV infection is highly prevalent in the criminal population, especially in individuals with a history of intravenous drug use (IDU). By virtue of the antisocial and violent tendencies of the criminal population, law enforcement and correctional department personnel often are subjected to injuries to the skin and are exposed to bodily fluids such as blood and saliva. Many police departments and correctional institutions have instituted HBV vaccination programs since the promulgation of the OSHA bloodborne pathogens standard, but these programs are not mandatory because these employees are not technically considered health care workers.

When law enforcement and correctional personnel are exposed to a source of bodily fluids in the line of work, it is often difficult (if not impossible) to test the source of the exposure in a timely manner. Often, the arrestee, suspect, or inmate (source) refuses voluntary testing for HBV, HCV, and HIV, and some states do not have statutory authority for the testing of bloodborne pathogens in the criminal population. When such authority exists, it is argued that the source's confidentiality is breached when the source is tested and the results revealed to law enforcement and correctional personnel. Because of the real threat of litigation against municipal and state law enforcement departments and correctional departments by the source for attempted testing, many departments have chosen not to aggressively pursue source testing. Often, the exposed law enforcement or correctional workers have to pursue legal action to test the source, either at their own expense or with the assistance of the labor union.

In these instances, the treating physician and the exposed law or correctional worker need to discuss the pros and cons of using HBIG. The theoretical risks and expense of HBIG passive immunization to that of contracting HBV (as well as postexposure prophylaxis for HIV) also should be discussed.

WORKERS IN LONG-TERM RESIDENTIAL FACILITIES

Historically, long-term residential facilities have been associated with diseases transmitted by the fecal/oral route, the respiratory route, fomites, and several other routes and vectors of transmission. Individuals residing in and those working in these facilities are at significant risk for contracting one of several communicable diseases. Contributing factors include poor hygiene, close living conditions, and individuals with overall poor health and/or physical conditioning.

HAV infection is common in day-care centers with children in diapers. In addition, among adults in crowded living conditions, where spread is a greater risk, transmission can be rapid if an infectious source/index case becomes available. This is often the situation in long-term residential facilities for the developmentally disabled.

HBV infection also has been linked to institutional clients and staff. HBV is transmitted most commonly via perinatal, sexual, and bloodborne routes. However, it also appears to be transmitted by household contacts. Thus HBV infection is also of concern in long-term residential facilities [7].

OTHER POPULATIONS AT RISK FOR ABRASIONS TO THE SKIN WHERE HBV IS PRESENT

Any situation in which an employee can sustain a cut or abrasion of the skin with subsequent exposure to blood or infectious bodily fluids at the portal of entry (e.g., cut, abrasion, or exposed mucous membrane) puts the individual at risk for HBV infection. Mevorach, Eliakim, and Brezis reported a case of horizontal transmission of HBV in Israeli meat cutters who shared knives in the butcher shop where they worked. These authors make the case that HBV vaccination should be universal and not reserved just for what historically have been considered high-risk groups [45].

Work Issues with Enteric Hepatitis (Hepatitis A and E)

Food handlers can transmit both HAV and HEV. Food handlers infected with HAV should not be allowed to prepare or serve food until they are no longer infectious. This is typically 7 days after the onset of jaundice [14]. Current CDC recommendations include IGIM treatment for other food handlers at the same location as the index case; IGIM administration to patrons also should be considered if the index-case food handler was involved in the preparation of foods to be eaten uncooked or was involved in the preparation or serving of foods after cooking and had diarrhea or poor hygiene practices. This assumes that the potentially exposed patrons can be identified within 2 weeks of exposure [9].

Because of the low prevalence of HEV infection in the United States, this disease is of less concern in this country. Individuals with HEV infection may be infectious for 14 days after the onset of jaundice (the period of infectivity has not been completely characterized). One should consider handling the worker infected with HEV using the well-established precautions for HAV infection.

HFV infection has not been well characterized. Until more is understood about this disorder, similar precautions should be followed as those for HAV infection.

Health care workers with HAV infection should be restricted from patient contact until 7 days after the onset of jaundice [14].

Work Issues with Bloodborne Hepatitis (Hepatitis B, C, and D)

In a work environment, individuals with HBV, HCV, or HDV infection may be of concern both to management and to co-workers. Those with acute infection are typically too ill to work. Special accommodations may be necessary for those who are able to work or who may be in the recovery or convalescent phase. Accommodation may be in the form of minimal exertion or an abbreviated workday.

Workers with acute and/or chronic infection who do not perform exposure-prone invasive procedures require no specific restrictions, provided that there is no epidemiologic link for transmission of infection to contacts [14]. Standard precautions should be used (see "Prevention" below) [46].

Workers with acute and/or chronic infection who perform exposure-prone invasive procedures require more careful work placement. These workers should not perform exposure-prone invasive procedures until counsel has been sought from an expert review panel that evaluates the particular disorder and skill level of the worker relevant to the specific procedure of concern [14]. Long-term accommodation may be necessary in these instances. These are often difficult decisions and reflect a balance between the rights of the infected employee and the duty to protect the public.

Prevention

As stated previously, preexposure vaccination against HAV and HBV is very effective in preventing these infections. There is currently no vaccine available for HCV, HDV, or HEV.

Because of the increasing recognition of the threat of bloodborne diseases, it is generally accepted that precautions should be used in health care settings, especially to prevent the transmission of currently known diseases for which there is no effective preexposure therapy.

Prior to the recognition of HIV-related illnesses, patients who were suspected of having communicable disease, such as hepatitis A or B, were placed on isolation. Those with suspected hepatitis A were placed on enteric precautions, and those with serum hepatitis (hepatitis B) were placed on blood precautions.

When etiologic factors associated with HIV infection were recognized, universal precautions were initiated for all HCWs who potentially could be exposed to patients' blood or bodily fluids. Universal precautions were applied only to those fluids known to transmit bloodborne diseases and to bodily fluids with visible blood. Universal precautions have since been replaced by standard precautions [46].

Standard precautions are now taken by HCWs when they are exposed to patients' blood, bodily fluids, secretions, and excretions (except for sweat) and when contacting patients' mucous membranes and nonintact skin.

Personal protective equipment that helps to prevent exposure to pathogens includes gloves, facial protection, and gowns. Hand washing is used after doffing gloves, between patients, and for any contact with blood, bodily fluids, secretions, or excretions. Hand washing, or use of hand sanitizers, is the single most effective way to interrupt the transmission of infections in health care settings.

Although standard precautions (a form of administrative control) and personal protective equipment provide some protection to the worker, engineering controls are clearly the most desirable means of preventing exposure. On that front, significant technological advances have been made in the design of needleless drug-delivery systems. Similarly, vascular access systems that minimize the risk of accidental needlesticks (self-sheathing systems) are also available. These should be used in an organized, methodical approach to preventing exposures.

In the United States during the period 1995–2006, the incidence of HAV infection declined by 90% to its lowest rate ever recorded (1.2 cases per 100,000 population). During 1990–2006, the incidence of HBV infection declined 81%, also to its lowest rate ever recorded (1.6 cases per 100,000 population). The decline in HAV infection was greatest in children in states where routine vaccination was recommended starting in 1999, resulting in an increase in the proportion of adult cases. The decline in HBV infection occurred in all age groups but was greatest in children. Higher rates occurred in adults, particularly males in the 25- to 44-year age range. HCV infection incidence peaked in the late 1980s, declined in the 1990s, and reached a plateau in 2003, with a slight increase in 2006, the incidence in that year being 0.3 cases per 100,000 population. For HCV infection, most cases occurred in adults, with injection drug use being the most common risk factor. These data reflect the successes of vaccination programs and likely other factors. A 2006 recommendation for routine HAV vaccination to include all children in the United States aged 12–23 months is expected to further reduce hepatitis A incidence. The data also reflect opportunities for further reduction of disease in other groups, such as adults with risk factors for HBV infection and injection drug users [48–50].

Future Challenges

In the past three decades, tremendous progress clearly has been made in the characterization and understanding of viral and nonviral hepatitides.

Our knowledge base has expanded from an understanding of the epidemiologic determinants of disease to characterization of the etiologic agents and the risks for infection and prevention of infection through immunobiologics. In addition, improved therapies are becoming available as a better understanding of the molecular biology of these diseases is gained. Furthermore, tremendous strides have been made in legislative protections for workers who are in the highest-risk groups. With the emergence and discovery of new agents of hepatic inflammation, challenges remain, however. This, coupled with continual development of improved treatments of infectious hepatitis, will continue to challenge occupational medicine physicians into the next millennium.

References

1. Dienstag JL, Isselbacher KJH. Acute viral hepatitis. In Fauci AS, Braunwald E, Isselbacher KJ, et al (eds), *Harrison's Principles of Internal Medicine*, 14th ed. New York: McGraw Hill, 1998, pp 1677–92.
2. Ockner RK. Acute viral hepatitis. In Bennett JC, Plum F (eds), *Cecil Textbook of Medicine*, 20th ed, Vol 1. Philadelphia: Saunders, 1996, pp 762–72.
3. Pagano JS, Blaser M, Buendia MA, et.al. Infectious agents and cancer: Criteria for a causal relation. *Semin Cancer Biol* 2004;14:453-471.
4. Liang T, Heller T. Pathogenesis of hepatits C-associated hepatocellular carcinoma. *Gastroenterology* 2004:127:S62–71.
5. Hollinger FB. Serologic evaluation of viral hepatitis. *Hosp Pract* 1987;15:101–14.
6. Carey WD, Patel G. Viral hepatitis in the 1990s: I. Current principles of management. *Cleve Clin J Med* 1992;59:317–25.
7. Benenson AS (ed). *Control of Communicable Diseases Manual,* 16th ed. Washington: APHA, 1995, pp 217–33.
8. Hepatitis A associated with consumption of frozen strawberries—Michigan, March 1997. *MMWR* 1997;46:288–95.
9. Prevention of hepatitis A through active or passive immunization: Recommendations of the Immunization Practices Advisory Committee (ACIP). *MMWR* 1996;45:1-25.
10. Outbreak of hepatitis C associated with intravenous immunoglobulin administration—United States, October 1993–June 1994. *MMWR* 1994;43:505–9.
11. Fleming DW. Immune globulin shortage—Health care provider information (letter, September 6, 1996). Document 221060. Atlanta: Centers for Disease Control and Prevention, October 9, 1996.
12. Swinker M. Occupational infections in health care workers: Prevention and intervention. *Am Fam Physician* 1997;56:2291–9.
13. Wood RC, MacDonald KL, White KE, et al. Risk factors for lack of detectable antibody following hepatitis B vaccination of Minnesota health care workers. *JAMA* 1993;270:2935–9.
14. Immunization of health-care workers: recommendations of the Advisory Committee on Immunization Practices (ACIP) and the Hospital Infection Control Practices Advisory Committee (HICPAC). *MMWR* 1997;46:3–8.
15. Hepatitis B virus: A comprehensive strategy for eliminating transmission in the United States through universal childhood vaccination. Recommendations of the Advisory Committee on Immunization Practices (ACIP). *MMWR* 1991;40:1-19.
16. Update on adult immunization: Recommendations of the Immunization Practices Advisory Committee (ACIP). *MMWR* 1991;40:9–10, 31, 47.
17. Jarrosson L, Kolopp-Sarda MN, Aguilar P, et al. Most humoral non-responders to hepatitis B vaccines develop HBV-specific cellular immune responses. *Vaccine* 2004;22:3789–96.
18. CDC. Hepatitis E among U.S. travelers, 1980–1992. *MMWR* 1993;42:1–4.
19. Bowden DS, Moaven LD, Locarnini SA. New hepatitis virus: Are there enough letters in the alphabet? *Med J Aust* 1996;164:87–9.
20. Ramazzini, B. *Diseases of Workers.* Thunder Bay, Canada: OH&S Press, 1993, pp 86–91. (Translated from the Latin text *De Morbis Artificium* of 1713 by Wilmer Cave Wright.)
21. Rylander R, Andersson K, Belin L, et al. Sewage worker's syndrome. *Lancet* 1976;28:478–9.
22. Updated US Public Health Service guidelines for the management of occupational exposures the HBV, HCV, and HIV and recommendations for postexposure prophylaxis. *MMWR* 2001;50:45-6. CDC last reviewed these guidelines November 21, 2006.
23. Szabo E, Lotz G, Paska C, et al. Viral hepatitis: New data on heaptitis C infection. *Pathol Oncol Res* 2003;9:215–21.
24. Wieland SF, Chisari FV. Stealth and cunning Hepatitis B and hepatitis C viruses. *J Virol* 2005;79: 9369–80.
25. Recommendations for follow-up of health-care workers after occupational exposure to hepatitis C virus. *MMWR* 1997;46:603–7.
26. Hsu HH, Feinstone SM, Hoofnagle JH. Acute viral hepatitis. In Mandell GL, Bennett JE, Dolin R (eds), *Principles and Practice of Infectious Diseases*, 4th ed. New York: Churchill Livingstone, 1994, pp 1136–53.
27. Moreno-Otero R. Therapeutic modalities in hepatitis C: Challenges an development. *J Viral Hepatitis* 2005;12:10–9.
28. Houghton M, Abrigani S. Prospects of a vaccine against the hepatitis C virus. *Nature* 2005;436:961–6.
29. Gaeta GB, Stornaiuolo G, Precone DF. Type B and D viral hepatitis: Epidemiologic changes in southern Europe. *Forum (Genova)* 2001;2:126–33.
30. Emerson S, Purcell R. Running like water: The omnipresence of hepatitis E. *N Engl J Med* 2004;351: 2367–8.

31. Stapleton JT. GB virus type C/hepatitis G virus. *Semin Liver Dis* 2003;23:137–48.
32. Akiba J, Umemura T, Alter HJ, et al. SEN virus: Epidemiology and characteristics of a transfusion-transmitted virus. *Transfusion* 2005;45:1084–8.
33. Liwen I, Januszkiewicz-Lewandowska D, Nowak J. Role of TT virus in pathogenesis of liver diseases: The prevalence of TTV in patients and healthy individuals. *Przegl Epidemiol* 2002;56:101–13.
34. Sumathipala RW, Morrison GW. *Campylobacter* enteritis after falling into sewage. *Br Med J* 1983; 286:1356.
35. Sehgal R, Mahajan RC. Occupational risks in sewage work. *Lancet* 1991;33:1404.
36. Skinhoj O, Hollinger FB, Hovind-Hougen K, et al. Infectious liver diseases in three groups of Copenhagen workers: Correlation of hepatitis A infection to sewage exposure. *Arch Environ Health* 1981;36: 139–43.
37. DeSerres G, Levesque B, Higgins R, et al. Need for vaccination of sewer workers against leptospirosis and hepatitis A. *Occup Environ Med* 1995;52:505–7.
38. Poole CJM, Shakespeare AT. Should sewage workers and carers for people with learning disabilities be vaccinated for hepatitis A? *Br Med J* 1993;306:1102.
39. Donoghue AM, Hancox B. Hepatitis A vaccination for sewage workers. *NZ Med J* 1995;108:235–6.
40. Longsen PJ. Hepatitis A vaccine. *Br Med J* 1992; 305:888.
41. Warken AA, Hoff GL. Hepatitis A in waste water treatment plant workers: Is vaccination necessary?. *J Occup Environ Med* 1998;40:515–7.
42. Maguire H. Hepatitis A virus infection: Risk to sewage workers unproved. *Br Med J* 1993;307:561.
43. California Department of Health. Illness in sewage workers/recommendations for prevention. *Calif Morbid* 1992;35/36:1.
44. Glas C, Hotz P, Steffen R. Hepatitis A in workers exposed to sewage: A systematic review. *Occup Environ Med* 2001;58:762–8.
45. Mevorach D, Eliakim R, Brezis M. Hepatitis B: An occupational risk for butchers? (Letter). *Ann Intern Med* 1992;116:428.
46. Garner JS. Guideline for isolation precautions in hospitals. *Infect Control Hosp Epidemiol* 1996;17:53–80.
47. Alberti A, Boccato S, Vario A, Benvegnu L. Therapy of acute hepatitis C. *Hepatology* 2002;36:S195–200.
48. Centers for Disease Control and Prevention. Surveillance for acute viral hepatitis—United States, 2006 (surveillance summaries). *MMWR* 2008;57:1–24.
49. Centers for Disease Control and Prevention. Prevention of hepatitis A through active or passive immunization: Recommendations of the Advisory Committee on Immunization Practices (ACIP). *MMWR* 2006;55:1–23.
50. Centers for Disease Control and Prevention. A comprehensive immunization strategy to eliminate transmission of hepatitis B virus infection in the United States: Recommendations of the Advisory Committee on Immunization Practices (ACIP): 2. Immunization of adults. *MMWR* 2006;55:1–23.

18 Occupational Gastroenteritis

Alain J. Couturier, Wendell Perry, and William E. Wright

Infectious gastroenteritis is a general term used to refer to infectious inflammation of the stomach, small intestines, and/or large intestines that typically results in symptoms related to the upper gastrointestinal tract (e.g., nausea, vomiting, abdominal cramps) and lower gastrointestinal tract (e.g., cramps and diarrhea that is often secretory). Fever and other constitutional symptoms may occur.

Infectious gastroenteritis is one of the most common types of infection throughout the world. There are no comprehensive data on incidence because the illness is often unreported or underreported. Its incidence is occupational groups is not clear, but it is thought to result in large numbers of absences in the United States and worldwide, along with lost productivity and medical expenses. Those who are charged with treating individuals with work-related gastroenteritis should have a good understanding of how the pathogens are transmitted and of risk factors for infection.

Epidemiology

RISK FACTORS FOR TRANSMISSION

The organisms most often involved in occupational gastrointestinal infections find their way to the host through a variety of routes. Most commonly, transmission is achieved through contaminated food or water, contact with a person who has infective gastroenteritis or with their excretions, or contact with fomites contaminated from these sources. The oral-fecal and person-to-person routes are important, and in some settings, large-droplet transmission or splashes of contaminated excretions play a role. A summary of the transmission factors for various organisms is given in Table 18-1 [1].

Workers especially likely to be affected by infectious gastroenteritis include hospital employees, nursing home workers, day-care employees, sewage and wastewater workers, military personnel confined to closed spaces, food handlers, animal handlers, abattoir workers, immigrants, migrants, those working with refugees, and travelers. Any work group that includes an ill individual with infectious gastroenteritis is at risk for an outbreak. Risk tends to be elevated especially if the work setting involves close contact among workers, crowded work conditions, lack of optimal hand hygiene, and suboptimal hygiene and sanitation. Work groups that have catered meal events or pot-luck celebrations in general work settings are at greater risk than average, particularly if food is brought to work, having been allowed to undergo transport or standing for long periods without either proper refrigeration or thorough reheating before serving.

Table 18-1
Modes of Transmission of Organisms that Cause Occupational Gastroenteritis

Organism	How Transmitted
Giardia lamblia	Fecal-oral, by contaminated food or water or person-to person
Listeria monocytogenes	Food-borne, by contaminated hospital equipment
Shigella	Fecal-oral, by contaminated food or person to person
Salmonella	Food-borne, fecal-oral, person to person; contaminated hospital equipment
E. coli 0157:H7 (EHECs)	Food-borne, water-borne, person to person
E. coli (ETECs)	Food-borne, water-borne
E coli (EIECs)	Food-borne
E coli (EPECs)	Food-borne, person to person
Cryptosporidium parvum	Food-borne, water-borne, fecal-oral, animal to person, and person to person
Vibrio cholerae	Water-borne, food-borne
Campylobacter jejuni	Food-borne, water-borne, animal to person
Helicobacter pylori	Oral-oral, fecal-oral, contaminated medical equipment
Clostridium difficile	Person to person
Yersinia frederiksenii	Food-borne, water-borne
Rotavirus	Fecal-oral, questionable water-borne, respiratory droplets
Hepatitis A virus	Fecal-oral, person to person, needle sharing
Norwalk virus	Fecal-oral, person to person

Infectious gastroenteritis occurs in all age ranges but tends to be more severe in the elderly, in children, in those with debility from other health conditions, and in those with immunodeficiency. Although healthy adults often can experience one of these infections as a self-limited illness with only brief incapacity, those just noted who are at the extremes of age or who have significant comorbidities can suffer severe complications and death. Acute viral infectious gastroenteritis has been estimated to account for 10–12% of hospitalizations among children in industrialized nations and for almost 3–6 million annual deaths among infants and children in developing countries; this population also experiences gastroenteritis as a more chronic and debilitating disease [2, 3].

The globalization of the world's food supply has contributed to international public health problems of food-borne disease. The World Health Organization (WHO) has responded by launching global *Salmonella* surveillance, instituting a sentinel-sites project to determine the burden of food-borne disease in regions lacking estimates, and supporting international collaboration related to the burden of illness from enteric diseases [4].

In 1996, the United States established the Food-borne Diseases Active Surveillance Network (Food-Net), an expansion of the previous food-borne-disease outbreak reporting and surveillance program as part of the U.S. Centers for Disease Control and Prevention's (CDC's) Emerging Infections Program. From 1998–2002, there were, on average, 1,329 outbreaks each year causing over 25,000 illnesses each year. Most outbreaks (55%) and cases were of bacterial origin, *Salmonella enteritidis* accounting for the largest number of outbreaks and number of cases, and *Listeria monocytogenes* accounting for the majority of deaths from any pathogen. Viruses, predominantly noroviruses, resulted in 33% of outbreaks and 41% of cases, with the proportion of outbreaks attributable to viruses increasing from 16% in 1998 to 42% in 2002 (perhaps owing in part to better detection methods). Parasitic illness accounted for 1% of outbreak and 1% of cases. Chemical agents accounted for 10% of outbreaks and 2% of cases [5]. The cited reference for these data includes an appendix that contains a CDC form used to report investigations of food-borne outbreak investigations to the CDC and an appendix containing guidelines for confirmation of food-borne-disease outbreaks.

Food-borne-disease outbreaks do not all result in gastroenteritis, and infectious gastroenteritis occurs outside food-borne-disease outbreaks. In the

United States, the burden of acute gastroenteritis has been estimated to be 0.72 episodes per person per year, accounting for 195 million yearly episodes [6]. Rates were highest in children (1.1 episodes per person-year) and lowest in those 65 years of age or older (0.32 episodes per person-year). *Salmonella* infection was estimated to account for 1.4 million cases of illness, 15,000 hospitalizations [4], and 400 deaths. Food-borne disease in the United States has been estimated to account for 76 million cases of gastroenteritis, 82% of which had an unknown cause [7]. A more recent estimate based on an expanded surveillance population in the United States is that bacterial food-borne disease affects about 0.36 per 1,000 population per year [8]. In England, an estimate was that 20% of the general population experienced acute gastroenteritis each year, most commonly owing to norovirus, with *Campylobacter,* rotavitus, and *Salmonella* (nontyphoidal) playing lesser roles. Acute gastroenteritis was estimated to result in 0.60 episodes per person per year in Northern Ireland and the Republic of Ireland (where food-borne sources were thought to account for about 32%). In The Netherlands, the acute gastroenteritis rate was reported to be 283 cases per 1,000 person-years [4].

Specific Illnesses

GENERAL CONSIDERATIONS

Infectious gastroenteritis can be classified in several ways. Some of the most common microbiologic agents related to infectious gastroenteritis that may be seen in the occupational setting are listed below by type of organism (i.e., viral, bacterial, protozoal, or helminthic). Another consideration for classification is based on how the organisms affect the bowel mucosa. Infectious diarrhea can be either noninflammatory (i.e., interference with fluid and electrolyte absorption) or inflammatory (i.e., invasion of mucosa eliciting an inflammatory response). In general, viruses and protozoans interfere with absorption, resulting in a noninflammatory secretory diarrhea with large volumes of liquid stool without prominent leukocytes in the stool. Many bacterial gastroenteritis infections result in inflammatory mucosal invasion with lower-volume diarrhea and prominent leukocytes and/or blood in the stool. Some bacteria can produce noninflammatory diarrhea owing to preformed toxins.

ILLNESS WITH SPECIFIC ORGANISMS: VIRAL GASTROENTERITIS

Viral gastroenteritis is the most common cause of gastroenteritis in industrialized countries. The most common form of viral gastroenteritis recognized in adults in the United States is caused by noroviruses (formerly called *Norwalk agent*), a group of small RNA caliciviruses that account for more than 90% of nonbacterial gastroenteritis in the United States. Disease can occur sporadically but commonly occurs in outbreaks. Norovirus infection is common in children and adults and is thought to be a major source of mild gastroenteritis in communities and a source of epidemic outbreaks worldwide. It is transmitted by the fecal-oral route, through eating shellfish grown in contaminated waters, from consuming other contaminated food or water, and from food contaminated by sick food handlers. Illness from noroviruses is sometimes called *winter vomiting disease* or *epidemic viral gastroenteropathy.* The incubation period tends to be about 12–48 hours. Nurses and nursing assistants who work in nursing homes have the highest incidence of occupational infection from this virus. During acute outbreaks, 30–50% of nursing home staff may be affected. One study describes an outbreak of Norwalk-like virus [small, round-structured virus (SRSV)] aboard a U.S. aircraft carrier where overcrowding was blamed for ease of transmission [9]. A number of norovirus outbreaks have been described on cruise ships [10]. One recent study attributed transmission of norovirus to school workers and students from a shared contaminated computer keyboard and mouse (of the fomite variety) [11].

Other viruses recognized to cause gastroenteritis primarily in children include RNA viruses such as group A rotoviruses of the family Reoviridae, sapovirus, astrovirus, and the DNA viruses, including adenovirus types 40 and 41. Of these, rotavirus in the most common cause of infectious diarrhea and gastroenteritis among infants and children worldwide. Especially in nonindustrialized countries, it is a leading cause of infant and childhood death. Most people who reach adulthood have been infected with rotavirus, but protective immunity is variable and often not complete. Adults can become ill from rotavirus or can be infected and have no symptoms, in which case they are able to spread this illness. Day-care and nursing home employees are particularly susceptible to rotavirus infections.

Hepatitis A virus (HAV), an RNA picronavirus, also can result in a mild gastroenteritis (i.e., abrupt onset of anorexia, nausea, and abdominal discomfort with fever and malaise), typically followed by jaundice after a few days. The incubation period is about 2–8 weeks. Fully 35–54% of nursing home staff, intensive care unit personnel, orphanage personnel, day-care workers, and other health care workers will test positive for past exposure to HAV. Janitorial staff are particularly vulnerable.

Entroviruses are a group of RNA viruses that are recognized to multiply in the gastrointestinal tract but do not have a prominent role in gastroenteritis. Members of the group include echoviruses, polioviruses, a number of coxsackieviruses, and others. Examples of illnesses they can cause in adults include aseptic meningitis and encephalitis, nonspecific febrile illnesses, common colds, and conjunctivitis.

Symptoms of viral gastroenteritis are typically rapid onset of nausea, vomiting, watery diarrhea, abdominal pain and cramping, clammy skin, and muscle and joint aches. Fever may occur, and rectal urgency or fecal incontinence can be a problem. Many adults work through this without seeking medical attention. Indications for medical atten-

tion for gastroenteritis (viral or bacterial) generally include sustained fever over 38.3°C (101°F), presence of bloody diarrhea, severe abdominal or chest pain, vomiting blood, aspiration of vomitus with respiratory distress, development of confusion, signs of dehydration such as orthostatic light-headedness or syncope, and persistence of vomiting and/or diarrhea for more than 1–2 days. Children, the elderly, immunosuppressed individuals, and those with comorbidities such as heart disease or diabetes mellitus should be encouraged to seek medical attention sooner. Table 18-2 reviews some of the major gastrointestinal pathogens and the symptoms associated with infection.

There is no specific treatment for viral gastroenteritis. Self-administration of antidiarrheal medications generally is not recommended. For adults, initial self-care is to avoid eating and drinking for a few hours and then gradually try to drink room-temperature liquids (avoid extremes of hot and cold) such as water, Gatorade, and/or dilute non-caffeinated beverages, avoiding milk and other dairy products, fruit juices, caffeinated beverages, and alcohol. After fluid intake has been established without inducing upper or lower gastrointestinal symptoms or distress, the diet can be expanded gradually to include soda crackers and toast while continuing oral hydration. The next step is to add cooled broths, gelatin, bananas, and rice and then nonfried chicken or baked potato. Until comfortable dietary intake is established, hot and cold liq-

Table 18-2
Signs and Symptoms Associated with Gastrointestinal Pathogens

Organism	Signs and Symptoms
Giardia lamblia	Nausea, epigastric distress, flatulence, nonbloody diarrhea
Listeria monocytogenes	Acute, mild febrile illness with influenza-like symptoms
Shigella	Early watery and then bloody diarrhea, tenesmus
Salmonella	Watery or bloody diarrhea with or without systemic symptoms
E. coli	Diarrhea with watery explosive onset, nausea, chills, and cramps
Cryptosporidium parvum	Crampy, profuse, watery diarrhea, sometimes with anorexia and vomiting
Vibrio cholerae	Abrupt, explosive rice water stool, severe electrolyte and fluid depletion, no abdominal pain or fever
Campylobacter jejuni	Prodrome of headaches, malaise, myalgias, fever, bloody diarrhea
Helicobacter pylori	Dyspepsia associated with epigastric or substernal "burning," early satiety, abdominal fullness
Clostridium difficile	Profuse watery diarrhea, fever, abdominal pain, leukocytosis
Yersinia frederiksenii	Simulates Crohn's disease and appendicitis, joint complaints
Rotavirus	Vomiting, watery diarrhea, fever, occasionally dehydration
Hepatitis A virus	Minor flulike illness: anorexia, malaise, nausea, vomiting, and fever
Norwalk virus	Diarrheal illness often severe enough to cause dehydration

uids, caffeine, alcohol, fatty foods, fluids or foods high in sugar content, highly seasoned foods, and milk or other dairy products should be avoided. If addition of a food results in recurrence of symptoms, then the dietary intake should not be advanced, and the offending item should not be consumed until the patient is well.

ILLNESS WITH SPECIFIC ORGANISMS: BACTERIAL GASTROENTERITIS

Bacterial gastroenteritis can be caused by a variety of pathogens, including *Escherichia coli* strains, *Salmonella*, *Shigella*, *Vibrio cholera*, *Campylobacter jejuni*, and other toxin-forming bacteria such as *Staphylococcus aureus*, *Bacillus cereus*, *Clostridium perfringens*, *C. difficile*, and *C. botulinum*. Heightened awareness of bioterrorism should include consideration that *Bacillus anthracis* infection can result in an acute abdominal syndrome with gastrointestinal complaints. Some of the more common forms of bacterial gastroenteritis are addressed here. Table 18-2 reviews some of the major gastrointestinal pathogens and the symptoms associated with infection.

Escherichia coli

This gram-negative bacillus has several forms that can result in gastroenteritis or severe diarrhea. Enterotoxigenic *E. coli* (ETEC) is a major cause of endemic diarrhea in developing countries and the most common cause of travelers' diarrhea. It is rare in the United States but has accounted for some food-borne outbreaks. Its effect is mediated by several toxins (e.g., LT-1 and STa) that result in watery diarrhea owing to extra fluid secretion in the small bowel. Symptoms are usually self-limited and commonly last up to 3 days. Enteropathic *E. coli* (EPEC) results in diarrhea in children and sometimes in hospital nurseries. It is uncommon in the United States. It can result in mucosal change (loss of villi) with mucus-containing diarrhea without blood, or chronic, persistent diarrhea. Enteroinvasive *E. coli* (EIEC) is noted to cause illness mostly in developing countries and among travelers. The initial secretory diarrhea is followed by an inflammatory colitis with fever, abdominal pain, and stools containing mucous and blood. It is a self-limited disease. It has occurred in food-related outbreaks in the United States. Enteroaggregative and diffusely adherent *E. coli* (EAEC and DAEC) are also diseases

primarily of developing countries that affect young children, resulting in mucosal changes and chronic watery diarrhea [12].

Shiga toxin–producing *E. coli* (STEC), sometimes referred to as *enterohemorrhagic E. coli* (EHEC), is an emerging pathogen that is found in cattle and their feces that are sometimes used to fertilize food crops. Contamination of meat can occur during processing. Unlike the other *E. coli* noted earlier, this one is more common in developed countries. This organism can result in hemorrhagic colitis and hemolytic-uremic syndrome (HUS) in 2–8% of cases, most often in young children and the elderly. The CDC has included HUS as a factor in surveillance of food-borne diseases, based on STEC likely accounting for more than 50% of the incident HUS in the United States. There are a number of serotypes of STEC, O157:H7 being the most common. They are all able to produce Shiga or related toxins that are ribosome-inactivating proteins. The incubation period is about 3–4 days, and the typically afebrile, self-limited illness is usually 5–10 days long. An initially secretory, watery diarrhea develops into a grossly bloody diarrhea in more than 90% of patients. HUS can develop 2 days to 2 weeks after the diarrhea. It may be related to an interaction of the toxin with vascular endothelial cells. Mortality with dialysis support is less than 10%. Treatment of STEC with antibiotics is not recommended because such treatment can increase the occurrence of HUS, thought to be related to increased release of the toxin [12]. In settings of beef processing and meat handling and in occupational or nonoccupational settings where there is the possibility of consuming inadequately cooked beef and drinking unpasteurized milk, workers are at increased risk for *E coli* infection from this strain of the bacteria. Fecal-oral human transmission also can occur.

Salmonella (Nontyphoid Strains)

These gram-negative bacilli produce an inflammatory acute enterocolitis with abdominal pain, fever, diarrhea, and sometimes nausea and vomiting. The incubation period is usually 12–36 hours but can vary beyond this span. The condition tends to be most severe in elderly, infirm, and immunosuppressed workers. Most common sources of infection include poultry, pigs, cattle, and their meat products; dairy products; and contamination of food by infected food handlers; sometimes pets such as chicks, turtles, iguanas, dogs, and cats can be carriers. In those who have normal immune function, most *Salmonella* gastroenteritis is self-limited and does not need antibiotic treatment, which has been found to be associated with relapses and a prolonged carrier state. Communicability generally lasts throughout the period of infection. Employees who staff hospitals, nursing homes, institutions for children, and restaurants are at higher risk for developing *Salmonella* infection.

Shigella

Shigella dysenteriae, a gram-negative bacillus, typically thrives in the distal small intestine and colon after ingestion and results in fever, nausea, vomiting, abdominal pain, tenesmus, and either watery diarrhea or bloody, mucus-containing dysentery. It occurs worldwide, and its reservoir is human. It is usually passed from an ill person or asymptomatic carrier by the fecal-oral route but can occur from ingestion of contaminated food or water. The incubation period ranges from 12 hours to 1 week, averaging about 1–3 days, and the illness is usually self-limited, lasting 4–7 days. Other *Shigella* strains, such as *S. sonnei* and *S. flexneri*, typically cause milder disease. Some forms are associated with arthropathy, as is the protozoan, *Giardia lamblia*. Shigellosis usually resolves without antibiotic treatment, but appropriate treatment can reduce carriage to a few days and prevent an asymptomatic carrier state. The disease can occur as a sporadic disease or in outbreaks, the outbreaks typically occurring in day-care facilities for children, prisons, refugee camps, mental hospitals, from a point source involved in food handling and preparation, or in situations of overcrowding when poor personal hygiene and proper sanitation are not maintained.

Helicobacter pylori

This gram-negative, spiral, flagella-equipped bacillus is found worldwide, primarily in humans. Infection is thought to occur in childhood, although the mode of transmission is not clear. It colonizes the stomach and is estimated to be present in about 30% of the U.S. population and up to 70–80% of people in developing countries. *H. pylori* is strongly associated with chronic superficial gastritis, duodenal ulcers, gastric ulcers, and stomach adenocarci-

noma and lymphoma. The organism can be spread nosocomially through contaminated, incompletely sterilized medical equipment. Endoscopists and their staff are at increased risk for contracting this infection mainly as a result of contact with contaminated medical equipment.

Campylobacter jejuni

These gram-negative bacilli are being identified as important causes of acute inflammatory gastroenteritis worldwide, with fever, abdominal pain, diarrhea with bloody stools, nausea, and vomiting. The enterocolitis can give the appearance of inflammatory bowel disease. In some populations, it is more common than *Salmonella* infection. The incubation period is typically 2–5 days. Sources are poultry, other birds, cattle, pigs, and pets (i.e., cats and dogs). Transmission is most often related to eating uncooked or undercooked contaminated food or raw milk or contact with infected animals. Symptoms typically last for less than a week; communicability typically lasts throughout the period of infection but can last for up to several weeks. Most cases require only supportive care. If antibiotics are given early (at the onset of illness), studies indicate that they can shorten illness duration. Increasing fluoroquinalone resistance has been found, particularly in Asia. Occurrence is probably highest among workers with the greatest risk of contact with uncooked or undercooked chicken, unpasteurized milk, and nonchlorinated water. Such workers include food factory processors and poultry handlers.

Clostridium difficile

This gram-positive anaerobic bacillus typically results in an antibiotic-associated diarrhea when the antibiotic disrupts normal colonic flora. Many people carry *C. difficile* asymptomatically, the proportion increasing after hospitalization. It can be a community-acquired illness or a nosocomial infection with institutional outbreaks. Particularly severe disease has been increasing, thought to be due to emergence of a strain with greater levels of specific toxin production (BI/NAP1) [13, 14]. *C. difficile* infection occurs most often after treatment with ampicillin, second- and third-generation cephalosporins, clindamycin, and fluoroquinolones. The illness can occur after a single dose of antibiotic or can occur after stopping treatment.

Mild self-limited illness can occur, but some people develop a severe pseudomembranous colitis (which can lead to colonic necrosis, toxic megacolon, shock, perforation, and death) or relapsing *C. difficile* diarrhea [3, 15]. Although infection with this organism is most frequently associated with patients receiving antibiotic therapy, hospital workers can be infected through contaminated materials and person-to-person contact.

Listeria monocytogenes

This gram-positive bacillus is prevalent worldwide and is thought to result in many subclinical infections. An asymptomatic fecal carrier state has been estimated to occur in about 10% of humans [16]. The organism can result in a mild febrile illness or more severe illness with nausea, vomiting, fever, septicemia, abscess formation, and meningoencephalitis. Pregnant women can transmit the infection to the fetus, which can result in miscarriage, still birth, or severe illness in the newborn. The estimated incubation period ranges from 3–70 days (median 3 weeks). The organism can be found in the soil, water, animal forage/silage, fowl, and domestic and wild mammals. It can occur in raw or contaminated milk, vegetables, soft cheeses, and meat products. Ripening soft cheeses contaminated with *Listeria* have resulted in outbreaks. Workers directly handling contaminated materials can develop papules on their hands and arms. Nosocomial infections can occur and are substantially more frequent in adults over 40 years of age. Abattoir workers and laboratory workers handling cultures are at risk. Workers who are immunosuppressed are at increased risk for infection and serious disease [16].

Yersinia enterocolitica

These gram-negative bacilli can produce an inflammatory acute enteritis with severe abdominal pain, ileitis, and bloody stools. *Y. pseudotuberculosis* can result in diarrhea and mesenteric lymphadenitis. *Y. enterocolitica* is the form most associated with disease in the adult human population. The infection can be followed by erythema nodosum and arthritis. These infections are a worldwide problem. The incubation period is generally 3–7 days. The infection can be self-limited, particularly in otherwise healthy people. Antibiotic treatment generally is recommended for severe cases or those involving

septicemia, particularly in the debilitated or immunosuppressed host. Pigs are the main reservoir, and human infection can occur through the oral route after handling or processing contaminated animals, fecal-oral route after contact with infected people, or after consuming contaminated water or contaminated uncooked or undercooked pork, particularly pork chitterlings. This infection can appear among hospital workers, and nosocomial spread has occurred.

Vibrio cholerae

This is a gram-negative bacillus that was essentially eliminated from the United States but now occurs occasionally from shellfish or imported food products. Cholera is still endemic in a number of parts of the world. Epidemic forms occur in Asia, Africa, and South America, but it is rarely a major risk for short-term travelers. It is the source of a number of historical pandemics. The organism produces a toxin that results in hypersecretion of fluid and electrolytes from the bowel, resulting in usually abrupt, explosive diarrhea (rice water stools). In its most severe form, vomiting, dehydration, leg cramps, shock, and death can occur. It is usually transmitted by food and water contaminated by feces of an infected person. The CDC does not recommend use of cholera vaccine, although one is available in some other countries (Duoral, SBL Vaccines) [17]. Cholera is a risk to health care personnel and others caring for its victims.

Other organisms that produce toxins involved in gastroenteritis include *S. aureus* (gram-positive cocci with heat-stable enterotoxin) and *B. cereus* (gram-positive bacilli), which grow when food storage is improper. These organisms typically cause nausea and vomiting about 8 or more hours after consuming the contaminated food. Typical foods involved are custards, other egg products, and potato salad (*S. aureus*) and fried rice (*B. cereus*). *C. perfringens*, a gram-positive bacillus that commonly resides in the human colon, can produce a toxin-related secretory diarrhea 8–16 hours after consumption of contaminated food [3]. *C. botulinum*, usually types A or B, can result in afebrile vomiting, diarrhea, and abdominal pain, but the most important symptoms are related to a neurotoxin attacking the peripheral nervous system at presynaptic nerve cells at the myoneural junction. Initial neurologic symptoms can include blurred vision, double vision, difficulty swallowing and speaking, fatigue, weakness, and a descending paralysis starting in the head and neck, then shoulders, moving down the arms, and then down the legs. Paralysis of respiratory muscles can occur, leading to death. *C. botulinum* can be found in soil, and botulism occurs worldwide as a food-borne illness related to preserved foods contaminated with heat-resistant spores that form toxin in an anaerobic environment. Although typically associated with home-canned or -jarred vegetables and fruit, outbreaks have occurred from commercial vegetable and meat products and from type E *C. botulinum* in fish and fish products. The incubation period is usually 12–36 hours but, depending on dose, can occur in a few hours or a few days. Transmission from person to person has not been identified.

V. parahaemolyticus is member of the same family of bacteria as the cholera *Vibrio*. It tends to reside in brakish seawater and can contaminate shellfish or cause skin infections in open wounds of those exposed to the water. The coastal waters of the United States and Canada can contain *V. parahaemolyticus,* and it is a common form of food-borne disease in Japan. Eating contaminated or raw shellfish can result in abdominal cramping, nausea, vomiting, fever, and chills, typically occurring within 24 hours of ingestion. Illness typically lasts 3 days. Antibiotic treatment is not recognized to reduce the severity or duration of illness, but in severe cases, antibiotics sometimes are used in addition to fluid replacement depending on the organism's sensitivity.

Travelers' diarrhea is estimated to be related to bacterial infection in 80–85% of cases, the most common bacteria noted by the CDC being ETEC [18]. About 15% of travelers' diarrhea includes vomiting and can resemble other forms of acute gastroenteritis. Prophylactic antibiotics have been tried but generally are not recommended because of increasing patterns of antibiotic resistance, suspected contribution of prophylaxis to emerging resistant organisms, and risk for adverse effects of antibiotic treatment. An exception for consideration is the individual who is immunosuppressed, taking a short trip, and at high risk for infection and complications. Travelers' diarrhea treatment is best done by targeting the specific organism. Empirical self-administered antibiotic treatment sometimes is provided, the current choices usually

being a fluoroquinolone such as ciprofloxacin or levofloxacin. However, increasing resistance to these drugs, particularly in Asia, makes them less useful. A nonabsorbable antibiotic, rifaximin, has been approved in the United States for treatment of travelers' diarrhea caused by noninvasive strains of *E. coli* [18, 19]. Prevention of travelers' diarrhea related to food and water is the same as for nontravel viral and bacterial gastroenteritis. These issues are covered in Chapter 27.

ILLNESS WITH SPECIFIC ORGANISMS: PROTOZOAL GASTROENTERITIS
Giardia lamblia

Infection with this protozoan is worldwide, and in some countries, the population prevalence in stool samples can be as high as 30%. It typically resides in the upper small intestine, and the presence of *G. lamblia* (*G. intestinalis, G. duodenalis*) in stools is usually asymptomatic. It can result in acute or chronic diarrhea with bloating, abdominal cramps, and malabsorption. Outbreaks typically occur in children or young adults in July to October in the United States. Transmission can occur from drinking unfiltered surface water, water from shallow wells, or contaminated community water supplies; swimming in freshwater; eating contaminated food; or via a person-to-person fecal-oral route. Incubation period averages 7–10 days but can be as short as 3 days or as long as 25 days [20]. Infection with this organism in occupational groups appears principally among day-care workers in the 25- to 39-year age group, outdoor workers who drink unfiltered surface water from streams, and occupational travelers who consume contaminated food or water. A number of other protozoans can cause gastroenteritis or severe diarrhea, including *Entamoeba histolyitica* (amoebiasis), *Cryptosporidium parvum* (prevalence of which in the general population is less than 1–4.5% in a survey of stool samples, but rates are higher for animal handlers, health care workers, and day-care employees), *Isospora belli*, microsporidian infections, and others. These protozoan infections are covered in more detail in Chapter 31.

ILLNESS WITH SPECIFIC ORGANISMS: HELMINTHIC GASTROENTERITIS

Many helminth infections can result in gastroenteritis and/or severe diarrhea; many have signs or symptoms related to other organ systems. The list includes *Schistosoma* infection (i.e., fever, abdominal pain, enteropathy with bleeding, diarrhea, and rarely, appendicitis), *Hymenolepsis nana* infection (common in day-care centers, orphanages, and conditions of crowding and poor hygiene), *Diphyllobothrium latum, Taenia saginata, Taenia solium, Anisakis marina, Gnathosoma spinigerum,* early *Trichinella spiralis* infection, and many others. These are of particular concern for occupational physicians who care for international travelers, immigrants to the United States, and migrants. These and other helminthic infections are covered in Chapter 30.

Occupational Risk Factors

Clearly, some vocations require that workers place themselves at increased risk for job-related gastroenteritis. These are discussed below.

HEALTH CARE WORKERS

The wide spectrum of health care occupations and professions includes physicians, nurses, nursing assistants, technicians, laboratory personnel, and housekeeping staff. As a broad category of workers, they are the most likely to contract infectious diseases, and gastrointestinal infections are no exception. Some reported incidents are outlined below; they provide a good overview of the organisms transmitted and the circumstances that contribute to their transmission [21].

Ironically, health care workers are one of the most uncooperative populations when it comes to appreciating the hazards to which they are exposed and taking appropriate precautions. One author cites the prevailing belief among hospital workers that their specialized knowledge and training is, in some way, armor against infectious diseases. In other cases, the zeal for research and medical advancement can blind some hospital workers to the personal dangers inherent in their profession. Gestal observes, "Despite the many serious dangers present in hospitals and medical research centres, health and safety regulations are frequently ignored" [22].

One article describes a hospital epidemic, principally among nursing staff, of a diarrheal illness owing to *Cryptosporidium* originating with a single immunocompromised patient. This case history looks retrospectively at the likely modes of transmission and possible breakdown of infection control standards. The authors conclude that although meticulous infection control procedures and equipment were in place at the facility, lapses in such matters as hand-washing techniques, use of protective clothing, and reporting of symptoms had occurred. Staff had not maintained rigid adherence to procedures. Conspicuous among the procedural violations were relaxed attitudes toward consuming food and drink at nursing stations. Since *Cryptosporidium* is transmitted by the fecal-oral route, there was a clear cause-and-effect consequence of these actions [23].

Another study looks at an outbreak of gastroenteritis caused by SRSV among hospital nursing staff. According to Caceres and Kim [24], these viruses "have been implicated frequently in closed communities, such as nursing homes, hospitals, cruise ships, and dormitories." This investigation demonstrated that SRSV infection can be transmitted person to person (the precise route was not established, but the respiratory route was a strong likelihood) as well as via food- or water-borne means. This study also showed that strictly observed infection control measures (including the use of gowns and gloves, use of face masks, frequent hand washing, and isolation of sick staff members) are effective in protecting patients. Even so, close person-to-person contact among infected staff members who relaxed their vigilance with each other resulted in an employee epidemic of gastroenteritis. The practical implications of this study led Caceres and Kim to two conclusions: (1) "casual contact between staff may spread SRSVs and cause gastroenteritis outbreaks in institutional settings" and (2) "staff should not work while ill with gastroenteritis and, optimally, should not return to work until completely free of symptoms" [24].

NURSING HOME PERSONNEL

The need to exclude ill employees from health care facilities is especially important in the case of nursing homes. Many nursing home residents are debilitated and suffer compromise of their immune system. This makes them particularly vulnerable to nosocomial infection, including gastroenteritis. In fact, each year more deaths owing to diarrhea occur among the elderly than among children. By the same token, the tendency of infectious diseases to be more widespread in nursing facilities makes employees proportionally susceptible to acquiring infections—and to transmitting them.

Epidemics of gastroenteritis in nursing homes can be swift and severe, affecting up to 50% of staff and residents. In one reported case, an outbreak of viral gastroenteritis in a nursing home accounted for 3 hospitalizations and 2 deaths among 121 residents. In this instance, 2 staff members continued to work while symptomatic. Some of the recommendations stemming from this study include "stopping new admissions and readmissions during the outbreak period, excluding symptomatic employees from patient care and food handling until 48 hours after resolution of diarrhea and vomiting, handling fecally contaminated laundry as little as possible and transporting such laundry in an enclosed and sanitary manner, wearing masks when cleaning vomitus or stool, and informing visitors of the outbreak." As always, this study reemphasizes the recurrent theme of strict adherence to good and frequent hand-washing techniques [25].

Gellert's study chronicles an unusually long (2-week) outbreak of acute gastroenteritis among staff and residents of a Los Angeles nursing home. The etiologic agent was identified as an SRSV related to Norwalk-like agents. The study was revealing in two ways. First, it raised the possibility that forms of acute gastroenteritis may be transmitted by airborne aerosolized vomitus as well as by the more commonly recognized person-to-person transmission. Second, the study gave rise to the novel recommendation that investigations of respiratory precautions be undertaken in such circumstances. It also underscored the time-honored infection control measure often echoed in these cases: To minimize personnel crossover from infected and uninfected wards, strict enforcement of employee sick leave during illness and careful hand washing are critical [26, 27].

In his study of a Norwalk virus outbreak in a nursing home, Stevenson emphasizes the importance of primary prevention; that is, eliminating the common source of the outbreak rather than simply implementing infection control measures once the epidemic has gained a foothold. In this instance, contamination of cold foods by kitchen staff was the etiologic event. Therefore, preventive measures such as exclusion of affected staff, good cleaning in the food-preparation area, reinforcement of

good hygiene practices, and elimination of higher-risk cold foods were stressed over isolation techniques and respiratory precautions. The author argued that once the outbreak became established, little could be done to prevent it from running its course. This line of thinking gained increasing popularity with Chadwick and other authorities, who came to believe that advocates of certain fastidious infection control methods had overstated their case [28–30].

WASTEWATER TREATMENT WORKERS

Studies that compare prevalence of infectious disease symptoms among various professions have shown that there is a statistically significant imbalance favoring gastrointestinal symptoms in wastewater workers. Clearly, workers who are exposed to the spectrum of wastewater products, from raw sewage to highly treated wastewater, encounter an impressive array of pathogens. Although specific bacterial, parasitic, fungal, and viral agents are not always recoverable from stool samples, manifestation of gastrointestinal symptoms—and possibly their subclinical disease counterparts—predominate in wastewater workers. Most studies have been disappointing in the yield of specific pathogens gathered from ill workers. There is, however, a strong relationship between level of exposure to wastewater and severity and frequency of symptoms such as abdominal bloating, cramping, and diarrhea [31].

MILITARY PERSONNEL

Military recruits in basic training have long been cited as examples of how infectious disease can spread rapidly among those confined to close spaces and subjected to overcrowding. Sharp and Hyams [13] provide an illustration of this phenomenon in a study examining an epidemic of gastroenteritis that swept through the enlisted spaces aboard a U.S. aircraft carrier. Significant findings from this study revealed that the outbreak of gastroenteritis—defined by nausea, vomiting, or watery stool—was more prevalent among those who had eaten in dining areas served by infected food handlers and two to three times greater among those who occupied berthing compartments accommodating more than 50 crew members. These data led the authors to allow for the possibility of both food- and water-borne transmission of disease, as well as spread through person-to-person contact. Not unimportant was the statistic that 1–2 work days were lost by ill crew members [9].

FOOD HANDLERS

As discussed previously, kitchen workers and food handlers in hospitals and nursing homes have been strongly implicated in the transmission of various gastrointestinal illnesses to fellow workers and residents. In the case of SRSV, a single ill worker can become a common infection source capable of contaminating food and water sources available to employees and institutional residents. Person-to-person transmission then can accelerate the epidemic. One interesting study [32] raised the possibility that a presymptomatic food handler shed SRSV in the kitchen of a hospital and contaminated cold lunch items that were subsequently consumed by both employees and residents who later became ill. Alternatively, the authors also were willing to consider the possibility that the virus was transmitted mechanically from the clothing of the worker who had handled a sick child at home. In any case, the heretofore overlooked possibility that presymptomatic kitchen workers were able to contaminate their work environment gave rise to infection control precautions never before implemented. For example, an educational program was created that emphasized awareness that employees could contaminate food *before* becoming symptomatic merely by coming into contact with a sick relative at home. That emphasis was designed to provide a rationale for taking particular care to follow good kitchen hygiene practices such as meticulous hand washing, changing into clean overclothing prior to beginning a shift, enforced sick leave for symptomatic workers, and destruction of food that symptomatic workers have handled [32].

In another notable case, a food-producing company instituted elaborate infection control and surveillance measures following a devastating outbreak of *Campylobacter* infection among workers at its plant [33]. Their new policy mandated that employees with gastrointestinal disturbances or anyone who had possible exposure to patients with such illnesses must have stool testing and must have follow-up and be cleared before returning to work. Anyone with positive stool specimens was barred from work with full pay. Moreover, when an employee has an episode of gastroenteritis symptoms, the worker is seen by a company physician, who takes a thorough history, aided by a detailed questionnaire [33].

ANIMAL HANDLERS

Gastrointestinal zoonoses (i.e., diseases that infect both humans and animals) are found in workers who come in contact with potentially infected animals, such as slaughterhouse (abattoir) workers and veterinarians. One illustration of how these infections can occur appears in a Swedish case in which abattoir workers contracted *Campylobacter* gastroenteritis during a particularly large holiday slaughter of poultry. Extenuating circumstances such as the youth and inexperience of the workers exacerbated what probably otherwise would have been only a minor outbreak [34].

A similar case in another Scandinavian country involved veterinary students who, in this instance, engaged in experimental work with calves intentionally injected with *Cryptosporidium*. Despite what they believed to be adequate protection through protective clothing and hand washing, all five students became infected and symptomatic with *Cryptosporidium* gastroenteritis, most probably through the fecal-oral route. The researchers conclude that cryptosporidiosis is a highly contagious cattle-borne zoonosis that "can certainly be considered an occupational risk for farmers, animal handlers, veterinary students and surgeons, laboratory personnel, and research workers . . . capable of crossing the interface between man and animals" [35]. As a footnote, other reports cite *Streptococcus suis* as a zoonotic pathogen occasionally seen in farmers who come into close contact with pigs. In humans, this disease is manifested as copious diarrhea that occasionally can result in acute dehydration.

WORKERS IN REMOTE LOGGING AND INDUSTRIAL CAMPS

Workers who are forced to operate in primitive, remote areas often enjoy less-than-hygienic work and living conditions. Most of these cases are "typical," and many of the circumstances are striking in their similarities. One case involved workers at a gas drilling rig in a remote wilderness area of British Columbia. There, 21 persons suffered a sudden attack of vomiting, abdominal cramps, and diarrhea.

Investigators determined that the water supply was situated 18 m from a crude, unlined sewage pit. It was surmised that contaminated drinking water was the culprit in this epidemic of gastroenteritis. Once water was transported from a municipal system and bacteriologic testing was implemented, there were no recurrences [36, 37].

TRAVELERS, IMMIGRANTS, MIGRANTS, AND REFUGEES

Occupational groups inclusive of these and similar categories of workers carry special risks for infectious gastroenteritis and importation of these and other diseases from endemic areas of countries of origin or countries and areas transited. Risk is especially high for some owing to overcrowding, lack of access to good hygiene and sanitation, and lack of control of food and water supplies and food preparation. Further information is available in the travel-related chapters of this book.

Prevention and Control

ADMINISTRATIVE CONTROLS AND EMPLOYEE EDUCATION AND TRAINING

Written plans or administrative controls that define policies to defeat the spread of infectious gastroenteritis in the workplace will have varying levels of effectiveness depending on the causative organism, mode of transmission, and occupation affected. Administrative plans for response and recovery related to occupational gastroenteritis should be part of the workplace's broader disaster management plan, which addresses bioterrorism and natural disasters. At a minimum, the content related to gastroenteritis outbreaks should address employee training, importance of hand washing and hygiene, contingency behaviors, and ideally, preventive measures such as symptom reporting, isolation of infected and uninfected employees, personal protective equipment, removal and cleanup practices, proper laundry and food handling, disease surveillance, and where practical, immunization. Ideally, such employee training should take place at the time of hiring and at regular intervals thereafter.

SAFE WORK PRACTICES AND ENGINEERING CONTROLS

The purpose of any rational engineering control strategy is to effectively separate the worker from any infectious agents (particularly those described earlier) that have become part of the work environment. Specific methodologies in this arena may include purely mechanical ones such as isolation of work processes and control of dissemination of contamination, supplemented by such approaches as use of protective clothing, hand washing, isolation techniques, food- and laundry-handling procedures, and cleanup and disinfection techniques. Approaches also may involve reporting sick contacts, preemptive notification of potential contacts, and elaborate surveillance methods.

It is difficult to be specific about some of these strategies because the many organisms incriminated in the etiology of infectious gastroenteritis possess unique properties. However, the key factors for prevention of many infectious gastrointestinal illnesses in the workplace are thorough and timely hand washing, especially after using toilet facilities, after handling potentially contaminated animals or their products, before touching the mouth or eating, and before touching shared potential fomites; decontamination of food-preparation surfaces during and after use; maintaining appropriate levels of refrigeration for food storage; cooking food thoroughly; and following regulations for the safety and health of food handlers.

PERSONAL PROTECTIVE EQUIPMENT

Personal protective equipment for standard, droplet, and airborne precautions has a role to play when a gastrointestinal pathogen may be present or has been documented—whether in an institutional setting or in a less controlled environment such as a logging camp. The need for personal protective equipment is often a tacit concession that engineering control methods and other preventive measures already have broken down. This is not to say that personal protective equipment is not a very useful tool standing between a vulnerable employee population and infection, particularly in the health care environment.

When examining our armamentarium of protective equipment, we must consider the entry points that an organism may exploit. Near-total coverage must include, at a minimum, gowns, caps, facemasks, footcovers, goggles, and gloves. Clearly, this whole array of protection is not practical in all situations, particularly not in non–health care settings such as remote camps and military bases. It does make sense, however, when the microbial "cat is out of the bag" in a given environment and risks to employees are high, for instance, in a research situation where a spill has occurred.

MEDICAL SURVEILLANCE AND BIOLOGIC TESTING

In most cases of occupational gastroenteritis, a retrospective look at epidemiologic and etiologic factors would not lead us to conclude that comprehensive medical monitoring or surveillance of employees would have been a practical or cost-effective preventive measure. Ongoing or frequently scheduled employee physical examinations and laboratory work in, for example, nursing homes, in the absence of suspicious symptoms or at least incriminating risk factors, would never pass the test of frugality in this cost-conscious medical culture. In any event, the efficacy of these strategies is as yet unproved for the prevention of rapidly spreading diseases such as the infectious forms of gastroenteritis.

A possible exception to this general statement may be the special circumstances of animal handlers who are constantly and chronically exposed to zoonoses that may be more readily detectable by methods such as complete blood count and determination of fecal leukocytes and fecal ova and parasites.

Similarly, well-intentioned biologic testing of potentially contaminated sources such as food and water supplies probably will not be sufficient to prevent such easily contagious and rapidly transmissible diseases as most forms of infectious gastroenteritis.

IMMUNIZATION AND PROPHYLACTIC MEASURES

Hepatitis A is susceptible to both pre- and postexposure chemoprophylaxis. HAV immune globulin (IG) has proved to be an effective agent of prevention when administered within 2 weeks of suspected exposure to the virus. Also, the recently developed vaccine against HAV would be a logical prophylactic choice for the wastewater worker who risks exposure to this virus on a daily basis. It is also recommended for health care workers and people who travel overseas.

An oral, live pentavalent rotavirus vaccine has been approved by the U.S. Food and Drug Admin-

istration (FDA) for use in the United States for prevention of rotavirus-associated gastroenteritis in infancy (RotaTeq, Merck). The three-dose schedule starts at 2 months of age and then at 4 and 6 months. The series is not to be started in infants older than 12 weeks, and it is not recommended for adults at the time of this writing. A monovalent rotavirus vaccine is available in some other countries (Rotarix, GlaxoSmithKline) [38, 39]. Unfortunately, technical and economic stumbling blocks have left few other preventive agents in the battle against occupational gastroenteritis. In short, the chemoprophylactic arsenal against this class of microbe is relatively meager. Our efforts should be focused on some of the preventive measures discussed earlier rather than on chemoprophylaxis. Prophylactic antibiotics have been used occasionally or recommended for prevention of travelers' diarrhea, but experience has resulted in detection of increasing antibiotic resistance to the agents used. Prophylactic antibiotics generally are not recommended, although they are sometimes considered for brief periods of use in immunosuppressed travelers who would have increased risk for infection and serious complications [18].

Differential Diagnosis

When reviewing the differential diagnosis of acute gastroenteritis, the common occupationally acquired organisms discussed earlier obviously must be considered, but to be thorough in the assessment of ill workers, other nonoccupational causes of gastrointestinal symptoms must be considered as well, including

- Laxative-induced diarrhea
- Antibiotic-induced diarrhea
- Other medication-induced diarrhea, such as that cause by iron- or manganese-containing compounds; high-dose salicylates, quinidine, nonsteroidal anti-inflammatory drugs (NSAIDs), beta blockers, methyldopa, digitalis, or phenothiazine
- Chemical toxin–mediated diarrhea
- Inflammatory bowel disease
- Irritable bowel syndrome
- Lactase deficiency
- Diabetes mellitus, autonomic neuropathy
- Hyperthyroidism

- Malabsorptive states
- Vascular, inflammatory, and physical abdominal problems requiring surgery

Diagnostic Evaluation

Very often the diagnosis of gastroenteritis is made without identification of the etiology. All diagnostic workups involve a detailed medical history (including travel and work history), physical examination, and laboratory evaluation.

In some settings, it has been useful to provide the ill employee with a detailed questionnaire chronicling sick contacts, work environments, adherence to preventive procedures, record of ingestions of food and fluids, prior illnesses, chronic illnesses, medications, etc. Obviously, this should never be used as a substitute for a thorough history taken by a medical professional.

The physical examination should focus on vital signs, which may show elevated temperature, extremes of blood pressure, respiratory distress, and tachycardia or arrhythmias. General appearance, alertness level, and listlessness may herald more serious complications, namely, electrolyte imbalance and dehydration. Evaluation of skin turgor, mucosal hydration, heart rate, peripheral capillary refill findings, and mental status may give clues to dehydration. The investigation should include checking for signs of upper and lower gastrointestinal bleeding and physical signs indicating a more serious or surgical abdominal problem.

In the laboratory workup, a complete blood count can be quite revealing in the areas of elevated polymorphonuclear leukocytes and/or depressed lymphocytes. These findings sometimes can point to a viral versus a bacterial cause. Helminthes typically can result in eosinophila, whereas protozoal infections typically do not. A basic electrolyte panel will reveal serious electrolyte imbalances caused by severe diarrhea and vomiting. Stool should be tested for blood and for leukocytes indicating inflammatory gastroenteritis. Stool studies are useful occasionally in determining the precise etiology of infective gastroenteritis. In general, however, they have been quite disappointing in identifying specific agents. A number of bacterial agents can be identified by culture; specific tests for toxins are available, and polymerase chain reaction testing is available for some agents. On occasion, acute and convalescent sera can identify an agent (see Chapter 2).

Treatment

Most bouts of acute gastroenteritis are short-lived and self-limited. These diseases often respond well to oral fluid replacement, as described in the section addressing viral gastroenteritis, and gastrointestinal "rest." Bland lactose-free diets and bismuth products are useful in providing symptomatic relief, but occasionally, a prolonged illness will require intervention with antibiotics and electrolyte supplements. Choice of antibiotics, parenteral fluid supplementation, and electrolyte replacement depends on the etiologic agent, severity of illness, degree of dehydration, assessment of electrolyte and pH status, and consideration of history of antibiotic allergies, pregnancy status, and comorbid conditions. Table 18-3 outlines proposed first-line antibiotics recommended for some specific infectious organisms. Severe disease may require additional antibiotics or combinations other than those described in the table. Owing to the ever-evolving nature of antibiotic resistance, current information on treatment should be consulted, and community patterns of disease and antibiotic resistance should be considered.

Occupational Considerations

Although infectious gastroenteritis is not an obvious topic for most discussions of occupational diseases, little imagination is required to identify several occupations where there is clear cause and effect between job responsibilities and employee infection. Prominent among these occupations are the health professions and their supporting staff. Fortunately, most health institutions have well-developed prevention and contingency plans to meet the challenges of occupational disease. This efficiency may be motivated as much by economic incentives as by humanitarian impulses. Long regarded as merely an annoying illness that offers no serious, long-lasting health risk to the host, gastroenteritis is taken seriously in the occupational setting, principally as a drain on employer resources.

The price of employee sick leave attributable to illness is a major expense for most health care facil-

Table 18-3
Antibiotics Recommended for Nonpregnant Adults for Specific Organisms

Organism	Antibiotic First Choice(s); Alternative
Giardia lamblia	Metronidazole, nitazoxanide
Listeria monocytogenes	Ampicillin alone or with gentamyin, TMSX[a]
Shigella	A fluoroquinolone, azithromycin, TMSX[a]
Salmonella (nontyphoid)	Cefotaxime or ceftriaxone or fluoroquinolone, ampicillin
E. coli (STEC/EHEC)[b]	Antibiotics contraindicated
E. coli (ETEC)[c]	Cefotaxime or ceftriaxone, cefepime or ceftazidime, ampicillin
Vibrio cholerae	A tetracycline, fluoroquinolone, TMSX[a]
Campylobacter jejuni	Erythromycin or azithromycin, fluoroquinolone, a tetracycline
Helicobacter pylori	Clarithromycin with PPI[d] and either ampicillin or metronidazole, other antibiotic combinations in concert with other agents (bismuth subsalicylate and PPI[d] or H₂-blocker)
Clostridium difficile	Metronidazole, vancomycin (each by oral route)
Yersinia enterocolitica	TMSX,[a] a fluoroquinolone, gentamycin, tobramycin, or amikacin

Note: Additional antibiotics or other combinations may be needed for severe disease.
[a]TMSX = trimethoprim-sulfamethoxazole.
[b]STEC = Shiga toxin–producing *E. coli,* EHEC = enterohemorrhagic *E. coli.*
[c]ETEC = enterotoxigenic *E. coli.*
[d]PPI = proton pump inhibitor.
Sources: Choice of Antibiotics, Treatment Guidelines from The Medical Letter. *Med Lett* 2007;5:33–50. For *Giardia lamblia,* ref. 3.

ities, and infectious gastroenteritis poses a particularly vexing set of problems. The frustrations in dealing with this disease entity are its unpredictability, rapid spread, and acutely debilitating symptoms. As noted earlier, chemoprophylaxis is not an important weapon against most of the causative organisms. In many cases, we have been forced to *react* to epidemics and hope that our efforts will stem a serious outbreak. This does not mean that prevention has no place in dealing with infectious gastroenteritis—quite the contrary. Prevention, of course, does not imply complete eradication of gastrointestinal illness in an institution for all time. Rather, it suggests somewhat smaller victories, such as reducing the frequency of occurrence and limiting the spread of disease. Implementation of routine preventive practices such as hand washing and hygienic food and water handling may obviate such heavy reliance on containment policies.

The health care industry in particular has gained valuable experience and subsequently provided leadership in controlling gastroenteritis outbreaks in their institutions. As outlined previously, most hospitals and nursing homes have developed some, all, or combinations of the following preventive techniques: (1) limitations on admissions to and discharge from wards where outbreaks are occurring, (2) involvement of the infection control department, (3) restrictions on visitors, (4) strict enforcement of staff sick leave, (5) thorough use of personal protective equipment, (6) frequent and thorough hand washing, including consideration of availability and use of alcohol-containing handwashing stations when soap and water are not readily available, (7) restriction of patient movements during an outbreak, (8) no cross-staffing between infected and uninfected wards, (9) liberal use of sodium hypochlorite disinfectant by dedicated cleaning staff, and (10) care in handling of soiled linen and other contaminated items [40].

Infective gastroenteritis is a ubiquitous health problem that has the potential to affect any worksite or occupational traveler. Each worksite should develop its own approach to preventing and containing outbreaks of occupational gastroenteritis. As a starting point, there are useful data and preventive approaches to borrow from the health care professions, Other work settings may benefit from adapting these approaches as applicable.

Other Resources

Center for Food Safety and Applied Nutrition, U.S. Food and Drug Administration. *The "Bad Bug Book": Foodborne Pathogenic Microorganisms and Natural Toxins Handbook.* Washington: FDA, 2007. (Not available in print but can be accessed and/or downloaded from www.cfsan.fda.gov.)

Surveillance for foodborne-disease outbreaks—United
Sates, 1998–2002. Surveillance summary. *MMWR*
2006;55:1–42.

References

1. Fleming LE. Unusual occupational gastrointestinal
   and hepatic disorders. *Occup Med State of the Art
   Revs* 1992;7:43.
2. Parashar UD, Glass RI. Viral gastroenteritis. In
   Kasper DL, Fauci AS, Longo DL, et al. (eds), *Harrison's Principles of Internal Medicine,* 16th ed. New
   York: McGraw-Hill, 2005, Chap 174, pp 1140–2.
3. Armitage KB, Salata RA. Infectious diarrhea and
   gastroenteritis. In Tan JS, File TM, Salata RA, et al.
   (eds), *Expert Guide to Infectious Diseases,* 2nd ed.
   Philadelphia: ACP Press, 2008, Chap 8, pp 143–
   67.
4. Flint JA, Van Duynhove YT, Anngulo FJ, et al.
   Estimating the burden of acute gastroenteritis, food-
   borne disease, and pathogens commonly transmitted by food: An international review. *Clin Infect Dis*
   2005;41:698–704.
5. Lynch M, Painter J, Woodruff R, et al. Surveillance
   for foodborne-disease outbreaks—United States,
   1998–2002. *MMWR* 2006;55:1–42.
6. Imhoff B, Morse D, Shiferaw B, et al. Burden of self-
   reported acute diarrheal illness in FoodNet surveillance areas, 1998–1999. *Clin Infect Dis* 2004;38:
   S219–26.
7. Mead PS, Slutsker L, Dietz V, et al. Food-related illness and death in the United States. *Emerg Infect Dis*
   1999;5:607–25.
8. Preliminary FoodNet data on the incidence of infection with pathogens transmitted commonly through
   food—10 states, 2006. *MMWR* 2007;56:336–9.
9. Sharp TW, Hyams KC. Epidemiology of Norwalk
   virus during an outbreak of acute gastroenteritis
   aboard a US aircraft carrier. *J Med Virol* 1995;45:61–
   7.
10. World Health Organization. *Sanitation on Ships:
    Compendium of Outbreaks of Foodborne and Water-
    borne Disease and Legionnaires' Disease Associated
    with Ships, 1970–2000.* Geneva: WHO, 2001.
11. Norovirus outbreak in an elementary school—Dis-
    trict of Columbia, February 2007. *MMWR* 56;2008:
    1340–3.
12. Russo TA. Diseases caused by gram-negative enteric
    bacilli. In Kasper DL, Fauci AS, Longo DL, et al
    (eds), *Harrison's Principles of Internal Medicine,* 16th
    ed. New York: McGraw-Hill, 2005, Chap 134, pp
    878–9.
13. McDonald LC, Killgore GE, Thompson A, et al. An
    epidemic, toxin gene-variant strain of *Clostricium
    difficile.* N Engl J Med 2005;353:2433–41.
14. Warny M, Pepin J, Fang A, et al. Toxin production by
    an emerging strain of *Clostridium difficile* associated
    with outbreaks of severe disease in North America
    and Europe. *Lancet* 2005;366:1079–84.
15. Treatment of *Clostridium difficile*–associated dis-
    ease. *Med Lett Drugs Ther* 2006;48:89–92.
16. Martin P. Listeriosis. In Heymann DL (ed), *Control
    of Communicable Diseases Manual,* 18th ed. Wash-
    ington: APHA, 2004, pp 309–12.
17. Centers for Disease Control and Prevention.
    Cholera FAQ. Division of Foodborne, Bacterial and
    Mycotic Diseases; available at www.cdc.gov/nczved/
    dfbmed/disease-listing/cholera.
18. Prevention of specific infectious diseases. In *CDC
    Health Information for International Travel 2008.*
    Available at wwwn.cdc.gov/travel, Chap 4.
19. DuPont HL, Jiang ZD, Ericsson CD, et al. Rifaximin
    versus ciprofloxacin for the treatment of travelers'
    diarrhea: A randomized, double-blind clinical trial.
    Clin Infect Dis 2001;33:1807–15.
20. Montresor A. Giardiasis. In Heymann DL (ed), *Con-
    trol of Communicable Diseases Manual,* 18th ed.
    Washington: American Public Health Association,
    2004, pp 229–31.
21. Sepkowitz KA. Occupationally acquired infections
    in health care workers, part II. *Ann Intern Med* 1996;
    125:917–28.
22. Gestal JJ. Occupational hazards in hospitals: Risk of
    infection. *Br J Ind Med* 1987;44:435–42.
23. Gardner G. An outbreak of hospital-acquired cryp-
    tosporidiosis. *Br J Nurs* 1994;3:152–8.
24. Caceres VM, Kim DK. A viral gastroenteritis out-
    break associated with person-to-person spread
    among hospital staff. *Infect Contr Hosp Epidemiol*
    1998;19:162–7.
25. Rodriguez EM, Parrott C. An outbreak of viral gas-
    troenteritis in a nursing home: Importance of ex-
    cluding ill employees. *Infect Contr Hosp Epidemiol*
    1996;17:587–92.
26. Standaert SM, Hutcheson RH. Nosocomial trans-
    mission of *Salmonella* gastroenteritis to laundry
    workers in a nursing home. *Infect Contr Hosp Epi-
    demiol* 1994;15:22–6.
27. Gellert GA, Waterman SH. An outbreak of acute
    gastroenteritis caused by a small round structured
    virus in a geriatric convalescent facility. *Infect Contr
    Hosp Epidemiol* 1990;11:459–64.
28. Stevenson P, McCann R. A hospital outbreak due to
    Norwalk virus. *J Hosp Infect* 1994;26:261–72.
29. Chadwick PR, McCann R. Transmission of a small
    round-structured virus by vomiting during a hospi-
    tal outbreak of gastroenteritis. *J Hosp Med* 1994;26:
    251–9.
30. Augustin AK, Simor AE. Outbreaks of gastroenteri-
    tis due to Norwalk-like virus in two long-term care
    facilities for the elderly. *Can J Infect Contr* 1995;
    10:111–3.
31. Khuder SA, Arthur T. Prevalence of infectious dis-
    eases and associated symptoms in wastewater treat-
    ment workers. *Am J Ind Med* 1998;33:571–7.
32. Lo SV, Connolly AM. The role of a presymptomatic
    food handler in a common source outbreak of food-
    borne SRSV gastroenteritis in a group of hospitals.
    Epidemiol Infect 1994;113:513–21.

33. Jones A. *Campylobacter* enteritis in a food factory. *Lancet* 1979;17:611.

34. Christenson B, Ringner A. An outbreak of *Campylobacter* enteritis among the staff of a poultry abattoir in Sweden. *Scand J Infect Dis* 1983;15:167–72.

35. Pohjola S, Okasanen H. Outbreak of cryptosporidiosis among veterinary students. *Scand J Infect Dis* 1986;18:173–8.

36. Glover D. Gastroenteritis outbreak at an industrial camp—British Columbia. *BC Dis Surveill* 1991;89:66–8.

37. Werner SB. Gastroenteritis following ingestion of sewage-polluted water: An outbreak at a logging camp on the Olympic Peninsula. *Am J Epidemiol* 1968;89:277–85.

38. Prevention of rotavirus gastroenteritis among infants and children: Provisional ACIP recommendations for use of rotavirus vaccine (RV). Available at *www.cdc.gov/nip;* accessed July 24, 2006.

39. RotaTeq: A New Oral Rotavirus Vaccine. *Med Let Drug Ther* 2006;48:61–3.

40. Russo PL, Spelman DW. Hospital outbreak of a Norwalk-like virus. *Infect Contr Hosp Epidemiol* 1997;18:576.

19

Occupational Tetanus

V. M. Voge, Philip E. Fisher, and William E. Wright

Given our present understanding of tetanus, the management of occupational tetanus infection is primarily an issue of prevention. If proper immunization practices are in place and prompt, proper wound care is administered, occupational tetanus could become a disease of the past. Although the bacterial culprit is ubiquitous, the unique mechanism of tetanus infection/disease permits several means of easy and effective intervention both prior to and following exposure to this potentially deadly pathogen.

The role of occupational accidents as a source of tetanus infection is not well known. During the period 1969–1985, 26% of tetanus cases in Finland were caused by occupational accidents; most of these were in forestry and agriculture, primarily in the summer and autumn. In 89% of the cases, the immunization status was either unknown or negative [1].

Epidemiology

INCIDENCE (GENERAL INFORMATION)

Tetanus infection remains the leading cause of neonatal death in developing countries [2]. In early 1998, the disease was estimated to kill well over half a million children each year in the developing world. Neonatal tetanus had a reported incidence of about 6 per 1,000 live births [3]. These neonatal infections are believed to result from the dressing of umbilical stumps with dung and from neonatal circumcision performed in primitive conditions. The infant mortality rate from tetanus in developing countries is reported to be 90% [4].

Tetanus is now extremely rare in Europe and North America because of better hygiene, improved wound care management, and higher immunization rates. It is increasingly becoming a disease of the elderly probably because of the impaired local responses to infection and to poorly maintained immunity [5]. The average annual incidence of tetanus in the United States during 1989–1990 was 0.02 per 100,000 people, or 90 new cases per year. Most of the cases involve individuals 55 years of age or older who have not been immunized or have been inadequately immunized. This is considerably less than the rate of 0.39 per 100,000 people reported in 1947. Similarly, the overall case-fatality rate for this same time period declined from 91% in 1947 to 24% in 1989–1990 [6, 7]. The incidence of tetanus in the United Kingdom also decreased markedly following introduction of a national tetanus immunization program in 1961. Only an average of 10 cases per year were reported in England and Wales between 1984 and 2000; 75% of these were over 45 years of age, with the highest annual incidence in those over 64 years of age. Sixty-three percent of the patients had never been immunized. The case-fatality rate in

England and Wales between 1984 and 2000 was 29% [8]. Given the considerable mortality rate that still exists today (untreated, the tetanus mortality rate is 70%), tetanus is clearly a disease that can and should be prevented [9].

RISK FACTORS FOR TRANSMISSION

Tetanus infection is not a contagious disease. The anaerobic spores of the *Clostridium tetani* organism, a Gram positive bacillus, reside in the soil and in the feces (gastrointestinal tract) of humans and domestic animals, such as horses and swine. The organism is found most commonly in warmer climates and in highly cultivated rural areas. The spores can survive in hostile conditions for long periods of time. Infection occurs when the spores are deposited into an anaerobic environment and then germinate into neurotoxin-producing organisms. The spores are typically introduced into deep puncture wounds. However, in many cases, no apparent wound is found, making it likely that very minor, unnoticed (and hence unreported) trauma can be the portal of entry. Decubitus ulcers also may become colonized and infected. Injection drug use (primarily intramuscular and subcutaneous) and abdominal surgery are also possible portals. Between 1995 and 2000, injection drug users accounted for between 15% and 18% of tetanus cases. Potential sources of *C. tetani* in drug users include contamination of drugs used, adulterants, paraphernalia, and the skin itself. The incubation period is usually from 3–21 days, although it may range from 1 day to several months depending on the character, extent, and localization of the entry point [8, 10]. The disease manifests itself when the organisms release their neurotoxin (tetanospasmin). The neurotoxin is a protein that diffuses from the infected wound, enters the circulation, and then travels along nerves to the spinal cord. There the neurotoxin binds to the inhibitory neurons, resulting in violent, spasmodic contraction of opposing muscle groups. Jaw muscles are commonly involved, giving rise to "lockjaw"—the common name for tetanus disease [11, 12].

Adding to the bacteria's virulence is the spore's ability to remain dormant in the infected tissue. It germinates later, producing and releasing the toxin after the initial wound has healed. Furthermore, the growth of other bacteria and/or the presence of foreign material, such as dirt or other types of foreign bodies, can enhance the anaerobic conditions that permit germination of the spores [12]. These considerations are important in the proper management and prevention of tetanus following any penetrating trauma.

OCCUPATIONAL RISK FACTORS

The single most important occupational risk factor for tetanus is lack of or inadequate immunization. It is imperative that every effort be made to initiate and maintain tetanus immunity among all at-risk employees.

Tetanus is a potential hazard in any outdoor occupation, especially those in which minor skin trauma is experienced. Occupational groups at risk include workers in contact with soils, groundwater, refuse, sewage, or animals or human and animal (including snake) bites; law enforcement personnel and other enforcement personnel (e.g., fish and wildlife officers, forest officers, etc.); medical and other trade personnel subject to cuts and puncture wounds and burns; laboratory animal technicians who handle rodents [13, 14]; and emergency medical personnel. Agricultural workers (including migrant workers) account for the largest percentage of exposed individuals in the United States, Canada, and France [10, 15, 16]. Flood and hurricane cleanup personnel may be at risk from contaminated soil or contaminated water entering broken skin (i.e., cuts, abrasions, or puncture wounds) [17, 18]. For recordkeeping purposes, the administration of tetanus shots or boosters is not considered medical treatment by the Occupational Safety and Health Administration (OSHA) [19].

Prevention and Control

ADMINISTRATIVE CONTROLS

All employers should develop a method for assessing the immune status of their at-risk employees at the time of hiring. Employers should arrange for the immediate correction of any immunization deficiencies before the worker begins employment. It is the employer's responsibility to track its employees and to notify them when the need arises (every 10 years) for booster immunizations. Recovery from tetanus may not result in immunity; vaccination following a tetanus infection is indicated [9, 20].

The best method to establish a safe workplace regarding tetanus is to prepare a tetanus prevention program [11]:

1. Prepare a written hazard assessment of worksites to identify existing or potential hazards.
2. Identify employees who are at risk of exposure.
3. Establish and regularly review written policies and procedures.
4. Provide training before an employee begins work and whenever changes are made affecting exposure.
5. Ensure that first aid and medical attention are available to employees.
6. Participate in hazard assessment and control, as well as training on biohazardous materials, controls, and procedures.
7. Follow precautions and procedures to minimize the risk of infection.

EMPLOYEE EDUCATION AND TRAINING

Employee training in tetanus prevention should focus on (1) the need for adequate immunization and (2) the importance of immediately reporting any work-related traumatic injury, particularly penetrating trauma or trauma associated with a high-risk or "dirty" wound. High-risk (tetanus-prone) wounds include [11, 14]

- Wounds for which more than 6 hours have elapsed between injury and treatment
- Wounds with retention of devitalized tissue or foreign bodies
- Any deep puncture wound
- Missile wounds
- Burns
- Frostbite
- Crush injuries
- Avulsion injuries

IMMUNIZATION AND PROPHYLACTIC MEASURES

Proper immunization involves both pre- and postexposure measures. Preexposure, all individuals ideally should have completed their initial immunization series, followed by a booster dose every 10 years for life. The initial immunization series ideally is begun in infancy (three doses of absorbed

tetanus toxoid given no less than 1 month apart, a booster given 12 months following the third dose, and a fifth dose on entering school) [5].

Following an injury, preventive measures include washing the area thoroughly with soap and water and may include surgery to remove dead tissue and any foreign bodies. In cases where the wound is considered "tetanus prone" (Table 19-1), prevention includes a booster toxoid immunization if it has been more than 5 years since the previous immunization, as well as the administration of human tetanus immune globulin. Table 19-1 also provides information on recent recommendations from the Centers for Disease Control and Prevention (CDC) for use of Tdap, which contains tetanus toxoid/reduced-dose diphtheria (Td) and acellular pertussis and is now given in response to increasing numbers of pertussis cases in adults [21, 22]. IG also should be given to patients with incomplete or

Table 19-1

Basic Guide to Tetanus Prophylaxis in Routine Wound Care in Nonpregnant Adults

Wound type:	Clean, minor wound		All other wounds	
History of tetanus immunization (doses)	Td[a]	TIG[b]	Td	TIG
Uncertain, or <3 previous doses:	Yes	No	Yes	Yes
Three or more previous doses:	No[c]	No	No[d]	No

[a]Tetanus toxoid/reduced-dose diphtheria for adolescent/adult formulation. *Note:* On October 26, 2005, the ACIP recommended a single dose of Tdap for adults aged 19–64 to replace the next booster dose of Td if they have not had a previous dose of Tdap. Tdap is Td with acellular pertussis.
[b]Tetanus immune globulin.
[c]Yes, if more than 10 years since previous dose.
[d]Yes, if more than 5 years since previous dose.
Note: A previously unimmunized adult with no contraindications can receive a three-dose primary series of Td, the first two doses being at least 4 weeks apart and the third dose 6–12 months after the second dose. Tdap can substitute for any one of the doses in the adult primary series [22]. In addition, the CDC, in Guidelines for Vaccinating Pregnant Women (May 2007) [22], states: "Although no evidence exists that tetanus and diphtheria toxoids are teratogenic, waiting until the second trimester of pregnancy to administer Td is a reasonable precaution for minimizing any concern about the theoretical possibility of such reactions" and "Data on safety, immunogenicity and the outcomes of pregnancy are not available for pregnant women who receive Tdap." These recommendations state if the person is pregnant and received the previous Td vaccination 10 or more years previously, a Td should be given during the second or third trimester; if the person received the previous Td vaccination less than 10 years ago, administer Tdap during the immediate postpartum period [22]. See also reference [25].
Source: Adapted from CDC and Vandelaer J. Tetanus. In Heymann DL (ed), *Control of Communicable Diseases Manual,* 18th ed. Washington: American Public Health Association, 2004, p 532.

unknown tetanus vaccine history and to patients with humoral immunosuppression, including human immunodeficiency virus (HIV) infection [13, 23, 24]. At the time of this writing the CDC has an early-release document available related to recommendations for vaccination for pregnant and postpartum women, which is not yet published. The practitioner should consult the final version when published [25].

Symptoms and Signs

Tetanus can present either as a local or a generalized infection. In local infections, muscle rigidity and painful spasms may be confined close to the site of injury or injection. Localized tetanus can last weeks or months, but it is more commonly a prodrome of generalized tetanus (the most frequently recognized form). It may take about 2 weeks for the infection to progress to generalized tetanus. Patients with generalized tetanus can present initially with either local tetanus or with symptoms of generalized tetanus. Generalized symptoms consist of restlessness, irritability, contraction of the muscles of the jaw (trismus, or "lockjaw"), abdominal rigidity, neck stiffness, generalized spasticity, severe dysphagia, respiratory difficulties, opisthotonos, autonomic dysfunction, and sometimes convulsions. Untreated, the pain is almost unbearable. The patient often dies of aspiration pneumonia [8, 11].

Once the tetanus neurotoxin has bound to the spinal neurons, any minor stimulus can trigger the simultaneous contraction of opposing muscle groups, giving rise to trismus ("lockjaw") or risus sardonicus ("sardonic smile") if the facial muscles are involved or opisthotonos (back arching) with back muscle involvement. With loss of sympathetic inhibition, the heart rate and blood pressure are both affected, giving rise to dangerous cardiovascular instability. The neurotoxin is unable to cross the blood-brain barrier, so the unmedicated patient's alertness and mentation remain intact throughout the course of the illness. The clinical presentation of tetanus has been divided into three categories [5, 8, 11]:

- *Mild tetanus.* Muscle rigidity that is either generalized or may affect only one limb (so-called local tetanus). There is often trismus and/or a

change in facial expression. Another form of localized tetanus is cephalic tetanus, which affects the cranial nerve musculature.
- *Moderate tetanus.* The rigidity is more severe, giving rise to risus sardonicus and opisthotonos. The diagnostic characteristic of a moderate case is dysphagia secondary to pharyngeal muscle involvement.
- *Severe tetanus.* There are intense reflex spasms. Untreated, these spasms can result in vertebral fracture(s). Back spasms are accompanied by laryngeal muscle spasms, as well as spasms of the diaphragm and intercostal muscles that may impede or prevent adequate ventilation. Severe tetanus frequently presents with varying degrees of autonomic dysfunction. Cardiovascular responses to stimuli, such as aspiration of secretions, become exaggerated. Systolic blood pressures in excess of 300 mmHg are not uncommon. There is profuse sweating and extreme peripheral vasoconstriction. Catecholamine levels rise; the sympathetic nervous system becomes grossly overactive and uncoordinated, giving rise to such cardiovascular complications as supraventricular tachycardia, multifocal ventricular ectopy, unresponsive hypotension, sudden bradycardia, and cardiac arrest.

Differential Diagnosis

There are few conditions that are similar clinically to tetanus. Poisoning with strychnine, an alkaloid which can result in irritability, hyperreflexia, muscle twitching, and violent, successive tonic/clonic spasm, is about the only true mimic. Phenothiazine overdose or sensitivity can be confused with tetanus; with these, one typically sees both grimacing and facial movements, with the jaw widely opened. Various acute central nervous system infections, such as meningitis, also may be confused with tetanus [5, 11].

Diagnostic Evaluation

Tetanus is a presumptive diagnosis based on history and physical examination (mild to moderate trismus plus one or more of the following: spasticity, dysphagia, respiratory embarrassment, spasms, and/or autonomic dysfunction). Three diagnostic laboratory tests are available: (1) tetanus toxin present in a serum sample (absence does not negate a clinical diagnosis; serum sample must be collected before IG treatment), (2) isolation of tetanus bacillus from the infection site (*C. tetani* very rarely is collected from infection site), and (3) tetanus toxin antibodies in the serum (low or absent antibody to tetanus toxin). The first two tests can provide laboratory confirmation of a tetanus infection. For the third test, samples need to be collected before IG treatment, and results can only support the presumptive diagnosis. Testing of drug samples or paraphernalia for tetanus spores also may be useful [8].

Treatment and Rehabilitation

Once the diagnosis of tetanus is suspected, attention should turn immediately to treatment. Once the tetanus neurotoxin binds to a neuron, the antitoxin will not neutralize its action. Consequently, it is imperative that the antitoxin be administered as soon as possible so that it can bind with and neutralize the neurotoxin before it has the opportunity to bind with the nerve cells. The management of a tetanus infection depends on the severity of the illness. In all cases, the physician must remain alert for symptom progression; hospitalization in an intensive care setting is always indicated [10].

Table 19-2 outlines tetanus management strategy. Clinical management includes intravenous or multiple-site intramuscular tetanus immunoglobulin administration; wound debridement; antimicrobials, including agents active against anaerobes (e.g., metronidazole); and vaccination with tetanus toxoid after recovery. A recent recommendation for antibiotic treatment of *C. tetani* infection includes metronidazole as the drug of first choice, with penicillin G or doxycycline being alternative drugs, the latter not generally being recommended for pregnant women or children less than 8 years old [26]. Ideally, one would endeavor to enlist the consultation services of an intensivist to assist in the management of the paralysis, mechanical ventilation, tracheostomy, cardiac instability, and the infectious process in general. Time is of the essence with regard to administrating the antitoxin. One should err on the side of giving it without delay in marginal situations. Human (not equine) tetanus

Table 19-2
Treatment of Tetanus (Summary)

1. Passive immunization (antitoxin): Human tetanus immunoglobulin (HTIG), 500 IU injected into the deltoid muscle STAT.

2. Active immunizations: Booster dose of tetanus toxoid (or initial of series if no previous), 0.5 mL Td injected into the deltoid muscle of the arm opposite that into which HTIG was injected.

3. Antimicrobials: Metronidazole, 500 mg intravenously or orally every 8 hours.

4. Symptomatic measures:

    a. Dysphagia/airway management: Intubate with a cuffed endotracheal tube on first suspicion of dysphagia; often, elective tracheostomy under general anesthesia is necessary.

    b. Muscle rigidity: Diazepam, 10 mg given intravenously every 3–4 hours.

    c. Paralyzed when intubated: Pancuronium is the agent of choice for critically ill patients requiring artificial ventilation [10].

    d. Anxiety (may be conscious although paretic): Benzodiazepines offer sedation, amnesia, and muscle relaxation in addition to their anxiolytic effects.

5. Wound debridement and/or excision: Do *after* giving antitoxin.

6. Nutrition:

    a. If mild, feed orally.

    b. If dysphagic, pass a nasogastric (NG) tube while under general anesthesia for tracheostomy, then NG feed (2,500 cal/day).

    c. If paralytic ileus, hyperalimentation.

7. Hydration: Complicated by heavy insensible fluid losses from sweating and unswallowed saliva.

    a. Weigh daily.

    b. Given enough fluid (orally and/or intravenously) to maintain a urine output of 1.5–2.0 L/day and a urine specific gravity ≤ 1.015.

8. Deep vein thrombosis/pulmonary embolism risk (owing to dehydration and prolonged immobilization once paralyzed): Anticoagulation therapy starting 24 hours after tracheostomy.

9. Autonomic and cardiovascular instability:

    a. Arterial and central venous pressure monitoring in an intensive care setting.

    b. No standardized approach proposed (owing to the lack of comparative trials and the limitations of case reports).

    c. Consider magnesium sulfate, 4 g intravenous bolus, then 2–3 g/hour [11].

    d. Consider adrenergic blocker—propranolol, 10 mg every 3–6 hours via NG tube until heart rate averages < 100.

    e. If hypertension persists, consider labetalol, 50–100 mg every 6 hours via NG tube or by continuous intravenous infusion (0.25–1.0 mg/min).

Sources: Refs 5, 8, 10, 27–29.

IG is much preferred. Severe and sometimes fatal anaphylactic reactions are relatively common with the equine IG; such reactions are extremely rare with human IG [2, 5, 8, 27–29].

References

1. Luisto M, Seppalainen AM. Tetanus caused by occupational accidents. *Scand J Work Environ Health* 1992;18:323–6.
2. Davies-Adetugbo AA, Torimiro SE, Ako-Nai KA. Prognostic factors in neonatal tetanus. *Trop Med Int Health* 1998;3:9–13.
3. Thayaparan B, Nicoll A. Prevention and control of tetanus in childhood (review). *Curr Opin Pediatr* 1998;10:4–8.
4. Ernst ME, Klepser ME, Fouts M, et al. Tetanus: Pathophysiology and management (review). *Ann Pharmacother* 1997;31:1507–13.
5. Wyngaarden JB, Smith LH (eds). *Cecil Textbook of Medicine,* 17th ed. Philadelphia: Saunders, 1985. Pp 1579–82.
6. Prevots R, Suter RW, Strebel PM et al. Tetanus surveillance—United States, 1989–1990. *MMWR* 1992;41:1–9.
7. Branch WT (ed). *Office Practice of Medicine,* 2nd ed. Philadelphia: Saunders, 1987. Pp 1256, 1259.
8. Health Protection Agency. *Tetanus: Information for Health Professionals,* HPA-CDSC, November 2003.
9. Environmental Biological Hazards at Fermilab, FESHM Chapter 5071, rev. February 2003.
10. Wald PH, Stave GM (eds). *Physical and Biological Hazards of the Workplace.* New York: Van Nostrand Reinhold, 1994. Pp 334–6.
11. Tierney LM Jr, McPhee SJ, Papadakis MA. *Current Diagnosis and Treatment,* 45th ed. New York: Lange Medical Books/McGraw-Hill, 2006. Pp 1409–10.
12. Nester EW, Roberts CE, Lidstrom ME, et al (eds). *Microbiology,* 3rd ed. Philadelphia: CBS College Publishing, 1983. Pp 583–85, 835.
13. Tetanus: Last review/update, April 11, 2005; available at www.pao.gov.ab.ca/health/bloworkerenv/appendix_10.htm.
14. Bemis PA. Animal Attack and Snakebite, Wild Iris Medical Education; available at www.nursingceu.com/courses/3/Index_nceu.html.
15. International Occupational Safety and Health Information Centre (CIS), Decree 75-863, September 1975 (Decree 55-806, June 171955), International Labor Organization.
16. France National Legislation, Decree 75-863, September 8, 1975 (Decree 55-806, June 17, 1955), International Labor Organization.
17. Occupational Safety and Health Administration, U.S. Department of Labor. Fact Sheet on Natural Disaster Recovery: Flood Cleanup, November 30, 2005; available at www.osha.gov.
18. National Multi-Agency Coordinating Group Memo, National Interagency Fire Center, Boise, Idaho, September 3, 2005.
19. U.S. Department of Labor, Occupational Safety and Health Administration. Recordkeeping Guidelines; available at www.osha.gov.
20. Lewy R, Brown T, Christenson WN, et al. American College of Occupational and Environmental Medicine Guidelines: Employee health services in health care institutions. *J Occup Med* 1986;28:518–23.
21. Preventing Tetanus, Diptheria, and Pertussis Among Adults: Use of Tetanus Toxoid, Reduced Diphtheria Toxoid and Acellular Pertussis Vaccine. Recommendations of the Advisory Committee on Immunization Practices (ACIP). *MMWR* 2006;55:1–37.
22. The Recommended Adult Immunization Schedule—United States, October 2007–September 2008, QuickGuide of October 19, 2007. *MMWR* 2007;56:Q1–4.
23. Animal Contact Medical Monitoring Program. *Animal Contact Program Handbook.* Gainesville: University of Florida Environmental Health and Safety, October 2005.
24. Cosens B, Grossman W. *Needle-Stick Guideline,* March 23, 2005; available at www.emedicine.com/emerg/topic333.htm.
25. Prevention of Pertussis, Tetanus, and Diphtheria Among Pregnant and Postpartum Women and Their Infants, Recommendations of the Advisory Committee on Immunization Practices (ACIP). *MMWR* 2008;57:1–47.
26. Choice of Antibacterial Drugs, Treatment Guidelines from *The Medical Letter* 2007;5:40–1.
27. Ceneviva Gd, Thomas NJ, Kees-Folts D. Magnesium sulfate for control of muscle rigidity and spasms and avoidance of mechanical ventilation in pediatric tetanus. *Pediatr Crit Care Med;*2003;4:480–4.
28. Shapiro BA, Warren J, Egol AB, et al. Practice parameters for sustained neuromuscular blockade in the adult critically ill patient: An executive summary. *Crit Care Med* 1995;23:1601–5.
29. Lipman J, James MF, Erskine J, et al. Autonomic dysfunction in severe tetanus: Magnesium sulfate as an adjunct to deep sedation. *Crit Care Med* 1987;15:987–8.

20 Occupational Rabies

Carl N. Zenz, Jr.

Although only a few cases of human rabies occur annually in the United States, the increase in international travel and foreign assignments, along with recent improvements in vaccines, has greatly enhanced pre- and postexposure strategies for this deadly virus. Rabies has plagued humankind for centuries. In the fourth century BC, Aristotle wrote "that dogs suffer from the madness. This causes them to become very irritable and all animals they bite become diseased" [1]. Hippocrates supposedly refers to rabies when he says that "persons in a frenzy drink very little, are disturbed and frightened, tremble at the least noise, or are seized with convulsions."

Aulus Comaelius Celsus, in 100 AD, contradicted Aristotle's assertion that humans were exempt from rabies and was the first to suggest treatment by excision and cautery of the bite inflicted by a rabid animal [2]. Girolamo Fra-castoro, a sixteenth-century Italian physician, wrote a description of the aspects of human disease. It was in 1804 that Zinke first demonstrated that rabies could be transmitted by saliva. Numerous researchers in the 1800s, such as Krugelstein and Ekstrom, studied the pathogenesis and treatment of rabies [3].

Pasteur discovered that the true infectious agent of rabies could be obtained and transmitted from the brains of animals dying of the disease. He published his first report in 1881. He reported induction of rabies by the central nervous system material and spinal fluid, thus demonstrating that the source of the virus was not limited to saliva. Pasteur noted that the virus was found not only in the lower centers of the brain but also in the spinal cord. He also differentiated "dumb rabies," characterized by paralysis, from "furious rabies," in which the animal attacked everything.

In 1884, Pasteur reported that the clinical signs produced were somewhat dependent on the dose of infective material and that infections with small amounts of virus did not produce immunity. He also reviewed the hypothesis of the passage of the virus from the periphery to the central nervous system via the nerves versus that of the distribution of the virus by the bloodstream. Additionally, he discussed the theoretical basis of immunizing injections [4].

Pasteur gave his first detailed report in 1885 to the Academy of Science on his method of rabies prophylaxis. The immunization was carried out by injecting a dog subcutaneously with a syringe of broth to which was added a small portion of rabid rabbit cord, beginning with one that was dried long enough to be avirulent and successively using more virulent material until a virulent cord was finally reached. The dog was then refractory to rabies.

During that summer, a 9-year-old boy was referred to him. The boy, who had been bitten 14 times by a rabid dog, was examined by Doctors Grancher and Valpian, who believed that he had received a fatal inoculation of rabies virus. Pasteur went on to say, "The death of this child seemed inevitable, and I decided not without lively and cruel doubts, as one can believe, to try in Joseph Meister, the method which had been successful in dogs. Consequently, on July 6 at 8:00 in the evening, 60 hours after the bites, in the presence of Doctors Valpian and Grancher, we inoculated under a skin fold in the right hypochrondrium of the little Meister a half syringe of the cord of a rabid rabbit preserved in a flask of dry air for 15 days." Thirteen successive inoculations were made with cords of increasing virulence. The patient survived [5]. These findings laid the foundation for a better understanding of the pathogenesis of the disease and development of improved vaccines.

The rabies virus belongs to the family Rhabdoviridae, genus *Lyssavirus*. The *Lyssavirus* genus is now considered to contain seven viruses, of which rabies is an enveloped, single, nonsegmented, negative-stranded RNA virus [6, 7].

The extremely poor prognosis for rabies encephalitis has hastened the development of vaccines to safely prevent the development of the disease, as well as to provide effective postexposure therapy. The importance of preventive measures remains the cornerstone for controlling rabies.

Epidemiology

INCIDENCE AND PREVALENCE

It is difficult to evaluate the true mortality rate owing to rabies worldwide. Most recent estimates by the World Health Organization (WHO) are about 55,000 deaths annually, with probable significant underreporting [8, 9]. The number of people worldwide receiving postexposure treatments for exposure to rabies-suspect animal bites is estimated to be 10 million per year [10]. An estimated 600,000 to 2 million dog bites occur yearly in the United States, and 30,000 people annually receive treatment for rabies prevention following potential exposures [11, 12]. Rabies in humans is rare in the United States. There are usually one to two human cases per year. The most common source of human rabies in the United States is bats. For example, among the 19 naturally acquired cases of rabies in humans in the United States from 1997–2006, 17 were associated with bats [13]. The only documented cases of rabies owing to human-to-human transmission occurred in patients who received corneal transplants from persons who died of undiagnosed rabies [14]. It has been estimated that

99% of all human deaths from rabies occur in the tropical zone [15].

TRANSMISSION RISK FACTORS

The transmission of the rabies virus to a human is usually through the bite of an infected animal. Other means include the inhalation of infected bat secretions, infected-animal licks on mucous membranes, and receiving corneal grafts from infected donors. The primary reservoirs of the virus are cats, dogs, foxes, coyotes, skunks, raccoons, jackals, wolves, and bats. In countries where domestic animal rabies has not been controlled adequately, dogs account for 90% or more of the reported cases in which there has been animal-to-human transmission. Within areas of good domestic-animal rabies programs (such as the United States, Canada, and European countries), dogs account for less than 5% of cases.

OCCUPATIONAL RISK FACTORS

Occupations that expose workers to potential infectious sources of this virus may be categorized into four groups based on risk. These categories are continuous, frequent, infrequent (but greater than the population at large), and rare (no greater than the population at large). Workers that fall into the continuous-risk category include rabies research laboratory workers and rabies biologics production workers. Other potentially exposed workers include veterinarians and staff, animal-control and wildlife workers in rabies-enzootic areas, rabies diagnostic laboratory workers, and mail delivery workers. Some situations have potential to result in episodic risk to people other than those working directly with animals, as occurred at a 2006 horse show in which a horse taken for rides on the grounds was later found to have rabies, resulting in notification of workers and about 150,000 attendees of rabies risk if horse-bite occurred, if one had contamination of a fresh open wound with horse saliva, or if one had eye, nose, mouth, or other mucous membrane contact with horse saliva [16]. Travelers, such as field engineers working in areas where rabies is enzootic and immediate access to adequate medical care (with biologics) is limited, are also at risk and should be immunized (Table 20-1) [17].

PREVENTION AND CONTROL

Education of potentially exposed workers with primary or preexposure vaccination is the key to

Table 20-1
Rabies Pre-exposure Prophylaxis Guide—United States, 1999

Risk Category	Nature of Risk	Typical Populations	Pre-exposure Recommendations
Continuous	Virus present continuously, often in high concentrations. Specific exposures likely vaccination if antibody to go unrecognized. Bite, nonbite, or aerosol exposure.	Rabies research laboratory workers[b]; rabies biologics production workers.	Primary course. Serologic testing every 6 months: booster vaccination if antibody titer below acceptable level.
Frequent	Exposure usually episodic, with source recognized. Bite, nonbite, or aerosol.	Rabies diagnostic lab workers,[a] spelunkers, Veterinarians and staff, and wildlife workers in rabies-enzootic areas.	Primary course. Serologic testing every 2 years: booster vaccination if antibody titer is below acceptable level[b] exposure.
Infrequent (greater than population at large)	Exposure nearly always episodic with source recognized. Bite or non-bite exposure.	Veterinarians and animal-control and wildlife workers in areas with low rabies rates. Veterinary students. Travelers visiting areas where rabies is enzootic and immediate access to appropriate medical care, including biologics, is limited.	Primary course. No serologic testing or booster vaccination.
Rare (population at large)	Exposure always episodic with source recognized. Bite or nonbite exposure.	U.S. population at large, including persons in rabies-epizootic areas.	No vaccination necessary.

[a]Judgment of relative risk and extra monitoring of vaccination status of laboratory workers are the responsibilities of the laboratory supervisor.
[b]Minimum acceptable antibody level is complete virus neutralization at a 1:5 serum dilution by the rapid fluorescent focus inhibition test. A booster dose should be administered if the titer falls below this level.
Source: Adapted from Centers for Disease Control and Prevention. Human rabies prevention—United States, 1999: Recommendations of the Advisory Committee on Immunization Practices (ACIP). *MMWR* 1999;48:1–21.

preventing this disease. Workers need to be aware of the transmission modes of the rabies virus, the need for immunization (depending on their job functions), and the necessity for immediate therapeutic intervention following an exposure incident.

Preexposure prophylaxis does not eliminate the need for additional therapy after exposure; however, it eliminates the use of rabies immune globulin (RIG) and decreases the number of doses needed. Additionally, if postexposure therapy is delayed, the primary series might protect those individuals.

IMMUNIZATION AND PROPHYLATIC MEASURES

Primary vaccination may be done via intramuscular or intradermal injections. Three 1.0-mL injections into the deltoid muscle of human diploid cell vaccine (HDCV), rabies vaccine adsorbed (RVA), or purified chick embryo cell vaccine (PCEC) on days 0, 7, and 21 or 28 may be used (Table 20-2).

The intradermal regimen of three 0.1-mL intradermal doses of HDCV on days 0, 7, and 21 or 28 is also used for preexposure vaccination. HDCV should not be administered intradermally to individuals receiving antimalarial chemoprophylaxis because this may inhibit antibody production.

Individuals who work in research laboratories or vaccine-production facilities are at high risk for inapparent exposures. These individuals should have rabies antibody tests every 6 months.

SYMPTOMS AND SIGNS

Human rabies evolves through five clinical phases: (1) incubation period, (2) prodrome, (3) acute neurologic phase, (4) coma, and (5) death or recovery [18]. Recovery is rare, and infected individuals usually succumb in the later stages of the disease. The development of rabies depends on the type of exposure, the animal involved, and pre- and postexposure treatment received. The rabies virus usually enters the body through skin broken by a bite

Table 20-2
Rabies Biologics—United States, 1999

Human Rabies Vaccine	Product Name	Manufacturer
Human diploid cell vaccine (HDCV)		Pasteur-Meneux Serum et Vaccins, Connaught Laboratories, Inc., phone: (800) VACCINE (822-2463)
Intramuscular	ImovaxG Rabies	
Intradermal	Imovax Rabies I.D.	
Rabies vaccine adsorbed (RVA)	Rabies vaccine adsorbed (RVA)	BioPort Corporation, phone: (517) 335-Ri 20
Purified chick embryo cell vaccine (PCEC), intramuscular	RaoAvert	Chiron Corporation, phone: (800) CHIRONE (244-7668)
Rabies immune globulin (RIG)	Imogam Rabies-HI	Pasteur-Meneux Serum et Vaccins, Connaught Laboratories, Inc., phone: (800) VACCINE (822-2463)
	BayRab	Bayer Corporation Pharmaceutical Div., phone: (800) 288-8370

Source: Adapted from Centers for Disease Control and Prevention. Human rabies prevention—United States, 1999: Recommendations of the Advisory Committee on Immunization Practices (ACIP). *MMWR* 1999;48:1–21.

or scratch; however, it also can enter through intact mucous membrane and may be inhaled as an aerosol or be transplanted through infected corneal grafts.

The incubation time in human rabies is variable. It may be as short as 9 days and as long as a year or more. The mean incubation period is 30–78 days. Approximately 14% of cases have longer incubations. Short incubation is seen in patients with more severe exposure and with bite exposures to the face and head [19]. The patient is asymptomatic during incubation.

PRODROMAL SYMPTOMS

The earliest symptoms of rabies generally are non-specific and may suggest another illness. Symptoms include malaise, headache, gastrointestinal symptoms, dyspnea, fatigue, and anorexia. Most patients are febrile: More than 50% in one series had a temperature greater than 101°F (38.3°C). Chills may accompany the fever. The most common early gastrointestinal symptoms include nausea, vomiting, abdominal cramping, and diarrhea. Other presenting symptoms may include sore throat, photophobia, headache, and dizziness. Pain or paresthesia at the site of the bite is the only relatively specific prodromal symptom. Itching may occur at the site of a healed bite wound or involve the whole bitten limb and may be so intense as to result in excoriation of the skin by scratching. The explanation for local paresthesia may be multiplication of the virus in the dorsal root ganglion of the sensory nerve supplying the area of the bite. Three of four patients

who had acquired rabies via corneal transplant noted pain referable to the eye receiving the infected cornea [20].

THE ACUTE NEUROLOGIC PHASE

This phase includes a wide variety of systemic disorders. The symptoms are varied and may include aerophobia and hydrophobia. The onset is 2–10 days after the prodromal symptoms; the individual develops signs of nervous system involvement, including hyperactivity, hallucinations, disorientation, seizures, nuchal stiffness, bizarre behavior, and paralysis. A period of marked hyperactivity may last from hours to days, with periods of agitation, thrashing, and biting; this is known as *furious rabies.* This hyperactivity may occur spontaneously or be precipitated by tactile, auditory, visual, or olfactory stimuli. Between episodes, the patient is usually lucid and cooperative but often is anxious.

Hydrophobia, the most characteristic symptom, occurs in up to 50% of patients. An intense psychic response, even terror, induced by attempts to drink or even the sight of water is typical. Severe, painful spasms of the pharynx and larynx produce choking, gagging, and fear. Inspiratory spasms lasting 5–15 seconds are part of the hydrophobic response, and these may lead to respiratory arrest or generalized fatal convulsions. Warrel and colleagues have suggested that the respiratory signs may be related to respiratory myoclonus and may be caused by brain stem lesions rather than occurring as a conditioned reflex arising from throat pain [21].

Abnormalities that may appear during this period of hyperactivity include muscle fasciculations (especially near the site of exposure), hyperventilation, hypersalivation, and focal or generalized convulsions. Most patients manifest signs of delirium. Other neurologic signs may include meningismus, cranial nerve pareses leading to diplopia, ptosis, dysphagia, and dysarthria. Limb paresis (at times with clear signs of pyramidal tract lesions) and reflex alterations also may be present.

Autonomic changes such as hyperpyrexia, hypotension, excessive sweating, piloerection, pupil dilatation, hypersalivation, and tachycardia frequently develop. In about 20% of patients, a second clinical form of rabies infection presents as paralysis. The entire clinical course is similar neurologically to the Landry-Guillain-Barré syndrome. This course of rabies has been described as *dumb rabies* (or *rage tranquil rabies*). The paralysis may be diffuse and symmetric or an ascending paralysis. The acute neurologic period usually lasts for 1 week.

COMA

During this phase of rabies, the previous signs of hydrophobia are replaced by irregular respiration and prolonged periods of apnea. Respiratory arrest resulting in death may occur during this time. The duration of coma may range from hours to months depending on the intensity of care the patient receives. Supplemental trials of corticosteroids, interferon, and other antivirals have not positively affected the outcomes.

RECOVERY

Very few patients have recovered from a documented rabies virus infection, even with aggressive treatment. In October 2004, a previously healthy female aged 15 years in Fond du Lac County, Wisconsin, received a diagnosis of rabies after being bitten by a bat approximately 1 month before symptom onset. This is the first documented recovery from clinical rabies by a patient who had not received either pre- or postexposure prophylaxis for rabies.

This case represents the sixth known occurrence of human recovery after rabies infection; however, the case is unique because the patient received no rabies prophylaxis either before or after illness onset [22]. This treatment approach has been termed the *Milwaukee protocol,* which consists of induction of therapeutic coma, waiting for an adaptive immune response to evolve to neutralize and clear the virus, and supportive antiviral and metabolic therapies [23]. Since then, several other uses of the Milwaukee protocol have not been successful [24–26].

Differential Diagnosis

Patients with encephalopathy of unknown origin should have rabies infection considered in the differential diagnosis, even without known exposure to the virus through an animal bite. In a review of all 32 rabies cases reported in the United States between 1980 and 1996, Noah and colleagues found that a lack of clinical suspicion of rabies delayed the diagnosis. Since no postexposure prophylaxis was received, all 32 individuals succumbed [27]. There is little to distinguish rabies from other viral encephalitides. A history of exposure is the most helpful diagnostic clue. Other possible conditions include poliomyelitis, Landry-Guillain-Barré syndrome, and hysterical reactions to animal bites (pseudohydrophobia). Neuroparalytic reactions from postexposure courses of rabies prophylaxis consisting of central nervous system tissue vaccines still may occur in parts of the world where this type of vaccine is used.

DIAGNOSTIC EVALUATION

Because laboratory diagnosis usually is not possible during the first week of illness, the appearance of symptoms and a history of exposure to a rabid animal strongly support the diagnosis of rabies. Individuals without a history of vaccination develop serum antibodies that are first detectable on the tenth day of illness (with a rapid rise thereafter to high levels). Detectable antibodies appear in the cerebrospinal fluid (CSF) later in the clinical course (approximately the third week). Since vaccination does not induce CSF antibodies, high CSF titers support the diagnosis.

Fluorescent antibody staining techniques enable the detection of rabies antigen in nuchal skin biopsies. Saliva and skin samples may be analyzed by reverse-transcriptase polymerase chain reaction (RT-PCR) assay. Rabies virus neutralizing antibody titers from serum and CSF samples can be obtained by the rapid fluorescent focus inhibition test (RFFIT). Virus isolation can be done to confirm other positive test results by tissue culture or intracerebral inoculation of mice [28].

Treatment

Postexposure prophylaxis following a possible exposure may be categorized into two groups: those with previous vaccinations and those without. Previously vaccinated persons are those who have received one of the recommend courses of HDCV, RVA, or PCEC. These individuals should receive two intramuscular doses (1.0 mL each) of vaccine, one immediately and one 3 days later.

Physicians need to evaluate each possible exposure to rabies and the need for rabies prophylaxis (Table 20-3).

Immediate washing of all bite wounds with soap and water and a virucidal agent (e.g., povidone-iodine solution) is important. Postexposure rabies vaccination should include both passive antibody and vaccine in previously unimmunized individuals. The recommended dose of human RIG is 20 IU/kg of body weight, and if feasible, the full dose should be infiltrated in the area around and into the wound. (Any remaining volume should be injected intramuscularly at a site distant from vaccine administration.) The first dose of a five-dose course (1 mL of HDCV, RVA, or PCEC) should be given intramuscularly as soon as possible after ex-

posure. The remaining doses should be given on days 3, 7, 14, and 28 after the first vaccination (Table 20-4).

Advances in the understanding of the immunology of the rabies virus have promoted the development of even more efficacious vaccines, along with an improved dosage schedule for both primary and postexposure immunizations. Routine preexposure vaccination should be contemplated for a variety of occupations depending on multiple issues, such as risk of exposure (as in laboratory workers) and location of the individual's work activities (as in the tropics). The availability of vaccines and RIG for follow-up treatment in certain parts of the world where rabies is endemic is another key consideration. For high-risk activities, serum antibody levels may be drawn to monitor the worker's protective levels. Owing to the extreme mortality rate associated with this virus, a high degree of employee awareness about the need for follow-up in postexposure situations is mandatory, as well as routine preventive administration of these vaccines for high-risk overseas workers.

Owing to the large global impact of rabies, an essentially lethal human disease amenable to preventive strategies, starting in 2006, the WHO and the Global Alliance for Rabies Control have united a number of organizations to mobilize awareness and resources to support human rabies prevention and animal rabies control. The programs and initiatives focus primarily on Africa and Asia, areas

Table 20-3
Rabies Postexposure Prophylaxis Guide—United States, 1999

Animal Type	Evaluation and Disposition of Animal	Postexposure Prophylax Recommendations
Dogs, cats, and ferrets	Healthy and available for 10 days' observation	Persons should not begin prophylaxis unless animal develops clinical signs of rabies.[a]
	Rabid or suspected rabid, unknown (e.g., escaped)	Vaccinate immediately. Consult public health officials.
Skunks, raccoons, foxes, and most other carnivores; bats	Regarded as rabid unless animal proven negative by laboratory tests[b]	Consider immediate vaccination.
Livestock, small rodents, lagomorphs (rabbits and hares), large rodents (woodchucks and beavers), and other mammals	Consider individually	Consult public health officials. Bites of squirrels, hamsters, guinea pigs, gerbils, chipmunks, rats, mice, other small rodents, rabbits, and hares almost never require antirabies postexposure prophylaxis.

[a]During the 10-day observation period, begin postexposure prophylaxis at the first sign of rabies in a dog, cat, or ferret that has bitten someone. If the animal exhibits clinical signs of rabies, it should be euthanized immediately and tested.
[b]The animal should be euthanized and tested as soon as possible. Holding it for observation is not recommended. Discontinue vaccine if results of immunofluorescence testing of the animal are negative.
Source: Adapted from Centers for Disease Control and Prevention. Human rabies prevention—United States, 1999: Recommendations of the Advisory Committee on Immunization Practices (ACIP). *MMWR* 1999;48:1–21.

Table 20-4
Rabies Postexposure Prophylaxis Schedule—United States, 1999

Vaccination Status	Treatment	Regimen[a]
Not previously vaccinated	Wound cleansing	All postexposure treatment should begin with immediate thorough cleansing of all wounds with soap and water. If available, a virucidal agent such as a povidone-iodine solution should be used to irrigate the wounds.
	RIG	Administer 20 IU/kg of body weight. If anatomically feasible, the full dose should be infiltrated around the wound(s) and any remaining volume should be administered intramuscularly at an anatomic site distant from vaccine administration. Also, RIG should not be administered in the same syringe as vaccine. Because RIG might partially suppress active production of antibody, no more than the recommended dose should be given.
	Vaccine	HDCV, RVA, or PCEC 1.0 mL intramuscularly (deltoid area[b], one dose each on days 0,[c] 3, 7, 14, and 28.
Previously vaccinated[d]	Wound cleansing	All postexposure treatment should begin with immediate thorough cleansing of all wounds with soap and water. If available, a virucidal agent such as a povidone-iodine solution should be used to irrigate the wounds.
	RIG	RIG should not be vaccine administered. HDCV, RVA, or PCEC 1.0 mL intramuscularly (deltoid area[b]), one dose each on days 0[c] and 3.

HDCV = human diploid cell vaccine; PCEC = purified chick embryo cell vaccine; RIG = rabies immune globulin; RVA = rabies vaccine adsorbed.
[a]These regimens are applicable for all age groups, including children.
[b]The deltoid area is the only acceptable site of vaccination for adults and older children. For younger children, the outer aspect of the thigh may be used. Vaccine should never be administered in the gluteal area.
[c]Day 0 is the day the first dose of vaccine is administered.
[d]Any person with history of preexposure vaccination with HDCV, RVA, or PCEC; prior postexposure prophylaxis with HDCV, RVA, or PCEC; or previous vaccination with any other type of rabies vaccine and a documented history of antibody response to the prior vaccination.
Source: Adapted from Centers for Disease Control and Prevention. Human rabies prevention—United States, 1999: Recommendations of the Advisory Committee on Immunization Practices (ACIP). *MMWR* 1999;48:1–21.

where most of the estimated 55,000 annual rabies deaths now occur.

References

1. Fleming G. *Rabies and Hydrophobia*. London: Chapman and Hall, 1872, p 7.
2. Smithcors JF. The history of some current problems in animal disease: VII. Rabies (part 1). *Vet Med* 1958;53:149.
3. Fernandez PJ. History of rabies and global aspects. In Baer GM (ed), *The Natural History of Rabies*, 2nd ed. Boca Raton, FL: CRC Press, 1991, pp 1–24.
4. Pasteur L, Chamferland CE, Roux M. Nouvelle communication sur la rage. *CR Acad Sci* 1884;98:457.
5. Pasteur L. Sur la rage. *CR Acad Sci* 1881;92:1259.
6. Plotkin SA, Rupprecht CE, Koprowski H. Rabies vaccine. In *Vaccines*, 3rd ed. Philadelphia: Saunders, 1999, pp 744–5.
7. Bourky H, Kissi B, Tordo N. Molecular diversity of the lyssavirus genus. *Virology* 1993;194:70–81.
8. Report from WHO Expert Consultation on Rabies. Geneva: WHO, October 5–8, 2004.
9. Wilde H, Mitmoonpitak C. Canine rabies in Thailand. *World Health Magazine* 1998;4:10–1.
10. World Health Organization. Rabies. Fact Sheet No. 99. Geneva: WHO, September 2006.
11. Hildreth EA. Prevention of rabies on the decline of Sirius. *Ann Intern Med* 1963;88:883–96.
12. Parish HM, Clark FB, Brobst D, et al. Epidemiology of dog bites. *Public Health Rep* 1967;82:1009–18.
13. Centers for Disease Control and Prevention. *Questions and Answers about Rabies and Bats in Summer Camps*. Atlanta: CDC, August 4, 2006.
14. Warrell DA, Warrell MJ. *Human Rabies and Its Prevention: An Overview, Reviews of Infectious Diseases*, Vol 10, Suppl 4. Chicago: University of Chicago Press, 1998.
15. Acha PN, Arambulo PV II. Rabies in the tropics: History and current status. In Kuwert E, Merieux C, Loprowski H, et al. (eds), *Rabies in the Tropics*. Berlin: Springer-Verlag, 1985, pp 343–59.
16. Centers for Disease Control and Prevention. Horse stabled at Tennessee Walking Horse 2006 National Celebration tested positive for rabies. *CDC, Rabies, News and Highlights,* September 9, 2006.
17. Centers for Disease Control and Prevention. Human rabies prevention—United States, 1999: Recommendations of the Advisory Committee on Immunization Practices (ACIP). *MMWR* 1999:48:1–21.
18. Robinson PA. Rabies virus. In Belshe RB (ed), *Textbook of Human Virology*, 2nd ed. St Louis: Mosby–Year Book, 1991, Chap 19.
19. Warrell DA. The clinical picture of rabies in man. *Trans R Soc Trop Med Hyg* 1976;70:188–95.
20. Centers for Disease Control and Prevention. Human-to-human transmission of rabies via corneal transplant—Thailand. *MMWR* 1981;30:472–4.

21. Miller A, Nathanson N. Rabies: Recent advances in pathogenesis and control. *Ann Neurol* 1977;2:511–9.

22. Centers for Disease Control and Prevention. Recovery of a patient from clinical rabies—Wisconsin, 2004. *MMWR* 2004;53:1171–3.

23. Willougby RE, Tieves KS, Hoffman GM, et al. Survival after treatment of rabies with induction of coma. *N Eng J Med* 2005;352:2508–14.

24. Centers for Disease Control and Prevention. Human rabies—Indiana and Califronia, 2006. *MMWR* 2007; 56:361–5.

25. Centers for Disease Control and Prevention. Human rabies—Alberta, Canada, 2007. *MMWR* 2008;57: 197–200.

26. Hemachudha T, Sunsaneewitayakul B, Desudchit T, et al. Failure of therapeutic coma and ketamine for therapy of human rabies. *J Neurovirol* 2006;12:407–9.

27. Noah D et al. Review of rabies cases reported in the U.S. between 1980 and 1996. *Ann Intern Med* 1998; 128:922–30.

28. Human rabies—Virginia, 1998. *MMWR* 1999;48: 95–7; *JAMA* 1999;281:891–2.

21

Occupational Infectious Diseases with Dermatologic Features

Dorothy J. Wawrose and Boris D. Lushniak

Occupational dermatology is the facet of dermatology that deals with skin diseases whose etiology or aggravation is related to some exposure in the workplace. The role of a medical practitioner involved in occupational dermatology is not only to diagnose and treat patients but also to determine the etiology of the occupational skin disease and to make recommendations for its prevention. Occupational dermatology covers a wide variety of skin diseases, including allergic contact dermatitis, irritant contact dermatitis, pigmentary disorders, skin cancer, and infectious diseases. Many general references on occupational skin disorders are available [1–3].

In general, the causes of occupational skin disorders can be grouped into the following categories:

1. Physical insults (e.g., friction, pressure, trauma, vibration, heat, cold, variations in humidity, ultraviolet/visible/infrared radiation, ionizing radiation, and electric current)
2. Chemical insults (e.g., water, soaps/detergents, inorganic acids, alkalis, salts of heavy metals, aliphatic acids, aldehydes, alcohols, esters, hydrocarbons, solvents, metallo-organic compounds, lipids, aromatic and polycyclic compounds, resin monomers, and proteins)
3. Biologic causes (e.g., plants, arthropods, bacteria, rickettsiae, viruses, fungi, and parasites)

Diseases in the biologic category include infectious diseases that have a major manifestation on the cutaneous surface and result from exposure to an infectious agent found in a workplace setting. This exposure can occur through direct skin contact (epicutaneous), inoculation (percutaneous), or the respiratory system (inhalational).

Epidemiology

Epidemiologic data specifically related to occupational dermatologic infectious diseases are very limited. Other than limited descriptions in case presentations, case studies, and epidemiologic investigation reports, little is known about the epidemiology of most of these diseases in the United States. In many cases it is difficult to prove definitively that the disease process is occupationally related. The accuracy of the diagnosis is related to the skill level, experience, and knowledge of the medical professional who makes the diagnosis and then confirms the relationship with a workplace exposure. The questions to be answered by the clinician include the following: (1) Is the patient's condition a dermatologic infectious disease? (2) Is the organism found in the patient's workplace environment? (3) Was there an opportunity for the worker to become infected in the workplace? (4) What other nonoccupational exposures (e.g., recreational activities) must be considered [4]?

The public health importance of a disease can be measured in several ways using statistical, clinical, and economic measures [5]. These measures include the absolute number of cases, the incidence rate, the prevalence rate, the prognosis and preventability of the disease, and the economic impact of the disease (e.g., medical costs and days away from work). There are many gaps in this information for occupational dermatologic infectious diseases.

As of 2005, 70 infectious diseases were designated as notifiable at the national level in the United States [6]. A notifiable disease is one for which regular, frequent, and timely information regarding individual cases is necessary for disease prevention and control. For the infectious diseases that are nationally reportable, it is impossible to determine what proportion are due to occupational exposures. Of the notifiable diseases that are discussed in this chapter, the following number of cases were reported for 2005: anthrax—0 cases; brucellosis—120; Lyme disease—23,305; measles—66; Rocky Mountain spotted fever—1,936; rubella—11; tularemia—154; and varicella—32,242 [6].

A study on the burden of skin diseases, which used a variety of data sources from 2004, concluded that in the United States the prevalence of herpes simplex and zoster was estimated to be over 188 million cases, with total direct and indirect costs of $1.6 billion [7]. The same study estimated over 58 million cases of human papillomavirus infection (total cost $1.1 billion) and over 29 million cases of cutaneous fungal infections (total cost $1.8 billion). Again, it is not possible to determine what proportion of these skin diseases may have been related to occupational exposures.

National occupational injury and illness data are available from the U.S. Bureau of Labor Statistics (BLS). The BLS conducts annual surveys of approximately 250,000 employers selected to represent all private industries in the United States [8]. The survey results then are projected to estimate the number and incidence rates of injuries and illnesses in the American working population. BLS data are limited in that they exclude self-employed individuals, small farms, and government agencies; depend on vague definitions of reportable occupational injuries and illnesses; rely to a large extent on employees reporting conditions to the employer; do not provide information on the etiology of the skin disease; and generally are considered underestimates of the true number of cases [5].

There is limited information on occupational dermatologic infectious diseases in the BLS data. In 2006, there were an estimated 41,400 cases of occupational skin diseases or disorders, or 4.5 per 10,000 workers [8]. Of these, 5,720 resulted in 1 or more days away from work. The majority of these cases with days away from work (60%) were due to the most common occupational skin disease—dermatitis. Infections of the skin and subcutaneous tissue accounted for 27% of the 5,720 cases, or 1,570 cases (0.2 per 10,000 workers). Most of these were listed as cellulitis and abscess (690 cases); the others included unspecified diseases (630), not elsewhere classified (180), and pilonidal cyst (40) [8]. The median time away from work for workers with these skin infections was 10 days. In 2006, under a separate category of infectious and parasitic diseases, the BLS recorded 2,550 cases that resulted in at least 1 day away from work [8]. The diagnoses with potential skin manifestations in this category included scabies/chiggers/mites—1,330 cases; viral diseases accompanied by exanthem—380; chickenpox—280; herpes zoster—40; dermatophytosis (including athlete's foot and tinea)—40; and Lyme disease—20.

Overview

Many of the occupational dermatologic infectious diseases result in not only cutaneous signs and symptoms but also systemic effects. The cutaneous manifestations will be stressed in this chapter. Infections such as impetigo, erysipelas, cellulitis, folliculitis, furuncles, carbuncles, and abscesses caused by common organisms such as group A streptococci or *Staphylococcus aureus* will not be discussed. An exception will be made to discuss issues related with methicillin-resistant *S. aureus* (MRSA).

Traumatic wounds or infestations secondarily infected with these common pathogens will not be emphasized in this chapter. Finally, sexually transmitted diseases, many of which have cutaneous manifestations and can be considered to be occupational diseases in the sex trades, will not be included here.

The occupational dermatologic infectious diseases covered in this chapter range from very common diseases in the United States, both in occupational and in nonoccupational settings (e.g., candidiasis and dermatophytosis), to very rare diseases in the United States (e.g., anthrax and tularemia), to diseases never seen in the United States. Some of these occur only outside the United States and are seen here only as rare cases of imported occupational diseases in workers exposed overseas.

In general, risk of infection can be associated with individual worker susceptibility (e.g., immune status or trauma to the protective barrier of the skin); the existence of the pathogen in the environment (e.g., endemic geographic locations); occupational exposure to the pathogen, its reservoir, and its fomites; and work conditions in which the pathogens thrive. Reservoirs and fomites of the pathogens include people (i.e., coworkers, clients, patients, or children), animals or animal products, soil or plant materials, ticks/insects, water, and marine life. Conditions in which pathogens can thrive and increase worker susceptibility include wet work and hot and humid environments. The occupational dermatologic infectious diseases associated with these sources and conditions are listed in Tables 21-1 through 21-6. In addition, laboratory workers are at risk of infection with the pathogens with which they are working.

The specific diseases will be described by pathogen category. Occupational dermatologic infectious diseases can be grouped by etiologic agent into the following disease categories: (1) bacterial (including rickettsiae), (2) viral, (3) superficial fungal, (4) subcutaneous fungal, (5) systemic fungal, and (6) parasitic.

Table 21-1
Occupational Dermatologic Infectious Diseases Associated with Exposures to Patients or Children

Cutaneous tuberculosis
Methicillin-resistant *Staphylococcus aureus*
Herpetic whitlow
Vaccinia
Warts
Measles
Rubella
Chickenpox
Herpes zoster (shingles)
Hand-foot-mouth disease
Erythema infectiosum (fifth disease)
Dermatophytes (anthropophilic)
Scabies

Table 21-2
Occupational Dermatologic Infectious Diseases Associated with Exposures to Animal and Animal Products

Anthrax
Brucellosis
Cat scratch disease
Erysipeloid
Mycobacterium bovis
Tularemia
Methicillin-resistant *Staphylococcus aureus*
Orf
Milker's nodules
Monkeypox
Warts
Dermatophytes (zoophilic)
Mites

Table 21-3
Occupational Dermatologic Infectious Diseases Associated with Exposures to Soil and Plants

Anthrax
Dermatophytes (geophilic)
Chromoblastomycosis
Mycetoma
Sporotrichosis
Blastomycosis
Paracoccidioidomycosis
Cutaneous larva migrans

Table 21-4
Occupational Dermatologic Infectious Diseases Associated with Exposures to Ticks and Insects

Lyme disease
Tularemia
Rocky Mountain spotted fever
Typhus
Leishmaniases

Table 21-5
Occupational Dermatologic Infectious Diseases Associated with Water, Marine, Fish, and Shellfish Exposures

Erysipeloid
Mycobacterium marinum granuloma
Tularemia
Vibrio vulnificus infection
Aeromonas hydrophila infection
Photobacterium (Vibrio) damsela infection
Vibrio parahaemolyticus infection
Pseudomonas aeriginosa infection
Warts
Cercarial dermatitides

Table 21-6
Occupational Dermatologic Infectious Diseases Associated with Exposures to Wet Work and Hot and Moist Environments

Candidiasis
Dermatophytoses
Tinea versicolor

BACTERIAL DISEASES
Anthrax

Anthrax is caused by *Bacillus anthracis,* a large, aerobic, spore-forming gram-positive rod. The disease is seen infrequently in most industrialized countries, but worldwide there are an estimated 20,000 to 100,000 cases of human anthrax annually [9]. Anthrax disease occurs after spores are introduced by cutaneous, inhalational, or gastrointestinal exposure. Cutaneous disease is the most common naturally occurring form and is a result of direct inoculation, usually through abrasions during contact with infected domestic and wild animals (e.g., cattle, sheep, goats, pigs, horses, and others) or animal products (e.g., hide, wool, hair, and bone) [10]. Infected animals shed the bacteria in hemorrhages or spilt blood. The spores can remain viable for years in soil, dried animal skin and hides, and animal products. High-risk occupations include abattoir (slaughterhouse) workers, farmers, hunters, laboratory workers, veterinarians, wildlife workers, upholsterers, wool workers, and any workers exposed to animal hair (especially goat hair), hides, or animal products, especially from the Middle East, Asia, Africa, South and Central America, and southern and eastern Europe [11,12]. These workers include longshoremen, freight handlers, and tannery workers. Inhalation or ingestion of

spores can cause severe respiratory disease (e.g., woolsorter's disease) or intestinal disease. In 2001, 22 cases of anthrax occurred in the United States as a result of a bioterrorism-related outbreak. Eleven of those cases were cutaneous [13].

The cutaneous form of the disease is usually seen on areas of exposed skin such as the head, forearms, and hands [10]. Two to three days after inoculation, a red patch appears that later becomes a painless, purplish-red, raised, boggy, vesicular or pustular nodule (*malignant pustule*). After a few days, this lesion becomes necrotic with an evident black eschar and surrounding edema. Satellite lesions can form around the primary lesion. After 1–2 weeks, the eschar loosens and falls off [14]. Systemic signs include high fever, malaise, and weakness. Regional lymph nodes may become enlarged, and septicemia is possible. Untreated cutaneous anthrax has a case-fatality rate of 5–20% [12]. The diagnosis is made by clinical signs, known exposures, serology, and Gram's stain and culture of the blood, lesion, or discharges. Polymerase chain reaction (PCR) is available at reference laboratories, and immunohistochemistry of pleural fluid or biopsy is useful if antibiotics have already been used [14]. Drugs of choice for initial treatment of cutaneous anthrax are ciprofloxacin or doxycycline owing to concerns over potential resistance to penicillins [15]. Antibiotics may be adjusted after results of susceptibility testing are known [15]. Preventive measures include immunizing high-risk workers, antibiotic prophylaxis, immunizing animals, sterilizing or disinfecting fomites, educating high-risk workers, controlling dusts and ventilating high-risk work areas, using protective clothing, and emphasizing workplace hygiene [12, 15–18].

Brucellosis

Brucellosis is caused by gram-negative coccobacillary rods found on animals or in animal products. It is the most common zoonotic disease globally with more than 500,000 new cases annually [19]. Human disease is caused by *Brucella abortus* (in cattle), *B. suis* (in pigs), *B. canis* (in dogs), or *B. melitensis* (in goats and sheep) [20]. The organisms are found worldwide, including the Mediterranean countries of Europe and Africa, the Middle East, India, central Asia, Mexico, and Central and South America. However, the epidemiology of human brucellosis has evolved over the past decade, with some endemic areas achieving control of the disease and the emergence of new endemic foci in central Asia [12, 19]. In the United States between 1993 and 2002, 1,056 cases were reported [19]. Most of these cases were caused by *B. melitensis* and affected people of Hispanic origin, and more than half were from Texas and California [19]. Humans are infected as a result of direct inoculation, usually through abrasions, during contact with infected domestic animals, their secretions, or animal products. Humans also can be infected by ingestion of unpasteurized milk or cheese and through inhalation of infected aerosolized particles [20]. High-risk occupations include the handling of infected animals or animal products, such as abattoir workers, meat packers, livestock handlers, dairy industry professionals, veterinarians, and laboratory workers. [12, 20–22].

The incubation period ranges from 1 week to several months, after which there is an onset of a febrile illness [12]. Systemic signs of infection can be severe and include chills, fever, headache, and weakness. Characteristic findings include lymphadenopathy, hepatosplenomegaly, and arthritis, but other manifestations, such as epididymoorchitis and endocarditis can occur [20]. The dermatologic manifestations are nonspecific and appear in less than 5% of those infected [23]. They include papulonodular and erythema nodosum–like lesions and papulopustular, maculopapular, urticarial, and vesicular eruptions, at times petechial or ulcerated. Skin manifestations may occur during both initial infection and relapse [23]. The diagnosis is confirmed by serology or culture. PCR tests have been developed, but clinical interpretation of results needs to be better understood [20]. Treatment is based on World Health Organization (WHO) guidelines and involves a drug combination of doxycycline and either streptomycin or rifampin; however, alternative regimens have been used [20]. Relapses can occur in approximately 10% of treated patients, usually in the first year after infection [20]. A human vaccine is not available. Preventive measures include eliminating infected animals, immunizing animals, educating high-risk workers, using protective clothing, and emphasizing workplace hygiene [12].

Cat Scratch Disease

Cat scratch disease is caused by *Bartonella* (formerly *Rochalimaea*) *henselae* and is usually a be-

nign, self-limited, disease. It can occur in animal handlers and veterinarians [12, 24, 25]. It usually occurs after a bite or scratch from a kitten or cat, although other sources such as dogs may play a role [26]. A papule, nodule, pustule, or ulceration develops after 3–14 days at the scratch or bite site, and this is followed by enlargement of the regional lymph nodes, which is the hallmark of the disease. The disease may be associated with systemic symptoms such as fever, malaise, and fatigue. Extranodal disease occurs in approximately 10% of patients and may include neurologic, ocular, musculoskeletal, and other manifestations [27, 28]. The diagnosis is made by history and clinical findings, culture, serology, and PCR [29]. The therapeutic effectiveness of antibiotics is unclear in immunocompetent patients. Treatment is recommended in immunocompromised patients with antibiotics such as erythromycin, doxycycline, or rifampin [29]. Preventive measures include educating high-risk workers, using protective clothing, and thorough cleaning of cat bites and scratches [12].

Erysipeloid

Erysipeloid is caused by *Erysipelothrix rhusiopathiae*, a gram-positive bacillus found in fish, crabs, and other shellfish in fresh- and saltwater environments and cattle, pigs, sheep, poultry, and some rodents [9, 30]. The disease occurs most often in the summer months and is the result of contact with infected animals, animal products, or contaminated objects. High-risk occupations include fishermen, butchers, cooks, poultry and farm workers, and veterinarians [30]. One to seven days after inoculation (usually on the hand), burning, itching, and pain develop, along with tender, erythematous, violet, or purplish plaques. Often there is slow peripheral spread and central clearing. Low-grade fever, malaise, lymphadenitis, and adjacent joint arthritis may occur [9, 30]. Lesion dissemination, septicemia, septic arthritis, and endocarditis are rare findings [9, 31, 32]. The diagnosis is made using clinical findings and culture. Molecular techniques have been used for confirmation [9]. Isolation of the pathogen may be difficult, often requiring full-thickness biopsies [30]. The treatments include systemic penicillin and cephalosporins. Recurrences may occur rarely. Preventive measures include the removal of decaying nitrogenous material and contaminated objects, worker education, and use of protective clothing [11, 30].

Methicillin-Resistant Staphylococcus aureus

Staphylococci are common causes of bacterial skin lesions such as impetigo, folliculitis, furuncles, carbuncles, and abscesses [12]. Methicillin-resistant *S. aureus* (MRSA) infections have occurred in health care settings since the 1960s, but recently, community-associated MRSA infections have increased in incidence [33]. The most frequently reported manifestation of community-associated MRSA is furunculosis [34]. Infection is usually localized to the skin and soft tissues, but life-threatening complications have been reported [34]. Diagnosis is confirmed by culture with antibiotic susceptibility testing and PCR [35]. Treatment should be based on antibiotic susceptibility testing, which often differs between health care–associated and community-associated strains of MRSA [36].

Workers at risk include health care personnel, and in addition, community-associated MRSA outbreaks have been reported in correctional facilities, athletic teams, day-care centers, and military facilities [37,38]. Specific strains of MRSA have been related to exposure to pigs or calves [39]. Prevention measures include education and emphasis on infection control strategies and personal hygiene [12]

Lyme Disease

Lyme disease, the most common tick-borne infection in North America and Europe, is caused by the spirochete *Borrelia burgdorferi,* which is transmitted by the bite of several species of *Ixodes* ticks [40, 41]. High-risk occupations include outdoor workers in endemic areas whose activities include farming, hunting, trapping, surveying, landscaping, brush clearing, forestry, and wildlife and parks management [42–45]. In the United States, cases occur most commonly in the northeastern, mid-Atlantic, and upper North Central regions, but cases have been reported in other regions, including the South and the West Coast [46]. Cases peak during the summer months.

Three stages of illness have been identified based on clinical manifestations. An initial manifestation, seen in up to 80% of patients and developing days to weeks after the tick bite, is a distinct lesion of erythema migrans [47]. This lesion begins as an erythematous macule or papule at the site of the tick bite that slowly enlarges in size and may develop central clearing. The untreated skin lesion can last up to several weeks. Systemic symptoms often occur in patients with the skin lesion and include fatigue, myalgia, arthralgia, headache, and fever [41]. Multiple lesions may develop after hematogenous dissemination of spirochetes. Lymphocytoma also may develop and is more common in Europe than in the United States [41]. Late manifestations of Lyme disease include neurologic disease, carditis, and arthritis [41]. In patients with erythema migrans in endemic areas, the diagnosis may be made on clinical criteria. Two-step serologic testing, culture, and PCR may aid in the diagnosis of later-stage disease [40, 41]. Treatments include doxycycline and ceftriaxone and depend on the stage of the disease [40]. Prevention strategies include worker education, avoidance of tick-infested habitats—usually wooded, brushy, or overgrown grassy areas, especially in spring and summer—use of repellants or insecticides (DEET or permethrin), use of protective clothing (e.g., long-sleeve shirts, boots, and high socks with pants tucked into socks), and prompt inspection for ticks and correct tick removal (grasp as close to the skin as possible with forceps and apply gentle traction) [48,49]. Antibiotic prophylaxis may be used in certain circumstances [40]. A licensed vaccine was withdrawn by the manufacturer in 2002 owing to its limited acceptance by the public and physicians [50].

Mycobacterium marinum *Granuloma*

M. marinum is an acid-fast photochromogen (Runyon group I) water-borne nontuberculous mycobacterium. It is the causative organism in a condition referred to as "swimming pool granuloma" or "fish tank granuloma" [51]. High-risk occupations include fishermen, butchers, fish tank workers, and those exposed to contaminated water [52–54]. A papule develops 2–6 weeks after trauma and exposure to the organism in water. This evolves into a warty or ulcerating nodule or plaque, usually on the hand, knee, or elbow, with some spread along the lymphatics (a sporotrichoid pattern). Delayed diagnosis or immunosuppression may contribute to invasive disease such as tenosynovitis, septic arthritis, or osteomyelitis [55]. Definitive diagnosis is by tissue culture; the organism grows best at 30–32°C. PCR may allow for detection from a biopsy specimen, but results need to be interpreted cautiously [56]. Recommended treatments include clarithromycin, doxycycline, trimethoprim-sulfamethoxazole, and rifampin or ethambutol [56]. Treatment with combination therapy may be required, and surgical excision may be indicated [57]. Preventive measures include worker education and use of protective clothing.

Cutaneous Tuberculosis

Cutaneous tuberculosis comprises less than 2% of tuberculosis cases [58]. The route of infection includes cutaneous inoculation, contiguous spread from adjacent underlying infection, or hematogenous dissemination of infection [59]. Cutaneous inoculation with *Mycobacterium tuberculosis* can cause primary inoculation tuberculosis (tuberculous chancre) or a verrucous condition in previously sensitized individuals called *tuberculosis verrucosa cutis* ("prosector's wart," "anatomic tubercle," or "necrogenic wart.") In both conditions, the pathogen can be introduced at the sites of minor abrasions or wounds. Tuberculous chancre can be found in health care workers, and tuberculosis verrucosa cutis historically had been seen in pathologists, morgue attendants, and physicians [60]. Similar lesions caused by *M. bovis* from cattle can affect veterinarians, butchers, and farmers [11].

Tuberculous chancre presents as a papule or scab that does not heal and develops into a large, painless ulcer with ragged edges weeks after inoculation [58]. Regional lymphadenopathy can follow the skin manifestations. Tuberculosis verrucosa cutis begins as a indurated nodule with a warty surface, which then extends in a serpiginous manner, resulting in a red-brown, warty plaque with central clearing. The diagnosis can be difficult; diagnostic options include acid-fast staining, culture of lesions or skin biopsies, and PCR of specimens; however, a negative result does not exclude the diagnosis [58]. The treatment of cutaneous tuberculosis is similar to that of pulmonary tuberculosis, and the possibility of multidrug-resistant or extensively drug-resistant tuberculosis should be considered [61, 62]. Prevention includes worker education, workplace hygiene, and the use of protective clothing.

Tularemia

The causative organism of tularemia is the gram-negative intracellular coccobacillus *Francisella tularensis.* It is transmitted by contact with infected animals or animal products, arthropod bite, contact with or ingestion of contaminated water or meat, or inhalation of infectious aerosols. In the United States, ticks account for approximately 75% of the cases, whereas other arthropod vectors include mosquitoes, deerflies, and fleas [63]. Animal reservoirs include rabbits, squirrels, skunks, beavers, muskrats, and other small mammals, including domestic cats [9, 63]. The disease is seen in North America, Europe, the former Soviet Union, China, and Japan. [12]. High-risk workers include abattoir workers, butchers, farmers, foresters, hunters (especially those skinning rabbit hides), and veterinarians.

There are six clinical manifestations—glandular, ulceroglandular, oculoglandular, typhoidal, pneumonic, and oropharyngeal [63, 64]. The most common manifestation is ulceroglandular tularemia, in which a tender papule develops 3–5 days after inoculation and progresses into an ulcer with black eschar. Infection is associated with fever, chills, and other systemic symptoms; regional lymphadenopathy; and splenomegaly [63, 64]. The diagnosis is made by serology or PCR [64]. Culture may be used for diagnosis, but owing to the high risk of infection of laboratory personnel, laboratories must be notified so that special safety procedures may be implemented when handling specimens [64]. Treatment is with streptomycin, gentamicin, doxycycline, or ciprofloxacin [63, 64]. Preventive measures include worker education, avoidance of tick-infested habitats and contaminated water, use of repellants and insecticides, and use of protective clothing and laboratory methods [12]. An investigational live attenuated vaccine is available for high-risk groups [63].

Other Water-Borne Infections

Vibrio vulnificus is an important water-borne pathogen that can cause severe wound infections with direct contact and a primary septicemia if ingested (usually in raw shellfish). The case-fatality rate can be up to 50% in disseminated disease [9]. The organism is found commonly in sediments in warm salt water and estuaries, in fish, and in shellfish. Fishermen, crabbers, shrimp workers, and those exposed to contaminated water are at risk, especially those who may have underlying immuno-compromising medical conditions such as liver disease [65]. Wound infections owing to *V. vulnifi-*

cus usually follow cuts on the hand while cleaning crabs or shrimp or from entry of the pathogen through an open wound exposed to seawater. Infections are endemic along the coast of the Gulf of Mexico and in warmer waters of the Pacific and Atlantic coasts [66, 67]. The wound infections can appear as pustules with cellulitis and lymphangitis; they may be rapidly progressive with extensive skin necrosis and gangrene [9,68]. The diagnosis is made by culturing the organism from blood or the wound. Treatment with both doxycycline and ceftazidime is recommended, along with early surgical evaluation for potential intervention [69]. Prevention strategies include worker education and protective clothing.

Similar wound infections sustained in freshwater, with manifestations of a bullous cellulitis, fasciitis, and myonecrosis, may be caused by *Aeromonas hydrophila* [68]. In addition, *Photobacterium (Vibrio) damsela* and *V. parahaemolyticus* also can induce wound infections after lacerations are exposed to shellfish or seawater [66, 70]. *Pseudomonas aeruginosa* folliculitis has been associated with the use of hot tubs, whirlpools, saunas, and swimming pools [71]. In addition, cases have been described in ocean divers [72–74] and at a cardboard manufacturing facility [75]. *Pseudomonas* also may be associated with moist environments such as laundry work, dishwashing, or metal working [76, 77].

Rocky Mountain Spotted Fever

Rickettsiae are coccobacillary obligate intracellular bacteria that are transmitted to humans by arthropods such as ticks, mites, fleas, and lice. These organisms are the cause of a variety of spotted fevers (usually with generalized rashes including lesions on palms and soles) and typhus (truncal rash).

The most common rickettsial infection in the United States is Rocky Mountain spotted fever, which is caused by *Rickettsia rickettsii.* In the United States, this infection is seen mainly in the southeastern and south-central regions, but it also can be found in Canada, Mexico, and Central and South America [12]. The main tick vectors in the United States are the American dog tick (*Dermacentor variabilis*) in the eastern and southern United States and the Rocky Mountain wood tick (*Dermacentor andersoni*) in the western United States [12].

Systemic symptoms such as fever, chills, myalgia, and headache develop 2–14 days after a tick bite,

with a rash occurring in 50% of patients by the third day of illness [78]. The rash begins as blanchable macules, often first appearing on wrists and ankles and spreading to palms and soles. Papules then develop, followed by petechiae or purpura. Rash is absent in approximately 10% of patients [79]. The diagnosis is confirmed by serology, PCR, and immunofluorescent staining of biopsy specimens [79]. The treatment is with doxycycline or chloramphenicol. Workers at high risk include outdoor workers such as farmers, foresters, rangers, trappers, hunters, construction workers, and surveyors [11]. Prevention strategies include worker education, avoidance of tick-infested habitats—especially in spring and summer—use of repellants and insecticides, use of protective clothing, and prompt inspection for ticks and correct tick removal [12].

VIRAL DISEASES
Herpetic Whitlow

Medical and dental professionals and staff are at risk for developing herpetic whitlow, caused by herpes simplex virus type I or type II [80, 81]. This condition presents 2–12 days after direct skin contact with a patient's lesion or with a carrier of herpes. The lesion usually occurs on a finger as a recurrent, painful vesicle(s) on an erythematous base. The diagnosis can be made clinically and confirmed by examining unroofed vesicle scrapings microscopically for multinucleated giant cells (Tzanck test) and by viral culture, serology, direct fluorescent antibody testing, and PCR. If left untreated, the lesions usually heal within 1–2 weeks but often reactivate. Antiviral oral medications such as acyclovir, famciclovir, and valacyclovir can shorten the course and induce long-term suppression. Antiviral medication also has been used prophylactically following percutaneous exposure [82]. Prevention is achieved by worker education, workplace hygiene, and protective clothing, especially gloves [12].

Orf and Milker's Nodules

Orf (ecthyma contagiosum) appears worldwide and is caused by a virus belonging to the genus *Parapoxvirus*. It is transmitted by direct contact with the lesions of infected sheep, goats, or other animals such as camels and deer [83]. Animals recently vaccinated with orf vaccine or contaminated objects such as fences, barn doors, feeding troughs, and shears also can transmit the virus [84, 85]. Milker's nodules are also caused by a *Parapoxvirus* and occur after contact with infected cattle. These viral infections can occur in abattoir workers, shearers, milkers, veterinarians, shepherds, and farm workers. Lesions of orf and milker's nodules are similar. After an incubation period of 3–7 days, infection results in a solitary, painless, flat, or dome-shaped papule, vesicle, or bulla with a central umbilicated crust, usually on the hands, fingers, and forearms. These lesions usually evolve over 1–2 months through a variety of stages, each lasting a week (maculopapular, targetoid, weeping, regenerative, papillomatous, and regressive stages) [11, 86]. Multiple lesions can occur as well, and there can be regional lymphadenopathy, fever, and malaise.

The diagnosis of orf and milker's nodules is based on clinical presentation and exposure history, along with viral culture, serology, electron microscopy, or PCR [84]. Lesions usually resolve within 2 months, and treatment is ordinarily not necessary. Persistent lesions may be electrodesiccated and curettaged or excised, and topical cidofovir and imiquimod have been used [83, 87]. Prevention strategies include worker education, maintaining cleanliness of animal housing areas, good personal hygiene, washing exposed areas with soap and water, and use of protective clothing [12].

Vaccinia and Monkeypox

Vaccinia is an orthopoxvirus that is used for smallpox vaccine. Smallpox was declared to be globally eradicated by the WHO in 1980; however, in response to concerns that smallpox potentially could be used as a bioterrorism agent, the United States initiated a limited smallpox vaccination program focusing on health care workers, first responders, and members of the military [88]. Vaccination is contraindicated in people with skin disease or in those who are immunocompromised or pregnant or close contacts of people with these conditions [89]. Those vaccinated and those potentially exposed to the virus, such as laboratory workers and close contacts of vacinees, are at risk for complications [90–92]. The adverse reactions of smallpox vaccination include eczema vaccinatum, generalized vaccinia, progressive vaccinia, inoculation of virus to other sites, encephalitis, and fetal vaccinia

[89]. Myopericarditis also has been reported [93]. Diagnosis of smallpox vaccine adverse reactions is based on history and clinical presentation and also may involve electron microscopy, immunofluorescence, and PCR [90–92]. While some postvaccination complications are self-limited, others may require vaccinia immune globulin and cidofovir [89]. Prevention includes education and infection control precautions.

Monkeypox is a rare orthopoxvirus that is usually found in Africa but was introduced into the United States recently through a shipment of small mammals that were transported to a pet distributor [94]. Common symptoms are rash (maculopapular progressing to vesicular and pustular), headache, sweats, fever, and lymphadenopathy [95, 96]. The disease seen in the United States generally was milder than that seen in Africa [94]. Fifty-nine percent of cases in one state occurred in persons exposed through their occupation and included veterinary staff, pet store employees, and animal distributors [95]. Diagnostic methods include virus isolation, electron microscopy, PCR, serology, and immunofluorescence, but many of these methods are nonspecific for monkeypox [96]. The role of vaccinia immune gobulin and cidofovir in the treatment of severe disease is unclear, and clinical consultation with state health departments or the Centers for Disease Control and Prevention (CDC) is recommended [97]. Vaccination with vaccinia virus, infection control practices, education, and proper animal care should be implemented as prevention strategies [96, 98].

Warts

Warts are caused by any of a variety of the over 100 human papillomaviruses (HPVs), which are found worldwide [99]. High-risk occupations include butchers of cattle and pigs, fish handlers, and poultry processing workers [11]. The warts of meat handlers are verrucous papules found most often on the hands and usually are caused by HPV type 7, but other types may be involved as well [100–103]. There is a suggestion that HPV type 7 is widely distributed in the environment, but an unknown factor in meat enhances viral replication [104]. Competitive athletes also may be affected by warts transmitted via common showers or skin-to-skin contact. The diagnosis of warts is usually made by clinical appearance, which can vary from dome-shaped papules to filiform papules to flat-topped papules or macules. There is no reliable cure for warts; most treatments rely on destruction (e.g., cautery and curettage, cryotherapy, keratolytics, laser, virucides, and immunotherapy) [105]. Prevention strategies include worker education and use of protective clothing. A licensed vaccine is available to protect against HPV types that cause cervical cancer and genital warts but not common cutaneous warts.

During destruction of warts using laser or electrosurgery, medical personnel may put themselves at risk because of exposure to aerosolized HPV, which can induce laryngeal warts [106, 107]. Facemasks and control of smoke through ventilation and work practices are recommended [108].

Other Viral Infections

Other viruses with important skin manifestations are usually seen in the pediatric population but may be important to susceptible health care, school, and day-care workers [109–115]. These include measles, rubella, chickenpox (varicellazoster), hand-foot-mouth disease, and erythema infectiosum. Transmission of these diseases is person to person through direct contact with secretions and via droplet and airborne routes. These diseases tend to be more severe in adults. Vaccinations are available for the first three diseases.

Measles (rubeola) is caused by infection with a paramyxovirus. Typical measles has a prodrome of 2–4 days of fever, respiratory congestion, conjunctivitis, and cough. This is followed by tiny white or blue-gray Koplik spots on the buccal mucosa and then by nonpruritic, erythematous papules that begin behind the ear, spread to the whole body, become confluent, and last from 4–7 days. Rubella is caused by a togavirus, which can cause a mild illness with a variable rash, usually a faint pink macular eruption that spreads from the face to the trunk and proximal extremities. Its most feared complication is congenital rubella syndrome. Varicella (chickenpox) is characterized by the abrupt onset of faint erythematous macules that progress to vesicles over 1–2 days, and lesions may be seen at all stages of development. Adults may experience a 2- to 3-day prodromal period. Older lesions crust over and fall off in 1–3 weeks. Perinatal disease can

be serious. Reactivation in adults can lead to herpes zoster (shingles), with painful vesicles occurring in dermatomal patterns. Hand-foot-mouth disease, caused by several coxsackievirus group A enteroviruses, is characterized by painful oral lesions and the abrupt onset of papules that progress to vesicles in an acral distribution. Although usually a benign disease, fatalities have been reported [116]. Erythema infectiosum (fifth disease) is caused by the human parvovirus B19. The typical presentation is the initial "slapped cheek" erythematous patches or plaques on the face, followed in 1–4 days by lacy, reticulated macules and papules on the extremities. The skin lesions may wax and wane for weeks to months. The clinical presentation of the adult infection may vary and may be confused with rubella or an allergic reaction. Fever, malaise, and headache may occur. The infection can cause arthritis in adults, particularly women, and can induce fetal death (hydrops fetalis) [117].

The diagnosis of these viral diseases is usually based on clinical manifestations and serology, virus isolation, or PCR. There is no specific treatment for measles, rubella, hand-foot-mouth disease, and erythema infectiosum, although immune globulin has been used for erythema infectiosum and for pregnant women exposed to rubella [118, 119]. Antiviral medications have been used in varicellazoster infections, and immune globulin has been used for postexposure prophylaxis in specific circumstances [120]. Prevention strategies include worker education, vaccination, reducing person-to-person contact (isolation), proper ventilation, and promotion of hygienic measures [12, 121].

SUPERFICIAL FUNGAL DISEASES
Candidiasis

Paronychial and interdigital candidal infection caused by *Candida albicans* is the most common fungal disease of occupational origin and can be seen in those engaged in wet work, such as food service personnel, dishwashers, housekeepers, and bartenders [11]. The presentation includes swollen, erythematous, tender skin in the nail folds or interdigital spaces, often with a serous or purulent discharge. In paronychial infections, malformation of the proximal nail plate can occur. Candidal infection also can occur in skin fold areas (intertrigo) in workers working in hot and humid environments.

The diagnosis of candidal infections can be made by microscopic examination of scale immersed in potassium hydroxide (KOH) or culture. Often, multiple organisms can be involved in paronychial infection, including *P. aeruginosa* and *S. aureus*. Treatment regimens include topical and oral antifungal agents. Patient education is very important to eliminate the predisposing factors (i.e., trauma, wet work, and hot and humid environments) and to introduce healing and prevention strategies. Keeping the hands dry through the use of appropriate gloves is key.

Dermatophytosis

Dermatophytosis, also known as *tinea* or *ringworm infections,* can be caused by a variety of species of *Epidermophyton, Microsporum,* and *Trichophyton.* These species can reside on humans (anthropophilic), animals (zoophilic), or in the soil (geophilic). Medical and dental workers, school and day-care workers, veterinarians, animal handlers, and agricultural and construction workers are at risk. Anthropophilic dermatophytes (e.g., *Trichophyton rubrum* and *T. mentagrophytes*) can cause fungal infection on the body or the feet. These can occur in medical or day-care environments or in workplaces in association with sweaty foot environments (e.g., use of protective boots) or where there are common shower areas [11, 122, 123]. *T. verrucosum* (cattle) and *Microsporum canis* (small animals), both zoophilic dermatophytes, can infect farmers, cattle handlers, veterinarians, and animal handlers [11, 124]. *M. gypseum,* found in clay or sandy soil, can infect agricultural and construction workers. The general clinical appearance of dermatophyte infections is that of annular, scaling, erythematous plaques, but presentations can vary by body site and can be highly inflammatory at times. Locations of involvement include the scalp (tinea capitis), the bearded areas (tinea barbae), general glabrous skin (tinea corporis), the groin (tinea cruris), the feet (tinea pedis), the hands (tinea manuum), and the nails (tinea unguium/ onychomycosis). The diagnosis can be made by microscopic examination of scale immersed in KOH or culture. Treatment regimens include topical and oral antifungal agents. Preventive measures include worker education, using fungicidal agents to clean showers and dressing rooms, maintaining personal hygiene including the use of fungicidal powders on feet and in shoes and socks, and using protective clothing [12, 122].

Tinea Versicolor

Tinea versicolor (pityriasis versicolor), a common skin disorder caused by *Malassezia* (most commonly *M. furfur, M. globosa,* and *M. sympodialis*), can be seen in workers who work in hot and humid environments [125]. Heat, humidity, occlusion, and sweat contribute to this condition. Clinically, it presents as asymptomatic, hypopigmented or hyperpigmented (color varies) macules or patches with fine, dustlike scales. The usual areas of involvement include the chest, neck, back, abdomen, and proximal extremities. The diagnosis can be made by microscopic examination of scale immersed in KOH, which gives the typical "spaghetti and meatballs" appearance of the hyphae and spores. Treatment regimens include topical and oral antifungal agents and selenium sulfide washes, but relapses are common. Prevention strategies are limited and include improving the ambient work conditions as well as selenium sulfide body washes.

SUBCUTANEOUS FUNGAL DISEASES
Chromoblastomycosis

Chromoblastomycosis (chromomycosis) is a chronic skin disease that results from traumatic implantation of the pathogenic agent from soil, plant debris, wood fragments, or other environmental debris into the skin [126]. The disease, which can be caused by a variety of dematiaceous (pigmented) fungi (including *Fonsecaea pedrosoi, Cladophialophora* (*Cladosporium*) *carrionii, F. compactum, Rhinocladiella aquaspersa,* and *Phialophora verrucosa*), can be found worldwide but is usually seen in tropical and subtropical areas. The disease usually affects the rural poor who are exposed to the soil in outdoor occupations such as laborers, lumberjacks, and agricultural workers [127]. The skin manifestations frequently are seen on the lower legs and feet and begin as pink, scaly papules that evolve into verrucous nodules and plaques with classic "black dots" (transepithelial elimination) on their surfaces. The diagnosis is confirmed through culturing the organism and skin biopsies (special fungal stains to look for sclerotic or Medlar bodies) [126]. Treatment can include wide excision and antifungal agents such as itraconazole, terbinafine, 5-fluorocytosine, and amphotericin B. Cryotherapy, heat therapy, and laser treatment have been used as well [128, 129]. Relapses and partial cures are common. Prevention strategies include worker education, personal hygiene, and protective clothing (especially shoes) [12].

Mycetoma

Mycetoma (Madura foot) is caused by either multiple species of aerobic actinomycetes (actinomycetoma) or true fungi (eumycetoma) found in soil [11]. After traumatic inoculation, usually into the foot, hand, or back (from carrying contaminated materials), slowly enlarging, painless, subcutaneous nodules form. Ultimately, these evolve into slowly progressive, chronic, indurated plaques with sinus tracts draining pus containing grains. The nodules connect to each other through deep abscesses, and osteomyelitis may occur [130]. Agricultural and other workers in tropical and subtropical areas are at risk [131]. The diagnosis is made by direct microscopic study of fine-needle aspiration or biopsy specimens and culture [132]. Serologic tests and PCR have been developed, and histopathology, magnetic resonance imaging (MRI), and ultrasound may aid in the diagnosis [130, 132, 133]. Treatment depends on the organism involved. Actinomycetoma has been treated with antibiotics such as streptomycin, cotrimoxazole, dapsone, amikacin, and imipenem, often using combination therapy. Relapse is not unusual. Eumycetoma is more difficult to treat and responds variably to antifungal agents and surgical excision [133]. Prevention strategies include worker education, personal hygiene, and protective clothing (especially shoes) [12].

Sporotrichosis

The organism causing sporotrichosis, *Sporothrix schenckii*, is a dimorphic fungus found in soil, timber, sphagnum moss, and other plant material, and it appears in most temperate and tropical climates of the world [134]. Agricultural and forestry workers, gardeners, florists, greenhouse workers, and miners are at risk. An epidemic among gold miners in South Africa affected over 3,000 workers; the source was fungus growing on mine timbers [12]. An outbreak in 1988 in the United States affected 84 people in 14 states; many of those infected were forestry or nursery workers handling sphagnum moss [135]. *S. schenckii* also infects animals, and

transmission to veterinarians has been reported [136]. The disease usually occurs weeks after traumatic implantation of the fungus through puncture or scratch. Sporotrichosis usually occurs in the skin and the lymph nodes and can be recurring if it is not treated. It most often presents as an ulcerating papule with nodules forming along the paths of the draining lymphatics (lymphocutaneous form with sporotrichoid spread). There is also a fixed form of the disease with no sporotrichoid spread. Extracutaneous sporotrichosis may occur but is less common [137]. The diagnosis can be confirmed through culturing the organism. Diagnosis from microscopic examination of skin biopsies is more difficult, and serology is not readily available [138]. Treatments include oral potassium iodide, itraconazole, ketoconazole, amphotericin B, and terbinafine [138]. Prevention strategies include worker education, decontamination of fomites with fungicides, and use of protective clothing [12, 139].

SYSTEMIC FUNGAL INFECTIONS

A number of systemic mycoses have rare cutaneous manifestations (usually in disseminated disease), including coccidioidomycosis, histoplasmosis, blastomycosis, and paracoccidioidomycosis. The most distinctive lesions can be seen in blastomycosis and paracoccidioidomycosis.

Blastomycosis

Blastomycosis is caused by the thermal dimorphic fungus, *Blastomyces dermatitidis*. The fungus is found in the soil or near the soil (decaying wood or animal manure). Most cases occur in the central and southeastern United States and Canada, but cases also have been reported in Africa, India, and the Middle East [12]. Farming, forestry, construction, and other outdoor workers may be at risk [11, 140]. The infection is usually acquired as a primary pulmonary infection, although cutaneous disease is its most common nonpulmonary manifestation, and direct cutaneous inoculation can occur [141]. The earliest lesions are papulopustules or nodules that progress to arciform, serpiginous plaques with a raised edge. These can ulcerate and form microabscesses. The diagnosis can be confirmed through culturing the organism (which is very difficult) and histopathologic examination of skin biopsies (using routine or special fungal stains). A urinary antigen test is also available [142]. Standard serologic antibody assays are available but generally are not helpful for clinical diagnosis. Treatments include azole antifungals and amphotericin B. There are no known successful prevention strategies for this disease.

Paracoccidioidomycosis

Paracoccidioidomycosis is caused by *Paracoccidioides brasiliensis,* which is found in the soil in tropical and subtropical areas of Mexico and Central and South America [12]. Farmers, laborers, construction workers, and other workers in contact with soil are at risk. The fungus is introduced into the lungs and disseminates to other organs such as the skin. The skin manifestations include painful ulcers in the mouth or around the mouth and nose. The diagnosis can be made by culture, microscopic examination of sputum, pus, or biopsied tissue, or serology. Treatments include azole antifungals, sulfonamides, and amphotericin B. There are no known successful prevention strategies for this disease.

PARASITIC DISEASES
Cercarial Dermatitis

Cercarial dermatitis ("swimmer's itch," "swamp itch," or "clam-digger's itch") is caused by avian schistosomes that penetrate the skin, causing a pruritic papular eruption [11]. This condition can occur worldwide, including in the Great Lakes region and the California coast, and can be seen in divers, lifeguards, and dock workers exposed to sea-level freshwater or brackish seawater. Outbreaks have been reported in rice farmers in Asia [143]. Infection results in urticarial papules on exposed skin surfaces that subside usually within weeks. The diagnosis is based on clinical appearance and exposure history. Treatment is symptomatic. Prevention strategies include worker education and protective clothing. Sea bather's eruption is often confused with swimmer's itch. This latter condition occurs only in salt water and is a very pruritic, macular, maculopapular, or vesicular eruption limited to areas covered by swimwear. It is not considered an infectious disease and is caused by larval forms of marine cnidarians [144].

Cutaneous Larva Migrans

Dog and cat intestinal hookworms, most commonly *Ancylostoma braziliense,* can produce mo-

bile, serpiginous, linear, pruritic plaques usually on the feet (creeping eruption). The organisms can migrate several centimeters in a day. Those at risk include workers exposed to contaminated sand or dirt on subtropical and tropical beaches, farmers, sewer workers, lifeguards, and construction workers. An outbreak was reported at a children's camp in Florida, with the likely source of infection identified as exposure to cat feces in a playground sandbox [145]. The diagnosis is usually made by clinical appearance of the lesion and a history of exposure. Treatment includes topical thiabendazole and oral albendazole or ivermectin [146]. Prevention strategies include worker education and protective clothing, especially shoes, and hookworm treatment for cats and dogs [145].

Other rare nematode-caused occupational skin diseases include trichinosis, dracunculiasis, filariasis, loiasis, onchocerciasis, enterobiasis, strongyloidiasis, and toxocariasis [11].

Leishmaniases

The leishmaniases are a variety of diseases caused by species of the protozoa *Leishmania,* transmitted from zoonotic or anthroponotic reservoir hosts to humans by sandflies (*Phlebotomus* and *Lutzomyia*) [147]. The infection is found in Asia, the Middle East, the Mediterranean region, sub-Saharan Africa, south-central Texas, Mexico, and Central and South America [12, 147]. Farmers and other outdoor workers working in forested areas are at risk, and military personnel deployed to endemic areas also may become infected [12, 148]. Forms of the disease include cutaneous (old world and new world) leishmaniasis, diffuse cutaneous leishmaniasis, visceral leishmaniasis, and mucocutaneous leishmaniasis. The skin lesions can vary and include pruritic papules, nodules, and ulcerated craters. The diagnosis is confirmed by identifying organisms in smears or biopsy specimens or by culture, PCR, or serology [149]. Lesions may be treated with pentavalent antimonials, amphotericin B, or other alternative treatments that have been described [147]. Prevention strategies include covering exposed skin and applying repellents and insecticides to minimize sandfly bites in endemic areas.

Mite Infestations

Human scabies is a contagious disease caused by the mite *Sarcoptes scabiei* and is spread by direct skin-to-skin contact and through fomites such as clothing and linen. High-risk groups include medical personnel, nursing home workers, and day-care workers [150]. Scabies is marked by intensely pruritic vesicles and burrows, usually found on interdigital webs, elbows, feet, genitalia, buttocks, and axillae. Other clinical forms include nodular and crusted (Norwegian) scabies. The diagnosis of scabies is made by demonstrating mites, eggs, or feces (scybala) on scrapings from affected skin. Treatment includes topical scabicides and oral ivermectin. Prevention strategies include worker education, good workplace hygiene, and protective clothing.

Mite infestations also may occur after an ecosystem disturbance such as a hurricane or flooding and were suspected to be the cause of papular urticaria diagnosed in construction workers using huts that had sustained flooding during Hurricane Katrina [151]. Mites that bite humans but do not generally infest the body include grain mites, straw mites, rat mites, fowl or avian mites, and dog/cat/rabbit mites [152]. These can produce pruritic papules or papular urticaria. Animal caretakers and agricultural workers are at risk.

Public Health Perspective

The clinician should view each patient with a potential occupational dermatologic infectious disease from a broader public health perspective. The worker with an occupational dermatologic infectious disease should be viewed as a "sentinel health event" [153–155]. This recognition and resulting action by the clinician, in consultation with public health authorities, can lead to potential disease prevention in other workers. This can only occur with proper diagnosis of the worker, a high level of suspicion on the part of the clinician in suspecting workplace exposures, ultimate confirmation of the association with workplace exposures that caused the disease, and finally, steps taken to modify those exposures [155]. If successful, this approach would lead to the prevention of relapses and of new cases of occupational dermatologic infectious diseases.

Other Resources

Pictures of a number of dermatologic conditions are available online at www.cdc.gov/niosh/ocderm .html. Slides 71–81 are the most relevant to this chapter.

Acknowledgment

Funding support: This chapter was written as part of the authors' official duties as government officers and thus cannot be copyrighted.

References

1. Adams RM, Fletcher J (eds). *Occupational Skin Disease,* 3rd ed. Philadelphia: Saunders, 1999.
2. Kanerva L, Elsner P, Wahleberg JE, et al. (eds). *Handbook of Occupational Dermatology.* New York: Springer, 2000.
3. Marks JG, Elsner P, DeLeo VA. *Contact and Occupational Dermatology,* 3rd ed. St Louis: Mosby–Year Book, 2001.
4. Di Salvo AF (ed). *Occupational Mycoses.* Philadelphia: Lea & Febiger, 1983.
5. Lushniak BD. The importance of occupational skin diseases in the United States. *Int Arch Occup Environ Health* 2003;76:325–30.
6. Centers for Disease Control and Prevention. Summary of notifiable diseases—United States, 2005. *MMWR* 2007;53:20–1.
7. The Society for Investigative Dermatology and the American Academy of Dermatology Association. *Report—The Burden of Skin Diseases 2005.* Cleveland, OH: The Lewin Group for the Society for Investigative Dermatolog and Washington, DC: The American Academy of Dermatology Association, 2005.
8. Bureau of Labor Statistics (BLS). *Occupational Injuries and Illnesses in the United States.* Washington: US Department of Labor, www.bls.gov, 2006.
9. Swartz MN, Weinberg AN. Miscellaneous bacterial infections with cutaneous manifestations. In Freedberg IM, Eisen AZ, Wolff K, et al. (eds), *Fitzpatrick's Dermatology in General Medicine,* 6th ed. New York: McGraw-Hill, 2003, pp 1918–32.
10. Inglesby TV, O'Toole T, Henderson DA, et al. Anthrax as a biological weapon, 2002: Updated recommendations for management. *JAMA* 2002;287: 2236–52.
11. Ancona A. Biologic causes. In Adams RM (ed), *Occupational Skin Disease,* 3rd ed. Philadelphia: Saunders, 1999, pp 86–110.
12. Heymann DL (ed). *Control of Communicable Diseases Manual,* 18th ed. Washington: American Public Health Association, 2004.
13. Jernigan DB, Raghunathan PL, Bell BP, et al. Investigation of bioterrorism-related anthrax, United States, 2001: Epidemiologic findings. *Emerg Infect Dis* 2002;8:1019–28.
14. Wenner KA, Kenner JR. Anthrax. *Dermatol Clin* 2004;22:247–56.

15. Bell DM, Kozarsky PE, Stephens DS. Conference summary: Clinical issues in the prophylaxis, diagnosis, and treatment of anthrax. *Emerg Infect Dis* 2002;8:222–5.

16. Briggs PM, Delta BG, Keener SR, et al. Human cutaneous anthrax—North Carolina, 1987. *MMWR* 1988;37:413–4.

17. Anonymous. Anthrax: Memorandum from a WHO meeting. *Bull WHO* 1996;74:465–70.

18. Hanna P. Anthrax pathogenesis and host response. *Curr Top Microbiol Immunol* 1998;225:13–35.

19. Pappas G, Papadimitriou P, Akritidis N, et al. The new global map of human brucellosis. *Lancet Infect Dis* 2006;6:91–9.

20. Pappas G, Akritidis N, Bosilkovski M, et al. Brucellosis. *N Engl J Med* 2005;352:2325–36.

21. Trout D, Gomez TM, Bernard BP, et al. Outbreak of brucellosis at a United States pork packing plant. *J Occup Environ Med* 1995;37:697–703.

22. Robichaud S, Libman M, Behr M, et al. Prevention of laboratory-acquired brucellosis. *Clin Infect Dis* 2004;38:e119–22.

23. Milionis H, Christou L, Elisaf M. Cutaneous manifestations in brucellosis: Case report and review of the literature. *Infection* 2000;28:124–6.

24. Zangwill KM, Hamilton DH, Perkins BA, et al. Cat scratch disease in Connecticut: Epidemiology, risk factors, and evaluation of new diagnostic test. *N Engl J Med* 1993;329:8–13.

25. Noah DL, Kramer CM, Verbsky MP, et al. Survey of veterinary professionals and other veterinary conference attendees for antibodies to *Bartonella henselae* and *B. quintana. J Am Vet Med Assoc* 1997;210:342–4.

26. Chomel BB, Boulouis HJ, Maruyama S, et al. *Bartonella* spp.: In pets and effect on human health. *Emerg Infect Dis* 2006;12:389–94.

27. Cunningham ET, Koehler JE. Ocular bartonellosis. *Am J Ophthalmol* 2000;130:340–9.

28. Maman E, Bickels J, Ephros M, et al. Musculoskeletal manifestations of cat scratch disease. *Clin Infect Dis* 2007;45:1535–40.

29. Lamps LW, Scott MA. Cat-scratch disease: Historic, clinical, and pathologic perspectives. *Am J Clin Pathol* 2004;121:S71–80.

30. Brooke CJ, Riley TV. *Erysipelothrix rhusiopathiae:* Bacteriology, epidemiology and clinical manifestations of an occupational pathogen. *J Med Microbiol* 1999;48:789–99.

31. Ruiz ME, Richards JS, Kerr GS et al. *Erysipelothrix rhusiopathiae* septic arthritis. *Arthritis Rheum* 2003;48:1156–7.

32. Nassar IM, de la Llana R, Garrido P, et al. Mitro-aortic infective endocarditis produced by *Erysipelothrix rhusiopathiae:* Case report and review of the literature. *J Heart Valve Dis* 2005;14:320–4.

33. Weber JT. Community-associated methicillin-resistant *Staphylococcus aureus. Clin Infect Dis* 2005;41:S269–72.

34. Zetola N, Francis J, Nuermberger EL, et al. Community-acquired methicillin-resistant *Staphylococcus aureus:* An emerging threat. *Lancet Infect Dis* 2005;5:275–86.

35. Stamper PD, Cai M, Howard T, et al. Clinical validation of the molecular BD GeneOhm StaphSR assay for direct detection of *Staphylococcus aureus* and methicillin-resistant *Staphylococcus aureus* in positive blood cultures. *J Clin Microbiol* 2007;45:2191–6.

36. Elston D. Methicillin-sensitive and methicillin-resistant *Staphylococcus aureus:* Management principles and selection of antibiotic therapy. *Dermatol Clin* 2007;25:157–64.

37. Centers for Disease Control and Prevention. Public health dispatch: Outbreaks of community-associated methicillin-resistant *Staphylococcus aureus* skin infections—Los Angeles County, California, 2002–2003. *MMWR* 2003;52:88.

38. Zinderman CE, Conner B, Malakooti MA, et al. Community-acquired methicillin-resistant *Staphylococcus aureus* among military recruits. *Emerg Infect Dis* 2004;10:941–4.

39. Van Rijen MM, Van Keulen PH, Kluytmans JA. Increase in a Dutch hospital of methicillin-resistant *Staphylococcus aureus* related to animal farming. *Clin Infect Dis* 2008;46:261–3.

40. Wormser GP, Dattwyler RJ, Shapiro ED, et al. The clinical assessment, treatment, and prevention of Lyme disease, human granulocytic anaplasmosis, and babesiosis: Clinical practice guidelines by the Infectious Diseases Society of America. *Clin Infect Dis* 2006;43:1089–134.

41. Hengge UR, Tannapfel A, Tyring SK, et al. Lyme borreliosis. *Lancet Infect Dis* 2003;3:489–500.

42. Goldstein MD, Schwartz BS, Friedman C. Lyme disease in New Jersey outdoor workers: A statewide survey of seroprevalence and tick exposure. *Am J Public Health* 1990;80:1225–9.

43. Schwartz BS, Goldstein MD, Childs JE. Antibodies to *Borrelia burgdorferi* and tick salivary gland proteins in New Jersey outdoor workers. *Am J Public Health* 1993;83:1746–8.

44. Schwartz BS, Goldstein MD, Childs JE. Longitudinal study of *Borrelia burgdorferi* infection in New Jersey outdoor workers, 1988–1991. *Am J Epidemiol* 1994;139:504–12.

45. Bowen SG, Schultze TL, Hayne C, et al. A focus of Lyme disease in Monmouth County, New Jersey. *Am J Epidemiol* 1984;120:387–94.

46. Centers for Disease Control and Prevention. Lyme disease—United States, 2003–2005. *MMWR* 2007;56:573–6.

47. Steere AC, Sikand VK. The presenting manifestations of Lyme disease and the outcomes of treatment. *N Engl J Med* 2003;348:2472–4.

48. Abele DC, Anders KH. The many faces and phases of borreliosis: I. Lyme disease. *J Am Acad Dermatol* 1990;23:167–86.

49. Corapi KM, White MI, Phillips CB, et al. Strategies for primary and secondary prevention of Lyme disease. *Nat Clin Pract Rheum* 2006;3:20–5.

50. Steere AC, Coburn J, Glickstein L. The emergence of Lyme disease. *J Clin Invest* 2004;113:1093–101.

51. Hautmann G, Lotti T. Atypical mycobacterial infections of the skin. *Dermatol Clin* 1994;12:657–68.

52. Miller WC, Toon R. *Mycobacterium marinum* in Gulf fishermen. *Arch Environ Health* 1973;27:8–10.

53. Cole G. *Mycobacterium marinum* infection in a mechanic. *Contact Dermatitis* 1987;16:283.

54. Kullavanijaya P, Sirimachan S, Bhuddhavudhikrai P. *Mycobacterium marinum* cutaneous infections acquired from occupations and hobbies. *Int J Dermatol* 1993;32:504–7.

55. Lahey T. Invasive *Mycobacterium marinum* infections. *Emerg Infect Dis* 2003;9:1496–8.

56. Rallis E, Koumantaki-Mathioudaki E. Treatment of *Mycobacterium marinum* cutaneous infections. *Exp Opin Pharmacother* 2007;8:2965–78.

57. Lewis FM, Marsh BJ, von Reyn CF. Fish tank exposure and cutaneous infections due to *Mycobacterium marinum*: Tuberculin skin testing, treatment, and prevention. *Clin Infect Dis* 2003;37:390–7.

58. Bravo FG, Gotuzzo E. Cutaneous tuberculosis. *Clin Dermatol* 2007;25:173–80.

59. Hay R. Cutaneous infection with *Mycobacterium tuberculosis*: How has this altered with the changing epidemiology of tuberculosis? *Curr Opin Infect Dis* 2005;18:93–5.

60. Barbagallo J, Tager P, Ingleton R, et al. Cutaneous tuberculosis. *Am J Clin Dermatol* 2002;3:319–28.

61. Centers for Disease Control and Prevention. Emergence of *Mycobacterium tuberculosis* with extensive resistance to second-line drugs—Worldwide, 2000–2004. *MMWR* 2006;55:301–5.

62. Furin J. The clinical management of drug-resistant tuberculosis. *Curr Opin Pulm Med* 2007;13:212–7.

63. Cronquist SD. Tularemia: The disease and the weapon. *Dermatol Clin* 2004;22:313–20.

64. Eliasson H, Broman T, Forsman M, et al. Tularemia: Current epidemiology and disease management. *Infect Dis Clin North Am* 2006;20:289–311.

65. Hsueh PR, Lin CY, Tang HJ, et al. *Vibrio vulnificus* in Taiwan. *Emerg Infect Dis* 2004;10:1363–8.

66. Bonner JR. Spectrum of *Vibrio* infections in a Gulf Coast community. *Ann Intern Med* 1983;99:464.

67. Hlady WG, Klontz KC. The epidemiology of *Vibrio* infections in Florida, 1981–1993. *J Infect Dis* 1996;173:1176–83.

68. Tsai YH, Hsu RW, Huang TJ, et al. Necrotizing soft-tissue infections and sepsis caused by *Vibrio vulnificus* compared with those caused by *Aeromonas* species. *J Bone Joint Surg* 2007;89A:631–6.

69. Bross MH, Soch K, Morales R, et al. *Vibrio vulnificus* infection: Diagnosis and treatment. *Am Fam Physician* 2007;76:539–44.

70. Durborow R. Health and safety concerns in fisheries and aquaculture. *Occup Med* 1999;14:373–406.

71. Centers for Disease Control and Prevention. *Pseudomonas* dermatitis/folliculitis associated with pools and hot tubs—Colorado and Maine, 1999–2000. *MMWR* 2000;49:1087–91.

72. Lacour JP, El Baze P, Castanet J, et al. Diving suit dermatitis caused by *Pseudomonas aeruginosa*: Two cases. *J Am Acad Dermatol* 1994;31:1055–6.

73. Ahlen C, Mandal LH, Iverson OJ. Identification of infectious *Pseudomonas aeruginosa* strains in an occupational saturation diving environment. *Occup Environ Med* 1998;55:480–4.

74. Ahlen C, Mandal LH, Iversen OJ. The impact of environmental *Pseudomonas aeruginosa* genotypes on skin infections in occupational saturation diving systems. *Scand J Infect Dis* 2001;33:413–9.

75. Hewitt DJ, Weeks DA, Millner GC, et al. Industrial *Pseudomonas* folliculitis. *Am J Ind Med* 2006;49:895–9.

76. Weinberg AN, Swartz MN. Gram-negative coccal and bacillary infections. In Freedberg IM, Eisen AZ, Wolff K, et al. (eds), *Fitzpatrick's Dermatology in General Medicine*, 6th ed. New York: McGraw-Hill, 2003, pp 1896–911.

77. Jaksic S, Uhitil S, Zivkovic J. Bacterial pollution of cutting fluids: A risk factor for occupational diseases. *Arh Hig Rada Toksikol* 1998;49:239–44.

78. Green JJ, Heyman WR. The rickettsioses and ehrlichioses. In Freedberg IM, Eisen AZ, Wolff K, et al. (eds), *Fitzpatrick's Dermatology in General Medicine*, 6th ed. New York: McGraw-Hill, 2003, pp 2152–62.

79. Parola P, Paddock CD, Raoult D. Tick-borne rickettsioses around the world: Emerging diseases challenging old concepts. *Clin Microbiol Rev* 2005;18:719–56.

80. Jones JG. Herpetic whitlow: An infectious occupational hazard. *J Occup Med* 1985;10:725–8.

81. Rowe N, Heine C, Kowalsky C. Herpetic whitlow: An occupational disease of practicing dentists. *JAMA* 1981;105:471–3.

82. Manian FA. Potential role of famciclovir for prevention of herpetic whitlow in the health care setting. *Clin Infect Dis* 2000;31:e18–9.

83. Erbagci Z, Erbagci I, Tuncel AA. Rapid improvement of human orf (ecthyma contagiosum) with topical imiquimod cream: Report of four complicated cases. *J Dermatol Treat* 2005;16:353–6.

84. Centers for Disease Control and Prevention. Orf virus infection in humans—New York, Illinois, California and Tennessee, 2004–2005. *MMWR* 2006;55:65–8.

85. Snyder RR, Diven DG. Orf (contagious pustular dermatitis, contagious ecthyma). In Freedberg IM, Eisen AZ, Wolff K, et al (eds), *Fitzpatrick's Dermatology in General Medicine*, 6th ed. New York: McGraw-Hill, 2003, pp 2110–4.

86. Bodnar MG, Miller OF, Tyler WB. Facial orf. *J Am Acad Dermatol* 1999;40:815–7.

87. Lowy DR. Milker's nodules. In Freedberg IM, Eisen AZ, Wolff K, et al (eds), *Fitzpatrick's Dermatology in General Medicine*, 6th ed. New York: McGraw-Hill, 2003, pp 2117–9.

88. Poland GA, Grabenstein JD, Neff JM. The US smallpox vaccination program: A review of a large

modern era smallpox vaccination implementation program. *Vaccine* 2005;23:2078–81.

89. Centers for Disease Control and Prevention. Smallpox vaccination and adverse reactions. *MMWR* 2003;52:1–28.

90. Lewis FM, Chernak E, Goldman E, et al. Ocular vaccinia infection in laboratory worker, Philadelphia, 2004. *Emerg Infect Dis* 2006;12:134–7.

91. Wlodaver CG, Palumbo GJ, Waner JL. Laboratory-acquired vaccinia infection. *J Clin Virol* 2004;29:167–70.

92. Centers for Disease Control and Prevention. Household transmission of vaccinia virus from contact with a military smallpox vaccine—Illinois and Indiana, 2007. *MMWR* 2007;56:478–81.

93. Halsell JS, Riddle JR, Atwood JE, et al. Myopericarditis following smallpox vaccination among vaccinia-naïve US military personnel. *JAMA* 2003;289:3283–9.

94. DiGiulio DB, Eckburg PB. Human monkeypox: An emerging zoonosis. *Lancet Infect Dis* 2004;4:15–25.

95. Croft DR, Sotir MJ, Williams CJ, et al. Occupational risks during a monkeypox outbreak, Wisconsin, 2003. *Emerg Infect Dis* 2007;13:1150–7.

96. Nalca A, Rimoin AW, Bavari S, et al. Reemergence of monkeypox: Prevalence, diagnostics, and countermeasures. *Clin Infect Dis* 2005;41:1765–71.

97. Centers for Disease Control and Prevention. Updated interim CDC guidance for use of smallpox vaccine, cidofovir, and vaccinia immune globulin (VIG) for prevention and treatment in the setting of an outbreak of monkeypox infections, 2003; available at www.cdc.gov/ncidod/monkeypox/treatmentguidelines.htm.

98. Centers for Disease Control and Prevention. Compendium of measures to prevent disease associated with animals in public settings, 2007. *MMWR* 2007;56:1–13.

99. Beutner KR. Nongenital human papillomavirus infections. *Clin Lab Med* 2000;20:423–30.

100. Rudlinger R, Bunney MH, Grob R, et al. Warts in fish handlers. *Br J Dermatol* 1989;120:375–81.

101. Jablonska S, Obalek S, Golebiowska A. Epidemiology of butcher's warts. *Arch Dermatol Res* 1988;280:S24–28.

102. Stehr-Green PA, Hewer P, Meekin GE, et al. The aetiology and risk factors for warts among poultry processing workers. *Int J Epidemiol* 1993;22:294–8.

103. Keefe M, al-Ghambi A, Coggon D, et al. Cutaneous warts in butchers. *Br J Dermatol* 1994;130:9–14.

104. Keefe M, al-Ghambi A, Coggon D, et al. Butchers' warts: No evidence for person-to-person transmission of HPV7. *Br J Dermatol* 1994;130:15–7.

105. Lipke MM. An armamentarium of wart treatments. *Clin Med Res* 2006;4:273–93.

106. Bergbrandt IM, Samuelsson L, Olofsson S, et al. Polymerase chain reaction for monitoring human papillomavirus contamination of medical personnel during treatment of genital warts with CO_2 laser and electrocoagulation. *Acta Derm Venereol (Stockh)* 1994;74:393–5.

107. Gloster HM, Roenigk RK. Risk of acquiring human papillomavirus from the plume produced by the carbon dioxide laser in the treatment of warts. *J Am Acad Dermatol* 1995;32:436–41.

108. National Institute for Occupational Safety and Health (NIOSH). *Hazard Controls—Control of Smoke from Laser/Electric Surgical Procedures.* DHHS (NIOSH) Publication 96-128. Cincinnati: U.S. Department of Health and Human Services, 1996.

109. Sepkowitz KA. Occupationally acquired infections in health care workers. *Ann Intern Med* 1996;125:826–34.

110. Memar O, Tyring SK. Cutaneous viral infections. *J Am Acad Dermatol* 1995;33:279–87.

111. Johnston JM, Burke JP. Nosocomial outbreak of hand-foot-mouth disease among operating suite personnel. *Infect Control* 1986;7:172–6.

112. Harrison J, Jones CE. Human parvovirus B19 infection in healthcare workers. *Occup Med* 1995;45:93–6.

113. Gillespie SM, Cartter ML, Asch S, et al. Occupational risk of human parvovirus B19 infection for school and day-care personnel during an outbreak of erythema infectiosum. *JAMA* 1990;263:2061–5.

114. Atkinson WL, Markowitz LE, Adams NC, et al. Transmission of measles in medical settings. *Am J Med* 1991;91:320S–4.

115. Valeur-Jensen AK, Pedersen CB, Westergaard T, et al. Risk factors for parvovirus B19 infection in pregnancy. *JAMA* 1999;281:1099–105.

116. Chong CY, Chan KP, Shah VA, et al. Hand, foot and mouth disease in Singapore: A comparison of fatal and non-fatal cases. *Acta Paediatr* 2003;92:1163–9.

117. Young NS, Brown KE. Parvovirus B19. *N Engl J Med* 2004;350:586–97.

118. Wiss K. Erythema infectiosum and parvovirus B19 infection. In Freedberg IM, Eisen AZ, Wolff K, et al. (eds), *Fitzpatrick's Dermatology in General Medicine*, 6th ed. New York: McGraw-Hill, 2003, pp 2054–8.

119. Vander Straten MR, Tyring SK. Rubella. *Dermatol Clin* 2002;20:225–31.

120. Centers for Disease Control and Prevention. Prevention of varicella. *MMWR* 2007;561–40.

121. Weber DJ, Rutala WA, Hamilton H. Prevention and control of varicella-zoster infections in healthcare facilities. *Infect Control Hosp Epidemiol* 1996;17:694–705.

122. Arnow PM, Houchins SG, Pugliese G. An outbreak of tinea corporis in hospital personnel caused by a patient with *Trichophyton tonsurans* infection. *Pediatr Infect Dis J* 1991;10:355–9.

123. Krejci-Manwaring J, Schulz MR, Feldman SR, et al. Skin disease among Latino farmworkers in North Carolina. *J Agr Saf Health* 2006;12:155–63.

124. Philpot CM. The role of animals in the spread of fungal skin infections in humans. In Marks R,

Plewig G (eds), *The Environmental Threat to the Skin.* London: Martin Dunitz, 1992, pp 377–80.

125. Schwartz RA. Superficial fungal infections. *Lancet* 2004;364:1173–82.

126. Al-Doory Y. Chromomycosis. In Di Salvo AF (ed), *Occupational Mycoses.* Philadelphia: Lea & Febiger, 1983, pp 95–122.

127. Lopez Martinez R, Mendez Trovar LJ. Chromoblastomycosis. *Clin Dermatol* 2007;25:188–94.

128. Bonifaz A, Paredes-Solis V, Saul A. Treating chromoblastomycosis with systemic antifungals. *Exp Opin Pharmacother* 2004;5:247–54.

129. Hira K, Yamada H, Takahashi Y, et al. Successful treatment of chromomycosis using carbon dioxide laser associated with topical heat applications. *J Eur Acad Dermatol Venereol* 2002;16:273–5.

130. Ahmed AO, van Leeuwen W, Fahal A, et al. Mycetoma caused by *Madurella mycetomatis:* A neglected infectious burden. *Lancet Infect Dis* 2004;4:566–74.

131. Maiti PK, Ray A, Bandyopadhyay S. Epidemiological aspects of mycetoma from a retrospective study of 264 cases in West Bengal. *Trop Med Int Health* 2002; 7:788–92.

132. Fahal AH. Mycetoma: A thorn in the flesh. *Trans R Soc Trop Med Hyg* 2004;98:3–11.

133. Ahmed AA, van de Sande WW, Fahal A, et al. Management of mycetoma: Major challenge in tropical mycoses with limited international recognition. *Curr Opin Infect Dis* 2007;20:146–51.

134. Goodman NL. Sporotrichosis. In Di Salvo AF (ed), *Occupational Mycoses.* Philadelphia: Lea & Febiger, 1983, pp 65–78.

135. England T, Kasten MJ, Martin R, et al. Multistate outbreak of sporotrichosis in seedling handlers, 1988. *MMWR* 1988;37:652–3.

136. Welsh RD. Sporotrichosis. *J Am Vet Med Assoc* 2003;223:1123–6.

137. Bustamante B, Campos PE. Endemic sporotrichosis. *Curr Opin Infect Dis* 2001;14:145–9.

138. Kauffman CA, Bustamante B, Chapman SW, et al. Clinical practice guidelines for the management of sporotrichosis: 2007 update by the Infectious Diseases Society of America. *Clin Infect Dis* 2007;45: 1255–65.

139. Hajjeh R, McDonnell S, Reef S, et al. Outbreak of sporotrichosis among tree nursery workers. *J Infect Dis* 1997;176:499–504.

140. Lenaway DD, Bailey AM, Smith H, et al. Blastomy-cosis acquired occupationally during prairie dog re-location—Colorado, 1998. *MMWR* 1999;48:98–100.

141. Gray NA, Baddour LM. Cutaneous inoculation blastomycosis. *Clin Infect Dis* 2002;34:e44–9.

142. Kauffman CA. Endemic mycoses: Blastomycosis, histoplasmosis, and sporotrichosis. *Infect Dis Clin North Am* 2006;20:645–62.

143. Nithiuthai S, Anantaphruti MT, Waikagul J, et al. Water-borne zoonotic helminthiases. *Vet Parasitol* 2004;126:167–93.

144. Tomchik RS, Russell MT, Szmant AM, et al. Clinical perspectives on seabather's eruption, also known as sea lice. *JAMA* 1993;269:1669–72.

145. Centers for Disease Control and Prevention. Outbreak of cutaneous larva migrans at a children's camp—Miami, Florida, 2006. *MMWR* 2007;56: 1285–7.

146. Caumes E. Treatment of cutaneous larva migrans. *Clin Infect Dis* 2000;30:811–14.

147. Reithinger R, Dujardin JC, Louzir H, et al. Cutaneous leishmaniasis. *Lancet Infect Dis* 2007;7:581–96.

148. Centers for Disease Control and Prevention. Update: Cutaneous leishmaniasis in U.S. military personnel—Southwest/Central Asia, 2002–2004. *MMWR* 2004;53:264–5.

149. Murray HW, Berman JD, Davies CR, et al. Advances in leishmaniasis. *Lancet* 2005;366:1561–77.

150. Jimenez-Lucho VE, Fallon F, Caputo C, et al. Role of prolonged surveillance in the eradication of nosoco-mial scabies in an extended care Veterans Affairs Medical Center. *Am J Infect Control* 1995;23:44–9.

151. Noe R, Cohen SD, Lederman E, et al. Skin disorders among construction workers following Hurricane Katrina and Hurricane Rita: An outbreak investigation in New Orleans, Louisiana. *Arch Dermatol* 2007;143:1393–8.

152. Krinski WL. Dermatoses associated with the bites of mites and ticks. *Int J Dermatol* 1983;22:75–91.

153. Newman LS. Occupational illness. *N Engl J Med* 1995;333:1128–34.

154. Landrigan PJ, Baker DB. The recognition and control of occupational disease. *JAMA* 1991;266:676–80.

155. Rutstein DD, Mullan RJ, Frazier TM, et al. Sentinel health events (occupational): A basis for physician recognition and public health surveillance. *Am J Public Health* 1983;73:1054–62.

22 Occupational Slow Virus Infection

Jonathan S. Rutchik and John W. Kephart

Slow infection is a term used to describe a group of illnesses in animals and humans that result from a transmissible prion protein, PrP. Known as *transmissible spongiform encephalopathies* (TSEs) [1], this group includes scrapies in sheep, bovine spongiform encephalopathy (BSE) in cattle, and Creutzfeldt-Jakob disease (CJD), Gerstmann-Straussler-Shenker syndrome (GSS), fatal familial insomnia (FFI), and atypical prion disease in humans. Prusiner and colleagues have demonstrated that PrP is a slowly infectious proteinaceous particle that is devoid of nucleic acid, resists the action of enzymes that destroy RNA and DNA, and has a structure that is unlike a virus [2]. The term *spongiform* refers to the classic neuropathologic changes found in the cerebral and cerebellar cortices at autopsy.

CJD is the most important of the TSEs in humans; GSS, FFI, and atypical prion disease are inheritable and extremely rare. CJD is a fatal dementing neurodegenerative illness that presents most commonly in late middle age. Neurologic and psychological symptoms are common, but clinical findings vary substantially.

Progressive dementia and myoclonus are the most constant clinical signs. When symptoms develop, however, death ensues within 1 year. CJD is predominantly sporadic, but prion disease has both infective and genetic properties. By injecting brain tissue from patients with this disorder, researchers have demonstrated that the agent responsible is transmissible from humans to primates [3]. CJD does not appear to be spontaneously contagious, but iatrogenic transmission has been reported in many instances [2]. Incubation periods for these cases have varied from months to decades [4]. Corneal transplantation, implantation of cerebral depth encephalography electrodes, implantation of dura mater grafts, and human growth hormone therapy [5] have been suggested as modes of transmission.

Occupations in which contact with human or animal neural tissues is common pose risk for exposure. These include histopathologists, laboratory technicians, veterinarian neuroscientists, pathologists, anatomists, neurosurgeons, and other surgeons, as well as morticians and others in health-related professions. Since CJD has been reported in animal handlers who may have been exposed to neural tissues, butchers and farmers also may have increased risk for exposure [6, 7]. Proper preparations, precautions, and handling techniques are discussed below.

In 1996, a new variant of CJD (vCJD) was first described in the United Kingdom. Discovered in younger patients (mean age 29 years), predominantly in the United Kingdom, vCJD has now spread to 10 other countries but is still found predominantly in the United Kingdom. This vCJD has been characterized by a specific pathologic profile as well as by the pathognomic spongiform changes found on histologic examination of the brain in patients with CJD [8]. Approximately 10 years prior to this, the United Kingdom experienced an epizootic BSE [9] thought to be secondary to exposure of calves to contaminated rendered cattle carcasses in the form of meat and bone-meal nutritional supplements. This has raised concerns over whether transmission from animal to humans may occur by means other than contact with neural tissues [10]. Subsequently, a U.K. government expert panel announced that the agent responsible for BSE might have spread to humans, based on the recognition of 10 persons with vCJD [11]. Since that time, several countries have established surveillance units to monitor new and suspected cases of vCJD. As of July 2006, there have been 192 confirmed cases of vCJD reported worldwide: United Kingdom—160; France—18; Ireland—4; Italy—1; United States—2; Canada—1; Saudi Arabia—1; Japan—1; the Netherlands—2; Spain—1; and Portugal—1. At least one case in the United States and cases in Canada and Japan and one person in Ireland had all lived in the United Kingdom at some point between the years 1980 and 1996; therefore, these cases are likely to be considered as U.K. infections [13]. In the United Kingdom, the National Creutzfeldt-Jakob Disease Surveillance Unit has reported three deaths from vCJD as of June 2006 [12].

Early research showed there to be no clear evidence supporting transmission by blood or bodily fluids or tissues from outside the central nervous system. Recently, however, there have been reports of two cases of probable iatrogenic vCJD transmission through blood transfusion. The first case was a 69-year-old man who presented with clinical symptoms typical of vCJD in late 2002. In 1996, the patient underwent surgery and was transfused with 5 units of nonleukodepleted packed red blood cells. One of the units was donated by an asymptomatic 24-year-old individual who developed vCJD symptoms approximately 3.5 years later and subsequently died in 2000 of pathologically confirmed vCJD. In late 2002, 6.5 years postoperatively, the patient began developing symptoms indicative of vCJD. The patient's condition deteriorated rapidly. The patient showed myoclonic jerks of the limbs and died 1 year after the onset of symptoms. On investigation, prion-protein typing confirmed deposition in the brain of type 2B prion protein, which is pathognomic of vCJD [14].

The second case was reported by Peden and colleagues [15] of the National Creutzfeldt-Jakob Disease Unit in the United Kingdom. The patient was an elderly woman who was a known recipient of a blood transfusion from an asymptomatic donor who subsequently developed vCJD. The patient, however, died from a nonneurologic disorder approximately 5 years after receiving the transfusion. On autopsy, protease-resistant prion protein (PrP^{res}) was detected by Western blot, paraffin-embedded tissue blot, and immunohistochemistry in the spleen but not the brain. The presence of PrP^{res} in the spleen is similar to that seen in the spleens of patients with clinical vCJD.

U.K. epidemiologists in one study have reported an increased incidence of CJD in dairy farmers in the United Kingdom and other countries. These authors underscore that mouse transmission studies presently underway will help to reveal whether the causative agent for BSE has infected humans [11].

As a result of these cases, the U.S. Food and Drug Administration (FDA), in January 2002, published guidance outlining a geography-based blood donor deferral policy to reduce the risk of bloodborne transmission of vCJD in the United States [16]. These cases highlight the importance of effective screening tools and protocols, as well as further highlighting the need to make certain whether all vCJD/BSE infections result in clinical disease or a subclinical carrier state may occur.

Incidence and Prevalence

The annual incidence of CJD has been reported to be 1–2 cases per 1 million population [2]. The incidence is higher in Israelis of Libyan descent, North African immigrants to France, and Slovakians. A small proportion (5–15%) of cases are familial, suggesting that some genetic susceptibility exists [17]. The high frequency in Libyan Jews is now known to be due to a codon 200 mutation in the PrP gene in affected families [18]. The Centers for Disease Control and Prevention (CDC) reported in 2005 that during 1979–1994, the annual death rate of CJD (not vCJD) had remained relatively stable at approximately 1 case per 1 million population [19]. The number of deaths attributed to CJD among those under 45 years of age ranged from 0 in 1984 to 8 in 1981 and 1993 [9]. However, risk of CJD does increase with age, and in persons over 50 years old, the annual rate is approximately 3.4 cases per 1 million population. In the United States, noniatrogenic CJD deaths (not vCJD) in persons under 30 years of age remain extremely rare (<1 case per 100 million per year). In contrast, in the United Kingdom, more than half of patients who died with vCJD were in this younger age group [19]. In 2004, however, the number of sporadic CJD deaths was lower than in the preceding three years. Furthermore, analysis of the incidence of vCJD onsets and deaths from January 1994 to December 2004 indicates that a peak has passed [20].

A statistically significant excess of cases among dairy farmers and their spouses and among people at increased risk of contact with live cattle infected with BSE was noted between 1970 and 1996 in a study performed in the United Kingdom [11]. This high incidence, however, was comparable with that observed in dairy farmers in countries where BSE is rare or nonexistent. The authors speculated that individuals in this occupation in countries where they collected data may be at increased risk of CJD for reasons other than exposure to the causative agent of the bovine disease. They also remarked, however, that the absolute risk was noted to be extremely low—well below 10 cases per million.

Transmission and Occupational Risk Factors

A European collaborative study group assessed occupational and historical risk factors retrospectively for 405 patients with definite or probable CJD between 1993 and 1995 in Belgium, France, Germany, Italy, the Netherlands, and the United Kingdom. They reported no increased risk in relation to a history of surgery or blood transfusion or an association between CJD and specific animal-source food consumption (not with beef, veal, lamb, cheese, or milk). No association was noted between CJD and occupational exposure to animals or leather. Positive findings were as follows: ingestion of raw meat [relative risk (RR) = 1.63, confidence interval (CI) = 1.18–2.23], ingestion of brain (RR = 1.68, CI = 1.18–2.39), frequent exposure to leather products (RR = 1.94, CI = 1.13–3.33), and exposure to fertilizer consisting of hoofs and horns (RR = 2.32, = CI 1.38–2.91). Also, the study found evidence of familial aggregation of

CJD with dementia owing to causes other than CJD [10].

CJD has been reported in 6 physicians and 24 health care workers, many of them with documented exposure to animal or human brain tissue [4]. A 61-year-old dairy farmer presented with atypical dementia and died 3 months after hospital admission. Postmortem neuropathologic examination identified spongiform changes typical of CJD. This patient had a documented case of BSE in his herd of cattle (the animal had been potentially exposed to contaminated feed before July 1988) but had no contact with the cow's internal organs or tissues. He had, however, drunk pooled milk from the herd. The authors suggested continued surveillance of specific occupational groups because of the risk of direct inoculation from bovine tissue, but they remarked that this was likely a chance finding and that a causal link was conjectural [6]. A 59-year-old cattle farmer was diagnosed with CJD. He also had a single case of BSE in the cattle on his farm in 1991. Sheep also were on the farm, but none were known to have scrapie. The farmer had been involved in calving and had assisted the veterinarian with cesarean sectioning. It was not known if he assisted with the BSE-infected cow, but he had otherwise not been involved in any other procedure with the animal. He had not had contact with meat or bone meal and denied ever tasting animal feed. He also denied drinking unpasteurized milk since before 1972. In this case, the clinical presentation and pathologic confirmation were consistent with the sporadic form of CJD, not with the new variant [7]. Other authors reiterated that two large epidemiologic surveys—one a French 15-year investigation [21] and the other a British case-control study conducted between 1980 and 1984 [22]—failed to find a link between occupation and CJD [23].

A 62-year-old woman had been employed in a neuropathology laboratory for 22 years. Her duties included rinsing formalin-fixed brains and processing, cutting, and staining sections of brain without participating in actual brain cutting. She became ill and died 1 year later. Autopsy confirmed a neuropathologic diagnosis of CJD [24]. Review of department log books revealed that she had worked on brain specimens of two persons who had been diagnosed with CJD. These cases were seen 16 and

11 years prior to the onset of her symptoms. The neuropathologist who worked on those brains remains healthy and active. The author of this case study acknowledged the occupational risks of the neuropathology profession but suspected a chance occurrence. A 75-year-old histologist developed CJD [25]. This was demonstrated and confirmed pathologically. Questioning of the patient's family revealed that he had worked with animal and human brains before 1969: In 1963 and 1964, he had performed sheep dissections. This author considered the occupational exposure a possible causative factor in the patient's illness.

The first pathologist diagnosed with CJD was reported in 1992. Records were not available to elucidate whether he had performed or assisted with any autopsies for which CJD was the diagnosis. The authors of this case study emphasized care and precautions in handling potential contaminated material at autopsy, especially for cadavers of patients with dementia of unknown or cytogenic origin [26].

A review article included a case report of an internist who had received 12 months of training in pathology in 1959 and died of CJD [27]. The patient's father had had Alzheimer's disease. The author of the article mentioned that it is unlikely that clinical illness invariably follows exposure to the infectious agent because there is a potentially high rate of exposure and only a small number of health care workers who have been reported to have had CJD. A genetic susceptibility may be required, however.

Prevention and Control

The pathogen responsible for CJD withstands many customary sterilization methods, including heat, formaldehyde, and ultraviolet radiation, which typically eradicate viral and bacterial pathogens [28]. Since many neurologic and psychological symptoms may herald CJD's clinical onset, pathologists and laboratory staff must exercise extreme caution when handling cadavers with unclear neurologic or psychiatric diagnoses.

It is possible to transmit CJD to nonhuman primates and small laboratory animals by intercerebral, subcutaneous, intraperitoneal, intramuscular, and intravenous inoculation and by ocular transplantation. Subcutaneous and intramuscular routes

of inoculation are said to be less efficient methods of inoculation than the intracerebral route in producing disease. Also, other tissues with a lower titer of infectivity are still transmissible, including liver, lung, lymph node, kidney, and leukocytes. Blood has been infectious in both human [29] and experimental CJD; urine also has been found to be infectious in humans. Saliva, external secretions, and stool have not been found to contain the pathogen. Conjugal cases, which have been reported, indicate a common source of infection rather than cross-contamination.

Many methods of disinfection have been tested [30]. Ineffective procedures include boiling, ultraviolet irradiation, ethylene oxide sterilization, ethanol, formalin, beta-propiolactone, detergents, quaternary ammonium compounds, Lysol, alcoholic iodine, acetone, and potassium permanganate. Formaldehyde, diluted to 10%, also has been shown to be ineffective. A 1.0 meq/L solution of sodium hydroxide bathed for 60 minutes and then steamed at 121°C for 30 minutes has proved effective in at least two studies [31, 32]. Steam autoclaving for 1 hour at 132°C is the other fully effective, recommended procedure. A more recent study instructs that instruments should be disposable or decontaminated by soaking in 1 N sodium hydroxide (40 g/L) or in undiluted sodium hypochlorite for 1 hour and then submitted to autoclaving at 134°C for 1 hour [33]. The study further describes that tissues should be blocked thinly for histologic analysis and soaked in concentrated formic acid for 1 hour and then in 4% formaldehyde solution for at least 48 hours. It is noteworthy that formalin-fixed tissues embedded in paraffin stored at room temperature may be infectious for years and thus always should be handled with caution.

The above-described disinfection procedures must be used for venipuncture needles, forceps, scissors, lumbar puncture needles, and any other instruments used on a patient with probable CJD. Discarded clothing worn during these procedures also should be collected and autoclaved. Specimens submitted to laboratories should be clearly marked as coming from patients with definite or suspected CJD. Disposable gloves should be worn, and skin contact with any possible infectious material should be followed by washing the skin with 1 N sodium hydroxide for several minutes. Universal precautions, including use of gown, glasses, masks, and gloves, should be used by those performing autopsy or necropsy on tissues possibly contaminated with PrP. The autopsy and brain-cutting work areas should be restricted to only those necessary to perform the work. Also, a manual saw should be used for cutting of the skull, taking care not to cut into the brain or spinal cord tissue. If an electric saw is used, a towel should cover it to reduce aerosolization. The autopsy drain should be closed and the water collected and decontaminated. The cadaver should be washed with 1 N of sodium hydroxide, the wash water sterilized, and appropriate precautions communicated to the mortician. Organs and trimmed tissues need to be meticulously collected and completely incinerated [30, 34].

If accidental puncture occurs, the wound should be cleaned with iodine (Betadine), phenolic antiseptic (hexachlorophene or 5% Lysol), or 0.5% sodium hypochlorite (Dakin's fluid or household bleach) or should be swabbed with a 1:3,000 solution of potassium permanganate [34].

Clearly, patients with CJD must not be blood or organ transplant donors or sources of human tissue for preparation of biologic products to be used in humans, such as dura mater, pituitary hormones, and human interferon.

Symptoms and Signs

Eighty percent of sporadic cases of TSE are diagnosed in persons between 50 and 70 years of age. TSE may be sporadic, infectious, or familial and has been reported recently in young adults. Both genders are equally affected. One third of a large series of patients had prodromal symptoms of fatigue, depression, weight loss, and disorders of sleep and appetite that lasted several weeks. Another third initially had neurologic symptoms such as memory loss, confusion, or uncharacteristic behavior, and one third initially had focal signs such as ataxia, aphasia, visual loss, hemiparesis, or amyotrophy. Early aspects of the disease vary greatly, but changes in behavior, emotional response, and intellectual function, together with abnormalities of cerebellar and visual function, are most common. Early symptoms may confuse the diagnostician. Progression, however, is rapid, and myoclonic contractions appear in all patients; this is associated

with a striking startle response. Ataxia and dysarthria also become prominent. Stupor and coma usually follow, and myoclonus often continues until death. Akinetic mutism is also common in the late stages of the disease [1, 35].

The electroencephalographic picture is often characterized by diffuse and nonspecific slowing accompanied occasionally by stereotypical high-voltage slow (1–2 Hz) and sharp-wave complexes on an increasingly slow and low-voltage background. The high-voltage sharp waves are synchronous with the myoclonus but may persist in its absence. Electroencephalogram (EEG) reveals this characteristic pattern in 60–90% of patients depending on the disease phase and the number of EEGs performed [36].

Blood and cerebrospinal fluid (CSF) are often normal. Specific diagnostic protein markers of the CSF, such as neuron-specific enolase, have been shown to be good diagnostic tools. CSF levels above 35 ng/mL were noted to be 80% sensitive and 92% specific for CJD [37]. Blood measurement of PrP, in conjunction with a clinical diagnosis, confirms the diagnosis of CJD owing to heritable causes.

The classic constellation of neuropathologic changes in CJD consists of spongiform degeneration, neuronal loss, and astrocytic gliosis. Only spongiform degeneration is specific for CJD, however. The disease usually affects the cerebral and cerebellar cortices diffusely. In some cases, occipitoparietal regions are involved almost exclusively; in others, the cerebellum is most seriously affected. Light microscopy of pathologic specimens typically leads to a definitive diagnosis. Immunohistochemistry using antibodies against the prion protein is preferable in all suspected cases of CJD and is mandatory whenever a routine histologic workup does not yield definitive results [36].

A description of features of vCJD was derived from a series of 10 patients in Great Britain. The mean age of onset was 29, and the median duration of illness was 14 months. All patients presented with early psychiatric symptoms, most often depression. Eight developed early sensory symptoms, which were persistent and painful. All patients developed ataxia and involuntary movements, and by the end, most had akinetic mutism. EEGs were abnormal in most, but none had characteristic features. Findings of cerebral imaging were normal [38]. Recently, PrP was found to be present in the biopsied tonsillary tissue of 20 patients with this clinical and pathologic variant of CJD; patients with the sporadic form of CJD were negative for tonsillary PrP. In late stages of vCJD, this biopsy technique may prove sensitive and specific [39].

Differential Diagnosis

Lithium intoxication, metabolic encephalopathies, carcinomatous meningitis, viral encephalitides, and diffuse central demyelinating disease, a type of multiple sclerosis called *Schilder's disease,* may mimic the presentation of TSE in the early aspects of the illness. Diffuse Lewy body disease and atypical Alzheimer's disease also may present with early mental changes and also may progress to myoclonus. Subacute sclerosing panencephalitis may resemble TSE but is seen mainly in children or young adults. Limbic encephalitis and acquired immune-deficiency syndrome (AIDS) dementia are also on the differential diagnostic list. Myoclonus and dementia may be present in cerebral lipidoses in children and young adults but are chronic and include retinal changes, which do not occur in TSE [1].

Because of the recent case reports of TSE in patients under age 45, a high index of suspicion is warranted for progressive atypical dementia in younger age groups.

Diagnostic Evaluation, Treatment, and Rehabilitation

Diagnostic evaluation for TSE includes a complete neurologic examination. Special attention should be given to assessment of mental status and visual and cerebellar function. Electroencephalography is suggested. MRI may not be helpful. Neuron-specific enolase may be useful if obtained from the CSF. Brain biopsy is diagnostic; the specimen should be taken from an area of the brain whose function reflects the prominent clinical features of the patient.

Because of the disease's rapidly progressive nature, no treatment or rehabilitation is possible. Recent studies, however, have shown substantial progress by demonstrating principal reversibility of the neuropathologic features and protection from clinical symptoms in animal models. In one study, possibly the only double-blind, placebo-controlled clinical trial for CJD treatment, researchers used flupirtine in treating CJD patients. The researchers believed that the *N*-methyl-D-aspartate antagonist properties of flupirtine might limit subsequent glutamate-induced neurotoxicity in progressing CJD [40]. They found that this treatment produced mild positive effects on cognitive function; however, no prolongation in survival time was observed in this study.

Gayrard and colleagues [41] discovered that the antiparasitic drug quinacrine is a very affective antiprion compound. Quinacrine, an acridine derivative, was reported to have marked in vitro antiprion action in mouse neuroblastoma cells. Because quinacrine was an already approved drug, it was administered to CJD patients on compassionate grounds despite the absence of preclinical in vivo studies to evaluate its efficacy. Some quinacrine-treated patients showed a transient improvement of arousal and akinetic symptoms; however, results from this investigation failed to show therapeutic benefits.

The rarity of patients has been a major problem for evaluating the therapeutic potential of lead compounds in CJD pharmacotherapy. Clinical trials, however, are underway at the Memory and Aging Clinic at the University of California, San Francisco, at the National Prion Clinic at the National Hospital for Neurology and Neurosurgery in London, and at the University of Ulm in Ulm, Germany [40].

References

1. Viral infections of the nervous system. In Adams RD, Victor M, Ropper AH (eds), *Principals of Neurology,* 6th ed. New York: McGraw Hill, 1997, Chap 33.
2. Prusiner SB. Genetic and infectious prion disease. *Arch Neurol* 1993;50:1129.
3. Gibbs CJ, Gadjusek DC, Asher OM. CJD (spongiform encephalopathy): Transmission to the chimpanzee. *Science* 1968;161:388–9.
4. Brown P. Iatrogenic CJD. *Aust NZ J Med* 1990;20: 633–4.
5. Billette de Villemeur T, Deslys JP, Pradel A, et al. CJD from contaminated growth hormone extracts in France. *Neurology* 1996;47:690–5.
6. Sawcer SJ, Yuill GM, Esmonde TF. CJD in an individual occupational exposed to BSE. *Lancet* 1993; 341:642.
7. Young GR, Fletcher NA, Zeidler M, et al. CJD in a beef farmer. *Lancet* 1996;348:610–11.
8. Will RG, Ironside JW, Zeidler M. A new variant of CJD in the UK. *Lancet* 1996;347:921–5.

9. Surveillance for CJD—United States. *MMWR* 1996; 45:665–8.
10. Van Duijn CM, Delasnerie-Laupretre N, Masulla C, et al. Case-control study of risk factors of CJD in Europe during 1993–1995. *Lancet* 1998;351:1081–5.
11. Cousens SN, Zeidler M, Esmende TF, et al. Sporadic CJD in the United Kingdom: Analysis of epidemiological surveillance data for 1970–1996. *Br Med J* 1997;315:389–96.
12. The National Creutzfeldt-Jakob Disease Surveillance Unit. Available at www.cjd.ed.ac.uk.
13. Belay ED, Sejvar JJ, Shieh W-J, et al. Variant Creutzfeldt-Jakob disease death, United States. *Emerg Infect Dis* 2005;11:1351–4.
14. Llewelyn CA, Hewitt PE, Knight RSG, et al. Possible transmission of variant Creutzfeldt-Jakob disease by blood transfusion. *Lancet* 2004;363:417–21.
15. Peden AH, Head MW, Ritchie DL, et al. Preclinical vCJD after blood transfusion in a PRNP codon 29 heterozygous patient. *Lancet* 2004;364:477–9.
16. Centers for Disease Control and Prevention. *Health Information for International Travel, 2005–2006.* Atlanta: US Department of Health and Human Services, Public Health Service, 2005, Chap 4.
17. Masters CL, Harris JO, Gadjusek DC, et al. CJD: Patterns of worldwide occurrence and the significance of familial and sporadic clustering. *Ann Neurol* 1979; 5:177.
18. Hsiao K, Meiner Z, Kahana E. Mutation of the prion protein in Libyan Jews with CJD. *N Engl J Med* 1991;324:1091–7.
19. Centers for Disease Control and Prevention. CJD (Cruetzfeld-Jakobs Disease, Classic). Atlanta: CDC, June 2005. Available at www.cdc.gov/ncidod/dvrd/cjd/index.htm.
20. The National CJD Surveillance Unit. *Thirteenth Annual Report 2004, Creutzfeldt-Jakob Disease Surveillance in the UK.* Edinburgh: Western General Hospital, 2004.
21. Brown P, Cathala F, Raubertas RF, et al. The epidemiology of CJD: Conclusions of a 15-year investigation in France and a review of the world literature. *Neurology* 1987;37:895–904.
22. Harries-Jones R, Knight R, Will RG. CJD in England and Wales, 1980–1984: A case-control study of potential risk factors. *J Neurol Neurosurg Psychiatry* 1988;51:1113–9.
23. Ridley RM, Baker RF. Occupational risk of CJD. *Lancet* 1993;341:641.
24. Miller DC. CJD in histopathology technicians. *N Engl J Med* 1988;318:853–4.
25. Sitwell L, Lach B, Atack E, et al. CJD disease in histopathology technician. *Neurology* 1988;318:854.
26. Gorman DG, Benson F, Vogel DG, et al. CJD in a pathologist. *Neurology* 1992;42:463.

27. Berger JR, David NJ. CJD in a physician: A review of the disorder in health care workers. *Neurology* 1993; 43:205–6.
28. Steelman VM. Creutzfeldt-Jakob disease: Recommendation for infection control. *Am J Infect Control* 1994;22:312–8.
29. Patry D, Curry B, Easton D, et al. CJD after blood product transfusion from a donor with CJD. *Neurology* 1998;50:1872–3.
30. Brown P, Gibbs CJ, Amyx HL, et al. Chemical disinfection of Creutzfeldt-Jakob disease virus. *N Engl J Med* 1982;306:1279–82.
31. Taguchi F, Tamai T, Uchida K. Proposal for a procedure for complete inactivation of the CJD agent. *Arch Virol* 1991;119:297–301.
32. Committee on Health Care Issues, American Neurological Association. Precautions in handling tissues, fluids and other contaminated materials from patients with documented or suspected CJD. *Neurology* 1986;19:75–7.
33. Budka H, Aguzzi A, Brown P, et al. Tissue handling in suspected CJD and other human spongiform encephalopathies (prion disease). *Brain Pathol* 1995; 5:319–22.
34. Gadjusek DC, Gibbs CJ, Asher DM, et al. Precautions of medical care of and in handling materials from patients with transmissible virus dementia (CJD). *N Engl J Med* 1977;297:1253–8.
35. Johnson RT, Gibbs CJ. Medical progress: CJD and related transmissible spongiform encephalopathies. *N Engl J Med* 1998;339:1994–2004.
36. Kreztschmar HA, Ironside JW, DeArmond SJ, et al. Diagnostic criteria for sporadic CJD. *Arch Neurol* 1996;53:913–20.
37. Zerr I, Bodemer M, Recker S. Cerebrospinal fluid concentration of neuron specific enolase in diagnosis of CJD. *Lancet* 1995;345:1609.
38. Zeidler M, Stewart GE, Barraclagh CR, et al. New variant CJD: Neurological features and diagnostic tests. *Lancet* 1997;350:903–7.
39. Hill AF, Butterworth RJ, Joiner S, et al. Investigation of variant Creutzfeldt-Jakob disease and other human prion diseases with tonsil biopsy sample. *Lancet* 1999;353:183–9.
40. Korth C, Peters PJ. Emerging pharmacotherapies for Creutzfeldt-Jakob disease. *Arch Neurol* 2006;63: 497–501.
41. Garard V, Picard-Hagen N, Viguie C, et al. A possible pharmacological explanation for quinacrine failure to treat prion disease: Pharmacokinetic investigations in an ovine model of scrapie. *Br J Pharmacol* 2005;144:386–93.

23 Occupational Meningitis

William E. Wright and Alain J. Couturier

This chapter is not meant to be a guide to current diagnosis and treatment. Owing to the shifting patterns of disease, emergence of new pathogens, and rapid evolution of resistant or multidrug-resistant organisms, current diagnostic and treatment information should be sought and used in consideration of local patterns of disease and antibiotic resistance. Many presentations of meningitis and meningoencephalitis are difficult to diagnose with certainty at first, and emergency use of empirical antibiotic therapy, the choice depending on local endemic and epidemic situations and special circumstances, is often essential. Decisions about whether to use corticosteroids need to be made. The reader should refer to current recommendations of the local infectious disease experts, treatment guidelines from the Infectious Disease Society of America (www.idsa.org) [1] or similar practice guidelines and other reputable sources [2, 3]. This chapter contains information on general types of meningitis and encephalitis, specific occupational concerns and emerging occupational issues, and resources for addressing concerns in the workplace.

A Common Occupational Medicine Dilemma

Meningitis in the practice of occupational medicine can become an issue of concern in different ways. One of the common ways that concerns arise is contact of the occupational physician by a business organization's manager or employee expressing concern that a case of meningitis has been reported as having occurred in a coworker. Depending on the business organization, a level of panic and disruption of work can ensue as word spreads that there is meningitis occurring at the workplace. This is a valid concern because meningitis can occur in epidemic form as well as in sporadic form, meningitis is a feared disease, some forms have been correctly publicized as being acute and deadly, and workplaces can involve crowding of people (including in living quarters), which increases the risk for spread of infectious illnesses. The occupational physician needs to be prepared to address the concerns quickly and efficiently using an orderly approach that is visible to the organization and protects medical confidentiality. The main concern is that a virulent person-to-person transmissible form of meningitis (e.g., *Neisseria meningitidis* meningitis) has occurred as a sentinel event or as part of a community- or organization-based outbreak in a limited population setting that would necessitate consideration of administration of chemoprophylaxis or vaccination of previously unvaccinated populations at increased risk for meningococcal disease [4, 5].

The potential that meningitis issues may arise this way is good reason for the occupational physician to have already established links with the local public health department and local hospital infection control professionals and to be aware of local, state, and regional disease occurrence and emerging infections. Knowledge of these data, particularly related to any reportable cases or outbreaks of meningitis that are community- or organization-based, will help the occupational health practitioner address concerns about meningitis and other potentially contagious illnesses that arise. The U.S. Centers for Disease Control and Prevention (CDC) defines an outbreak as organization-based if it involves the occurrence of three or more confirmed or probable cases of meningococcal disease of the same serogroup in 3 months or less among persons who have a common affiliation but no close contact with each other, resulting in a primary disease attack rate of 10 or more cases per 100,000 persons [5].

The steps to address these issues should be based on the occupational health organization's written policies and procedures related to preventive services and emergency preparedness, which includes approaches to risk assessment in various situations. The operating procedures may be part of a broader emergency preparedness and response plan. The plan may include alert thresholds, action thresholds, and/or epidemic thresholds. In the occupational medicine setting, the approaches used need to be respectful of medical confidentiality, must be applied equally to like-type situations, and when addressing or touching on return to work, fitness for work, or infectious disease risks at work, must be aligned with the Americans with Disabilities Act and concepts of imminent harm, which are covered in Chapter 6. A number of organizations have developed and published plans that address high-level community-based or occupational preparedness and response, the impetus for some being the specter of bioterrorism, and some plans specifically target meningitis [6–10].

For the worksite meningitis example raised earlier, which can occur relatively commonly, the first action is to gather information related to the reported case from the person who raises the concern. Often the information is vague and incomplete but usually it will include the identity of the suspected index patient. Organizational resources should be able to confirm whether the individual is at work or absent. Contact needs to be made with the individual and/or family members to determine whether the report is rumor or fact. Cooperation is facilitated by sympathetically explaining the reason for the inquiry and that concern is not related to the individual's illness per se, because that is his or her personal information, but rather is related to whether there is a risk to public health from a contagious disease. One can inquire whether the treating health care provider has advised about risk to others or public health risk and how the treating provider can be contacted to help address the public health concern. A similar approach can be taken with the health care provider, who has a duty to advise about risks to public health. Depending on the answer, the occupational physician may need to coordinate an approach with the local or state health department. Feedback to the business organization's designee for these issues should involve advice about whether any public health risk has been identified and whether a business organization-based approach is needed for follow-up or prevention.

There are variations on this approach depending on the business organization, its size and location, and the occupational physician's relationship with the employer. If the index individual is unwilling to help clarify the situation or unavailable, the occupational physician can query the local health department about reportable cases and patterns of meningitis and whether its surveillance efforts include workplace organization-based concerns or patterns. A role of the occupational physician is to communicate information on public health risk and risk management simply and clearly to the people who need to know this in ways that will result in logical, focused approaches that will help to prevent panic and dysfunctional approaches, and prevent disease.

Meningitis and Encephalitis

There are many microorganisms that can result in meningitis, which is a syndrome of inflammation of the subarachnoid fluid and membranes covering the brain and spinal cord usually owing to infection. Meningitis can occur with or without inflammation of the brain (encephalitis), which usually also has an infectious cause. In adults, meningitis most commonly presents with fairly abrupt onset of fever, severe headaches, photophobia, and neck and/or back stiffness. Nausea, vomiting, drowsiness, and confusion may occur. Sometime pharyngitis may be present. Cranial nerve palsies, other focal neurologic signs, and local or generalized seizures may occur. These same symptoms may occur with encephalitis, although stiff neck and back are less common in pure encephalitis, and irritability, poor control of temper, inflexibility, memory loss, impaired judgment, indecisiveness, withdrawal, speech problems, confusion, disorientation, drowsiness, abnormal reflexes, clumsiness, gait disturbances, and seizures tend to be more common. A mixed clinical picture can occur that may be termed *meningoencephalitis*. When this range of presentations of illness is considered, the potential causes are numerous. Both meningitis and encephalitis can have either bacterial or viral causes, which are the most common causes in the United States. Other types of organisms can result in meningoencephalitis, and some noninfectious materials (e.g., drugs) and diseases can present clinically with features of meninoencephalitis.

Meningitis is sometimes thought of as either aseptic meningitis (usually viral) or bacterial meningitis. This distinction is blurred because a number of bacterial pathogens can cause a clinical picture of aseptic meningitis, and the initial clinical presentation of aseptic meningitis, viral meningitis, and bacterial meningitis sometimes can be indistinguishable. Based on cerebrospinal fluid (CSF) analyses, five factors have been found to predict bacterial infection with high certainty: (1) glucose concentration of less than 34 mg/dL, (2) CSF:blood glucose ratio of less than 0.23, (3) protein concentration of more than 2.2 g/L, (4) white blood cell count of more than 2000/mm^3, and (5) neutrophils more than 1180/mm^3 [11]. None of these factors can rule out bacterial meningitis with absolute certainty [12].

ASEPTIC MENINGITIS

The term *aseptic meningitis* is sometimes loosely used to denote viral meningitis, but aseptic meningitis is a syndrome that can result from infection with viral, bacterial, or other pathogens and noninfectious conditions. The CDC defines aseptic meningitis as a syndrome of acute onset of meningeal symptoms, fever, and CSF pleocytosis with absence of bacteria and fungi on standard microbiologic stains and cultures [13].

In addition to viral causes, acute aseptic meningitis syndromes have been reported in infections with *Leptospira*, *Borrelia burgdorferi*, other *Borrelia* species, *Mycoplasma*, *Nocardia*, *Mycobacterium tuberculosis*, *Treponema pallidum*, *Brucella* species, *Actinomycetes*, various fungi and parasites, and *Chlamydia* and *Rickettsia* [14]. An occupational case of concurrent infection with *B. burgdorferi* and *Ehrlichia* in a logger with reticulate erythematous rash on the upper torso, fever, thrombocytopenia, and meningoencephalitis has been reported [15]. Many of the pathogens listed in this paragraph are covered in pathogen-specific chapters of this book, travel-related chapters, or others.

The aseptic meningitis syndrome also can result from partially treated bacterial meningitis, a parameningeal focus of infection, viral postinfectious syndromes, some medications, postvaccination syndromes, intracranial tumors, brain abscess, carcinomatous meningitis, leukemia, and systemic illnesses, particularly granulomatous diseases, connective tissue diseases, and vasculitides [14].

Some industrial materials can result in symptoms and signs, some of which are shared with acute aseptic meningitis syndromes. These include poisoning with lead, mercury, bismuth, aluminum, some organic and halogenated organic solvents, and some insecticides [16]. A recent case report introduced zinc oxide–related metal fume fever as a consideration for differential diagnosis of aseptic meningitis [17].

VIRAL MENINGITIS

The most common cause of meningitis in the United States is viral, which frequently produces a syndrome of aseptic meningitis. The incidence of aseptic meningitis is uncertain owing to underreporting, lack of recognition, or lack of hospitalization of many patients. One survey estimated that aseptic meningitis affects at least 300,000 people in the United States annually [18]. A study of hospitalizations for viral meningitis in the United States estimated an annual average of 36,000 admissions per year, a rate of 14 hospitalizations per 100,000 population per year, at an estimated annual hospitalization cost of up to $310 million per year [19].

About 90% of viral meningitis in the United States is caused by enteroviruses, the main types being coxsackieviruses and echoviruses. Many people who become infected with these viruses may have no symptoms or have symptoms of a cold or flu with fever and/or a rash or mild intestinal illness. The enteroviruses can be transmitted by direct contact with saliva, respiratory secretions, or stool, which can occur through hand-to-hand contact, droplets, or fomites. Incubation periods are typically from 3 days to a week, and the ability to spread the virus usually starts 3 days after infection to about 10 days after developing symptoms. Control and prevention require good hand hygiene, not sharing eating utensils and beverage containers, avoidance of direct and airborne contact with respiratory secretions, and decontamination of surfaces and objects with soap and water or weak bleach solution. Viral meningitis, particularly cases related to enteroviruses, is primarily a disease of the summer months and autumn in the United States. Echovirus has been implicated in meningitis related to use of a swimming pool [20].

Other non-arthropod vector-related causes of viral meningitis include Ebstein-Barr virus (EBV), mumps, measles, rubella, some adenoviruses, varicella-zoster virus (VZV), and poliovirus. Pathogens also include lymphocytic choriomeningitis virus (primarily in North America, South America, and Europe) caused by an arenavirus transmitted by a reservoir of house mice, *Mus musculus,* through handling them, their excertia, or contaminated areas and dust (this also has been an issue in research laboratories handing hamsters); herpes simplex virus 1 (HSV-1), a common cause of sporadic encephalitis in the United States and a common infection throughout the world, which can result in meningoencephalitis, sometime with focal neurologic signs (as a primary infection or from recrudescence); human immunodeficiency virus (HIV), which can have its initial presentation as meningitis in about 10–15% of cases; and cytomegalovirus (CMV), primarily in immunosuppressed hosts. HSV-2 is a common sexually transmitted disease in the United States that can occur as a primary infection and recurrences. It can result in aseptic meningitis with radiculitis.

Some cases of viral meningitis or encephalitis are transmitted by mosquito or tick bites. An emerging vector-borne meningoencephalitis infection in the United States is West Nile virus (WNV), a flavivirus. In North America, it is transmitted to humans by some *Culex* and *Aedes* mosquitoes. This pathogen was recognized as having widespread endemicity in Africa and was apparently unintentionally introduced to the United States in 1999. Since then, it has spread across the continental United States and Canada. Increases in U.S. cases are sometimes preceded by die-off of birds, particularly American crows [21, 22]. However, in an aseptic meningitis epidemic occurring in relation to an avian epizootic in the United States, no WNV was found in human cases. Polymerase chain reaction (PCR) testing identified enterovirus as the pathogen in the human epidemic, serotyped as echoviruses 13 and 18, emphasizing that enteroviruses are an important cause of aseptic meningitis [23]. As of this writing, for 2007, the CDC received reports of 3,598 cases of WNV disease. West Nile fever accounted for 65% of cases, and meningitis/encephalitis accounted for about 34% of cases. The overall case-fatality rate for all reported cases was about 3.4% [24]. This virus is also present in areas of Europe, the Middle East, and India. WNV is covered in more detail in Chapters 28 and 37. Other important vector-borne illnesses that can present with meningitis/encephalitis syndromes in the United States include Colorado tick fever, which is a febrile illness with neutropenia and thrombocytopenia, sometime with rash, typically occurring in spring and early summer in people bitten by infected *Dermacentor andersoni* ticks that reside at high altitude (over 1,500 m) in the Rocky Mountains; eastern equine encephalitis (EEE, Togaviridae, *Alphavirus*) occurring in the United States, Canada, the Caribbean, and Central and South America and transmitted to humans by *Aedes* or *Coquillettidia* mosquitoes; western equine encephalitis (WEE, Togaviridae, *Alphavirus*) occurring in the United States, Canada, and South America and transmitted to humans by *Culex tarsalis* mosquitoes; St. Louis encephalitis (SLE, a flavivirus) occurring in most of the United States, Canada, Central America, and northern South America and transmitted by *Culex* mosquitoes; LaCrosse encephalitis (a bunyavirus) in the central to eastern United States and carried by *A. triseriatus;* snowshoe hare encephalitis (bunyavirus) in Canada, China, and the Russian Federation; and California encephalitis (a bunyavirus) carried by *Aedes* mosquitoes. Venezuelan equine encephalitis (VEE), caused by Togoviridae, *Alphavirus,* is transmitted to humans by *Culex, Aedes,* and other mosquitoes from rodent reservoirs. VEE is endemic in northern South America and Central America and spread temporarily to the southern United States in 1971 [25]. Some of these diseases may need to be distinguished from phlebotomine-borne viral fevers and dengue hemorrhagic fever, the latter being an emerging global infection with presence in the United States.

Seen worldwide and important in relation to residents and travelers to endemic countries are Japanese encephalitis (a flavivirus), found in western Pacific Islands, Asia, northern Australia, and the Middle East and transmitted by *Culex* mosquitoes; yellow fever (a flavavirus), transmitted by *Aedes* or *Haemogogus* mosquitoes in northern South America and Africa; and Murray Valley encephalitis (a flavivirus), transmitted by *Culex* mosquitoes in Australia. Flaviviruses are also involved in tick-borne encephalitides in Europe, the Russian Federation, and Asia. These are primarily *Ixodes* ticks and include Far Eastern, Central Euopean, louping ill, and Powassan virus tick-borne encephalitides. Powassan also occurs in Canada and the United States.

Other arthropod-borne viral diseases with potential for meningitis/encephalitis syndromes, usually spread to humans by mosquitoes, include Oropouche virus (a Simbu group bunyavirus) in northern South America and Central America; Rift Valley fever (a phlebovirus), which occurs in sheep and other animals and can result in human outbreaks as an arthropod vector-borne disease or by butchering or handling infected animal tissue; Kunjin virus (a flavivirus) in Australia and Papua New Guinea; and others. Many of these can occur as asymptomatic infection or mild febrile illness. Of non-arthropod vector-borne encephalitides, rabies (rhabdovirus, genus *Lyssavirus*) is a major problem in developing countries worldwide and is covered in Chapters 20 and 28.

Any meningitis is a serious disease, but viral meningitis tends to be milder than bacterial meningitis, is rarely fatal (except for rabies), and tends to resolve without specific treatment. All cases of suspected meningitis should be treated as a medical emergency that requires prompt diagnosis, usually with examination of CSF, CSF culture, and blood cultures, because viral and bacterial meningitis may present similarly initially, but bacterial meningitis tends to be much more severe, has greater mortal-

ity and residual morbidity, including permanent damage to the brain, and requires specific treatment. Aseptic meningitis and viral meningitis are often not the subject of specific viral diagnosis, but diagnosis of many types can be made using PCR testing, acute and convalescent serum titers, and isolation of the virus from stool.

BACTERIAL MENINGITIS (SELECTED TYPES)
Streptococcus pneumoniae

Streptococcal meningitis is the most common form of meningitis in adults in the United States and is also a prominent cause of this illness in children. An estimated 15,000 cases occur annually in the United States. *S. pneumoniae*, a gram-positive coccus (formerly called *pneumococcus*) is the causative organism. Risk for this streptococcal meningitis is increased with recent pneumonia or upper respiratory infection, recent otitis media, advanced age, history of splenectomy, diabetes mellitus, chronic alcohol use, artificial heart valves, and injury or trauma to the head, particularly with CSF leak. The onset of meningitis is typically rapid, with high fever, tachycardia, severe headache, stiff neck, photophobia, nausea, vomiting, and confusion. Case mortality is typically around 20%, and of those who survive, more than half have serious long-term sequelae such as deafness, muscle paralysis, mental changes, hydrocephalus, and subdural accumulations of fluid.

Diagnosis is usually made by examination of CSF, which typically shows white blood cells, elevated protein, and low glucose and may show gram-positive cocci, and by CSF culture. Blood cultures also may grow this organism. Computed tomographic (CT) scan of the brain is usually normal. Rapid initiation of treatment is critical and should precede culture-proven diagnosis. Treatment depends on local patterns of microbial drug resistance. For pneumococcus generally, the choice of antibiotics depends on the penicillin-related minimal inhibitory concentration (MIC) for the organism. Serious infections are usually treated with parenteral penicillin G. For meningitis from organisms of high-level resistance, *The Medical Letter* 2007 recommendation for first choice is vancomycin plus ceftriaxone or cefotaxime with or without rifampin [3]. Owing to changing patterns of resistant organisms, the reader should consult a local infectious disease expert and current treatment guidelines. For adults, vaccination with pneumococcal vaccine is recommended for people at high risk and for everyone over age 55 years.

Neisseria meningitidis

Meningococcal meningitis is the second most common form of bacterial pneumonia in adults in the United States and is the major form of bacterial meningitis in children. The illness is caused by *N. meningitidis*, a gram-negative diplococcus. The clinical disease was first described in the early 1800s related to a serious outbreak that swept through Geneva, Switzerland. The meningococcus was identified as the causative agent of such outbreaks in 1887.

Nasopharyngeal carriage of *N. meningitidis* is a common precursor to disease, but most carriers don't get meningitis from it. Worldwide, it has been estimated that 10–25% of the population carries *N. meningitidis* at any given time. The carriage rate can be higher in some areas and much higher when epidemics occur [26]. Cigarette smokers have been found to have higher carriage rates [27]. Meningitis can occur when the body defenses allow invasive growth with septicemia.

The main risk factors for meningococcal meningitis are recent upper respiratory tract infection and recent exposure, with close contact and exposure to respiratory secretions of someone with meningococcal meningitis. Household members of patients have been found to be at particularly high risk, the risk being hundreds-fold greater than the general population [28, 29]. Outbreaks can occur related to close living quarters, such as can occur in households, boarding schools, college dormitories, jails and prisons, military barracks, pilgrimages, and other work settings that bring people together to live in close quarters. Specific occupational concerns also have included health care workers, particularly those closely and heavily exposed to respiratory secretions, those doing tracheal intubations or servicing tracheostomy tubes, paramedics [30], medical laboratory workers [31–33], laboratory researchers [34], and travelers, including those with aircraft passenger exposures [35–38].

The reservoir for *N. meningitidis* is human, and the average incubation period is 4 days, ranging from 2–10 days. This form of meningitis occurs more in the winter and spring months. It carries a case-morality rate of 5–15%, even when antibiotic therapy is given, and among survivors, up to 15% will have long-term sequelae. *N. meningitidis* meningitis can result in death in 24–48 hours of onset of disease, even when antibiotic therapy is given [26]. A 2002 epidemic caused by the W-135 strain in Burkina Faso affected 13,000 people and resulted in 1,500 deaths [26].

As with streptococcal pneumonia, the onset of this illness may be very rapid, with high fever, severe headache and malaise, stiff neck, photophobia, nausea, vomiting, and mental changes. However, meningococcal meningitis is more likely to also involve a petechial rash and purpura. As with streptococcal meningitis, the CSF typically shows increased white blood cells, high protein, and low glucose, but Gram stain may show gram-negative cocci. CSF and blood cultures grow *N. meningitidis*. CT scan is usual normal.

Vaccination is available for protection from meningococcal meningitis. Vaccines may not provide adequate protection for 10–14 days after injection [26]. The currently available quadravalent vaccines in the United States cover serogroups A, C, Y, and W-135 based on the antigenicity of the polysaccharide capsule of meningococcus. However, they does not cover meningococcus serogroup B, which has resulted in outbreaks in the United States, Canada, and Europe. Type A causes most of the serious large-scale epidemics in the world and most meningococcal disease in Africa and Asia. Types B and C are more common in Europe and South America, and type C has been increasing in the United States. Serogroup W-135 is an emerging pathogen that has increased its claim in the proportion of meningococcal disease and has been linked to epidemics in the Middle East and Africa. In some areas of the world, infection with serogroup Y is also increasing, including the United States, with types C, Y, and W-135 accounting for about two-thirds of cases during 1994–1998 [39]. The current CDC recommendations for use of the quadravalent meningococcal polysaccharide-protein conjugate vaccine (MCV4, Menactra, Sanofi Pasteur, Inc.) include vaccination of people aged 19–55 years who are at increased risk. The groups at increased risk are identified as college freshmen living in dormitories, microbiologists routinely exposed to *N. meningitidis* isolates, military recruits, travelers to or residents of countries in which *N. meninitidis* meningitis is hyperendemic or epidemic, persons with terminal complement component deficiencies, and people with anatomic or functional asplenia. Vaccination is also recommended for all people aged 11–18 years with one dose of MCV4 at the earliest opportunity. For this age group, the MCV4 should be given with Tdap (tetanus toxoid, reduced diphtheria toxoid, and acellular pertussis) if both vaccines are indicated and available. The CDC noted some reports of Guillain-Barré syndrome (GBS) after use of MCV4, advising that a history of GBS is a relative contraindication to receiving MCV4 [5, 40]. The CDC identifies areas at high risk overseas as including the sub-Saharan African "meningitis belt" from Mali to Ethiopia (peak serogroup A meningococcal disease occurring regularly in the dry season from December through June and in major epidemics about every 8–12 years) and Saudi Arabia in association with the Hajj pilgrimage and Ramadan Umrah visits, for which Saudi Arabia now requires visitors to obtain a tetravalent vaccine (covering types A, C, Y, and W-135) at least 10 days prior to arrival in the country [26]. Related to these pilgrimages, there were epidemics in 2000 and 2002, with infections occurring in returning pilgrims and their families in a number of countries including the United States [41].

There is also a quadravalent meningococcal polysaccharide vaccine (MPSV4, also Sanofi Pasteur) available in the United States that covers the same serogroups as MCV4. MCV4 is expected to be more effective in children and to confer longer-lasting protection. MPSV4 is recommended among people older than 55 years and as an acceptable alternative for those aged 2–55 years, particularly for short-term protection (i.e., 3–5 years). Both vaccines are contraindicated in people known to have severe allergic reactions to any component of the vaccines, including diphtheria toxoid (for MCV4), or to dry natural-rubber latex. The CDC reports that studies of MCV4 in pregnant woman have not been done, and studies of MPSV4 during pregnancy have not documented adverse events in either the women or the neonates [5, 40].

As with any suspected bacterial meningitis, early diagnosis and treatment are crucial. Treatment is commonly given prior to central nervous system and blood culture confirmation. The reader should check for current recommendations for empirical antibiotic therapy for meningitis. At the time of this writing, the first-choice antibiotic for treatment of confirmed meningococcal disease is penicillin G. The choice may vary based specific sensitivity testing and local patterns of antibiotic resistance. Alternative choices for treatment include cefotaxime, deftizoxime, ceftriaxone, and chloramphicol [3, 12].

Carriage of *N. meningitidis* is more common among close contacts of people who have had meningococcal disease, and contacts, particularly household contacts, have a higher risk for invasive disease. It is recommended that carriers receive antibiotic chemoprophylaxis to eliminate nasopharyngeal carriage [5, 42]. For prophylaxis after close contact with infected patients, a fluoroquinolone or rifampin has been recommended [3]. Until 2007–2008, meningococcal disease resistant to ciprofloxacin had been described only in Argentina, Australia, China, France, India, and Spain. A February 22, 2008, report from the CDC identified a cluster of cases in North Dakota and Minnesota with fluoroquinolone-resistant serogroup B *N. meningitidis.* [42]. Other recommendations for elimination of nasopharyngeal carriage for close household contacts of an initial case of meningococcal disease (including household or day-care center personnel and medical personnel in direct close contact with the patient) include rifampin as a first choice (80–90% effective in eliminating asymptomatic nasopharyngeal carriage), less desirable alternatives being single-dose oral ciprofloxacin and intramuscular ceftriaxone [12]. Minocycline also has been found to be effective in eliminating carriage but is not used commonly owing to vestibular side effects.

Haemophilus influenzae

This gram-negative bacillius occurs in several serotypes and is a commensal of the human upper respiratory tract. The most important serotype in human disease, particularly meningitis, is *H. influenzae* serotype b (Hib). This serotype is present worldwide and used to be a much more common form of meningitis in some countries, including the United States, prior to the advent of effective vaccination and implementation of vaccination programs. Several vaccines are available and are used for widespread vaccination of infants. The CDC reports that use of vaccine for Hib has resulted in a 95% reduction in Hib among children in the United States. Rates in adults have remained stable, Hib still causing about 5–10% of bacterial meningitis in adults. Long-term efficacy and post-vaccination antibody persistence are unclear [43].

The reservoir for *H. influenzae* is human, transmission is from droplets and discharge from the nose and throat of infected people, and the incubation period is probably 2–4 days. Even with early treatment, death can occur, 20% of those infected may experience some hearing loss, and some may have permanent brain damage. It is recommended that all nonimmunized family contacts of individuals with this type of meningitis begin chemoprophylaxis as soon as possible [44].

At the time of this writing, first-choice treatment for meningitis and other serious *H. influenzae* infections is cefotaxime or ceftriaxone, alternatives being ciprofloxacin, erythromycin, chloramphenicol, and meropenem [3]. Rifampin has been used in adults to eliminate nasal carriage of Hib.

Hib continues to be a leading cause of meningitis in countries that do not have effective or global vaccination programs. It is also a leading cause of bacterial pneumonia deaths in children. It has been estimated to result in an annual burden of 3 million cases of meningitis and severe pneumonia worldwide, with 386,000 deaths, mostly in children. The World Health Organization and the Global Alliance for Vaccines and Immunizations, along with other partners, are leading an initiative to provide Hib vaccine to identified low-income nations worldwide [45].

Streptococcus suis

Streptococcal meningitis also can be caused by *S. suis*, an alpha-hemolytic gram-positive coccus that is a zoonosis mainly reported in pig-rearing and pork-consuming countries. *S. suis* serotype 2 can live as a commensal organism in the tonsils of pigs, its natural host, and there are now about 35 recognized serotypes, many of which can be pig-related. A recent study in Asia estimated that based on data from hospitalizations, the general population incidence of *S. suis* infection is 0.9 cases per 100,000 population and 32 cases per 100,000 population for people with occupational exposure to pigs and raw pork [46]. About half of these infections resulted in meningitis, the remainder of infections were septicemia or endocarditis, and the case-fatality rate was 5%. A report from the People's Republic of China related severe disease outbreak with meningitis and streptococcal toxic shock-like syndrome from serotype 7, with 38 deaths observed in 215 cases (about 18% mortality) [47]. This outbreak had an occupational component in that the person who processed the infected pig from the herd and the person who processed the meat became infected. Another report related a case of peritonitis owing to *S. suis* serotype 16 in a pig keeper who regularly consumed pig meat [48].

The most common disease manifestation of *S. suis* in humans is a purulent meningitis, which often involves cochleovestibular signs and residual damage expressed as hearing loss and ataxia. It has been a rare but emerging disease, with fewer than 150 cases reported between about 1971 and 2001. This can be an occupational disease for those who work with domestic pigs or their meat products. It has been reported in a butcher [49], a pig breeder [50], and a meat-processing worker [51]. Although it is found most commonly in northern Europe and southern Asia, recent case reports include cases of occupational exposure in Spain, Italy, South America, and the United States [52–56]. The latter cited report involved an individual who returned to the United States from an extended stay in the Philippines. In the Netherlands, a poacher contracted *S. suis* meningitis after killing and butchering a wild boar [57].

Another emerging pig-processing-related neurologic illness has been reported recently in the United States. Part of the CDC working case definition is that this consists of new onset of bilateral and relatively symmetric flaccid weakness/paralysis of the limbs that also may involve cranial nerve-innervated muscles. Reduced or absent deep tendon reflexes are reported in the affected limbs. In a number of cases, the legs are more affected than the arms. CSF findings have included elevated protein levels with no or minimal pleocytosis. This appears to be a progressive inflammatory neuropathy (PIN) and has not been linked to an infectious etiology. Risk is highest for workers at pig-processing head tables, where, in some plants, the work process of "blowing brains" involved application of compressed air through the foramen magnum to liquefy the brains for easier removal, resulting in generation of aerosolized small droplets and splatter. As of this writing, the investigation of swine slaughterhouses is ongoing, and no food-borne infectious risk has been identified for workers or the general population. A hypothesis is that PIN represents an autoimmune peripheral neuropathy induced by pig neural protein [58].

Listeria monocytogenes

Infection with this gram-positive rod and several of its serovars can present with meningitis, meningoencephalitis, or encephalitis. Meningitis is the most common form of central nervous system infection related to *L. monocytogenes,* and this organism has a predilection for causing central nervous system infections in the elderly and in those with impaired cellular immunity. It may be difficult to diagnose because only about half the patients will have positive Gram stains in CSF. This infection also has the capacity to present as encephalitis with red blood cells in CSF, mimicking herpes simplex virus encephalitis (HSV-1). CSF lactic acid tends to be high in *L. monocytogenes* encephalitis but not in HSV-1 encephalitis [59]. *L. monocytogenes* meningoencephalitis has been reported to present atypically with fever, altered consciousness, and seizures with no headache or meningeal signs [60]. The bacterium is present in soil, water, and forage material and causes infection in many animals. Humans can have asymptomatic fecal carriage. Transmission can occur through contaminated food, milk and milk products, soft cheeses, vegetables, processed foods and meats, contact with infected people, and direct contact with domestic or wild mammals and fowl or handling their carcasses. Incubation can range from 3–70 days, but the median is several weeks. As of this writing, drugs of first choice are usually ampicillin with or without gentamycin, an alternative being trimethoprim-sulfamethoxazole [3].

Mycobacterium tuberculosis

Tuberculosis and its complications are most often seen in the United States in immigrants, refugees, migrant workers, and people who are immunosuppressed. Complicated tuberculosis is a much larger problem in developing countries. Meningeal disease related to tuberculosis is covered in Chapter 9.

PROTOZOAL MENINGITIS

Malarial infection, particularly *Plasmodium falciparum* malaria, has the capacity to result in severe meningitis. The occurrence of fever in an individual who has traveled to an area in which malaria is endemic, even if the person took appropriate antimalarial prophylaxis and is up to 1 year after the end of the travel period, should be checked for malaria. Malaria is covered in Chapter 25. Other protozoal illnesses that can have meningitis or meningoencephalitis in their clinical presentation include infection with *Entamoeba histolytica, Naegleria fowleri* (primary amebic meningoencephalitis), *Acanthamoeba* species (granulomatous amebic encephalitis), and *Trypanosoma* species. These are covered in Chapter 31.

FUNGAL MENINGITIS

A number of fungi can affect the central nervous system and result in meningitis. These infections are more common in people whose immune systems are impaired. Among the fungi that can affect the central nervous system are *Coccidioides immitis, Blastomyces dermatitidis, Histoplasma capsulatum, Sporothrix schenkii, Cryptococcus neoformans,* the Mucorales order of fungi including *Rhizopus arrhizus* and others (zygomycosis), and others. Please see Chapter 32 for more details.

HELMINTHIC MENINGITIS

Many helminthic infections are characterized by eosinophilia. Eosinophilic meningitis, characterized by an eosinophilic pleocytosis in CSF, is a rare form of meningitis. Worldwide, the rat lungworm, *Angiostrongylus cantonensis,* is the most common infectious cause. An outbreak occurred in the United States in 2004–2005 [61]. Other helminthes with a life cycle in humans that can result in meninglencephalitis syndromes include *Gnathostoma spinigerum, Baylisascaris procyonis, Toxocara canus* and *T. cati, Schistosoma* species, *Spirometra mansoni, Echinococcus granulosus, Taenia* species, *Paragonimus* species, and others. These are covered in Chapter 30.

Occupational Considerations and Conclusion

As mentioned in the first sections of this chapter, the occupational physician may be involved in meningitis issues in a number of different ways. These include fielding administrative issues related to alerts about possible meningitis in the workforce, emergency preparedness, training employees (including travelers) about causes and prevention of meningitis, recognizing meningitis risks in the workplace and helping develop safe work practices and surveillance, recognizing meningitis syndromes, arranging for immediate proper care, reporting disease occurrence, and dealing with prophylaxis and prevention issues related to sporadic cases, outbreaks, and epidemics.

Based on the foregoing pages, it is clear that many occupational groups are at risk for this disease and that the level of risk in specific work groups can vary over time. In the occupational setting, the likelihood of meningitis occurrence, either common or uncommon forms, above the general population's incidence figures depends on the type of work done, the immune status of the workers, the ages of workers, community patterns of illness, types of occupational travel, and other factors. Some specific occupational groups at risk include abattoir workers, butchers and other handlers of meat and animal products, farmers, ranchers and animal handlers, veterinarians and their staff, workers involved in disturbance of soil, health care professionals (including emergency medical technicians), other first responders and those who give cardiopulmonary resuscitation to infected individuals, child care workers (which may result in risks to other workers if child day care is housed within another type of workplace), medical laboratory workers, research laboratory workers dealing with cultures or animals, outdoor workers in areas of specific endemic tick- and mosquito-borne pathogens, migrant workers and others housed in rodent-infested quarters, military personnel, college and university students and personnel, prison workers, refugee aid workers, those working in overcrowded conditions, those working in a setting with close contact with someone who has meningitis, travelers in confined quarters or overcrowded areas with others, travelers on airline flights, travelers to endemic, hyperendemic, or epidemic areas, those consuming inadequately treated or contaminated food and water, those on pilgrimages and those whose work involves pilgrims and immigrants from endemic areas, those whose work involves recreational water activities, and others.

Workplace practices that can limit the effects of meningitis in the workplace include administering vaccinations according to standard schedules (see Chapter 5); educating employees about the risks, control, and prevention of infectious diseases; being aware of patterns of disease and emerging pathogens in the community; recognizing soil-, water-, food-, animal-, arthropod-, and travel-related sources of infection related to the worksite; and encouraging administrative, engineering, personal protective equipment, and personal practice measures to limit exposures (see Chapters 27, 34, and 35); recognizing and reporting cases early; using case incident-related prophylaxis and vaccinations according to guidelines; encouraging ill workers to take absence leaves; avoiding contact with respiratory secretions; providing for convenient disposal of items soiled with respiratory secretions; encouraging thorough hand-washing precautions in response to soiling or potential contamination and prior to eating or touching facial areas; avoiding overcrowding and close contact, including sharing of eating utensils and beverage containers; and carrying out prompt decontamination of potentially contaminated areas. Many of these suggestions are commonsense approaches that help with prevention and control of many types of illnesses. Please refer to other chapters for more detail.

References

1. Tunkel AR, Hartman BJ, Kaplan SI, et al. Practice guidelines for the management of bacterial meningitis. *Clin Infect Dis* 2004;39:1267–84.
2. *The Medical Letter on Drugs and Therapeutics* (serial publication).
3. Choices of antibacterial drugs. *Treatment Guidelines from The Medical Letter* 2007;5:33–50 (updated periodically).
4. Centers for Disease Control and Prevention. Control and prevention of meningococcal disease and control and prevention of serogroup C meningococcal disease: Evaluation and management of suspected outbreaks. Recommendations of the Advisory Committee on Immunization Practices (ACIP). *MMWR* 1997;46:1–21.
5. Prevention and control of meningococcal disease: Recommendations of the Advisory Committee on Immunization Practices (ACIP). *MMWR* 2005;54:1–21.
6. Queen Mary College. Meningitis Policy: Procedure for Dealing with Outbreaks of Meningitis, Incorporating Guidance form UK Universities on Managing Meningococcal Disease (Septicaemia Or Meningitis) in Higher Education Institutions, January 2005; available at www.ohs.qmul.ac.uk/Queen%20-%20 Meningitus%20Policy.

7. Centers for Disease Control and Prevention. Cholera, meningitis and yellow fever—Still threats to public health. Epidemic Preparedness and Response, Data for Decision Making (Refers to and links to disease specific technical guidelines, workshops, strategies). Atlanta: CDC, available at www.cdc.gov/cogh/dgphcd/modules/ddm/national.htm. Accessed May 22, 2008.

8. Centers for Disease Control and Prevention. Business Emergency Management Planning, Emergency Preparedness for Business (various links to documents). Atlanta: CDC, available at www.cdc.gov/niosh/topics/prepared/. Accessed May 22, 2008.

9. Agency for Healthcare Research and Quality. Community-Based Mass Prophylaxis: A Planning Guide for Public Health Preparedness. Washington: AHRQ, 2004; available at www.ahrq.gov.

10. University of St. Andrew. Outbreak of Meningitis Protocol, September 2006; available at www.st-andrews.ac.uk/staff/policy/Healthandsafety/Publications.

11. Schuchat A, Robinson K, Wenger JD, et al. Bacterial meningitis in the United States in 1995. Active Surveillance Team. *N Engl J Med* 1997;337:970–6.

12. Ramirez-Ronda CH, Ramirez-Ramirez CR. Bacterial meningitis. In Tan JS, File TM, Salata RA, et al. (eds), *Expert Guide to Infectious Diseases,* 2nd ed. Philadelphia: ACP Press, 2008, Chap 3, pp 55–65.

13. Centers for Disease Control and Prevention. Case definitions for infectious conditions under public health surveillance. *MMWR* 1997;46:43–4.

14. Gopalakrishna KV, Ahlu/Walia MS. Viral meningitis and viral encephalitis. In Tan JS, File TM, Salata RA, et al. (eds), *Expert Guide to Infectious Diseases,* 2nd ed. Philadelphia: ACP Press, 2008, Chap 4, pp 80–9.

15. Ahkee S, Ramirez J. A case of concurrent Lyme meningitis with ehrlichiosis. *Scand J Infect Dis* 1996; 28:527–8.

16. Harbison RD (ed). *Hamilton & Hardy's Industrial Toxicology,* 5th ed. St Louis: Mosby, 1998.

17. Hassaballa HA, Lateef OB, Bell J, et al. Metal fume fever presenting as aseptic meningitis with pericarditis, pleuritis and pneumonitis. *Occup Med (Lond)* 55;2005:638–41.

18. Parasuraman TV, Deverka PA, Toscani MR. Estimating the economic impact of viral meningitis in the United States. *Infect Med* 2000;17:417–27.

19. Khetsuriani N, Quiroz ES, Holman RC, et al. Viral meningitis–associated hospitalizations in the United States, 1988–1999, *Neuroepidemiology* 2003;22:345–52.

20. Surveillance for waterborne disease and outbreaks associated with recreational water—United States, 2003–2004. *MMWR* 2006;55:13.

21. Julian KG, Eidson M, Kipp AM, et al. Early season crow mortality as a sentinel for West Nile virus disease in humans, northeastern United States. *Vector Borne Zoonotic Dis* 2002;2:145–55.

22. Guptill SC, Julian KG, Campbell GL, et al. Early-season avian deaths from West Nile virus as warnings of human infections. *Emerg Infect Dis* 2003;9:483–4.

23. Julian KAG, Mullins JA, Olin A, et al. Aseptic meningitis epidemic during a West Nile virus avian epizootic. *Emerg Infect Dis* 2003;9:1082–8.

24. Centers for Disease Control and Prevention. 2007 West Nile Virus Activity in the United States (Reported to CDC as of March 4, 2008): West Nile Virus, Surveillance, Statistics, and Control. Atlanta: CDC, 2008.

25. Shope R, Mackenzie J. Arthropod-borne viral fevers, and arthropod-borne viral encephalopathies. In Heymann DL (ed), *Control of Communicable Diseases Manual,* 18th ed. Washington: American Public Health Association, 2004, pp 43–52.

26. World Health Organization. Meningococcal meningitis. Fact sheet no 141. Geneva: WHO, 2003.

27. Stuart JM, Cartwright KAC, Robinson PM, et al. The effect of smoking on meningococcal carriage. *Lancet* 1989;2:723–5.

28. De Wals P, Hetoghe L, Borlee-Grimee I, et al. Meningococcal disease in Belgium: Secondary attack rate among household, daycare nursery, and pre-elementary school contacts. *J Infect* 1981;3:S53.

29. Meningococcal Disease Surveillance Group. Analysis of endemic meningococcal disease serogroup and evaluation of chemoprophylaxis. *J Infect Dis* 1976; 134:201.

30. Whisman K, Spivak L, Tarman J, et al. Case conference: EMS response to meningococcal meningitis. *Emerg Med Serv* 2004;33:120–2.

31. Centers for Disease Control and Prevention. Laboratory-acquired meningococcal disease—United States, 2000. *MMWR* 2002;51:141–4.

32. Sejvar JJ, Johnson D, Popovic T, et al. Assessing the risk of laboratory-acquired meningococcal disease. *J Clin Microbiol* 2005;43:4811–4.

33. Kessler AT, Stephens DS, Somani J. Laboratory-acquired serogroup A meningococcal meningitis. *J Occup Health* 2007;49:399–401.

34. Athlin S, Vikerfors T, Fredlund H, et al. Atypical clinical presentation of laboratory-acquired meningococcal disease. *Scand J Infect Dis* 2007;39:911–3.

35. Centers for Disease Control and Prevention. Exposure to patients with meningococcal disease on aircrafts—United States, 1999–2001. *MMWR* 2001;50:485–9.

36. Wilder-Smith A, Memish Z. Meningococcal disease and travel. *Int J Antimicrob Agents* 2003;21:102–6.

37. O'Connor BA, Chant KG, Binotto E, et al. Meningococcal disease: Probable transmission during an international flight. *Commun Dis Intell* 2005;29:312–4.

38. Wilder-Smith A. Meningococcal disease in international travel: Vaccine strategies. *J Travel Med* 2005; 12S1:522–9.

39. Centers for Disease Control and Prevention. Meningococcal disease and college students: Recommendations of the Advisory Committee on Immunization Practices (ACIP). *MMWR* 2000;49:11–20.

40. Centers for Disease Control and Prevention. Notice

to readers: Revised recommendations of the Advisory Committee on Immunization Practices to vaccinate all persons aged 11–18 years with meningococcal conjugate vaccine. *MMWR* 2007;56: 794–5.

41. Meningococcal disease. In CDC, *Health Information for International Travel 2008*, Chap 4; available at www.n.cdc.gov/travel/yellowBook/.

42. Centers for Disease Control and Prevention. Emergence of fluoroquinolone-resistant *Neisseria meningitidis*—Minnesota and North Dakota, 2007–2008. *MMWR* 2008;57:173–5.

43. Division of Bacterial and Mycotic Diseases, Centers for Disease Control and Prevention. *Haemophilus influenzae* Serotype b (Hib) Disease. Atlanta: CDC, 2008; available at www.cdc.gov/ncidod/dbmd/diseaseinfo/haeminfluserob_t.

44. Meningitis—*H. influenza*, Medline Plus, National Library of Medicine, National Institutes of Health; available at www.nlm.nih.gov/.

45. Progress toward introduction of *Haemophilus influenzae* type b vaccine in low-income countries—Worldwide, 2004–2007. *MMWR* 2008;57:148–51.

46. Ma E, Chung PH, So T, et al. *Streptococcus suis* infection in Hong Kong: An emerging infectious disease? *Epidemiol Infect* 2008;1–7.

47. Ye C, Zhu, X, Jing H, et al. *Streptococcus suis* sequence type 7 outbreak, Sichuan, China. *Emerg Infect Dis* 2006;12; available at www.cdc.gov/ncidod/EID/vol12no08/06-0232.htm.

48. Hghia HDT, Hoa NT, Linh LD, et al. Human case of *Streptococcus suis* serotype 16 infection. *Emerg Infect Dis* 2008;14; available at www.cdc.gov/EID/content/14/1/155.htm.

49. Braun S, Jechart G, Emmerling U, et al. Meningitis caused by *Streptococcus suis*. *Dtsch Med Wochenschr* 2007;132:1098–100.

50. Matsuo H, Sakamoto S. Purulent meningitis caused by *Streptococcus suis* in a pig breeder. *Kansenshogaku Zasshi* 2003;77:340–2.

51. Ibaraki M, Fujita N, Tada M, et al. A Japanese case of *Streptococcus suis* meningitis associated with lumbar epidural abscess. *Rinsho Shinkeigaku* 2003;43:176–9.

52. Geffner Sclarsky DE, Moreno Munoz R, Campillo Alpera MS, et al. *Streptococcus suis* meningitis. *Ann Med Interna* 2001;18:317–8.

53. Camporese A, Tizianel G, Bruchetta G, et al. Human meningitis caused by *Streptococcus suis:* The first case report from northeastern Italy. *Infez Med* 2007; 15:111–4.

54. Lopreto C, Lopardo HA, Bardi MC, et al. Primary *Streptococcus suis* meningitis: First case in humans described in Latin America. *Enfrm Infecc Microbiol Clin* 2005; 23:110.

55. Willenburg KS, Sntochnik DE, Zakods RN. Human *Streptococcus suis* in the United States. *N Engl J Med* 2006;354:1325.

56. Lee GT, Chiu CY, Haller BL, et al. *Streptococcus suis* meningitis, United States. *Emerg Infect Dis* 2008;14; available at www.cdc.gov/EID/content/14/1/183.htm.

57. Halaby T, Hoitsma E, Hupperts R, et al. *Streptococcus suis* meningitis: A poacher's risk. *Eur J Clin Microbiol Infect Dis* 2000;19:943–5.

58. Centers for Disease Control and Prevention. Investigation of progressive inflammatory neuropathy among swine slaughterhouse workers—Minnesota, 2007–2008. *MMWR* 2008;57:122–4.

59. Cunha BA, Fatehpuria R, Eisenstein LE. *Listeria monocytogenes* encephalitis mimicking herpes simplex virus encephalitis: The differential diagnostic importance of cerebrospinal fluid lactic acid levels. *Heart Lung* 2007;36:226–31.

60. Itaya K, Ohno H, Kawase Y. *Listeria monocyogenes* meningoencephalitis lacking meningeal signs. *No To Shinkei* 2006;58:621–4.

61. Hochberg NS, Park SY, Blackburn BG, et al. Distribution of eosinophilic meningitis cases attributable to *Angiostrongylus cantonensis*, Hawaii. *Emerg Infect Dis* 2007;13; available at www.cdc.gov/EID/content/13/11/1675.htm.

24 HIV in the Workplace

Alan L. Williams and Richard J. Thomas*

Over 25 years have elapsed since the first cases of what would become known as the *acquired immune deficiency syndrome* (AIDS) were reported in 1981 [1]. The complex interactions between the human immunodeficiency virus (HIV) and the workplace are still being defined and understood. While occupationally acquired infections from HIV are of much individual concern, they are rare events [2]. HIV is neither the most common nor the most infectious bloodborne pathogen. In the United States, seroconversion related to employment has been documented in health care workers and in those who occupationally engage in sexual contact [3–5]. The medical response to HIV exposure has been addressed by various health organizations [6–8]. Because of the currently incurable nature of HIV infection, seroconversion after an exposure to human blood is often the foremost concern for an employee. Prompt treatment following an HIV exposure can decrease the chances of seroconversion. Therefore, evaluation and treatment of potential exposures are urgent medical matters. Occupational medicine providers should be prepared to evaluate and treat or promptly refer employees who present following such an exposure. This chapter will deal primarily with exposure to HIV from nonsexual contact with infectious material. Occupational HIV surveillance, workplace limitations, and employment restrictions, if any, for HIV-positive employees and candidates are also reviewed.

Occupational Exposure to Bloodborne Pathogens: A Brief History

Previous experience with viral hepatitis has provided a framework for response to HIV. Hepatitis B, previously known as *serum hepatitis,* was noted to occur via parenteral infection. Cases arose from blood transfusions, sharing of needles from illicit drug use (e.g., during the Vietnam War), and through immunizations, including 200,000 cases associated with infected lots of yellow fever vaccine among U.S. forces in the 1940s [9]. The identification of the MS-1 (hepatitis A) and MS-2 (hepatitis B) strains by Krugman and colleagues [10] in the Willowbrook studies preceded the detection of the Australia antigen (now referred to as the *hepatitis B surface antigen*) in the late 1960s by Blumberg and colleagues [11]. More complete understanding of hepatitis B pathophysiology was followed by routine serologic testing of blood transfusion units and patients infected with hepatitis and the eventual development of the hepatitis B vaccine. Because of the similar nature of their occupational risks and the timing of a fuller understanding of pathogenesis, the groundwork in the global

*The opinions expressed by the authors do not reflect the policy of the Department of Health and Human Services, the Department of the Navy, or the Department of Defense.

response to occupational risks for hepatitis B has shaped the response to HIV.

The magnitude of the number of health care workers (HCWs) exposed to bloodborne pathogens via occupational needlestick injuries became clearer by the mid-1970s. Preventive strategies for needlestick exposure in HCWs were proposed as early as 1981 [12], the same year as the first case report of AIDS [1]. In 1982, Dienstag and Ryan demonstrated a correlation between the intensity and duration of human blood and body fluid exposure and the likelihood of hepatitis B conversion [13]. The 1983 version of the U.S. Centers for Disease Control and Prevention (CDC) Guidelines for Isolation Precautions in Hospitals was the last to have a specific category for blood and body fluid precautions [14]. The emergence of AIDS cases in the early 1980s and subsequent identification of HIV [15–17] prompted the National Institute for Occupational Safety and Health (NIOSH) and other parts of the CDC to reconsider the utility of having a specific category of blood and body fluid precautions [18,19]. The phrase *universal precautions* has been promoted to raise awareness of potential infectious risks within health care systems. Each patient encounter is a potential risk; therefore, appropriate precautions must be universally applied. The first occupational HIV infection, the result of a needlestick injury, was reported in late 1984 [20]. By 1987, the CDC had reports of six cases of occupationally acquired HIV in the United States. Four of the six had needlestick exposures, whereas the remaining two had extensive blood or body fluid contact from an HIV-infected patient [21]. Use of single-agent antiretroviral postexposure therapy was discussed in a 1989 publication by Henderson and Gerberding [22]. The CDC developed the National Surveillance System for Health Care Workers (NaSH) to track occupationally related disease. In 1991, the U.S. Occupational Safety and Health Administration (OSHA) released legal guidelines to protect employees in an attempt to reduce or mitigate the effects of the estimated 800,000 needlestick injuries that occur in the United States annually [23, 24].

HCWs face a wide range of workplace hazards, including needlestick injuries and mucous membrane exposures. The total number of exposures is unknown but may increase owing to increasing numbers of workers at risk. The health care field in the United States was the largest industry in 2006, employing over 14 million workers. Women represent nearly 80% of the health care workforce in America [25]. Worldwide, there are conservatively estimated to be 35 million HCWs, but this estimate does not include the millions of support staff who also are at risk for occupational exposure [26]. Police, firefighters, sanitation workers, and many others have lower but real occupational risks for accidental exposure to human blood or body fluid [27]. Most research and prevention measures have focused on HCWs, especially in the hospital setting. The results of these efforts have been mixed [28]. A recent anonymous survey of 582 surgical residents at 17 medical centers reported that 99% of surgeons in training experienced a needlestick at some time during their training. Only 51% of the most recent needlestick injuries were reported [29].

The effectiveness of highly active antiretroviral therapy (HAART) for HIV has increased the life expectancy of persons living with HIV/AIDS, thus increasing the number of HIV-positive sources. These therapies have lowered viral load in many of these same individuals, making exposure to their blood or body fluids potentially less likely to result in infection. Table 24-1 shows the CDC statistics for reported occupational HIV infections in HCWs in the United States through 2006 [3]. Whether the result of improved prophylaxis, safety devices, employee education, or underreporting, no occupationally related HIV infections have been reported to the CDC since 2001.

HIV/AIDS Surveillance

The CDC performs HIV/AIDS surveillance for the United States and issues annual reports, most recently providing data through 2005. General trends show a steady increase in the estimated number of persons living with AIDS in the United States— 421,873 at the end of 2005. Because it may take a decade or more for an HIV-positive individual to develop AIDS, and because universal testing is not the norm, it is not known precisely how many individuals in the United States are infected. The CDC estimates that over 1 million people in the United States are HIV-positive and that a quarter of them are unaware of their HIV status. The general trends indicate that an increasing number of persons are

Table 24-1
Number of U.S. Health Care Workers with Documented and Possible Occupationally Acquired HIV Infection, Reported through December 2006

Occupation	Documented Transmission	Possible Transmission
Dental worker, including dentist	0	6
Embalmer/morgue technician	1	2
Emergency medical technician/paramedic	0	12
Health aide/attendant	1	15
Housekeeper/maintenance worker	2	13
Laboratory technician, clinical	16	17
Laboratory technician, nonclinical	3	0
Nurse	24	35
Physician, nonsurgical	6	12
Physician, surgical	0	6
Respiratory therapist	1	2
Technician, dialysis	1	3
Technician, surgical	2	2
Technician/therapist, other than those listed above	0	9
Other health care occupations	0	6
Total	57	140

Source: Adapted from Centers for Disease Control and Prevention. *Surveillance of Occupationally Acquired HIV/AIDS in Healthcare Personnel, as of December 2006;* available at *www.cdc.gov/ncidod/dhqp/pdf/bbp/fact_sheet_clearance_revised_090507Dec2006.pdf.*

living with HIV/AIDS owing to both new cases of infection and lengthened life expectancy [30].

Pathophysiology of HIV

HIV is an RNA-based retrovirus of the subfamily Lentivirus, a group of viruses that cause chronic cytopathic infections of the immune system of various vertebrate species. HIV is closely related to the immunodeficiency viruses of nonhuman primates. With the extraordinary growth in the human population in the last half of the twentieth century, human penetration into remote forest habitats, and rapid transit, this virus appears to have made a successful species jump in the relatively recent past. It has been rapidly propagated and amplified by human behavior and susceptibility [31–33].

Humans are the only known reservoir of HIV. Transmission requires intimate contact between susceptible host target cells and free virus or virus contained in inflammatory cells either suspended in human blood or present in other body fluids or tissues. Transmission does not occur via vectors or fomites, intact skin to intact skin contact, the airborne-respiratory route, or the fecal-oral contact. The dominant and characteristic form of ongoing viral infection and pathogenesis occurs with binding of the virus-specific envelope protein complex, gp120/gp 41, to the CD4 molecule expressed on the surface of helper T-lymphocytes as part of T-cell responsiveness to foreign antigens [34]. Binding then initiates the next stages of the viral life cycle: penetration, conversion of the RNA genome to DNA by the unique viral enzyme reverse transcriptase, and integration of viral DNA with host cell DNA. Resting CD4+ T cells may harbor proviral DNA without progressing forward in the viral replication process [35]. CD4+ T cells that are immunologically activated either before or after initial binding of HIV will continue the replication process via expression of viral messenger RNA, formation of viral proteins, followed by virion assembly and budding from the cell membrane. The specific cause of the immunologic activation has not yet been identified and may vary from patient to patient. Figure 24-1 demonstrates a simplified life cycle of HIV. In addition to CD4, coreceptors that play a role in HIV entry into host cells have been identified and are targets for pharmacologic intervention [36].

HIV Treatment

HIV treatment is a rapidly evolving field. Figure 24-1 also lists the classes of HIV medication and indicates their sites of action. The Food and Drug Administration (FDA)–approved medications for the treatment of HIV, as of early 2008, are listed in Table 24-2 [37]. Each drug generally has two to three names, which can complicate the understanding of an HIV source's medication history. Entry and fusion inhibitors work by preventing the processes involved with HIV gaining entry into CD4+ cells. Because of their action early in the process, there is promise for these drugs in acute postexposure treatment [38]. However, their use is not currently recommended without expert consultation [8]. Another recently added category of anti-HIV medication, the integrase inhibitors, acts

Figure 24-1
Simplified life cycle of the HIV virus

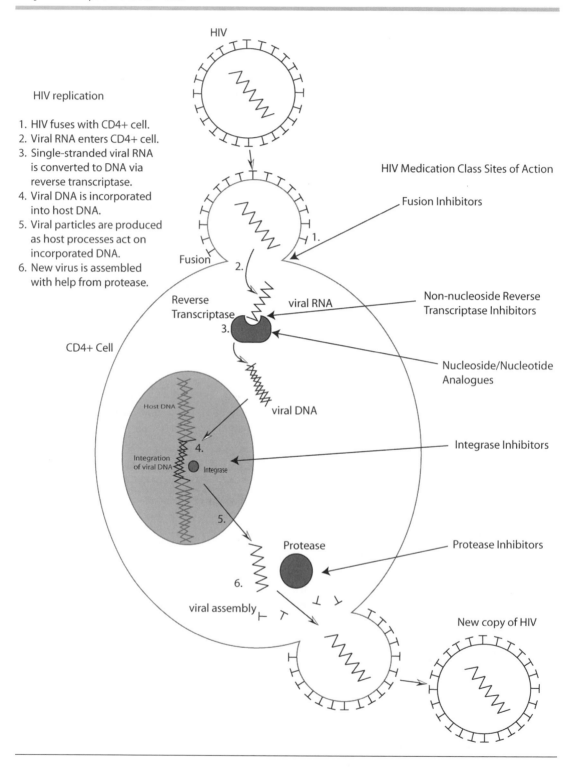

HIV

HIV replication

1. HIV fuses with CD4+ cell.
2. Viral RNA enters CD4+ cell.
3. Single-stranded viral RNA is converted to DNA via reverse transcriptase.
4. Viral DNA is incorporated into host DNA.
5. Viral particles are produced as host processes act on incorporated DNA.
6. New virus is assembled with help from protease.

HIV Medication Class Sites of Action

Fusion Inhibitors

Fusion

1.

2.

Reverse Transcriptase

viral RNA

Non-nucleoside Reverse Transcriptase Inhibitors

3.

Nucleoside/Nucleotide Analogues

CD4+ Cell

Host DNA

viral DNA

4.

Integrase Inhibitors

Integration of viral DNA

Integrase

5.

Protease

Protease Inhibitors

6.

viral assembly

New copy of HIV

Table 24-2
FDA-Approved HIV Drugs, Early 2008 (Generic Name, Trade Name, Other Identifiers)

Entry/Fusion Inhibitors
  Enfuvirtide, Fuzeon, ENF, T-20
  Maraviroc, Selzentry, UK-247, 857
Nonnucleoside Reverse-Transcriptase Inhibitors
  Delavirdine, Rescriptor, DLV
  Efavirnez, Sustiva, EFV
  Etravirine, Intelence, TMC125
  Nevirapine, Viramune, NVP
Nucleoside/Nucleotide Reverse-Transcriptase Inhibitors
  Abacavir, Ziagen, ABC
  Didanosine, Videx, dideoxyinosine, ddI
  Emtricitabine, Emtriva, FTC
  Lamivudine, Epivir, 3TC
  Stavudine, Zerit, d4T
  Tenofovir DF, Viread, TDF
  Zalcitabine, Hivid, dideoxycytidine, ddC
  Zidovudine, Retrovir, ZDV, azidothymidine, AZT
Integrase Inhibitors
  Raltegravir, Isentress, RGV, MK-0518
Protease Inhibitors
  Atazanavir, Reyataz, ATV
  Darunavir, Prezista, DRV
  Fosamprenavir, Lexiva, FOSAPV, FPV
  Indinavir, Crixivan, IDV
  Lopinavir LPV
  Nelfinavir, Viracept, NFV
  Ritonavir, Norvir, RTV
  Saquinavir, Invirase, SQV
  Tipranavir, Aptivus, TPV
Combination Medications
  Atripla: efavirnez, emtricitabine, tenofovir
  Combivir: lamivudine, zidovudine
  Epzicom: abacavir, lamivudine
  Kaletra: lopinavir, ritonavir
  Trizivir: abacavir, lamivudine, zidovudine
  Truvada: emtricitabine, tenofovir

to prevent the integration of viral DNA into the host cell chromosomes. The role of this agent in postexposure prophylaxis (PEP) is not yet established. The nucleoside/nucleotide analogues and the nonnucleotide reverse-transcriptase inhibitors interfere with reverse-transcriptase conversion of genomic RNA to the proviral DNA. The protease inhibitors interfere with the final steps that produce infective viral units.

Because HIV undergoes essentially continuous replication via an error-prone reverse transcriptase, an individual with chronic infection typically har-

bors a pool of circulating virus with many different mutations. Clinically, it has been observed that a single drug in an infected individual is likely to select for a preexisting resistant virus. Because monotherapy has demonstrated rapid onset of viral resistance, the institution of highly active antiretroviral therapy (HAART), which combines three or more drugs from different classes, has become the standard of care for individuals being treated for HIV/AIDS [39].

Acute HIV Infection

Clinically, the likelihood of transmission depends on the viral titer of the source and the volume and mode of contact of the infectious material. Virus can be recovered eventually from most body fluids and tissues, but only blood products, sexual fluids, breast milk, and visibly bloody fluids have been associated with transmission [40–43]. Based on these data, the CDC has issued a list of body fluids considered to be infectious (Table 24-3) [8]. Viral titer is determined by the natural stage of infection, treatment, treatment failure, and individual viral

Table 24-3
CDC Definition of Blood or Body Fluid Potential for HIV Infection

Potentially Infectious
  Blood
  Human tissue
  Cerebrospinal fluid
  Synovial fluid
  Pleural fluid
  Peritoneal fluid
  Pericardial fluid
  Amniotic fluid
  Semen
  Vaginal secretions
  Any visibly bloody body fluid
Not Considered to Be Infectious
  Feces
  Nasal secretions
  Saliva
  Sputum
  Sweat
  Tears
  Urine
  Vomitus

Source: From Updated U.S. Public Health Service guidelines for the management of occupational exposures to HIV and recommendations for postexposure prophylaxis. *MMWR* 2005;54(RR-9):1–17.

setpoint. In general, it is highest about 3–4 weeks after infection and increases again in late-stage infection or when a particular antiviral regimen is failing [44, 45]. Not surprisingly, clinical and epidemiologic observations document that transmission occurs more often from contact with infected individuals just prior to seroconversion, in late-stage disease, or with a persistent high viral load despite treatment [46, 47].

About 80% of newly antibody-positive individuals recall a brief mononucleosis-like illness, the so-called acute retroviral syndrome, which can occur shortly after transmission and 10–21 days before seroconversion. The clinical manifestations of HIV infection associated with chronic and progressive immunocompromise are not expected for at least many months, more commonly years, and occasionally, a decade or more [44].

Percutaneous exposure is consistently reported to result in seroconversion in about 1 in 300 contacts. However, the risk of actual contacts clearly varies with exposure factors and can be as high as 1 in 20 with penetration of highly infective material into highly vascular tissue [2, 48] (Table 24-4). In the health care setting, blood splashes to oral mucosa and nonintact skin have been rarely associated with transmission [49]. The normal concentration of inflammatory cells in the human mouth could be expected to support receptive transmission, but saliva itself is inhibitory to virus. The rare reports of transmissions owing to bites emphasize both the extent of inflammatory disease and the presence of blood in the mouth of the biter [50]. HIV transmission following a punch to the mouth of a sus-

pect has been reported in a police officer [51]. Isolated HIV transmission has not been associated with ocular mucosal contact alone.

Prevention of Blood Exposure for Health Care Workers

Occupational medicine professionals play a significant role in the ongoing implementation of a comprehensive exposure control plan. Their role in defining the plan will vary depending on the size and needs of a given institution. Table 24-5 contains the essential elements of a prevention program for employees who work with or who potentially may be exposed to bloodborne pathogens. OSHA provides a template exposure control plan to be modified to reflect local specifics [52]. A robust surveillance system for bloodborne pathogen incidents evaluates the potential for occupational exposures among all workers in a medical treatment facility. This may involve employees (both full and part time), temporary employees, contract employees (e.g., contract vendors, agency pools, per-diem employees, and individual service providers), volunteers (including adults and students of high school and college age) and medical, nursing, and other professional students.

A workplace program to evaluate potential employee exposures must be available 24 hours a day. This can occur either on-site or at a referral facility. Regardless of where the evaluation is performed, surveillance data detailing the specifics of exposure

Table 24-4
Factors Predicting Transmission of HIV to Health Care Providers after Percutaneous Exposure

	Adjusted Odds Ratio[a]	Factor (95% CI)[b]
Deep (intramuscular) injury	16.1	6.1–44.6
Visible blood on sharp device	5.2	1.8–17.7
Needle used to enter blood vessel	5.1	1.8–14.8
Source patient with terminal AIDS	6.4	2.2–18.9
Zidovudine prophylaxis used	0.2	0.1–0.6

[a]All were significant at $p < 0.01$.
[b]Confidence interval.
Source: Adapted from Centers for Disease Control and Prevention. Case-control study of HIV seroconversion in health care workers after percutaneous exposure to HIV-infected blood—France, United Kingdom, and United States, January 1988–August 1994 *MMWR* 1995;50:931.

Table 24-5
Essential Elements of an Exposure Control Plan

Determination of employee exposure
Implementation of various methods of exposure control, including
    Universal precautions
    Engineering and work practice controls
    Personal protective equipment
    Housekeeping
Hepatitis B vaccination
Postexposure evaluation and follow-up
Communication of hazards to employees and training
Recordkeeping
Procedures for evaluating circumstances surrounding exposure incidents

Source: From Model Plans and Programs for the OSHA Bloodborne Pathogens and Hazard Communications Standards, 2003; available at *www.osha.gov/Publications/osha3186.html.*

need to be collected. These data should protect the identity of the employee. In addition to complying with the OSHA sharps log requirement, this ensures timely feedback and identification of worksites where training and procedure review need to be restarted owing to a turnover of personnel or need to be reemphasized to existing employees. An important task is to develop a culture of safety within the entire medical treatment facility and a climate where employees feel that they will be seen promptly and without retribution.

Training

The required elements of bloodborne pathogen (BBP) training are outlined in the OSHA bloodborne pathogen standard [53]. Initial training at the onset of at-risk work and follow-up annual refresher training are required for all personnel at risk for bloodborne pathogen exposure. This may be accomplished with a variety of media, including small or large group presentations, Web-based programs, and written training guides. A written or Web-based copy of the facility specific exposure control plan must be available at the worksite with clear directions on what to do in the case of a potential BBP incident. Preemployment evaluations offer an opportunity to remind future employees of the first aid and response plan to blood or body fluid exposures and to emphasize the benefits of prompt reporting.

Personal Protective Equipment, Engineering Controls, and Work Practices

The most important part of universal precautions is the use of personal protective equipment (PPE) by all employees at all appropriate times. Table 24-6 provides a sample PPE precautions guideline. Engineering controls are the physical objects that isolate or eliminate a BBP hazard. Sharps boxes, self-sheathing needles, and needleless access systems are examples that have been used successfully [54–56]. The revised OSHA standard clarifies the need for employers to select safer needle devices and to involve employees in identifying and choosing those devices. Work practice controls (e.g., prohibiting two-handed recapping of needles) are those institutional changes in the manner a task is performed that decrease the chances of an injury.

Table 24-6
Sample Personal Protective Equipment Precautions

All employees using PPE must observe the following precautions:

Wash hands immediately or as soon as feasible after removing gloves or other PPE.

Remove PPE after it becomes contaminated and before leaving the work area.

Used PPE may be disposed of in [list appropriate containers for storage, laundering, decontamination, or disposal].

Wear appropriate gloves when it is reasonably anticipated that there may be hand contact with blood or OPIM and when handling or touching contaminated items or surfaces; replace gloves if torn, punctured, or contaminated or if their ability to function as a barrier is compromised.

Utility gloves may be decontaminated for reuse if their integrity is not compromised; discard utility gloves if they show signs of cracking, peeling, tearing, puncturing, or deterioration.

Never wash or decontaminate disposable gloves for reuse.

Wear appropriate face and eye protection when splashes, sprays, spatters, or droplets of blood or OPIM pose a hazard to the eye, nose, or mouth.

Remove immediately or as soon as feasible any garment contaminated by blood or OPIM in such a way as to avoid contact with the outer surface.

Source: From Model Plans and Programs for the OSHA Bloodborne Pathogens and Hazard Communications Standards, 2003; available at *www.osha.gov/Publications/osha3186.html.*

Proper handling and disposal of sharps and procedures for handling contaminated laundry and clean-up of spills involving blood or other body fluids are important to avoid exposure of coworkers. Although not always clearly considered in the areas at highest risk for BBP incidents, housekeeping and laundry personnel must have appropriate training, including how and where to report an exposure. This training needs to be in an understandable language for the employee.

Institutional commitment to universal precautions, engineering and work practice controls, and PPE can decrease the number of occupational exposures substantially [56]. A clear, well-communicated, and easily accessible plan is crucial to achieve the goal of employees presenting for prompt postexposure evaluation and potential prophylaxis.

Blood Exposure Evaluation

The evaluation of a worker with a potential exposure to HIV should be considered an urgent medical matter that requires prompt attention. The range of psychological reactions by those exposed to HIV can be quite broad. Extreme anxiety can complicate evaluation and treatment decisions. Likewise, denial, anger, or complacency can lead employees to make decisions that they later regret, specifically declining postexposure prophylaxis (PEP) or delaying presentation. These factors necessitate expert medical interviewing skills to assess the employee's state of mind while at the same time assessing the nature of the exposure to formulate a medical plan that is tailored to both the employee and the exposure. Long-term psychological consequences of HIV exposure have been reported, even in the absence of subsequent chronic infection [57].

In the event of human blood or body fluid exposure in a health care setting, traditional labels can become confusing when discussing the case with the employee or with consultants. Clear language is critical to avoid any misunderstandings. One suggested approach is to identify the *source* as one entity and the *employee* as the person exposed. This allows one to have a conversation with the employee about the results of the source's laboratory values without unnecessary confusion. The word *patient* could be applied to either the source or the employee and is potentially the most confusing in a health care setting.

First Aid

When a percutaneous injury or mucosal splash occurs with potentially HIV-infected blood or body fluids, the first step is copious irrigation. If blood can be expressed from a puncture wound, it may be useful both to assess the depth of the wound and to potentially express transmitted virus, but this procedure should not be prolonged at the expense of washing. Wounds should be cleansed with at least soap and water, but some advocate more aggressive decontamination. Povidone-iodine and chlorhexidine at concentrations lower than found in common clinical solutions will effectively kill HIV [58]. Pouring isopropyl alcohol into open wounds or otherwise damaging tissue is not advised. Mucosal exposures such as mouth or eyes should be irrigated for several minutes with tap water or sterile normal saline. The protocol at the National Institutes of Health Occupational Medical Service (NIH OMS) is 15 minutes of gentle scrubbing with a surgical sponge and povidone-iodine for injuries and 15 minutes of irrigation with sterile saline for mu-

cous membrane exposures. This approach is used for consistency and ease of staff training and to ensure adequate first aid in the absence of convincing science about the best approach.

Blood or body fluid on intact skin should be quickly cleansed, but this does not constitute an HIV exposure. There has never been a reported HIV infection following an exposure to intact skin alone. However, previously open wounds (e.g., cuts, abraded skin, or skin condition that results in a disrupted epidermis) that become contaminated with potentially infectious material constitute an exposure and warrant evaluation [8]. While the risk is lower than with other types of exposures, a punch or a bite may necessitate both individuals being evaluated as source and employee for each other if both have broken skin integrity and bleeding.

Because of the emotional stress experienced as a result of an exposure, first aid provided by the employees themselves before reporting to the occupational medical provider may be inadequate. One way to ensure adequate first aid is to repeat the scrubbing after presentation. Care should be taken not to further abrade the skin while performing the scrub. Because of the time-sensitive nature of initiating PEP, as much data about the source and the exposure should be collected while first aid is administered.

Figure 24-2, based on the 2005 CDC guidelines for PEP, outlines the general approach to occupational human blood or body fluid exposure [8]. See Table 24-7 for important historical information that should be gathered. The elapsed time since exposure may drive decisions about the utility of PEP or scrubbing in that delay may render them futile. This information also can identify opportunities for education of employees unaware of the importance of prompt reporting of exposures. The nature of the exposure, the quantity of material, and the history of the source will determine the relative risk of HIV infection. Table 24-7 and Figure 24-2 outline the higher-risk exposures. Recording of safety measures in place at the time of exposure can reveal organizational, equipment, or training lapses that should be addressed either individually or as a part of an ongoing exposure control plan.

Evidence for Postexposure Prophylaxis

The data that support the use of PEP are based on a case-control study in HCWs, indirectly from

Figure 24-2
General approach to occupational human blood or body fluid exposure

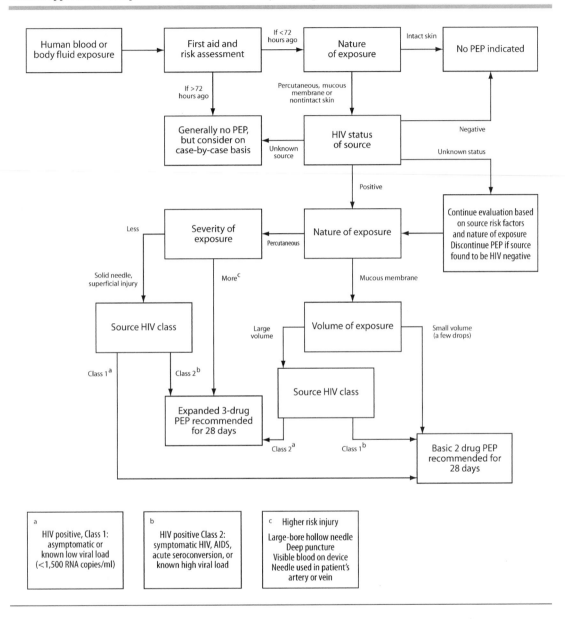

maternal-fetal HIV studies, and animal research. In one case-control study of HCWs exposed to HIV, the risk of HIV infection was reduced by the use of single-agent PEP (AZT) [2]. Studies demonstrate in a primate model that the earlier PEP is initiated, the more effectively it prevents retrovirus infection. Ideally, treatment should begin within the first few hours of exposure. While 72 hours is a general cut-off for no longer offering PEP, there are no absolute limits. Animal data also suggest that short-duration PEP is not as effective as longer treatment [59,60]. Following an HIV exposure, PEP should be given for 28 days [8].

A recent Cochrane review of PEP for occupational HIV exposure acknowledges the limited evidence for PEP and the fact that a randomized, controlled trial is neither ethical nor practical and emphasizes that HCWs should be counseled that

Table 24-7
Important Historical Facts Surrounding a Human
Blood or Body Fluid Exposure

Time of exposure

Nature of exposure (needlestick, splash, etc.)

Safety measures used at time of exposure

Quantity and type of potentially infectious material

Factors influencing infectivity of material (time elapsed
between source to employee, concentrated virus versus fixed
tissue, etc.)

Type and timing of first aid delivered

Known source diagnoses

Social history of source

Medication history of source

Medical history of employee

Current employee medications and allergies

PEP is not 100% effective in preventing HIV seroconversion [61]. None of the HIV medications approved by the FDA have a specific indication for
PEP.

Medical Decision Making for Postexposure Prophylaxis

Several world organizations have addressed PEP in
HCWs exposed to HIV [6–8]. The use of PEP for
nonoccupational exposures also has been addressed
[62]. These guidelines are helpful to formulate a
general plan, but there is no one-size-fits-all approach.

Because the medical decisions involved in providing PEP can be very complicated, expert consultation is often necessary. The University of
California, San Francisco, National Clinician's Postexposure Hotline (1-888-448-4911) has been set up
to assist U.S. providers who have questions about
postexposure evaluation and PEP. This is particularly helpful for those providers who only rarely
deal with HIV exposures. In addition to help with
the decision to initiate PEP, the hotline consultants
also can help with issues of viral resistance, medication selection, and side-effect management.

Testing of the source for hepatitis B, hepatitis C,
and HIV should be performed as soon as possible,
following local requirements for informed consent.
If the source is known to be positive for any of these
infections, repeat testing for antibody is not necessary. Expert consultation for positive sources is recommended because the decisions about further

source testing require detailed knowledge of the
source medical history.

Figure 24-2 addresses the general approach to
PEP decision making based on current CDC guidelines [8]. Table 24-8 lists potentially useful references for clinicians seeking up-to-date guidance on
HIV exposure and PEP.

In cases where the source is unknown (e.g., a
needle in the sharps box), the decision to initiate
PEP should be determined by an assessment of the
kind of work performed in that area, the age of the
sharp, and the general risk of potential sources for
HIV. HIV can survive in a syringe for days to weeks
depending on the volume of blood and viral titer
[63]. However, HIV has been shown to be sensitive
to drying and does not survive well under typical
environmental conditions [64]. HIV RNA was
recovered from only 3.8% of syringes used for intramuscular and subcutaneous injections on HIV-
positive patients [65].

Because viral load is a measure of free virus, it is
only an indirect measure of total body viral burden.
It is still possible to transmit HIV in the face of an
undetectable viral load. Presumably, an undetectable viral load corresponds to a source less
likely to result in HIV infection after an exposure,
but a low viral load should not be the sole determining factor in deciding not to offer PEP [8].

HIV exposure to a source during acute seroconversion presents a clinical challenge. During this
time, viral load and total body viral burden, which
are not detected by antibody measurement, would
be high. There have been no case reports in the

Table 24-8
Resources for Postexposure Prophylaxis and HIV
Treatment

PEPline (for clinical consults regarding PEP, medication side
effects, and viral resistance): www.ucsf.edu/hivcntr/Hotlines/
PEPline; telephone: 888-448-4911

HIV/AIDS Treatment Information Service (drug information,
PDA guidelines, HIV information): http://aidsinfo.nih.gov

HIV Antiretroviral Pregnancy Registry (voluntary reporting of
pregnant women exposed to antiretroviral agent): www
.apregistry.com/index.htm

Food and Drug Administration (for reporting unusual or severe toxicity to antiretroviral agents): www.fda.gov/medwatch;
telephone: 800-332-1088

Centers for Disease Control and Prevention (for reporting HIV
infections in HCP and failures of PEP): telephone: 800-893-
0485

United States of an HCW acquiring infection in this way. However, in the adult film industry, transmission during this "window period" has been documented [4]. In addition, cases of HCW exposure during the window period that were treated with PEP and did not result in seroconversion have been reported abroad [66]. While the authors of that report recommend HIV antigen testing, this is not performed routinely following an exposure. As more sophisticated HIV laboratory testing becomes available, the types of HIV testing performed on sources may change. Increasing availability of rapid HIV antibody testing has made it possible in many places to preliminarily determine a source HIV antibody status within 1 hour. This has decreased the number of doses of PEP given to HCWs while awaiting laboratory results [67]. HIV antigen or HIV RNA testing are not available routinely in all health care settings, and each has its own limitations. Issues arising from false-positive tests must be considered when determining which source laboratory tests to perform. These concerns and routine availability drive the CDC recommendation for HIV antibody testing with reflex confirmatory testing of initial positives. At this time, the CDC does not recommend the routine use of HIV antigen testing following an occupational exposure [8]. The decision to obtain advanced testing or to initiate PEP while awaiting further test results is determined individually based on the specifics of the source history and the nature of the exposure.

The CDC recommends an expanded three- or more-drug PEP regimen for all high-risk exposures. Low-risk exposures from a lower-risk HIV-positive source can be treated with a basic two-drug PEP regimen (see Figure 24-2). European guidelines recommend three-drug therapy for all exposures in contrast to the CDC guidelines [7]. The rationale behind the CDC decision is that the rate of PEP discontinuation is high owing to side effects. The rate is higher for three- or more-drug regimens than for the basic two-drug regimens [68,69]. The majority of human data about PEP come from single-agent prophylaxis, so there is some efficacy for less than triple-drug therapy. The decision comes down to which prevents more occupational infections: a larger percentage of employees completing a possibly less efficacious two-drug regimen or a smaller percentage of employees completing a possibly more efficacious

three- or more-drug regimen. When one also considers the drug-drug interactions, toxicity, and cost, the decision making becomes all that more complex. Finally, because as clinicians we deal with one patient at a time, the applicability of population analyses and statistics to an individual case is often challenging. A group may experience 30% nausea or have a 0.3% risk of infection, but an individual patient either does or does not get infected, have side effects, or discontinue treatment.

PEP Regimens and Side Effects

When PEP was recommended initially by the CDC, there were substantially fewer options available for treatment of HIV. Highlighting the rapidly changing field of anti-HIV therapeutics, the most recent CDC guidelines have a total of eight different basic (two-drug) regimens and seven different expanded (three- or more-drug) regimens [8]. As new drugs become available and more data are added to the literature, it is inevitable that recommendations regarding HIV PEP will change.

The employee's medical history, medication allergies, current prescription and nonprescription drug use, the nature of the exposure, and the source's medication and laboratory history all have an impact on the decision of which PEP regimen to use. An employee should be asked about pregnancy prior to determining PEP regimen. While pregnancy does not preclude the use of PEP, it may influence regimen selection. Pregnancy testing should be offered, if necessary. Efavirenz and nelfinavir are specifically noted for their teratogenic effects on animals. Their use for PEP in pregnancy is contraindicated. Rapid availability of medication is also a factor because the goal is to initiate therapy as quickly as possible following an exposure. In a setting where one anticipates that exposures may occur, having a short-term supply of PEP on hand is recommended.

The basic two-drug regimen currently recommended by CDC guidelines consists of two nucleotide/nucleoside reverse-transcriptase inhibitors (NRTIs) given for 28 days. Either zidovudine or tenofovir is recommended for the first agent, combined with lamivudine or emtricitabine. The availability of fixed-combination tablets has simplified the administration of two of these regimens. Combivir contains 300 mg zidovudine and 150 mg lamivudine and is dosed one tablet twice a day. Truveda contains 300 mg tenofovir and 200 mg emtricitabine and is dosed one tablet a day. The combination of zidovudine and emtricitabine and the combination of tenofovir and lamivudine are the other basic regimen combinations recommended by the CDC. Alternate basic regimens that consist of other combinations of two NRTIs are listed in the CDC guidelines [8]. Common side effects of NRTIs used for PEP include diarrhea, nausea, and fatigue. Serious toxicity (e.g., severe anemia, neutropenia, lactic acidosis, etc.) is rare when NRTIs are used for 28 days.

If an exposure warrants more expanded treatment (see Figure 24-2), the CDC recommends adding drugs to a basic regimen. The preferred expanded regimen includes the addition of lopinavir/ritonavir to the two NRTIs. The combination pill Kaletra contains 200 mg lopinavir and 50 mg ritonavir and is dosed two tablets twice a day. Alternate expanded regimens that consist of adding one or two protease inhibitors to a basic regimen are listed in the CDC guidelines. In addition to the side effects mentioned earlier, patients on Kaletra may develop severe hyperlipidemia. Drug-drug interactions are more common than with the basic regimen [8]. All PEP regimens should be scrutinized for any known drug interactions with the employee's current prescription and nonprescription medications.

HIV viral resistance in the source is a concern if recent drug regimens have failed to lower the viral load or if the source has been intermittently compliant. Expert consultation is recommended for cases in which viral resistance is suspected. The results of HIV viral resistance tests take several days to weeks to obtain. Unless coincidentally available, they would not be useful for PEP regimen decisions. The newer classes of HIV medications have been used anecdotally for PEP [38]. There is theoretical potential for the use of these agents in PEP, but the significance of individual case reports must be determined in light of the rarity of seroconversion without intervention. Current guidelines suggest use of alternative classes of HIV medications for PEP only after expert consultation [8].

HCWs receiving PEP have been shown to have a higher rate of side effects than HIV-positive patients treated with the same medications [70]. It has been reported that about a third of HCWs with an HIV exposure started on PEP will elect to discontinue the medications owing to side effects. Commonly reported side effects were nausea, vomiting, fatigue, headache, diarrhea, dizziness, myalgias, and arthralgias. While the discontinuation rate for PEP was high, only 1–3% of HCWs experienced serious adverse effects [68, 71, 72]. The common side effects of the chosen medications should be discussed with the employee. A plan for side-effect treatment, which may involve additional prescription medications and lifestyle modification (e.g., timing and size of meals, etc.), should be developed.

After initiating PEP, new information may become available that is significant enough to force a change in the regimen. The employee should be scheduled for frequent follow-up appointments to assess medication side effects and compliance, to review patient education, and to discuss any new clinical information.

Laboratory Evaluation and Follow-up

In addition to baseline HIV antibody testing, it is recommended that an employee exposed to HIV receive repeat HIV antibody tests at 6 weeks, 12 weeks, and 6 months following exposure, even if the employee elects not to receive PEP. More frequent or prolonged testing could be determined by the clinical situation surrounding each unique exposure. Testing at 12 months for HIV antibody is specifically recommended for exposures to sources that are co-infected with HIV and hepatitis C [8].

Additional laboratory testing may be necessary to monitor for side effects of PEP. These would be determined by the specific regimen employed but often include complete blood counts, liver function testing, blood chemistries, bilirubin determination, and urinalysis.

All persons exposed to HIV should be counseled to avoid blood or tissue donation while receiving interval antibody testing. The risks of pregnancy and breast-feeding from either HIV or PEP should be discussed, if relevant. Repeating education after the initial stress has improved may be helpful for some employees. The NIH OMS protocol for follow-up of employees on PEP includes scheduled appointments at 72 hours, 2 weeks, and 4 weeks after exposure, with telephone support and additional appointments as need. Every employee is offered referral to a social worker who is experienced in cases of occupational exposure.

Medical Surveillance and Biologic Testing

A number of large institutions have experience with ongoing HIV surveillance in an occupational setting. Serologic testing for HIV was standardized by the U.S. military by the late 1980s [73]. The combination of an enzyme-linked immunosorbent assay (ELISA) for screening and the Western blot electrophoretic assay for confirmation provided overall sensitivity and specificity of greater than 99% [74]. At the National Institutes of Health, the Occupational Medical Service offers a voluntary program for at-risk employees to monitor the potential for seroconversion to the primary retroviruses under study in laboratory and clinical research programs in the various institutes. The mainstay of such a program is periodic testing—yearly for clinical staff and semiannually for laboratory personnel working directly with the viruses. Any institution wishing to establish such a program must be prepared to organize data and maintain records with the most stringent confidentiality and attention to detail. This involves clear understanding and planning for follow-up of both positive and "indeterminate" Western blot results, including communication, counseling, and when necessary, referral of involved employees.

PEP protocols and surveillance programs both generate data on repeat, periodic serologic testing. Large institutions such as the U.S. military and the NIH are able to depend on dedicated computer databases. Steps to ensure the preservation and confidentiality of these databases are integral to these programs. They also permit statistical review and analysis. However, outside these major institutions, it may be much more difficult to collect or to make appropriate use of data regarding occupational HIV infection. For-profit health care institutions may be particularly shy about overtly generating data that might be reviewed to their legal or financial disadvantage. HIV reporting by name is now a requirement in 48 states, the District of Columbia, Guam, Puerto Rico, and the U.S. Virgin Islands. Hawaii and Vermont have code-based reporting. Written HIV consent for testing is re-

quired in 35 states, whereas 28 states require pretest counseling. Any occupational medical service or practitioner planning HIV exposure surveillance can and should explore community, state, and CDC public health data-collection processes and requirements for support.

Employees confirmed as HIV antibody positive, whether or not as a result of occupational exposure, must be referred promptly for appropriate evaluation and follow-up. However, the emotional support and the treatment appropriate for HIV infection are beyond the capabilities of most occupational medical services. Further, attempting to provide appropriate care for HIV infection in a work-based setting may pose an unacceptable violation of privacy.

The HIV-Infected Worker, Americans with Disabilities Act (ADA), and Clearance for Work

As HAART continues to increase the asymptomatic period and overall life expectancy for persons living with HIV, there will be more HIV-infected employees. Because HIV is not transmitted by casual contact, saliva, or fomites, there is no need for work restriction for the majority of asymptomatic HIV-positive workers. As an employee's health declines, comorbid medical illness or treatment side effects may affect the employee's performance or safety. Routine occupational health procedures should be followed to ensure on-the-job safety of the employee and his or her coworkers. Employees who, by the nature of their job and health status, may expose others to their infectious blood or body fluid have been restricted from high-risk activities, but there is no blanket national policy. The American College of Surgeons (ACS) issued a statement against routinely limiting credentials for HIV-infected surgeons [75]. The CDC [76], ACS, and others [77] have provided opinions about how best to address the issue of infected physicians and other HCWs performing similarly invasive procedures.

HIV-positive employees generally should not receive live-virus vaccines, which would preclude work for which such vaccines are required. Asymptomatic HIV infection has been accepted as a disability under the ADA [78]. Decisions about work restrictions for HIV-positive employees should balance realistic estimates of risk. Public opinion about HIV-infected HCWs demonstrates the need for ongoing education about this virus and its transmission [79].

Conclusion

Prevention of occupational HIV exposures can be accomplished with simple, effective, and readily available measures to stop human blood and body fluid exposures. In the hopefully rare event that these universal precautions do not prevent exposure, prompt first aid and PEP can further reduce the chances of an employee becoming infected. Being infected with HIV has transitioned in the past 25 years from a death sentence to a lifelong chronic disease for which treatment is available. It remains a global crisis, and much remains to be done to combat this insidious infection more effectively.

References

1. *Pneumocystis* pneumonia—Los Angeles. *MMWR* 1981;30:250–2.
2. Cardo DM, Culver DH, Ciesielski CA, et al. A case-control study of HIV seroconversion in health care workers after percutaneous exposure. Centers for Disease Control and Prevention Needlestick Surveillance Group. *N Engl J Med* 1997;337:1485–90.
3. Centers for Disease Control and Prevention. Surveillance of Occupationally Acquired HIV/AIDS in Healthcare Personnel, as of December 2006. Atlanta: US Department of Health and Human Services, September 2007; available at www.cdc.gov/ncidod/dhqp/bp_hcp_w_hiv.html#2
4. Brooks JT, Robbins KE, Youngpairoj AS, et al. Molecular analysis of HIV strains from a cluster of worker infections in the adult film industry, Los Angeles 2004. *AIDS* 2006;20:923–8.
5. HIV transmission in the adult film industry—Los Angeles, California, 2004. *MMWR* 2005;54:923–6.
6. World Health Organization. HIV Post-Exposure Prophylaxis for Occupational and Non-Occupational Exposure to HIV Infection. Geneva: WHO, September 2005; available at www.who.int/hiv/topics/arv/HIV-PEPflyer081606.pdf.
7. Puro V, Cicalini S, De Carli G, et al. Post-exposure prophylaxis of HIV infection in healthcare workers: Recommendations for the European setting. *Eur J Epidemiol* 2004;19:577–84.
8. Panlilio AL, Cardo DM, Grohskopf LA, et al. Updated U.S. Public Health Service guidelines for the management of occupational exposures to HIV and recommendations for postexposure prophylaxis. *MMWR* 2005;54:1–17.
9. Dean JA, Ognibene AJ Hepatitis. In Ognibene AJ, Barrett O (eds), *Internal Medicine in Vietnam,* Vol II: *General Medicine and Infectious Diseases.* Washington: Office of the Surgeon General US Army, 1982, pp 397–441.
10. Krugman S. The Willowbrook hepatitis studies revisited: Ethical aspects. *Rev Infect Dis* 1986;8:157–62.
11. Blumberg BS, Sutnick AI, London WT. Australia antigen and hepatitis. *JAMA* 1969;207:1895–6.
12. McCormick RD, Maki DG. Epidemiology of needlestick injuries in hospital personnel. *Am J Med* 1981;70:928–32.
13. Dienstag JL, Ryan DM. Occupational exposure to hepatitis B virus in hospital personnel: Infection or immunization? *Am J Epidemiol* 1982;115:26–39.
14. Centers for Disease Control and Prevention. Universal Precautions for Prevention of Transmission of HIV. Atlanta: CDC, 1996 available at www.cdc.gov/ncidod/dhqp/bp_universal_precautions.html.
15. Barré-Sinoussi F, Chermann JC, Rey F, et al. Isolation of a T-lymphotropic retrovirus from a patient at risk for acquired immune deficiency syndrome (AIDS). *Science* 1983;220:868–71.
16. Gallo RC, Montagnier L. The discovery of HIV as the cause of AIDS. *N Engl J Med* 2003;349:2283–5.
17. Broder S, Gallo RC. A pathogenic retrovirus (HTLV-III) linked to AIDS. *N Engl J Med* 1984;311:1292–7.
18. Recommendations for preventing transmission of infection with human T-lymphotropic virus type III/lymphadenopathy-associated virus in the workplace. *MMWR* 1985;34:681–6, 691–5.
19. Recommendations for prevention of HIV transmission in health-care settings. *MMWR* 1987;36:1–18S.
20. Needlestick transmission of HTLV-III from a patient infected in Africa. *Lancet* 1984;2:1376–7.
21. Update: Human immunodeficiency virus infections in health-care workers exposed to blood of infected patients. *MMWR* 1987;36:285–9.
22. Henderson DK, Gerberding JL. Prophylactic zidovudine after occupational exposure to the human immunodeficiency virus: An interim analysis. *J Infect Dis* 1989;160:321–7.
23. OSHA. Needlestick Injuries. Healthcare Wide Hazards Module—Bloodborne Pathogens; available at www.osha.gov/SLTC/etools/hospital/hazards/bbp/bbp.html#Ninjuries.
24. OSHA, 29 CFR, Section 1910.1030, Bloodborne Pathogens. www.osha.gov/pls/oshaweb/owadisp.show_document?p_table=STANDARDS&p_id=10051.
25. U.S. Department of Labor Bureau of Labor Statistics, www.bls.gov/oco/cg/cgs035.htm.
26. Prüss-Ustün A, Rapiti E, Hutin Y. Estimation of the global burden of disease attributable to contaminated sharps injuries among health-care workers. *Am J Ind Med* 2005;48:482–90.
27. Rischitelli G, Harris J, McCauley L, et al. The risk of acquiring hepatitis B or C among public safety workers: A systematic review. *Am J Prevent Med* 2001;20:299–306.

28. Henderson DK. How're we doin'? Preventing occupational infections with blood-borne pathogens in healthcare. *Infect Control Hosp Epidemiol* 2004;25:532–5.

29. Makary MA, Al-Attar A, Holzmueller CG, et al. Needlestick injuries among surgeons in training. *N Engl J Med* 2007;356:2693–9.

30. Centers for Disease Control and Prevention. HIV/AIDS Surveillance Report, 2005. Vol. 17, rev ed. Atlanta: US Department of Health and Human Services, 2007; available at www.cdc.gov/hiv/topics/surveillance/resources/reports/.

31. Sharp PM, Li WH. Understanding the origins of AIDS viruses. *Nature* 1988;336:315.

32. Myers G, MacInnes K, Korber B. The emergence of simian/human immunodeficiency viruses. *AIDS Res Hum Retroviruses* 1992;8:373–86.

33. McCutchin FE. Global diversification of HIV. In Crandall KA (ed), *The Evolution of HIV*. Baltimore: Johns Hopkins University Press, 1999, pp 41–101.

34. Barker E, Barnett SW, Stamatatos L, et al. The human immunodeficiency viruses. In Levy JA (ed), *The Retroviridae*, Vol 4. New York: Plenum Press, 1995, pp 1–67.

35. Pope M, Haase AT. Transmission, acute HIV-1 infection and the quest for strategies to prevent infection. *Nat Med* 2003;9:847–52.

36. Emmelkamp JM, Rockstroh JK. CCR5 antagonists: Comparison of efficacy, side effects, pharmacokinetics and interactions—Review of the literature. *Eur J Med Res* 2007;12:409–17.

37. *FDA-Approved HIV AIDS Drugs;* available at www.fda.gov/oashi/aids/virals.html.

38. Méchai F, Quertainmont Y, Sahali S, et al. Postexposure prophylaxis with a maraviroc-containing regimen after occupational exposure to a multiresistant HIV-infected source person. *J Med Virol* 2008;80:9–10.

39. Panel on Antiretroviral Guidelines for Adult and Adolescents. Guidelines for the Use of Antiretroviral Agents in HIV-1-Infected Adults and Adolescents. Washington: US Department of Health and Human Services, January 29, 2008, pp 1–128; available at www.aidsinfo.nih.gov/ContentFiles/AdultandAdolescentGL.pdf.

40. Levy JA. The transmission of HIV and factors influencing progression to AIDS. *Am J Med* 1993;95:86–100.

41. Royce RA, Seña A, Cates W, et al. Sexual transmission of HIV. *N Engl J Med* 1997;336:1072–8.

42. Gershon RR, Vlahov D, Nelson KE. The risk of transmission of HIV-1 through non-percutaneous, non-sexual modes: A review. *AIDS* 1990;4:645–50.

43. Hughes SC. HIV and pregnancy: Twenty-five years into the epidemic. *Int Anesthesiol Clin* 2007;45:29–49.

44. Zetola NM, Pilcher CD. Diagnosis and management of acute HIV infection. *Infect Dis Clin North Am* 2007;21:19–48, vii.

45. Buckheit RW. Understanding HIV resistance, fitness, replication capacity and compensation: Targeting viral fitness as a therapeutic strategy. *Exp Opin Invest Drugs* 2004;13:933–58.

46. de Vincenzi I. A longitudinal study of human immunodeficiency virus transmission by heterosexual partners. European Study Group on Heterosexual Transmission of HIV. *N Engl J Med* 1994;331:341–6.

47. Dickover RE, Garratty EM, Herman SA, et al. Identification of levels of maternal HIV-1 RNA associated with risk of perinatal transmission: Effect of maternal zidovudine treatment on viral load. *JAMA* 1996;275:599–605.

48. Baggaley RF, Boily M, White RG, et al. Risk of HIV-1 transmission for parenteral exposure and blood transfusion: A systematic review and meta-analysis. *AIDS* 2006;20:805–12.

49. Do AN, Ciesielski CA, Metler RP, et al. Occupationally acquired human immunodeficiency virus (HIV) infection: National case surveillance data during 20 years of the HIV epidemic in the United States. *Infect Control Hosp Epidemiol* 2003;24:86–96.

50. Bartholomew CF, Jones AM. Human bites: A rare risk factor for HIV transmission. *AIDS* 2006;20:631–2.

51. Abel S, Césaire R, Cales-Quist D, et al. Occupational transmission of human immunodeficiency virus and hepatitis C virus after a punch. *Clin Infect Dis* 2000;31:1494–5.

52. OSHA. Model Plans and Programs for the OSHA Bloodborne Pathogens and Hazard Communications Standards, 2003; available at www.osha.gov/Publications/osha3186.html.

53. Occupational exposure to bloodborne pathogens—OSHA. Final rule. *Fed Reg* 1991;56:64004–182.

54. Beekmann SE, Vlahov D, Koziol DE, et al. Temporal association between implementation of universal precautions and a sustained, progressive decrease in percutaneous exposures to blood. *Clin Infect Dis* 1994;18:562–9.

55. Haiduven DJ, DeMaio TM, Stevens DA. A five-year study of needlestick injuries: Significant reduction associated with communication, education, and convenient placement of sharps containers. *Infect Control Hosp Epidemiol* 1992;13:265–71.

56. Azar-Cavanagh M, Burdt P, Green-McKenzie J. Effect of the introduction of an engineered sharps injury prevention device on the percutaneous injury rate in healthcare workers. *Infect Control Hosp Epidemiol* 2007;28:165–70.

57. Worthington MG, Ross JJ, Bergeron EK. Posttraumatic stress disorder after occupational HIV exposure: two cases and a literature review. *Infect Control Hosp Epidemiol* 2006;27:215–7.

58. Harbison MA, Hammer SM. Inactivation of human immunodeficiency virus by Betadine products and chlorhexidine. *J Acquir Immune Defic Syndr* 1989;2:16–20.

59. Grob PM, Cao Y, Muchmore E, et al. Prophylaxis

against HIV-1 infection in chimpanzees by nevirap-ine, a nonnucleoside inhibitor of reverse transcrip-tase. *Nat Med* 1997;3:665–70.

60. Tsai CC, Emau P, Follis KE, et al. Effectiveness of postinoculation (*R*)-9-(2-phosphonylmethoxy-propyl) adenine treatment for prevention of persis-tent simian immunodeficiency virus SIVmne infection depends critically on timing of initiation and duration of treatment. *J Virol* 1998;72:4265–73.

61. Young TN, Arens FJ, Kennedy GE, et al. Antiretrovi-ral post-exposure prophylaxis (PEP) for occupa-tional HIV exposure. *Cochrane Database Syst Rev* 2007;1:CD002835.

62. Smith DK, Grohskopf LA, Black RJ, et al. Antiretro-viral postexposure prophylaxis after sexual, injec-tion-drug use, or other nonoccupational exposure to HIV in the United States: Recommendations from the U.S. Department of Health and Human Services. *MMWR* 2005;54:1–20.

63. Heimer R, Abdala N. Viability of HIV-1 in syringes: implications for interventions among injection drug users. *AIDS Read* 2000;10:410–7.

64. Tjøtta E, Hungnes O, Grinde B. Survival of HIV-1 activity after disinfection, temperature and pH changes, or drying. *J Med Virol* 1991;35:223–7.

65. Rich JD, Dickinson BP, Carney JM, et al. Detection of HIV-1 nucleic acid and HIV-1 antibodies in nee-dles and syringes used for non-intravenous injec-tion. *AIDS* 1998;12:2345–50.

66. Giulieri S, Schiffer V, Yerly S, et al. The trap: profes-sional exposure to human immunodeficiency virus antibody negative blood with high viral load. *Arch Intern Med* 2007;167:2524–6.

67. Landrum ML, Wilson CH, Perri LP, et al. Usefulness of a rapid human immunodeficiency virus-1 anti-body test for the management of occupational ex-posure to blood and body fluid. *Infect Control Hosp Epidemiol* 2005;26:768–74.

68. Wang SA, Panlilio AL, Doi PA, et al. Experience of healthcare workers taking postexposure prophylaxis after occupational HIV exposures: Findings of the HIV Postexposure Prophylaxis Registry. *Infect Con-trol Hosp Epidemiol* 2000;21:780–5.

69. Bassett IV, Freedberg KA, Walensky RP. Two drugs or three? Balancing efficacy, toxicity, and resistance in postexposure prophylaxis for occupational expo-sure to HIV. *Clin Infect Dis* 2004;39:395–401.

70. Quirino T, Niero F, Ricci E, et al. HAART tolerabil-ity: Post-exposure prophylaxis in healthcare workers versus treatment in HIV-infected patients. *Antivir Ther* 2000;5:195–7.

71. Kiertiburanakul S, Wannaying B, Tonsuttakul S, et al. Tolerability of HIV postexposure prophylaxis among healthcare workers. *J Hosp Infect* 2006;62: 112–4.

72. Lee LM, Henderson DK. Tolerability of postexpo-sure antiretroviral prophylaxis for occupational ex-posures to HIV. *Drug Saf* 2001;24:587–97.

73. Brown AA, Brundage JF, Tomlinson JP, et al. The US Army HIV testing program: The first decade. *Milit Med* 1996;161:117–22.

74. Damato JJ, O'Bryen BN, Fuller SA, et al. Resolution of indeterminate HIV-1 test data using the Depart-ment of Defense HIV-1 testing program. *Lab Med* 1991;22:107–13.

75. American College of Surgeons Statement on the surgeon and HIV infection. Revised May 2004; available at www.facs.org/fellows_info/statements/st-13.html.

76. Recommendations for preventing transmission of human immunodeficiency virus and hepatitis B virus to patients during exposure-prone invasive procedures. *MMWR* 1991;40:1–9.

77. Reitsma AM, Closen ML, Cunningham M, et al. In-fected physicians and invasive procedures: Safe practice management. *Clin Infect Dis* 2005;40:1665–72.

78. *Bragdon* v. *Abbott* (97-156) 107 F.3d 934, vacated and remanded. http://supct.law.cornell.edu/supct/html/97-156.ZO.html.

79. Tuboku-Metzger J, Chiarello L, Sinkowitz-Cochran RL, et al. Public attitudes and opinions toward physicians and dentists infected with bloodborne viruses: Results of a national survey. *Am J Infect Control* 2005;33:299–303.

25 Occupational Malaria

Bruce A. Barron and Mark J. Utell

Malaria is a tropical parasitic infection that has successfully evaded scientific advances in prevention, control, and treatment. Although the incidence of vector-borne malaria in the United States is exceptionally low, international travelers account for more than 1,000 imported cases annually [1–3]. Imported malaria has become a growing health concern in geographic regions where the disease has been eradicated previously, for example, North America and Europe. In 2003, there were 10 cases of malaria acquired in the United States, whereas 4 individuals were infected in 2004 [3, 4]. Occupational malaria, for the most part, is an acquired illness resulting from travel to malaria-endemic regions of the world (Figure 25-1). Employees (both military and civilian) traveling to regions having high transmission rates, drug-resistant parasites, and/or insecticide-resistant mosquitoes are at the greatest risk of contracting this disease [5].

Malaria was first described by Hippocrates during the fourth century BC, and despite its long history, the etiology and natural course of the disease were not completely delineated until the early twentieth century. Clear delineation of the malaria parasite life cycle also has been crucial to our understanding of transmission risk factors (Table 25-1), which are both complex and multifactorial. Ultimately, transmission risks depend on a delicate balance between the *Plasmodium* agent, mosquito vector, susceptible human host, and environmental conditions, as shown in Figure 25-2. Each facet of this balance is reviewed in this chapter.

Plasmodium Organisms

The *Plasmodium* life cycle follows a pattern of asexual reproduction in the human host and sexual reproduction in the mosquito vector. There are four species of the *Plasmodium* agent that naturally infect humans: *P. falciparum, P. vivax, P. ovale,* and *P. malariae.*

P. falciparum is the most virulent of the species. It accounts for nearly half the world's malaria infections and more than 95% of deaths owing to malaria [6]. *P. falciparum* is most abundant in sub-Saharan Africa, New Guinea, and Haiti [6, 7]. *P. vivax* predominates in the Indian subcontinent, Middle East, and Central America [6, 7]. The prevalence of these two species is similar in Southeast Asia, Oceana, and South America. *P. malariae* and *P. ovale* infections are relatively unusual outside Africa [6, 7]. *P. malariae* is remarkable because this species has the ability to persist in the circulatory system for years without causing symptoms. These infectious agents have gained renewed public health interest as a result of the recent emergence of drug-resistant strains, which have precipitated in an increased incidence and geographic distribution of the disease [8].

Figure 25-1
Approximate Geographic Distribution of Malaria

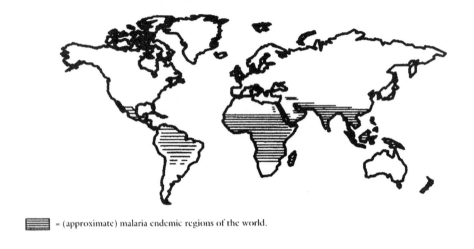

= (approximate) malaria endemic regions of the world.

Figure 25-2
Major Factors Affecting Malaria Transmission in Travelers (Transmission risk depends on the interactions and relative balance of each factor. See text for details.)

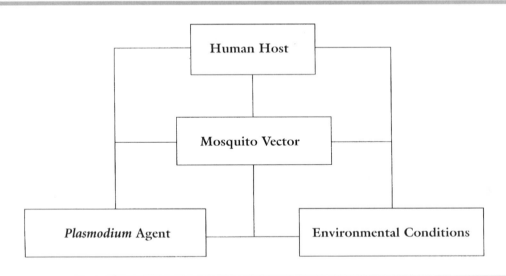

There are no free-living forms of this parasite. Human hosts represent the only significant reservoir for the organism [9]. Although other primate malarias can infect humans, natural transmission is extremely rare [10]. Transmission of malaria from infected mosquitoes to humans is strongly dependent on the sporozoite rate (i.e., the ratio of infective to noninfective female anopheline mosquitoes), whereas the sporozoite rate depends on the mosquito vector's susceptibility to parasitic infection, in vivo parasite replication, vector longevity, and vector population densities [11].

As a host, humans serve an important role in the life cycle of the malaria parasite. Even though malaria can be transmitted congenitally [12], through blood transfusions [13], and through exposure to bloodborne pathogens [14, 15], the preponderance of the disease is transmitted through

Table 25-1
Malaria Transmission Risk Factors in Traveling
Employees

Environmental
  Geographic region (high to low risk)
  West Africa
  East Africa
  Indian subcontinent
  Far East
  South America
  Central America
  Rainy seasons
  Regions with poor pest control
  Ambient temperatures between 16 and 33°C
  Elevations less than 2,000 m
Mosquito vector
  A. gambiae, A. arabiensis, and *A. funestus*
  Mosquito vector population densities (high)
  Mosquito vector longevity (prolonged)
  Mosquito insecticide resistance
Plasmodium **agent**
  P. falciparum (greater than non-*falciparum* forms)
  Plasmodium drug resistance
  Sporozoite rates (high)
Human host
  Repeated or prolonged trips to malaria-endemic areas
  Repeated or prolonged nighttime exposure in malaria-
  endemic areas
  Inadequate antimosquito measures and chemoprophylaxis
  Poor compliance with antimosquito measures and chemo-
  prophylaxis
  Poor health status/preexisting systemic illness
  Sensitivities/allergies to chemoprophylactic and therapeutic
  agents
  Nonimmune status
  Pregnancy

the bite of an infective female *Anopheles* species mosquito. This mosquito is the only known vector for malaria [9, 16]. Although these mosquitoes feed from dusk until dawn, their feeding activity may vary considerably throughout the night depending on the species [7, 16, 17]. Conversely, it is important for occupational physicians to realize that mosquitoes that bite during the day do not transmit malaria [16, 17]. *A. gambiae* mosquitoes are effective vectors because this species is ubiquitous, long-lived (5–25% daily mortality rate), and anthropophilic (have a preference for human hosts) [9, 18]. These factors make them especially effective vectors [19, 20].

There are other highly anthropophilic and long-lived anophelines, such as *A. dirus,* found in Southeast Asia. Fortunately, *A. dirus* mosquitoes breed in small forest pools and usually are not a problem in domestic environments. This is unlike *A. gambiae,* which are well adapted to human habitats. Studies suggest that rural villagers living in high-transmission areas may be bitten 50–100 times per night by *A. gambiae* mosquitoes (having a 5% sporozoite rate). Since these mosquitoes rest after blood meals on house walls (i.e., endophilic), they are susceptible to malaria vector control measures (e.g., spraying the house with a residual insecticide) [21]. *Anopheles* mosquitoes also have a broad geographic distribution. This species still can be found in the United States and has been implicated recently in three outbreaks of vector-borne malaria from infected migrant workers in Texas, New Jersey, and California [1, 3, 22, 23].

Malaria transmission depends on a number of environmental factors, including geographic location, season, climate, deforestation, irrigation, and pest control measures. Unfortunately, many anopheline mosquitoes have developed resistance to chlorinated insecticides, organophosphates, and carbamates [24]. Ambient temperature and ground elevation are also important determinants of transmission risk because sporogeny cannot take place in temperatures below 16°C or above 33°C or in extremely arid climates, heavy rains, or altitudes above 2,000 m [9, 14, 15]. Transmission rates are higher during the rainy seasons because the moisture fosters mosquito breeding sites [15, 25].

Plasmodium Life Cycle

The *Plasmodium* life cycle begins when a female *Anopheles* mosquito ingests infected human blood containing the sexual stages of the parasite (gametocytes), as depicted in Figure 25-3. Male and female gametocytes unite to form the ookinete inside the mosquito's stomach. The ookinete subsequently penetrates the stomach wall and forms a cyst containing thousands of sporozoites on its outer surface. This process requires 8–35 days depending on the species of parasite and the vector's ambient temperature. Sporozoites migrate to the salivary glands and other organs of the infected mosquito, rendering them infective for life. Infective mosquitoes inject 5–100 motile sporozoites into the human host during a blood meal. The sporozoites

Figure 25-3
The *Plasmodium* Life Cycle. (The left side of the figure summarizes the sexual [mosquito] phase and the right side of the figure summarizes the asexual [human] phase of the life cycle.)

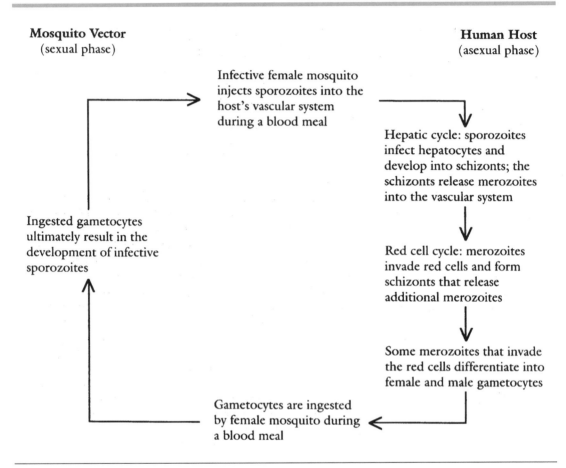

rapidly invade hepatocytes and develop into exo-erythrocytic schizonts. After the sporozoites mature, the hepatocytes rupture and release between 10^5 and 10^6 asexual parasites (merozoites) into the hepatic sinusoids and vascular system.

In *P. vivax* and *P. ovale* infections, a small number of organisms lie dormant in the liver for several months to years before multiplying. These sleeping forms of the parasite (known as *hypnozoites*) can cause either delayed primary attacks or relapses in the future [26]. It is for this reason that *P. vivax* and *P. ovale* infections have been labeled *relapsing malarias*. Conversely, *P. falciparum* and *P. malariae* do not form hypnozoites, and as a result, relapses do not occur.

The merozoites (released by hepatocyte rupture) quickly invade susceptible circulating red blood cells, where they grow and multiply cyclically [27]. Most of the merozoites develop into asexual forms. Merozoites differentiate from early trophozoites (ring forms) to mature blood schizonts that rupture the red blood cell, releasing 8–30 free merozoites, which invade other red blood cells. This process takes 48 hours for *P. falciparum*, *P. vivax*, and *P. ovale* infections (tertian fevers) and 72 hours for *P. malariae* infections (quartan fever). Clinical symptoms parallel the rupture of red blood cell schizonts.

After 3–15 days, red blood cell merozoites that did not differentiate into asexual forms may develop into male (microgametocyte) or female (macrogametocyte) sexual forms. Gametocytes do not cause symptoms. These sexual forms may circulate for months to years in the bloodstream until they are ingested by an anopheline mosquito during a blood meal. Within the mosquito's midgut, thousands of new infective sporozoites are formed, and the life cycle begins again [9, 14].

In summary, the mosquito must feed twice on humans to transmit malaria. They must first ingest human blood infected with the sexual stages of the parasite, survive 8–35 days for the gametocytes to mature to sporozoites, and then bite another susceptible human host to transmit the disease [19, 20].

Epidemiology

Its global impact on morbidity and mortality makes malaria one of the most important tropical diseases. This parasitic disease is endemic in more than 100 countries, and nearly 40% of the world's population lives in endemic tropical regions [10]. Malaria has an estimated prevalence of 300–500 million persons and accounts for more than 1 million deaths annually [6, 7]. Although malaria has been eradicated from North America, Europe, and Russia, the emergence of drug-resistant parasites and pesticide-resistant mosquitoes has resulted in a resurgence of the disease in the tropics [28–30]. Despite significant advances in malaria prevention and control, the burden of disease has increased dramatically over the past several decades [31–33].

Each year about 8 million U.S. civilians travel to malaria-endemic countries, and nearly 30,000 contract malaria [34–36]. Longitudinal studies of North American and European travelers in Africa reveal an incidence of 15 cases per 1,000 travelers per month and a 2–4% mortality rate [5, 37–40]. Malaria in the United States is, for the most part, limited to imported cases in travelers, military personnel, and immigrants from malaria-endemic countries [41]. Nonimported infections in the United States have been acquired rarely through the bite of an infected *Anopheles* mosquito entering the country in aircraft returning from malaria-endemic regions (airport malaria) [42–45], congenitally from an infected mother, iatrogenically through blood transfusion (induced malaria), and by local transmission (autochthonous malaria) from persons with imported disease who serve as the reservoir for local vector mosquitoes [1, 3, 22, 23]. From an occupational perspective, individuals at highest risk include military personnel, traveling federal employees, foreign-service diplomats, cor-

porate travelers, expatriated business executives, commercial airline crews, airport employees, and maritime employees.

Prevention and Control

It is important to remember that occupational malaria is a preventable disease. The risk of contracting this disease within a given geographic region depends on the presence of malaria parasites, vector mosquitoes, susceptible human hosts, and favorable environmental conditions. Interventions designed to eliminate or control one or more of these risk factors significantly decrease the incidence of disease in the occupational setting.

Although both genetic resistance and immunity decrease the morbidity of malaria, these traits are unlikely to be significant factors in the prevention of occupational malaria. Resistance to infection occurs in employees who have sickle cell trait, hereditary ovalocytosis, or absent Duffy blood group antigen on their red blood cells, but this population represents a small proportion of the traveling workforce at any given point in time [46, 47]. Natural immunity in U.S. travelers is also unlikely because this requires prolonged residence in hyperendemic regions and repeated infections. Natural immunity is species-specific, strain-specific, and stage-specific (asexual forms of the parasite), and it is acquired gradually [48]. Natural immunity confers only partial immunity (semi-immunity), and subsequent attacks still can occur, albeit at decreased frequency and severity. Most tropical residents have asymptomatic infections by 10 years of age through the development of antitoxic immunity or premunition (a state in which an active low-grade infection establishes resistance to reinfection). Since the nonimmune traveler usually lacks genetic resistance, partial homologous immunity (immunity derived from members of a single species), and premunition, occupationally acquired infections are more likely to be fulminant and lethal.

Education, training, and appropriate application of antimosquito measures are important factors in preventing occupational malaria. Since anopheline mosquitoes are endophilic and bite from dusk to dawn, traveling employees should be encouraged to observe the following antimosquito measures [49]:

- Remain in air-conditioned and/or well-screened facilities after sunset.
- Avoid the use of perfumes that would attract mosquitoes.
- Wear protective long-sleeved clothes (sprayed with permethrin insecticide when feasible).
- Apply a topical insecticide such as 30–35% diethyltoluamide (DEET) to exposed skin areas [7, 16].
- Use bed nets impregnated with permethrin [16, 17, 50, 51].
- Spray living areas with pyrethrum-containing insecticide before bedtime.

Chemoprophylaxis is another measure that may be effective in the primary prevention of occupational malaria. Commonly prescribed chemoprophylactic agents are summarized in Table 25-2 [7, 14–17, 35]. The goal of chemoprophylactic agents is to prevent the occurrence of infection (causal prophylaxis) and/or abort clinical disease (suppressive prophylaxis).

It is interesting to note that the most frequently used chemoprophylactic agents (i.e., chloroquine, mefloquine, and doxycycline) do not kill sporozoites or liver forms of the parasite and, as such, do not actually prevent malaria infections. They eradicate asexual blood forms, which subsequently aborts clinical manifestations of the disease [52]. Chemoprophylaxis (except for doxycycline) is usually started 1–2 weeks before entering a malaria-endemic area to allow sufficient time for adequate blood levels to develop; however, this procedure has never been validated [53]. The major rationale for initiating these agents prior to entering a malaria-endemic area is to establish the habit of taking the

Table 25-2
Medications Commonly Used in the Prevention of Malaria

Chemoprophylactic agents (choice depends on local *Plasmodium* sensitivities)

Chloroquine salt, 500 mg/week

Doxycycline, 100 mg/day

Mefloquine salt, 250 mg/week

Proguanil, 200 mg/day, in combination with chloroquine weekly

Terminal prophylaxis (*P. vivax* and *P. ovale*)

Primaquine base, 15 mg orally once daily for 14 days, or 45 mg orally weekly for 6–8 weeks after exposure

medication and to identify adverse drug effects prior to departure. Chemoprophylactic agents should be continued during the exposure and for a 4-week period after departure from the malaria-endemic area. This allows sufficient time for the incubating liver forms to mature and be released into the bloodstream, where suppressive drugs are biologically active [10, 16–18, 35].

Chloroquine is the prophylactic agent of choice for travel to countries not exhibiting chloroquine-resistant parasites [10, 16, 18, 35, 54]. It has a serum half-life of 7–10 days, and the usual dose is 500 mg chloroquine phosphate (300 mg base) once weekly. Chloroquine's exact mechanism of action has not been fully elucidated; however, this drug appears to exert its antimalarial activity on the hemoglobin-containing digestive vesicles of the parasite. Although chloroquine is usually well tolerated, adverse health effects are dose-related and have been reported in 23% of travelers [40]. The most frequent adverse drug effects include mild nausea, abdominal discomfort, and diarrhea. Less frequent side effects include headache, light-headedness, fatigue, emesis, pruritus, and erythema [40, 55]. Rare side effects include photosensitization, myopathy, and aplastic anemia. Prophylactic doses of chloroquine also have been reported to cause neuropsychiatric toxicity (e.g., toxic psychosis, hallucinations, and disorientation) [40, 56]. The incidence of severe adverse reactions necessitating physician consultation or hospitalization has been estimated to be 1 in 7,000 travelers who have taken chemoprophylaxis [40].

Mefloquine, 250 mg salt once weekly, is the chemoprophylactic agent of choice for employees traveling to geographic regions harboring chloroquine-resistant *P. falciparum* and *P. vivax*. It should be started 1–2 weeks prior to travel and taken weekly during the exposure and for 4 weeks after departure from the malarious area. Although mefloquine initially had been reported to be 90–95% effective in preventing malaria [7, 15, 54, 57], a meta-analysis reported significantly lower efficacy rates [58]. The rate of adverse drug effects (e.g., depression, dreams, fatigue, headache, insomnia, anorexia, abdominal discomfort, nausea, vomiting, fever, and pruritus) and drug discontinuance were high in most of the studies analyzed. The authors concluded that this outcome was likely to impair mefloquine's effectiveness and preclude its routine use for chemoprophylaxis in travelers [58]. It is important to note that chemoprophylactic doses of mefloquine may cause the same severe neuropsychiatric effects found in therapeutic doses, but much less frequently (1 in 10,000 travelers) [40, 56].

Doxycycline, 100 mg daily, is reportedly 88–100% effective in preventing malaria and is the preferred chemoprophylactic agent for individuals unable to take mefloquine (e.g., pilots and mefloquine-intolerant employees) who are traveling to geographic regions with chloroquine-resistant malaria. It is also the drug of choice for travelers to Thailand, where *P. falciparum* is mefloquine-resistant. Doxycycline should be taken 2–3 days before travel, daily during the exposure, and for 4 weeks after exposure. The most commonly reported side effects are nausea, epigastric distress, and vaginal candidiasis. Doxycycline may cause severe photosensitivity reactions; therefore, it should be prescribed in conjunction with a sunscreen. Pregnant women and other travelers who are unable to take doxycycline or mefloquine should be advised not to travel to geographic regions of chloroquine or mefloquine resistance because there are no safe and effective chemoprophylactic alternatives [7, 16–18, 35].

Atovaquone-proguanil is a combination drug that was approved by the U.S. Food and Drug Administration (FDA) in the year 2000 for the prevention and treatment of acute, uncomplicated *P. falciparum* malaria. Atovaquone is a selective inhibitor of parasite mitochondrial electron transport. Proguanil, through its metabolite cycloguanil, acts as a dihydrofolate reductase inhibitor. For chemoprophylaxis, the dose is one adult tablet taken once daily. The first dose should be taken 1–2 days prior to travel in malaria-endemic areas such as Africa, South America, the Indian subcontinent, Tajikistan, Asia, and the South Pacific. The traveler should continue the once-daily regimen during travel in the malaria-endemic region and for 7 days after departure. The most commonly reported side effects include abdominal pain, nausea, vomiting, and headache. Atovaquone-proguanil is contraindicated in individuals with known hypersensitivity to any of its components and severe renal insufficiency, as well as in women who are pregnant or breast-feeding infants weighing less than 11 kg (25 lb) [59].

Since chloroquine, mefloquine, doxycycline, and atovaquone-proguanil are not active against hypnozoites, travelers to areas of the world where *P. vivax* and *P. ovale* are indigenous species must follow these agents with a 2-week course of primaquine (terminal prophylaxis) to prevent relapse [7, 15–17, 54, 59]. Relapses can occur weeks or months after discontinuing schizonticidal drugs; thus terminal prophylaxis should at least partially overlap the terminal weeks of chloroquine, mefloquine, or doxycycline prophylaxis. When atovaquone-proguanil is used for prophylaxis, primaquine may be taken either during the last 7 days of the atovaquone-proguanil regimen and then for an additional 7 days or for 14 days after atovaquone-proguanil prophylaxis is completed. Although primaquine is usually well tolerated, the most common adverse drug effects include abdominal discomfort, nausea, headache, and pruritus. Since primaquine is a potent oxidant, it can cause severe hemolytic anemia in persons with glucose-6-phosphate dehydrogenase (G-6-PD) deficiency. Similarly, pregnant women should not be prescribed primaquine because the G-6-PD status of the fetus is unknown. This is primaquine's most common serious adverse effect; therefore, the G-6-PD status of an employee must be established prior to its administration. This drug should be taken at a dose of 30 mg daily (26.3-mg primaquine phosphate tablets are equivalent to 15-mg primaquine base tablets) for 14 days.

According to Behrens and Curtis, the efficacy of chemoprophylactic agents measured in terms of percent risk reduction compared with unmedicated controls was 66% for chloroquine and 61% for doxycycline, assuming 100% compliance [60]. One should note that these efficacy calculations assumed 100% compliance and that compliance itself was a major confounder of the data. Studies assessing drug compliance have yielded high *noncompliance* rates ranging from 23% in travelers visiting West Africa [61], to 72% in hospitalized patients with confirmed malaria [60], to 75% in airline flight attendants [62]. Compliance in U.S. travelers also has been reportedly low [63]. Some 62% of American travelers who developed malaria did not take chemoprophylaxis, whereas another 15% did not take the appropriate prophylactic regimen suggested by the Centers for Disease Control and Prevention (CDC). Furthermore, only two-thirds of travelers continued chemoprophylaxis for a full 4 weeks after their departure from malaria-endemic regions [40].

The emergence of drug-resistant parasites and insecticide-resistant vectors has made vaccine development more compelling. As a result, there has been a considerable amount of research and funding directed toward vaccine development during the past two decades. Although initial clinical trials are currently in progress and have demonstrated promising results, vaccine licensing still appears to be several years away. Many vaccines in current use have been developed against diseases for which natural infection confers lifelong immunity; however, malaria infections do not routinely confer such prolonged immunity. The partial immunity conferred by infection is not only temporary but also species-, strain-, and stage-specific [18, 64]. Ultimately, a vaccine that proves effective most likely will stimulate both humoral and cell-mediated immunity and contain antigens from all three malarial stages: sporozoite, merozoite, and gametocyte. In fact, CDC scientists are in the process of developing multistage, multiple-target artificial proteins for vaccine candidates (FALVAC) using selected antigenic targets (epitomes) from different lifecycle stages [65]. Other future directions for malaria prevention and control include the sequencing of the entire P. falciparum genome to identify opportunities to improve diagnostic methods and to develop new antimalarial drugs and vaccines [66]. There are also current efforts to develop transgenic mosquitoes that are incapable of becoming infected by and transmitting malaria.

Symptoms and Signs

The early recognition and diagnosis of malaria can be quite challenging because the initial symptoms are nonspecific and similar to those of many other infections (e.g., fever, chills, general malaise, fatigue, headache, myalgias, and mild abdominal discomfort). The acute symptoms of malaria typically occur after an incubation period of 8–16 days. The average time interval between infective bites and onset of symptoms is approximately 7–14 days for P. falciparum, 7–30 days for P. malariae, and 8–14 days for P. vivax and P. ovale. Infected employees may complain of fatigue, headache, myalgias, arthralgias, vague abdominal discomfort, and dys-

phoria [67–69]. To those unfamiliar with the disease (e.g., nonimmune patients and nontropical physicians), these nonspecific symptoms frequently are attributed to flulike illnesses, whereas semi-immune persons often recognize them as an early prodrome of the disease.

The classic malarial paroxysm has three stages: (1) The chill stage begins with a sudden shaking chill that lasts 15–90 minutes, (2) the hot stage is associated with temperature spikes up to 42°C, and (3) the sweating stage begins as the temperature falls below 39°C and the victim sweats profusely. The paroxysm usually subsides 4–8 hours later and is followed by fatigue and sleep. Table 25-3 summarizes the most common signs and symptoms of imported malaria observed in military and civilian tropical travelers [10]. Nearly all travelers complained of fever, chills, rigors, diaphoresis, and headache, but only one-third presented with classic paroxysms.

Complicated malaria is almost always caused by P. falciparum. The risk of complicated malaria increases as parasitemias rise above 2% in nonimmune or pregnant employees and above 5% in semi-immune hosts. The most frequent complications include coma, seizures, renal failure, hemoglobinuria (blackwater fever), noncardiogenic pulmonary edema, profound hypoglycemia, bleeding, coagulopathy, and jaundice [10]. The

Table 25-3
Common Clinical Manifestations of Imported Malaria

Symptoms (decreasing order of frequency)
  Fever
  Chills and sweats
  Headache
  General malaise, fatigue, and anorexia
  Arthralgias and myalgias
  Nausea, vomiting, diarrhea, and abdominal pain
  Dyspnea
  Chest pain
  Altered mental status
  Rash
Signs (decreasing order of frequency)
  Elevated temperature
  Splenomegaly
  Hepatomegaly
  Orthostatic hypotension
  Jaundice
  Abdominal tenderness

mortality rate for patients with complicated malaria exceeds 30% even when treated in intensive care units [18]. Table 25-4 summarizes clinical and laboratory findings associated with high mortality rates [70, 71].

Special emphasis should be placed on the early recognition and treatment of cerebral malaria because this complication can be fatal within 6–24 hours after the onset of fever. The mortality rate in those who develop this complication is almost 100% in untreated and 20% in treated individuals [71]. Approximately 3% of survivors experience permanent sequelae (e.g., mental retardation, cortical blindness, deafness, cerebellar ataxia, hemiparesis, and spasticity) such that their quality of life and employability are severely impaired [72]. Clinically, this complication resembles a toxic encephalopathy, and as such, meningismus and nuchal rigidity do not occur. Focal and lateralizing neurologic signs are uncommon. Delirium, stupor, hypertonicity, extensor plantar responses, brain stem dysfunction, frontal lobe release signs, and retinal hemorrhages may be present, but papilledema is notably absent [71]. Lumbar puncture, which should be performed to exclude bacterial meningitis, is usually unremarkable except for increased lactate and protein levels. Similarly, computed tomographic (CT) scanning and magnetic resonance imaging (MRI) may show mild cerebral edema, but cerebral hemorrhages and infarctions are quite rare [18].

DIFFERENTIAL DIAGNOSIS

Malaria mimics many infectious diseases, and therefore, the differential diagnosis is quite exten-

Table 25-4
Clinical and Laboratory Prognostic Indicators of Death

Clinical prognostic indicators
Hemodynamic shock
Coma
Recurrent seizures
Concomitant bacterial superinfections
Laboratory prognostic indicators
Parasitemias greater than 500,000/mL
Lactic acidosis
Hypoglycemia
Azotemia
Severe anemia
Coagulopathy

sive (Table 25-5) [73–75]. Although malaria is a relatively common disease among tropical travelers, the diagnosis is frequently missed by nontropical physicians [10, 37, 67, 69]. Studies have shown that fever in returning travelers rarely represents an unusual tropical disease; therefore, a positive travel history should be enough to prompt nontropical clinicians to include malaria in the differential diagnosis [73–75]. This point was substantiated by investigators at the McGill Centre for Tropical Diseases, who reported the following diagnoses in 587 febrile travelers: malaria (32%), hepatitis (6%), viral upper respiratory infection (6%), pyelonephritis (4%), pneumonia (3%), dengue (2%), enteric fever (2%), shigellosis (2%), nontyphoidal salmonellosis (2%), infectious mononucleosis (2%), and acute bronchitis (2%) [75].

DIAGNOSTIC EVALUATION

Timely and accurate diagnosis starts with a comprehensive health history and physical examination. A negative travel history (recent and remote), transfusion history, and illicit drug history and residence more than 2 miles from an international airport or migrant housing render the diagnosis of malaria highly unlikely [3, 22, 42–45]. Conversely, a positive travel history should prompt the occupational physician to order thick and thin blood smears in tropical travelers presenting with fever or flulike syndromes.

Thick and thin blood smears are minimally invasive, simple, and cost-effective. Their sensitivity and specificity exceed 90% in most instances [14, 18, 20]. It is essential for these smears to be interpreted by experienced personnel who are able to differentiate species through the visualization of distinct morphologic features. Clinically, the most important aspect of species identification is the differentiation of *P. falciparum* from *P. vivax, P. ovale,* and *P. malariae.* The thin smear is also useful in quantifying the percentage of parasitized red blood cells because this finding has important prognostic implications. A single set of negative thick and thin blood smears does not exclude malaria. Thick and thin blood smears should be repeated every 6–12 hours for 48 hours [14, 35]. The probability of malaria becomes quite low when repeated thick and thin blood smears remain negative [18].

In addition to thick and thin blood smears, molecular probes have been developed recently for

Table 25-5
Differential Diagnosis of Fever in Tropical Travelers (Partial List)

Common causes
  Viral syndrome
  Upper respiratory infections
  Gastroenteritis
  Food-related illnesses and toxins
  Infectious mononucleosis
  Hepatitis A
  Drug fever
Cyclic fever
  African trypanosomiasis
  Brucellosis
  Dengue
  Endocarditis
  Malaria
  Relapsing fever
  Sepsis
  Visceral leishmaniasis
Fever and splenomegaly
  Babesiosis
  Brucellosis
  Endocarditis
  Enteric fever
  Epidemic typhus
  Infectious mononucleosis
  Leptospirosis
  Malaria
  Relapsing fever
  Schistosomiasis (acute)

  Toxoplasmosis
  Visceral leishmaniasis
Fever and hepatomegaly
  Amebic liver abscess
  Cytomegalovirus infection
  Hepatitis A, B, C, D, E
  Lassa fever
  Leptospirosis
  Malaria
  Q fever
  Relapsing fever
  Yellow fever
  Visceral leishmaniasis
Fever and anemia/thrombocytopenia
  AIDS (acute)
  Cytomegalovirus infection
  Dengue
  Drug fever
  Endocarditis
  Enteric fever
  Hemorrhagic fever
    Infectious mononucleosis
  Malaria
  Meningococcemia
  Q fever
  Sepsis
  Visceral leishmaniasis

rapid diagnosis. These probes were designed to detect parasitic DNA and protein antigens. The rapid antigen detection tests (RDTs) are the most practical of the newer testing techniques. These tests can detect parasitic proteins in blood from finger-prick samples; however, they currently are limited to the detection of *P. falciparum* and *P. vivax* [76]. Other shortcomings include their inability to quantify parasitemia, suboptimal test performance with low-level parasitemia, and unreliability as tests of cure. Polymerase chain reaction (PCR) tests are both sensitive (>90%) and highly specific (~100%) [77]. Unfortunately, the turnaround times for PCR tests are too long for the tests to be of use clinically. Despite the initial interest and promising results of molecular probes, blood smears remain the test of choice for diagnosis, species differentiation, and parasite counts.

    Serologic testing for malaria is useful from an epidemiologic but not a diagnostic perspective be-cause it cannot differentiate acute from chronic infection and protective from nonprotective antibody [48]. Although *P. falciparum* parasites can be cultured in vitro to test for drug sensitivities, cultures are not used for diagnostic purposes.

Treatment

Occupational health professionals must consider the diagnosis of malaria in all traveling employees who develop flulike symptoms or fever on return to the United States because a delay in diagnosis and treatment could be fatal in 12–24 hours [37, 38]. Studies have shown that with the advent of rapid transmeridian flight, approximately 90% of transient tropical travelers become symptomatic on return to the United States [38, 73, 78–81]. The potential for suboptimal clinical outcomes is further compounded by the fact that nontropical physicians have been shown to misdiagnose malaria almost 40% of the time in fatal cases [37]. Until an accurate diagnosis has been established, a presumptive diagnosis of malaria should be considered in all tropical travelers who present with fever, flulike symptoms, or systemic illness.

The treatment of malaria can be quite complex because it depends on the type of infection, severity of infection, level of parasitemia, presence of malarial complications, probability of parasite drug resistance, and host health status (e.g., age, allergies, medications, and confounding medical conditions) [54]. Some basic treatment strategies include (1) treating as a *P. falciparum* infection until proven otherwise, (2) assuming chloroquine resistance until drug sensitivities are known, and (3) assuming chloroquine and mefloquine resistance in travelers to Southeast Asia until drug sensitivities are known.

All nonimmune and pregnant employees with *P. falciparum* malaria should be admitted to the hospital. Nonimmune employees with *falciparum* parasitemias greater than 2%, semi-immune employees with *falciparum* parasitemias greater than 5%, and any employee with complicated malaria should be admitted to an intensive care unit. Reliable semi-immune adults with mild *P. vivax*, *P. ovale*, or *P. malariae* infections may be treated on an outpatient basis, provided daily parasite counts can be obtained until the infection has been controlled adequately [9, 14, 18, 35, 82].

There are a substantial number of therapeutic agents in the antimalarial drug armamentarium. They can be categorized by medication class and mechanism of action, as depicted in Table 25-6 [9, 14, 15, 82]. Treatment strategies for stand-by treatment (SBT), uncomplicated malaria, uncomplicated drug-resistant malaria, and complicated malaria are summarized in Tables 25-7 and 25-8 [14, 35, 54, 82]. The therapeutic agents most commonly used in the United States are discussed briefly in the following paragraphs.

STAND-BY TREATMENT

SBT, as defined by the World Health Organization (WHO), is the self-administration of antimalarial medication for treatment of fever or flulike symptoms when prompt medical attention is unavailable [83]. The CDC refers to SBT as presumptive self-treatment of malaria. The risks of adverse drug effects are ostensibly mitigated because self-

Table 25-6
Categorization of Antimalarial Drugs

Drug classification schema
Quinoline-related compounds
   Chloroquine
   Halofantrine
   Mefloquine
   Primaquine
   Quinidine
   Quinine
Antifolates
   Proguanil
   Pyrimethamine
Qinghaosu/artemisinin derivatives
   Arteether
   Artemether
   Artesunate
Antimicrobial agents
   Azithromycin
   Clindamycin
   Dapsone
   Sulfonamides
   Tetracycline
Mechanism of action schema
   Blood schizonticides (eradicate parasites in red cells)
   Fast-acting/potent
      Artemisinin
      Chloroquine
      Halofantrine
      Mefloquine
      Quinidine
      Quinine
   Slower-acting (added for synergism)
      Clindamycin
      Doxycycline
      Sulfonamides
      Tetracycline
   Hepatic schizonticides (eradicate intrahepatic parasites)
      Primaquine
      Proguanil
      Pyrimethamine
   Gametocides (eradicate blood sexual form of parasite)
      Primaquine
      Pyrimethamine

treatment is considered a lifesaving intervention in complicated *falciparum* infections. Therefore, employees must be well educated regarding prodromal symptoms and indications for presumptive self-treatment. SBT should not be considered during the first week of exposure because the incubation period for malaria is at least 7 days. Employees also

Table 25-7
Stand-by Treatment for Nonimmune Travelers

Indications for stand-by treatment (SBT)

1. SBT without chemoprophylaxis

   Low-risk areas having limited medical availability

   Short-term travelers in which the efficacy of chemoprophylaxis is not clearly defined

   Brief repeated exposures in which the risks of long-term chemoprophylaxis are not acceptable

2. SBT with chemoprophylaxis

   High-risk areas

Stand-by treatment (regimen depends on parasite type, parasite drug resistance, transmission risks, drug toxicities, and employee health status)

1. Chloroquine-sensitive malaria–endemic areas

   Chloroquine, 1,000 mg orally initially, followed by 500 mg orally 6 hours later, then 500 mg orally once daily for 2 days

2. Chloroquine-resistant malaria–endemic areas

   Mefloquine, 500 mg orally followed by 500 mg orally 12 hours later, or fansidar, 3 tablets orally as a single dose, or halofantrine, 500 mg orally every 6 hours for three doses

3. Multidrug-resistant malaria–endemic areas

   Quinine, 650 mg \orally every 8 hours for 7 days, or doxycycline, 100 mg orally once daily for 7 days

---

should be advised that symptoms may first develop after leaving malaria-endemic zones and on return to the United States. As soon as possible after initiating SBT, definitive medical attention must be sought for further evaluation and treatment, as indicated. SBT may be used separately or in conjunction with chemoprophylaxis. Recommended SBT indications and therapeutic agents are summarized in Table 25-7 [84].

UNCOMPLICATED MALARIA

Chloroquine is the drug of choice for all uncomplicated chloroquine-sensitive infections. The usual dosage is 25 mg base per kilogram administered over a 72-hour period, as summarized in Table 25-8. Cure rates exceed 95% when this regimen is employed [54]. Chloroquine must be followed by a 2-week course of primaquine to eradicate *P. vivax* and *P. ovale* hypnozoites and prevent relapse (radical cure) [54, 82]. As noted previously, primaquine may cause severe oxidant hemolysis in employees with G-6-PD deficiency. Although primaquine is contraindicated in severe G-6-PD deficiency, it may be administered once weekly to employees with

---

Table 25-8
Medications Commonly Used in the Treatment of Malaria

Therapeutic agents (choice depends on sensitivities and drug availability)

Uncomplicated malaria infections

Chloroquine base, 10 mg/kg orally (600 mg max), followed by 5 mg/kg orally (300 mg max) at 6, 24, and 48 hours

Quinine sulfate, 10 mg/kg (usually 650 mg) orally three times daily for 7 days *plus*

Tetracycline, 250 mg orally four times daily for 7 days, *or*

Clindamycin, 10 mg/kg orally (900 mg max) every 8 hours for 3–5 days, *or*

Pyrimethamine, 25 mg/sulfadoxine 500 mg (per tablet), three tablets orally as a single dose

Mefloquine base, 15 mg/kg orally (usually 750 mg), followed by 10 mg/kg orally (usually 500 mg) 6–8 hours after the initial dose (maximum recommended total dose is 1,250 mg)

Halofantrine base, 8 mg/kg orally every 6 hours for three doses (500 mg maximum/dose); repeat after 7 days for nonimmune employees

Artesunate, 4 mg/kg orally once daily for 3 days, *plus* mefloquine or tetracycline

Complicated malaria infections (plus other adjunctive agents and modalities as indicated)

Chloroquine base, 10 mg/kg intravenously over 8 hours (600 mg max), then 15 mg/kg intravenously over 24 hours (900 mg max)

Quinidine gluconate base, 10 mg/kg intravenous load over 1–2 hours, followed by 0.02 mg/kg/min intravenously until parasitemia is less than 1% and employee can tolerate oral medications

Artemether, 3.2 mg/kg intramuscularly, followed by 1.6 mg/kg intramuscularly every 24 hours until employee can tolerate oral medications

Artesunate, 2.4 mg/kg intravenous load, followed by 1.2 mg/kg intravenously at 12 and 24 hours, then 1.2 mg/kg intravenously every 24 hours until employee can tolerate oral medications

Exchange transfusion for parasitemias greater than 10% in conjunction with altered mental status

mild deficiency under close observation for a period of 6–8 weeks [82].

UNCOMPLICATED DRUG-RESISTANT MALARIA

Uncomplicated chloroquine-resistant *P. falciparum* malaria is best treated with quinine sulfate plus tetracycline, doxycycline, or clindamycin (the latter for pregnant women) or atovaquone-proguanil [54, 59, 85]. In geographic regions where pyrimethamine-sulfadoxine resistance is uncontrolled, chloroquine-resistant *P. falciparum* infections should be treated with quinine sulfate plus tetracycline, mefloquine, or halofantrine [54, 86]. Nonimmune travelers to Thailand, other parts of Southeast Asia, or the Amazon should receive a full 7-day course of treatment because *P. falciparum* parasites are less sensitive to quinine in those geographic regions [86–88].

Clinicians should be aware that despite reportedly high cure rates, the effectiveness of these therapeutic agents is often limited by adverse drug effects. Some of the more notable adverse effects include (1) quinine—bitter taste, cinchonism, and hyperinsulinemic hypoglycemia [9, 52, 54]; (2) pyrimethamine-sulfadoxine—severe exfoliative dermatitis, erythema multiforme, and Stevens-Johnson syndrome [18, 52]; (3) mefloquine—emesis, dysrhythmia, and toxic encephalopathy [52, 54, 88, 89]; and (4) halofantrine—dose-dependent atrioventricular conduction delay, QTc prolongation, and sudden death [89, 90].

Chloroquine-resistant *P. vivax* can be treated effectively with mefloquine or quinine sulfate plus tetracycline. Pyrimethamine-sulfadoxine has proved to be less effective [18, 54, 82], and higher doses of pyrimethamine (22.5–30 mg base per day for 14 days) are required to eradicate hypnozoites and prevent relapses [54, 91].

UNCOMPLICATED MULTIDRUG-RESISTANT MALARIA

Quinine sulfate plus tetracycline (clindamycin in pregnant employees) is recommended for the treatment of uncomplicated mefloquine-resistant *P. falciparum* infections [52, 54, 88]. Although the artemisinin compounds are fast-acting and effective, they have not been licensed for use in the United States. These compounds have been highly effective in the treatment of multidrug-resistant *falciparum* infections and have become the drugs of choice for quinine-resistant *P. falciparum* elsewhere in the world [52, 92–94].

COMPLICATED MALARIA

The treatment of choice for complicated malaria is strongly dependent on parasite sensitivities. Parenteral chloroquine is the drug of choice for severe chloroquine-sensitive malaria infections [35, 54]. Quinidine gluconate is recommended for treatment of severe chloroquine- and mefloquine-resistant *P. falciparum* infections because parenteral quinine dihydrochloride is no longer available in the United States [54, 95]. Although a number of regimens have proven effective, the one most commonly employed in the United States is quinidine gluconate 10 mg/kg intravenously over 1–2 hours, followed by a continuous infusion of 0.02 mg/kg per minute. The rate of infusion must be titrated according to clinical response, and the rate should be decreased by 30–50% after 48 hours in hyperparasitemic patients [54]. Major toxicities include hypotension, dysrhythmias, and hyperinsulinemic hypoglycemia [54].

In many countries, parenteral artemisinin and tetracycline or mefloquine are recommended for treatment of quinine-resistant *P. falciparum;* however, in the United States, parenteral quinidine plus tetracycline, doxycycline, or clindamycin remains the treatment of choice because artemisinin agents are not available [54, 93].

Whether complicated or uncomplicated, malaria treatment interventions must be closely monitored. Most employees with uncomplicated or drug-sensitive malaria show marked clinical improvement within 48 hours and defervesce within 96 hours [14, 18, 35]. Examination of thick and thin blood smears every 12 hours is recommended until the parasitemia proportion is less than 1% [18]. Drug resistance is indicated by parasitemia levels that fail to decline by 75% after 48 hours or persist beyond 8 days of treatment [18, 82]. The presence of circulating gametocytes during the treatment phase does not indicate drug resistance or treatment failure [82].

Since the risk of death from malaria is directly proportional to the degree of parasitemia [70,96], exchange transfusion (ET) should be considered in all critically ill patients who have not responded adequately to other therapeutic interventions [61, 97]. Although ET has not been shown to improve survival rates in randomized clinical trials, it is currently recommended as an adjunct in patients with *P. falciparum* parasitemias exceeding 10%, coma, respiratory failure, coagulopathy, or renal failure [98]. Once initiated, ETs should be continued until parasitemia levels have fallen to less than 5%.

Severe malaria should be managed in an intensive care unit to monitor and maintain fluid and electrolyte balance [71]. In addition to ET, other therapeutic interventions previously shown to be clinically effective in the treatment of complicated malaria include acetaminophen for fever [18], prophylactic phenobarbital to prevent seizures [99], benzodiazepines to treat seizures [82], early hemodialysis or peritoneal dialysis for oliguric renal failure [100], positive-pressure ventilation for noncardiogenic pulmonary edema [101], and glucose supplementation for hypoglycemia [18].

Occupational Considerations

In summary, in the United States and other nonendemic malaria areas, occupational malaria is primarily a concern in employees and military personnel traveling to malaria-endemic geographic regions. Pretravel health assessments are recommended at least 1 month prior to departure to identify preexisting medical conditions that may adversely impact the employee's health and safety while in a travel status. It is paramount for the occupational health professional to be adequately informed regarding travel itineraries because methods of prevention must be tailored on an individual basis. The occupational health professional also must closely monitor CDC and WHO preventive and treatment recommendations because of frequent changes in the distribution of malaria and parasite drug resistance. Additionally, it is important to realize that evolving environmental changes such as global warming may alter the geographic distribution of malaria and vectorial densities significantly in the future [102]. As noted previously, allergic, pregnant, and other employees who are unable to take or comply with chemoprophylactic regimens recommended by the CDC, WHO, or U.S. Public Health Service should not be medically

cleared for travel to high-risk areas unless there are mitigating circumstances.

It is also strongly recommended that pretravel health assessments include employee education and training regarding the risks of malarial disease, antimosquito measures, malaria chemoprophylaxis (including terminal prophylaxis), signs and symptoms of disease, stand-by treatment, postexposure procedures and prophylaxis, and the necessity to comply with preventive recommendations as delineated in Table 25-9. Additionally, employees should be encouraged to minimize exposure risks whenever feasible because it is possible to acquire malaria despite the appropriate application of antimosquito measures and the use of chemoprophylactic agents. As a final measure, employees who become ill after returning to the United States should be instructed to inform their physicians that they have been traveling and potentially exposed to malaria parasites. Current information regarding malaria prevention, diagnosis, and treatment is available on the CDC website (www.cdc.gov).

Since occupational malaria usually results from employee travel to malaria-endemic zones on business, most cases will be compensable, and appropriate claims will need to be filed. Compensability

Table 25-9
Employee Personal Protective Measures

Antimosquito measures
    Wear long-sleeved shirts and trousers.
    Apply DEET to exposed areas at dusk.
    Spray "knock-down" insecticide in living and sleeping areas at dusk.
    Use electrically operated insecticide generators containing pyrethroids or mosquito coils.
    Stay in air-conditioned/screened rooms after sunset.
    Use permethrin-impregnated bed nets.

Employee behavior patterns
    Limit activities in malaria-endemic areas when feasible.
    Avoid unprotected nighttime exposures when feasible.
    Comply with recommended chemoprophylaxis and stand-by treatment.
    Pregnant females and employees who are unable to comply with recommended preventive measures owing to medication allergies or poor health should not travel to malaria endemic areas unless absolutely necessary.
    Employees should be well educated regarding the signs and symptoms of malaria.
    Employees should be aware that malaria symptoms may start during or after exposure.

may be more difficult to ascertain in rare situations such as runway malaria and airport malaria; however, these and other possibilities (e.g., autochthonous malaria) should be considered when a causal link is not obvious during the disability case review [42–45, 103–106].

Finally, there is very little in the scientific literature regarding malaria-associated disability in traveling employees; however, uncomplicated imported malaria infections typically defervesce after 2–3 days of hospitalization [107]. Most employees return to work in approximately 1 week, depending on workplace demands and premorbid health status, without permanent impairment or disability [106]. Conversely, complicated infections (usually *P. falciparum*) may result in prolonged hospitalizations, extended disability, permanent impairment, and death. Therefore, early recognition and treatment are critical in preserving employee health, performance, and productivity.

References

1. Centers for Disease Control and Prevention. Mosquito-transmitted malaria—California and Florida, 1990. *MMWR* 1991;40:106–8.
2. Centers for Disease Control and Prevention. Summary of notifiable diseases—United States, 1990. *MMWR* 1991;39:55–61.
3. Centers for Disease Control and Prevention. Malaria surveillance—United States, 2004. *MMWR* 2006;55:645–648.
4. Centers for Disease Control and Prevention. Malaria surveillance—United States, 2003. *MMWR* 2005;54:25–40.
5. Steffen R, Fuchs E, Schildknecht J, et al. Mefloquine compared with other malaria chemoprophylaxis regimens in tourists visiting East Africa. *Lancet* 1993;341:1299–1303.
6. World Health Organization. World malaria situation in 1993. *Wkly Epidemiol Rec* 1996;71:17–24.
7. Centers for Disease Control and Prevention. *Health Information for International Travel—1995.* Atlanta: CDC, 1995.
8. Barat LM, Bloland PB. Drug resistance among malaria and other parasites. *Infect Dis Clin North Am* 1997;11:969–87.
9. Miller LH. Malaria. In Warren KS, Mahmoud AAF (eds), *Tropical and Geographical Medicine.* New York: McGraw-Hill, 1994. Pp 223–39.
10. Stanley J. Malaria. *Emerg Med Clin North Am* 1997;15:113–55.
11. Beier JC, Copeland RS, Mtalib R, et al. Ookinete rates in Afrotropical mosquitoes as a measure of

human malaria infectionousness. *Am J Trop Med Hyg* 1992;47:41–6.
12. Quinn TC, Jacobs RF, Mertz GJ, et al. Congenital malaria: A report of four cases and a review. *Clin Lab Obstet* 1982;10:229.
13. Bruce-Chwatt LJ. Transfusion malaria revisited. *Trop Dis Bull* 1982;79:827–40.
14. Zucker JR, Campbell CC. Malaria: Principles of prevention and treatment. *Infect Dis Clin North Am* 1993;7:547–67.
15. Schwartz IK. Prevention of malaria. *Infect Dis Clin North Am* 1992;6:313–31.
16. Centers for Disease Control and Prevention. Recommendations for the prevention of malaria among travelers. *MMWR* 1990;39:1–10.
17. Advice for travelers. *Med Lett* 1995;37:99–108.
18. White NJ. Malaria. In Cook GC (ed), *Manson's Tropical Diseases,* 2nd ed. Philadelphia: Saunders, 1996. Pp 1087–164.
19. MacDonald G. *The Epidemiology and Control of Malaria.* London: Oxford University Press, 1957. Pp 5–35.
20. Jones C, Grab B. The assessment of insecticidal impact on the malaria mosquito's vectorial capacity from data on the proportion of parous females. *Bull WHO* 1965;31:71–86.
21. Curtis CF. Introduction: I. An overview of mosquito biology, behaviour and importance. In Bock GR, Cardew G (eds), *Olfaction in Mosquito-Host Interactions.* New York: Wiley, 1996, pp 3–7.
22. Brook JH, Genese CA, Blotand PB, et al. Brief report: malaria probably locally acquired in New Jersey. *N Engl J Med* 1994;331:22–3.
23. Brillman J. *Plasmodium vivax* malaria in Mexico—A problem in the United States. *West J Med* 1994;147:469–73.
24. Wyler DJ. Malaria—Resurgence, resistance, and research. *N Engl J Med* 1983;308:875–8.
25. Harries AD. Malaria: Keeping the mosquitoes at bay. *Lancet* 1993;342:506–7.
26. Krotoski WA. Discovery of the hypnozoite and a new theory of malaria relapse. *Trans R Soc Trop Med Hyg* 1985;79:1–11.
27. White NJ, Ho M. The pathophysiology of malaria. *Adv Parasitol* 1992,31:34–173.
28. Wernsdorfer WH. Epidemiology of drug resistance in malaria. *Acta Trop* 1994;56:143–56.
29. World Health Organization. Insecticide resistance and vector control. Seventeenth report of the WHO Expert Committee on Insecticides. WHO Technical Report Series no 443. Geneva: WHO, 1970.
30. Krogstad DJ. Malaria as a reemerging disease. *Epidemiol Rev* 1996;18:77–89.
31. Centers for Disease Control and Prevention. Epidemic malaria—Tadjikistan. *MMWR* 1996;45:513–6.
32. Quinn TC, Plorde JJ. The resurgence of malaria. *Arch Intern Med* 1981;141:1123–4.
33. Brillman J. *Plasmodium vivax* malaria from

Mexico—A problem in the United States. *West J Med* 1994;147:469–73.

34. Freedman DO. Imported malaria—Here to stay. *Am J Med* 1992;93:239–42.

35. Hoffman SL. Diagnosis, treatment, and prevention of malaria. *Med Clin North Am* 1992;76:1327–55.

36. Zucker JR, Barber AM, Paxton LA, et al. Malaria surveillance—United States, 1992. *MMWR* 1995;44:1–17.

37. Greenberg AE, Lobel HO. Mortality from *Plasmodium falciparum* malaria in travelers from the United States, 1959–1987. *Ann Intern Med* 1990;113:326–7.

38. Lobel HO, Campbell CC, Schwartz, et al. Recent trends in the importation of malaria caused by *Plasmodium falciparum* into the United States from Africa. *J Infect Dis* 1986;152:613–7.

39. Lobel HO, Phillips-Howard PA, Brandling-Bennett AD, et al. Malaria incidence and prevention among European and North American travellers to Kenya. *Bull WHO* 1990;68:209–15.

40. Steffen R, Heusser R, Machlon R, et al. Malaria chemoprophylaxis among European tourists in tropical Africa: Use, adverse reactions, and efficacy. *Bull WHO* 1990;68:313.

41. Olliaro P, Cattani J, Wirth D. Malaria, the submerged disease. *JAMA* 1996;275:230–3.

42. Holvoet G, Michielsen P, Vandepitte J. Airport malaria in Belgium. *Lancet* 1982;ii:881–2.

43. Smeaton MJ, Slater PJ, Robson P. Malaria from a "commuter" mosquito. *Lancet* 1984;i:845–6.

44. Whitefield D, Curtis CF, White GB, et al. Two cases of *falciparum* malaria acquired in Britain. *Br Med J* 1984;289:1607–9.

45. Isaacson M. Airport malaria: A review. *Bull WHO* 1989;67:737–43.

46. Miller LH, Mason SJ, Clyde DF, et al. The resistance factor to *Plasmodium vivax* in blacks. *N Engl J Med* 1976;295:302–4.

47. Nagel RL, Roth EF. Malaria and red cell genetic defects. *Blood* 1989;74:1213–21.

48. Deans JA, Cohen S. Immunology of malaria. *Ann Rev Microbiol* 1983;37:25–49.

49. Wolfe MS. Protection of travelers. *Clin Infect Dis* 1997;25:177–86.

50. Beach RF, Ruebush TR, Sexton JD. Effectiveness of permethrin-impregnated bed nets and curtains for malaria control in a holoendemic area of western Kenya. *Am J Trop Med Hyg* 1993;49:290–300.

51. D'Alessandro U, Olaleye BO, McGuire W, et al. Mortality and morbidity from malaria in Gambian children after introduction of an impregnated bed-net programme. *Lancet* 1995;345:479–83.

52. Kain KC. Chemotherapy and prevention of drug-resistant malaria. *Wilderness Environ Med* 1995;6:307–24.

53. Navy Medical Department. *Guide to Malaria Prevention and Control.* Norfolk, VA: Navy Environmental Health Center, 1995. Pp 62–9.

54. Drugs for parasitic infections. *Med Lett* 1995;37:99–108.

55. Harries AD, Chugh KS. Chloroquine-induced pruritus in Nigerian medical and nursing students. *Ann Trop Med Parasitol* 1986;80:479–80.

56. Phillips-Howard PA, terKuile FO. CNS adverse events associated with antimalarial agents—Fact or fiction? *Drug Safety* 1995;12:370–83.

57. Magill AJ, Smoak BL. Failure of mefloquine chemoprophylaxis for malaria in Somalia. *N Engl J Med* 1993;329:1206.

58. Croft A, Garner P. Mefloquine to prevent malaria: A systematic review of trials. *Br Med J* 1997;315:1412–6.

59. Centers for Disease Control and Prevention. Retrieved from www.cdc.gov/travel/malariadrugs.htm on October 17, 2005.

60. Behrens RH, Curtis CF. Malaria in travelers: Epidemiology and prevention. *Br Med Bull* 1993;49:363–81.

61. Phillips-Howard PA, Radalowicz A, Mitchell J, et al. Risk of malaria in British residents returning from malarious areas. *Br Med J* 1990;300:499–503.

62. Steffen R, Holdener F, Wyss R, et al. Malaria prophylaxis and self-therapy in airline crews. *Aviat Space Environ Med* 1990;61:942–5.

63. Centers for Disease Control and Prevention. Malaria surveillance—United States, 1992. *MMWR* 1995;44:SS-5:1–17.

64. Wyler DJ. Malaria—Resurgence, resistance, and research. *N Engl J Med* 1983;308:875–8.

65. Vaccine development and evaluation. Available at www.cdc.gov/malaria/cdcactivities/research.htm; accessed on December 25, 2007.

66. Fletcher C. The *Plasmodium falciparum* genome project. *Parasitol Today* 1998;14:342–4.

67. Froude JRL, Weiss LM, Tanowitz HB, et al. Imported malaria in the Bronx: Review of 51 cases recorded from 1986–1991. *Clin Infect Dis* 1992;15:774–80.

68. Gordon S, Brennessel DJ, Goldstein JA, et al. Malaria: A city hospital experience. *Arch Intern Med* 1988;148:1569–71.

69. Wiest PM, Opal S, Romulo RL, et al. Malaria in travelers in Rhode Island: A review of 26 cases. *Am J Med* 1990;91:30–6.

70. Field JW. Blood examination and prognosis in acute falciparum malaria. *Trans R Soc Trop Med Hyg* 1949;43:33–68.

71. Warrell DA, Molyneaux ME, Beales PF. Severe and complicated malaria. *Trans R Soc Trop Med Hyg* 1990;84:1–65S.

72. Brewster DR, Kwiatowski D, White NJ. Neurological sequelae of cerebral malaria in children. *Lancet* 1990;336:1039–43.

73. Svenson JE, Gyozrkos TW, MacLean JD. Diagnosis of malaria in the febrile traveler. *Am J Trop Med Hyg* 1995;53:518–21.

74. Gasser RA, Magill AJ, Oster CN, et al. The threat of infectious disease in Americans returning from Operation Desert Storm. *N Engl J Med* 1991;324:857–64.

75. Strickland GT. Fever in the returned traveler. *Med Clin North Am* 1992;76:1375–92.

76. Moody A. Rapid diagnostic tests for malaria parasites. *Clin Microbiol Rev* 2002;15:66–78.

77. Snounou G, Viriyakosol S, Jarra W, et al. Identification of the four human malarial species in field samples by polymerase chain reaction and detection of a high prevalence of mixed infections. *Mol Biochem Parasitol* 1993;58:283–92.

78. Maegraith B. Unde venis. *Lancet* 1963;1:401–4.

79. Baker PB, Dronen SC. *Vivax* malaria. *Am J Emerg Med* 1986;4:52–8.

80. Stair T, Ricci R, Pedicano J, et al. Malaria in the emergency department. *Ann Emerg Med* 1983;12: 422–5.

81. Kain KC, Harrington MA, Tennyson S, et al. Imported malaria: Prospective analysis of problems in diagnosis and management. *Clin Infect Dis* 1998;27: 142–9.

82. White NJ. The treatment of malaria. *N Engl J Med* 1996;335:800–6.

83. World Health Organization. Health risks and their avoidance. In *International Travel and Health.* Geneva: WHO, 1993.

84. World Health Organization. Development of recommendations for the protection of short-term travellers to malaria endemic areas: Memorandum from two WHO meetings. *Bull WHO* 1988;66:177–9.

85. Dobertslyn EB, Phintuyothim P, Noeypatimondh S, et al. Single-dose therapy of *falciparum* malaria with mefloquine or pyrimethamine-sulfadoxine. *Bull WHO* 1979;57:275–9.

86. Watt G, Loesuttiribool L, Shanks GD, et al. Quinine with tetracycline for the treatment of drug resistant *falciparum* malaria in Thailand. *Am J Trop Med Hyg* 1992;47:108–11.

87. Looareesuwan S, Charoenpan P, Ho M. Fatal *Plasmodium falciparum* malaria after an inadequate response to quinine treatment. *J Infect Dis* 1990;161: 577.

88. Patchen LC, Campbell CC, Williams SB. Neurologic reactions after a therapeutic dose of mefloquine. *N Engl J Med* 1989;321:1415–6.

89. terKuile FO, Dolan G, Nosten F, et al. Halofantrine versus mefloquine in treatment of multidrug resistant falciparum malaria. *Lancet* 1993;341:1044–9.

90. Nosten F, terKuile FO, Luxemburger C, et al. Cardiac effects of antimalarial treatment with halofantrine. *Lancet* 1991;341:1054–6.

91. Krotoski WA. Frequency of relapse and primaquine resistance in Southeast Asian *vivax* malaria. *N Engl J Med* 1980;303:587–92.

92. Hien TT, White NJ. Qinghaosu. *Lancet* 1993;341: 603–8.

93. White NJ. Artemisinin: Current status. *Trans R Soc Trop Med Hyg* 1994;88:3–4S.

94. Looareesuwan S, Wiravan C, Vanijanonta S, et al. Randomized trial of artesunate and mefloquine alone and in sequence for acute uncomplicated *falciparum* malaria. *Lancet* 1992;339:821–4.

95. Miller KD, Greenberg AE, Campbell CC. Treatment of severe malaria in the United States with a continuous infusion of quinidine gluconate and exchange transfusion. *N Engl J Med* 1989;321:65–70.

96. Marik PE. Severe *falciparum* malaria: Survival without exchange transfusion. *Am J Trop Med Hyg* 1989;1:627–9.

97. Phillips P, Nantel S, Benny WB. Exchange transfusion as an adjunct to the treatment of severe *falciparum* malaria: Case report and review. *Rev Infect Dis* 1990;12:1100.

98. Miller KD, Greenberg AE, Campbell CC. Treatment of severe malaria in the United States with a continuous infusion of quinidine gluconate and exchange transfusion. *N Engl J Med* 1989;321:65–70.

99. White NJ, Looareesuwan S, Phillips RE, et al. Single-dose phenobarbitone prevents convulsions in cerebral malaria. *Lancet* 1988;2:64–6.

100. Tran TMT, Nguyen HP, Ha V, et al. Acute renal failure in patients with severe *falciparum* malaria. *Clin Infect Dis* 1992;15:874–80.

101. Brooks MH, Kiel FW, Sheehy TW, et al. Acute pulmonary edema in *falciparum* malaria: A clinicopathological correlation. *N Engl J Med* 1968;279: 732–7.

102. Intergovernmental Panel on Climate Change, Working Group II. *Summary for Policymakers: Scientific-Technical Analyses of Impacts, Adaptations, and Mitigation of Climate Change.* Cambridge, England: Cambridge University Press, 1995.

103. Conlon CP, Berendt AR, Dawson K, et al. Runway malaria. *Lancet* 1990;335:472.

104. Bada JL, Cabezos J, Fernandez-Roure JL. Runway malaria. *Lancet* 1990;335:881.

105. Connor MP, Green AD. Runway malaria in a British serviceman. *J R Soc Med* 1995;88:415–6P.

106. Oswald G, Lawrence EP. Runway malaria. *Lancet* 1990;335:1537.

107. *Official Disability Guidelines, 1998.* Corpus Christi, TX: Work-Loss Data Institute, 1997. Pp 125–6.

26 Occupational Lyme Disease

William E. Wright

Lyme disease in North America is caused by a spirochete, *Borrelia burgdorferi sensu stricto*, which is a genetic subspecies of the broader category of related genospecies, the *Borrelia burgdorferi sensu lato* complex. It was identified as the causative agent in U.S. cases of Lyme disease in 1982. The spirochete is transmitted to humans by bites of ticks from the *Ixodes ricinus* family. The deer tick, *I. scapularis,* is the most important vector in the northeastern and midwestern United States. The western black-legged tick, *I. pacificus,* is the most important vector on the West Coast. These ticks may be co-infected with *Anaplasma phagocytophilum* (previously called *Ehrlichia phagocytophilia*) or *Babesia microti*.

Epidemiology

A potentially multisystem and multistage disease, Lyme disease has become the most common vector-borne infection in the United States. It accounts for more than 95% or all reported vector-borne diseases [1]. In 2004, there were 19,804 cases of Lyme disease reported to the Centers for Disease Control and Prevention (CDC), and in 2005, 23,305 cases were reported. The national average incidence rates for those years were about 6.7 cases and 7.86 cases per 100,000 population per year, respectively. The geographic distribution is broad. For the period 1994–2005, except for Montana, cases were reported from all states and the District of Columbia. Case identification is concentrated in specific areas [2, 3]. Thirteen states (i.e., DE, CT, NJ, MA, PA, NY, WI, MD, NH, ME, MN, VT, and RI) accounted for 95.4% of the 2005 reported U.S. cases. These states had an average annual incidence rate of 29.6 cases per 100,000 population per year. These states are listed here in order of their 2005 incidence rates, which range from Delaware's high of 76.58 cases per 100,000 population per year to Rhode Island's 3.62 cases per 100,000 population per year. In 2003, Rhode Island had the highest annual incidence rate in the United States (68.39 cases); in 2004, Delaware took over that distinction (40.83 cases). Ten of these 13 states (excepting NH, ME, and VT) are listed in *Healthy People 2010* as "Lyme disease reference states," where Lyme disease is endemic [4]. The only other state-level reporting units with incidence rates above 2 cases per 100,000 population per year in 2005 were Virginia (3.62 cases), West Virginia (3.36 cases), and Iowa (3.0 cases). In the 2003–2005 time period, no cases were reported from Arkansas, Colorado, Hawaii, and Montana [3]. Within states, rates can vary significantly from county to county and from urban to suburban and rural areas. Actual rates may be much higher than the reported rates. Peak illness onset in the United States is in June, July, and August. The lowest occurrence of new cases is in the period from December to March [1–4].

Lyme disease cases have been reported in Europe, Russia, China, Japan, Canada, and Australia. In Europe, the *Borrelia* genomic groups *B. burgdorferi sensu stricto, B. garinii,* and *B. afzelii* have been identified, along with other strains, including *B. bissetti* and *B. valaisiana,* that have been associated with the disease. *B. afzelii* is associated with cutaneous sequelae (e.g., lymphadenosis benigna cutis and acrodermatitis chronica atrophicans). *B. garinii,* which tends to predominate in Europe, is associated with neurologic disease [5, 6].

The common vectors for disease transmission are *I. ricinus* in Europe and *I. pesculatus* in Asia [7–9]. Models have predicted that current trends in global climate change may result in expansion of the *I. scapularis* tick's range in North America [10].

A recent report from Brazil describes an illness termed *Lyme disease-like syndrome* or *Lyme disease-imitator syndrome,* with erythema migrans-like lesions and osteoarticular and neurologic symptoms. This is described as a zoonosis transmitted by ticks of the genus *Amblyomma.* Blood under dark-field examination shows mobile uncultivatable spirochete-like bacteria, which also have been identified in central nervous system fluid. Polymerase chain reaction (PCR) has been negative for *B. burgdorferi sensu stricto* and the *Borrelia* genus; other testing indicates these are not in the genera *Borrelia, Leptospira,* or *Treponema* [11].

Vector and Transmission

The *Ixodes* arthropod vectors of Lyme disease are arachnids (not insects) and are much smaller than common dog and cattle ticks (Figures 26-1 and 26-2). The *Ixodes* ticks vary in size and shape depending on their maturity and blood-meal status (Figure 26-3). The figures are provided to help practitioner correctly identify *Ixodes* ticks. The ticks seek host animals from the tips of tall grasses and shrubs and transfer to animals or people who brush against the vegetation. Questing ticks can attach to any body part but often crawl to more hidden or hairy areas, such as the groin, armpits, and scalp. Ticks feed on blood by inserting their mouthparts into the host's skin. A complete meal can take several days. As they feed on the blood, infected ticks may transmit the spirochete to the host. Transmission of the Lyme disease spirochete to the human

Figure 26-1
From left to right, an *Ixodes scapularis* larva, nymph, adult male tick, and adult female tick.

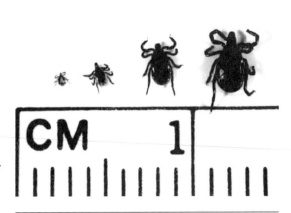

host usually requires 24–48 hours of feeding. The infected tick appears to need the blood meal for the spirochete to circulate in the tick and be transmitted.

Risk for transmission of the spirochete is related to the life cycle of the tick. Ticks pass through four stages—egg, larva, nymph, and adult. Tick larvae rarely carry the infection at the time of feeding. The most important vector of the disease is the nymph, which appears during the spring. Its appearance coincides with the time of year when people tend to increase their outdoor activity and wear fewer layers of clothing. The nymph is difficult to detect because of its small size (<2 mm). Infected adult ticks also can transmit the disease.

The tick has a 2-year life cycle. Adult ticks feed and mate on large animals, especially deer, in the fall and early spring. The recent growth of the white-tailed deer (*Odocoileus virginianus*) population in the East Coast of the United States, combined with suburban sprawl into farm and wooded areas, has increased the sharing of habitat between deer and the expanding human population. This is thought to be a factor related to increase in Lyme disease cases in some areas. Female ticks drop off the deer or other animal host to lay eggs on the ground. An adult female may lay as many as several thousand eggs. During the summer, eggs hatch into larvae. Larvae feed on mice, other small mammals,

Figure 26-2
Types of Ticks and their Relative Sizes.

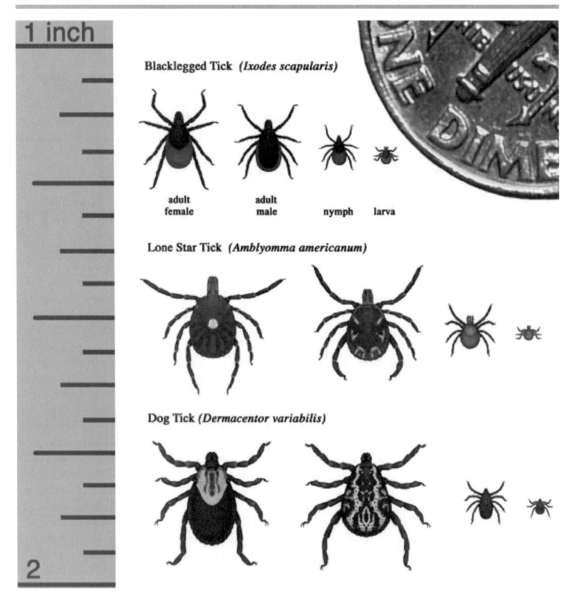

Figure 26-3
Ixodes scapularis ticks showing changes in blood engorgement after various durations of attachment. Nymphal stage.

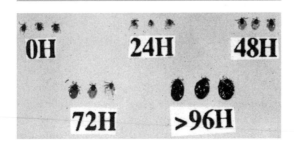

and birds in the summer and autumn. They are then inactive until the next spring when they molt into nymphs. Nymphs feed on small rodents, other mammals, and birds in the late spring and summer and then molt into adults in the autumn, completing the 2-year life cycle. Ticks acquire *B. burgdorferi* when they feed on infected animals, most important of which is the white-footed mouse, which is the key reservoir of the disease in nature. Proportions of *Ixodes* ticks infected with *B. burgdorferi* vary greatly depending on the degree of endemicity. Figures of 25–30% for nymphs and 50% or more for adult ticks have been reported. Humans are incidental hosts.

The proportion of people developing Lyme disease after a deer tick bite in a Lyme disease—endemic area has been reported to be about 1–3%. Risk is highest for ticks that are attached for more than 24 hours [12].

Removal of Ticks

Owing to the circulation of spirochetes during the tick's feeding cycle, ticks are thought to not transmit *B. burgdorferi sensu stricto* until after 1–2 days of attachment. Early removal of ticks is therefore recommended to limit the spread of Lyme disease. The procedure recommended for tick removal is designed to limit the potential for breaking off head and mouthparts at the site of the attachment because these can be related to local irritation or wound infection [13, 14]. Care should be taken to avoid crushing the tick's body, which could spread contamination. This can best be achieved by approaching the head of the tick from the side (perpendicular to the longitudinal axis of the tick's body) rather than by grasping the body longitudinally (Figure 26-4). The procedure recommended is to (1) grasps the tick with forceps or fine-tipped tweezers as close to the skin as possible, (2) pull the tick straight out with gentle, firm pressure without twisting or jerking, (3) dispose of the tick by drowning in alcohol or flushing down a drain, (4) wash hands with soap and water, and (5) apply an antiseptic to the bite site. One of the references given here is a patient handout on Lyme disease with a picture showing tick removal, which may be photocopied noncommercially by physicians and other health care professionals to share with patients; bulk reprints are also available [14].

If tweezers or forceps are not available, fingers can be used to remove the tick, but they should be protected with gloves, tissue, or a paper towel to avoid potential contact of pathogens with broken skin. Removal of ticks by applying nail polish, petroleum jelly, alcohol, a cigarette lighter, a hot match, or a burning cigarette is not considered to be effective or safe.

Employees who are subject to tick bites often ask about testing ticks that they have removed. Some state and local health departments may offer tick identification and testing on a research or community service basis. Testing of ticks generally is not

Figure 26-4
Proper Removal of a Tick.

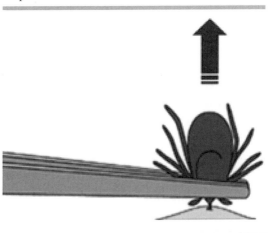

useful for deciding medical treatment of individuals. If testing of ticks is done, the sensitivity and specificity of the test method should be considered [15].

Occupational Factors

A number of studies in the United States and from around the world have assessed occupational risks for Lyme disease [16–44]. Many of these are cross-sectional studies, and some have used volunteers. Early studies frequently were designed to identify prevalence of seropositivity rather than clinically confirmed symptomatic Lyme disease. Some of the more recent studies have included clinical disease measures. Most studies used an occupational category of workers as a surrogate for occupational exposure, not taking into account duration of outdoor work activity, residence, and avocational opportunities for exposure or personal preventive behaviors to avoid or limit tick attachments. Especially in the early studies, the laboratory tests used to determine serologic status were enzyme-linked immunosorbent assays (ELISAs), which may have overestimated prevalence. Some later studies have included confirmatory Western blot tests. Some studies included comparison work groups such as office workers but did not take into account their avocational exposure or residence history. In studies that included clinical histories, it was not unusual for seropositive individuals to not recall tick bites or symptomatic illness consistent with Lyme disease. Crossreactivity of the test with non-*Borrelia* organisms or other forms of *Borrelia* may have occurred. Each of these factors raise questions about the accuracy of estimates of illness prevalence and risk. However, the available documentation appears to support that occupational risks for seropositivity and Lyme disease are present in some groups. Risk for seropositivity may be as high as sixfold or higher.

Occupational groups at risk include outdoor workers and animal handlers in endemic areas, particularly in wooded areas or sites with leaves, brush, and grasses. Work populations that may be at risk include forestry workers, park workers, farmers, migrant farm workers, lawn care workers, gardeners, landscapers, groundskeepers, utility line workers, construction workers, military personnel, surveyors, veterinarians, field biologists, kennel workers, law enforcement personnel, firefighters, emergency medical technicians, and others who have similar access to the outdoors or to animals.

Cattle may carry deer ticks. Dogs that enter tick habitats also can carry *Ixodes* (deer ticks) and become infected [45]. In some parts of the United States, 50% or more of unvaccinated dogs have been reported to have Lyme borreliosis [46, 47]. Determination of occupational causation may be complicated by avocational hunting, fishing, hiking, camping, gardening, property maintenance, golfing, or other activities related to the outdoors and to outdoor pets in endemic areas.

Clinical Description

Lyme disease can have a range of manifestations including skin rash, fever, fatigue, arthralgias, myalgias, carditis, and neurologic involvement. A distinction is usually made between early localized infection, early disseminated infection, and late manifestations. Sometimes these distinctions are labeled stages 1, 2, and 3.

EARLY LOCALIZED INFECTION, ERYTHEMA MIGRANS (EM)

Early localized infection generally is considered to be the first 30 days of infection. Diagnosis during this period usually is made based on the presence of EM alone or with other symptoms, without laboratory confirmation. Available laboratory tests are usually negative in the first weeks of infection and may take up to 6–8 weeks to become positive. IgM antibodies usually peak in the third to sixth week of infection. IgG antibodies can be detectable within 6–8 weeks after infection, peak around 4–6 months, and can be elevated indefinitely. A history of tick bite is not usually required to make a diagnosis because many tick attachments may not be noticed [48].

The classic skin lesion of Lyme disease is EM, which was formerly called *erythema chronicum migrans*. EM is a red macule or papule that, in the course of days to weeks, expands to form a circle, often with central clearing. The EM lesions can be single or multiple and can develop satellite lesions. EM has been reported to occur in about 60–80% of clinically recognized cases of Lyme disease [7, 48].

To establish uniform national case surveillance and reporting for the Centers for Disease Control and Prevention (CDC), the EM lesion must be 5 cm or more in diameter to be considered significant [48]. The surveillance case definitions should not be used as the only criteria for establishing a clinical diagnosis or deciding on medical care for any individual. EM can be accompanied by fatigue, fever, headache, mild neck stiffness, arthralgias, or myalgias. These may occur within days to a week of infection and can resolve spontaneously. The EM rash usually fades in 3–4 weeks.

In some cases of EM, there is no central clearing. The inflammatory response sometimes can be so intense that it is not easily distinguishable from cellulitis. Some individuals may develop an annular erythematous lesion within several hours of a tick bite, which is thought to represent a hypersensitivity reaction and does not qualify as EM for reporting purposes [48].

Hematogenous spread of *Borrelia* is thought to be important in its pathogenesis but has been difficult to confirm by usual blood culture methods. A study of culture methods in people with EM concluded that plasma is a better culture source than whole blood or serum, noting successful plasma culture in more than 40% of cases. The hematogenous spread was noted to be symptomatic usually, but it could occur subclinically, the genotype of *B. burgdorferi* and age at initiation of Lyme disease greater than 55 years being factors associated with risk of dissemination [49].

An EM-like rash, very similar to that seen in Lyme disease (a red, expanding bull's-eye lesion around the site of a lone-star tick bite), also has been reported in southern tick-associated rash illness (STARI) and is transmitted by *Amblyomma americanum* ticks [50]. The adult female lone-star tick is distinguished by a white dot on her back (a "lone star"). The rash usually begins within a week of the tick bite and grows to 8 cm or more. The rise of this disease, like that of Lyme disease, human monocytic (or monocytotropic) ehrlichiosis and *Erlichia ewingii* ehrlichiosis, also has been attributed to the explosion of growth of white-tailed deer in the eastern United States, the white-tailed deer being a host for all stages of lone-star ticks [51]. One case of STARI had *B. lonestari* detected in skin, but many cases have had no sign of *B. lonestari* in-

fection. To date, the cause of STARI is considered to be unknown [50]. The acute illness with rash may be accompanied by fatigue, fever, headache, muscle aches, and joint pains. The condition responds to oral antibiotics and is not recognized to have any arthritis or neurologic or chronic symptoms. The lone-star tick resides in Texas and Oklahoma and ranges to the east through the southern states and along the Atlantic coast to Maine [50]. STARI is the subject of a CDC investigational protocol, and the CDC encourages physicians seeing a patient with a recent lone-star tick bite and an expanding rash of 5 cm in diameter to contact CDC at 970-221-6400.

EARLY DISSEMINATED INFECTION

These manifestations may occur weeks to months after the appearance of EM and are attributed to hematologic or lymphatic dissemination of the spirochete. Diagnosis of Lyme disease based on one or more manifestations of early disseminated or late illness is usually made by demonstration of diagnostic IgM or IgG antibodies to *B. burgdorferi* in serum or cerebrospinal fluid (CSF). The neurologic manifestations can include cranial nerve palsies (particularly facial palsy, which may be bilateral), mononeuritis multiplex, meningitis, or painful radiculoneuropathy. A meningoradiculoneuritis with CSF lymphocytic pleocytosis and severe pain, usually worse at night, is more common in European forms of Lyme disease (Bannwarth syndrome). Intense inflammatory responses in the central nervous system (CNS) related to Lyme disease may mimic CNS lymphoma or leukemic meningeal infiltration [52, 53].

Early disseminated illness also can be expressed as carditis. Fever and atrioventricular block may occur. The level of block may fluctuate and can include second- and third-degree block. Temporary pacing may be required.

Another not-well-known effect of infection is borrelial lymphocytoma, usually a single bluish red, mildly uncomfortable papule that can measure up to a few centimeters in diameter. It occurs most commonly near the site of a previous tick bite and can occur in an area affected by EM (uncommon) or previously affected by EM (more commonly occurring after EM and lasting longer, up to a year). This lesion occurs most commonly on the earlobe in children and on the breast in adults. Particularly in adults it can mimic malignancy, and histologic evaluation is recommended. Histology is typically a polyclonal, predominantly B-lymphocyte infiltration of skin and subcutaneous tissue, frequently with germinal centers [54, 55]. This manifestation of Lyme disease has been recognized primarily in Europe and may be the only manifestation of Lyme disease, or it may occur with other signs [55]. Some reports of borrelial lymphocytoma have come from outside Europe [56, 57].

Intermittent joint pain and swelling in one or more joints may occur. The episodes may last a few weeks and recur at intervals of several months, total duration lasting sometimes for years. Inflammatory arthritis may develop. The severity of recurrent episodes usually lessens as time passes. A recent report related occurrence of temporomandibular joint involvement in two Western blot–confirmed acute *B. burgdorferi* infections that resolved after intravenous treatment with ceftriaxone and resulted in no long-term symptoms or radiographic signs of persistent inflammation [58].

LATER MANIFESTATIONS

Six months or more after EM, and sometimes years after the initial infection, individuals may develop episodes of swelling and pain in large joints. Chronic arthritis that is usually pauciarticular may occur. Treatment-resistant Lyme arthritis appears to be a consequence of disseminated *B. burgdorferi* infection, affecting up to 10% of infected individuals. It may occur over several years and resolve. Onset appears to correlate with IgG reactivity to outer surface protein A (Osp-A) and does not appear to be related to persistence of the spirochete. The arthritis correlates with major histocompatability (MHC) class II alleles, including HLA-DR4, and may be caused by a T-cell autoimmune response owing to cross-reactivity between Osp-A and a human leukocyte function-associated antigen (hLFA-1α_L) in susceptible individuals [7, 59, 60]. Chronic paresthesias, radicular pain, and chronic meningoencephalitis have been reported, the latter being more common in Europe than in the United States. One European case report noted left arm paresthesias, dysphagia, and dysphonia owing to *B. burgdorferi*–related brain stem arteritis [61].

Seen primarily in Europe, acrodermatitis chronic atrophicans typically occurs several years after Lyme disease infection. It can occur after infection with any *Borrelia* species but most commonly follows *B. afzelii* infection. It usually affects the extensor surfaces of the hands and feet, starting with edema and bluish red discoloration and progressing to skin atrophy over months to years, with a prominent lymphoplasmacellular infiltrate of skin and sometimes subcutaneous tissue. It may be associated with peripheral neuropathy [55].

Some primary cutaneous B-cell lymphomas have been reported to demonstrate *B. bergdorferi*-specific DNA on PCR testing. Some have been reported to respond/regress after antibiotic therapy for Lyme disease, suggesting a response similar to that seen with borrelial lymphocytoma, but one recent report notes a lack of regression of a primary cutaneous marginal zone B-cell lymphoma after antibiotics [62].

PERSISTENT SUBJECTIVE COMPLAINTS

Sometimes people who have had well-documented treatment for Lyme disease have persistent musculoskeletal pain, neurologic symptoms, dysesthesias, or cognitive difficulties, often associated with fatigue. Evaluations have not found signs of persistent *B. burgdorferi* infection or co-infection with other tick-borne pathogens [63]. Sometimes these patients are labeled as having *chronic Lyme disease* or *post-Lyme disease syndrome*. These labels appear to describe a heterogeneous group rather than to represent a specific diagnostic condition. Many infectious and noninfectious conditions may share some or all of these symptoms. This may result in an overdiagnosis of Lyme disease in some situations [64]. The general population prevalence of fatigue and/or arthralgias of more than 10% complicates consideration of these issues [65]. The Infectious Diseases Society of America has issued a proposed definition of post-Lyme disease syndrome as a framework for future research and to reduce ambiguity of study populations [55].

BABESIOSIS

Babesiosis shares a tick vector with Lyme disease and can occur as a co-infection. Babesiosis occurs worldwide and is caused most commonly by *Babesia microti* in the eastern and midwestern United States, by *Babesia* type WA1 in the western coastal United States, and by *B. divergens* in Europe. Its incubation is typically longer than that of Lyme disease (1–8 weeks), and most infections are sub-clinical. However, severe or fatal disease can occur. The illness is characterized by fever, chills, myalgias, fatigue, mild to severe hemolytic anemia, and jaundice. It can be severe enough to mimic *falciparum* malaria. Diagnosis is made by either serologic studies and/or recognition of typical pear-shaped parasites in red blood cells [66]. More information on this condition is presented in Chapter 31.

ANAPLASMOSIS/EHRLICHOSIS

Anaplasmataceae infections (ehrlichioses) also can share a tick vector with Lyme disease and can occur as a co-infections. Anaplasmataceae are small obligate intracellular pleomorphic bacteria that can live and grow in phagosomes of the human host's mononuclear and polymorphonuclear blood cells. This group of bacteria formerly was classified as members of the Rickettsiaceae family. The group includes an organism that results in human monocytotropic ehrlichiosis (*Ehrlichia chaffeensis*) in the middle to southern tiers of the United States; one that results in human granulocytic anaplasmosis (*Anaplasma phagocytophilum*), which is an emerging infectious disease in North America (Lyme disease–endemic areas), Europe, and Asia; an organism that tends to be found in neutrophils of immunocompromised hosts (*E. ewingii* causing the disease ehlichiosis ewingii); the organism *E. muris,* found in Japan and Russia, which results in a monocytropic form of ehrlichiosis; and *Neorickettsia sennetsu,* found in Japan, which results in a mononucleosis-like illness (Sennetsu fever) with sore throat, cervical and postauricular adenopathy, atypical circulating lymphocytes, fever, chills, malaise, headache, myalgias, and joint pain. Illness from these organisms ranges from mild to severe or (except for *E. ewingii* and *E. muris*) fatal. The clinical syndrome can include fever, headache, anorexia, and myalgia. Nausea and vomiting may occur. Meningoencephalitis can be seen in about 20% of cases owing to *E. ewingii* and *E. muris* but is rare with *A. phagocytophilum*. This latter condition has a 7- to 14-day incubation period, and findings also may include thrombocytopenia, leukopenia, and elevated transaminases levels in blood. Diagnoses are usually confirmed with antibody testing, immunohistochemistry testing, identifying typical white blood cell inclusions on peripheral blood smears, culture, or PCR. Doxycycline is usually the drug of choice for treatment of nonpregnant adults with these bacterial illnesses [67].

Diagnosis and Laboratory Testing

The diagnosis of Lyme disease generally is based on consideration of symptoms, physical findings (e.g., EM, facial palsy, arthritis, and carditis), a history of possible exposure to infected ticks, and laboratory testing. Not all these need be present in a specific case. Symptoms and physical findings are usually most important for choosing treatment options.

Available validated laboratory tests rely on detecting antibodies made in response to infection. As noted in the clinical description of EM earlier, it generally takes several weeks to develop an antibody response, so standard testing likely will be negative in early localized infection (EM). Laboratory testing is more useful and reliable for early disseminated infection and late manifestations [15, 68, 69]. The CDC defines exposure as "having been (less than or equal to 30 days before onset of EM) in wooded, brushy, or grassy areas (i.e., potential tick habitats) in a county in which Lyme disease is endemic. A history of tick bite is not required" [48]. The CDC definition for endemicity of Lyme disease in a county is having a history of at least two confirmed cases being acquired there or having established populations of a tick vector infected with *B. burgdorferi*.

General guidelines for laboratory testing for Lyme disease involve a two-tiered approach that can be done using the same blood sample. The first step is to use a highly sensitive enzyme-linked immunosorbent assay (ELISA) or immunofluorescent antibody (IFA) test. The ELISA or IFA will identify most people with Lyme disease but also may be positive in people without the disease (e.g., may be positive with syphilis, relapsing fever, Rocky Mountain spotted fever, leptospirosis, HIV infection, herpes simplex type 2 infection, mononucleosis, lupus, or rheumatoid arthritis) [7, 70]. If the ELISA or IFA is negative, then no further testing is recommended. An indeterminant result on ELISA or IFA can be followed up with a repeat test after a few weeks. The second step is to use a highly specific Western blot test. Western blot tests are designed to assess either IgM or IgG antibody responses. The technology and sensitivity of Western blots for *B. burgdorferi* have improved with use of recombinant antigens, particularly with V1sE for IgG antibody detection and Osp-C for IgM antibody detection. Detection rates may vary from 20–50% for early localized illness (stage 1), to 70–90% for early disseminated illness (stage 2), to near 100% for late manifestations (stage 3) [71]. Thus, if the Western blot is negative, then the positive ELISA or IFA is likely a false-positive test, but the Western blot can be negative in some confirmed cases.

The CDC and the U.S. Food and Drug Administration (FDA) have advised caution related to use of Lyme disease testing by commercial laboratories in the United States, Canada, and Europe using assays that do not have adequately established accuracy and clinical usefulness [72]. These tests may include urine antigen tests, immunofluorescent staining for cell wall–deficient forms, lymphocyte transformation tests, and PCR tests for *B. burgdorferi* DNA on inappropriate specimens (e.g., blood and urine) or interpreting Western blot tests using unvalidated criteria [72].

Laboratory diagnosis of nervous system Lyme disease is done by documenting intrathecal antibodies. The spirochete is difficult to isolate from biopsy samples. The *sensu stricto* form can be grown in Barbour-Stoenner-Kelly medium [7]. PCR may be available in specialized laboratories and can identify spirochete genetic material in tissue, blood, urine, and cerebrospinal and synovial fluid. The role of PCR in diagnosis and management of patients is not well established; it may have a role in tissue and fluid analysis of complex late-stage illness [71].

As noted previously, ticks carrying *B. burgdorferi* also can carry *A. phagocytophilum* and *B. microti*. Co-infections may occur, the Lyme disease patient presenting with or later developing human granulocytic anaplasmosis and/or babesiosis. Specific clinical testing is needed to identify these infections.

Treatment

Some treatment issues related to Lyme disease have been controversial, particularly during the period after a tick bite, in chronic stages, and in patients with persistent subjective complaints. Treatment approaches continue to evolve, but some current recommendations for regimens are available [7, 55, 63, 65]. Adjustments in treatment protocol may be

needed depending on an individual's clinical presentation and course. Complete clinical and subjective response may not occur during the treatment period, and relapse may occur with any of these regimens. A second course of treatment may be needed when objective evidence of relapse is seen. However, early disease and most of the later disseminated manifestations are curable with antibiotics, resulting in long-term cure with no adverse sequelae [55, 63, 73].

Pregnant employees represent special situations for treatment, particularly avoidance of doxycycline and other antibiotics of that class. The CDC advises that "studies of women infected during pregnancy have found that there are no negative effects on the fetus if the mother receives appropriate treatment for her Lyme disease" [74]. It is advisable for pregnant employees to discuss treatment options with their own health care provider.

The treatment recommendations below apply to adults only. The recommendations reflect expert and consensus advice at the time of this writing and, in this dynamic area of medicine, can be expected to change. The antibiotic treatment recommendations are those published in *The Medical Letter* [63] and the 2006 Infectious Diseases Society of America (IDSA) guidelines [55]. The latter publication contains a great deal of detail covering the background for recommending their evidence-based guidelines, and the entire article is well worth reading before dealing with the clinical and therapeutic issues related to Lyme disease. These two publications differ from each other very little in terms of antibiotics and doses recommended. One difference is that the IDSA guidelines include as an alternative parenteral regimen penicillin G, 18–24 million units/day intravenously divided into every-4-hour doses (with dose reduction for impaired renal clearance).

The IDSA guidelines also list a number of treatments *not* recommended for Lyme disease. These include multiple, repeated courses of antimicrobials for the same episode of Lyme disease, doses or durations of therapy in excess of IDSA recommendations, combination antimicrobial therapy, pulsed dosing (antibiotics given on some days but not on others), first-generation cephalosporins, benzathine penicillin G, fluoroquinolones, carbapenems, vancomycin, metronidazole, tinidazole, trimethoprim-sulfamethoxazole, amantadine, ketolides, isoniazid, fluconazole, empirical therapy for babesiosis, anti-*Bartonella* therapies, hyperbaric oxygen, fever therapy, intravenous immunoglobulins, ozone, cholestyramine, intravenous hydrogen peroxide, vitamins or nutritional managements, and magnesium or bismuth injections.

PROPHYLAXIS

Using antibiotic treatment in response to tick bites, without evidence of EM or other Lyme disease manifestations, has been controversial. One study used a randomized, double-blind, placebo-controlled approach employing a single 200-mg dose of doxycycline or placebo in 482 people who had ticks removed within the previous 72 hours. EM developed at the site of the tick bites in a significantly smaller proportion of the group treated with doxycycline rather than placebo (0.4% versus 3.2%, $p < 0.04$) [75]. The study was done in an area of New York that is hyperendemic for Lyme disease. EM occurred in 9.9% (8 of 81 bites) of untreated nymphal tick bites when the nymphs were at least partially engorged with blood, but in none of the bites in which flat or unfed nymphs were removed.

A current recommendation is that the strongest indication for antibiotic prophylaxis is when there is reliable identification of the tick being an *I. scapularis* adult or nymph that has been attached for more than 36 hours (based on degree of engorgement of the tick or on certainty of time of exposure), when the tick bite occurred in a highly endemic areas where more than 20% of ticks are infected with *B. bergdorferi*, when doxycycline is not medically contraindicated, and when treatment can be started within 72 hours of the time of tick removal. If these conditions can be met, then the recommended dose of doxycycline is 200 mg orally taken once. If the criteria are not met, then observation is recommended [55, 63]. The IDSA guidelines specify that this recommendation is for tick bites in the United States.

ERYTHEMA MIGRANS

Oral antibiotic therapy shortens the duration of EM and generally prevents late sequelae. One of three drugs is usually used for the early stage of the disease. Current recommendations are doxycycline 100 mg PO bid for 10–21 days, amoxicillin 500 mg PO tid for 14–21 days, or cefuroxime axetil 500 mg PO bid for 14–21 days [63]. Of these three, only doxycycline is also effective against *A. phagocytophilum* (formerly *Ehrlichia*). Doxycycline should not be used in pregnant employees. A double-blind, controlled trial in patients with EM indicated that a 10-day course of doxycycline was as effective as a 20-day course. One patient in the 10-day treatment group developed meningitis [63]. Some sources recommend 2 weeks of treatment for isolated EM and 3–4 weeks of treatment for early disseminated infection [7]. The current recommendation for treatment of borrelial lymphocytoma is to use the same treatment regimens used for EM [55].

Current antibiotic resistance profiles of the patient's locale should be considered in making treatment decisions. Amoxicillin generally appears to be as effective as doxycycline. Macrolides appear to be less effective, and fluoroquinolones are not effective (see previous list covering treatments not recommended by the IDSA) [55]. If bacterial cellulitis cannot be excluded from the diagnosis of EM, then treatment with cefuroxime axetil or amoxicillin–clavulanic acid is recommended by *The Medical Letter* because these are active against *B. burgdorferi*, *Streptococcus pyogenese*, and most community-acquired *Staphylococcus aureus* [63].

NEUROLOGIC AND CARDIAC DISEASE

In complex situations, including neurologic, cardiac, or late disease, it may be of value and prudent to consult a specialist in infectious diseases or in the specialties of the organ systems affected. Practice parameters for treatment of neurologic manifestations of Lyme disease have been published recently, and these should be consulted [76]. The general conclusion was that nervous system infection responds well to penicillin, ceftriaxone, cefotaxine, and doxycycline (level B recommendation); most studies used parenteral regimens for neuroborreliosis, but some European studies support use of oral doxycycline in adults with meningitis, cranial neuritis, and radiculitis (also level B recommendation), reserving parenteral regimens for parenchymal CNS infection, other severe neurologic symptomatology, or failure of response to oral agents [76].

The 2007 recommendations for adults from *The Medical Letter* cover some of these situations [63]:

1. For treatment of facial nerve palsy (without other neurologic involvement) or first-degree atrioventricular block (PR interval <300 ms) [77], treatment with either oral doxycycline (100 mg bid) or oral amoxicillin (500 mg tid) for 14–21 days is usually effective.

2. For more severe neurologic manifestations of Lyme disease, ceftriaxone (2 g once per day, that is, every 24 hours intravenously) for 10–28 days is recommended. This same dose schedule can be used for 14–21 days for more severe cardiac disease. In some severe cases of cardiac disease, a temporary pacemaker may be necessary, but on resolution of heart block with stable cardiac function, oral treatment may be used. For the more severe forms of neurologic or cardiac disease, cefotaxime (2 g intravenously every 8 hours) for 14–28 days may be substituted for ceftriaxone. The IDSA guidelines include as an alternative parenteral regimen penicillin G (18–24 million units/day intravenously) divided into every-4-hour doses (with dose reduction for impaired renal clearance) [55].

LATE DISEASE, ARTHRITIS

The arthritis of late Lyme disease may take months to respond to the recommended treatment regimen of doxycycline 100 mg PO bid for 28 days or amoxicillin 500 mg PO tid for 28 days. If the arthritis is persistent or recurrent, then a second course of oral antibiotics can be given. If these treatments fail to result in response, ceftriaxone 2 g once daily (every 24 hours) intravenously for 14–28 days can be used. Cefotaxime 2 g intravenously every 8 hours for 14–28 days may be used as an alternative to ceftriaxone [63]. The IDSA guidelines include as an alternative parenteral regimen penicillin G, 18–24 million units/day intravenously divided into every-4-hour doses (with dose reduction for impaired renal clearance) [55].

Treatment recommended for acrodermatitis chronica atrophicans is with oral antibiotics usually used for Lyme disease [55].

PERSISTENT SUBJECTIVE COMPLAINTS

One randomized, placebo-controlled trial treated subjects who had persistent subjective complaints with either a 90-day course of intravenous and oral antibiotics or intravenous and oral placebo [78]. Antibiotic treatment consisted of intravenous cef-

triaxone 2 g daily for 30 days followed by 60 days of oral doxycycline at 200 mg daily. The 90-day treatment protocol did not improve symptoms more than placebo. Additional antibiotic therapy is not recommended for patients with persistent subjective complaints if their Lyme disease has been treated appropriately; additional antibiotic treatment has not been found to be of clinical benefit [55, 63].

A more recent study report describes a randomized, placebo-controlled trial of 10 weeks of intravenous ceftriaxone for previously diagnosed and antibiotic-treated Lyme disease patients with memory impairment, which was evaluated and followed with neurocognitive testing [79]. The investigators reported a generalized, moderate improvement in the antibiotic-treated subjects at the 12-week point, but relapse in cognition occurred after antibiotic treatment stopped (as measured at 24 weeks). Complications of treatment for the antibiotic treatment group were about 3.6 times those of the intravenous placebo group.

RELAPSES AND RECURRENCES

Relapses may occur with the recommended treatment protocols. In endemic areas, consideration should be given to whether the apparent relapse is a reinfection resulting from another *Ixodes* bite. Reinfection after successful treatment often can be recognized clinically by development of a repeat episode of EM at a different location on the skin during months when the tick vectors are abundant [80]. Relapses and recurrences also raise the issue of possible preexisting co-infection or new infection with a different pathogen. In tick-endemic areas, consideration should include (but not be limited to) babesiosis, Rocky Mountain spotted fever, *A. phagocytophilum* (*Ehrlichia*), Colorado tick fever, tularemia, Southern tick–associated rash illness (*B. lonestari*) [50], and relapsing fever (*B. recurrentis*) [7]. Treatment should be tailored to the clinical presentation, laboratory confirmations, and course of the disease.

Vaccine

A vaccine was approved by the FDA in 1998 as safe and effective for prevention of Lyme disease (LYMErix). This vaccine used an outer surface protein A (Osp-A) of *B. bergdorferi sensu stricto* in a recombinant form (r-Osp-A). The vaccine was pulled from the market by the manufacturer in 2002. Issues related to the vaccine included cost, a three-dose schedule for primary vaccination (first administration followed by additional doses at 30 days and 1 year), level of protection, need for booster doses, and concern that in some situations vaccination may be related to immune-mediated rheumatologic problems, particularly antibiotic-resistant forms of Lyme arthritis in people with HLA-DR4 and related alleles [59, 81]. Currently, no vaccine is commercially available in the United States for use in humans. Further research has been related to identifying other antigens, such as Osp-C, terminal Osp-A, and recombinant preparations of genes from the OspA/B locale, that may be effective and develop serologic responses with low potential for cross-reactivity with human tissue antigens [59, 82, 83]. One approach that conferred protection in mice from challenge with *B. burgdorferi* involved linking Osp-A and Osp-C to particulate carriers capsid-like particles (CLPs) from hepatitis B virus [84].

Personal Protection

An effective approach for protection from tick bites is to avoid tick-infested areas to the extent feasible, especially during the spring and summer months. The CDC [13] recommends that people take other precautions prior to, during, and after leaving potentially tick-infested areas:

1. Wear light-colored clothing so that you can see ticks crawling on clothing.
2. Tuck pant legs into socks or boots, and tuck shirt into pants.
3. Use insect repellent containing *N,N*-diethyl-*m*-toluamide (DEET) on clothes and exposed skin (avoid face).
4. Use permethrin on pants, socks, and shoes. Permethrin can repel and kill ticks.
5. Walk in the center of trails to avoid grasses and overhanging brush.
6. After being outdoors, remove clothing, and search clothing for ticks.
7. Inspect body carefully for ticks. Use a mirror to check hard-to-see areas.
8. Remove attached ticks. Use tweezers to grasp the tick as close to the skin as possible, and pull straight back with a slow, steady force to avoid crushing the tick's body.
9. Use high temperatures for washing and drying clothing.

Additional recommendations are to not use repellants on skin that is under clothing or on cuts, wounds, or irritated skin. Treated skin should be washed with soap and water after leaving the tick-infested area. If a rash or other reaction develops to an insect repellant, then stop using it, wash the treated areas with soap and water, and seek medical attention, taking the insect repellant container with you.

Picaridin (KRB 3023) is an insect repellant now available in the United States in a 7% solution. It has been used in Europe and Australia for years in higher concentrations. It offers some advantages over DEET in that it is odorless, nonoily, less irritating to the skin, and does not damage synthetic materials. Its 20% solution appears to be comparable to DEET in protection from mosquitoes. One study on African ticks (*Amblyomma hebraeum*) found Picaridin to be protective but not as effective as DEET 2 or more hours after application [85]. Further evaluation is needed to identify what protection Picaridin can provide against *Ixodes* ticks and Lyme disease in the United States.

Tick Control

Many occupations at risk for Lyme disease may be involved in outdoor activities episodically or in a variety of locations, some of which are either vast or involve property not under their direct control (e.g., farm workers, foresters, surveyors, utility linemen, lawn and garden workers, construction workers, surveyors, military personnel, emergency medical technicians, law enforcement personnel, field biologists, and veterinarians). In these situations, environmental control of ticks and animal reservoirs by the involved occupational group may be impractical or impossible.

Some employers may have lawns or grounds areas that are frequented by employees. General recommendations for grounds keeping to reduce tick populations in yard-type areas are to keep grass well trimmed, minimize damp microhabitats, remove leaf debris, clear brush, maintain a dry wood chip or gravel border between woods and lawns, remove plants that attract deer, and install barriers to discourage deer from entry [13].

In nonoccupational settings, attention has been given to other methods to reduce tick populations, limit *B. burgdorferi* penetration into those populations, and control host reservoirs of the spirochete. Broadcast of chemical insecticides or acaricides can be effective in reducing nymph and adult tick populations in the area of application, but the duration of their effects is limited, and frequent reapplications may be required. Treated areas can become reinfested as a result of traversing of the area by host mammals and dilution or degradation of the chemical treatment. Landowners and communities may be reluctant to broadcast chemicals with potential adverse health and environmental effects. Some alternative approaches, such as vaccination of mouse reservoirs, application of acaricides directly to white-tailed deer at feeding stations or to rodents at bait boxes, treatment of mice with a fungus that is toxic to *Ixodes* larvae, or introduction of nematodes that attack ticks are under study [86–89]. A study of reduction of deer density in New Jersey over three seasons documented an about 46% reduction from 45.6–24.3 deer/km^2, but no effect was found on numbers of questing *I. scapularis* subadults or overall numbers of host-seeking ticks, and no clear trend in incidence of Lyme disease was identified [90].

Other *Borrelia*-Related Illnesses: Tick- and Louse-Borne Relapsing Fevers

The occupational medicine provider also may need to consider or deal with *Borrelia*-related illnesses other than Lyme disease and the potentially related illnesses noted earlier. Relapsing fever is an illness that is transmitted to from one infected human to another by lice (*Pediculus humanus,* variant *corporis*) or as a zoonotic disease transmitted to humans from rodents or lagamorphs by ticks (particularly argasid ticks, genus *Ornithodoros*). Louse-borne (epidemic) relapsing fever (LBRF) is caused by *B. recurrentis* and occurs in areas of Asia, eastern Africa, and the highlands of central Africa and South America. Tick-borne relapsing fever (TBRF) is usually caused by *B. hermsii* or *B. turicatae* in North America (typically in the western U.S. states and western Canada) and by other *Borrelia* species in other parts of the world. In addition

to occurring in North America, TBRF occurs in tropical Africa, India, the Middle East, Portugal, Spain, and other limited areas in Europe (*B. hispanica* being the typical agent for relapsing fever in Europe), North Africa, central Asia, and South America. The typical pattern is that ticks emerge at night to quest and feast on sleeping humans. In the United States, TBRF typically occurs most often in spring and summer and may be associated with sleeping in outdoor settings, rustic homes, or infested vacation homes. Worldwide, LBRF is particularly related to periods of war and famine, forced population migrations owing to these factors, and conditions of poverty, overcrowding, and lack of hygiene, sanitation, and clothes washing [91, 92]. The illnesses can be related to occupational travel, the LBRF being an issue particularly for military and for relief workers.

Illness from LBRF and TBRF occurs after an incubation period of about 7 days (range 2–18 days). The organism spreads hematogenously from the bite site. Onset is typically sudden with fever (usually 40°C or higher), headache, shaking chills, sweats, myalgias, and arthralgias. The illness worsens over several days to a week and can resolve by crisis involving rising temperature with rigors (chill phase) followed by falling temperature and diaphoresis (flush phase). Crisis is associated with disappearance of the spirochete from the circulation; the organism can sequester in the liver, spleen, bone marrow, and CNS during remission. Without treatment, spirochetemia and return of symptoms can occur about 7–9 days later. Further relapses can occur. The illness can be associated with abdominal pain, vomiting, agitation, confusion, delirium, dry cough, pleurisy, hemopsysis, epistaxis, eye pain, photophobia, neck pain (meningismus), cranial nerve palsies, lymphocytic meningitis, splenic rupture, coma, or death [91]. The overall case-fatality rate of untreated cases is about 2–10% [92]. In 2004–2005, three cases of TBRF were reported to involve acute respiratory distress syndrome [93]. *B. hermsii* was confirmed in two of the three patients. The report noted that *Ornithodoros hermsii* ticks typically feed for less than 30 minutes, and most patients do not recall being bitten. Differential diagnosis of TBRF and LBRF includes considerations of dengue, malaria, arboviral infections, viral hemorrhagic fevers, tuberculosis, leptospirosis, Colorado tick fever, typhus, and typhoid [91].

Diagnosis can be made based on the clinical picture (which may mimic viral hemorrhagic fevers and other serious diseases); detection of spirochetes in blood, bone marrow, or CSF on dark-field examination; detection of spirochetes on Wright or Giemsa stains of peripheral blood; enzyme immunoassays for antibody; or immunofluorescent antibody tests; culture is done with Barbour-Stoenner-Kelly (BSK-II) medium. Blood-borne organisms are likely to be highest during episodes of high fever and may be absent between relapses. [91, 92].

Antibiotic treatment of LBRF and TBRF is usually very effective. Jarisch-Herxheimer reactions can occur within the first 4 hours of the first dose. Recommended treatment for nonpregnant adults includes tetracyclines as the drug of first choice, alternatives drug choices for adults being penicillin G or erythromycin [94]. Single-dose oral regimens of tetracycline, doxycylcine, erythromycin, or chloramphenicol may be sufficient therapy for LBRF; oral treatment for 7 days is recommended for TBRF [91]. Parenteral treatment may be needed when oral treatment is not tolerated.

Conclusion

Lyme disease has become an important concern for some occupational groups in the United States and abroad, particularly for those who work outdoors in endemic areas. Most of the manifestations of the illness can be treated successfully with antibiotics. In some occupational situations, employee education and training about Lyme disease, personal protection, and early removal of ticks are approaches that can help to reduce the risk of illness. Evolving issues relate to treatment, diagnostic testing, second-generation vaccines, and vector-based control technologies. One evolving issue in Connecticut is an investigation of possible antitrust violations in connection to the IDSA Lyme disease guidelines, particularly related to what some call "chronic Lyme" disease. While the current guidelines remain in place, an agreement has prompted further review to see if revision is needed [95, 96].

References

1. U.S. Department of Labor, Occupational Safety and Health Administration. Potential for Occupational Exposure to Lyme Disease. Safety and Health Information Bulletin. Washington: OSHA, February 11, 2003.
2. Centers for Disease Control and Prevention, Division of Vector-Borne Infectious Diseases. Lyme Disease Statistics. Atlanta: CDC, October 25, 2005; available at www.cdc.gov/ncidod/dvbid/lyme/ld_statistics.htm.
3. Bacon RM, Kugeler KJ, Griffith KS, et al. Lyme disease—United States, 2003–2005. MMWR 2007;56:573–6.
4. Healthy People 2010 (conference ed., in 2 vols). Washington: US Department of Health and Human Services, 2000; available at www.health.gov/healthypeople.
5. Weber K. Aspects of Lyme borreliosis in Europe. Eur J Clin Microbiol Infect Dis 2001;20:6–13.
6. Gern L, Mumair PF. Ecology of Borrelia burgdorferi sensu lato in Europe. In Gray JS, Kahl O, Lane RS, et al. (eds), Lyme Borreliosis: Biology, Epidemiology and Control. New York: CABI Publishing, 2002. Pp 149–74.
7. Hulinska D. Lyme disease. In Heymann DL (ed), Control of Communicable Disease Manual, 18th ed. Washington: American Public Health Association, 2004. Pp 315–20.
8. Miyamoto K, Masuzawa T. Ecology of Borrelia burgdorferi sensu lato in Japan and East Asia. In Gray JS, Kahl O, Lane RS, et al (eds), Lyme Borreliosis: Biology, Epidemiology and Control. New York: CABI Publishing, 2002. Pp 201–22.
9. Saito K, Ito T, Asashima N, et al. Case report: Borrelia valaisiana infection in a Japanese man associated with traveling to foreign countries. Am J Trop Med Hyg 2007;77:1124–7.
10. Ogden NH, Maarouf A, Barker IK, et al. Climate change and the potential for range expansion of the Lyme disease vector Ixodes scapularis in Canada. Int J Parasitol 2006;36:63–70.
11. Mantovani E, Costa IP, Gauditano G, et al. Description of Lyme disease–like syndrome in Brazil: Is it a new tick-borne disease or Lyme disease variation? Braz J Med Biol Res 2007;40:443–56.
12. Cooper JD, Feder HM. Inaccurate information about Lyme disease on the Internet. Pediatr Infect Dis J 2004;23:1105–8.
13. Centers for Disease Control and Prevention. Tick Tips. Atlanta: CDC, May 16, 2005, available at www.cdc.gov/ncidod/ticktips2005/
14. Zeller JL. Lyme disease. JAMA 2007;297:2664.
15. Centers for Disease Control and Prevention, Division of Vector-Borne Infectious Disease. Lyme Disease Diagnosis. Atlanta: CDC, October 7, 2005; available at www.cdc.gov/ncidod/dvbid/lyme/ld_humandisease_diagnosis.htm
16. Zhioua E, Rodhain F, Binet P, et al. Prevalence of antibodies to Borrelia burgdorferi in forestry workers of Ile de France, France. Eur J Epidemiol 1997;13:959–62.
17. Rath PM, Ibershoff B, Mohnhaupt A, et al. Seroprevalence of Lyme borreliosis in forestry workers

from Brandenburg, Germany. *Eur J Clin Microbiol Infect Dis* 1996;15:372–7.

18. Ahkee S, Ramirez J. A case of concurrent Lyme meningitis with ehrlichiosis. *Scand J Infect Dis* 1996;28:527–8.

19. Ikushima M, Kawahashi S, Okuyama Y, et al. The survey of prevalence of Lyme borreliosis in forestry workers in Saitama prefecture. *Kansenshogaku Zasshi* 1995;69:139–44.

20. Nakama H, Muramatsu K, Uchikama K, et al. Possibility of Lyme disease as an occupational disease: Seroepidemiolgical study of regional residents and forestry workers. *Asia Pacific J Public Health* 1994;7:214–7.

21. Moll van Charante AW, Groen J, Osterhaus AD. Risk of infections transmitted by arthropods and rodents in forestry workers. *Eur J Epidemiol* 1994;10:349–51.

22. Rees DH, Axford JS. Evidence for Lyme disease in urban park workers: A potential new health hazard for city inhabitants. *Br J Rheumatol* 1994;33:123–8.

23. Schwartz BS, Goldstein MD, Childs JE. Longitudinal study of *Borrelia burgdorferi* infection in New Jersey outdoor workers, 1988–1991. *Am J Epidemiol* 1994;139:504–12.

24. Nuti M, Amaddeo D, Crovatto M, et al. Infections in an Alpine environment: Antibodies to hantaviruses, *Leptospira, Rickettsiae,* and *Borrelia burgdorferi* in defined Italian populations. *Am J Trop Med Hyg* 1993;48:20–5.

25. Kuiper H, van Dam AP, Moll van Charante AW, et al. One-year follow-up study to assess the prevalence and incidence of Lyme borreliosis among Dutch forestry workers. *Eur J Clin Microbiol Infect Dis* 1993;2:413–8.

26. Parrott C, Johnson K, Strauss S, et al. Lyme disease in outdoor workers on Assateague Island: High tick exposure but low disease risk. *MD Med J* 1993;42:165–8.

27. Kuiper H, de Jongh BM, Nauta AP, et al. Lyme borreliosis in Dutch forestry workers. *J Infect* 1991;23:279–86.

28. Schwartz BS, Goldstein MD. Lyme disease in outdoor workers: Risk factors, preventive measures, and tick removal methods (see Comments). *Am J Epidemiol* 1990;131:877–85.

29. Moll van Charante AW, Groen J, Mulder PG, et al. Occupational risks of zoonotic infections in Dutch forestry workers and muskrat catchers. *Eur J Epidemiol* 1998;14:109–16.

30. Arteaga F, Golightly MG, Garcia Perez A, et al. Disparity between serological reactivity to *Borrelia burgdorferi* and evidence of past disease in a high-risk group. *Clin Infect Dis* 1998;27:1210–13.

31. Arteaga Perez F, Garcia-Monco Carra JC. Risk factors associated with the presence of antibodies against *Borrelia burgdorferi. Rev Clin Esp* 1999;199;136–41.

32. Ikushima M, Yamada F, Kawahashi S, et al. Antibody response to OspC-I synthetic peptide derived from outer surface protein C of *Borrelia burgdorferi* in sera from Japanese forestry workers. *Epidemiol Infect* 1999;122:429–33.

33. Werner M, Nordin P, Arnholm B, et al. *Borrelia burgdorferi* antibodies in outdoor and indoor workers in southwest Sweden. *Scand J Infect Dis* 2001;33:128–31.

34. Piacentino JD, Schwartz BS. Occupational risk of Lyme disease: An epidemiologic review. *Occup Environ Med* 2002;59:75–84.

35. Reimer B, Erbas B, Lobbichler K, et al. Seroprevalence of *Borrelia* infection in occupational tick-exposed people in Bavaria (Germany). *Int J Med Microbiol* 2002;291:S215.

36. Niscigorska J, Skotarczak B, Wodecka B. *Borrelia burgdorferi* infection among forestry workers: Assessed with an immunoenzymatic method (ELISA), PCR and correlated with the clinical state of the patients. *Ann Agric Environ Med* 2003;10:15–19.

37. Santino I, Cammarata E, Franco S, et al. Multicentric study of seroprevalence of *Borrelia burgdorferi* and *Anaplasma phagocytophila* in high-risk groups in regions of central and southern Italy. *Int J Immunopathol Pharmacol* 2004;17:219–23.

38. Cinco M, Barbone F, Grazia-Ciufolini M, et al. Seroprevalence of tick-borne infections in forestry rangers from northeastern Italy. *Clin Microbiol Infect* 2004;10:1056–61.

39. Baker BC, Croft AM, Crwinfield CR. Hospitalisation due to Lyme disease: Case series in British Forces Germany. *J R Army Med Corps* 2004;150:182–6.

40. Letrilliart L, Ragon B, Hanslik T, et al. Lyme disease in France: A primary care-based prospective study. *Epidemiol Infect* 2005;133:935–42.

41. Cisak E, Chmielewska-Badora J, Zwolinski J, et al. Risk of tick-borne bacterial diseases among workers of Roztocze National Park (southeastern Poland). *Ann Agric Environ Med* 2005;12:127–32.

42. Rojko T, Ruzic-Sabljic E, Strle F, et al. Prevalence and incidence of Lyme borreliosis among Slovene forestry workers during the period of tick activity. *Wien Klin Wochenschr* 2005;117:219–25.

43. Tomao P, Ciceroni L, D'Ovidio MC, et al. Prevalence and incidence of antibodies to *Borrelia burgdorferi* and to tick-borne encephalitis virus in agricultural and forestry workers from Tuscany, Italy. *Eur J Clin Microbiol Infect Dis* 2005;24:457–63.

44. Sarwari AR, Strickland T, Pena C, et al. Tick exposure and Lyme disease at a summer camp in Maryland. *W V Med J* 2005;101:126–30.

45. Rabinowitz PM, Gordon Z, Odofin L. Pet-related infections. *Am Fam Physician* 2007;76:1314–22.

46. Stone EG, Lacombe EH, Rand PW. Antibody testing and Lyme disease risk. *Emerg Infect Dis* 2005;11:722–4.

47. Littman MP. Lyme disease: Diagnosis and treatment. *ACVIM Proc* 2004.

48. Centers for Disease Control and Prevention. Lyme Disease (*Borrelia burgdorferi*) 1996 Case Definition.

Atlanta: CDC, updated November 15, 2005; available at www.cdc.gov/epo/dphsi/casedef/lyme_disease_current.htm.

49. Wormser GP. Hematogenous dissemination in early Lyme disease. *Wien Klin Wochenschr* 2006;118:634–7.

50. Centers for Disease Control and Prevention, Division of Vector-Borne Infections Disease. Southern Tick–Associated Rash Illness. Atlanta: CDC, updated July 27, 2006; available at www.cdc.gov/ncidod/dvbid/stari/index.htm.

51. Paddock CD, Yabsley MJ. Ecological havoc, the rise of white-tailed deer, and the emergence of *Amblyomma americanum*–associated zoonoses in the United States. *Curr Top Micrbiol Immunol* 2007;315:289–324.

52. Bahrain H, Laureno R, Krishnan, et al. Lyme disease mimicking central nervous system lymphoma. *Cancer Invest* 2007;25:336–9.

53. Schweighofer CD, Fätkenheuer G, Staib P, et al. Lyme disease in a patient with chronic lymphocytic leukemia mimics leukemic meningeosis. *Onkologie* 2007;30:564–6.

54. Stanek G, Strle F. Lyme borreliosis. *Lancet* 2003;362:1639–47.

55. Wormser GP, Dattwyler RJ, Shapiro ED, et al. The clinical assessment, treatment, and prevention of Lyme disease, human granulocytic anaplasmosis, and babesiosis: Clinical practice guidelines by the Infectious Diseases Society of America. IDSA Guidelines. *Clin Infect Dis* 2006;43:1089–1134.

56. Finkel MF, Johnson RC. *Borrelia* lymphocytoma: A possible North American case. *Wisconsin Med J* 1990;89:683–6.

57. Yoshinari N, Spolidorio M, Bonoldi VL, et al. Lyme disease–like syndrome–associated lymphocytoma: First case report in Brazil. *Clinics* 2007;62:525–6.

58. Lesnicar G, Zerdoner D. Temporomandibular joint involvement caused by *Borrelia bergdorferi*. *J Craniomaxillofac Surg* 2007;35:397–400.

59. Willett TA, Meyer AL, Brown EL, et al. An effective second-generation outer surface protein A–derived Lyme vaccine that eliminates a potentially autoreactive T cell epitope. *Proc Natl Acad Sci USA* 2004;101:1303–8.

60. Drouin EE, Glickstein LJ, Steere AC. Molecular characterization of the OspA(161–175) T-cell epitope associated with treatment-resistant Lyme arthritis: Differences among the three pathogenic species of *Borrelia burgdorferi sensu lato*. *J Autoimmun* 2004;23:281–92.

61. Habek M, Mubrin Z, Brinar VV. Avellis syndrome due to borreliosis. *Eur J Neurol* 2007;14:112–4.

62. Monari P, Farisoglio C, Calzavara P. *Borrelia burgdorferi*–associated primary cutaneous marginal-zone B-cell lymphoma: A case report. *Dermatology* 2007;215:229–32.

63. Treatment of Lyme disease. *Med Lett* 2007;49:49–51.

64. Hsu VM, Patella SJ, Sigal LH. "Chronic Lyme disease" as the incorrect diagnosis in patients with fibromyalgia. *Arthritis Rheum* 1993;36:1489–92.

65. Wormser GP, Nadelman RB, Dattwyler RJ, et al. Practice guidelines for the treatment of Lyme disease. *Clin Infect Dis* 2000:31:S1–14.

66. Meslin F, Western K. Babesiosis. In Heymann DL (ed), *Control of Communicable Disease Manual*, 18th ed. Washington: American Public Health Association, 2004. Pp 61–63.

67. Walker DH, Dumler JS. Ehrlichioses. In Heymann DL (ed), *Control of Communicable Disease Manual*, 18th ed. Washington: American Public Health Association, 2004. Pp 187–90.

68. Kulie T, Vogt K, Sevetson E, et al. When should you order a Lyme titer? *J Fam Pract* 2005;54:1084–88.

69. DePietropaolo DL, Powers JH, Gill JM, et al. Diagnosis of Lyme disease. *Am Fam Physician* 2005;72:297–304.

70. Strasfeld L, Romanzi L, Seder RH, et al. False-positive serologic test results for Lyme disease in patient with acute herpes simplex virus type 2 infection. *Clin ID* 2005;41:1826–7

71. Wilske B. Epidemiology and diagnosis of Lyme borreliosis. *Ann Med* 2005;37:568–79.

72. Notice to readers: Caution regarding testing for Lyme disease. *MMWR* 2005;54;125.

73. Shapiro ED. Lyme disease. *Adv Exp Med Biol* 2008;609:185–95.

74. Centers for Disease Prevention and Control, Division of Vector-Borne Infectious Diseases. Lyme Disease Treatment and Prognosis. Atlanta: CDC, October 10, 2005; available at www.cdc.gov.

75. Nadelman RB, Nowskowski J, Fish D, et al. Prophylaxis with single-dose doxycycline for the prevention of Lyme disease after an *Ixodes scapularis* tick bite. *N Engl J Med* 2001;345:79–84.

76. Halperin JJ, Shapiro ED, Logigian E, et al. Practice parameter: treatment of nervous system Lyme disease (an evidence-based review): Report of the Quality Standards Subcommittee of the American Academy of Neurology. *Neurology* 2007;69:91–102.

77. Correction: Lyme disease (*Med Lett Drugs Ther* 2007;49:49). *Med Lett Drugs Ther* 2007;49:64.

78. Kempner MS, Hu LT, Evans J, et al. Two controlled trials of antibiotic treatment in patients with persistent symptoms and a history of Lyme disease. *N Engl J Med* 2001;345:85–92.

79. Fallon BA, Keilp JG, Corbera KM, et al. A randomized, placebo-controlled trial of repeated IV antibiotic therapy for Lyme encephalopathy. *Neurology* 2007; epub ahead of print, available at PubMed, www.ncbi.nlm.nih.gov; accessed March 20, 2008.

80. Nadelman RB, Wormser GP. Reinfection in patients with Lyme disease. *Clin Infect Dis* 2007;45:1032–8.

81. Hanson MS and Edelman R. Progress and controversy surrounding vaccines against Lyme disease. *Exp Rev Vaccines* 2003;2:683–703.

82. Koide S, Yang X, Huang X, et al. Structure-based

design of a second-generation Lyme disease vaccine based on a C-terminal fragment of *Borrelia bergdorferi* OspA. *J Mol Biol* 2005;350:290–9.

83. Wallich R, Jahraus O, Stehle T, et al. Artificial-infection protocols allow immunodetection of novel *Borrelia burgdorferi* antigens suitable as vaccine candidates against Lyme disease. *Eur J Immunol* 2003;33:708–19.

84. Nassal M, Skamel C, Vogel M, et al. Development of hepatitis B virus capsids into a whole-chain protein antigen display platform: New particulate Lyme disease vaccines. *Int J Med Microbiol* 2008;298:135–42.

85. Picaridin: A new insect repellant. *Med Lett* 2005;47:46–47.

86. Patrican LA, Allan SA. Application of desiccant and insecticidal soap: Treatments to control *Ixodes scapularis* (Acari: Ixodidae) nymphs and adults in a hyperendemic woodland site. *J Med Entomol* 1995;32:859–63.

87. Tsao JI, Wootton JT, Bunikis J, et al. An ecological approach to preventing human infection: Vaccinating wild mouse reservoirs intervenes in the Lyme disease cycle. *Proc Natl Acad Sci USA* 2004;101:18159–64.

88. Hornbostel VL, Ostfeld RS, Benjamin MA. Effectiveness of *Metarhizium anisopliae* (Deuteromycetes) against *Ixodes scapularis* (Acari: Ixodidae) engorging on *Peromnyscus leucopus*. *J Vector Ecol* 2005;30:91–101.

89. Suszkiw J. Tackling ticks that spread Lyme disease. *Agric Res* 1998;22–24.

90. Jordan RA, Schuze TL, Jahn MB. Effects of reduced deer density on the abundance of *Ixodes scapularia* (Acari: Ixodidae) and Lyme disease incidence in a northern New Jersey endemic area. *J Med Entomol* 2007;44:752–7.

91. Dennis DT, Hayes EB. Relapsing fever. In Kasper DL, Fauci AS, Longo DL, et al (eds), *Harrison's Principles of Internal Medicine,* 16th ed. New York: McGraw-Hill, 2005, Chap 156. Pp 991–5.

92. Hulinská D. Relapsing fever. In Heymann DL (ed), *Control of Communicable Disease Manual,* 18th ed. Washington: American Public Health Association, 2004. Pp 450–3.

93. Murphy FK, Parker S, Stokich D, et al. Acute respiratory distress syndrome in persons with tickborne relapsing fever—Three states, 2004–2005. *MMWR* 56;2007:1073–6.

94. Choice of antibacterial drugs. *Treatment Guidelines from The Medical Letter* 2007;5:33–50.

95. From the President: IDSA Stands Up For Lyme Disease Guidelines, 2007: Available at: www.idsociety.org.

96. Collins D. Doctors to reassess antibiotics for "chronic Lyme" disease. 2008. The Associated Press. Available at: www.nl.newsbank.com/nl-search/.

Occupational Travel

27

Occupational Travel and Prevention of Infectious Diseases

William E. Wright

Many published resources describe model travel medicine programs, their essential elements, and administration. These include the U.S. Centers for Disease Control and Prevention (CDC) [1], the World Health Organization (WHO) [2], and the International Society of Travel Medicine [3]. This chapter is not intended to be a comprehensive resource for general management of travel medicine programs. Its focus is on general principles and approaches to prevention, specifically related to infectious diseases. It can be used for service planning and employee education. It also provides guideposts to other chapters in this book that cover details of specific infectious diseases.

Scope of Infectious Disease Issues in Occupational Travel

The nature of populations of humans, animals, and insects is that they move and adapt to local and global conditions. The nature of microorganisms is their unique ability to rapidly shift their own population's capabilities to adjust to local conditions and take advantage of changes in vector, reservoir, and host populations. These are the challenges of infectious disease and travel medicine that makes these fields dynamic. A strategy to deal with these challenges is to continually update our epidemiologic understanding of local and world populations. The CDC Health Alert Network [4] and the WHO's Epidemic and Pandemic Alert and Response (EPR) [5] are resources that can help the practitioner keep up with changing and emerging patterns of disease. The U.S. Department of State also posts country-specific information, Travel Warnings when travel to a country is recommended to be deferred owing to civil unrest, other dangerous conditions, or lack of diplomatic relations with a country that could make it very difficult to assist Americans in distress, and Travel Alerts about terrorist threats and other relatively short-term or transnational conditions that could pose a risk to American travelers. These can be accessed at www.travel.state.gov.

Human population shifts can be small and short term, like most business travel. The business traveler's movements can overlap and interact with larger-scale and longer-term shifts that include holiday travel, immigration, and refugees from war and natural disasters. The inexorable worldwide expansion of human populations into rural or forested areas where they share habitats with animal and insect vectors of disease has an impact on business travelers. Migration and displacement of reservoirs and vectors, either because of changes of seasons, global climate change, or human activity, also can have an impact. These overlaps of population movements often are unplanned and/or poorly controlled [6]. The WHO notes that the number of people traveling internationally increases every year and in 2005 exceeded 800 million. Business travel accounted for 16% (125 million). Fifty percent of international travel arrivals were for leisure, recreation, and holiday. Twenty-six percent were for visiting friends and relatives, religious purposes/pilgrimages, and health treatments [7]. In the United States in 2003, business travel accounted for 18% (about 210 million person-trips) of all U.S. domestic person-trips [8].

A role of the occupational physician is to understand shifts in populations of people, animals, insects, and microbes and help employers and employees to assess the risks and address concerns about the advisability of business travel abroad. Globalization has brought increases in U.S. business travel to developing countries. Commercial travelers increasingly are exposed to endemic infectious disease and have the potential to be targets of bioterrorism (see Chapter 39), pandemic disease (see Chapter 11), and rapidly changing patterns of infectious diseases (see Chapter 37). Sometimes the weight of these factors and expectations for expenses for medical care of illness, hospitalizations, lost work time, medical evacuations, and potential quarantine influence companies to reduce travel abroad and use alternative methods, such as telecommuting, teleconferencing, and other electronic means or using agents to connect to business partners and manage relationships.

Although the term *travel medicine* in the United States often refers to citizens traveling abroad, this is a limited concept of travel medicine in the occupational setting. Many businesses work with visiting business travelers who come to the United States from other nations. Immigrants, refugees, and other documented or undocumented aliens also travel from their nations of origin to the United States for work. These workers can bring special health concerns (and unusual infectious disease risks) to work. These workers may have been medically underserved, may lack current resources, may not be familiar with ways to appropriately access medical care, and may have social and language barriers that influence their choices to

seek medical care. There is good reason to include these workers when considering provisions for travel and infectious disease-related medical services in the occupational setting. Toward the end of this chapter, issues of immigrants, refugees, and migrants are covered in more detail.

Prevention During Pretravel Preparation

VACCINATIONS

The role of vaccination is a critical element of primary prevention that helps travelers stay healthy. An assessment of vaccination status is part of pretravel preparation. The basic protection for the traveler should include basic childhood immunizations (given age-related considerations) with appropriately completed booster doses for tetanus, diphtheria, measles, mumps, rubella, varicella, and poliomyelitis (see Chapter 5 and specific diseases in other chapters).

In addition to the usual childhood vaccinations, a traveler's further travel-related vaccination plan should consider issues including itinerary, length of stay, type of occupational activity during travel, plans to visit relatives or friends in the destination country (which increases the risk for illness above that of a traveler who does not do such visits), likelihood of entry into rural or rustic environments, current patterns of disease incidence and prevalence, personal habits, presence of immune deficiency, presence of and likelihood of pregnancy, and presence of asplenia or other comorbidities. Vaccinations against influenza, hepatitis A, and hepatitis B are recommended for most travelers. Special consideration should be given to preexposure prophylaxis for rabies, meningococcal vaccination, pneumococcal polysaccharide vaccination, typhoid, yellow fever, and other vaccinations depending on the profile of the traveler and his or her travel plans (see Chapter 5).

PROPHYLAXIS

Antimalarial prophylaxis should be prescribed if the traveler is scheduled to enter areas where malaria is endemic. The traveler should understand the necessity to take antimalarial medication as prescribed, including during the pre- and post-travel periods as indicated. See Chapter 25 for further details. The traveler may need to consult a health care provider regarding advisability of using prophylaxis for travelers' diarrhea or carrying a supply of prophylactic antibiotics for his or her rheumatic or other valvular heart disease or prostheses.

OTHER

Tuberculosis occurrence is increasing in many countries. Tuberculin testing to establish pretravel status is advisable (see Chapter 9). Other pretravel preparations include risk and medical care considerations related to chronic illness. Infectious disease issues of particular importance are hepatitis immune status and chronic liver disease (see Chapter 17), chronic respiratory disease, current or recent treatment of malignancy, posttransplant status, other use of immunosuppressive drugs, syndromes of immunodeficiency, and infection with human immunodeficiency virus (HIV) [9]. Some countries required HIV testing of entering travelers, particularly those with plans to reside in country long term [10] (see Chapters 24 and 28).

Travelers should be counseled and provided with appropriate methods for dealing with travelers' diarrhea [11, 12] (see Chapter 28). Consideration should be give to providing antibiotics with instructions for presumptive treatment of anticipated conditions (such as malaria) based on the individual's medical profile. Contact lens wearers should be counseled to use only purified water for rinsing contact lenses and to use glasses for correction when hygienic conditions cannot be maintained [13]. Consideration should be given to providing the contact lens wearer with antibiotic drops or ointment to use for early treatment of eye inflammation in situations in which medical treatment is either unavailable or not easily accessible. These can be included in a traveler's kit of first aid items, which can include a supply of familiar over-the-counter medications known by the traveler to be well tolerated, antifungal and antibiotic ointments or creams, antidiarrheal treatments, a full trip-long supply of usual prescription medication (with copies of prescriptions), vaccination records, water purification supplies, and other items [14] (Table 27-1). Travelers who require use of needles and syringes for self-treatment should carry their own supply, along with a health care provider's letter verifying their medical necessity. Pregnancy should be considered when advising female travelers about travel and risks (see Chapter 33).

The increasing risks for bioterrorism, pandemic illness, and endemic or epidemic infectious diseases create a need for travel-related occupational health programs to also assist employers and employees with plans for travelers' health insurance for travel to areas where health risks are significant and where medical care is expensive or not readily available, medical care, hospitalization, evacuation abroad, and emergency repatriation for health reasons. Medical evacuations can cost more than $50,000 and are not typically covered by U.S. medical insurance. The CDC and the U.S. State Department Web sites can provide guidance on these issues [1, 15]. Currently, the CDC encourages travelers to prepare for emergencies by providing travel itineraries, contact information, and emergency contact/next-of-kin information to the airline used for travel if that airline provides this type of registration process [16]. The Department of State now offers free travel registration service to all U.S. citizens traveling or living abroad to facilitate State Department assistance in case of an emergency [17].

Employers should be prepared to address payment issues for hospitalizations abroad. In some developing countries, hospitalized travelers from the United States have been held hostage in the hospital, not to be released until full payment for services is received in U.S. funds. Employers' programs also should be prepared to address issues for disabled travelers and workers' compensation related to infectious diseases. In some situations, employers may want to make contingency arrangements for medical care overseas, including evacuations, particularly related to travel in countries with political disruptions/unrest and in developing countries with high or unusual infectious disease risks. The Department of State or the International Association for Medical Assistance to Travelers (IAMAT) can be helpful with such planning [15, 18]. If travelers who are U.S. citizens become seriously ill overseas, the local U.S. consulate can be contacted for assistance in locating appropriate medical services. The prepared traveler should have the local contact information in hand.

If a worker is traveling with service dogs, special attention needs to be given to possible restrictions for entry to destination countries, quarantine/vaccination requirements, and housing arrangements. The traveler should check in advance with the embassy or consulate of the destination countries.

Table 27-1
Travelers' Health Kit

There are a number of travelers' health kits available commercially for care of minor health problems while traveling. Similar kits can be assembled at home. Contents of a personalized kit depend on the individual's medical condition and destination, duration, and type of travel. The following is a basic kit for adults recommended by the U.S. Centers for Disease Control and Prevention. The occupational health professional or individual traveler may want to modify this list based on consideration of personal experience, medical needs, personal physician's advice, other information in chapters in this book, or other sources of travel advice.

Medications
- Personal prescription medications in original containers with a copy of each prescription, including generic names of medications; have a note from the prescribing physician on letterhead stationery for controlled substances and injectable medications.
- Antimalarial medications, if applicable
- Over-the-counter (OTC) antidiarrheal medication (e.g., bismuth subsalicylate, loperadmide)
- Antibiotic for self-treatment of moderate to severe diarrhea
- Antihistamine
- Decongestant, alone or in combination with antihistamine
- Anti–motion sickness medication
- Acetaminophen, aspirin, ibuprofen, or other medication for fever and pain
- Mild laxative
- Cough suppressant/expectorant
- Throat lozenges
- Antacid
- Antifungal and antibacterial ointments or creams
- 1% Hydrocortisone cream
- Epinephrine autoinjector (e.g., EpiPen, especially if history of severe allergic reaction)

Other Important Items
- Insect repellant containing DEET (up to 50%)
- Sunscreen (preferably SPF 15 or greater)
- Aloe gel for sunburns
- Digital thermometer
- Oral rehydration solution packets
- Basic first aid items (e.g., adhesive bandages, gauze, Ace wrap, antiseptic, tweezers, scissors, and cotton-tipped applicators)
- Antibacterial hand wipes or alcohol-based hand sanitizer containing at least 60% alcohol
- Moleskin for blisters
- Lubricating eye drops
- First aid quick reference card

Other Items That May Be Useful in Certain Circumstances
- Mild sedative (e.g., zolpidem) or other sleep aid
- Antianxiety medication
- High-altitude preventive medication
- Water purification tablets
- Commercial suture/syringe kits (to be used by local health care provider; these items also will require a letter from the prescribing physician on letterhead stationery)
- Latex condoms
- Address and phone numbers of area hospitals or clinics

Note: This list is similar to that published in another recommended source: World Health Organization. Health risks and precautions: General considerations. In *International Travel and Health, 2007*. Geneva: WHO Press, 2007, Chap 1, pp 4–5.
DEET = *N,N*-diethyl-*m*-toluamide; SPF = sun protection factor.
Source: Travelers' health kit. In *Pre- and Post-travel General Health Recommendations: CDC Health Information for International Travel 2008*. Atlanta: CDC, 2008, Chap 2.

Information on requirements and restrictions is also available at http://travel.state.gov. Some certificates, including inoculation certificates, may need to be translated from English to the destination country's language. The traveler also should consult a veterinarian for information on disease risks, maintaining animal health during travel, vaccinations, medications, and certificates.

The employer or the occupational medicine resource also should be prepared to deal with the death of employees overseas, including those related to bioterrorism, pandemics, or serious epidemic or endemic infectious agents. Importing uncremated human remains into the United States is covered by federal quarantine regulations [19]. The CDC can restrict importation of remains if necessary to prevent the spread of disease. Special

procedures need to be followed if the traveler is known to have died from or is suspected of dying from diseases such as cholera, diphtheria, infectious tuberculosis (TB), plague, smallpox, yellow fever, viral hemorrhagic fevers, or severe acute respiratory syndrome (SARS). With these conditions, permission to import remains must be requested and obtained from the CDC's Division of Global Migration and Quarantine. Permission depends on assurances related to proper handling of remains, use of a hermetically sealed casket, and plans for proper interment. The remains must be cleared by a CDC Quarantine Officer at the port of arrival based on review of the Division of Global Migration and Quarantine—signed permission and the death certificate, translated into English, which addresses the cause of death [19]. People who need to use these procedures should seek assistance from the U.S. consulate in the country where the remains reside. Additional information is available from the Department of State [20].

Travelers also will benefit from counseling that covers the infectious disease risk specific to their itineraries, avoidance of risk for injuries that create opportunities for infection or need for invasive medical care, and the general behavioral techniques for controlling or limiting infectious disease risks, which are covered below.

Behavioral Prevention of Infectious Disease During Travel

A goal of occupational travel is to work effectively and efficiently. Staying healthy is an important factor in achieving this goal. The occupational traveler should be aware of the potential for infectious disease to disrupt work and how to prevent this from occurring. The infectious disease risks of travel can be classified according to routes of exposure, which is a convenient way to provide training for travelers. This section covers some standard behavioral precautions that can limit risk of infectious diseases during travel.

ORAL ROUTE

Food and water are common sources of infection during travel. The agents that result in infection through the oral route include bacterial, viral, protozoan, and helminthic organisms. These are addressed in detail in the five travel-related chapters that follow and in chapters that address specific microorganisms or conditions (e.g., Chapter 18).

An important aspect of preventing oral-route contamination is to avoid hand-associated fecal-oral transmission. Travelers should be reminded of the importance of hand washing with soap and water or with alcohol-based fluids or wipes (with more than 60% alcohol content) after activities such as using toilet facilities; shaking hands; covering sneezes or coughs with tissues or hands; handling children, their toys, diapers, or other sources of human feces; contacting or dressing wounds, sores, rashes, or secretions/excretions of others; touching animals, their secretions, or feces; after working in any other situations during which hand contamination may occur; before, during, and after food preparation; prior to dressing wounds, taking

or giving medication, handling contact lenses, touching own facial areas, and eating or handling food; and when hands look dirty. Hand washing should involve thorough coverage of the backs of the hands, fingertips, and interdigital areas, as well as palmar surfaces, and be of adequate duration (at least 20 seconds, approximating the time it takes to completely sing "Happy birthday to you . . ." twice (CDC An Ounce of Prevention campaign 2007). Naturally, the hand washer also should use water-conservation practices so that tap water is not run unless being actively used to wet or rinse.

In some rural and remote travel settings frequented by employees I have cared for, latrines/privies and/or pit privies have been available with no water source; others have had access to one flush-toilet used by many people that had water for flushing available only 1 hour each day; toilet paper, if available at all, was used by the local people according to their custom, which was to place used toilet tissue on the floor so that it could be reused by others. In these situations, good hygiene is very difficult to maintain. The traveler who may even occasionally enter this type of situation or who wants to be prepared for scarce paper resources would be well advised to carry some toilet paper or a substitute for it (e.g., tissues) and alcohol-based wipes and/or hand cleaning fluids.

As a general precaution, in areas with inadequate hygiene and sanitation, raw food should be avoided. This includes salads, vegetables (unless cooked), fruit (unless washed with clean water and peeled sanitarily by the consumer), unpasteurized milk and milk products (including cheeses), and uncooked or undercooked meat, fish, or shellfish. This advice also applies to sushi and sashimi unless it is prepared in a reputable establishment by experienced chefs likely to maintain a high standard of hygiene. For more information on fish-related diseases, including anisakiasis (which is increasingly related to sushi/sashimi ingestion), *Dioctophyma renale* infection, diphyllobothritis, and others, see Chapter 30. Some helminthes survive undercooking, pickling, freezing, air drying, cold smoking, or kippering. Even thoroughly cooked food, if allowed to stand or cool, can allow for bacterial growth. It this happens, then the food should be reheated/recooked thoroughly before eating. The general guideline here is to eat hot cooked food while it is still hot. In some cultures, I have observed well-cooked food being placed in fly-infested holding areas to await serving. The finer restaurants aimed electric fans on the platters of waiting food to reduce the fly population on it. This also cools hot food rapidly.

The guideline to "eat hot food hot" is often accompanied by the rule "eat cold food cold." While this can be a good practice, in areas with inadequate sanitation and hygiene or uncertain supplies of electricity for reliable refrigeration, it is wise to avoid eating products that require refrigeration, particularly if they contain milk or milk products. Moreover, travelers should not try to transport perishable food with them during travel.

Special situations that arise during travel can present risks of infection. Exotic fare, such as "bush meat" in Africa, may include the flesh of primates and increases the risk for disease [21, 22]. Street vendors' and street-vending open markets' wares of food or beverage often can increase the risk of illness; in one study [23], about 45% of sampled taco dressings contained fecal contamination; such dressings may be prepared the day before sale and left unprotected. Table items, such as salsa, have been found to carry an increase risk of contamination with *Escherichia coli* in the United States and abroad [24]; fecal contamination was found in 66% of table sauce samples in Guadalajara, Mexico, and in 40% of samples in Houston, Texas. The guidelines for safe eating in developing countries also should apply to food and water provided by commercial airlines, particularly for fresh and uncooked items, nonbottled water, ice, and milk-based products if they are likely to have been obtained in developing countries where unsanitary circumstances and refrigeration requirements are issues.

In areas where sanitation and hygiene are inadequate, tap water, ice made from the general water supply, and glasses of water brought to the table should not be consumed at all. This applies to use of ice in drinks and water for brushing teeth. In these circumstances, safe beverages generally are those made from boiled water, such as coffee and tea, and served hot. Canned and bottled beverages such as sodas and carbonated mineral water generally are safe, recognizing that if the containers are cooled by immersion in water or ice, then their exteriors are likely to be contaminated. Cleaning the containers with soap and hot water is advisable before drinking from them. Sealed cans or bottles of

water that are opened in the traveler's presence (i.e., containers unlikely to have been used previously and refilled under unsanitary conditions) generally are safe. Beer, wine, and liquor (with no water or ice) are likely to be safe from contamination by infectious agents, but their ability to dehydrate the body should be recognized and their use limited or avoided, particularly in hot climates or when hydration is needed. Care should be taken to not pour potentially safe beverages into contaminated containers for consumption; drinking from the bottle's or can's cleaned surface is safer. In many venues, cleaning the drinking surface of the beverage's container is a good idea because containers are not usually the subject of strict sanitation, may have been cooled in contaminated ice/water, may have been stored in rodent-infected areas, and likely have been handled without hand-washing precautions.

The most reliable way to prepare potentially contaminated water for drinking is to boil it. The general rule is to bring the water to a rolling boil for 1 minute and let it cool to room temperature before drinking [25, 26]. Ice should not be added to cool it, and the prepared water should not be poured into containers likely to be contaminated. At altitudes above 2000 m, water should be boiled for 3 minutes instead of one; if boiled for only 1 minute at these altitudes, chemical disinfection of the boiled water is recommended.

Chemical treatment with tincture of iodine (2% USP) or other commercial iodine-containing products is the most reliable alternative to boiling. The manufacturer's instruction should be followed, adjusting the dose according to the temperature and cloudiness of the available water and observing posttreatment standing time prior to consuming the treated water. For use of iodine 2% USP, 5 drops per liter or quart of clear water (10 drops, which is 0.5 mL, per liter or quart of cold or cloudy water) is recommended, followed by a minimum of a 30-minute period of stand time before drinking the treated water [25, 26]. For each 10°C below 25°C (77°F) of water temperature, the standing time after disinfection should double before drinking. This method results in a residual iodine taste that some may consider unpleasant. The taste can be masked by adding small amounts of powdered commercial products that are used for electrolyte replacement or noncaffeinated sports drinks, such as Gatorade mix and others, or powdered iced-tea mix, which are fairly easy for travelers to carry. (I have no financial interest in mentioning a commercial product but note one here as a type, having found it to be available in many travel locations and available in powder form useful for travel.) Tincture of iodine is usually sold with a wand affixed to the inside of the bottle cap, intended for application as an antiseptic. If it is to be used by the traveler for water treatment, the traveler should be equipped with several eye droppers because it is very difficult and messy (at least in my experience—perhaps I'm just uncoordinated) to use the wand to accurately measure out drops for water treatment. Iodine treatment is not effective for killing *Cryptosporidium*. In addition, iodine treatment is recommended only for short-term use (i.e., 2–3 weeks) and is not recommended for pregnant women, people with thyroid problems, or people hypersensitive to iodine-containing materials. Portable chlorination products are considered to be less reliable than iodine methods. The CDC guidance refers to a variety of commercial products and to methods one can use to make a crystalline iodine saturated solution for a disinfectant supply. Iodine in sufficient dose is a poison; it should be consumed only in properly diluted solutions and should be kept away from children [26].

Portable water filtration is an evolving technology, and there are many products available that provide different levels of protection. The most effective filters tend to be expensive. The size of the device needed for quick filtration of large amounts of water, particularly for multiple people, can be a limit to their utility for travelers (average usual water intake for adults, including water in food, is 1600–2200 mL/per day; fever, vomiting, and diarrheal illness increase needs for fluid replacement; activity in hot environments can result in 1- to 3-L fluid loss per hour) [27]. Further limits include the need to change contaminated filters, clogging of filters by particulate in water supplies, filter failure, and difficulty identifying when filters deteriorate or degrade over time. A guide to water filters can be found at www.cdc.gov. Some devices can filter out *Cryptosporidium, Giardia,* and most diarrhea-causing bacteria, but these filters with absolute pore sizes of 0.1–1.0 μm will miss viruses smaller than the pore size. For these filters, iodine treatment is recommended after filtration [26, 28].

In the event of significant diarrhea or gastroenteritis, the traveler should be prepared to maintain or reestablish adequate hydration using a source of uncontaminated or treated water as the basis for rehydration solutions. The WHO's current recommendation for rehydration solution is for all causes of diarrhea in all age groups and is lower in osmolarity (245 mOsmol/L) than its previously recommended 311 mOsmol/L solution. Each liter of the currently recommended oral rehydration fluid should contain 2.6 g sodium chloride, 13.5 g anhydrous glucose, 1.5 g potassium chloride, and 2.9 g trisodium citrate dihydrate. This new solution reduced the need for supplemental intravenous therapy in children and resulted in less vomiting and lower stool output than other reduced-osmolarity solutions [29]. The WHO recommends that adults drink this oral hydration fluid freely as required and stop treatment when diarrhea stops; it is recommended that any remaining solution be discarded after 24 hours has elapsed since preparation [29]. The recommended dose for infants is stated on the WHO labeling as 1 L over 24 hours; for children, the labeling indicates 1 L over an 8- to 24-hour period according to age. This new WHO formula is different from the formula currently listed in Chapter 4 of the 2008 CDC Yellow Book, which differs by listing 3.5 g/L of sodium chloride and 20.0 g/L of glucose; these amounts reflect prior WHO-recommended oral replacement fluid content. WHO's original 311 mOsmol/L oral rehydration fluid contained sodium carbonate instead of citrate. The citrate-containing fluid was recommended in 1984 because it was more stable in hot and humid climates. Historically, both these fluids were effective in rehydration and reduction of morbidity and morality.

Packets of oral rehydration salts can be purchased prior to travel and are also available in stores in many developing countries. They should not be taken without proper dilution. If packets of oral rehydration salts are not available to the traveler, oral rehydration should be carried out with the most appropriate option available. Chapter 29 contains a recipe for a homemade solution that approximates the old WHO formula. If the traveler lacks all the recipe items, other alternatives can be used. The glucose content of many sports drinks is high enough so that they can osmotically pull water into the bowel. However, glucose facilitates sodium absorption from the bowel, and if available, such drinks can be diluted for use as part of the rehydration regimen. The goal of oral rehydration is best achieved if one avoids extremes of hot and cold in oral fluid replacement and avoids alcohol, milk and milk products, and potentially irritating beverages such as coffee.

PERCUTANEOUS AND MUCOUS MEMBRANE ROUTES

The skin and mucous membranes can be very important routes of exposure during travel, particularly in areas where hygiene and sanitation are inadequate. The agents that result in infection through skin and mucous membrane routes include bacterial, viral, protozoan, fungal, and helminthic organisms and arthropod- and tick-borne infections. These are covered in the travel chapters that follow. See also Chapter 21, the chapters for specific agents, and Chapter 36.

The traveler should be briefed on general care of the skin and the risks to it. High heat and humidity can lead to maceration. The skin's protective barrier also may be breeched or degraded by cuts, abrasions, blisters, punctures (e.g., mechanical injury, plant spines, or questing insects and arachnids), plant toxins and sensitizers, chemical injury, or burns from thermal or radiant energy. A general guideline for travelers is to be equipped with soap and water and a topical antiseptic and to use these early on, even for what ordinarily may be minor injuries, particularly when in unsanitary environments or tropical areas. Proper foot care is essential. This includes traveling with comfortable footwear that has been "broken in" to avoid tissue injury, using a supply of clean socks, avoiding contact of the foot and other skin with soil particularly in areas where helminths are endemic, avoiding maceration and allowing time for airing of feet and footwear, using drying powders, and using foot coverings in hotel rooms, bathrooms, and showers.

Behavioral monitoring and modification are important in avoiding infection from skin and mucous membrane exposures. The traveler should be advised about precautions for blood-borne pathogens and their transmission by contact with blood, including blood transfusions, sexual contact, shared paraphernalia for injection of drugs, and exposure to inadequately sterilized equipment used for dental, medical, acupuncture, body piercing, or tattoo procedures. In populations with a high prevalence of chronic hepatitis B virus (HBV) infection, open sores and wound exudates can be a source of HBV transmission. If sexual contact is likely during travel, condoms should be used, but with the understanding that no device can provide complete safety. Travelers should be reminded that flavored condoms are available commercially for a good reason—because oral sex is not without risks.

When traveling to areas in which mosquito, fly, tick, or other arthropod/insect-borne disease are endemic, the traveler should be well versed in the questing/feeding habits of the specific disease vector in terms of time of day (e.g., dusk and dawn, evening). Dress should limit skin exposure (e.g., hats, long-sleeved shirts tucked into long pants, and pant legs tucked into socks). In heavily infested areas, head netting can be used to avoid insects, including moisture-seeking flies that prefer travelers' mouths, noses, eyes, and ears; the most comfortable head nets are those that fit over a broad-brimmed hat, which helps to keep the netting off the user's face. Habitats such as rodent-infested quarters/areas or outside areas with tall grasses or brush should be avoided when possible. Mosquito netting with a mesh size of less than 1.5 mm is recommended [30]. Mosquito netting should be used so that it is well tucked under the mattress to prevent mosquito entry. The netting should be installed so that it does not come in contact with the individual during use. Further protection can be obtained by treating the mosquito netting with permethrin. Netting should be checked for holes, tears, and other deterioration with each use. Small holes sometimes can be everted successfully and tied off as a temporary measure, but netting damaged beyond effective repair should be replaced. The traveler may be able to further reduce the mosquito threat by eliminating standing water that may be a breeding place for mosquitoes in the work area and in or around living quarters. Those who travel to risk areas for extended stays for work should make sure that doors and windows fit snugly, holes in living quarters are repaired, and doors, windows, and porches are protected with screens using 16–18 mesh screening material [30]. Insect bites should receive first aid treatment as for any other puncture wounds or small breaks in the skin. The traveler should be trained to remove attached ticks in ways that avoid leaving insect mouthparts in the wound (see also Chapter 26). In essence, the technique is to avoid touching or handling the tick; approach the tick head from the side with tweezers, grasp the head/mouth area as close to the skin as possible, and then pull away from the skin in the direction of the longitudinal axis of the tick's body with a steadily increasing pressure to remove it. If mouthparts remain, they also should be removed with tweezers. The tweezers then should be cleaned with alcohol. Scratching sites of bites can produce further damage to the skin and increase the likelihood of local infection. If an insect bite develops unusual redness, swelling, bruising, or pain, the traveler should seek medical advice.

Travelers, employers, and aircraft/airport employees should be aware that malaria-bearing mosquitoes can be transported by aircraft. Although countries may require disinfection of aircraft arriving from malaria and yellow fever areas, cases of malaria are reported in people who live or work in the vicinity of airports [31].

There are a number of effective insect repellants on the market, and their use should be encouraged in travelers to risk areas. The most commonly used are preparations containing *N,N*-diethyl-*m*-toluamide (DEET). It should be applied to clothes and exposed skin (avoid face) according to manufacturer's instructions. Long-acting preparations are available. Higher concentrations give protection for longer periods of time, but concentrations over 50% do not appear to provide added protection. A relatively new insect repellant, Picaridin (KBR 3023), which has been used in Europe and Australia in a 20% solution, is now available in the United States in a 7% solution. The CDC recommends DEET or Picaridin as the most effective mosquito repellants [32]. Picaridin is odorless, nonsticky, and less likely than DEET to irritate the skin. No published studies are available on the efficacy of the 7% solution, but studies of the higher concentrations have shown Picaridin to be about as effective as 20–35% DEET for mosquitoes. One study showed less efficacy of Picaridin compared with DEET several hours after application [33]. In my own experience, a 92.8 g/L solution of Picaridin was fairly effective against aggressive, annoying Australian flies but not as effective as a head net (see above). Insect repellants such as DEET-containing materials and Picaridin should not be used under clothing or applied to broken skin. On coming inside,

treated areas of skin should be washed with soap and water. Permethrin also can be used. It can repel and kill ticks and mosquitoes. It can be applied to the outside of clothing, such as hats, pants, socks, and shoes, but is not recommended for use on skin. Permethrin can bind to clothing, which can retain residual insect repellant activity after multiple washings. Permethrin-treated hats, socks, shirts, and other clothing with long-lasting insect repellant properties are now being marketed. Protection levels diminish after multiple washings; manufacturers' guidelines should be consulted. This type of clothing may be one part of a protection plan but should not be the sole protection used. If a repellant appears to be causing a rash or irritation, the areas of application should be washed with soap and water, and use of the repellant should be stopped. Further information on insect repellants and their safety is available at www.epa.gov.

Bat-infested quarters, buildings, and locales should be avoided, and the traveler should be briefed before travel on what steps to take if exposed to bats, dogs, or other animals potentially infected with rabies (see Chapters 20 and 28).

RESPIRATORY ROUTE

The respiratory route is a major route for exposure to infectious agents during travel and is very difficult to protect. The agents that result in infection through the respiratory route include bacterial, viral, fungal, and—through water or water droplet exposures—protozoan organisms. Theses microorganisms are covered in the following travel chapters and chapters that address specific pathogens. See also Chapters 13, 14, 23, and 36. Further information on respiratory protection is presented in Chapter 14.

The nature of most travel is that it results in either contacting or sharing spaces with people who may have respiratory symptoms and infection. The shared spaces may be confining for long periods and without optimal ventilation (e.g., airplanes, trains, buses and metro public transportation, ships, airports, hotels, restaurants, and meeting rooms). Many people in such spaces do not use good respiratory hygiene practices. Although aircraft may recirculate up to 50% of their air through HEPA filters with a total change of air 20–30 times per hour, there is still a potential for spread of illness from coughs, sneezes, and through direct contact with part of the aircraft touched by other passengers or contaminated with their secretions.

The respiratory hygiene practices of importance to the traveler include thorough hand washing before touching facial areas, limiting contact to the extent possible with those who have overt respiratory symptoms, covering coughs and sneezes with tissues or sleeve at the elbow, and encouraging others to do likewise.

Many people are interested in whether surgical masks provide protection from infection during travel. Adequate studies on their effectiveness for general populations are lacking. Surgical masks may be placed on patients with communicable diseases to help contain respiratory droplets and reduce spread of infectious particles. The traveler may wish to wear such a mask when ill. However, surgical masks are not considered to be adequate protection against infections such as severe acute respiratory syndrome (SARS) or other serious infections. These masks may serve as a barrier to droplets, but they do not protect against aerosols and small particles, they allow leakage around the mask on inspiration, and they cannot be fit-tested [34]. They are used by health professionals in situations of high risk only when more effective respiratory protection is unavailable.

The N-95 filtering facepiece respirator is designed to screen out particles from inhaled air. N-95 or equivalent-type respirators are used in hospitals to protect against infection. This type is the least or lowest level of protection recommended for health care providers to use for protection against infection. Their use in the workplace is regulated by the Occupational Safety and Health Administration (OSHA), which requires education and training in use, maintenance, and care of the respirator and fit-testing to ensure a proper seal between the respirator's sealing surface and the user's face. The N-95 or equivalent-type respirators are not effective in blocking virus-sized particles but can limit some aerosol and droplet transmission if used properly [35].

Travelers should be concerned about the risk for respiratory infections and should be educated in the methods and importance of hand hygiene as a primary prevention strategy. Hand-washing guidance was provided earlier in this chapter in the section on oral-route transmission. The traveler should understand that respirators are complex tools that have limitations and are difficult and uncomfortable to wear properly for extended periods. They interfere with communication and eating and can increase the work of breathing. During travel, it may be difficult to tell when infectious disease threats to the respiratory system are occurring. Respirators can be ineffective if too many particles are in the air. Respirators can be degraded by oils and other materials in the ambient air. They can collect infectious materials and become fomites that can transmit disease. These factors make them unlikely to be acceptable, convenient, or effective for the usual business traveler.

MIXED-EXPOSURE ROUTES

Assignment of microbes to one of three routes of exposure was done to give examples of preventive practices and as a convenience for employee training. Clearly, this does not provide the traveler with a realistic view of risk for some pathogens. The traveler should understand that a number of microbes can infect humans through more than one route (e.g., *Staphylococcus* and *Streptococcus* species, *Yersinia pestis*, *Bacillus anthracis*, *Brucella* species, rabies, and many others). The plague, anthrax, and rabies examples are particularly important to explain to travelers because of the seriousness and lethality of these diseases.

Some human activities are particularly prone to offering multiple exposure routes to microbes. Swimming is a form of recreation that can involve ingestion of water as well as percutaneous and respiratory exposures. In many parts of the world, ocean water, lakes, canals, and rivers may be contaminated with sewage, animal feces, urine, carcasses and carrion, wastewater runoff, industrial effluent, and thermal pollution. In some settings human corpses may also be present in bodies of water. Some bodies of water also may contain trash, industrial and construction debris, broken glass, and discarded sharps that can result in serious wounds. Swimming or wading in contaminated water can result in diarrhea; skin, eye, and ear infections; respiratory infections; helminth infections such as *Schistosoma* aquatic forms (see Chapter 30); and fatal amebic meningoencephalitis (see Chapter 31). Travelers should avoid swimming when they have diarrhea or cuts or abrasions of the skin. If swimming in potentially contaminated or untreated water, it is prudent to not submerge the head, to avoid swallowing water, and to wear nose plugs. Swimming pool water treated by chlorination may be safe, but this depends on whether the chlorination is maintained properly. Even with proper chlorination of pools, water still may harbor *Cryptosporidium* or *Giardia lamblia* (see Chapter 31), hepatitis A, or noroviruses (see Chapter 28), so precautions should be taken to avoid oral and nasopharyngeal exposure [25].

Prevention During the Posttravel Period

About half of U.S. travelers to the developing world will become ill during their travels [36]. Occupational health programs need to determine who will receive posttravel debriefings and/or medical screening depending on travel itineraries, duration of travel, expected standards of living accommodations, personal risk factors, occupational risk factors, vaccination history and schedules, prophylactic medication requirements, and occurrence of outbreaks or changes in patterns of disease occurrence during the travel period.

Debriefing after travel to malaria-endemic areas is very important to reinforce when and how continuation of prophylaxis should occur in the posttravel period. Malarial illness may not become manifest for up to a year and can occur even if antimalarial prophylaxis has been taken as prescribed. The traveler returning from malaria-endemic areas should be reminded to see a health care provider promptly if fever occurs during the year after return to the United States and should be instructed to relate to that health care provider the history of travel and increased risk for malaria. Unexplained fever posttravel should be a red flag for early consultation with a specialist in infectious or tropical diseases [37].

Depending on the timing of exposure and incubation periods, the returning traveler may be well on return to the United States or even for 12 weeks or longer before becoming ill from a pathogen obtained overseas. The most frequent problem in returning ill travelers is persistent or intermittent diarrheal illness, which may affect as many as 10% of travelers. In many cases, the primary gastrointestinal illness will have passed, but postinfectious lactose intolerance or irritable bowel syndrome may linger [38, 39]. Evaluation may include tests for intestinal parasites, particularly if symptoms do

not resolve within 2 weeks of normalization of diet [40]. Abdominal pain, unintentional weight loss (10% or more of body weight), hematochezia, and dehydration should be flagged for immediate attention. It is advisable to consult a specialist in infectious disease or tropical medicine, particularly for travelers with diarrheal problems who have lived overseas, because they are at risk for co-infection with multiple parasites. Other less frequent problems of returning travelers are skin lesions and rashes, respiratory infections, and fever. Posttravel screening for tuberculosis (TB) using tuberculin testing, if indicated, generally should be done 8–12 weeks after potential exposure.

In addition to the issues just noted, questions about animal contact, bites, or the presence of bats in living quarters during sleep can provide critical information about rabies risk. The posttravel debriefing should address consistency of use of preventive behaviors recommended for travel. Screening for hepatitis, HIV, and/or other sexually transmitted disease should be considered if the travel history includes unsafe sexual practices, invasive medical treatments, dental procedures, injections, sharing of paraphernalia for intravenous drug use, tattoos, acupuncture, or body piercing.

Immigrant and Migrant Worker Infectious Disease Issues

For the occupational physician, immigrants and workers of nonresident, nonimmigrant status often pose infectious disease issues that are different from those of other workers. There are numerous categories that can apply to non-U.S.-born individuals who are in the United States. Some of these categories include

- *Immigrants.* These are people admitted to the United States as lawful permanent residents (lawful permanent residence is sometimes referred to as "having a green card"). They may be issued immigrant visas by the Department of State overseas or, if already in the United States, may be adjusted to permanent resident status by the Immigration and Naturalization Service. Most immigrant visas are based on family relations or employment.
- *Refugees.* These are people who are outside their country of nationality (but not in the United

States) and who are unable or unwilling to return to that country owing to persecution, well-founded fear of persecution, or issues of race, religion, political opinion, or other characteristics.

- *Asylees.* These are people who are foreign nationals in the United States who make a claim for refugee protection here.
- *Parolees.* These are people who normally would not be admissible to the United States but are allowed to enter temporarily for humanitarian, medical, and legal reasons. This represents temporary admission status rather than formal admission to the United States.
- *Nonimmigrant residents.* Theses are foreign nationals legally admitted temporarily to the United States for a specific period of time (e.g., students or temporary workers).
- *Business visitors.* The United States has a visa waiver program to waive nonimmigrant visas for nationals of 27 countries.
- *Temporary visitors.* People in this category may be in the United States for business or other purposes on a nonimmigrant visa.
- *Internally displaced persons.* These are people who have fled home for the same reasons as refugees but who have not crossed an internationally recognized border.
- *Unauthorized immigrants.* These are foreigners who immigrate across a country's national boundary in a way that violates the immigration laws of the destination country or who entered legally but overstayed their visa. This status is sometimes referred to as an "undocumented or illegal alien" in common language.
- *Migrant workers.* This is not an immigration category; it is a general term for those who choose to migrate for remunerated work and covers a broad category of workers who may or may not be legal residents. One migrates when one crosses the boundary of a political or administrative unit in a way that changes social ties and membership. Migration can occur within a country or internationally between nation-states. The United Nations Educational, Scientific, and Cultural Organization refers to a migrant worker as one who is engaged, has been engaged, or is to be engaged in a remunerated activity in a state of which he or she is not a national [41]. The worker chooses to migrate as a

convenience and so is not a refugee. Migrant workers may enter the nation of work legally (e.g., under a visa), such as guest workers, overseas contract workers, or highly skilled business migrants, or may be in a category of "irregular migrants" (e.g., undocumented/illegal migrants), people who enter a country, usually in search of employment, without the necessary documents and permits.

In the United States, of major current social concern are the irregular migrants/migrant workers, many of who are crop farm workers or in non-farm contract labor jobs. Of the crop farm workers, many are foreign-born, mostly from Mexico and Central America, speak only Spanish, an estimated one-third are undocumented, and most are young men with average to low levels of formal education. Many live in substandard and/or overcrowded housing, they may lack access to a treated water supply and/or toilets at home or at work, and many earn so little that they and their families live in poverty [42].

In the United States, more than one and one quarter million immigrants were granted permanent residence status in 2006. Most of these immigrants came from Asia (33%), North America (32%), Europe (13%), South America (11%), and Africa (9%). Most legal immigrants arriving from North America and Asia settle initially either in California, New York, Florida, Texas, New Jersey, or Illinois. Overall, about 12.6% of all immigrants received employment-based preferences for immigration [43]. In 2005, legal immigrants accounted for about 38% of the annual increase in the U.S. population [44]. In addition, there were about 700,000 who became naturalized citizens in 2006. In 2004, the United States received about 2 million temporary visitors for business purposes on nonimmigrant visas and 2.2 million business visitors under the visa waiver program. In addition, 148 million Mexican and Canadian citizens visited the United States without nonimmigrant visas [45]. Figures vary on occupational aspects of legal immigrants, but most are of working age, and about half list occupations in professional or technical areas. Since 2000 in the United States, about 50,000 refugees have entered each year from various areas of the world [43]. After a year in the United States, refugees can apply for status as legal permanent residents.

Estimates of the unauthorized immigrant population vary. In 2000, the U.S. Immigration and Naturalization Service estimated the number to be 7 million, with the most common country of origin being Mexico (4.8 million, or 69%), followed by El Salvador, Guatemala, Colombia, Honduras, China, and Ecuador. California was estimated to have the largest share of unauthorized immigrants (32%), followed by Texas, Illinois, Arizona, Georgia, and North Carolina. The growth of the unauthorized immigrant population was estimated to be about 350,000 per year in the 1990s. A January 2006 estimate is that there are 11.6 million unauthorized immigrants living in the United States, about 57% from Mexico; California is estimated to have about 2.8 million unauthorized immigrants, Texas 1.6 million, Florida 0.98 million, and in descending population order from 550,000 to 280,000: Illinois, New York, Arizona, Georgia, New Jersey, North Carolina, and Washington, other states accounting for about 3 million unauthorized immigrants [46].

U.S. immigration laws require that overseas medical screening of immigrants and refugees must be carried out. This screening includes infectious disease issues, but this is not the exclusive focus. In addition to communicable diseases of public health significance, the screening checks for physical and mental disorders associated with harmful behavior, drug abuse and addiction, and factors indicating that the person may become a ward of the state. The protocols for examination are established by the CDC. Typically the infectious disease focus for adults includes screening for TB with skin testing, chest radiograph, and sputum smears if needed; blood testing for syphilis and HIV infection; and a general physical examination with screening for leprosy and sexually transmitted diseases (e.g., syphilis, chancroid, gonorrhea, granuloma inguinale, and lymphogranuloma venereum). Additional testing is at the discretion of the examiner or is used to confirm a diagnosis. Examinations overseas are done by panel physicians selected by the U.S. Department of State. In 2007, the CDC announced that new technical instructions for TB screening are under review and should be implemented in the next several years.

People with immigrant status are legally required to be vaccinated based on the Advisory Committee on Immunization Practices (ACIP) before entering the United States. Ordinarily, immigrants may enter the United States from overseas having had the initial vaccination of recommended series. This requirement for predeparture vaccinations does not apply to U.S.-bound refugees, although outbreak-related vaccinations may occur. Refugees entering the United States are required to have mandatory medical examinations. If, after a year, the refugee applies to change status to legal permanent resident, he or she is then required to be vaccinated according to recommendations of the ACIP. For this adjustment of legal status to permanent residency, the person is referred to designated civil surgeons, who are doctors in the United States who perform medical examinations for this purpose. A list of civil surgeons is available from the U.S. Citizenship and Immigration Service at www.uscis.gov/portal/site/uscis. Health departments in the United States receive a blanket designation as civil surgeons for vaccination assessment of refugees if the health department has a physician meeting the legal definition of civil surgeon and accepts the designation. Currently, the United States has no requirement for medical examinations for visitors to the United States in nonimmigrant, short-term transit or other status such as migrants entering with or without proper documentation. However, aliens applying for nonimmigrant (temporary admission) visas may be required to have a medical examination at the discretion of the overseas consular officer or an immigration officer at the U.S. port of entry if there is reason to suspect an inadmissible health-related condition is present [47]. If an immigration applicant has an excludable infectious disease medical condition, such as syphilis or TB, he or she is required to be treated to achieve a noninfectious state before the visa is issued. HIV-positive applicants must be granted a waiver from the Immigration and Naturalization Service to continue the immigration process. On the basis of overseas screening, public health departments are notified of arrivals of individuals from overseas who need prompt medical follow-up. These include people with excludable conditions (class A conditions) or class B conditions. These conditions are shown in Table 27-2.

The CDC has published listings of recent infectious disease outbreaks among U.S.-bound refugees from Africa and Asia. From 2004–2007, outbreaks of hepatitis A, typhoid, polio, and varicella, rubella, measles, malaria, meningitis, and mumps have

Table 27-2

Overseas Classifications of Infectious Disease
of Immigrants/Refugees

Class A: Conditions that preclude a refugee from entering the
United States, but refugee may be given approval waivers for
entry with a requirement of immediate follow-up on arrival.

Tuberculosis, active, infectious

HIV infection

Syphilis, untreated

Chancroid, untreated

Gonorrhea, untreated

Granuloma inguinale, untreated

Lymphogranuloma venereum, untreated

Leprosy

Class B: Significant health problems requiring follow-up soon
after arrival in the United States.

Tuberculosis (B1, active, not infectious)

Tuberculosis (B2, inactive, old)

Tuberculosis (B3, any possible past TB disease)

Syphilis, treated

Other sexually transmitted diseases

Leprosy, treated, tuberculoid, borderline, or paucibacillary

Other significant physical disease, defect, or disability

Note: Among noninfectious diseases, class A also includes some classes of
substance addiction or abuse and physical or mental disorders with
harmful behavior or a history of such behavior with likelihood that the
behavior will recur. Among noninfectious diseases, class B includes pregnancy, some classes of substance addiction or abuse in remission, and
mental or physical disorders without harmful behavior or a history of
such behavior considered unlikely to recur.
HIV = human immunodeficiency virus; TB = tuberculosis.
Source: Immigrant, Refugee and Migrant Health, Division of Global Migration and Quarantine, Centers for Disease Control and Prevention.
Class A and B Conditions. CDC Domestic Refugee Health Program: Frequently Asked Questions. Atlanta: CDC, 2007; available at www.cdc.gov.

been documented. Recent articles point out the
risks for importation of vaccine-preventable diseases, cost/benefits of carrying out vaccinations
overseas, and issues related to this approach [48,
49].

The foregoing emphasizes a number of infectious disease concerns related to immigrant,
refugee, and migrant health. The Internet and other
resources related to these issues are vast. Many state
health departments have programs to address these
concerns, with protocols for examinations; TB
screening; stool testing for ova and parasites; HIV
testing; malaria smears; syphilis, *Strongyloides,*
Schistosoma, and *Plasmodium* serology; gonorrhea
probes/culture; *Chlamydia* probe; immunization
procedures, and other evaluations and requirements. Some of these programs may be useful as
models for occupational medicine programs so

that they deal with these issues in a way that inte-
grates well with the state and local health department approaches. Medical evaluations need to be
based on considerations of country of origin; history of residence or transit through countries prior
to entry into the United States; history of migrant
activity in the United States, which may involve infection risks from outbreaks or endemic areas;
work history and activities; family, medical, and
vaccination history; current health status; and cultural factors [50].

For reasons including cultural differences, language barriers, decisions about use of health care
resources, poverty, and migrant lifestyle, infectious
disease problems among many immigrant groups
are likely underreported. Studies have shown that
migrant farm workers have higher rates of diarrheal illness than the urban poor, increased incidence of intestinal parasitic infections, higher
prevalence and incidence of TB, and in some
groups, higher HIV-1 prevalence than the general
U.S. population [42]. Many of these workers and
nonfarm workers who work outdoors may have increased risks for other illnesses such as dengue,
West Nile virus infection, Lyme disease, other vector-borne diseases, soil-related fungal infections,
parasitic disease, and other illnesses related to their
current work. The occupational physician needs to
have a plan for consideration of health issues of immigrants, refugees, and migrants to help maintain
and improve the health of all employees.

Conclusion

The integration of travel medicine services into occupational medicine practice offers the health care
provider with opportunities to assist with services
related to education, training, and primary prevention. Many employees and employers need and appreciate these preventive services and advice for
safe travel. These services can have profound effects
on the health, productivity, and risk control for employees, their families, coworkers, and employers.

References

1. Centers for Disease Control and Prevention, www
   .cdc.gov/travel.
2. World Health Organization, www.who.int/ith.
3. International Society of Travel Medicine, www.istm
   .org.

4. Health Alerts, Advisories, and Updates. Available for e-mail distribution via Health Alert Network, Centers for Disease Control and Prevention, Atlanta.

5. World Health Organization. Epidemic and Pandemic Alert and Response (ERP), ERP Factsheets and Disease Outbreak News; available at who.int/csr/don/en/.

6. World Health Organization. Human Health under Threat from Ecosystem Degradation: Threats Particularly Acute in Poorer Countries. WHO Media centre, news release 2005; available at www.who.int/mediacentre/news/releases/2005/pr67/en/.

7. World Health Organization. Health risks and precautions: General considerations. In *International Travel and Health, 2007.* Geneva: WHO Press, 2007, Chap 1.

8. Travel Industry Association. *Domestic Travel Market Report, 2004.* Washington: Travel Industry Association, 2004 (tia.org).

9. Centers for Disease Control and Prevention. The immunocompromised traveler. In *Advising Travelers with Specific Needs: Health Information for International Travel, 2005–2006.* Atlanta: CDC, 2006, Chap 9.

10. U.S. Department of State, Bureau of Consular Affairs. Human Immunodeficiency Virus (HIV) Testing Requirements for Entry in Foreign Countries, July 2004; available at www.travel.state.gov/travel/tips/brochures/brochures_1230.html.

11. DuPont HL. Travellers' diarrhoea: Contemporary approaches to therapy and prevention. *Drugs* 2006; 66:303–14.

12. Adachi JA, DuPont HL. Rifaximin: A novel nonabsorbed rifamycin for gastrointestinal disorders. *Clin Infect Dis* 2006;42;541–7.

13. Donzis PB. Corneal ulcers from contact lenses during travel to remote areas. *N Eng J Med* 1998;383: 1629–30.

14. Centers for Disease Control and Prevention. Travelers' health kit. In *Pre- and Post-travel General Health: Health Information for International Travel, 2008.* Altanta: CDC, 2008, Chap 2.

15. U.S. Department of State. List of Travel Insurance and Medical Evacuation Companies; available at www.travel.state.gov/travel/index.html.

16. Centers for Disease Prevention and Control. Registration of Traveler Emergency Contact and Itinerary Information: Traveler's Health. Atlanta: CDC, 2008; available at www.cdc.gov/travel/contentRegisterContactInfo.aspx.

17. U.S. Department of State. Travel Registration; available at www.travelregistration.state.gov/ibrs/ui/.

18. IAMAT, www.iamat.org.

19. Death overseas: Importation or exportation of human remains. In *Conveyance and Transportation Issues: Health Information for International Travel, 2005–2006.* Atlanta: Centers for Disease Control and Prevention, 2006.

20. U.S. Department of State, www.travel.state.gov/family/issues_death.html.

21. Peeters M, Courgnaud V, Abela B, et al. Risk to human health from a plethora of simian immunodeficiency viruses in primate bushmeat. *Emerg Infect Dis* 2002;5; available at www.cdc.gov/ncidod/EID/vol8no7/02-0157.htm.

22. Apetrei C, Metzger MJ, Richardson D, et al. Detection and partial characterization of simian immunodeficiency virus SIVsm strains from bush meat samples from rural Sierra Leone. *J Virol* 2005;79: 2631–6.

23. Estrada-Garcia T, Lopez-Saucedo C, Zamarripa-Ayala B, et al. Prevalence of *Escherichia coli* and *Salmonella* spp. in street-vended food of open markets (tianguis) and general hygienic and trading practices in Mexico City. *Epidemiol Infect* 2004;132: 1181–4.

24. Adachi JA, Mathewson JJ, Jiang ZD, et al. Enteric pathogens in Mexican sauces of popular restaurants in Guadalajara, Mexico, and Houston, Texas. *Rev Gastroenterol Disord* 2003;3:884–7.

25. Centers for Disease Control and Prevention. Risks from food and water. In *Pre- and Post-travel General Health Recommendations: Travelers' Health* (Yellow Book). Available at www.ncid.cdc.gov.

26. Centers for Disease Control and Prevention. Water Treatment Methods: Travelers' Health: Filters and Bottled Water. Fact Sheet, Parasitic Disease Information, Division of Parasitic Diseases, CDC, Atlanta, 2005; available at www.cdc.gov/ncidod/dpd/parasites/cryptosporidiosis/factsht_crypto_prevent_water.

29. World Health Organization and UNICEF. *Oral Rehydration Salts: Production of the New ORS.* Geneva: WHO Press, 2006.

30. United States Department of Agriculture, Agricultural Research Service. Protection and Prevention: General Recommendations, Personal Protection, 2006; available at www.ars.usda.gov/Research/docs.

31. Chapter 2 in *International Travel and Health.* Geneva: World Health Organization, 2005.

32. Centers for Disease Control and Prevention. West Nile Virus, Questions and Answers, Insect Repellant Use and Safety; available at www.cdc.gov.

33. Picaridin—A New Insect Repellant. *Med Lett Drugs Ther* 2005;47:46–47.

34. NIOSH. Respirator Fact Sheet: What You Should Know in Deciding Whether to Buy Escape Hoods, Gas Masks, or Other Respirators for Preparedness at Home and Work. Washington: National Personal Protective Technology Laboratory, 2006. Available at www.cdc.gov/niosh/.

35. NIOSH. Understanding Respiratory Protection Against SARS. National Personal Protective Technology Laboratory, 2006; available at www.cdc.gov/niosh/.

36. Steffen R, DuPont HL. Travel medicine: What's that? *J Travel Med* 1994;1:1–3.

37. American Society of Tropical Medicine, www.astmh.org.

38. McKendrick MW, Read NW. Irritable bowel syndrome: Post-*Salmonella* infection. *J Infect Dis* 1994; 29:1–3.

39. Conner BA, Landzberg BR. Persistent travelers' diarrhea. In Keystone JS, Kozarsky PE, Freedman DO, et al. (eds), *Travel Medicine.* Philadelphia: Saunders, 2004, pp 503–15.

40. Connor BA. Persistent travelers' diarrhea. In DuPont HL, Steffens RS (eds), *Textbook of Travel Medicine and Health,* 2nd ed. Hamilton, NY: BC Decker, 2001, pp 177–83.

41. UNESCO. Migration Glossary, Migrant—Social Transformations, Social and Health Sciences, International Migration and Multicultural Policies. UNESCO, 2008; available at www.portal.unesco.org.

42. Villarejo D, Baron SL. The occupational health status of hired farm workers. *Occup Med State Art Rev* 1999;14:613–35.

43. Office of Immigration Statistics, U.S. Department of Homeland Security. *Yearbook of Immigration Statistics: 2006.* Washington: US Government Printing Office, 2007.

44. U.S. Census Report, 2006; available at www.census.gov.

45. U.S. Citizenship and Immigration Services, U.S. Department of Homeland Security. *Temporary Migration to the United States, Nonimmigrant Admissions under U.S. Immigration Law. U.S. Immigration Report Series,* Vol. 2. Washington: US Government Printing Office, January 2006.

46. Hoffer M, Rytina N, Campbell C. Estimates of the Unauthorized Immigrant Population Residing in the United States—January 2006. Population Estimates, August 2006. Office of Immigration Statistics, U.S. Department of Homeland Security. Available at www.dhs.gov.

47. Centers for Disease Control and Prevention. *Medical Examination for Immigration—Frequently Asked Questions (FAQs): Global Migration and Quarantine.* Atlanta: CDC, 2007; available at www.cdc.gov/ncidod/dq/refugee/faq.

48. Bagga S, Posey D. Cost of vaccinating refugees overseas versus after arrival in the United States, 2005. *MMWR* 2008;57:229–32.

49. U.S.-incurred costs of wild poliovirus infections in a camp with U.S.-bound refugees—Kenya, 2006. *MMWR* 2008;57:232–5.

50. Department of Public Health, Commonwealth of Massachusetts. Refugee and Immigrant Health Program, 2002; available at www.mass.gov/dp.

28 Viral Travel-Related Infections

William E. Wright

This chapter addresses a selection of viral infections out of a myriad of viruses with the potential to be related to travel. The conditions selected represent a balance of considerations such as incidence, high endemicity, severity of consequences, potential for impact on employee health and productivity, and employee concern owing to high public visibility.

Other viral infections may be of concern to individual travelers, either based on their itinerary or because global patterns of viral disease and public health concerns can shift rapidly. Two sources for checking current recommendations for travelers for these and other viral illnesses are the online sites of the World Health Organization (WHO) and the U.S. Centers for Disease Control and Prevention (CDC) [1, 2]. Detailed information on vaccines is covered in Chapter 5 and in some of the disease-specific chapters. General principles of travel medicine programs are covered in Chapter 27 of this book. Information on treatment in these chapters reflects that available at the time of writing but is likely to change. The reader should check authoritative sources for current treatment.

Acute Respiratory Illness

ACUTE VIRAL RHINITIS

The common cold is a frequent cause of absence from work. It occurs worldwide and can affect those traveling for work. Two RNA viruses, rhinoviruses (family Picornaviridae) and coronaviruses, cause most common colds in adults. The incubation period is usually about 1–2 days. The period of communicability begins shortly before symptoms develop through about the first 5 days of illness. Transmission can occur from direct contact with discharges from the nose and throat or from airborne droplets. Virus may be recoverable on plastic surfaces for several hours. Symptoms usually last 2–7 days and include rhinorrhea, sneezing, nasal congestion, and sore throat. Hoarseness, sinusitis, otitis, bronchitis, and exacerbation of either asthma or chronic lung disease may occur. In tropical areas, the incidence of common colds coincides with the rainy season. In more temperate zones, the incidence is greatest in the autumn, winter, and spring [3]. Travelers should be trained to practice hand hygiene, cover coughs and sneezes, dispose of oral and nasal secretions safely, and maintain adequate hydration. They may benefit from traveling with their familiar over-the-counter preparations to remediate symptoms as needed.

INFLUENZA

Influenza occurs worldwide and in all seasons. In temperate zones, it is most common in late autumn and winter months. In tropical zones, it is most common during rainy seasons. Influenza viruses can result in serious individual infections, epidemics, and pandemics. They have the potential to incapacitate individual travelers, cause fatal illness, and disrupt commerce on a broad scale. Concerns are high regarding a potential pandemic related to an H5N1 avian influenza that is now spreading from Asia to Europe and Africa in birds and is resulting in human cases with a high proportion of fatalities. Employers and travelers should be made aware of the risks and be encouraged to receive annual influenza vaccine as recommended by the CDC. Detailed information on influenza viruses is given in Chapters 11A (which contains a 2008 update), 11B, and 37. Occupational physicians who deal with international travelers also should consult online resources for current information. These include the WHO (www.who.int/csr/disease/influenza/pandemic/en), the U.S. Department of Health and Human Services (www.hhs.gov/pandemicflu/plan), and the CDC (www.cdc.gov/flu/).

SEVERE ACUTE RESPIRATORY SYNDROME (SARS)

SARS was first recognized in China in 2003, related to cases that likely began occurring in late 2002. It then spread to 29 countries in Asia, the Americas, Europe, Africa, and the Middle East before the global outbreak was contained [4]. The syndrome had about a 10% overall case fatality and 50% case fatality in elderly victims. It included occupation-related deaths. The outbreak was contained as a result of international cooperation in public health efforts, including rapid case detection, contact investigations, patient isolation, and community quarantine.

SARS is caused by an RNA virus designated *SARS-associated coronavirus* (SARS-CoV) that appears to be of animal-host origin. The virus appears to be transmitted by close person-to-person contact (e.g., living with, kissing, sharing utensils for food and drink, and close conversation within 3 ft of a person with SARS) or contact with respiratory secretions, droplets, or aerosols and possibly fomites. The virus can be viable in urine and stool for up to 4 days. The CDC advises that "to date, all diagnosed cases and cases under investigation have been linked to chains of transmission involving close personal contact with an identified case. There is no evidence of wider transmission in the community" [5]. The CDC and WHO monitor the SARS situation globally [6]. The most recently identified SARS case activity is from an April 2004 outbreak related to a laboratory-acquired (occupational) infection in China. As of a May 3, 2005 notice, there was no SARS transmission anywhere in the world [7], and this continues to be the case at the date of this writing in 2008. The CDC and WHO should be contacted online for further updates and guidance.

The CDC website has a document available that relates public health guidance for community-level preparedness and response to SARS and includes issues related to international travel, many principles of which can be applied to outbreaks from similar microorganisms [8].

Guidance for occupational groups, such as airline flight crews, cargo and cleaning personnel, and personnel interacting with arriving passengers, is also available at the CDC Web site. General practices include notifying authorities (U.S. Quarantine Station) if an ill person matching SARS-like illness is arriving in the United States by plane (airline captain's responsibility), keeping ill people separated from close contact with others as much as possible, encouraging the ill person to wear a surgical mask to limit droplet spread, having workers practice good hand hygiene, using disposable gloves for contact with the ill person's blood or body fluids (which does not take the place of good hand hygiene, particularly after removing and disposing of the gloves), notifying cleaning and ground crews, using nonsterile disposable gloves when cleaning the airline cabin and lavatories, washing hands after disposal of gloves, avoiding cleaning practices that could aerosolize material (such as use of compressed air), wiping down toilet facilities and case/passenger-related adjacent surfaces (e.g., armrests, tray tables, seatbacks, cabin walls, seat belt latches, and light and air controls) with a low- to intermediate-level U.S. Environmental Protection Agency (EPA)–registered germicide (see Figure 3-11 and related text for more information on germicides), seeking health care if exposed to SARS or when having SARS-like symptoms instead of going to work, and reporting illnesses occurring within 10 days of exposure to the ill persons or involvement in clean-up processes. The CDC does not recommend routine use of respirators, gloves, or surgical masks for protection from

SARS unless the worker is a health care worker caring for a patient with confirmed or possible SARS [9].

The incubation period of SARS-CoV is from 3–10 days. Common presenting symptoms are fever (>38°C), chills, headache, malaise, myalgia, and sometimes mild respiratory symptoms. Dyspnea and dry, nonproductive cough develop rapidly (within 2–7 days) and sometimes are followed by pneumonia and respiratory failure. Diarrhea, lymphopenia, and thrombocytopenia may develop. The diagnosis is confirmed by polymerase chain reaction (PCR) detection of SARS-CoV RNA, immunofluorescent assays, or enzyme-linked immunosorbent assays on sequential or multiple body fluid samples or isolation in cell culture of SARS-CoV from a clinical specimen. The case-fatality rate increases with age and comorbidity, averaging about 6–15% for adults aged 24–64 and 50% or more for people age 65 and older. In addition to age, the level of lactate dehydrogenase in the blood at presentation appears to predict mortality, perhaps because it is a measure of tissue damage [10].

There is no commercially available vaccine for SARS; some vaccine studies have been done in rodents, and an inactivated SARS-CoV vaccine was used in some clinical trials in China, but safety issues were raised related to its use [11].

Gastroenteritis

EPIDEMIC VIRAL GASTROENTEROPATHY

Norwalk-like viruses (now in the *Norovirus* genus) are the most common cause of outbreaks of nonbacterial gastroenteritis. Noroviruses, sometimes referred to by the broader family name, caliciviruses, are RNA viruses that occur worldwide. Most adults in the United States have antibodies to them by age 50. Humans are the only known reservoir. These agents are thought to be transmitted by person-to-person spread (e.g., fecal-oral contact, aerosols, or contamination from vomitus), contaminated food (most often from infected food handlers), and water or shellfish (contaminated with sewage). Outbreaks have been noted in restaurants, cruise ships, schools, institutions, and other settings involving catered meals or food prepared or handled by ill food handlers [12]. A recent CDC investigation of a BII subtype *Norovirus* outbreak in an elementary school in the United States reported an attack rate of about 38% among students and 36% among staff. In addition to noting likely person-to-person transmission, *Norovirus* contamination was found on a computer keyboard and computer mouse shared by staff and students in the only classroom independently associated with illness, suggesting transmission by a shared computer equipment fomite [13].

The incubation period is usually 24–48 hours but may be shorter (median in outbreaks 33–36 hours). The illness is characterized by 24–60 hours of a combination of symptoms such as sudden, forceful vomiting, abdominal cramps, and watery, nonbloody diarrhea. Symptoms also may include anorexia, nausea, malaise, low-grade fever, headache, and myalgias. Affected individuals may be able to transmit the infection during the acute phase of illness and for several days after diarrhea stops [14].

Noroviruses can be identified in stool or emesis samples using reverse transcriptase polymerase chain reaction (RT-PRC). Availability of testing may be limited to government public health laboratories in some areas. A rise in specific antibody of fourfold or more in acute and convalescent blood samples also can be used to diagnose the illness.

Prevention includes use of proper hand hygiene, safe disposal of human feces, hygienic preparation of food, chlorination of water, thorough cooking of shellfish and other foods, exclusion of food handlers from food preparation who have gastroenteritis, and exclusion of sick children and infants from areas where food is prepared. Areas contaminated with vomitus should be cleaned and disinfected with bleach solution. When illness occurs, treatment involves replacement of fluids and electrolytes as needed. No long-term sequelae have been noted. No vaccine is available commercially for adults, and no specific antiviral treatments are recommended. The U.S. Food and Drug Administration (FDA) has approved an oral live pentavalent rotavirus vaccine to prevent rotavirus-associated gastroenteritis in infancy (RotaTeq, Merck). The vaccine covers the most prevalent human serotypes of the virus (G1, G2, G3, G4, and P1) [8]. This has been recommended as part of routine immunizations and is given in three doses, at ages 2, 4, and 6 months (series not to be begun in infants older than 12 weeks). A monovalent vaccine is available in some other countries (Rotarix, GlaxoSmithKline) [15, 16].

Viral gastroenteritis, with vomiting and typically nonbloody diarrhea, also can occur from infection with other viruses. Kaplan [17] proposed epidemiologic criteria for identifying the likely viral etiology of gastroenteritis outbreaks. These include no bacterial pathogenic agent found on stool culture, mean or median incubation period of 24–48 hours, mean or median illness duration of 12–60 hours, and 50% or more of affected people with vomiting. Besides *Norovirus,* the main viruses implicated include RNA-based rotoviruses (the most common cause of childhood diarrhea in the United States), sapoviruses, astroviruses, and DNA-based adenoviruses (typically types 40 or 41). These are usually easily transmissible with low doses of viral particles [18]. In tropical climates, these illnesses occur throughout the year; in the continental United States and other temperate areas, they occur more often in cooler months and are sometimes called *winter vomiting disease,* a term also used for some *Norovirus* infections or other outbreaks. The incubation period for viral gastroenteritis is typically 1–2 days and may last from 1 day to more than a week. These viral infections can be transmitted by sewage-contaminated water or food (particularly contaminated shellfish), food contaminated by ill foodhandlers, or close contact with infected adults or children (including fecal-oral contact, sharing eating utensils, etc.). Food and water sanitation, proper disposal of human feces, prompt disinfection of contaminated surfaces, prompt cleaning of soiled clothes, and good hand hygiene are essential elements of prevention. There is no specific treatment for these illnesses, but maintaining adequate hydration is essential to avoid serious complications. Antibiotic treatment and use of agents to reduce gut motility are generally not recommended.

Hepatitis

HEPATITIS A AND E

Hepatitis A virus (HAV) is an RNA picornavirus that is endemic in developing nations. It causes a vaccine-preventable hepatitis in travelers and occurs in community outbreaks. It is transmitted by the fecal-oral route from direct contact, sewage contamination of shellfish or water, or contamination of fruit, vegetables, or other uncooked food during growth, harvesting, or handling. Sharing of

paraphernalia for injecting drugs also has the potential to transmit hepatitis A.

Countries or regions with intermediate or high endemicity of HAV include eastern Europe, Asia, Africa, Mexico, Central and South America, the western Pacific islands, New Zealand, and Greenland. The CDC recommends HAV vaccination for all nonpregnant travelers to these areas. The occupational physician should consider the risks of HAV infection for the pregnant female's travel itinerary and confer with her own health care provider because the safety of the vaccine during pregnancy has not been determined [19]. Prophylactic treatment with immune globulin also could be considered. Other issues and precautions related to HAV vaccination are covered in Chapter 5.

The monovalent, inactivated HAV vaccines (currently available as Havrix, GlaxoSmithKline, and VAQTA, Merck) are given in a two-dose series that may take from up to 6–18 months to complete [19]. The first dose ordinarily results in protective antibody in 94% or more of vaccinated people after 1 month. The combined hepatitis vaccine with hepatitis A and B (Twinrix, GlaxoSmithKline, with half the dose contained in Havrix and hepatitis B represented by a recombinant surface antigen protein) can be given in a three-shot series at 0, 1, and 6 months. A booster is recommended at 1 year [19]. If an unvaccinated traveler or newly vaccinated traveler (departing fewer than 2 weeks after vaccination) is leaving for an intermediate- or high-risk area, prophylactic treatment with immune globulin (0.02 mL/kg of body weight, or 2 mL for adults) should be considered (the same dose as recommended for postexposure prophylaxis). Higher doses are recommended for the unvaccinated traveler with plans to travel to risk-prone areas for more than 3 months (0.06 mL/kg of body weight or 5 mL for adults), to be repeated every 4–6 months if travel exposure continues. Immune globulin also can be used for postexposure prophylaxis for unvaccinated individuals within 2 weeks of exposure to HAV and for household and sexual contacts of infected individuals. Active immunization with HAV vaccine can be given simultaneously. Postexposure prophylaxis for workplace contacts is not recommended except for food-handling coworkers if a food handler is diagnosed with hepatitis A during a common-source outbreak. In some programs, determining hepatitis A immune status by blood testing prior to deciding on vaccination may be an appropriate and cost-effective approach [19].

HAV infection may be unapparent or range from mild illness to severe liver inflammation. The incubation period averages 28 days (range 15–50 days). Onset of clinically apparent infection is often abrupt, with fever, malaise, anorexia, and jaundice. Nausea and abdominal pain may occur. Illness may last several weeks. The period of infectivity usually runs from 1–2 weeks prior to symptoms through the first few days of jaundice. HAV does not result in chronic infection, but some case may be prolonged for up to 9 months. Case-fatality rate increases with age, being 1.8% in adults older than 50 years (population case-mortality proportion usually 0.1–0.3%) [20].

The most effective prevention of HAV infection is vaccination. Vaccination does not preclude the need for the traveler to use proper hand-washing practices, safe preparation of food and beverages, and sensible choices of foods during travel. No specific antiviral treatment is recommended for hepatitis A. Treatment is usually supportive, with activity encouraged as tolerated.

Hepatitis E virus (HEV) is an RNA virus of the Caliciviridae family. It causes hepatitis that is clinically indistinguishable from hepatitis A, except by serologic testing. A distinctive feature is that it carries a high case-fatality rate (about 20%) for pregnant women in their third trimester. Overall case-fatality rate is about 0.5–4%. Like hepatitis A, it is transmitted by the fecal-oral route and is most common in regions with inadequate environmental sanitation. Sporadic cases and epidemics occur in Asia, the Middle East, Africa, and Mexico. In the United States, it is primarily a travel-related disease, but recently, a small number of cases have been identified in people who did not recently travel internationally [21]. The mean incubation period is 26–42 days (range 15–64 days). The period of communicability is unknown [21]. There is no specific treatment for hepatitis E and no commercially available vaccine. Treatment is supportive. Food, water, and behavioral precautions are the same as for hepatitis A.

HEPATITIS B AND D

Hepatitis B virus (HBV) is a DNA hepadnavirus with eight main genotypes, all of which can cause hepatitis B infection. It occurs worldwide and is endemic in many areas. Acute infection can be unapparent (about 30% of cases). It can be fulminant and fatal in about 1%. In adults who become infected, up to 10% may develop a chronic HBV infection. Acute infection at early ages results in a much higher proportion of cases of chronic infection (90% in infants infected at birth, 20–50% in children aged 1–5 years) [20]. Immunocompromised individuals are at increased risk for chronic HBV infection. About 15–25% of chronic HBV infections result in death from cirrhosis or hepatocellular cancer.

The CDC recommends preexposure prophylactic hepatitis B vaccine for unvaccinated people traveling to areas of the world where HBV is at intermediate or high endemicity, defined as active or chronic HBV infection as measured by hepatitis B surface antigen (HBsAg) prevalence greater than 2%, who will have either close contact with the local population (i.e., sexual contact or daily physical contact) or medical or dental treatment locally [21]. Traveling to live in these endemic areas for more than 6 months is another criterion for vaccination [20]. International travelers whose duties abroad involve health care, public safety, or disaster relief, with potential exposure to blood and body fluids, are also at risk and should be vaccinated.

HBV vaccine dose schedules and details are covered in Chapter 5. The 6- to 12-month vaccination periods have resulted in some using accelerated schedules for travelers who do not have time to complete the standard vaccination schedule prior to travel (e.g., doses on days 0, 7, and 21) [22]. Dose schedules with more than one dose in a given month are not approved by the FDA [21].

Training for employees who travel should include knowledge of the greatest risks of HBV, which include sexual contact and other potential bloodborne pathogen exposures. HBV can remain viable on environmental surfaces for a week or more. In populations with a high prevalence of chronic HBV infection, open sores and wound exudates can be a source of HBV transmission.

Current areas of highest endemicity (chronic HBV > 8%) are Africa, Southeast Asia (including China), the Philippines, the Middle East (except for Israel), South Pacific and Western Pacific islands, the interior Amazon Basin, Haiti, and the Dominican Republic. Areas of intermediate prevalence (2–7%) include south central and southwestern

Asia, Israel, Japan, eastern and southern Europe, Russia, most areas around the Amazon Basin, Honduras, and Guatemala [21].

The incubation period's usual range is 45–180 days (average 60–90 days) but can be shorter or longer depending on the dose and mode of viral transmission and host factors. Blood can transmit infection for weeks before clinical illness occurs, during the acute illness, and during chronic infection. Acute symptomatic HBV illness is usually characterized by fatigue, anorexia, and vague abdominal pain, which can be followed by jaundice after 1–2 weeks. Mild fever, nausea, vomiting, skin rashes, and arthralgias or arthritis may occur. Constitutional symptoms usually begin to resolve on onset of icterus, but liver enlargement and abdominal pain may become more prominent. Clinical and biochemical resolution occurs in most patients 3–4 months after onset of icterus. Serologic parameters for diagnosis of acute and chronic infection are covered in Chapter 17.

The best ways to prevent HBV infection is through use of the HBV vaccine and avoidance of behaviors that increase risk. In cases of unimmunized individuals who have percutaneous or mucous membrane exposure to blood or sexual contact with an HBV-infected person, postexposure treatment with HB immune globulin (HBIG) and initiation of the primary vaccination series are recommended. HBIG treatment should be given within at least 24 hours of a high-risk needle stick and within 14 days of such sexual contact. There is no specific treatment for acute HBV infection. Further information on HBV vaccination is presented in Chapters 5 and 17. Several drugs are available in the United States that are used for treatment of active chronic HBV infection. These include adelfovir, entecavir, lamivudine, and telbivudine [23].

Hepatitis D virus (HDV, delta hepatitis virus) is an RNA-based particle thought to be a defective virus or new "satellite" family of subvirions. It is coated with hepatitis B surface antigen and has a unique internal delta antigen. It occurs worldwide and exists in three genotypes: I is the most widespread, II was isolated in Japan and Taiwan, and III was isolated in the Amazon basin. HDV is unable to cause hepatitis on its own. When it co-infects with HBV, it can cause severe infection but is usually self-limited. When HDV superinfects a person with HBV infection, it can cause fulminant infection (particularly genotype III) and lead to chronic hepatitis. Incubation period is about 2–8 weeks. Infectivity is present prior to symptoms and probably indefinitely thereafter. HDV shares transmission factors (i.e., blood and sexual contact) with HBV. It is most prevalent in regions with the highest levels of HBV endemicity. Diagnosis is made by identifying HDV antigen by enzyme immunoassay. There is no specific treatment for hepatitis D and no commercially available vaccine. Controlling hepatitis B through vaccination and education about risk behaviors helps to limit hepatitis D infection [20, 24].

HEPATITIS C

Hepatitis C virus (HCV) is an RNA virus of the genus *Hepacavirus,* of which more than a hundred subtypes exist. It occurs worldwide. The human population is its reservoir. An estimated 2–3% of the world's population is infected with hepatitis C. HCV is the most common chronic bloodborne pathogen in the United States [25, 26]. It is transmitted by contact with blood, including blood transfusions, sexual contact, sharing of paraphernalia for intravenous injection of drugs, and exposure to inadequately sterilized equipment used for dental, medical, acupuncture, body piercing, or tattoo procedures. Travelers who avoid these factors are at low risk for hepatitis C. The virus is most prevalent in human populations of Egypt (>15%) and is also prevalent in the western Pacific regions, Africa, Asia, and the Middle East, with the overall population prevalence in the world being estimated at 3% [20, 26, 27].

Acute HCV infection is often mild or unapparent. Incubation period can be from 2 weeks to 6 months (average 6–9 weeks). Period of communicability begins a few weeks before symptoms and lasts indefinitely. A small proportion of people (about 20%) who become infected may have classic symptoms of hepatitis, such as anorexia, nausea, fatigue, abdominal discomfort, and jaundice. Diagnosis is usually made by detecting antibodies to HCV using enzyme immunoassays or recombinant immunoblot assay. An estimated 75–85% of people infected with hepatitis C develop chronic infection, and more than half with chronic infection develop chronic liver disease. Cirrhosis or hepatoma may occur after 20 or more years of chronic infection [27, 28]. No vaccine is available for hepatitis C; immunoglobulin treatment has not been protective. There is no specific treatment for acute hepatitis C. Chronic hepatitis C can be treated with ribavirin and pegylated interferons.

Acquired Immune Deficiency Syndrome (AIDS)

Human immunodeficiency virus (HIV) is an RNA retrovirus with two serotypes (HIV-1 and HIV-2). Both serotypes produce a decline in cellular immunity that can be sufficient to result in AIDS, characterized by fewer than 200/μL CD4+ T cells or less than 14% of lymphocytes and by the occurrence of opportunistic infections, other indicator diseases, or cancers [29,30]. The CDC listed 23 conditions in the 1986 case definition (e.g., *Pneumocystis carinii* (now *Pneumocystis jiroveci*) pneumonia, *Mycobacterium avium*, various lymphomas, Kaposi's sarcoma, etc.) and in 1993 added *M. tuberculosis*, recurrent pneumonia, and invasive cervical cancer [30]. HIV-1 occurs worldwide. HIV-2, which tends to produce less aggressive illness, is prevalent in western Africa. The incubation period generally is about 1–3 months. The initial HIV infection may be unapparent or produce a mild illness consisting of fever, sore throat, and cervical lymphadenopathy. As the virus replicates, CD4+ T cells decline. After about 1–15 years, AIDS can develop. Without antiretroviral treatment, about 90% of HIV-infected people develop AIDS; most die in about 3–5 years. These figures have improved dramatically with current treatments. HIV infection and AIDS are manageable with combinations of antiretroviral drugs.

The areas of the world with the highest HIV prevalence are in sub-Saharan Africa, the Caribbean Islands, and south and southeastern Asia, but risk of transmission is present anywhere in the world depending in large part on personal behaviors while traveling [31]. Transmission modes of concern to travelers include sexual contact, contact with blood or blood-containing body fluids, shared use of paraphernalia for injecting drugs, blood or blood component transfusions that have not been screened adequately, and exposure to medical, dental, tattooing, or body-piercing procedures with instruments that have been reused without adequate decontamination.

Travelers will find that some countries require long-term visitors (e.g., students and workers) to have HIV testing as part of a medical examination prior to entry. This class of traveler should check with their destination country's embassy or representative in Washington, DC, regarding requirements. Information on requirements is also available online at the U.S. Department of State, but the information is subject to change. The July 2004 listing included 57 countries with requirements related to HIV. The list included Australia, United Kingdom, Canada, Russia, Greece, India, Taiwan, Republic of Korea, People's Republic of China, Saudi Arabia, Syria, Lebanon, and Panama [32]. Some countries accept testing done in the United States.

The traveler with HIV infection or AIDS faces increased risk for infections, risk of unusual severity of infections, and potential need for complicated medical treatment and its monitoring. These factors need to be considered by the traveler and the travel medicine physician to help ensure that resources match the employee's needs.

Zoonoses

RABIES

Rabies in humans is an almost uniformly fatal encephalomyelitis. It is caused by a bullet-shaped RNA virus of the genus *Lyssavirus*, family Rhabdoviridae. When first isolated in Africa, *Lyssavirus* was thought to be a unique virus. *Lyssavirus* is now categorized into two phylogroups (I and II) that are made up of genotypes that share a broad antigenic crossreactivity. Four new isolates are under study for characterization as new genotypes. Classic rabies is caused by genotype 1 (RABV) of phylogroup I, which occurs worldwide. This is the standard vaccine strain. Other phylogroup I viruses include Duvenhage virus (DUVV), which originated in southern Africa; European bat lyssavirus types 1 and 2 (EBLV-1 and EBLV-2); and Australian bat lyssavirus (ABLV). These five genotypes involve bats as their exclusive vector, except for RABV, which also includes terrestrial animals. Experimental evidence indicates that the standard genotype I vaccine does not protect against infection by the two phylogroup II lyssaviruses that originated in sub-Saharan Africa, Lagos bat virus (LBV), and Mokola virus (MOKA). The vector for LBV is the frugivorous bat. The vector for MOKA is unknown.

These viruses vary in their pathogenicity, but each can cause a rabies-like illness [33].

Most fatal cases of rabies occur in Africa and Asia. These continents have been estimated to have about 55,000 human deaths from canine rabies per year [90% confidence interval (CI) 24,500–90,800] [33]. In contrast, in 2004 in the United States, 8 cases of human rabies were reported, and 7 of the 8 patients died. Two of the cases were acquired outside the United States, and four were linked to receipt of transplanted organs or an arterial segment from an infected man [34]. Europe has recently reported fewer than 50 rabies deaths annually.

Worldwide, most rabies in humans is caused by bites of endemically infected dogs. However, geographic areas may contain other animals that can be infected with rabies. These include bats, foxes (particularly in Europe), raccoons (particularly in the eastern United States), cats, cattle, coyotes, beavers, skunks, and the mongoose. People often associate risk of rabies with bites from sick animals. An important point for employee education is that animals can carry and shed the virus for substantial periods before showing signs of illness (from 3–7 days for dogs and cats, 8 days for skunks, 12 days for bats, and 14 days for strains in Ethiopian dogs). Data on rabies in animals and humans are available electronically from the WHO, including interactive global or country maps and information on local conditions through Rabnet [35].

Recommended initial treatment of bite wounds should include flushing and cleaning with soap or detergent and water, followed by application of 70% ethanol, tincture of iodine, or povidone-iodine. Ordinarily, the wound should not be sutured. Infiltration of the wound as soon as possible with human or equine rabies immune globulin (HRIG or ERIG) is recommended, followed by vaccination at a different site. The risk for serum sickness from ERIG can be as high as 40% depending on the preparation [36, 37]. It is less expensive than HRIG and may be the only rabies immune globulin available in some countries.

Preexposure vaccination is recommended for veterinarians, animal handlers, people working in laboratories with rabies virus, wildlife workers, and travelers residing in high-risk areas. It is probably prudent for people who travel to do disaster response work to also receive preexposure vaccination. An important training point for employees who receive preexposure vaccination for rabies is that it does *not* avoid the need for postbite treatment. It makes postexposure treatment simpler and prolongs the window of time to arrange for effective treatment. The latter issue is important for workers in deep jungle areas, rural areas, and areas of civil unrest or social disruption, in which usual services and transport may not be readily available. The incubation period can be very short if a bite is severe, contains large amounts of infected saliva, and/or occurs near the central nervous system (e.g., head and neck). Preexposure vaccine may allow the bitten individual time to get effective postexposure vaccine treatment. Those receiving preexposure vaccine whose potential for exposure to rabies virus continues should have serum tested every 2 years for neutralizing antibody and get booster doses of vaccine as needed. Chapters 5 and 20 have more information on rabies vaccination.

The rabies virus cannot penetrate intact human skin. It usually infects humans through bites or direct contact with wounds or mucosal surfaces. The teeth of bats can be small enough to result in bites that may be unapparent, especially if people are bitten during sleep. If one is not protected by bed netting and awakes with a bat in the room, medical attention should be sought. The incubation period usually is 3–8 weeks but can be as short as 9 days or as long as 7 years [36]. The virus can replicate in nonnervous tissue or enter peripheral nerves and travel in retrograde fashion to the central nervous system (CNS).

The initial symptom of rabies in humans is usually pain at the site of the infected wound. The course of the illness usually lasts about 2–6 days. Death is often from respiratory paralysis. The clinical signs of encephalomyeloradiculitis can present in two forms: furious (excited) or paralytic. The classic disease is nonparalytic, with onset of pain at the site of a previous bite, fever, headache, malaise, and apprehension. Spasms develop in response to tactile, auditory, visual, or olfactory stimuli, along with hydrophobia (spasms of muscles of deglutition in response to attempts to swallow), aerophobia (spasms of muscles of inspiration during inhalation or spontaneously), and alternating periods of agitation, lucidity, and confusion. Late illness can include delirium and convulsions. The paralytic form of illness can be associated with myoedema at percussion sites on the chest or large muscles of the proximal arms or legs. Nonclassic or atypical rabies encephalomyelitis is reported increasingly. The WHO recommends consideration of rabies as a cause of illness in anyone who presents with signs of encephalitis [33].

The diagnosis of rabies is usually made initially based on clinical presentation and course of illness. An expert in rabies treatment should be consulted. Fluorescent antibody staining of brain tissue or frozen skin sections taken from the back of the neck at the hairline (hair follicles containing elements of peripheral nerves) can aid in diagnosis during early illness, as can virus isolation or neutralization in mice or cell culture. Saliva, spinal fluid, and tears can be used to diagnose rabies, but shedding of virus may be intermittent, and results may be falsely negative. Samples should be refrigerated according to the receiving laboratory's guidelines. Precautions should be taken to properly label, protect, and package body fluid and tissue samples during transport to laboratories to prevent further human exposure. Magnetic resonance imaging (MRI) with widespread ill-defined, mildly hyper-signal T2 images in the CNS deep cortical white matter, gray mater, brain stem, hypothalamus, and hippocampus is consistent with rabies [33, 36].

Generally, later treatment is supportive, with sedation and avoidance of invasive procedures once the diagnosis is confirmed. Recommendations for protection of health care workers providing treatment include using universal precautions, including gowns, gloves, goggles, masks, and other barriers appropriate to the situation. Rabies virus is usually not present in the blood but may be seen in tissue, saliva, tears, urine, and CNS fluid. Laboratories generally use biosafety level 2 (BSL-2) practices but may use BSL-3 precautions when working with large concentrations of virus, performing procedures that may produce aerosols, or dealing with new rabies viruses. Biosafety levels are covered in Chapter 3. See Chapter 20 for more information and updates.

HANTAVIRUS

The term *Hantavirus* refers to about 25 antigenically distinct species of RNA viruses of the family Bunyaviridae. These viruses infect rodents (e.g., field rodents, voles, deer mice, pack rats, and chipmunks) worldwide and are transmitted to humans through aerosolized rodent excretions (i.e., urine, feces, and saliva). Humans are accidental hosts. *Hantavirus* infection in humans can increase vascular permeability and result in hypotension, shock, and hemorrhage. Asymptomatic infection can occur, but clinically apparent serious *Hantavirus* infections are usually classified according to whether the primary target organ is the kidney [usual form hemorrhagic fever with renal syndrome (HFRS)] or the lung [hantavirus pulmonary syndrome (HPS)] [38].

Incubation period usually averages 2–4 weeks but can be as short as a few days or as long as 2 months. Severe illness with HRFS has been associated with the Hantaan virus of Asia and the Dobrava virus in the Balkans. HPS was first recognized in the western United States in 1993 and has occurred in parts of the United States, Canada, and South America. Worldwide, over 150,000 cases of these syndromes are reported annually [39].

The renal syndrome is characterized by abrupt onset of fever, low back pain, headache, malaise, anorexia, and petechiae with thrombocytopenia. This phase of illness generally lasts 3–7 days, followed by a period of defervescence and hypotension for up to 3 days, and then periods of oliguria (3–7 days), diuresis, and weeks to months of convalescence. The case-fatality proportion is usually 5–15%, with most deaths occurring during the hypotensive and oliguric phases.

The pulmonary form of *Hantavirus* illness is characterized by fever, myalgia, and gastrointestinal complaints, followed by sudden onset of respiratory distress and hypotension, leading to respiratory failure and shock. Radiographic signs of interstitial pulmonary edema can progress to severe bilateral alveolar infiltrates and pleural effusions. Case-fatality proportions approach 40–50%. Thrombocytopenia is often present but not usually hemorrhagic manifestations and kidney problems.

Prevention depends on avoiding rodents and their excretia and controlling rodent access to living quarters. There is no commercial vaccine for hantaviruses. Specific antiviral treatment is under study. Treatment generally is supportive, with attention to avoiding hypoxia, maintaining blood pressure, and consideration of extracorporeal oxygenation if respiratory failure occurs. Broad-spectrum antibiotics typically are given early while waiting for confirmation of diagnosis. See Chapter 16 for more information.

Viral Hemorrhagic Fevers

DENGUE

Dengue viruses are RNA genotype flaviviruses. They occur in four serotypes, numbered DEN-1 through DEN-4. The virus cycles between humans and mosquitoes. Infected *Aedes aegypti* and other *Aedes* mosquitoes are vectors. These mosquitoes are "day feeders," most commonly questing for blood meals during the several hours after sunrise and before sunset. In some areas of Asia and Africa, monkeys also may be part of the reservoir. The viruses are endemic in tropical regions. Travelers to Africa, Asia, western Pacific islands, Central and South America, Caribbean Islands, northern Australia, and the southern United States (particularly Texas) are at risk. These viruses have the capacity to produce three clinical syndromes: dengue fever (DF), dengue hemorrhagic fever (DHF), and dengue shock syndrome (DSS). The incubation period in humans is generally 4–7 days but can be as long as 2 weeks [40].

DF (breakbone fever) consists of sudden onset of high fever (39–40°C or higher), intense, usually frontal headache, retroorbital pain, myalgias, and arthralgias. Nausea and vomiting may occur. The fever may be bimodal, lessening after several days and then rising. Defervescence can occur in 2–7 days, at which time a generalized maculopapular rash may develop. Bleeding also may occur in the form of petechiae, epistaxis, gingival bleeding, or bleeding from underlying conditions (e.g., gastrointestinal bleeding from peptic ulcers). Lymphadenopathy and thrombocytopenia are common. Recovery is usually complete but may be characterized by months of weakness and profound fatigue.

DHF and DSS are more severe forms of DF and occur most commonly with serotypes DEN-2 and DEN-3. Prior DF infection appears to be a risk factor. DHF is characterized by postdefervescent increased vascular permeability (with possible ascites or pleural effusion), hemorrhagic manifestations (e.g., petechiae, purpura, hematemesis, melena, or other bleeding), and thrombocytopenia of less than 100,000/mm^3. A more than 20% drop in hematocrit after volume replacement can occur. When hypovolemic shock occurs in this setting, the condition is labeled DSS. Some forms of epidemic DHF are accompanied by severe liver damage and encephalopathy. Case mortality in severe disease usually depends on timely recognition and effective treatment of shock and can ranged from 1–50% [41, 42].

In the United States, dengue is not a reportable disease, but voluntary reports from clinicians to state health departments are sent to the CDC (passive surveillance), which then does diagnostic testing of patient specimens. For the period 2001–2004, 366 serum samples from people suspected of having dengue were sent to the CDC. Of these, 77 were laboratory-diagnosed as acute dengue infections, 183 patients had negative dengue testing, and the rest were either indeterminant (lacking a convalescent serum sample) or had testing suggestive of *Flavivirus* infection or vaccination (e.g., yellow fever) [43]. A report on dengue cases in 2005 related 96 laboratory-diagnosed cases, including death in a 28-year-old woman who spent a week in Mexico [44]. These data suggest either a sharp upturn in U.S. travel-related cases, improved voluntary reporting of cases, or both.

There is no commercially available vaccine for dengue viruses. The traveler to endemic and epidemic areas needs to exercise caution regarding mosquito exposure and seek medical treatment as soon as symptoms of DF or DHF occur. Use of aspirin, other platelet inhibitors, or ulcerogenic medications may worsen hemorrhagic fevers.

YELLOW FEVER

Yellow fever virus is an RNA *Flavivirus*. The virus cycles between nonhuman primates and mosquitoes in its sylvatic form in tropical Africa and South America, sometimes infecting humans. In its urban form, the virus cycles between humans and *A. aegypti* or other *Aedes* mosquitoes.

Yellow fever is endemic in equatorial Africa and South America. A 30% increase in cases has occurred in past 5 years in West Africa, where outbreaks continue to occur [45]. Yellow fever and other mosquito-borne viral illnesses (e.g., West Nile virus, Japanese encephalitis, and dengue) are spreading geographically in part owing to population growth and urbanization of rural endemic areas [46]. Yellow fever is not known to be present in Asia.

The incubation is from 3–6 days. The illness can be mild, but the classic disease results in abrupt onset of high fever, chills, headache, backache, myalgias, nausea, and vomiting. The fever can lessen and then recur (bimodal), and sometimes Faget's sign (slow pulse with elevated temperature) is present. Most cases resolve after about the fifth day. Jaundice is a predictor of poor outcome, being associated with a 20–50% case-fatality rate [47]. It can be present early and worsen during the illness. In severe disease, hematemesis, melena, gingival bleeding, epistaxis, and renal and/or hepatic failure may occur.

Prevention depends on vaccination programs [48], reduction of mosquito breeding sites, wearing protective clothing, and using mosquito netting and insect repellants. See Chapter 5 for more details on vaccination. As vaccination programs expand, there is concern about the very rare occurrence of yellow fever vaccine-associated viscerotropic disease (YEL-AVD), which can result in a yellow fever-like illness with multiple-organ failure and death in a matter of days [49].

EBOLA AND MARBURG VIRAL HEMORRHAGIC FEVERS

Ebola virus and Marburg virus are RNA viruses of the Filviridae family. Their reservoir is unknown, but they have caused outbreaks primarily in Central Africa and in some areas where infected nonhuman primates have been transported [50]. The WHO reports recent outbreaks of Marburg virus (e.g., Democratic Republic of the Congo 1998–2000 and Angola 2005) and Ebola (e.g., from 2000–2007, outbreaks occurred in Uganda, Gabon, Republic of the Congo, Sudan, and Democratic Republic of the Congo) with devastatingly high mortality [51].

These viruses are rare and notorious for causing outbreaks of serious hemorrhagic disease with high mortality (50–90%). Incubation period is from 2 days to 3 weeks (usually 5–10 days). Illness starts abruptly with fever, headache, myalgias, and malaise. Pharyngitis, gastrointestinal disturbances, and maculpapular rash (most prominent on the chest, back, and abdomen) follow around the fifth day. The illness proceeds to hemorrhagic manifestations with renal failure, confusion/delirium, liver and multiorgan dysfunction, and shock. Person-to-person transmission is through contact with blood, saliva, urine, or other secretions/excretions, with greatest risk during late phases of illness. International travelers would be at greatest risk if exposed

to nonhuman primates (from the countries noted earlier), to their corpses or body fluids, or to the blood, secretions, or semen (for months after illness) of infected people either directly or on fomites during an outbreak. Specialized ELISA and PCR tests have been used to identify these viruses early in the disease process. There are no vaccines available commercially for these viruses and no specific treatment. Treatment is supportive with strict adherence to recommended precautions for contact, blood-borne pathogens, droplet transmission, and airborne transmission. In laboratory settings, monkeys can be infected via small-particle aerosols, but such transmission has not been confirmed in human cases to date [52].

Mosquito- and Tick-Borne Arboviral Encephalitides

A number of arthropod-borne viruses can result in meningitis, encephalitis, or meningoencephalitis. Incubation periods usually range from 5–15 days. A number of strains of mosquitoes are involved. The viruses usually exist in a mosquito/animal cycle with rodents, horses, birds, reptiles, other local wildlife, or domesticated mammals. Some mosquitoes are infected transovarially. The health risk for travelers is determined by the geographic distribution of the infected mosquito and seasons. For instance, in temperate areas, Japanese encephalitis occurs in summer and early autumn; in tropical areas, it occurs more during rainy seasons [53].

Many of these viruses cause asymptomatic or mild infections lasting less than a week. Mild infections are usually characterized by fever, headache, and malaise. Onset of illness may be abrupt with high fever, chills, severe (usually frontal) headache, retroorbital pain, nausea, vomiting, and pharyngitis. Severe infections usually have high fever, severe headache, and meningeal signs, followed by somnolence or disorientation, coma, or focal or generalized convulsions with primarily spastic, but sometimes flaccid, paralysis. A broad range of other neurologic deficits also can occur with encephalitis, including aphasia, hemiparesis, cranial nerve palsies, myoclonic jerks, tremors, and temperature dysregulation. Case-fatality rates range from 1–60%. Postinfection residual neurologic impairments can be severe, particularly with Eastern equine encephalitis, which also carries a high mortality proportion (usually over 50% in clinically apparent infections). The distribution of these diseases can shift, and outbreaks can occur. For detailed information on vaccines, refer to Chapter 5 and online information from the WHO and CDC.

Venezuelan, Eastern, and Western equine encephalitidies (VEE, EEE, and WEE) are caused by RNA alphaviruses (Togaviridae) and are carried by a variety of mosquitoes, including *Culex* and *Aedes*. VEE occurs in northern South America, Central America, and Trinidad. It also has occurred in the southern United States. Occurrence is increasing in urban areas, possibly owing to increased urbanization and destruction of rain forest habitats [54]. EEE occurs in the eastern half of the continental United States and Canada, the Caribbean islands, and Central and South America. WEE occurs in the central and western United States, Canada, and South America. A vaccine for VEE is available for adults at high risk.

Japanese encephalitis (JE), Murray Valley encephalitis (MVE), and St. Louis encephalitis (SLE) are caused by RNA flaviviruses transmitted by a variety of *Culex* mosquitoes. JE occurs primarily in southern and Southeast Asia, the western Pacific islands, and northern Australia. Its geographic reach is also spreading. MVE is sometimes called *Australian encephalitis*, occurring there and in Papua New Guinea. SLE occurs primarily in the Brazil, Central America, most of the United States, and Canada. Vaccine is available commercially for JE [53].

Tick-borne encephalitidies of the Central European, Far Eastern, Powassan virus (CEE, FE, and POW), and Louping ill forms are RNA flavivirus illnesses transmitted by *Ixodes* ticks (some of which also may be vectors for Lyme disease) primarily in rural or sylvan areas. Incubation periods are usually 1–2 weeks. Deer and goats are the mammal hosts for Louping ill virus, primarily in the United Kingdom, Ireland, and western Europe, which usually causes mild illness. Hosts for the other tick-borne encephalitidies are usually rodents and birds. CEE occurs in Europe. FE occurs in eastern areas of the former Soviet Union. Some outbreaks of CEE have been linked to consumption of unpasteurized dairy products from sheep and goats. PE is found in the United States, Canada, and Russia.

Colorado tick fever (CTF, an RNA coltivirus), mosquito-borne West Nile virus (WNV, a flavi-

virus), Rift Valley fever (RVF, an RNA phlebovirus), and Oropouche virus (a bunyavirus), cause febrile illnesses that can result in meningoencephalitis. Incubation periods are about 3–12 days for the mosquito-borne illnesses and 4–5 days for CTF. WNV is present in Africa, Europe, the Middle East, India, and the United States. RVF occurs in Africa and, recognized for the first time in 2000, in the Middle East (Saudi Arabia and Yemen). It primarily affects cattle and other domesticated herd animals. The case-fatality proportion is about 1% in humans [55]. A vaccine is under study for RVF. Oropouche virus occurs in Central and South America and Trinidad. CTF occurs in the mountains of the western United States and Canada. It can display a biphasic or triphasic fever pattern [56].

WNV was unintentionally imported into the United States in New York City in 1999, resulting in bird kills and human illness ranging from a mild febrile illness to meningoencephalitis. Since then, it has spread to birds in every state of the continental United States (with cases of the human neuroinvasive form being reported in about 90% of states) [57] and Canada. Infection with WNV is an underreported disease in the United States. Most infections in humans are asymptomatic or subclinical; about 20% of reported cases involve fever, headache, muscle aches, and muscle or joint pains. About 1% can result in meningitis or encephalitis that can be fatal. As of this writing, for 2007, the CDC received reports of 3,598 cases of WNV disease. West Nile fever (clinical disease without neurologic involvement), a notifiable disease, accounted for about 65% of reported cases, and meningitis/encephalitis accounted for about 34% of reported cases. The overall case-fatality rate for all reported cases was about 3.4% [58]. The reported cases for 1999–2001 averaged about 50 per year, rose to 4,156 in 2002, peaked at 9,862 cases in 2003, and rose from 2,539 in 2004 to 4,269 in 2006 [58].

Occupational risk groups for WNV and similar insect-borne diseases include outdoor workers, such as outdoor construction, repair, and maintenance workers; telephone, cable, and electrical linemen; laborers; foresters; gardeners; landscapers; heavy equipment operators; entomologists and field workers; and health care workers or biologists exposed to human or avian tissues or body fluids.

Worker education, protection, and reporting of symptoms consistent with WNV or other diseases listed here are important elements of workplace safety programs. See also Chapters 8 and 27.

Smallpox, Varicella, and Monkeypox

Since worldwide eradication of smallpox from human populations in 1979 and storage of the Variola virus in designated laboratories, concern about this viral illness has recurred because of its potential use as a bioterrorism agent in a world population that is increasingly unimmunized. As with other potential microbiologic bioterrorism agents, travelers could be selected for primary exposure so that bioterrorists could avoid having to enter the target country to deliver the microbiologic weapon. Occupational physicians and others who manage travel medicine programs should be aware of the potential for bioterrorism and be vigilant for unusual illnesses, such as smallpox, in returning travelers. Related information is presented in Chapter 39.

Variola is a DNA virus, an *Orthopoxvirus* that occurs in two types, variola major and variola (alastrim) minor. They are transmitted by respiratory droplets, aerosols, or skin inoculation. The incubation period is about 1–2$\frac{1}{2}$ weeks. Illness onset is abrupt, with high fever (40°C), headache, backache, abdominal pain, vomiting, malaise, and prostration. Then 2–4 days after this prodrome fever falls, sores develop in the mouth and break down, and a centrifugal rash occurs and then evolves over a 3- to 4-week period. The rash is initially macular but progresses through papular, to multilocular noncollapsing vesicular lesions that may develop a central depression, to deep pustular lesions, and then to scabs. The rash, initially occurring on the face and limbs (also can affect palms and soles), spreads to the trunk. In any given area, skin lesions are in the same stage of development. Mortality from variola minor is about 1%; for variola major, it is 20–50% in unvaccinated people. Variola major also can present in a hemorrhagic form that is uniformly fatal and a usually fatal malignant form in which skin lesions remain soft, and flat pustules do not develop [59–61]. People vaccinated for smallpox may experience the prodrome but have limited numbers of atypical lesions that heal relatively quickly.

Chickenpox (varicella) may resemble smallpox. However, it tends to produce less fever, a less severe prodrome, and a centripetal rash. The varicella rash first affects the trunk in a maculopapuar form and, after a few hours, becomes vesicular. Unlike smallpox, the rash can affect the apex of the axilla and is characteristically superficial and itchy. In chickenpox, vesicles tend to be unilocular and collapse when punctured, and skin lesions in the same area tend to be pleomorphic.

Monkeypox (caused by another *Orthopoxvirus*) occurs in central and western Africa and is related to a nonhuman primate and squirrel reservoir in the rainforests. It also can infect rats, mice, and rabbits. Travelers who work handling animals in these areas, have contact with ill residents, or are involved in animal export/import activities can be at risk. The first human case was reported in 1970. Outbreaks have occurred in Africa and in the United States. A 2003 U.S. outbreak has been attributed to contact with pet prairie dogs that were sick with the virus. The illness resembles smallpox and may be modified by previous vaccination for smallpox. The incubation period is typically about 12 days, and the illness starts with fever, headache, muscle aches, and backaches. The rash starts at least 1 day after the fever, often starting on the face, and then spreads, but it can start on other parts of the body. Vesicles develop, get crusty, and form scabs that fall off. Generally, the illness lasts about 2–4 weeks. Those not previously vaccinated for smallpox face a case-mortality rate of 1–14% for monkeypox. Pleomorphism and cropping of skin lesions can occur, as seen in chickenpox, and lymphadenopathy tends to be more prominent than in smallpox and occurs early in the illness [62]. Based primarily on expert opinion, the CDC published guidance for treatment and prevention of monkeypox during outbreaks, including consideration of use of smallpox vaccine, cidofovir, and vaccinia immune globulin (VIG) [63]. The guidance supports smallpox vaccination for investigators of suspected monkeypox cases, health care workers involved in the care of suspected or confirmed cases, and household members and those with close or intimate contact (*close* being defined, as for smallpox, as 3 or more hours of direct exposure within 6 ft) if not medically contraindicated. Ideally, the vaccine should be given within 4 days of initial direct exposure and considered for those within 2 weeks of most recent exposure. Health care workers are instructed to use standard contact and airborne infection control precautions, including an N-95 or comparable respirator, even if vaccinated. There are currently no data on use of VIG or cidofovir for treatment or prophylaxis, although some think that these may be useful. If faced with an outbreak, current guidance and recommendations should be sought from the state health department and CDC (1-877-554-4625) [63].

Common Viral Diseases of Childhood

Measles (rubeola: *Morbillivirus,* Paramyxoviridae family), mumps (*Rubulavirus,* Paramyxoviridae family), rubella (*Rubivirus,* Togaviridae family), poliomyelitis (*Enterovirus* genus), and chickenpox (varicella-zoster virus, human [alpha] herpesvirus type 3) are sometimes referred to as *viral diseases of childhood* because of their epidemiology. They are the targets of childhood vaccination programs. Throughout the world in populations that are not immunized, outbreaks occur. These can affect travelers who are naive to these viruses, inadequately immunized, or immunosuppressed. It is important that travelers be up to date on primary vaccinations and recommended boosters for these viruses. Related information is available in Chapters 5 and 35. The reader also should check the current recommendations from the Advisory Committee on Immunization Practices (ACIP), CDC updates on vaccines and travel advisories, or similar resources of the WHO and specific nations' advisories.

Rubella (German measles, sometimes called *three-day measles*) carries substantial risks for pregnant women because of its ability to produce fetal loss or birth defects, particularly when infection occurs during the first half of pregnancy. In the United States, vaccination efforts have virtually eliminated rubella and congenital rubella syndrome [64]. This is not a reason to not continue using the measles, mumps, rubella (MMR) vaccine and vaccinating the population for this disease, particularly women with an unreliable vaccination history and women who lack laboratory evidence of immunity, particularly if of child-bearing age. Rubella and its complications occur in many countries in which vaccination programs have not achieved an adequate level of population coverage. In general, it is a mild respiratory illness with low-grade fever followed by the appearance of a maculopapular rash that lasts about 3 days. Many subclinical infections occur. The Pan-American Health Organization is carrying out a program to eliminate rubella.

Measles is a highly contagious disease that can be a serious disease in older adult travelers, involving pneumonia or encephalitis, and a major contributor to mortality and morbidity in those who lack protective immunity. The illness typically begins with a prodrome of fever, cough, conjunctivitis, and coryza. After 3 days to a week, a red, blotchy rash typically first appears on the face and spreads to the rest of the body, lasting about 4–7 days. During the prodrome, characteristic Koplik spots may be seen on the buccal mucosa (i.e., red-based lesions with a central white to bluish white area). Among children, particularly among the very young in areas with poor nutrition and vitamin A deficiency, the case-mortality rate can reach 30%, and morbidity can be severe [65]. The WHO and the United Nations Children's Fund (UNICEF) are carrying out a comprehensive strategy of immunization, surveillance, and clinical management (including attention to nutrition, particularly vitamin A deficiency) to reduce mortality from measles in 47 countries (primarily in Africa, Asia, the Middles East, and Pacific nations) that experience the greatest global burden of measles disease. This is related to a World Health Assembly's Global Immunization Vision and Strategy goal for global measles control, which includes reduction of measles mortality by 90% by 2010. By 2005, the process goals were being exceeded, and a 60% reduction in measles-related mortality was reported [66]. Endemic measles was eliminated in the WHO's Pan-American Health Organization region in 2002.

Measles is no longer considered to be endemic in the United States, and measles in U.S. residents is typically related to cases imported by visitors or by U.S. travelers abroad, which can result in outbreaks in the United States. In a recent outbreak of measles (genotype G5) in Japan, which appears to be the imported source of a U.S. outbreak in Pennsylvania, Michigan, and Texas in 2007, the index case was a Japanese youth who attended an international sporting event in Pennsylvania. The CDC investigation included review of air flight passenger manifests and contact of passengers seated in rows nearby the U.S. index case [67,68]. Other outbreaks have occurred in the United States recently [69, 70]. People born before 1957 are considered to be immune to measles owing to natural infection. Adults born during or after 1957 should receive one or more doses of measles vaccine, if not contraindicated, unless they have had a physician-confirmed diagnosis of measles, a documented immunization, or laboratory evidence of immunity. A second dose of measles vaccine is recommended for adults who have been exposed recently to measles, are in an outbreak setting, had previously received killed measles vaccine or an unknown type of measles vaccine during 1963–1967, are students in postsecondary educational institutions, work in health care facilities, or plan international travel [71].

Recent mumps outbreaks in the United States have been of concern. An outbreak of genotype G strain in Iowa in 2005 affected many young adults who were documented to have been vaccinated for mumps. This outbreak spread to other states. The disease may be asymptomatic or subclinical, but it typically starts with headache, malaise, and fever and within 1 day development of salivary (predominantly parotid) gland swelling. Orchitis, oophoritis, meningitis, and deafness may occur. There has been an ongoing epidemic of mumps (genotype G) in England that has affected more than 70,000 people [72]. Adults born prior to 1957 are generally considered to be immune owing to natural infection, but if they are health care workers and show no signs of immunity, consideration of a single dose of vaccine is recommended, with a second dose recommended if a local outbreak of mumps occurs. If not in these groups, then adults are recommended to receive one dose of MMR vaccine, if not medically contraindicated. If adults are in an age group affected by a mumps outbreak are students in a postsecondary educational institution, are health care workers, or plan international travel, then a second does is recommended [71, 73].

Chickenpox can be serious disease in older adult travelers, involving pneumonia or encephalitis. See the earlier section on smallpox, varicella, and monkeypox for a description of the disease. Vaccination is recommended for all adults if not medically contraindicated. Special priority groups include those with close contact with persons at high risk for severe disease, health care personnel, family contacts of immunosuppressed people, teachers, day-care employees, residents and staff of institutional settings and correctional facility settings, college students, military personnel, adolescents and adults living in households with children, nonpregnant women of childbearing age, and international travelers [71]. Older travelers or those with malignancies or immunosuppression are susceptible to reactivation of latent varicella infection (shingles), with pain and paresthesias that can impair work function during travel. The current Advisory Committee on Immunization Practices (ACIP) recommends a single herpes zoster vaccination for all adults aged 60 years or older, if not medically contraindicated, regardless of whether they report a previous episode of herpes zoster [74].

Further information on viral infections that may affect occupational travel is presented in Chapters 11A, 11B, 14, 16, 17, 18, 20, 23, 24, and 37.

References

1. World Health Organization, www.who.int/en/.
2. U.S. Centers for Disease Control and Prevention, www.cdc.gov.
3. Acute viral rhinitis: Common cold. In Heymann DL (ed), *Control of Communicable Diseases Manual*, 18th ed. Washington: American Public Health Association, 2004. Pp 454–6.
4. Heymann D. Severe acute respiratory syndrome. In Heymann DL (ed), *Control of Communicable Diseases Manual*, 18th ed. Washington: American Public Health Association, 2004. Pp 480–7.
5. Centers for Disease Control and Prevention. Current SARS Situation, May 3, 2005.
6. World Health Organization. WHO Guidelines for the Global Surveillance Of Severe Acute Respiratory Syndrome (SARS), updated October 2004; available at www.who.int/csr/resources/publications.
7. Centers for Disease Control and Prevention. Basic Information about SARS (Fact Sheet), May 3, 2005; available *at* www.cdc.gov/ncidod/sars.
8. Centers for Disease Control and Prevention. Managing international travel-related transmission risk. In *Public Health Guidance for Community-Level Preparedness and Response to Severe Acute Respiratory Syndrome (SARS)*, version 3, supplement E, May 3, 2005; available at www.cdc.gov/ncidod/sars/guidance/E/index.htm.
9. Centers for Disease Control and Prevention. Guidance about SARS for Airline Flight Crews, Cargo and Cleaning Personnel, and Personnel Interacting with Arriving Passengers, May 3, 2005; available at www.cdc.gov/ncidod/sars/airpersonnel.htm.
10. Choi KW, Chau TN, Tsang O, et al. Outcomes and prognostic factors in 267 patients with severe acute respiratory syndrome in Hong Kong. *Ann Intern Med* 2003;139:715–23.

11. Marshall E, Enserink M. Medicine: Caution urged on SARS vaccines. *Science* 303;2004:944–6.
12. Centers for Disease Control and Prevention. Norovirus: Technical Fact Sheet, January 1, 2005.
13. Norovirus outbreak in an elementary school—District of Columbia, February 2007. *MMWR* 2008;56:1340–3.
14. Fontaine O. Epidemic viral gastroenteropathy. In Heymann DL (ed), *Control of Communicable Diseases Manual*, 18th ed. Washington: American Public Health Association, 2004. Pp 227–9.
15. Prevention of Rotavirus Gastroenteritis among Infants and Children: Provisional ACIP Recommendations for Use of Rotavirus Vaccine (RV), 2005; available at www.cdc.gov/nip.
16. RotaTeq: A new oral rotavirus vaccine. *Med Lett Drug Ther* 2006;48:61–3.
17. Kaplan JE, Feldman R, Campbell DS, et al. The frequency of a Norwalk-like pattern of illness in outbreaks of acute gastroenteritis. *Am J Public Health* 1982;72:1329–32.
18. Parashar UD, Glass RI. Viral gastroenteritis. In Kasper DL, Fauci AS, Longo DL, et al (eds), *Harrison's Principles of Internal Medicine*, 16th ed. New York: McGraw-Hill, 2005, Chap 174. Pp 1140–1.
19. Hepatitis, viral, type A. In *Health Information for International Travel, 2008* (Yellow Book). Atlanta: CDC, 2008, Chap 4; available at www.cdc.gov/travel/yb.
20. Lavanchy D. Viral hepatitis. In Heymann DL (ed), *Control of Communicable Diseases Manual*, 18th ed. Washington: American Public Health Association, 2004. Pp 247–68.
21. Hepatitis, viral. In *Health Information for International Travel, 2008* (Yellow Book). Atlanta: CDC, 2008, Chap 4; available at www.cdc.gov/travel/yb.
22. Keystone JS. Travel-related hepatitis B: Risk factors and prevention using an accelerated vaccination schedule. *Am J Med* 2005;118:63–8S.
23. Telbivudine (Tyzeka) for chronic hepatitis B. *Med Lett Drug Ther* 2007;49:11–2.
24. Viral hepatitis D, www.cdc.gov/ncidod/diseases/hepatitis/d.
25. Chou R, Clark EC, Helfand M. Screening for hepatitis C virus infection: A review of the evidence for the U.S. Preventive Services Task Force. *Ann Intern Med* 2004;140:465–79.
26. Alter MJ, Kruszon-Moran D, Nainan OV, et al. The prevalence of hepatitis C virus infection in the United States, 1988 through 1994. *N Engl J Med* 1999341:556–62.
27. Hepatitis, viral, type C. In *Health Information for International Travel, 2008* (Yellow Book). Atlanta: CDC, 2008, Chap 4; available at www.cdc.gov/travel/yb.
28. Herrine SK. Approach to the patient with chronic hepatitis C virus infection. *Ann Intern Med* 2002;136:747–57.
29. 1993 Revised classification system for HIV infection and expanded surveillance case definitions for AIDS among adolescents and adults. *MMWR* 1992;41:RR-17.
30. Centers for Disease Control and Prevention. Acquired Immunodeficiency Syndrome, 1993 Case Definition; available at www.cdc.gov/eo/dphsi/prints/aids1993htm.
31. Acquired immunodeficiency syndrome (AIDS). In *Health Information for International Travel, 2008* (Yellow Book). Atlanta: CDC, 2008, Chap 4; available at www2.ncid.cdc.gov/travel/yb.
32. U.S. Department of State, Bureau of Consular Affairs. Human Immunodeficiency Virus (HIV) Testing Requirements for Entry in Foreign Countries, July 2004; available at travel.state.gov/travel/tips/brochures/brochures_1230.html.
33. World Health Organization. *WHO Expert Consultation on Rabies.* WHO Technical Report Series 931, First Report. Geneva: WHO, 2005.
34. Krebs JW, Mandel EJ, Swerdlow DL, et al. Rabies surveillance in the United States during 2004. *JAMA* 2005;227:1912–25.
35. World Health Organization. Rabnet; available at *www.who.int/rabies/rabnet/*.
36. Meslin F. Rabies. In Heymann DL (ed), *Control of Communicable Diseases Manual*, 18th ed. Washington: American Public Health Association, 2004. Pp 438–47.
37. Human rabies prevention—United States, 1999: Recommendations for the Advisory Committee on Immunization Practices (ACIP). *MMWR* 1999;48:1–21.
38. Khan AS, Kitsutani PT, Corneli AL. Hantavirus pulmonary syndrome in the Americas: The early years. *Semin Respir Crit Care Med* 2000;21:313–22.
39. Khaiboullina ST, Morzunov SP, St Jeor SC. Hantaviruses: Molecular biology, evolution and pathogenesis. *Curr Mol Med* 2005;5:773–90.
40. Dayal-Drager R. Dengue fever, dengue hemorrhagic fever, dengue shock syndrome. In Heymann DL (ed), *Control of Communicable Diseases Manual*, 18th ed. Washington: American Public Health Association, 2004. Pp 146–52.
41. World Health Organization. Fact Sheet on Dengue Fever and Dengue Haemorrhagic Fever, updated July 23, 2004.
42. Centers for Disease Prevention and Control, Division of Vector-Borne Infectious Diseases. Dengue Fever, August 22, 2005; available at www.cdc.gov/ncidod/dvbid/dengue/.
43. Beatty ME, Vorndam V, Hunsperger EA, et al. Travel-associated dengue infections—United States, 2001–2004. *MMWR* 2005;54:556–8.
44. Travel-associated dengue—United States, 2005. *MMWR* 2006;55:700–2.
45. World Health Organization. Increased Risk of Urban Yellow Fever Outbreaks in Africa: Epidemic and Pandemic Alert and Response, 2008: available at www.who.int/csr/disease/yellowfev/.
46. Petersen LR, Marfin AA. Shifting epidemiology of Flaviviridae. *J Travel Med* 2005;12:S3–11.

47. Roth C, Shope R. Yellow fever. In Heymann DL (ed), *Control of Communicable Diseases Manual,* 18th ed. Washington: American Public Health Association, 2004. Pp 595–600.

48. Pugachev KV, Guirakhoo F, Monath TP. New developments in flavivirus vaccine with special attention to yellow fever. *Curr Opin Infect Dis* 2005;18:387–94.

49. Gerasimon G, Lowry K. Rare case of fatal yellow fever vaccine–associated viscerotropic disease. *South Med J* 2005;98:653–6.

50. CDC Assists in Public Health Response to Marburg Hemorrhagic Fever in Angola, May 24, 2005; available at www.cdc.gov/nicdod/dvrd.

51. World Health Organization. Ebola and Marburg Viruses, Epidemic and Pandemic Alert and Response (EPR), 1998–2007.

52. Centers for Disease Control and Prevention. Interim Guidance for Managing Patients with Suspected Viral Hemorrhagic Fever in U.S. Hospitals, May 19, 2005; available at www.cdc.gov/ncidod/dhqp/bp_vhf_interimGuidance.html.

53. Inactivated Japanese encephalitis virus vaccine: Recommendations of the Advisory Committee on Immunization Practices. *MMWR* 1993;42:1–22.

54. Aguilar PV, Greene IP, Coffey LL, et al. Endemic Venezuelan equine encephalitis in northern Peru. *Emerg Infect Dis* 2004; available at www.cdc.gov/ncidod/EID/vol10no5/03-0634.htm.

55. Centers for Disease Control and Prevention. Rift Valley Fever Fact Sheet, 2005; available at www.cdc.gov/ncidod/dvrb.

56. Attoui H, Jaafar FM, deMicco P, et al. Coltiviruses and seadornaviruses in North America, Europe, and Asia. *Emerg Infect Dis* 2005;11; available online at www.cdc.gov/ncidod/EID/vol11no11/o5-0868.htm.

57. West Nile virus update—United States, January 1–November 13, 2007. *MMWR* 2007;56:1191–2.

58. Centers for Disease Control and Prevention. 2007 West Nile Virus Activity in the United States (Reported to CDC as of March 4, 2008), West Nile Virus, Surveillance, Statistics, and Control; available at www.cdc.gov/ncidod/westnile/surv&control/CaseCount07_detailed.htm.

59. Inglesby TV, Henderson DA, Bartlett JC. Consensus statement: Smallpox as a biologic weapon: Medical and public health management. *JAMA* 1999;281:2127–37.

60. World Health Organization, *www.who.int/csr/disease/smallpox/en;* accessed February 17, 2006.

61. Centers for Disease Control and Prevention. Smallpox Disease Overview; available at www.bt.cdc.gov/agent/smallpox/overview/disease-facts.asp.

62. Centers for Disease Control and Prevention. Questions and Answers About Monkeypox, November 4, 2003; available at www.cdc.gov/ncidod/monkeypox.qa.htm.

63. Centers for Disease Control and Prevention. Updated Interim CDC Guidance for Use of Smallpox Vaccine, Cidofovir, and Vaccinia Immune Globulin (VIG) for Prevention and Treatment in the Setting of an Outbreak of Monkeypox Infections. Monkeypox Guidelines and Resources, June 25, 2003; available at www.cdc.gov/ncidod/monkeypox/treatmentguidelines.htm.

64. Achievements in public health: Elimination of rubella and congenital rubella syndrome—United States, 1969–2004. *MMWR* 2005;54:279–81.

65. Hersh B. Measles. In Heymann DL (ed), *Control of Communicable Diseases Manual,* 18th ed. Washington: American Public Health Association, 2004. Pp 347–8.

66. Progress in global measles control and mortality reduction, 2000–2006. *MMWR* 2007;56:1237–41.

67. Hunt E, Lurie P, Lute J, et al. Multistate measles outbreak associated with an international youth sporting event—Pennsylvania, Michigan, and Texas, August–September 2007. *MMWR* 2008;57;169–72.

68. Amornkul PN, Takahashi H, Bogard AK, et al. Low risk of measles transmission after exposure on an international airline flight. *J Infect Dis* 2004;189:S81–5.

69. Postexposure prophylaxis, isolation, and quarantine to control an import-associated measles outbreak—Iowa, 2004. *MMWR* 2004;53:969–71.

70. Parker AA, Staggs W, Dyan GH, et al. Implications of a 2005 measles outbreak in Indiana for sustained elimination of measles in the United States. *N Engl J Med* 2006;355:447–55.

71. Recommended adult immunization schedule—United States, October 2007–September 2008, *MMWR* 2007;56:Q1–4.

72. Mumps epidemic—United Kingdom 2004–2005. *MMWR* 2006;55:173.

73. Mumps outbreak recommendations. *Med Lett Drugs Ther* 2006;48:45.

74. Recommended adult immunizations schedule—United States, October 2007–September 2008. *MMWR* 2007;56:1072–1100.

29 Bacterial Travel-Related Infections

Karin E. Byers

As other countries have become increasingly accessible, Americans are traveling in greater numbers to remote areas of the world, where they may be exposed to infections that are endemic to those regions. It is estimated that more than 8 million North Americans travel to developing countries each year for vacations, study, business, or providing service. In order to prevent infections, travelers need to take specific precautions both before and during their travels. Clinicians also must be able to recognize illnesses that are associated with travel.

One-third of persons who travel abroad develop travel-related illness. The most common illness is diarrhea, affecting up to half the travelers from industrialized countries who visit the developing world. Health care workers, those working with animals, military personnel, and those working for prolonged periods of time in remote areas may be exposed to more unusual pathogens. This chapter provides an overview of the more common bacterial illnesses affecting travelers. Many of the diseases discussed are reviewed in greater detail in other chapters.

A number of things can be done to prevent illness when traveling. The most important considerations are immunizations, food and water precautions, and avoiding mosquitoes and ticks.

Immunizations

When planning on traveling, people often think about the exotic vaccines that they will require. But they also need to make sure that they are up to date on all their routine immunizations, including diphtheria, tetanus, pertussis, meningococcus, pneumococcus, and influenza vaccines. Outside the usual indications, the meningococcal vaccine also should be given to travelers who are going to high-risk destinations such as India and for travelers who go to Saudi Arabia for the Hajj. While most vaccines are voluntary, some countries require specific immunizations prior to entry. A list of the requirements for each country is available in *Health Information for International Travel,* published by the Centers for Disease Control and Prevention (CDC). An up-to-date version is also available on the CDC website at www.cdc.gov/travel/index .com. These vaccinations must be documented in the International Certificate of Vaccination and validated by a stamp issued by state health departments and designated centers such as traveler's clinics and some physician offices.

In general, inactivated vaccines can be given simultaneously at separate sites without changing their efficacy or the risk of adverse events. An inactivated vaccine can be given with a live-virus vaccine, but injected live-virus vaccines should be separated by at least 28 days. This may require some advance planning for travelers who require multiple immunizations. If a dose is missed, the vaccine series can be resumed without adding any additional doses. The exception is the oral typhoid vaccine.

Live, attenuated vaccines should be avoided in persons who are immunocompromised or if a household member is significantly immunocompromised, including having an illness such as human immunodeficiency virus (HIV) infection, leukemia, lymphoma, generalized malignancy, or prolonged therapy with corticosteroids [1, 2].

Specific Vaccines for Bacterial Diseases

Typhoid fever is endemic in much of the developing world. It can be prevented with food and water precautions in fastidious travelers, but the vaccine is suggested for travelers to developing countries with prolonged exposure to potentially contaminated food and water. These vaccines are not 100% effective, so this is not a substitute for taking standard food and water precautions. Both oral and parenteral vaccines are available. The oral live, attenuated Ty21 vaccine (Vivotif Berna) is administered as one capsule every other day for a total of four doses. It must be refrigerated. Because it is a live vaccine, the patient must not be taking antibiotics during the time of the vaccination. Its efficacy ranges from 33–66%. It does not require a booster until 5 years have relapsed since the previous dose. It does not appear to have significant side effects.

The older parenteral vaccine (Typhoid Vaccine) is a heat- and phenol-inactivated vaccine that requires two doses that are separated by at least 4 weeks. This may be difficult for patients who present for their immunizations shortly before they leave. It is 51–77% effective. It can cause significant side effects, including fevers, headaches, and severe pain or swelling at the injection site. About 21–24% of vaccinees will miss school or work owing to side effects. Boosters are required every 3 years if there is ongoing or a new exposure.

The newest vaccine (Typhim Vi) is a parenteral polysaccharide that is made up of the capsular polysaccharide that the organism produces, also known as the *virulence* (Vi) *antigen*. It is 55–74% effective after a single dose. It provides protection for 2 years, and it is better tolerated than the two-dose parenteral vaccine [3–5].

The cholera vaccine is no longer recommended for U.S. travelers, and it is not available. The risk of cholera is negligible among those who follow standard food and water precautions.

Neisseria meningitidis epidemics frequently occur in sub-Saharan Africa during the dry season, between December and June. Outbreaks are also common among pilgrims going to Mecca, Saudi Arabia, during the annual Hajj. Many outbreaks are due to serotypes A and C, which are included in the quadrivalent polysaccharide vaccine. The vaccine is recommended for travelers going to sub-Saharan Africa, Nepal, parts of India, Mongolia, Saudi Arabia, and East and Central Africa. Saudi Arabia requires proof of immunization from all visa applicants. This vaccine is effective against serotypes A, C, Y, and W-135. Serotype B causes some outbreaks and is prevalent in the United States, but there is no effective vaccine [2, 3].

Streptococcal pneumonia is not a disease that is limited to travelers, but it is still the most common cause of pneumonia, and penicillin-resistant *Streptococcus pneumoniae* is an international problem. Vaccination with the pneumococcal vaccine should be considered for those at increased risk for infection or for serious complications of infection. This includes those with chronic pulmonary disease, advanced cardiovascular disease, diabetes mellitus, alcoholism, cirrhosis, chronic renal insufficiency, cerebrospinal fluid (CSF) leak, and all those older than 65 years of age. Persons in an immunocompromised state, such as those with splenic dysfunction or asplenia, multiple myeloma, lymphoma, Hodgkin's disease, or HIV infection and those who have had organ transplantation also should be immunized.

The influenza vaccine also should be considered for patients in the previously mentioned groups. While influenza occurs almost exclusively in the winter months (December to April) in the northern hemisphere, it occurs most often between May and September in the southern hemisphere. Influenza not only may cause morbidity and mortality owing to the viral illness but also may predispose to secondary bacterial infections.

The tetanus and diphtheria vaccine should be given to all Americans, with a booster at 10-year intervals. In 2005, a tetanus toxoid, reduced diphtheria toxoid, and acellular pertussis vaccine (Tdap) was licensed in the United States. (ADCEL). This should replace one of the booster immunizations that normally would have been given with the diphtheria toxoid vaccine (dT). If vaccinations are not up to date, travelers should be revaccinated prior to travel rather than risk needing the vaccine in areas where either it may not be available or the safety of needles is in question. In recent years, there has been an outbreak of diphtheria in Russia and the new independent states of the former Soviet Union, and travelers to these regions must be protected [3].

Food and Water Precautions

There are several commonsense rules for avoiding food-borne illness. Although many travelers are cautious about the source of their drinking water, it is easy to forget that ice, salad bars, and brushing teeth may be other sources of contaminated water. Boiling water is the most reliable method of purifying it for drinking. Water should be brought to a vigorous boil for 1 minute. When the altitude is above 2 km (6,526 ft), water should be boiled for 3 minutes, or a chemical disinfectant should be used [1].

Chemical disinfection can be performed with iodine or chlorine. Iodine is preferred because the efficacy of chlorine depends on the temperature, pH, and organic content of the water. However, iodine cannot kill *Cryptosporidium* unless the water is allowed to sit for 15 hours before drinking it. Five drops (0.25 mL) of 2% tincture of iodine should be added to each quart or liter of water. If the water is cold or cloudy, the amount should be doubled. Alternatively, iodine can be added in the form of hydroperiodide tablets (e.g., Globaline, Porta-Aqua, and Coghlan's). These should be added according to the manufacturer's instructions [1].

Filters provide protection against many organisms, but their efficacy is variable. Reverse-osmosis filters provide the best protection against bacteria, viruses, and protozoa, but they are expensive and cumbersome. The small pores in these filters also may become clogged quickly with cloudy water. Microstrainer filters with pores in the 0.1- to 0.3-μm range may filter bacteria and protozoa effectively, but they are not effective against viruses. If these are used, viruses may be killed with the addition of iodine or chlorine [1]. In general, drinks should be limited to carbonated and bottled soft drinks, beer, and wine. Bottled water *may* be safe, but it is sometimes bottled from a local source and thus may not be pure.

Travelers should be advised to avoid any food that may have been contaminated by water and food that is uncooked. Unpasteurized milk and milk products, such as cheese, also should be avoided. Food should be well cooked and eaten right after preparation. Even cooked food that has been allowed to sit at room temperature for several hours may not be safe, and it should be reheated. Only fruits and vegetables that the traveler can peel should be eaten. Homemade sauces and mayonnaise should be avoided. The general rule is "Boil it, peel it, cook it, or forget it."

Diarrhea

Diarrhea is the most common travel-related illness, affecting 30–50% of travelers to developing countries [6]. High-risk areas include Latin America, Africa, the Middle East, and Asia. Intermediate-risk areas include most of the southern European countries and a few of the Caribbean Islands. Low-risk areas include Canada, northern Europe, Australia, New Zealand, the United States, and a number of the Caribbean Islands [1]. Greater than 80% of cases are due to bacteria, predominantly *Escherichia coli* [7]. However, because most traveler's diarrhea is a self-limited illness, it is usually not necessary to make a specific diagnosis. The duration of traveler's diarrhea, without treatment, is usually 3–4 days. Sixty percent of patients recover within 48 hours [8]. Ten percent of cases persist for longer than 1 week and 2% for longer than 1 month. Approximately 2–10% have diarrhea accompanied by fevers, bloody stools, or both [1]. Table 29-1 lists the common causes of diarrhea.

Travelers with fever or bloody diarrhea should seek medical care. Bloody diarrhea and abdominal pain suggest amebic dysentery (*Entamoeba histolytica*) or bacterial dysentery (*Shigella dysenteriae, Campylobacter jejuni,* or *Plesiomonas shigelloides*). If the medical history reveals recent antibiotic use, *Clostridium difficile* should be considered. Ingestion of raw or undercooked meat followed by bloody diarrhea suggests *Escherichia coli* 0157:H7, which may cause hemolytic-uremia syndrome.

If diarrhea is severe, patients may require oral rehydration. One of the best oral rehydration solu-

Table 29-1
Bacterial Causes of Diarrhea

Noninflammatory	Inflammatory
Bacillus cereus	*Aeromonas hydrophila*
Campylobacter species	*Campylobacter* species
Clostridium perfringens	Enteroaggregative *E. coli*
Enteropathogenic *E. coli* (EPEC)	(EaggEC)
Enterotoxigenic *E. coli* (ETEC)	Enterohemorrhagic *E. coli*
Salmonella species	(EHEC)
Vibrio cholerae	Enteroinvasive *E. coli* (EIEC)
Vibrio parahemolyticus	*Plesiomonas shigelloides*
	Shigella species
	Yersinia enterocolitica

tions is the WHO formula. This comes in packets that can be easily ordered. A homemade version would include 1 L of clean water, $\frac{1}{2}$ tsp salt, $\frac{1}{4}$ tsp salt substitute (for potassium), $\frac{1}{2}$ tsp baking soda (for bicarbonate), and 2–3 tbsp sugar. Ingestion of glucose is important to promote water and sodium absorption from the gut. Too much glucose, however, can inhibit water absorption by its osmotic pull of water into the intestinal lumen. The ideal glucose concentration is 20 g/L. Apple juice, Gatorade, or cola drinks should be avoided because of their high sugar content but can be used in dilute form (50% in clean water) if better alternatives are not available.

One cause of traveler's diarrhea that deserves special attention is cholera. Cholera is endemic in more than 60 countries. Fortunately, the disease rarely poses any risk to short-term travelers because outbreaks are usually well localized and are not usually in areas near tourist attractions. It is caused by *Vibrio cholerae*. While most *V. cholerae* infections are asymptomatic or result in mild diarrhea, the infected individual may have profuse, watery diarrhea. Patients with severe disease can die in several hours if they are not properly treated. Early symptoms cannot be distinguished from other causes of traveler's diarrhea, and self-therapy is identical [9]. In severe cases, intravenous hydration and antibiotics may be necessary. Resistance to antimicrobials has been developing rapidly, but in most regions, traveler's diarrhea can be treated with tetracycline or doxycycline. Antibiotics decrease the duration of symptoms, the excretion of live cholera bacteria, and the volume of fluid lost, but they are not necessary for successful treatment.

Salmonella species can result in food-borne gastroenteritis with inflammatory diarrhea, abdominal pain, and fever. Although associated with food-borne outbreaks in industrialized countries, it is not a frequent cause of travelers' diarrhea worldwide. Clinically significant bacteremia is rare in healthy adults, and most patients do not require antibiotic treatment. However, when the victim is very young, elderly, or immunosuppressed, the illness tends to be more severe and requires antibiotics. Drugs of first choice for salmonellosis (excluding typhoid fever) are cefotaxime, ceftriaxone, or a fluoroquinolone; alternatives include ampicillin or amoxicillin, trimethoprim-sulfamethoxazole, or chloramphenicol [10].

Prolonged diarrhea suggests a nonbacterial infection, such as giardiasis. In patients who have taken antibiotics, *C. difficile* should be considered. Finally, not all diarrhea in travelers represents travel-related illness. If the evaluation does not reveal any pathogens and there is no response to empirical treatment, noninfectious causes of diarrhea, such as lactose intolerance or inflammatory bowel disease, also should be considered.

Antibiotics for prophylaxis generally are not necessary because traveler's diarrhea (TD) is generally self-limited, increasing resistance to antibiotics used prophylactically has occurred, and the risk of side effects, including drug allergies, photosensitivity, yeast vaginitis, and *C. difficile* infection, is a concern. For those who do take prophylaxis, agents such as bismuth subsalicylate (Pepto Bismol) are preferred over antibiotics. Bismuth subsalicylate has been shown to decrease the incidence of traveler's diarrhea by 60%, reducing the occurrence from about 40% to 14% [1], but it must be used with caution in patients with aspirin allergy, renal insufficiency, or gout and in those who are taking anticoagulants, probenicid, or methotrexate. Because of the risk of salicylate toxicity, bismuth subsalicylate is also contraindicated in persons who are already taking aspirin. It should *not* be given to anyone with a viral syndrome because of the risk of Reye's syndrome. Travelers should be advised that it may turn their tongue or their stools black, and occasionally it may cause nausea or constipation. The usual dose is 2 oz or two tablets four times per day. Because consuming this volume of the liquid can become cumbersome, it is easier for most people to take the tablets [1].

If diarrhea occurs, it usually can be ameliorated quickly by a combination of dietary restraint (rest of the bowel by consuming clear, nonirritating liquids and avoiding very hot or very cold liquids, solid food, fatty foods, and dairy products) and, if necessary for severe diarrhea, use of an over-the-counter antidiarrheal medication such as loperamide. If this is not effective, given that most traveler's diarrhea is due to bacteria, a short course of empirical antibiotics may help. Some physician's provide travelers with an antibiotic for treatment of presumed *E. coli*-related severe diarrhea, the treatment depending on the individual's health status and local patterns of bacterial resistance. The 2008 CDC Yellow Book [1] states that "Antibiotics are the principal element in the treatment of TD," and agents for control of symptoms are considered adjuncts. Empirical antibiotic first-line choices include fluoroquinolones (i.e., ciprofloxacin or levofloxacin), except in Thailand and Nepal, where fluoroquinolone-resistant *Campylobacter* has been found. Alternatives include trimethaprim-sulfamethoxazole, azithromycin, and rifaximin (Table 29-2). Adjunctive treatment also could include bismuth subsalicylate (Pepto Bismo), diphenoxylate (Lomotil), or loperamide (Imodium).

Respiratory Infections

Prolonged air travel and crowded conditions predispose travelers to respiratory infections. The low humidity of airplane cabins dries out mucous membranes, impairing an important defense mechanism. Also, cabin air is recirculated during flights, which may promote the spread of airborne diseases, including tuberculosis. Restriction in close quarters during flights or on arrival increases the likelihood of spreading other airborne illnesses, such as influenza, *Neisseria meningitidis,* and diphtheria.

The evaluation of respiratory infections in recent travelers is similar to that of patients presenting from the general population. Underlying illnesses and vaccination status must be considered. However, tuberculosis (TB) also should be considered, especially in travelers returning from areas where tuberculosis is prevalent or among those who had prolonged exposure to residents. Teachers, health care workers, volunteer relief workers, and students are at particular risk. Transmission also has occurred during travel on commercial aircraft [11]. If tuberculosis is suspected, chest radiography, sputum culture for common respiratory pathogens and *Mycobacterium tuberculosis,* and a tuberculin skin test should be obtained. If hospitalization is required, the patient should be placed in respiratory isolation until TB can be excluded. Treatment depends on the likelihood of multidrug-resistant TB. See Chapter 9.

Exposure to influenza depends on the time of year and the destination. Influenza can occur year round in the tropics. In temperate regions of the southern hemisphere, influenza activity is greatest between May and September. Travelers also may be exposed to influenza during the summer, when traveling with large groups that include persons from parts of the world where the influenza virus is circulating. Influenza and other viral causes of respiratory infection can be complicated by a variety of secondary bacterial pathogens. See Chapters 11A and 11B.

Table 29-2
Drug Regimens for the Treatment of Traveler's Diarrhea

Drug	Adult Dose	Comments
Bismuth subsalicylate (Pepto Bismol)	20 mL or 2 tablets every 30 minutes for 8 doses	Maximum 240 mL (16 tablets) per day
Loperamide (Imodium)	2 caplets; then 1 caplet after each loose stool	Maximum 8 caplets (16 mg) per day
Ciprofloxacin (Cipro)	500 mg twice daily or 750 mg as one dose	Contraindicated in pregnant women and those under age 18
Levofloxacin (Levaquin)	500 mg PO daily	Contraindicated in pregnant women and those under age 18
Azithromycin	500 mg PO daily	Rarely causes nausea or vomiting
Rifaximin	200 mg three times/day	Not for invasive *E. coli.* Don't use if fevers or bloody stools

Meningitis

In certain parts of the world, *N. meningitidis* is an important cause of meningitis. It is endemic in the "Meningitis Belt," which stretches across sub-Saharan Africa to northern India and Nepal. When an individual who returns from travel to any of these areas exhibits symptoms and/or signs of meningitis, the possibility of *N. meningitidis* infection is an important consideration. This organism is contagious, and patients with suspected meningococcal infection should be put into isolation. Many of the systemic illnesses discussed below also may present with severe headaches and, rarely, meningitis. Table 29-3 lists other systemic illnesses that also may have cutaneous manifestations. More details are presented in Chapter 23.

Systemic Illnesses

Malaria must be considered in any traveler who returns with a systemic febrile illness. Malaria owing to *Plasmodium falciparum* is a medical emergency. All febrile patients who have traveled to endemic areas must be considered to have malaria until proven otherwise. This disease is caused by a parasite and is discussed in greater detail in Chapter 25. Travelers with systemic febrile illness may have a bacterial infection, but it is important to consider malaria as a diagnosis if they traveled to a malaria zone within the past year or otherwise could have been exposed.

ENTERIC FEVER

Enteric fever is caused most often by the gram-negative bacillus *Salmonella typhi*, although it also

Table 29-3
Common Systemic Bacterial Infections Associated with Skin Lesions

Bartonellosis
Brucellosis
Gonococcemia
Leptospirosis
Lyme disease
Meningococcemia
Rat-bite fever
Rickettsial infections
Syphilis
Typhoid fever

may be caused by *S. paratyphi*. Although typhoid and paratyphoid fever are acquired through the enteral route, diarrhea is not a common presenting symptom. Patients usually present with high fever, prostration, and abdominal pain. Enteric fever is seen most commonly in those who are returning from developing countries. Although immunization decreases the likelihood of contracting this infectious disease, it does not exclude the diagnosis because none of the available vaccines offers 100% protection. Enteric fever may have an insidious or abrupt onset. The incubation period ranges from 5–21 days depending on the size of the inoculum and the underlying health of the traveler. Presenting symptoms are nonspecific but typically include high fevers (38–39°C) and may include diarrhea, abdominal pain, constipation, headache, anorexia, cough, and muscle pain. Approximately 5–10% of patients develop neuropsychiatric manifestations, which may include psychosis and confusion. Thirty percent of patients develop "rose spots." This is classically a salmon-colored maculopapular rash on the trunk. The lesions contain organisms that can be cultured from punch biopsy specimens.

The diagnosis of enteric fever depends on isolation of *S. typhi* or *S. paratyphi* from the patient. Cultures of blood, stool, urine, rose spots, bone marrow, and gastric and intestinal secretions may be useful. In more than 90% of patients, bacteria are isolated from blood, bone marrow, or intestinal secretions. If only blood cultures are performed, the sensitivity is 50–70%. Bone marrow cultures are 90% sensitive in making the diagnosis. Stool cultures are often negative.

Resolution of fever and most symptoms occurs in 90% of patients by the fourth week of infection without antibiotic therapy. However, weakness, weight loss, and debilitation may persist for months. If the infection is treated with antibiotics, symptoms usually resolve in 3–5 days. Antibiotic therapy depends on regional susceptibility. Historically, reasonable antibiotic choices include beta-lactam antibiotics, chloramphenicol, fluoroquinolones, or trimethoprim-sulfamethoxazole [12]. At the time of this writing, the first choice for treatment of typhoid fever is a fluoroquinolone (none are recommended for children or pregnant women) or ceftriaxone; the other historical choices are alternatives [10].

RICKETTSIAL INFECTIONS

Rickettsial infections include the spotted fevers, typhus fever, and Q fever. This group of infections is characterized by the abrupt onset of fever and headache. Except for Q fever, vectors (usually ticks) carry these illnesses.

The spotted fevers are often recognized by the tache noire, or eschar, at the site of the tick bite. The disease is transmitted by a tick bite and is caused by various *Rickettsia* species. The initial symptoms are fevers, myalgias, and headaches. A tache noire may be identified by careful examination. Severe cases may resemble Rocky Mountain spotted fever and result in disseminated vascular infection.

Murine typhus, which is caused by *R. typhi*, occurs after inoculation of infected flea feces into a fleabite wound. The presentation is nonspecific; patients usually have fever, headache, chills, myalgias, and nausea. Only 18% of patients have a rash at the onset of illness, but 50% develop a rash during the course of the illness. Most of the clinical findings are due to vasculitis, which may affect any organ [13].

Scrub typhus is caused by *R. tsutsugamushi* and is transmitted by the bite of larval-stage trombiculid mites (chiggers). It is found in eastern Asia and the western Pacific region. The vector predominantly lives in scrub, which is the vegetation in the transitional area between forest and clearings. Awareness of the vector's habitat is important for both military personnel and local residents. If an eschar and regional adenopathy are present, this strongly suggests the diagnosis. Symptoms begin 6–18 days after the bite. The most prominent findings are fever, severe headache, and myalgias. Lymphadenopathy is common [14].

Q fever is caused by *Coxiella burnetii*. The important reservoirs for this infection are cattle, sheep, and goats. The organism can be shed in urine, feces, milk, or birth products. The incubation period is approximately 20 days, and symptoms usually include severe headache, fever, chills, fatigue, and myalgias. Unlike the cutaneous involvement associated with other rickettsial infections, rash is rare in patients with Q fever. When it does occur, it is generally due to an immune complex vasculitis, which may result from chronic disease [15].

Rickettsial illnesses can be treated with tetracycline, doxycycline, or chloramphenicol. Fluoroquinolones also may be useful.

LEPTOSPIROSIS

Leptospirosis is found worldwide and is caused by *Leptospira interrogans* serovars. It is acquired after exposure to the urine of infected animals. Rats are the most important source of infection (typically the serovar *icterohaemorrhagiae*), although dogs (*canicola*), swine (*pomona*), cattle (*hardjo*), and raccoons (*autumnalis*) can be sources. Leptospirosis usually causes a mild, self-limited disease. However, it may cause a biphasic illness including a septicemic phase followed by a temporary decline in fever and then an immune phase. The septicemic phase begins 7–12 days after exposure and it is characterized by high fevers (38° to 40°C), headache, nausea, vomiting, diarrhea, cough, pharyngitis, myalgias and conjunctival suffusion. These symptoms last for about 1 week. Leptospires can be isolated from blood, urine, CSF and most tissues during this phase but meningeal signs are not prominent.

When the immune phase occurs, it is often more severe than the septicemic phase. Symptoms are variable but the most common one is aseptic meningitis (in up to 80% of cases). Some of these patients will also have delirium. Other findings may include jaundice, myalgias, conjunctival suffusion with or without hemorrhage, adenopathy and hepatosplenomegaly. Severe disease, or icteric leptospirosis, results in fulminant hepatic failure, or Weil's disease, characterized by jaundice and renal failure. During the immune phase, the organism still can be found in the kidney, urine, and aqueous humor. The diagnosis is often made retrospectively with serologic tests. Treatment with penicillin, tetracycline, or doxycycline during the first few days of the initial phase may shorten the duration of fever and reduce the incidence of renal, hepatic, meningeal, and hemorrhagic complications.

BRUCELLOSIS

Brucellosis, or undulant fever, is found worldwide, especially in the Mediterranean Basin, the Arabian Peninsula, the Indian subcontinent, and in parts of Mexico and Central and South America. It is caused by *Brucella* species (biovars of *B. abortus, melitensis, suis,* and *canis*) and occurs after direct or indirect contact with animals, in particular cattle, goats, sheep, swine, and dogs. The disease is seen most commonly in abattoir (slaughterhouse) workers, veterinarians, livestock industry workers, and laboratory workers. Most commonly, bacteria enter the body through abrasions in the skin or after accidental inoculation into the conjunctiva. *B. melitensis* is often ingested in unpasteurized milk. Symptoms begin 2–8 weeks after inoculation. Patients present with nonspecific symptoms of fever, sweats, malaise, anorexia, headache, and back pain. If brucellosis is not treated, the patient may develop an undulant fever pattern. Because it is a systemic disease involving the reticuloendothelial system, patients often have lymphadenopathy, splenomegaly, and/or hepatomegaly. Isolating the bacteria from blood, bone marrow, or other tissues can make the diagnosis. Alternatively, serologic tests can be used to make a presumptive diagnosis. Because of the high rate of relapse associated with use of a single drug, combination treatment generally is recommended. Doxycycline is given in combination with rifampin or an aminoglycoside. With appropriate treatment, most patients recover within weeks to months.

ANTHRAX

Anthrax, a disease of herbivores that come into contact with spores in the soil, is caused by *Bacillus anthracis*. In its spore form, *B. anthracis* can persist for years. Anthrax is found worldwide but is endemic in South America, Central America, Iran, and Russia. It is spread to humans by direct contact with skin, inhalation, or ingestion. Contaminated animal hides and wool can be a source of infection. Ninety-five percent of infections are cutaneous, and 5% involve the respiratory tract. Gastrointestinal anthrax also has been reported [16]. In humans, cutaneous illness presents as a painless papule, usually on exposed areas of the head, neck, or arms. The lesion becomes vesicular with an ulcerated center and then develops the characteristic black eschar.

Pulmonary anthrax occurs when spores are inhaled. In the past, outbreaks had been reported among wool sorters. This is the type of anthrax that is most severe and would be most likely after exposure to weapons-grade anthrax. This is a biphasic illness. The initial symptoms of malaise, fatigue, myalgias, fever, and a nonproductive cough often resemble those of a mild upper respiratory infection. After 2–4 days, the patient may show some improvement, but this initial phase is followed by the sudden onset of severe respiratory distress. Patients soon become hypotensive, and death usually occurs within 24 hours.

Intestinal anthrax occurs after ingestion of contaminated food and results in nausea, vomiting, anorexia, and fever. Abdominal pain, hematemesis, and bloody diarrhea also may develop. With further progression, shock, cyanosis, and death may occur 2–5 days after the initial ingestion. Oropharyngeal infection, resulting in edema and tissue necrosis in the area of the cervical spine, also may occur. The main clinical features are sore throat, dysphagia, fever, regional lymphadenopathy, and toxemia. Most patients with oropharyngeal infection die [16].

Infected patients almost always have an apparent source of exposure. Anthrax bacilli often can be isolated from vesicular fluid or blood, and the serologic findings of a fourfold rise in acute and convalescent titers or a single titer greater than 1:32 confirms the diagnosis. While cutaneous anthrax can be treated successfully with very little mortality, if it is untreated, 20% of cutaneous cases result in death. Penicillin G is the drug of choice; fluoroquinolones, erythromycin, tetracyclines, and chloramphenicol are alternatives. Excision of the lesion is contraindicated. Dressings removed from the lesion should be treated as biohazardous waste [16]. If someone has inhalational or gastrointestinal anthrax, he or she should be treated with a combination of antibiotics.

BARTONELLOSIS

Bartonellosis is caused by *Bartonella bacilliformis*, which is found only in river valleys of the Andes Mountains (i.e., Columbia, Peru, and Ecuador) at altitudes between 2,000 and 8,000 ft. The only proven vector is the sandfly. *B. bacilliformis* organisms invade red blood cells and cause intravascular hemolysis and fever. The organism then can invade the reticuloendothelial system [17].

The acute form of bartonellosis, Oroya fever, occurs after an incubation period of about 3 weeks. Patients may present with anorexia, headache, malaise, and a slight fever. In more severe cases, the initial presentation includes high fever, chills, headache, and confusion. Patients may become jaundiced because of rapid hemolysis. Other possible findings are myalgias, arthralgias, dyspnea, insomnia, delirium, and in terminal cases, coma. Generalized lymphadenopathy and thrombocytopenic purpura also may occur. If patients survive this stage, the convalescent stage begins. The organisms disappear from the red blood cells, and there is a decrease in fever and an increase in the number of erythrocytes. Intercurrent infection is common at this stage and may be an important cause of mortality [17].

The diagnosis often can be made by eosin/thiazine stain of blood smears during the acute phase. IgM antibodies may be present but are nonspecific. Treatment is with chloramphenicol, penicillin, or fluoroquinolones. Fever often disappears within 24 hours of starting treatment. Patients with severe anemia may require blood transfusions [17].

An eruptive cutaneous form known as *verruga peruana* may occur after resolution of Oroya fever, or it may occur without prior symptoms in those with previous episodes of bartonellosis. Joint pains and low-grade fever often present in the preeruptive stage. Nodules (verrugas) develop over a period of 1–2 months and may persist for months to years. The verrugas appear most often on exposed parts of the body. Cutaneous lesions vary from red to purple and appear in crops. Individual lesions may reach 1–2 cm in diameter, and the organism may be cultured from the lesions. There is a variable response to antibiotics. Secondary infections may require surgery or antimicrobial therapy [17].

Prevention requires control of the sandfly. Dwellings may be sprayed with DDT and insect repellents. Use of bed netting is important [17].

MELIOIDOSIS

Melioidosis is caused by *Burkholderia pseudomallei*. This disease is endemic in Southeast Asia, with the largest concentration of cases in Vietnam, Cambodia, Laos, Thailand, Malaysia, Myanmar, and northern Australia. It has been reported in latitudes between 20 degrees north and south of the equator and has been reported rarely in the western hemisphere. In endemic areas, the organism is found in surface water, mud, rice paddies, and market produce. Clinical disease is rare except in northeast Thailand, where it accounts for 40% of deaths from community-acquired septicemia [18]. The disease can recur months or years after apparent cure, or it may break out after many years of latency. The clinical manifestations are variable. The most common presentation is acute pulmonary infection, but melioidosis may cause transient bacteremia, asymptomatic pulmonary infiltration,

acute localized suppurative infection, septicemia, or a chronic suppurative infection. The disease should be suspected in persons returning from an endemic area if symptoms of respiratory failure or multiple pustular or necrotic skin or subcutaneous lesions develop, or if there is a radiographic appearance consistent with tuberculosis but no mycobacteria can be isolated. The diagnosis can be made by culturing the organism or by serologic testing. When treatment is necessary, it should be based on the results of susceptibility testing. Combination therapy is recommended for severely ill patients.

PLAGUE

Plague is caused by the bacterium *Yersinia pestis* (see Chapter 15). It is found worldwide, with most of the human cases reported from developing countries in Asia and Africa. Plague is primarily a zoonotic infection. Humans become infected from contact with rodents and their fleas. The most common presentation is *bubonic plague,* which is characterized by the sudden onset of fevers, chills, weakness, headache, and painful regional lymphadenitis. The most common site of lymphadenitis is the groin, but axillary and cervical buboes also occur. Buboes are 1–10 cm in length and are extremely tender. They occur in 90% of cases of plague. *Septicemic plague* is defined as plague without a bubo, which often progresses rapidly to shock. Patients with septicemic plague have high-grade bacteremia; a blood smear may reveal the characteristic bipolar-staining gram-negative, ovoid, "safety pin"–appearing bacilli. The case-fatality rate is 33%. *Pneumonic plague* is most often a secondary pneumonia in a patient with bubonic plague. It also can occur in cases of human-to-human contact. The pneumonia is necrotizing and is invariably fatal if antibiotic therapy is delayed by more than 1 day. Plague meningitis is a rare complication of inadequately treated bubonic plague; it results from hematogenous spread and has a high mortality rate [19].

The diagnosis of plague should be suspected in febrile patients who have been exposed to rodents or other mammals in the known endemic areas of the world. A diagnosis often can be made quickly with a smear and culture of a bubo aspirate. In patients with negative cultures, a fourfold or greater increase in titer or a single titer of at least 1:16 provides a presumptive diagnosis. Streptomycin is the drug of choice; tetracycline, fluoroquinolones, and chloramphenicol are effective alternatives [19].

Prevention depends on controlling rodent and flea reservoirs. Proper disposal of food and refuse, removal of unused outbuildings and woodpiles, and periodic treatment with pesticides are important. Buildings should be rat-proof. In high-risk areas, the formalin-killed vaccine should be considered. This is given as a primary series of two injections, with a 1- to 3-month interval between them, followed by boosters every 6 months [18]. See Chapter 15.

TULAREMIA

Tularemia is caused by *Francisella tularensis*. Although widely distributed, it is primarily a disease of the northern hemisphere. Rodents and lagomorphs are important reservoirs. Transmission to humans occurs after an insect bite, direct contact with contaminated animal products, or inhalation. High-risk occupations include veterinarians, farmers, sheep workers, hunters and trappers, cooks or meat handlers, and laboratory workers [20].

The incubation period for *F. tularensis* generally is 3–5 days but may be as short as 1 day or as long as 3 weeks. Clinical symptoms usually start abruptly with fever, chills, headache, malaise, anorexia, and fatigue. Without treatment, fever lasts an average of 1 month, and adenopathy may persist for several months. The presentation is often classified as ulceroglandular, glandular, oculoglandular, pharyngeal, typhoidal, or pneumonic. Ulceroglandular disease is most common and is characterized by tender localized lymphadenopathy. The inciting skin lesion may appear before, with, or after the lymphadenopathy. It generally starts as a painful red papule and then undergoes necrosis, leaving a tender ulcer. Glandular disease is similar but without an apparent skin lesion. Oculoglandular tularemia occurs when the organism gains entry through the conjunctiva. Patients may have photophobia, excessive lacrimation, and a painful conjunctivitis, with small yellow conjunctival ulcers or papules in some patients. Typhoidal tularemia is a febrile illness without prominent lymphadenopathy. This form is the most difficult to diagnosis. Pneumonic tularemia presents with predominantly pulmonary symptoms. It may occur after inhalation or from hematogenous spread to the lung. The most common complication is suppuration of involved lymph nodes. Patients with severe disease may have disseminated intravascular coagulation, renal failure, rhabdomyolysis, jaundice, and hepatitis [20].

The diagnosis depends on clinical suspicion. *F. tularensis* may be recovered from various sites in the body, and it is a significant risk to laboratory workers. The diagnosis can be confirmed with serologic studies. The drug of choice for treatment is streptomycin; gentamicin, ciprofloxacin, and doxycycline are reasonable alternatives [20].

The best preventive measure is avoidance of exposure to the organism. Wild animals should not be skinned or dressed using bare hands or when the animal appears ill. Gloves, masks, and protective eyewear should be worn. Wild game should be cooked thoroughly. Water that is contaminated by dead animals should not be used. When working in high-risk areas with large numbers of ticks, clothing that covers most of the body should be worn. Tick repellents also should be considered [20].

LEPROSY

Leprosy is caused by an acid-fast bacillus, *Mycobacterium leprae,* that cannot be grown in bacteriologic medium or cell cultures. Transmission requires close contact, and the organism is thought to be transmitted from the nasal mucosa to the skin or respiratory tract or by close contact with skin lesions. The reservoir is essentially limited to humans, and incubation periods can range from 9 months to 20 years. The two main forms of leprosy are lepromatous (multibacillary) and tuberculoid (paucibacillary), although borderline (bipolar/labile) and indeterminate forms occur. Lepromatous leprosy, with an average incubation period of about 8 years, is characterized by symmetric, bilateral skin lesions (more than five and typically numerous) comprising nodules, papules, macules, and infiltrates. The classic disease shows involvement and destruction of nasal mucosa, keratitis, and iritis. Tuberculoid leprosy, with an average incubation period of about 4 years, is characterized by five or fewer well-demarcated skin lesions (often single; by definition, five or fewer) that are hypoesthetic or anesthetic, with asymmetric involvement of peripheral nerves. The diagnosis of leprosy is usually made on clinical grounds in endemic areas without laboratory confirmation, although examination of scrape/incision skin harvesting can show acid-fast bacilli.

The story of leprosy is one of the world's recently emerging public health success stories. Leprosy used to be a much-feared disease that resulted in extreme social ostracism of its victims. Historically, it was endemic in ancient civilizations of India, China, and Egypt and was spread to Europe and other areas by travelers pursuing trade or conquest, thus having an occupational travel component (see Chapter 1). In current times, leprosy represents little to no risk for most travelers because of initiatives of the World Health Organization (WHO), philanthropic foundations, and many participating countries committed to elimination of this disease. In 1981, the WHO recommended that single-drug treatment with dapsone be replaced by multidrug therapy (MDT) consisting of dapsone, rifampin, and clofazimine, a combination that is thought to prevent transmission after the first dose and result in cure within 6–12 months depending on the type of leprosy treated. In 1991, the World Health Assembly resolved that leprosy should be eliminated as a public health problem, and since 1995, the WHO has provided free MDT for all leprosy patients in the world. This effort has resulted in eliminating leprosy as a health problem (defined as prevalence less than 1 case per 10,000 population) in more than 113 countries, the 1985 global disease burden of about 5.2 million cases having decreased to less than 300,000 in 2004. The disease is still a public health problem in some parts of the world, the large majority of new cases occurring in Brazil, India, Madagascar, Mozambique, Nepal, and the United Republic of Tanzania [21, 22].

Sexually Transmitted Diseases

Medical professionals who care for travelers often underestimate exposure to sexually transmitted diseases (STDs). There is evidence that travel increases the risk of acquiring STDs, although this may be due to overall high-risk behavior of individuals who have casual sex during travel [23]. The prevalence of STDs is much higher in developing countries than in the United States. Those most likely to engage in unprotected sexual intercourse with a new partner while abroad are business travelers and young men traveling for long periods of time alone. Chlamydia and gonorrhea are the most common causes of urethritis in men and cervicitis in women. However, the differential diagnosis for genital ulcerative diseases is fairly large, including syphilis (*Treponema pallidum*), chancroid (*Haemophilus ducreyi*), lymphogranuloma venereum (*Chlamydia trachomatis*), and granuloma inguinale (donovanosis, *Calymmatobacterium granulomatis*). In assessing the individual with an STD, one must consider that simultaneous infection with multiple organisms may be present, including HIV and herpes simplex virus (HSV-2). Chapters 24 and 35 present some information for employees regarding prevention of these diseases.

Syphilis is generally categorized by phase: (1) an incubation period lasting about 3 weeks, (2) primary syphilis with a painless ulcer (chancre), regional adenopathy, and early bacteremia, (3) secondary syphilis, which is characterized by generalized mucocutaneous lesions and adenopathy, (4) latent syphilis, and (5) in a small proportion of patients, tertiary syphilis, which most often involves the ascending aorta and the central nervous system (CNS).

Primary syphilis begins as a single painless papule that quickly erodes and becomes indurated to form a smooth, painless ulcer without any exudate (chancre). During this stage, dark-field microscopy can be used to make the diagnosis. The chancre usually resolves within 3–6 weeks. Secondary syphilis begins 2–8 weeks after the appearance of the chancre. During this period, the spirochete is widely disseminated. Macular, maculopapular, papular, and/or pustular lesions may appear on the body, including the palms of the hands and soles of the feet. Mucous patches may be seen in the mouth. Plaques, known as *condyloma lata*, also may be seen; these are highly contagious. There are often constitutional symptoms, and the CNS is frequently involved. Syphilis then may enter a latent stage without any clinical evidence of disease, but it may recur later as late syphilis with endarteritis obliterans of vaso vasorum resulting in aortic aneurysm or coronary ostium stenosis or neurosyphilis (i.e., acute meningitis, meningovascular syphilis, Argyll Robertson pupils, general paresis, tabes dorsalis, or Charcot's joints).

In primary and secondary syphilis, the diagnosis can be made with the dark-field microscopy. However, the diagnosis is made most often with serologic tests. These tests are not reliable in primary syphilis but are usually positive by the time a patient develops secondary syphilis. Screening is usually performed with one of the nonspecific tests: a rapid plasma reagin test (RPR) or venereal disease research laboratory test (VDRL). These tests are inexpensive, rapid, and convenient, but there are many false-positive test results. When results are positive, the diagnosis can be confirmed with one of the specific treponemal tests. These include the fluorescent treponemal antibody absorption test (FTA-ABS) and the *T. pallidum* hemagglutination assay (TPHA). Penicillin G is the drug of choice, doxycycline or ceftriaxone being alternatives [10].

Chancroid is found worldwide and is associated with low socioeconomic status and poor hygiene. Only 10% of reported cases are in women. The incubation period is generally 5–7 days. Lesions begin as tender papules that become pustular and then erode to form an ulcer. The typical ulcer is painful, nonindurated, ragged, and undermined with an erythematous halo. The base bleeds easily and may be covered with a necrotic exudate, which can be up to 20 mm in size. Approximately half of patients have inguinal lymphadenopathy that is unilateral and tender and may require drainage.

The diagnosis of chancroid is difficult to make clinically. A culture specimen should be obtained with a swab from the purulent ulcer base or by aspiration of the bubo. Gram staining may show large numbers of gram-negative coccobacilli. Patients with suspected chancroid also should be evaluated for syphilis because the infections may be difficult to differentiate, and patients may be co-infected. Most patients respond to treatment with erythromycin, azithromycin, ceftriaxone (unless they are co-infected with HIV), and amoxicillin–clavulonic acid.

Lymphogranuloma venereum (LGV) is endemic in Africa, India, Southeast Asia, South America, and the Caribbean. The primary lesion appears 3–30 days after infection. It is a small papule or ulcer that produces few, if any, symptoms. Days to weeks later, patients develop lymphadenopathy and systemic symptoms, including fever, headache, and myalgias. Initially, the lymph nodes are discrete and tender and have overlying erythema; then the inflammation spreads into the surrounding tissue, forming an inflammatory mass (bubo). Abscesses, fistulas, or sinus tracts may develop within this mass. Rupture of the bubo occurs in a third of patients and

relieves pain and fever, although sinus tracts may continue to drain pus for several weeks or months. As the disease progresses, fibrosis of the lymph nodes develops, and elephantiasis of the genitalia may occur in both genders.

The clinical diagnosis of LGV rests on the presence of painless ulcers and matted unilateral lymph nodes. Unlike herpes, in LGV there is usually just one lesion, which is painful. Indurated margins and bilateral adenopathy suggest syphilis. Large ulcers that are multiple and extremely tender suggest chancroid. *C. trachomatis* can be recovered from bubo aspirates, genital tissue, or rectal tissue in a third of patients. Histopathologic changes in LGV, combined with serologic tests (e.g., immunofluorescence, enzyme immunoassays, DNA probe, or polymerase chain reaction) in an appropriate setting, or culture of aspirate is sufficient to make the diagnosis. Doxycycline or erythromycin is used to treat this infection. A fluctuant bubo also may require aspiration to prevent rupture and formation of sinus tracts.

Granuloma inguinale is a chronic, progressive ulcerative disease. It is reported most commonly in southeast India, New Guinea, the Caribbean, and parts of South America. It also has been recorded in Zambia, Zimbabwe, the Natal Region of South Africa, Southeast Asia, and among aborigines in Australia. After an incubation period of 8–80 days, the gram-negative bacillus typically results in a small painless papule or indurated nodule appears. This soon ulcerates to form a beefy-red, granulomatous ulcer with rolled edges and a characteristic satin-like surface that bleeds easily. Multiple lesions may coalesce to form large ulcers, and new lesions may form from autoinoculation. The ulcers are painless, unless there is severe secondary infection. The disease spreads subcutaneously and may become destructive. In severe cases, patients may develop lymphedema with elephantiasis of the external genitalia. The diagnosis is usually made clinically and can be confirmed histologically by punch biopsy of the edge of active lesions or a crush preparation of granulation tissue. The demonstration of typical intracellular Donovan's bodies is the "gold standard" for making the diagnosis. Trimethoprim-sulfamethoxazole is considered the drug of first choice; other options include doxycycline and ciprofloxacin with or without gentamycin.

Gonococcal infection with the gram-negative diplococcus, *N. gonorrhoeae,* typically results in acute purulent urethral discharge in males after an incubation period of 2–7 days. Of the two main serotypes identified by outer membrane protein type, Por1A is typically associated with disseminated gonococcal infection (DGI strains); Por1B typically results in local genital infections and is more likely to be asymptomatic, a feature that helps to facilitate transmission. Diagnosis usually can be confirmed based on the history and Gram stain findings of typical diplococci in the purulent urethral fluid. In females, a mucopurulent cervicitis may be asymptomatic or, less often, may present with the salpingitis and/or endometritis of pelvic inflammatory disease. Gonococcal infection also can be manifest by epididymitis, proctitis, pharyngitis, or conjunctivitis; the DGI strains may result in a joint-localized septic joint (typically affecting one or two joints of the knees, wrists, ankles, or elbows) or a more widespread bacteremia with high fever and chills, tenosynovitis, arthritis-dermatitis syndrome (i.e., arthralgias, tenosynovitis, and hemorrhagic papular and/or pustular skin lesions with purpuric centers, primarily in the distal limbs), perihepatitis, meningitis, or endocarditis. Plasmid-related resistance to penicillin and tetracycline is widespread, and strains from Asia, which now affect many parts of the world, show widespread resistance to fluoroquinolones. The drug of first choice for treatment is ceftriaxone, with alternatives including cefixime, cefotaxime, and penicillin G [10], but owing to the evolution of resistant organisms, practitioners should be aware of current local patterns of resistance.

References

1. Centers for Disease Control and Prevention. *Health Information for International Travel 2008.* Atlanta: CDC, 2008.
2. Jong EC. Immunizations for international travel. *Infect Dis Clin North Am* 1998;12:249–66.
3. Wolfe MS. Protection of travelers. *Clin Infect Dis* 1997;25:177–86.
4. Miller SI, Hohmann EL, Pegues DA. *Salmonella* (including *Salmonella typhi*). In Mandell GL, Bennett JE, Dolin R (eds), *Principles and Practices of Infectious Diseases,* 4th ed. New York: Churchill Livingstone, 1995. Pp 2024–6.
5. Typhoid immunization recommendations of the Advisory Committee on Immunization Practices. *MMWR* 1994;43:1–7.
6. National Institutes of Health Consensus Conference. Traveler's diarrhea. *JAMA* 1985;253:2700–4.
7. Kozarsky PE, Lobel HO, Steffen R. Travel medicine 1991: New frontiers. *Ann Intern Med* 1991;115:574–5.
8. Hill DR, Pearson RD. Health advice for international travel. *Ann Intern Med* 1988;108:839–52.
9. Haburchak DR, Felz MW. Diseases associated with foreign travel. *Compr Ther* 1997;23:19–24.
10. Treatment guidelines. *Med Lett* 2007;5:57.
11. Centers for Disease Control and Prevention. Exposure of passengers and flight crew to *Mycobacterium tuberculosis* on commercial aircraft, 1992–1995. *MMWR* 1995;44:137–40.
12. Miller SI, Hohmann EL, Pegues DA. *Salmonella* (including *Salmonella typhi*). In Mandell GL, Bennett JE, Dolin R (eds), *Principles and Practices of Infectious Diseases,* 4th ed. New York: Churchill Livingstone, 1995, pp 2020–1.
13. Dumler JS, Walker DH. Murine typhus. In Mandell GL, Bennett JE, Dolin R (eds), *Principles and Practices of Infectious Diseases,* 4th ed. New York: Churchill Livingstone, 1995. Pp 1737–9.
14. Saah AJ. *Rickettsia tsutsugamushi* (scrub typhus). In Mandell GL, Bennett JE, Dolin R (eds), *Principles and Practices of Infectious Diseases,* 4th ed. New York: Churchill Livingstone, 1995. Pp 17340–1.
15. Marrie TJ. *Coxiella burnetti* (Q fever). In Mandell GL, Bennett JE, Dolin R (eds), *Principles and Practices of Infectious Diseases,* 4th ed. New York: Churchill Livingstone, 1995. Pp 1727–35.
16. Lew D. *Bacillus anthracis* (anthrax). In Mandell GL, Bennett JE, Dolin R (eds), *Principles and Practices of Infectious Diseases,* 4th ed. New York: Churchill Livingstone, 1995. Pp 1885–9.
17. Roverts NJ. *Bartonella bacilliformis* (bartonellosis). In Mandell GL, Bennett JE, Dolin R (eds), *Principles and Practices of Infectious Diseases,* 4th ed. New York: Churchill Livingstone, 1995. Pp 2209–10.
18. Chaowagul W, White NJ, Dance DAB, et al. Melioidosis: A major cause of community-acquired septicemia in northeastern Thailand. *J Infect Dis* 1989;159:890–9.
19. Butler T. *Yersinia* species (including plague). In Mandell GL, Bennett JE, Dolin R (eds), *Principles and Practices of Infectious Diseases,* 4th ed. New York: Churchill Livingstone, 1995. Pp 2070–8.
20. Penn RL. *Francisella tularensis* (tularemia). In Mandell GL, Bennett JE, Dolin R (eds), *Principles and Practices of Infectious Diseases,* 4th ed. New York: Churchill Livingstone, 1995. Pp 2060–8.
21. Heymann DL (ed). *Control of Communicable Diseases Manual,* 18th ed. Washington: American Public Health Association, 2004. Pp 302–6.
22. World Health Organization. *Leprosy Today and Leprosy Fact Sheet.* Geneva: WHO, 2008.
23. Arvidson M, Hellberg D, Mardh PA. Sexual risk behavior and history of sexually transmitted diseases in relation to casual travel sex during different types of journeys. *Acta Obstet Gynaecol Scand* 1996;75:49.

30 Helminthic Travel-Related Infections

Jeffrey G. Jones

Although helminthic infections receive relatively little attention in the United States, they represent a significant burden of suffering throughout the world. In fact, some authors estimate that up to 25% of the world's populace is infected with helminths. As the world rapidly becomes more accessible to more people, helminthic infections are becoming more common in the United States. Groups at special risk for these infections include international workers, students and travelers, migrant laborers, refugees, children of foreign adoptions, and the homeless. Environmental factors include substandard housing, crowding, breakdown of hygienic standards, and inaccessible medical care, all of which are risks for contracting helminthic infections.

Parasites in general and worm infections specifically are looked on in the United States with abhorrence. Thus there is a strong social stigma associated with these infections, which may or may not be warranted by their detriment to health. The practitioner must keep this in mind when working with patients who have these infections. Unlike many other types of infections, helminthic infections are often diagnosed primarily through microscopic detection of helminth eggs or larval stages. For this reason, the practitioner is encouraged to have ready access to a high-quality atlas of parasites [1].

The helminths are composed of three groups. The first includes nematodes, or roundworms. These may be intestinal, in the blood or tissues, or zoonotic. The second includes the trematodes, or flukes, and the third, the cestodes, or tapeworms.

Adult Nematoda Residing in the Human Gut

These are the most prevalent of all nematodes. They are found primarily in tropical and subtropical climates. In general, their presence reflects the sanitary and socioeconomic conditions of the environment. To varying degrees, these are all found in the United States and worldwide.

ASCARIS LUMBRICOIDES

Ascaris lumbricoides is the largest intestinal nematode, measuring up to 30 cm in length. This nematode has the appearance of an earthworm but is white or light pink in color. It is the worm that frequently causes panic in the individual who passes one in the stool or coughs up or vomits one.

The prevalence of human *Ascaris* infection, which, as mentioned previously, may occur worldwide, is thought to be greater than 1.2 billion. This corresponds to approximately one-fifth the world's population [2]. Point prevalence varies widely

539

according to geographic variations and is highest in East Africa, sub-Sharan Africa, India, China, Latin America, and the Caribbean [3]. Approximately 10.5 million disability-adjusted life years (DALYs) are lost owing to *Ascaris* infection and its complications [4]. *Ascaris* infections are responsible for more than 20,000 deaths per year. Transmission is by oral contact with fecally contaminated soil, either directly or via food stuff. Occupational and environmental risk factors include work in and around soil, especially clay soil because it is especially well suited for survival of the organism's eggs [5]. Workers who are exposed to sewage also are at risk for this infection, especially because eggs may survive treatment of sewage [6].

The life cycle begins when an infected human passes eggs with the feces into the soil, where the eggs embryonate and become infective over a 2- to 4-week period [7]. They contaminate the environment and reach another human through the oral route. Under the proper circumstances, eggs can survive in the soil for up to a decade [7]. The embryonated egg must be swallowed for the life cycle to be completed because the egg needs the bile salts and alkaline enteric juices to go through its next stage of development [8]. The adult worm can live 12–18 months. After ingestion, the eggs hatch in the intestine. There is a phase of transit through the lung. The larval forms then are coughed up and swallowed, and the mature worm ends up in the small intestine. The worms then lay eggs, which are passed with the feces, thus completing the cycle.

Techniques involved in effective prevention of infection include hand washing and proper hygienic precautions when working around fecally contaminated soil. Engineering controls include hygienic disposal of human feces. Respiratory protection when working in dusty, fecally contaminated soils is the primary personal protective measure. Surveillance includes screening families who are at risk for this infection and examining stool samples for ova and parasites. This should be done with adequate time for the eggs to be in the stool after exposure (2–3 months). Stool assessment for ova and parasite generally is thought to be most useful in assessing the adequacy of a preventive program.

Clinical Features and Diagnostic Evaluation

Most people with *Ascaris* infection are asymptomatic; others may develop vague abdominal dis-

comfort. *Ascaris* may cause malnutrition through a variety of mechanisms [9]. Occasionally, some people develop signs of obstruction as a result of a bolus of worms, which can produce a mechanical small bowel obstruction [10]. Biliary colic, hepatitis, and pancreatitis are other possible presentations. Löffler's pneumonia, the complex of substernal burning, cough, dyspnea, and wheezing and rales during the larval migration through the lungs, may cause the brief appearance of perihilar infiltrates on chest radiograph. During this time, Charcot-Leyden crystals and larvae may be present in the sputum and eosinophilia in the blood. If the patient is reinfected, the pulmonary phase may take on the appearance of an allergic asthmatic reaction [11]. Obstruction of the liver or pancreatic ducts may be present [12]. If a barium study is performed, one may see a thin column of barium in the worm's body [5]. Several stimuli, including anesthesia, fever, illness, or ingestion of spicy foods, may cause the worm to exit via the mouth, nose, or rectum [13].

The infection is usually diagnosed through the identification of characteristic eggs in the stools, but sometimes the infection can be diagnosed by viewing an adult worm that the patient has passed. An enzyme-linked immunosorbent assay (ELISA) serologic test is available but usually is reserved for epidemiologic studies.

Treatment

One must remember that medications are not active against migrating larvae [5]. Treatments of choice for adults are mebendazole (Vermox), 100 mg orally twice daily for 3 days or 500 mg as a single dose, ivermectin, 150–200 μg/kg by mouth once, or albendazole as a single dose of 400 mg [14]. Drugs and dosages are the same for children. In high-transmission areas, periodic, age-targeted chemotherapy is cost-effective [15] and has the greatest effect in decreasing DALYs [16]. Because chronic helminth infection may have an adverse effect on immune response to vaccines, there is much interest in treatment of infected patients prior to giving vaccinations [17].

ENTEROBIUS VERMICULARIS

Enterobius vermicularis, also known as *oxiuriasis, seatworms, pinworms,* or *threadworms,* is the most common helminth seen by primary care practitioners in North America. It is estimated that more than 290 million people are infected [12]. The infection is seen most commonly in children; adults are apparently less susceptible to the infection [8]. Transmission is by the fecal-oral route, and humans are the only source of the infection [18]. The eggs can be ingested in food, dust, and fomites or from environmental contamination. Autoinfection (anus-to-mouth transfer of eggs by fingers) permits the infection to continue indefinitely and to be amplified [5]. People who work in day-care or institutional settings are at increased risk for this infection. Once the eggs are in the environment, they are quite hardy; they are not killed by chlorination of water in swimming pools [5]. The infection is cosmopolitan in distribution. It is more common in temperate than in tropical climates, a somewhat unusual feature of distribution. The life cycle is human to human.

Prevention and Control

Administrative controls such as personal hygiene standards are critical to controlling this infection. The cleaning and trimming of fingernails of children is very helpful. Washing clothing and bedding on a regular basis also helps to kill the eggs, which may remain viable for up to 13 days under optimal conditions [5]. Hand washing is the primary personal protective measure. The use of gloves when dealing with the hygienic needs of children in an institutional setting is also warranted. Families who have this infection need to understand that it is not considered evidence of poor hygiene and that reinfections are quite common. Surveillance of institutionalized children, along with periodic mass retreatment if infection continues to be a problem, is a reasonable option. Retesting children represents the best method of assessing adequacy of control and prevention.

Clinical Features

Eggs laid on the perianal skin become infective in approximately 6 hours [12]. The prepatent period, or time from egg ingestion to egg production by the female worm, is 1–2 months [18]. Retroinfection, in which the eggs actually hatch on the perianal skin and return to the large intestine through the anus, is possible. Pruritus ani, perianal eczema, dermatitis, insomnia, enuresis, gastrointestinal (GI) disturbance, genitourinary infections (in girls), and vulvovaginitis are all potential symptoms. The infection often causes intense itching secondary to

the development of hypersensitivity to the worm proteins. The infection also may be asymptomatic; it rarely causes serious lesions. Females can develop inflammation of the genital tract, and *Enterobius* infection has been associated with cervicitis, endometritis, salpingitis, and oophoritis [19]. It also may cause vulvovaginitis and predispose to urinary tract infections [20].

Diagnostic Evaluation

The diagnosis generally is made most easily from visualization of characteristic eggs on the "Scotch tape" test. In this test, the sticky side of clear cellulose tape is pressed up against the perianal skin and then attached to a microscope slide, where it is scanned under low power. The eggs are not generally seen in stools collected for ova and parasite analysis. During the night, adult worms, which are approximately 1 cm in length, may be visualized in the perianal area. Laboratory findings are usually not helpful unless there is tissue invasion, which is unusual but is associated with eosinophilia [5].

Treatment

Simultaneous treatment—treating the whole family—with either pyrantel pamoate, 11 mg/kg as a single dose up to a maximum dose of 1 g, mebendazole, 100 mg as a single dose, or albendazole, 400 mg as a single dose, is effective therapy [14]. Treatment must be repeated 2 weeks after initial therapy. The doses are the same for adult and pediatric patients.

TRICHURIS TRICHIURA

Trichuris trichiura, also known as *whipworm,* is the second most common soil-transmitted helminth worldwide [21]. Nine hundred million cases are thought to occur worldwide and are responsible for 6.4 million lost DALYs [4]. Although other species of *Trichuris* are found in animals, host specificity is generally the rule, and these are not usually zoonotic infections. Transmission is by the fecal-oral route. Embryonated eggs are usually ingested with food or fluid or from fingers contaminated with soil that contains the eggs. The primary occupational risk factor is contact with soil. The life cycle is human to environment (soil) to human.

Prevention centers around hygienic treatment of sewage so as to avoid introduction of the eggs into the food chain. This is especially important in areas where sewage is used as fertilizer. The eggs are relatively resistant to chemical disinfectants, making hygienic practices of key importance. Hand washing is the primary personal protective measure. Surveillance can be done by obtaining stools for ova and parasite analysis. Chemoprophylaxis in the form of group treatment (e.g., treatment of all school-age children in a geographic area) may be warranted in situations in which there is a high prevalence of infection. This results in improved growth and physical fitness of school children [22].

Clinical Features

The incubation period is 2–3 months from the time of egg ingestion until eggs are present in the stool, but symptoms may start before this time. The infection is usually asymptomatic, although there may be vague abdominal symptoms. Tenesmus, owing to mucosal swelling of the rectal tissue, may occur, and protracted tenesmus occasionally causes rectal prolapse in very heavy infections in infants [23]. Also seen with heavy infection are bloody diarrhea, hemorrhagic ulcerations of the colon, perforation, and peritonitis. Chronic infection may be responsible for growth stunting and malnutrition in children. Rarely, a worm bolus can cause obstruction. The mucosal damage caused by *Trichuris* may facilitate invasion by other pathogens.

Diagnostic Evaluation

Differential diagnosis includes other intestinal parasites, including amebic dysentery, and inflammatory bowel disease. Diagnosis is made by identification of the distinctive bipolar-plugged eggs in the stool. Charcot-Leyden crystals also may be seen. Low-grade eosinophilia and iron-deficiency anemia may be seen, especially if infections are heavy [23]. The erythrocyte sedimentation rate (ESR) usually remains normal.

Treatment

Treatment options include mebendazole, 100 mg orally twice daily for 3 days or 500 mg orally in a single dose, or albendazole, 400 mg daily for 3 days [14]. Regimens are the same for adults and children.

HOOKWORM

Hookworm infections are caused by *Ancylostoma duodenale* or *Necator americanis* and are also called *tropical anemia* and *uncinariasis*. There is a geographic distribution of hookworm, with *N. americanis* predominating in the Americas and sub-Saharan Africa and *A. duodenale* usually occurring in Southeast Asia and the Mediterranean area [24]. There are exceptions to this generalization, however. The species can be differentiated microscopically by the characteristic morphology of the head capsule, but they are clinically indistinguishable. Approximately 900 million people are infected worldwide. Because these worms feed on intestinal mucosa and blood, they are a common cause of tropical anemia and have a disproportionately high effect on lost DALYs (22.1 million DALYs lost) [4]. Although infectious larvae can penetrate intact skin, they usually enter through hair follicles. The larvae can survive in soil for several months under optimal conditions. Risk factors include walking barefoot or having other skin-to-soil contact. This sort of infection is common in people who work in crawl spaces or other shady, moist areas. The life cycle is from humans to humans via soil.

Prevention

Administrative requirements to wear shoes and avoid skin-to-soil contact are the best methods for preventing infection in employees who work in contaminated areas. Sanitary disposal of human feces as an engineering control is warranted. Education regarding the risk factors for hookworm infection is helpful to reinforce the need to wear shoes. A hookworm vaccine is thought to be feasible, and one is currently in clinical trials [25].

Clinical Features

Symptoms may be seen 1–2 days after contact with the eggs. The time from skin penetration until eggs are passed in the feces is 4–6 weeks. *Ancylostoma* organisms also can infect if ingested or through transmammary or transplacental passage [11]. The classic acute signs of infection are ground itch, in which a pruritic maculopapular rash appears at the site of skin penetration. The second type of presentation is pulmonary and is due to the migratory phase of the worms as they pass through the lungs. This presentation is similar to that seen in patients with *Ascaris* infection. Shortness of breath, mucus production, and occult blood in the sputum are common during this phase. The GI phase is usually associated with vague complaints, although a more severe GI phase, known as *Wakana disease,* may occur if large numbers of larvae are ingested. This causes nausea, vomiting, dyspnea, and eosinophilia [26]. A major clinical feature of hookworm is iron-deficiency anemia, resulting directly from chronic blood loss. Since the adult worms may live up to 15 years, the blood loss is significant; often up to 0.26 mL of blood per day per worm may be lost. In people with low iron intake, even small numbers of worms may result in iron-deficiency and anemia [27].

Diagnostic Evaluation

Diagnosis is made by visualization of eggs in the feces. Species cannot be determined by egg appearance, however. There is often a high level of eosinophilia that begins 2–3 weeks after skin penetration. Stools are often heme-positive. Hypoalbuminemia is not uncommon.

Treatment

Treatment consists of medications to kill the worms and, afterward, iron replacement therapy. Effective regimens are mebendazole, 100 mg orally twice daily for 3 days or 500 mg as a single dose, pyrantel pamoate, 11 mg/kg up to a maximum dose of 1 g/kg for 3 days, or albendazole, 400 mg as a single dose [14]. The drugs and dosages are the same for children.

STRONGYLOIDES

Strongyloides infections may be caused by *S. stercoralis* or, rarely, *S. fulleborni*. Approximately 200 million infections occur worldwide. Transmission can occur either through the transdermal route after contact with fecally contaminated soil or sexually. Occupational groups at risk include those who have contact with soil, especially miners in temperate climates. The geographic distribution is worldwide [24], but the infection is especially prevalent in Southeast Asia and Brazil. There is an endemic focus in Appalachia, with approximately 3% of Kentucky school children [28] and 6% of Tennessee Veterans Administration inpatients [29] testing positive for this infection. *S. fulleborni* is seen only in Africa and Papua New Guinea.

Prevention

Systems to hygienically dispose of human feces are key to avoiding this infection. Also, it is necessary to avoid direct skin contact with contaminated soil and infected animals. Wearing gloves when handling patients with hyperinfection or autoinfectious cycles is preventive for health care workers. Surveillance of patients, especially before instituting corticosteroid or other immunosuppressive treatments, is critical because it helps to prevent hyperinfection and dissemination of the infection.

Clinical Features

The time from skin penetration until rhabditiform larvae appear in the feces is 2–4 weeks. As with hookworm, there may be an initial cutaneous phase, which is characterized by an itchy eruption at the site of larval penetration. Although uncommon, there also may be a pulmonary phase as larvae pass through the lungs. The GI phase may be asymptomatic or cause mild to severe abdominal symptoms, including acute steatorrhea or weight loss. Autoinfective *Strongyloides* occurs when rhabditiform larvae transform into the infective filariform stages within the host and then reinfect the same host by penetration of either the perianal skin or the bowel wall. These larvae then migrate through the tissues and the lung, after which they reestablish themselves in the intestine as new adult worms. This allows the infection to persist for years after the original exposure. If autoinfective cycles are present, migrating larvae may cause larva currens, serpiginous wheals surrounded by a flare. These wheals come and go in the course of a few hours and are usually seen on the trunk. Hyperinfection occurs when the body loses its defenses against the autoinfectious cycle and enormous numbers of filariform larvae reinvade the host. This is common if the host is taking corticosteroids, is malnourished, or is immunosuppressed. Curiously, human T-lymphocytic virus type 1 (HTLV-1) but not human immunodeficiency virus (HIV) predisposes to *Strongyloides* hyperinfection [30, 31], in which diarrhea, paralytic ileus, gram-negative septicemia, peritonitis, pulmonary symptoms, and even brain involvement occur. Eosinophilia is not associated with hyperinfection. In compromised hosts, hemorrhage, inflammation, and necrosis of any organ may result.

Diagnostic Evaluation

The differential diagnosis includes other intestinal parasites, especially hookworm. Other causes of eosinophilic pneumonia and cutaneous larva migrans also must be ruled out. The diagnosis of *Strongyloides* infection is often difficult. Demonstration of larvae in the stool or duodenal fluid often requires concentration techniques for examining stool samples [32]. Fecal culture, in which stool is mixed with water and charcoal and left to incubate at room temperature, is often helpful [33]. Serologic diagnosis does have a high sensitivity [32].

Treatment

For adults and children, the treatment regimen is ivermectin, 200 mg/kg per day for 2 days [14]. An alternative is albendazole, 400 mg orally twice a day for 7 days. The doses are the same in children. Because treatment failures are not unusual, a test of cure after treatment should be done with repeat serology at 3 months [34] and/or decreased eosinophilia [35].

Adult Nematoda Residing in the Blood, Lymphatics, or Subcutaneous Tissue

This section discusses filarial infections, including guinea worm infection. The human filarial parasites infect up to 140 million people worldwide. There are great similarities in the life cycles, in that the infective larval stage is carried by an insect, and the adult worm is found either in the lymph nodes, adjacent lymphatic vessels, or subcutaneous tissue. The microfilariae (MF) either circulate in the blood or migrate through the skin and then can be ingested by the appropriate arthropod, where they develop into the infective larvae, thus completing the cycle. The adults are long-lived, whereas the MF tend to live 3 months to 3 years. They differ in nucleoli patterns and presence of a sheath [1]. Filarial

worms exhibit a trait known as *periodicity*. This implies that the MF are present and active only during certain times. These periodicity traits are shown in Table 30-1. The clinical manifestations of filarial worm infection develop slowly, and the clinical picture varies according to whether the individual has had previous exposure. Previously unexposed individuals tend to have more acute onset of symptoms.

Although there are eight types of filarial worms, it is useful to consider them according to their clinical presentations. Thus they are discussed in this chapter as lymphatic filariasis, onchocerciasis, loa loa, *Mansonella* infections, and guinea worm infections.

LYMPHATIC FILARIASIS

Three filarial worms are associated with lymphatic filariasis: *Wuchereria bancrofti, Brugia malayi,* and *B. timori.* These three threadlike worms all live in the lymphatic channels or lymph nodes of the host and may remain alive for more than 20 years. Lymphatic filariasis is the second leading cause of permanent long-term disability [36].

W. bancrofti is the most widely distributed of the filarial worms and causes more than 90% of lymphatic filariasis. It is present in Africa, in portions of South and Central America, in the Caribbean Basin, in Southeast Asia, and in the Pacific islands [24]. *W. bancrofti* is estimated to have a prevalence of greater than 100 million people [37]. *B. malayi* is present in China, India, Indonesia, Japan, Korea, Malaysia, and the Philippines. *B. timori* has been described as present only in specific islands in Indonesia. Although the lymphatic filarial worms usually exhibit nocturnal periodicity, there are also subperiodic forms of both major types. This im-

Table 30-1
Selected Traits of Filarial Worms

Species	Periodicity	Vector	Adult Location	Microfilaria Location	Sheath on MF
Wuchereria bancrofti	Nocturnal	Mosquito	Lymphatics	Blood	Present
Brugia malayi	Nocturnal	Mosquito	Lymphatics	Blood	Present
Brugia timori	Nocturnal	Mosquito	Lymphatics	Blood	Present
Onchocerca volvulus	None	Black fly	Subcutaneous	Skin, eye	Absent
Loa loa	Diurnal	Deer fly	Subcutaneous	Blood	Present
Mansonella streptocerca	None	Biting midge	Subcutaneous	Skin	Absent
Mansonella ozzardi	None	Biting midge, black fly	Subcutaneous	Blood	Absent
Mansonella perstans	None	Biting midge	Body cavities, mesentery, perirenal	Blood	Absent

plies that the MF are present in blood at all times but are maximal in number in the afternoon. Humans are the natural reservoir for infection, although *B. malayi* can be a natural infection in cats and monkeys. Risk factors for infection include geographic factors and mosquito exposure.

Prevention and Control

Any engineering or administrative interventions that lessen the risk for the presence of mosquitoes are likely to lessen the risk for lymphatic filarial infections. Personal protective measures, including the use of insect repellents and netting, are likely to be helpful in lessening the problem. Education about the relationship between mosquito bites and the disease is also likely to be helpful. Surveillance is generally helpful only for populations who are not routinely exposed. In the routinely exposed, the use of diethylcarbamazine (DEC), either alone [38] or with either ivermectin or albendazole [37, 39], is helpful in interrupting transmission of the filarial worms. For the person who is not exposed routinely, insect precautions, along with doxycycline 100 mg/day chemoprophylaxis, may be a consideration [40].

Clinical Features

The usual incubation period for lymphatic filariasis is 5–18 months. Symptoms may occur prior to the appearance of MF in peripheral blood. The range of time from infection to the appearance of symptoms is a minimum of 1–3 months to a maximum of years. Early symptoms tend to be related to dilatation of the lymphatics and thickening of the vessel walls, along with damage to valves within the lymphatic vasculature, and often consist of scrotal symptoms in men, lymphatic inflammation, and obstruction. Even asymptomatic patients may have lymphatic abnormalities, which show up only on lymphoscintigraphy [41]. Lymphangitis, lymphadenitis, orchitis, urticaria, and epididymitis all may occur. Filarial fever, which typically recurs 6–10 times per year and lasts for 3–7 days at a time, is more common in native populations.

Tropical pulmonary eosinophilia is an uncommon form of acute filariasis that is associated with the rapid clearance of MF as they pass through the lungs. Patients who have this syndrome are usually males (4:1 predominance) in their third decade of life. Clinical features of tropical pulmonary

eosinophilia are paroxysmal cough, nocturnal wheezing, weight loss, fever, adenopathy, and extremes of peripheral blood eosinophilia. Chest radiography usually reveals increased bronchovascular markings. Pulmonary function studies show restrictive abnormalities, which may be accompanied by obstructive defects. If the disease is not treated, pulmonary damage may result in chronic fibrosis.

Chronic findings include lymphedema of the legs, arms, and scrotum. There may be associated hyperplastic changes of the skin or elephantiasis, which may predispose the patient to secondary bacterial infection. If the lymphatic vessels rupture into the renal pelvis, chyluria may occur.

Diagnostic Evaluation

Differential diagnosis of lymphatic filarial infections includes deep venous thrombosis, infection, and trauma. Definitive diagnosis of the disease requires demonstration of MF. This can be done in blood and usually is accomplished after some sort of concentration process such as filtration through a Nuclepore filter or in a 2% formalin solution (Knott's concentration technique) [42]. Most serologic tests are useful only for individuals who are not native to the endemic area because native populations may have positive serology owing to exposure to infected mosquitoes but not actually have the infection. Polymerase chain reaction (PCR)–based assays for lymphatic filarial infections are also available. Evaluation via lymphoscintigraphy can provide information about lymphatic function. In males, evaluation of the scrotum by ultrasonographic techniques may reveal nodules, evidence of lymphatic dilatation, or even active worm motion [43]. Since some individuals with filariasis are not microfilaremic, the diagnosis sometimes may need to be made on clinical grounds alone.

Treatment

Diethylcarbamazine is the treatment of choice for lymphatic filarial infections. Pretreatment with antihistamines or corticosteroids may be required to decrease the possibility of allergic reactions owing to disintegration of the MF in these infections. If MF are present in the blood, a slow increase in dosing is warranted. On day 1, 50 mg is given orally, followed by 50 mg orally three times daily on day 2. On day 3, 100 mg orally three times daily is given.

On days 4–14, 6 mg/kg per day is given in three divided doses [14]. These doses are identical for pediatric patients. If no MF are present, full doses can be given from the first day [14]. Ivermectin is useful for killing the MF but does not kill the adult worms. Care should be taken to rule out *Onchocerca* infection prior to DEC treatment because a potentially serious Mazzotti reaction could result. (The Mazzotti reaction is the appearance of an acute rash owing to death of MF in the skin within 2–24 hours of a test dose of DEC; this is sometimes used as a test for onchocerciasis.) Treatment of the chronic lymphatic obstruction should be directed at management of the lymphedema, including measures such as limb elevation, support stockings, and local skin care. Surgical decompression may be necessary in severe cases of elephantiasis. Hydroceles may be drained or managed surgically.

ONCHOCERCA VOLVULUS

Onchocerca is a tissue-dwelling nematode, the MF of which are found primarily in the skin and eye. Its prevalence has decreased slowly as a result of mass campaigns to destroy the larvae with insecticides as well as the use of chemotherapy to decrease the pool of filariae in human hosts. Transmission occurs as a result of the black fly (*Simulium* species).

The primary environmental risk factor is living or working in an endemic area. Geographic distribution of onchocerciasis tends to be in western Africa and some areas of eastern Africa [24]. There is a small endemic area in Yemen and southwest Saudi Arabia. In the western hemisphere, onchocerciasis is present in Central and South America in selected foci [24].

The uses of vector control via insecticide spraying has been beneficial in some sites but is not suitable for broad control. The community-wide use of ivermectin has become the primary strategy used for control of onchocerciasis. This technique is thought to be most effective in breaking the transmission cycle worldwide [44].

Clinical Features

The incubation period of onchocerciasis is usually 1–2 years. MF usually first appear between 3 and to 15 months after exposure. Adult worms can survive for up to 15 years. The MF may persist for 2–3 years. Usual signs and symptoms include dermatitis, subcutaneous nodules, eye findings, and lymphadenopathy. The most common manifestation of the dermatitis is pruritus, which may be incapacitating and is usually generalized. With long-term infections, this dermatitis results in exaggerated and premature wrinkling of the skin with loss of elastic fibers and epidermal atrophy. It also may result in hypo- or hyperpigmentation of the skin. This condition is sometimes called *leopard skin* [24]. Subcutaneous nodules usually are palpable and are commonly found over the lower back, hips, and iliac crests. The most serious clinical finding associated with onchocerciasis is the resulting visual impairment. This is usually seen in persons with moderate to heavy infections. Lesions can occur in all parts of the eye. The most common early finding is photophobia and conjunctivitis. In the cornea, so-called snowflake opacities are common [24]; these are caused by a tissue reaction to dead MF in the cornea. Sclerosing keratitis is the most common cause of blindness in patients with onchocerciasis. Anterior uveitis and iridocyclitis are not uncommon and may result in secondary glaucoma. Following damage to the anterior segments of the eye, choroidoretinal lesions occur frequently, with resulting optic atrophy. Lymphadenopathy, particularly in the inguinal and femoral areas, is common. The enlarged nodes may become dependent, causing what is commonly called *hanging groin*. In persons with heavy infections, generalized weakness and loss of adipose tissue and muscle mass are common. This is partly responsible for the increased mortality in people who are blind as a result of onchocerciasis.

Diagnostic Evaluation and Treatment

Diagnosis involves identification of MF in skin snips or of an adult worm from an excised nodule. Skin-snip techniques involve the use of a corneoscleral punch biopsy device or a skin shave [45]. Slit-lamp examination frequently reveals MF in the anterior eye chamber. Commercially available serologic assays are sensitive but have low specificity and cannot distinguish among the filarial species or distinguish active infections.

Treatment of onchoceriasis is aimed at avoiding permanent damage owing to the infection and alleviating nuisance symptoms. Nodules, especially if present over the head, should be excised in order to lessen the chances of eye problems secondary to proximity of the adult worm. However, chemotherapy with ivermectin remains the treatment of choice for onchocerciasis. For both adults and children, ivermectin as a single dose of 150 µg/kg is given initially and repeated in 6–12 months [14].

LOA LOA

Loaiasis, also called *African eye worm* and *Calibar swelling,* is common in the rain forests of west and central Africa [46]. Transmission is through the bite of a deer fly, also called the *Tabanid fly.* The adult worms can live for longer than 10 years in their human hosts. People who work in the African rain forest are at risk for this infection. The life cycle is from human to human via the Tabanid fly (*Chrysops dimidiata* or *C. silacea*).

Prevention

Because of the ample number of breeding places for this fly, control of the vector is difficult. Engineering controls, such as placing screens over windows, may be helpful. Personal protective measures, such as the use of insect repellents and wearing of long sleeves and pants, also may be helpful. In workers who are at high risk, weekly dosing with DEC at 300 mg per week has been shown to act as chemoprophylaxis for this agent [47].

Clinical Features

The incubation period for loa loa is 1 year or more. The infection and production of MF are fairly well tolerated. The appearance of the adult worm in the subconjunctival eye space is a frequently disturbing aspect of this infection. Allergic complications tend to cause most symptoms. Localized pruritus and swelling are common. The swelling, also called *Calibar swelling,* results from hypersensitivity and is migratory. Nephropathy is thought to be caused by immune complex mechanisms [48]. The brisk humeral and cell-mediated immune response, sometimes referred to as the *hyperresponsive syndrome,* also may cause episodes of inflammation or allergic symptoms, especially in expatriates [49]. In returning travelers, the most common presenting symptoms are (in decreasing order of frequency) pruritis (generalized or localized), Calabar swellings, urticaria, myalgias, arthralgias, and edematous conjunctivitis [45].

Diagnostic Evaluation

Other filarial infections and gnathostomiasis are in the differential diagnosis. The diagnosis can be made based on identification of the adult worm in the eye or identification of MF in the blood, but these are rarely detected [45]. The infection is generally accompanied by high-grade eosinophilic and elevated levels of serum IgE. PCR and serum antibodies to the L1-SXP-1 antigen represent improved sensitivity and specificity in diagnosing this infection [50, 51].

Treatment

Treatment includes surgical removal of the worm as it crosses the eye, if possible. The primary therapy is a DEC regimen, however. In patients with MF, pretreatment with antihistamines or corticosteroids may help to prevent allergic reactions related to disintegration of the MF, along with a slow increase in the DEC dose. The usual protocol for DEC is 50 mg on the first day, 50 mg three times daily on the second day, 100 mg three times daily on the third day, and 9 mg/kg per day in three divided doses on days 4–21 [14]. The schedule is similar in children. In heavy infections with loa loa, rapid killing of MF can provoke an encephalopathy. In this circumstance, apheresis or albendazole may be considered. If no MF are present, full doses of DEC may be used from the onset. Since DEC may precipitate severe ocular side effects, including blindness, in patients who have onchocerciasis, it should be used very cautiously in filarial infections acquired where both loa loa and onchocerciasis coexist.

MANSONELLIASIS

Mansonella species include *M. streptocerca, M. perstans,* and *M. ozzardi.* These filarial worms are all transmitted by the biting midge (*Culicoides* species), although *M. ozzardi* also can be transmitted by black fly (*Simulium* species). The primary occupational or environmental risk factor is living or working in a geographic area where these midges or filarial worms are found. For *M. streptocerca,* this area is the tropical forest belt of Africa. For *M. perstans,* it is the center of Africa and northeastern part of South America. *M. ozzardi* is restricted to Central and South America, as well as selected Caribbean islands [46]. Humans act as the reservoir for these infections, and the life cycles are all similar in that the human-to-human transmission is either the biting midge and, in the case of *M. ozzardi,* the black fly. Humans are the hosts, but *M. streptocerca* also can be found in nonhuman primates. Avoiding bites from the arthropod vectors is the principal method of prevention.

Clinical Features

Data on the incubation period for *Mansonella* infections are lacking. The usual signs and symptoms of *M. streptocerca* are skin pruritus, papular rashes, and changes in pigmentation. Most individuals with this infection also have inguinal adenopathy. The parasites and resulting cutaneous symptoms tend to be present across the shoulders and upper torso [52]. Most patients with *M. perstans* are asymptomatic, although a transient angioedema and pruritus, with swellings that are like the Calibar swellings of loaiasis, may occur. Fever, headache, arthritis, right upper quadrant pain, and occasional pericarditis or hepatitis may occur. With *M. ozzardi* infection, it is not clear whether the organism is truly pathogenic. Symptoms may be similar to those attributed to other *Mansonella* infections.

Diagnostic Evaluation

The differential diagnosis includes other filarial infections, especially onchocerciasis. In cases of *M. streptocerca,* because of the hypopigmented macules, one also must rule out leprosy. The diagnostic test of choice for *M. streptocerca* is the skin snip, wherein the characteristic unsheathed MF may be seen. In *M. ozzardi* and *M. perstans* infections, identification of the MF in blood or other body fluids is usually sufficient for diagnosis.

Treatment

Treatment for *M. streptocerca* infection is generally with DEC, which is usually effective. This is usually given as a dose of 6 mg/kg per day for 12 days. As with other filarial infections, urticaria, arthralgia, myalgia, abdominal discomfort, and headache may occur in response to treatment. Ivermectin, 150 µg/kg as a single dose, also can be used [14]. For *M. perstans,* albendazole, 400 mg orally twice a day for 10 days, and mebendazole, 100 mg orally twice daily for 30 days, are effective [14]. For *M. ozzardi,* DEC is thought to be ineffective, but ivermectin,

200 µg/kg by mouth as a single dose, has been reported to be effective [53].

DRACUNCULUS MEDINENSIS

Dracunculus medinensis, or the guinea worm, has declined rapidly in prevalence secondary to global eradication strategies [54]. This worm, which normally resides in the subcutaneous tissues, is acquired through ingestion of contaminated water. The geographic distribution for this infection is the Sudan and western Africa. There are progressively fewer cases in the Middle East and Indian subcontinent. After a human (terminal host) ingests water containing *Cyclops* (intermediate host, a minute, free-swimming, freshwater copepod crustacean sometimes called a *water flea*) infected with guinea worm larvae, the larvae migrate from the *Cyclops* and penetrate the human host's GI tract. Here, the larvae develop into adults and mate. The female worm then migrates to the subcutaneous tissues of the human host, usually toward the lower extremities, where a blister forms. The migration may take up to 1 year. When the human host enters a body of water, the blister breaks, releasing a large number of rhabditiform larvae, which may then infect more *Cyclops,* thereby perpetuating the worm's life cycle. Later, at the site of the blister on the human host, an ulcer forms, and it is from this ulcer that the worm emerges.

Prevention

Engineering provisions for safe water through water treatment, filtering, or drilled wells all serve to lessen the risk for this infection. Filtering individual drinking water with a 100-µm pore-size filter is also an effective method of preventing the infection.

Clinical Features

The incubation period is usually about 1 year, or until the worm emerges. During this time, vague symptoms associated with the migration may occur. The infection is usually asymptomatic until just before the blister forms. Then, fever and generalized allergic symptoms such as wheezing, urticaria, and periorbital swelling have their onset. The emergence of the worm is associated with pain and swelling. Multiple worms may emerge. Aberrant locations of the worms are not unusual.

Arthritis may result if a joint is infected. The ulcer that results from the emergence of the worm can easily become secondarily infected and can act as a portal for tetanus [55]. There is no protective immunity after being infected with the worm, and reinfection is common.

Diagnostic Evaluation

Diagnosis is usually clinical, based on the presentation of the adult worm as it emerges. One can identify the discharged motile larvae microscopically. Treatment is usually the gradual extraction of the worm by winding a few centimeters of it on a stick each day.

Treatment

No drug or vaccine is available to treat or prevent dracunculiasis. The treatment of choice is the slow extraction of the worm, wound care, and pain management [56].

Zoonotic Nematodes

Zoonoses are infections in humans by parasites that usually live in animals. In the nematodes discussed in this section, humans are dead-end hosts. It is for this reason that these nematodes do not mature into adults but rather cause problems because of their larval stages. A vast array of zoonotic nematodal infections occurs, but only the most important ones are discussed in detail.

ADULT ZOONOTIC NEMATODES RESIDING IN THE GI TRACT
Capillaria philippinensis

C. philippinensis, a parasite of aquatic birds that feed on fish, produces a clinical condition called *intestinal capillariasis.* This organism is unique in that it can reproduce within the host and, in this capacity, resembles the autoinfectious cycle of *Strongyloides.* The adult worms resemble those of *Trichonella.* Transmission is from eating raw or undercooked freshwater fish. The geographic distribution is primarily the Philippines and parts of Thailand. A few cases have been reported from other parts of Southeast Asia and the Middle East. The reservoir is thought to be aquatic birds, whereas fish act as intermediate hosts [57].

Prevention. The most important prevention technique is the avoidance of eating raw or undercooked fish. Hygienic methods for disposal of feces can help to disrupt the cycle of reinfection of fish.

Clinical Features. The incubation period for intestinal capillariasis is thought to be approximately 1 month. The primary symptom is rampant diarrhea, which is associated with malaise, anorexia, and vomiting. With time, the severe diarrhea causes electrolyte disturbances, malabsorption, and protein-wasting enteropathy [58]. The chronic aspects of this disease—cachexia, congestive heart failure, and secondary bacterial infections—are thought to be responsible for its 10% mortality rate [59].

Diagnostic Evaluation. Characteristic laboratory findings include persistent eosinophilia and low albumin levels. Differential diagnosis includes *Strongyloides,* giardiasis, cryptosporidiosis, isosporidiosis, and the malabsorption seen in patients with tropical sprue. The diagnosis depends on finding eggs or living larvae in hosts. The eggs resemble those of *Trichuris.*

Treatment. Treatment includes replacement of fluid and electrolytes, along with nutritional support. The treatment of choice is mebendazole, 200 mg orally twice daily for 20 days, although albendazole, 400 mg daily for 10 days, is also effective [14]. The same regimens are used for pediatric patients. All infected patients should be treated because of the high risk of autoinfection.

Trichinella spiralis

T. spiralis, the etiologic agent of trichinosis, is capable of infecting all mammals. Its prevalence in the United Sates is thought to be about 4% on the basis of autopsy studies [11]. This infection is unusual in that the L1 larval form both causes the pathology and is the infectious form. Transmission occurs through ingestion of raw or undercooked infected meat. Risks for infection are dietary. If undercooked or uncooked pork, bear, or horse is eaten, the risk increases. Geographic distribution is worldwide among meat-eating populations. It is less common in the tropics. The life cycle is animal to animal; humans are an incidental host. Other species, including *T. native* and *T. pseudospiralis* also may cause infection in humans [60, 61].

Prevention. Administrative controls generally consist of cooking refuse that is fed to pigs, thus stopping the cycle of propagation caused by feeding meat scraps to pigs. Personal protective measures include adequate cooking of meat [62]. It may be prudent to avoid homemade sausage and ensure the thorough cooking of all game.

Clinical Features. The incubation period of trichinosis is 10–20 days. Early symptoms include diarrhea, vomiting, abdominal pain, headache, and fever. Later, during the migration phase, fever, blurred vision, facial edema, cough, and eosinophilia develop. This phase may last up to 1 month. The muscular phase, characterized by muscle pain, follows. If the myocardium is involved, myocarditis may occur, and abnormal electrocardiograms (ECGs) may be seen. Central nervous system (CNS) involvement may occur with petechial hemorrhages of the brain. One also may see petechial hemorrhages in the conjunctivae and under the nails.

Diagnostic Evaluation. Differential diagnosis includes allergic reaction, Katayama fever, visceral larva migrans, and eosinophilia-myalgia syndrome. The diagnosis is characterized by laboratory studies through massive eosinophilia (>5,000 cells/mm^3) but a low erythrocyte sedimentation rate (ESR). Enzyme-linked immunosorbent assay (ELISA) is positive 2–4 weeks after infection. Muscle biopsy may show encysted larvae. Other laboratory findings include an elevated creatine kinase (CK) and lactate dehydrogenase (LDH).

Treatment. Treatment consists of steroids plus albendazole, 400 mg twice a day for 8–14 days, or, as an alternative, mebendazole, 200–400 orally three times daily for 3 days, followed by 400–500 mg orally three times daily for 10 days [14]. Early treatment kills the adults that reside in the gut. These are normally excreted over 2–3 months, so early treatment may help to avoid excessive production of larvae. Corticosteroids are especially helpful for severe symptoms. The larval stages, which encyst in muscles as "nurse cells," are difficult or impossible to eradicate but tend not to cause symptoms and eventually calcify and die.

Trichostrongylus Species

Trichostrongylosis, also called *pseudo–hookworm infection* [63], behaves much like infection with the common hookworm. *Trichostrongylus* worms are found in a variety of herbivorous animals. Living or working around infected animals is a risk factor for this infection. Geographic distribution of the disease in humans is primarily in Asia, although it is also seen in Europe, Africa, and especially rural Iran and Iraq. Animal infection is seen throughout the world. The life cycle is one of animal to animal via the environment. Humans act as incidental hosts, but the life cycle can be completed within humans.

Prevention. Ingestion of food or water contaminated with animal feces is the most common form of acquisition [5]; thus hygienic food practices are preventive. As with hookworm, *Trichostrongylus* worms can penetrate skin, so wearing of shoes is also a wise preventive measure.

Clinical Features. The incubation period of trichostrongyloides is thought to be about 3 weeks. The disease is usually asymptomatic, although mild GI symptoms may occur. In patients with severe infection, anemia or occult blood in the stool also may occur.

Diagnostic Evaluation and Treatment. Differential diagnosis includes infections with other intestinal parasites, especially hookworm. Diagnosis is based on the identification of eggs in the stool or duodenal aspirates. Stool culture to recover larvae is also a useful technique. For both adult and pediatric patients, treatment is with pyrantel pamoate, 11 mg/kg as a single dose (maximum of 1 g), mebendazole, 100 mg orally twice daily for 3 days, or albendazole, 400 mg as a single dose [14].

Oesophagostomum Species

The *Oesophagostomum* species are nematodes related to and resembling hookworms. Infection with these worms has a variety of synonyms, including *helminthoma, pimplygut,* and *nodular worm* [12]. Unlike hookworm, transmission is by the fecal-oral route, and percutaneous infection does not occur. Close proximity with the zoonotic reservoirs of this infection is the risk factor. The geographic distribution is primarily Africa. The life cycle generally is animal to animal, although humans also may permit completion of the transmission cycle and transmit the infection to other humans [64]. The normal animal hosts are sheep, goats, pigs, and some primates. Although these infections occur worldwide, the primary area of human infection has been Africa.

Prevention. Prevention of this infection is primarily through personal protective measures such as hand washing prior to eating and hygienic food practices. Hygienic disposal of human feces is especially important in areas where human-to-human transmission occurs.

Clinical Features. Symptoms commonly occur 2–3 weeks after ingestion of eggs. Then 30–40 days after ingestion, eggs may appear in the stool. The infection may be asymptomatic, although right lower quadrant abdominal pain and fever may occur. Complications of the infection include abscess formation, fistula formation, hemorrhage, and perforation.

Diagnostic Evaluation and Treatment. Characteristic laboratory findings include low-grade eosinophilia. Differential diagnosis includes tumors of the GI tract, ameboma, schistosomal granuloma, appendicitis, and ileocecal tuberculosis. The diagnosis is made by the identification of eggs in the feces, which strongly resemble hookworm eggs. Additionally, ultrasonography can be useful in detecting colonic wall pathology [65]. Treatment includes surgical resection of the nodule or pharmacologic treatment with albendazole, 400 mg as a single dose [66]. Uncommon zoonotic nematode infections in the GI tract are listed in Table 30-2 [1].

MARINE NEMATODES

Anisakiasis is the term given to infection with marine nematodes of the *Anisakis* or *Pseudoterranova* genera. Common names include *herring worm, whale worm, cod worm,* and *seal worm.* Prevalence is tied to the frequency of eating sushi or sashimi and appears to be increasing with the growing popularity of these foods. Transmission is oral, through

the ingestion of the larval form of the nematode in infected fish. Although most reported cases are from Japan, there has been an increasing number worldwide. The life cycle involves marine vertebrates and invertebrates. Hosts of the worm are marine mammals, including whales, seals, and dolphins. They pass eggs into the sea water, which are taken up by small crustaceans and progress through the food chain. Many kinds of fish have been implicated in carrying the larval stages [57].

Prevention

The primary preventive measure is avoidance of eating lightly cooked or raw fish. The larval form can be killed by thorough cooking or freezing of fish. There are some species that have been relatively resistant to freezing, however. Professional sushi chefs often can identify the parasites and avoid them if they are pigmented [67].

Clinical Features

Although anisakiasis may be asymptomatic, the most common presentation is related to the attachment of the larval worm to the gastric mucosa. This results in severe abdominal pain, nausea, vomiting, and diarrhea 1–12 hours after eating the larva-infected fish. Since the larvae can attach anywhere in the GI tract, tingling sensations in the throat may be experienced secondary to attachment there. Intestinal infection usually produces symptoms (e.g., abdominal pain, nausea, and vomiting) 1–2 weeks after ingestion. The worm may become invasive and penetrate the gastric or intestinal mucosa and

Table 30-2
Uncommon Zoonotic Nematode Infections of the Human GI Tract

Name	Geographic Location	Animal Host	Disease Diagnosis	Symptoms	Transmission
Genus *Physaloptera*	Africa	Primates	Eggs in feces	Similar to ascaris	Accidental ingestion of insects (intermediate host)
Gongylonema species	Worldwide	Ruminants, monkeys	Eggs in feces	Local irritation in GI tract	Accidental ingestion of beetle or cockroach
Ternidens diminutus	South Africa	Simian primates	Fecal culture; eggs	Similar to hookworm	Fecal oral
Macracanthorhynchus hirudinaceus	China	Wide range of vertebrates, especially pigs	Eggs in feces	GI symptoms, gut perforation, ulceration	Accidental ingestion of beetle
Moniliformis moniliformis	Worldwide	Wide range of vertebrates, especially rats	Eggs in feces	GI symptoms, ulceration, perforation	Accidental ingestion of beetle

then migrate to the omentum, pancreas, liver, or lung. Characteristic laboratory findings includes eosinophilia and leukocytosis. Differential diagnosis includes noninfectious causes. The gastric form of anisakiasis resembles peptic ulcer disease, gastritis, or pancreatitis. The intestinal form resembles appendicitis, diverticulitis, or inflammatory bowel disease [68]. Diagnosis is usually based on clinical grounds, although upper GI or barium enema may reveal threadlike filling defects at areas of thickened or obstructed bowel wall [12]. Eggs and larval forms are not found in the feces. Treatment is through removal of the worm, usually by means of an endoscopic procedure. Occasionally, during surgery for presumed acute abdomen, a worm is discovered and removed. There is some evidence that albendazole, 400 mg twice a day for 3–5 days, is helpful [69].

CUTANEOUS LARVA MIGRANS

Also called *creeping eruption,* cutaneous larva migrans (CLM) is actually a distinctive type of dermatitis that results from infection with larval stages of various animal nematodes. The larvae generally are confined to the epidermal layers of the skin but may go deeper. This condition is caused most commonly by *Ancylostoma braziliense,* although a number of other nematodes may cause this syndrome (Table 30-3). Transmission occurs through contact with contaminated soil, and any occupation that requires frequent exposure to soil may be in danger of this condition. The condition is especially common on hands, feet, knees, and buttocks. There is no predilection for age, race, or gender. The organisms causing CLM are ubiquitous and endemic to geographic areas most hospitable to the larval forms, namely, those with warm, humid climates.

The life cycle involves the passing of rhabditiform larvae with the feces of infected animals. These develop in the soil through a series of molts into filariform larvae, which then enter a host through hair follicles or intact skin via digestive enzymes. Humans are dead-end hosts.

Prevention

Since it is quite difficult to dispose of animal feces, protection of skin from fecally contaminated soil is the most practical way of avoiding CLM. Wearing shoes is especially important.

Clinical Features

The usual incubation period for CLM is 2–7 days. The syndrome usually includes a pruritic serpiginous papulovesicular lesion that becomes linear, the tract lengthening daily. There may be associated wheezing and urticaria, especially if there has been previous sensitization. In these cases, vesicles and marked edema may be present. Some nematodes may invade deeper tissues. *A. caninum* can cause an eosinophilic enteritis [70]. Although rare, Loeffler's syndrome can be seen occasionally with CLM [71]. In these more invasive forms of CLM, eosinophilia is a characteristic laboratory findings, but it may not be seen in all cases.

Diagnostic Evaluation and Treatment

Although a biopsy is not usually necessary, it reveals a mild perivascular dermal infiltrate composed primarily of polymorphonuclear cells and eosinophils. On chest radiograph, one may see migratory pulmonary infiltrates in up to 50% of patients. The differential diagnosis includes cercarial dermatitis, scabies, cutaneous filariasis, human

Table 30-3
Causes of Cutaneous Larva Migrans

Organism	Animal Host	Location	Incidence
Ancylostoma braziliense	Cats, dogs	Skin	Most common
A caninum	Dogs	Skin	Common
A tubaeformis	Cats	Skin	Rare
Uncinaria stenocephala	European dogs	Skin	Rare
Bunostomum phlebotum	Cattle	Skin	Rare
Pleodora strongyloides	Free living	Skin	Rare
Anatrichosoma species	Monkeys, opossum	Skin, nasal and oral mucosa	Rare
Thelazia species	Dogs, rabbits	Conjunctival sac, cornea	Rare

hookworm, and *Strongyloides*. Human hookworm tends to have a more transient ground itch. *Strongyloides*, which causes larva curens, is more routinely associated with urticaria, and its symptoms are more intermittent. The diagnosis of CLM is made on clinical grounds. For both adult and pediatric patients, treatment consists of ivermectin, 200 μg/kg orally per day for 1–2 days, or albendazole, 400 mg orally every day for 3 days [14].

VISCERAL LARVA MIGRANS

Visceral larva migrans (VLM) is a clinical syndrome caused by the prolonged wanderings of the larvae of various zoonotic nematodes as they migrate throughout the human body. Since the human is a dead-end host, the larvae never mature into adults. During their movements, the larvae produce inflammatory reactions, which can cause diverse clinical syndromes depending on their location. This can be the viscera or the eye—ocular larva migrans (OLM)—or the central nervous system (CNS)—neural larva migrans (NLM). Most cases of VLM are due to *Toxocara canus* and *T. cati*, which are the common large round worms of dogs and cats, respectively. Other causative organisms are addressed separately. VLM is a common infection: Serosurveys suggest that 2–3% of the world's population is infected, primarily children and people with pica [5]. Transmission is through ingestion of embryonated eggs, either from contaminated soil or from foods contaminated with the eggs. This could be an occupational risk factor for people working in contaminated soils, but practically speaking, VLM is a disease of young children. The geographic distribution is worldwide, but larvae tend to survive best in warm, moist clay soils. Although the larvae cannot mature into adults in the human host, they may remain viable for up to 10 years.

Prevention

Preventive techniques include control of dog and cat feces. For parents, such techniques include keeping covers over sand piles, a favored place of defecation for cats, careful attention to worming of domestic pets, and avoidance of pet feces in play areas. Personal protective measures include hand washing and other means of avoiding transmitting contaminated fomites to the mouth. Education should include the danger of pica.

Clinical Features

The incubation period of visceral larva migrans is approximately 1 month. The signs and symptoms are quite variable, and the patient may be asymptomatic. The most common symptoms are fever, cough, wheezing, abdominal pain, myalgia, and a large and tender liver and/or spleen [72]. Other symptoms reflect the location of the larvae. If they are in the CNS, seizures and encephalopathy are possible complications. In the heart, myocarditis may occur. In the eye, OLM may cause leukochoria, strabismus, decreased visual acuity, and fundal mass.

Diagnostic Evaluation

Characteristic laboratory findings include a high-grade, persistent eosinophilia unless there is an isolated OLM, in which case there is no eosinophilia. Liver function tests tend to be elevated, and a liver biopsy usually reveals eosinophils and granulomas. IgG levels are elevated, and there is leukocytosis. On chest radiographs, about a third of patients have an infiltrate. Differential diagnosis includes invasive helminth infections of any type. For OLM, it also includes retinoblastoma; cases of OLM have resulted in enucleation because of an assumed diagnosis of retinoblastoma. Diagnosis is best made with ELISA, which is relatively sensitive and specific. Identification of larvae in the tissue may provide a diagnosis, but this is not routine. Note should be made that eggs and parasites are not found in the feces.

Treatment

Treatment often involves the use of corticosteroids to suppress the intense manifestations of the inflammatory reaction. Albendazole, 400 mg orally twice daily for 5 days, or mebendazole, 100–200 mg orally twice daily for 5 days, is the treatment of choice [14]. Some people treat for up to 20 days. Regimens are the same for pediatric patients.

BAYLISASCARIS PROCYONIS

B. procyonis, the common raccoon roundworm, is an increasingly recognized cause of visceral larva migrans (VLM), found primarily in North America. The baylisascaral syndrome differs from *Toxicara* in that it is caused by more aggressive larvae and has a much greater likelihood of causing neurologic disease, especially in patients with heavy infections. Clinical findings range from mild to devastating CNS involvement [73]. This often develops quickly, over 2–4 weeks, and progresses rapidly. *Baylisascaris* also can cause subacute neuroretinitis. In children with known exposure to raccoon feces or contaminated soil, prophylactic treatment with albendazole, 25 mg/kg per day for 20 days, is recommended [74]. Unfortunately, the prognosis for patients with established disease is grave, with or without treatment, because of the extensive neurologic damage done by the time the diagnosis is made.

GNATHOSTOMA SPINIGERUM

Gnathostomiasis is caused most commonly by *Gnathostoma spinigerum*, although several other species may infect humans [75]. *G. spinigerum* is a parasite that affects a number of mammals, including cats, dogs, and mongeese, and has intermediate hosts, including cyclops, birds, freshwater fish, snakes, and frogs. This nematode is present throughout Southeast Asia (especially Thailand) and parts of South America. Humans become infected by ingesting the intermediate host and may develop subcutaneous swellings, ocular larva migrans, and eosinophilic meningitis. The acute phase generally begins 1–2 days after ingestion of the larvae. Systemic symptoms include nausea, vomiting, pruritus, urticaria, and abdominal pain. After 3–4 weeks, the chronic stage begins. It is characterized by symptoms caused by movement of the parasite through various tissues, including the skin or, more rarely, the central nervous system or eye. A migrating red rash, a sign of subcutaneous involvement, is the most common manifestation of this disease. Rarely, the worm migrates to the CNS, where it may cause a variety of CNS syndromes. Diagnosis is aided with a sensitive serologic test using an immunoblot [76]. Treatment is with albendazole, 400 mg twice a day for 21 days, or ivermectin, 200 µg/kg per day for 2 days. Surgical removal sometimes may be feasible [14].

ANGIOSTRONGYLUS SPECIES

A. cantonensis results from the ingestion of the third-stage larvae of the rat lungworm. After ingestion, the larvae migrate to the brain, spinal cord, and eye, where they cause a variety of symptoms depending on their specific location. They are generally acquired through the ingestion of uncooked or undercooked slugs or snails or vegetables contaminated by the slime of these mollusks. The incubation period is usually 2 weeks. Patients often have a severe headache, stiff neck, and low-grade to moderate fever. A variety of paresthesias, paralyses, or cranial nerve palsies may occur [77]. With eye involvement, decreased vision, extraocular muscle paralysis, and exophthalmus may occur. Laboratory findings include eosinophilia of the cerebrospinal fluid (CSF) and peripheral blood. Treatment is supportive. Surgery may be used to remove larvae that enter the anterior chamber of the eye. Corticosteroids are useful for severe meningitis, but antihelminthics are not effective and may exacerbate neurologic symptoms [78].

The geographic distribution of *A. costaricensis* is Central and South America. The primary difference between it and *A. cantonensis* is that, after being ingested, *A. costaricensis* larvae tend to develop in the lymphatics of the abdominal cavity and then migrate to the mesenteric arteries, where they deposit eggs in the intestinal wall. This causes granulomatous and eosinophilic inflammatory reactions that manifest as a variety of gastrointestinal symptoms [79]. Infected individuals frequently present with acute abdomen. If the spermatic artery is involved, testicular necrosis may be a complication. Larvae and eggs are not found in the stool examination. Treatment is generally supportive, and surgery may be necessary if perforation or obstruction occurs.

ZOONOTIC FILARIAL INFECTIONS

Dirofilarial infections are common in animals. *Dirofilaria immitis* causes the dog heartworm, whereas other species of *Dirofilaria*, including *D. tenuis* (in raccoons), *D. repens* (in cats and dogs), and *D. ursi* (in bears) cause subcutaneous infections both in the host and in humans, who are incidental hosts. *D. immitis* can cause a pulmonary dirofilariasis in humans, whereas the other species cause a subcutaneous dirofilariasis [80]. *D. immitis* is acquired in humans from the bite of a mosquito that has bitten an animal host. It is most common in the Americas, Australia, Europe, China, India, and Japan. The other *Dirofilaria* species have been reported on all continents. *D. immitis* is apparently not rare in humans. Serosurveys suggest that up to 5% of people in the United States may be infected. The incubation period is 2–3 months. *D. immitis* larvae occlude a small pulmonary artery, causing a sharply defined infarct. This tissue contains the worm, necrotic material, granulomas, and eosinophils. The tissue may calcify, allowing it to be seen on routine chest radiograph [81]. The clinical presentation is usually cough, chest pain, low-grade fever, and rarely, hemoptysis. If eosinophilia is present, it is usually low grade. The differential diagnosis for *D. immitis* primarily involves ruling out a tumor or a granuloma-producing infection. The diagnosis is usually made from surgical biopsy of the necrotic material, although fine-needle biopsy has been used in some cases. Treatment generally consists of surgical removal.

For the other species of *Dirofilaria*, the mosquito is also the vector, with the exception of *D. ursi*, for which it is the blackfly. Clinically, these other species tend to cause subcutaneous nodules, which are usually single [82]. Rarely, these parasites may be found in the eye. Current studies indicate that the human prevalence of dirofilarial infections is increasing [83]. The diagnosis of the other *Dirofilaria* species is usually through biopsy. In all *Dirofilaria* infections, microfilaremia is absent in humans. Treatment is surgical removal.

NEMATODES OF OTHER ORGAN SYSTEMS

Dioctophyma renale is the organism responsible for giant kidney worm disease. This is a rare infection resulting from ingestion of the larval form in raw or undercooked fish or frogs. The ingested larvae penetrate the intestinal wall, enter the peritoneal cavity, and migrate to the kidney, where they destroy the kidney, leaving only the capsule. Cases have been reported in Asia, the Americas, and Europe. The usual animal hosts are minks and dogs, which shed eggs when they urinate. If urination is near bodies of water, the eggs are then ingested by an aquatic worm, which is in turn ingested by fish or frogs [12]. Proper cooking of seafood and frogs prevents the infection.

Clinical Features

The usual incubation time between ingestion of larvae and appearance of eggs in the urine is 3–6 months. Symptoms include flank pain, renal colic, and hematuria. Rarely, there may be a subcutaneous mass [84]. Urinalysis, which usually shows hematuria, is helpful in making the diagnosis. If the worm is a female, eggs can be identified in the urine. In the case of male worms, only surgical re-moval of the nematode makes the diagnosis. Treatment is surgical removal of the parasite.

Human infection with larval nematodes of the genus *Eustrangylides* is rare. Risk factors for infection with *Eustrongylus* species are similar to those for dioctophymiasis. In nearly all cases, patients have reported the curious habit of swallowing live bait minnows [85]. Clinical symptoms tend to start within 24 hours and consist of intense abdominal pain, which is often localized in the right lower quadrant. Appendicitis is generally suspected in these patients. During surgery, large blood-red worms are found in the peritoneal cavity. Anisakiasis is one of the differential diagnoses for both these infections.

Capillaria hepatica, a rat-liver parasite that is also found in a number of other mammals, causes the disease hepatic capillariasis [8]. Humans may develop the infection after ingestion of embryonated eggs, which may be present in contaminated soil. The eggs hatch, and the worms migrate to the portal circulation of the liver, where they are nourished by the liver tissue. If enough worms are present, the host may suffer liver failure and die. The parasite is common in rats, but reports of human infection are rare. They have been seen in Africa, the Americas, Asia, and Europe. Eggs are hardy, remaining viable in the soil for some months. Prevention requires food and drink hygiene.

Diagnostic Assessment

Incubation is usually 3–4 weeks, and symptoms include fever, a tender, enlarged liver, splenomegaly, and often a transient pneumonitis. Laboratory studies include eosinophilia and abnormal liver function tests. The diagnosis is made by biopsy of the liver for identification of the parasite or eggs [86]. The eggs are not found in the intestine. Unfortunately, no treatment has been developed. Prevention is a matter of food and drink hygiene.

Trematodes

All the medically important trematodes, including blood flukes, intestinal flukes, and tissue flukes, are in the order Digenea.

SCHISTOSOMA

Schistosoma, which are blood flukes, exist as separate sexes but live *in copula*. Schistosomiasis, also called *bilharziasis* or *swamp fever,* affects more than 200 million people worldwide. Globally, this corresponds to 4.5 million DALYs lost [4]. Transmission of *Schistosoma* can be either by drinking infested water or by invasion of intact skin by a motile aquatic form called a *cercaria*. A cercaria can penetrate intact skin and is transformed into a schistosomum, which migrates through the lungs and systemic circulation, slowly finding its way to the portal venous system, where it matures into an adult and resides for years. Eggs excreted by these adults find their way back to the environment via feces or urine and hatch in the water, releasing miracidia, which penetrate the snail, which then develops over 4–6 weeks into a cercaria, thus completing the cycle [87]. Each species of *Schistosoma* has an associated species of snail. The main occupational and environmental risk factor is working in areas where freshwater ingestion or exposure is commonplace. Even brief exposures to infested waters, such as fording a stream or rafting [88], may result in schistosomiasis. Schistosomiasis occurs in more than 70 countries, but a distinctive geographic distribution of the major species is present. *S. mansoni* is the only species of schistosome that occurs in the western hemisphere, where it appears in parts of Brazil, Suriname, Venizuela, Dominican Republic, and Puerto Rico. It is widely prevalent in Africa. *S. nicum* is common throughout Asia, including the Philippines, China, and Japan. *S. haematobium* is also widely distributed throughout most of Africa and extends into southern Europe and western Asia [89]. Humans are the definitive hosts for all of the major *Schistosoma* species, although monkeys and baboons may act as hosts for *S. mansoni* and *S. haematobium*. In the case of *S. japonicum*, water buffalo and cattle also may serve as hosts.

Prevention

Hygienic handling of urine and feces and assurance of a safe water supply are most important methods of preventing schistosomiasis. The use of molluscocidal agents to eliminate snails also may be an important administrative practice. Personal protective measures include wearing rubber boots to prevent skin contact with fresh water. Lipodeet lotion applied to the skin is said to prevent cercarial penetration [90].

Clinical Features

The incubation period of schistosomiasis varies with the clinical presentation. Cercarial dermatitis may develop within hours of exposure. For the acute form of schistosomiasis, Katayama fever, incubation is generally from 2–10 weeks. For the chronic syndromes, it may take weeks to years for the disease to present. Clinical presentations are highly variable. Cercarial dermatitis is more common with zoonotic schistosomal infections, those that attack birds and small mammals, and does not produce other pathology. This dermatitis, which occurs in areas of skin not covered by bathing suits, results in a hypersensitivity reaction that causes a maculopapular pruritic rash. This condition, also called *swimmer's itch,* is self-limited but can be treated with antihistamines and topical corticosteroids.

Acute schistosomiasis, or Katayama fever, occurs in a minority of patients. It results from an allergic reaction during larval migration and early oviposition by adult worms [91]. It usually occurs 2–12 weeks after skin penetration. The symptoms are quite variable but may include nocturnal fever, sweats, cough with wheezing, abdominal pain, urticaria, headaches, and diarrhea. There may be hepatosplenomegaly and lymphadenopathy. Laboratory tests are positive for marked peripheral eosinophilia. This, along with the travel history, usually makes the diagnosis. At this phase, eggs may not be present. Treatment is with praziquantel, as in the chronic disease. The addition of corticosteroids is often warranted. Artemisinin coumpounds are being investigated for use in acute schistosomiasis.

The chronic aspects of schistosomiasis are mediated by the granulomatous response to the eggs. Many eggs are trapped in the host and never reach the external environment. There are several types of reactions, including intestinal, hepatic, urinary tract, and ectopic egg syndromes.

Intestinal schistosomiasis is seen commonly in all types of chronic schistosomal infections. The primary symptoms relate to the associated enteropathy and accompanying protein and blood loss. Signs include the presence of pseudopolyps with focal areas of hemorrhage. Schistosomal appendicitis also may occur.

Hepatic lesions result from the body's response to the eggs in the liver, which is initially due to a granulomatous process but followed by a fibrotic response. The most severe of these conditions results in the clay pipestem fibrosis of Symmers [87], which causes portal hypertension and its associated complications. Liver function studies are usually normal until very late in the disease process. Liver changes can be detected by ultrasonography, which has been used successfully for field diagnosis [92]. With the advent of mass chemotherapy and public educational intervention, the most severe forms of the hepatic fibrosis are becoming more rare [93].

Urinary tract schistosomiasis is most common with *S. haematobium.* More than half the *S. haematobium* eggs are present in the urinary tract, and as with other organ systems, the pathology results from the body's reaction to the eggs. This leads to hematuria, dysuria, secondary urinary tract infections, and obstructive uropathy. Because of this, simple urine dipstick tests have been valuable for field identification of patients at high risk for the infection [94]. Chronic urinary schistosomiasis correlates with bladder cancer [95].

Ectopic egg syndromes result from the embolization of eggs to other organ systems. Most serious of these is brain and spinal cord involvement. The brain is more commonly involved with *S. japonicum,* whereas spinal cord involvement (especially transverse myelitis) is most commonly due to *S. haematobium* and *S. mansoni* [12].

There is an association between schistosomiasis and *Salmonella* infections that causes prolonged typhoid fever with accompanying chronic anemia and splenomegaly. This probably results from *Salmonella*'s presence in the *Schistosoma* themselves and usually requires simultaneous antibiotic and antihelminthic treatment [96].

Clinical Features and Diagnosis

Characteristic laboratory findings include a marked eosinophilia early in the course of schistosomiasis, which may decrease with time. In the case of *S. haematobium,* radiographs of the genitourinary tract show linear calcifications in the submucosa of the bladder and ureters. Differential diagnosis includes VLM, liver flukes, the migratory phase of *Strongyloides,* and other helminth infections in the acute stage. Diagnosis usually depends on identification of viable eggs in the stool, urine, rectal biopsy specimen, or other tissues. Serologic tests traditionally have been useful to detect a response to the *Schistosoma* but not to distinguish active from inactive infections; however, newer techniques may not have this problem [97]. Serologic tests are available through the Centers for Disease Control and Prevention (CDC). The diagnosis can be especially difficult to make early, before eggs are produced.

Treatment

Treatment is with praziquantel. The dosage is a function of the type of schistosomiasis. For *S. japonicum* and *S. mekongi,* a dose of 60 mg/kg per day in three divided doses for 1 day is therapeutic in both adults and children [14]. For *S. haematobium* and *S. mansoni,* the dose is 40 mg/kg per day in two doses for 1 day for both adults and children [14]. Oxamniquine is an alternative treatment for *S. mansoni* and may be preferable for treatment of patients in some areas of Africa, where praziquantel may be less effective [98]. In this case, the regimen for oxamniquine in adults is 15–60 mg/kg in a single dose. For pediatric patients, it is 20 mg/kg per day in two divided doses for 1 day. The dosage varies with the specific country of acquisition.

INTESTINAL TREMATODES

The intestinal trematodes, or intestinal flukes, are not highly prevalent throughout the world, although there are pockets where they are quite common [24]. The transmission of all these flukes is similar in that the metacercarial stages are typically encysted in freshwater fish, mollusks, or aquatic vegetation. After ingestion, they take up residence in the intestine of the human host. The eggs generally pass with the feces, where freshwater snails act as an intermediate host. Risk factors for infection are primarily dietary. Details about geographic distribution and other aspects of infections are presented in Table 30-4. There are a number of other flukes of animals in Southeast Asia that have been reported to cause zoonotic infections in humans. When present, they tend to be asymptomatic or cause mild inflammatory changes with associated diarrhea and colicky pain. These intestinal flukes tend to have a short lifespan, and symptoms are limited. They include the following: *Pygidiopsis summa, Haplorchis* species, *Gymnophylloides seoi,*

Table 30-4
Intestinal Trematodes

Scientific/ Common Name	Geographic Location	Acquisition	Reservoir	Incubation	Major Disease Manifestations	Diagnosis
Fasciolopsis buski (giant intestinal fluke)	Southeast Asia, Indian subcontinent	Ingestion of water plants: water caltrop, water chestnut, watercress, water bamboo	Humans, pigs, dogs, rabbits	2–3 months until eggs in feces; symptoms may start earlier	Most asymptomatic; occasional appearance of worms in feces; in heavy infection, diarrhea and edema, even obstruction; impaired vitamin B_{12} absorption; may migrate to other organs	Detection of large operculate eggs in feces; eosinophilic leukocytosis
Echinostoma species	China, Southeast Asia, other scattered areas; high prevalence in Thailand	Ingestion of raw or undercooked fishes or mollusks; drinking water; water plants	Humans, mammals, birds	1 month	Abdominal cramps and pain, bloating, diarrhea, edema if heavy infection	Eggs in stool
Heterophyes heterophyes (dwarf fluke)	East and Southeast Asia, India, southern Europe (Spain), North Africa (Nile River delta), Turkey	Ingestion of raw or undercooked fish; salted or pickled fish also a risk	Birds, mammals	1–2 weeks	Most asymptomatic or mild diarrhea, cramps, nausea; rarely may migrate to heart or brain	Eggs in feces
Metagonimus yokogawai (Yokogawa's fluke infection)	East and Southeast Asia, former Soviet states, southern Europe, Balkan states	Ingestion of raw or undercooked freshwater fish	Birds, mammals	2 weeks	Most asymptomatic	Eggs in feces
Nanophyetus salmincola (salmon poisoning in dogs)	North America, eastern Siberia	Ingestion of raw or undercooked fish or roe; common in salmon; can survive in salted or smoked fish	Raccoons, skunks, dogs, foxes, coyotes, birds	1 week	Usually asymptomatic or mild episodic diarrhea, abdominal pain, bloating; may co-transmit *Neorickettsia helmintheca*, a rickettsia	Identification of eggs (number is small)
Gastrodiscoides hominis (Gastrodisciasis)	India, Southeast Asia, former Soviet states	Ingestion of aquatic vegetation	Humans, pigs	Unknown	Diarrhea in heavy infection	Characteristic eggs

Centrocestus formosanus, Prosthodendrium molen-kampi, Stellantchasmus falcatus, Phaneropsolus bonnei, and *Neodiplostomum seoulense* [1].

Treatment for all these intestinal flukes is with praziquantel. For all but *Nanophyetus salmincola,* the dosage is 75 mg/kg per day in three divided doses for 1 day for both adult and pediatric patients. For *N. salmincola,* it is 60 mg/kg per day in three doses for 1 day [14].

LIVER FLUKES

Liver flukes have a life cycle similar to that of the other trematodes. It involves an appropriate freshwater snail as the first intermediate host and either fish or contaminated water plants as the source of acquisition for humans. An exception to this generalization is *Dicrocoelium dendriticum,* for which a terrestrial snail is the intermediate host, and ants who eat the slime from this snail are the vector to humans [1]. Clinical symptoms are variable and often include abdominal pain and colic. Eosinophilia is common [99, 100] Specific information about the liver flukes is provided in Table 30-5.

Treatment

Treatment for *Fasciola hepatica* in both adult and pediatric patients is triclabendazole, 10 mg/kg once or twice. An alternative is bithionol, 30–50 mg/kg on alternate days for 10–15 doses [14]. For the other liver flukes, the treatment is praziquantel, 75 mg/kg per day in three doses for 1 day, for both adult and pediatric patients [14]. For *Clonorchis sinensis,* an alternative treatment for adult patients is albendazole, 10 mg/kg per day for 7 days.

LUNG FLUKES

Paragonimus westermani and other *Paragonimus* species are responsible for human lung fluke infections. Their life cycle is similar to that of other trematodes in that there is an obligatory snail intermediate host. The species are found in Southeast Asia and the Indian subcontinent. The other fluke species cause infections in the Americas, Asia, and Africa. The infection is acquired through ingestion of raw or undercooked freshwater crayfish, crabs, and shrimp. It also may be caused, although rarely, by the ingestion of undercooked wild boar meat. A number of mammals serve as reservoirs, including foxes, tigers, pigs, cats, and dogs. Incubation for the pulmonary symptoms is generally 6 months,

whereas for CNS symptoms it can be 12–16 months. The lung findings usually start insidiously with cough, hemoptysis, and rusty sputum. Later, wheezing, fever, and pleuritic pain may appear [101]. Lung flukes have the radiographic appearance of tuberculosis and can present an especially confusing picture if they coexist with tuberculosis. The flukes may migrate to other areas, where they can cause a variety of symptoms. In less than 1% of patients, they migrate to the CNS. When this happens, eosinophilic meningitis, along with a number of other neurologic symptoms, may occur. Migrating larvae can reach any part of the body, and subcutaneous masses are not uncommon. Peripheral eosinophilia is a common laboratory finding [102]. Sputum may contain Charcot-Leyden crystals. Chest radiographs commonly show effusions, diffuse infiltrates, nodules, cavities, and calcifications [103], frequently resembling tuberculosis, except that the apices are usually spared. Diagnosis is made by identification of eggs in sputum, feces, pleural fluid, or cerebrospinal fluid; the eggs also may be present in the feces because of swallowed sputum. Serologic studies may be useful and are available through the CDC. The treatment of choice is praziquantel, 75 mg/kg per day in three divided doses for 2 days [14], or, alternatively, bithionol, 30–50 mg/kg per day on alternate days for 10–15 doses [14]. The regimen is the same for adults and children.

Cestodes

Cestodes are parasitic tapeworms that can be quite large and are composed of a head, or scolex, and a long segmented portion, the strobilia. The scolex, which is the only point of attachment to the host, uses suckers, hooks, or grooves for this purpose. The rest of the body, or strobilia, is composed of the segmented sections, the proglottids, which are anatomically independent and contain both male and female sex organs. These proglottids also may be independently motile. Cestodes tend to have a complex life cycle, consisting of adult and larval stages. The pathology of cestode infections depends on whether humans act as hosts for the adult or larval stage of the tapeworm. The larval stages tend to be associated with much more invasive and serious disease. In general, adult tapeworms do not cause many symptoms. The adult tapeworms discussed

Table 30-5
Liver Flukes

Scientific/ Common Name	Geographic Location	Acquisition	Reservoir	Incubation	Major Disease Manifestations	Diagnosis
Fasciola hepatica (sheep liver fluke disease)	Worldwide in sheep and cattle-raising areas	Contaminated water, watercress, dandelion greens, lettuce	Sheep, cattle	3–4 months	Live in bile duct; asymptomatic or mild fever, liver pain, diarrhea, jaundice, cholangitis, cholecystitis; may migrate to other sites such as brain, orbits, subcutaneous, rare pharyngeal fasciolitis if raw liver	Abnormal liver function tests; anemia if heavy; filling defect in biliary tree; eosinophilia; eggs in stool or duodenal aspirate; serologic tests
Fasciola gigantic	Southeast Asia and Africa	Contaminated water, aquatic vegetation	Herbivorous mammals, especially cattle	3–4 months	Human infection rare; similar to *F hepatica*	Serodiagnosis, large eggs in feces
Clonorchis sinensis (Oriental liver fluke)	China, Japan, Korea, Taiwan; not uncommon in shipped fish	Raw or pickled freshwater fish or crayfish	Many, especially dogs and cats	3–4 weeks	Early—fever, epigastric and RUQ pain, diarrhea, malaise Chronic—may be asymptomatic, cholecystitis, pancreatitis, cholangiocarcinoma	High-grade eosinophilia; increased alkaline phosphatase; identification of eggs in feces or duodenal aspirate
Opisthorchis felineus	Eastern Europe, especially Poland, western Russia; Philippines, India, Japan, Vietnam	Raw or pickled freshwater fish or crayfish	Many wild and domestic animals	3–4 weeks	Same as *C sinensis*	Same as *C sinensis*
Opisthorchis viverrini	Thailand, Laos	Raw or pickled freshwater fish or crayfish	Cats, dogs	3–4 weeks	Same as *C sinensis*	Same as *C sinensis*
Opisthorchis guayaquilensis	Ecuador	Raw or pickled freshwater fish or crayfish	Cats, dogs	3–4 weeks	Same as *C sinensis*	Same as *C sinensis*
Metorchis conjunctus (North American liver fluke)	Canada	Raw fish, especially white sucker			Abdominal pain, anorexia, liver function abnormalities	Eggs in feces
Dicrocoelium dendriticum	Europe, former Soviet states, North Africa, northern Asia, Far East, Western Hemisphere	Ingestion of ants harboring metacercariae; terrestrial snails are intermediate hosts	Sheep, deer, cattle, other herbivores		Usually mild GI symptoms; if heavy, biliary symptoms	Eggs in feces; ingestion of infected liver may result in spurious passage of eggs

in this chapter include *Taenia saginata, T. solium, Diphyllobothrium* species, *Hymenolepis nana, H. diminuta,* and *Diplylidium caninum.*

TAENIA SAGINATA

The human is the definitive host for *T. saginata,* the beef tapeworm. Cattle act as intermediate hosts and become infected by grazing in pastures contaminated with eggs from human feces. The disease occurs worldwide in beef-eating countries. Acquisition is through ingestion of cysticerci in raw or undercooked beef. This infection also can occur in reindeer and camels.

The incubation period after consumption of the cysticerci is usually 10–14 weeks, after which proglottids can be found in the stool. Symptoms may occur earlier than this and may include epigastric discomfort, weight loss, nausea, vomiting, and diarrhea. The most common complaint is the passage of motile proglottids through the anus [5]. The proglottids may be found in the perianal area, in underclothing, or in bedding. Usually, only one worm is present. It may live for 25–30 years in the human intestine. Eosinophilia is not usually prominent, although IgE may be elevated. If a GI barium study is performed, one may see a ribbon-like defect. The diagnosis is made by identification of either proglottids or eggs in the stool. The Scotch tape test may be useful in detecting these forms. The eggs of *T. saginata* are not morphologically distinct from those of *T. solium.* For both adult and pediatric patients, the treatment of choice is praziquantel, 5–10 mg/kg as a one-time dose to kill the adult worm [14]. Alternatively, niclosamide, 2 g by mouth once in adults (50 mg/kg in children), can be used.

TAENIA SOLIUM

The life cycle of *T. solium* is the same as that of *T. saginata.* The major distinction is that humans also may serve as the intermediate host, causing cysticercosis (see below). As with *T. saginata* infection, usually only a single worm is present and causes little tissue reaction. The disease is widely distributed, but in the United States it is seen primarily in immigrants from endemic areas [104]. Humans acquire the infection through ingestion of raw or undercooked pork that is infected with the cysticerci.

It usually takes 8–12 weeks from ingestion of cysticerci to the presence of proglottids or eggs in the stool of the human. The worm usually does not cause symptoms, although vague GI symptoms, including epigastric discomfort, nausea, and diarrhea, may occur [105]. Finding proglottids or eggs in fecal specimens is diagnostic for *Taenia* infection. Laboratory technicians or anyone handling fecal specimens must exercise caution because eggs are infective and could cause cysticercosis if accidentally ingested. Treatment is the same as for the beef tapeworm.

DIPHYLLOBOTHRIUM LATUM

Diphyllobothritis, or fish tapeworm infection, may result from ingestion of a large variety of fresh- or saltwater fish [12]. The human is the definitive host, although other fish-eating mammals can be infected. The distribution of the disease is determined by the temperature requirements of the water, which are some 15–25°C. Specific copepods are necessary to act as intermediate hosts. Acquisition is through ingestion of raw or undercooked fish or fish products. Pickling, kippering, cold smoking, and air drying do not reliably kill the parasites.

It takes 4–6 weeks from ingestion of infected fish until eggs appear in the feces. The adult worm may live some 30–40 years. The infection is usually mild or asymptomatic, although if symptoms are present, they may be nonspecific, including abdominal pain, distention, flatulence, and diarrhea [106]. Rarely, megaloblastic anemia may result from vitamin B_{12} deficiency produced by the tapeworm's competition within the host for absorption of essential nutrients [107]. Also rare are complications resulting from mechanical obstruction. Diagnosis is made by identification of characteristic eggs or proglottids in the feces. Treatment for both adults and children is the same as for *T. saginata.*

HYMENOLEPIS NANA

Humans act as the definitive and intermediate hosts for the dwarf tapeworm, *H. nana.* Acquisition of the infection is through the fecal-oral route owing to food, water, or fomites or by accidental ingestion of infected arthropods. *H. nana* is unique among cestodes in that it is able to autoinfect its host. Geographic distribution is worldwide, although infections are most common in conditions of crowding and poor hygiene. *H. nana* is the most common tapeworm in the United States [57]. The incidence of infection is quite high in institutions such as day-care centers, orphanages, and institutions for the mentally impaired.

It generally takes 2–4 weeks after ingestion for eggs to appear in the stool. Because of the capacity for autoinfection, the infection may be sustained indefinitely. Symptoms are usually mild, if present at all. Severe infections may be noted in immunocompromised patients. Signs and symptoms of heavy infection include diarrhea, epigastric pain, nausea, vomiting, irritability, anorexia, weight loss, headache, and weakness. Eosinophilia may occur in up to 30% of patients. Diagnosis is based on identification of the characteristic eggs in the stool. The treatment is praziquantel, 25 mg/kg as a single dose, or, alternatively, nitazoxanide, 500 mg twice a day for 3 days [14]. In children, nitazoxanide is dosed by age.

HYMENOLEPIS DIMINUTA

Infection with *H. diminuta*, the rat tapeworm, is rare [12]. Infection with *H. diminuta* usually occurs in children and is acquired through ingestion of arthropods containing the infective cysticercoid stage—usually mealworms or grain beetles that infest food. Although the rat tapeworm is present worldwide, human cases are reported primarily in areas with poor rodent control.

It usually takes 2–4 weeks from ingestion of the larva until eggs appear in the stool. The disease is usually mild. If symptoms are present, they tend to be nonspecific, but eosinophilia does accompany infection. Diagnosis requires identification of the eggs in feces [108]. Treatment is the same as for *H. nana*.

DIPLYLIDIUM CANINUM

D. caninum is the organism that causes dipylidiasis, dog tapeworm infection, which occurs worldwide. It is a common tapeworm of cats as well as dogs. Humans act as an incidental host, after ingestion of flea- or louse-contaminated food or water containing the larvae. Most infections occur in infants or young children [109]. The infection is relatively rare.

It takes 3–4 weeks after ingestion until proglottids appear in the stool. The infection is usually asymptomatic or mild. The proglottids, which re-

semble cucumber seeds, may migrate from the anus to the perianal area. Diagnosis is made from identification of the proglottids or from eggs. Eggs may be seen in packets, which contain 8–15 eggs [1]. Hooks often may be seen within each egg. Treatment is with praziquantel at the same dosage as that for *T. saginata*.

UNCOMMON CESTODE PARASITES

A number of cestodal zoonotic infections may occur in humans. *Bertiella* species occur in monkeys and may be transmitted by mites, which serve as intermediate hosts. *Bertiella* infection usually occurs in humans who work closely with or live with monkeys [110]. *Mesocestoides* commonly causes infections in monkeys, foxes, raccoons, and rodents. Cases of this infection are occasionally reported throughout the United States as well as Europe and Asia [111]. *Inermicapsifer* species are primarily parasites of rodents but may be transmitted to humans through accidental ingestion of arthropod intermediate hosts [1]. The proglottids are passed in the feces and resemble grains of rice when dried. *Diplogonoporus grandis* is a whale tapeworm, but human cases have been reported in Japan. Marine fishes are thought to serve as intermediate hosts [112].

Larval Cestode Infections

CYSTICERCOSIS

Cysticercosis is the human infection with the larval stage of *T. solium*, the pork tapeworm. In this infection, humans act as an intermediate host. Cysticercosis is a common cause of neurologic diseases, especially seizures, in many parts of the world. Areas with the most cases with cysticercosis include Central and South America, parts of Asia, and Africa [113]. Southern and eastern Europe also have had some cases of this infection. The acquisition is through ingestion of egg-contaminated food or water or eggs on fomites. Reverse peristalsis associated with vomiting potentially could allow eggs from intestinal parasites to reach the upper GI tract, where they could hatch and start the cysticercosis cycle. More commonly, humans acquire cysticercosis by ingesting eggs from their own feces as a result of lapses in personal hygiene.

The time from egg ingestion to the occurrence of symptoms is usually at least 2 years. During this time, embryos hatch from ingested eggs, penetrate the gut wall, and disseminate via the circulation. They may lodge in a number of tissues but are found most commonly in subcutaneous tissue, brain, eye, and skeletal muscle. These cysticerci cause little host reaction while alive, but when they start to degenerate, they may provoke granulomatous changes and other pathologic reaction. Cysts in the muscles tend to calcify with time. Signs and symptoms of cysticercosis of the CNS, or neurocysticercosis, are varied and include seizures, intracranial hypertension, alteration of mental status, neurologic deficit, meningitis, and encephalitis. Neurocysticercosis involving the spinal cord is not uncommon, nor is ocular involvement. Nodules may appear in the skin and soft tissues and are usually about 2 cm in diameter.

Radiographic evaluation may reveal calcified cysticerci in muscle. Computed tomographic (CT) scanning or magnetic resonance imaging (MRI) of the head will reveal the cysts, often appearing as ring-enhanced cystic lesions. Blood studies with the enzyme-linked immunotransfer blot are highly specific [114], and peripheral eosinophilia is usually absent. Diagnosis is usually made by a combination of serologic tests and the biopsy of tissue.

Treatment of cysticercosis is complicated and varies with the location of the larvae. Initial treatment of symptomatic neurocysticercosis should focus on antiseizure medication. In addition, treatment with albendazole or praziquantel is useful. In adults, the dosage for albendazole is 400 mg twice daily for 8–30 days; in children, it is 15 mg/kg per day to a maximum of 800 mg given in two daily doses for 8–30 days [14]. The dosage for praziquantel is 100 mg/kg per day in three doses for 1 days, followed by 50 mg/kg per day in three doses for 29 days in both adult and pediatric patients [14]. Concurrent corticosteroid administration is often used to blunt the inflammatory response to dying parasites, which might exacerbate neurologic findings. The treatment of patients with cysticercosis must be individualized because the antiparasitic drug treatment of ocular or spinal cysts may cause irreversible sequelae. Surgical treatment also may be warranted, and management of symptoms with anticonvulsant medications or ventricular shunting may be necessary.

ECHINOCOCCOSIS

Echinococcosis, or hydatid disease, is caused by the larval stage of *Echinococcus granulosus*. In this infection, dogs are the definitive hosts; sheep, other animals, and humans may serve as intermediate hosts. Environmental and occupational risk factors for the disease are living and working closely with dogs. Acquisition of infection is through ingestion of infective eggs via food and water contamination or fomites. The infection is present on all continents but is concentrated in sheep-raising areas [115].

It usually takes several years from ingestion of eggs to manifestation of the disease state. Signs and symptoms vary with the number and size of cystic lesions, but they are usually related to mechanical pressure of the mass or to allergic reactions to the foreign proteins. Cysts commonly involve the liver and lung. Other sites, including the kidney, spleen, heart, bones, muscle, and CNS, may be involved. Anaphylactic reaction may accompany leakage of cyst fluids. Laboratory studies show peripheral eosinophilia in approximately one-third of patients. This is associated with leakage of fluid. Single or multiple lesions can be visualized by ultrasonography, CT scan, or other imaging techniques. Definitive diagnosis is usually made by microscopic identification of the parasite in surgically removed specimens. Serology is also useful.

Treatment of adults is usually albendazole, 400 mg twice daily for 1–6 months; the pediatric dose is 15 mg/kg per day for 1–6 months [14]. Puncture, aspiration, injection, and reaspiration (PAIR) is a technique that, in skilled hands, provides an effective nonsurgical option for treatment [116].

ECHINOCOCCUS MULTILOCULARIS

This infection, also called *alveolar hydatid disease,* is similar to *E. granulosis* but has a higher fatality rate. It is associated with a rapidly enlarging mass that is invasive, and hematologic dissemination may lead to metastatic infection [116]. Often the disease is inoperable by the time the diagnosis is made. Laboratory tests are usually unremarkable, and imaging studies usually show a solid mass with central cavitation. Radical surgical resection may be curative if diagnosis is made early. Albendazole, 20 mg/kg per day, which is only parasitostatic against *E. multilocularis,* should be used for 2 years following the surgery [116].

ECHINOCOCCUS VOGELI

E. vogeli infection causes polycystic hydatid disease and is also similar to *E. granulosis* infection. Human cases have been reported only in Central and South America. Clinical symptoms usually are related to a liver mass. Treatment is usually a combination of surgical resection and albendazole [117]. The severity of this infection is usually intermediate—between that of *E. granulosis* and *E. multilocularis*.

COENUROSIS

Coenuriasis is a larval tapeworm infection caused by one of several species of *Taenia*, including *T. multiceps, T. serialis,* and *T. brauni*. (Some authors believe that these parasites belong to the genus *Multiceps*.) In this infection, dogs are the definitive hosts, and sheep are usually the intermediate hosts, although humans may act as incidental intermediate hosts. The infection results from ingestion of the eggs from contaminated food, water, or fomites. Human infection is rare, although the tapeworm is common in areas where sheep are present. In sheep, the infection is called *gid* or *staggers* [12].

After ingestion, onchospheres escape from the eggs, hatch, and penetrate the intestinal wall. Then they are spread hematogenously to various tissues, where they form cysts. Common sites of larval encystment include the CNS, eye, subcutaneous tissue, and muscle. The clinical features depend on the location of these cysts. When the CNS is involved, common symptoms include drowsiness, headache, vomiting, papilledema, seizures, and hemiparesis [118]. A number of ocular findings are seen in response to encystment of the eye [119]. Subcutaneous coenuri may or may not be painful and are commonly confused with lipomas, ganglions, and neurofibromas. The diagnosis is usually made on the basis of microscopic identification of coenuri. If the eye is involved, slit-lamp examination may be used to make direct diagnosis. Eosinophilia is not usually a feature. Treatment generally involves surgical excision of the cerebral, ophthalmic, or subcutaneous coenuri. Medications do not appear to be useful [12].

SPARGANOSIS

Sparganosis is caused by larval infection with a *Spirometra* species, usually *S. mansoni*. The defini-

tive hosts for this infection are dogs and cats. There are two intermediate hosts, including a cyclops and a vertebrate. Humans may be incidental intermediate hosts; they usually acquire this infection through ingestion of cyclops-contaminated water; ingestion of larvae in undercooked frog, snake, poultry, or pork; or application of raw frog flesh as a poultice [120]. Although the infection is common in animals, it is rare in humans [12].

The incubation period varies greatly depending on the route of acquisition. The clinical features, although usually mild, relate to the number of parasites and the areas the larvae reach during migration. Migrations may be subcutaneous, ocular, or neural. One may see either nonproliferative or proliferative sparganosis. Nonproliferative sparganosis is more common and is characterized by the presence of one solitary discrete lesion that contains the tapeworm [121]. Proliferative sparganosis tends to occur with *S. proliferum* and is highly invasive. It tends to proliferate and metastasize throughout the body by a process of branching and budding. Dissemination can occur anywhere but is most common in the CNS, skeletal muscle, subcutaneous tissue, and internal organs [122]. The diagnosis is usually made by serologic tests and pathologic specimens. Treatment of nonproliferative cases is surgical excision of the entire sparganum. Drug therapy does not appear to be helpful. There is no effective treatment for proliferative sparganosis.

References

1. Ash LR, Orihel TC. *Atlas of Human Parasitology,* 5th ed. Chicago: American Society of Clinical Pathologists, 2007.
2. de Silva NR, et al. Soil-transmitted helminth infections: Updating the global picture. *Trends Parisitol* 2003;19:547–51.
3. Hotez PJ, Molyneux DH, Fensick A, et al. Control of neglected tropical diseases. *N Engl J Med* 2007;357:1018–27.
4. Chan MS. The global burden of intestinal nematode infections—Fifty years on. *Parasitol Today* 1997;13:438–43.
5. Wilson ME. *A World Guide to Infections: Diseases, Distribution, Diagnosis.* New York: Oxford University Press, 1991.
6. Bryan FD. Diseases transmitted by foods contaminated by waste water. *J Food Protein* 1977;40:45–56.
7. Seltzer E, Barry M, Compton DWT. Ascariasis. In Guerrant RL, Walker DH, Weller PF (eds), *Tropical*

Infectious Diseases: Principles, Pathogens, and Practice, 2nd ed. New York: Elsevier, 2006. Pp 1257–64.

8. Despommier DD, Gwadz RW, Hotez PJ, Knirsch CA. *Parasitic Diseases,* 4th ed. New York: Springer-Verlag, 2000.

9. Crompton DWT. Chronic ascariasis and malnutrition. *Parasitol Today* 1985;1:47–52.

10. Teneza-Mora NC, Lavery EA, Chun HM. Partial bowel obstruction in a traveler. *Clin Infect Dis* 2006;43:214.

11. Leventhal R, Cheadle R. *Medical Parasitology: A Self-Instructional Text,* 4th ed. Philadelphia: FA Davis, 1996.

12. Part VI: Helminthic infections. In Connor DH, Chandler FW, Schwartz DA, et al (eds), *Pathology of Infectious Diseases.* Stamford, CT: Appleton & Lange, 1997. Pp 1305–1588.

13. Maguire JH. Intestinal nematodes (roundworms). In Mandell EL, Bennett JE, Dolin R (eds), *Mandell, Douglas, and Bennett's Principles and Practice of Infectious Diseases,* 6th ed. New York: Elsevier, 2005. Pp 3260–67.

14. Drugs for parasitic infections. *Treatment Guidelines from the Medical Letter* 2007; 5:e1–14.

15. Albonico M, Montresor A, Crompton DWT, Savioli L. Intervention for the control of soil-transmitted helminthiasis in the community. In Molyneux DH (ed), *Control of Human Parasitic Diseases.* London: Academic Press, 2007. Pp 311–48.

16. Warren KS, Bundy DA, Anderson RM, et al. Helminth infections. In Jamison DJ (ed), *Disease Control Prevention in Developing Countries.* New York: Oxford University Press, 1993, Pp 131–60.

17. Elias D, Britton S, Kassu A, et al. Chronic helminth infections may negatively influence immunity against tuberculosis and other diseases of public health importance. *Exp Rev Anti-Infect Ther* 2007;5: 475–84.

18. American Academy of Pediatrics. Pinworm infestation. In Peter G (ed), *Red Book: Report of the Committee on Infectious Diseases,* 27th ed. Elk Grove Village, IL: American Academy of Pediatrics, 2006.

19. Beckman EN, Holland JB. Ovarian enterobiasis: A proposed pathogenesis. *Am J Trop Med Hyg* 1981;30: 74–6.

20. Burkhart CN, Burkhart CG. Assessment of frequency, transmission, and genitourinary complications of enterobiasis (pinworms). *Int J Dermatol* 2005;44:837–40.

21. Bethony J, Brooker S, Albanico M, et al. Soil-transmitted helminth infections: Ascariasis, trichariasis and hookworm. *Lancet* 2006;367:1521–32.

22. Stephenson LSM, Latham NC. Treatment with a single dose of albendazole improves growth of Kenyan school children with hookworm, trichuris and ascaris infections. *Am J Trop Med Hyg* 1989;41: 78–87.

23. Gilman RH, Chang YH, David C, et al. The adverse consequence of having trichuris infection. *Trans R Soc Trop Med Hyg* 1983;7:432–8.

24. Peters W, Pasvol G. Atlas of *Tropical Medicine and Parasitology,* 6th ed. London: Mosby-Elsevier, 2007.

25. Loukas A, Bethony J, Brooker S, et al. Hookworm vaccines: Past, present and future. *Lancet Infect Dis* 2006;6:733–41.

26. Hotez PJ, Brooker S, Ethony JM, et al. Current concepts: Hookworm infection. *N Engl J Med* 2004;351: 799–807.

27. Stolzfus RJ, Albonico M, Chwaya HM, et al. Hemoquant determination of hookworm-related blood loss and its role in iron deficiency in African children. *Am J Trop Med Hyg* 1996;55:399–404.

28. Walzer PD, Milder JE, Banwell JG, et al. Epidemiologic features of *Strongyloides stercoralis* infections in an endemic area of the United States. *Am J Trop Med Hyg* 1982;31:313–9.

29. Berk SL, Verghese A, Alvarez J, et al. Clinical and epidemiologic features of strongyloidiasis: A prospective study in rural Tennessee. *Arch Intern Med* 1987; 147:1257–60.

30. Gotuzzo E, Terashima A, Alvarez H, et al. *Strongyloides stercoralis* hyperinfection associated with human T-cell lymphotropic virus type 1 infection in Peru. *Am J Trop Med Hyg* 1999;60:146–49.

31. Petithory JC, Derouin F. AIDs and *Strongyloides* in Africa. *Lancet* 1987;1:921.

32. Conway DJ, Lindo JF, Robinson RD, et al. Towards effective control of *Strongyloides. Parasitol Today* 1995;11:420–4.

33. Koga K, Kasuya S, Khamboonruang C, et al. A modified agar plate method for detection of *Strongyloides stercoralis. Am J Trop Med Hyg* 1991;45:518–21.

34. Kobayashi J, Sato Y, Toma H, et al. Application of encyme immunoassay for postchemotherapy evaluation of human strongyloidiasis. *Diagn Microbiol Infect Dis* 1994;18:19–23.

35. Nuesch R, Zimmerli L, Stockli R, et al. Imported strongyloidosis: A longitudinal analysis of 31 cases. *J Trav Med* 2005;12:80–4.

36. Sunish IP, Rajendran R, Mani TR, et al. Evidence for the use of albendazole for the elimination of lymphatic filariasis. *Lancet Infect Dis* 2006;6:125–6.

37. Ottesen EA, Duke BOL, Karam M, et al. Strategies and tools for the control/elimination of lymphatic filariasis. *Bull WHO* 1997;75:491–503.

38. Bockaire MJ, Tisch DJ, Kastens W, et al. Mass treatment to eliminate filariasis in Papua New Guinea. *N Engl J Med* 2002;347:1841–8.

39. Ramzy RMR, Setouly ME, Helmy H, et al. Effect of yearly mass drug administration with diethylcarbamizine and albendazole on bancroftian filariasis in Egypt. *Lancet* 2006;367:992–99.

40. Taylor MJ, Hoerauf A. A new approach to the treatment of filariasis. *Curr Opin Infect Dis* 2001;23:401–9.

41. Freedman DO, Almeida Filho PJ, Besh S, et al. Lymphoscintigraphic analysis of lymphatic abnormalities in symptomatic and asymptomatic human filariasis. *J Infect Dis* 1994;170:927–33.

42. Leggat PA, Melrose W, Durrheim DN. Could it be lymphatic filariasis? *J Trav Med* 2004;11:56–60.

43. Faris R, Hussain O, Setouhy ME, et al. Bancraftian filariasis in Egypt: Visualization of adult worms and subclinical lymphatic pathology in scrotal ultrasound. *Am J Trop Med Hyg* 1998;59:864–67.

44. Boatin BA, Richards FO. Control of onchocerciasis. In Molyneux DH (ed), *Control of Human Parasitic Diseases.* London: Academic Press, 2007. Pp 349–94.

45. Ryan ET, Felsenstein D, Aguino SL, et al. Case 39-2005: A 63-year old woman with a positive serological test for syphilis and persistent eosinophilia. *N Engl J Med* 2005;353:2697–705.

46. Klion AD, Nutman TB. Loiasis and *Mansonella* infections. In Guerrant RL, Walker DH, Weller PF (eds), *Tropical Infectious Diseases: Principles, Pathogens, and Practice.* New York: Elsevier, 2006. Pp. 1163–75.

47. Nutman TB, Miller KD, Mulligan M, et al. Diethylcarbamazine prophylaxis for human loiasis: Results of a double-blind study. *N Engl J Med* 1988;319:752–6.

48. Klion AD, Massougbodji A, Sadeler B-C, et al. Loiasis in endemic and nonendemic populations: Immunologically mediated differences in clinical presentation. *J Infect Dis* 1991;163:1318–25.

49. Nutman TB, Miller KD, Mulligan M, et al. Loa loa infection in temporary residents of endemic regions: Recognition of hyperresponsive syndrome with characteristic clinical manifestations. *J Infect Dis* 1986;154:10–4.

50. Toure FS, Kassambara L, Williams T, et al. Human occult loiasis: Improvement in diagnostic sensitivity by the use of nested polymerase chain reaction. *Am J Trop Med Hyg* 1998;59:144–49.

51. Klion AD, Vijaykumar A, Oei T, et al. Serum immunoglobulin G_4 antibodies to the recombinant antigen, L1-SXP-1, are highly specific for loa loa infection. *J Infect Dis* 2003;187:128–33.

52. Meyers WM, Connor DH, Harman LE, et al. Human streptocerciasis: A clinicopathologic study of 40 African (Zairians) including identification of the adult filaria. *Am J Trop Med Hyg* 1972;21:528–45.

53. Gonzales AA, Chadee DD, Rawlins SC. Ivermectin treatment of mansonellosis in Trinidat. *W Ind Med J* 1999;48:231–34.

54. Barry M. The tailend of Buinea worm: Global eradication without a drug or a vaccine. *N Engl J Med* 2007;356:2561–64.

55. Centers for Disease Control and Prevention. Progress toward global eradication of dracunculiasis, January 2005–May 2007. *MMWR* 2007;56:813–17.

56. Greenaway C. Dracunculiasis (guinea worm disease). *Can Med Assoc J* 2004;170:495–500.

57. Heymann DL (ed). *Control of Communicable Diseases Manual,* 18th ed. Baltimore: United Book Press, 2004.

58. Watten RH, Beckner WM, Cross JH, et al. Clinical studies of *Capillaria philippinensis. Trans R Soc Trop Med Hyg* 1970;66:828–32.

59. Cross JH. Intestinal capillariasis. *Clin Microbiol Rev* 1992;5:120–9.

60. Centers for Disease Control and Prevention. Trichinellosis associated with bear meat—New York and Tennessee, 2003. *MMWR* 2004;53:606–10.

61. Ranque S, Faugere B, Pozio E, et al. *Trichinella pseudospiralis* outbreak in France. *Emerg Infect Dis* 2000; 6:543–7.

62. Most H. Trichinosis: Preventable yet still with us. *N Engl J Med* 1978;298:1178–80.

63. Markell EK. Pseudohookworm infection—trichostrongyliasis: Treatment with thiabendazole. *N Engl J Med* 1968;278:831–2.

64. Krepel HP, Baeta S, Polderman AM. Human *Oesophagostomum* infection in northern Togo and Ghana: Epidemiological aspects. *Ann Trop Med Parasitol* 1992;86:289–300.

65. Storey PA, Spannbrucker N, Yelifar L, et al. Ultrasound detection and assessment of preclinical oesophagostomum bifurcum-induced colonic pathology. *Clin Infect Dis* 2001;33:166–70.

66. Zlem JB, Ketltenis IMJ, Bayita A, et al. The short term impact of albendazole treatment on oesophagostomum bifurcum and hookwork infections in northern Ghana. *Ann Trop Med Parasitol* 2004;98:385–90.

67. Zvejnieks PA, Lichtenstein KA, Koneman EW. Luminal anisakidosis due to *Pseudoterranova decipiens. Clin Infect Dis* 1998;26:1222–3.

68. Bouree P, Paugam A, Petithory JC. Anisokidosis: Report of 25 cases and review of the literature. *Comp Immunol Microbiol Infect Dis* 1995;18:75–84.

69. Moore DAJ, Girdwood RWA, Chiodini PL. Treatment of anisakiasis with albendazole. *Lancet* 2002; 360:54.

70. Prociv P, Croese J. Human eosinophilic enteritis caused by dog hookworm *Ancylostoma caninum. Lancet* 1990;335:1299–1302.

71. Soo JK, Vega-Lopez F, Stevens HP, et al. Cutaneous larva migrans and beyond: A rare association. *Trav Med Infect Dis* 2003;1:41–43.

72. Schentz PM, Glickman LT. Current concepts in parasitology: Toxocaral visceral larva migrans. *N Engl J Med* 1978;298:436–9.

73. Sorvillo F, Ash LR, Berlin OGW, et al. *Baylisascaris procyonis:* An emerging helminthic zoonosis. *Emerg Infect Dis* 2002;8:355–9.

74. Murray WJ, Kazacos KR. Raccoon roundworm encephalitis. *Clin Infect Dis* 2004;39:1484–92.

75. Rusnak JM, Lucey DR. Clinical gnathostomiasis: Case report and review of the English-language literature. *Clin Infect Dis* 1993;16:33–50.

76. Moore DAJ, McCroddan J, Dekumyoy P, et al.

Gnathostomiasis: An emerging imported disease. *Emerg Infect Dis* 2003;9:647–50.

77. Re VL, Gluckman SJ, Eosinophilic meningitis due to *Angiostrongylus cantenensis* in a returned traveler: Case report and review of literature. *Clin Infect Dis* 2001;33:e112–115.
78. Slom TJ, Cortese MM, Gerber SI, et al. An outbreak of eosinophilic meningitis caused by *Angiostrongylus cantonensis* in travelers returning from the Caribbean. *N Engl J Med* 2002;346:668–75.
79. Loría-Cortés R, Lobo-Sanahuja JF. Clinical abdominal angiostrongylosis: A study of 116 children with intestinal eosinophilic granuloma caused by *Angiostrongylus costaricensis*. *Am J Trop Med Hyg* 1980; 29:538–44.
80. Orihel TC, Eberhard ML. Zoonotic filariasis. *Clin Microbiol Rev* 1998;11:366–
81. Risher WH, Crocker EF Jr, Beckman EN, et al. Pulmonary dirofilariasis. *J Thorac Cardiovasc Surg* 1989;97:303–8.
82. Weissman BW. Raccoon heartworms causing a facial mass. *South Med J* 1992;85:845–6.
83. Kramer LH, Kartasher VV, Grandi G, et al. Human subcutaneous dirofilariasis, Russia. *Emerg Infect Dis* 2007;13:150–2.
84. Gutierrez Y, Cohen M, Machicao CN. Dioctophyine larva in the subcutaneous tissues of a woman in Ohio. *Am J Surg Pathol* 1989;13:800–2.
85. Wittner M, Turner JW, Jacquette G, et al. Eustrongylidiasis: A parasitic infection acquired by eating sushi. *N Engl J Med* 1989;320:1124–6.
86. Attah EB, Nagarajan S, Obineche EN, et al. Hepatic capillariasis *Am J Clin Pathol* 1983;79:127–30.
87. Gryeels B, Polman K, Clerinex J, et al. Human schistosomiasis. *Lancet* 2006;368:1106–18.
88. Stuiver PC. Acute schistosomiasis among Americans rafting the Omo River, Ethiopia. *JAMA* 1984;251:508–10.
89. Blanchard TJ. Schistosomiasis. *Trav Med Infect Dis* 2004;2:5–11.
90. Salafsky B, Ramaswamy K, He YX, et al. Development and evaluation of Lipodeet, a new long-acting formulation of N,N-diethyl-m-tolumide (DEET) for the prevention of schistosomiasis. *Am J Trop Med Hyg* 1999;61:743–50.
91. Ross AG, Vickers D, Olds GR, et al. Katayama syndrome. *Lancet Infect Dis* 2007;7:218–24.
92. Friis H, Ndhlovu P, Kaondera K, et al. Ultrasonographic assessment of *Schistosoma mansoni* and S. *haematobium* morbidity in Zimbabwean schoolchildren. *Am J Trop Med Hyg* 1996;55:290–4.
93. World Health Organization. Report of the WHO Expert Committee on the Control of Schistosomiasis. WHO Technical Report Series. Geneva: WHO, 1991.
94. Hammad TA, Gabr NS, Talaat MM, et al. Hematuria and proteinuria as predictors of *Schistosoma haematobium* infection. *Am J Trop Med Hyg* 1997;57:363–7.
95. Schwartz DA. Helminths in the induction of cancer: *Schistosoma haematobium* and bladder cancer. *Trop Geogr Med* 1981;33:1–7.
96. Rocha H, Kirk JW, Hearey CD. Prolonged *Salmonella* bacteremia in patients with *Schistosoma mansoni* infections. *Arch Intern Med* 1971;128:254–7.
97. Valli LCP, Kanamura HY, DaSilva RM, et al. Efficacy of an enzyme-linked immunosorbent assay in the diagnosis of and serologic distinction between acute and chronic *Schistosoma mansoni* infections. *Am J Trop Med Hyg* 1997;57:356–62.
98. Stelma FF, Sall S, Daff B, et al. Oxamniquine cures *Schistosoma mansoni* infection in a focus in which cure rates are unusually low. *J Infect Dis* 1997;26:95–106.
99. Lun ZR, Gasser RB, Lai DH, et al. Clonorchiasis: A key foodborne zoonosis in China. *Lancet Infect Dis* 2005;5:31–41.
100. A-Harris NL, McNeely WF, Shepard JO, et al. Case records of the Massachusetts General Hospital. Case 12-2002. *N Engl J Med* 2002;346:1232–39.
101. Singh TS, Mutum SS, Razaque MA. Pulmonary paragonimiasis: Clinical features, diagnosis and treatment of 39 cases in Manipur. *Trans R Soc Trop Med Hyg* 1986;80:967–71.
102. Robertson KB, Janssen WJ, Saint S, et al. Clinical problem solving: The missing piece. *N Engl J Med* 2006;355:1913–8.
103. Johnson RJ, Johnson JR. Paragonimiasis in Indochinese refugees: Roentgenographic findings with clinical correlations. *Am Rev Respir Dis* 1983;128:535–8.
104. Despommier DD. Tapeworm infection: The long and short of it. *N Engl J Med* 1992;327:727–8.
105. Garcia HH, Gonzalez AE, Evans CAW, et al. *Taenia solium* cysticercosis. *Lancet* 2003;362:547–56.
106. Turner JA, Sorvillo FJ, Chin J, et al. Diphyllobothriasis associated with salmon—United States. *MMWR* 1981;30:31–2, 37.
107. Nyberg W, Gräsbeck R, Saarni M, et al. Serum vitamin B_{12} levels and incidence of tapeworm anemia in a population heavily infected with *Diphyllobothrium latum*. *Am J Clin Nutr* 1961;9:606–12.
108. Hamrick HJ, Bowdre JH, Church SM. Rat tapeworm (*Hymenolepis diminuta*) infection in a child. *Pediatr Infect Dis J* 1990;9:216–9.
109. Ratiere CR. Dog tapeworm (*Dipylidium caninum*) infestation in a 6-month-old infant. *J Fam Pract* 1992;34:101–2.
110. Panda DN, Panda MR. Record of *Bertiella studeri* (Blanchard, 1891), an anaplocephalid tapeworm, from a child. *Ann Trop Med Parasitol* 1994;88:451–2.
111. Schiltz LF, Roberto RR, Rutheford GW, et al. *Mesocestoides* (cestoda) infection in a California child. *Pediatr Infect Dis J* 1992;11:332–4.
112. Nakamura N, Nakayama J, Shimazu T, et al. First two cases of diplogonoporiasis grandis from Nagano prefecture, Japan. *Jpn J Parasitol* 1993;42:434–7.

113. Carpio A. Neurocysticercosis: An update. *Lancet Infect Dis* 2002;2:751–62.

114. White AL Jr. State-of-the-art: neurocysticercosis: A major cause of neurologic disease worldwide. *Clin Infect Dis* 1997;24:101–13.

115. Craig PS, McManus DP, Lightowlers MW, et al. Prevention and control of cystic echinococcosis. *Lancet Infect Dis* 2007;7:385–94.

116. McManus DP, Zhang W, Li J, et al. Echinococcis. *Lancet* 2003;362:1295–304.

117. Meneghelli UG, Martinelli ALC, Llorach Velludo MAS, et al. Polycystic hydatid disease (*Echinococcus vogeli*): Clinical, laboratory, and morphologic findings in nine Brazilian patients. *J Hepatol* 1991;14:203–10.

118. Pau A, Perria C, Turtas S, et al. Long-term follow-up on the surgical treatment of intracranial coenurosis. *Br J Neurosurg* 1990;4:39–43.

119. Ibechukwu BF, Onwukeme KE. Intraocular coenurosis: A case report. *Br J Ophthalmol* 1991;75:430–1.

120. Wiwanitkit V. A review of human sparganosis in Thailand. *Int J Infect Dis* 2005;9:312–6.

121. Norma SH, Kreutnew A Jr. Sparganosis: Clinical and pathologic observations in ten cases. *South Med J* 1980;73:297–300.

122. Nakamura T, Hara M, Matsuoka M, et al. Human proliferative sparganosis: A new Japanese case. *Am J Clin Pathol* 1990;94:224–8

31 Protozoan Travel-Related Infections

John Ellis

During a relatively short period of time on earth in geologic terms, humans have acquired over 70 species of protozoa of an estimated number in the tens of thousands. Most protozoa are free-living in soil and water. Of the relatively few protozoa that humans carry, only a few cause serious clinical disease. However, for these relative few, an immense burden of illness and death has been borne on every continent. Most occur in the tropics, and the study of protozoal infections is much of tropical medicine. The advent of acquired immune deficiency syndrome (AIDS) and disorders of induced immunosuppression [as in chronic disease states, steroid therapy, or after transplants or from human immunodeficiency virus (HIV) infection] has added yet another dimension to the impact of these unique organisms. Many of these diseases can remain asymptomatic for years, only to reactivate with immunosuppression.

Protozoa are among the earliest life forms and are termed *eukaryotic,* meaning that they have a membrane-bound nucleus compared with bacteria, which do not. Because bacteria lack such membranes and some other cytoplasmic features of protozoa, they are termed *protokaryotic,* indicating a more primitive state.

Protozoa also have specialized organelles, also membrane-bound, that are assigned essential functions such as respiration or photosynthesis (e.g., the chloroplasts in plant protozoal cells). Some protozoa divide sexually, either full or part time, making them suited for potentially more rapid evolutionary adaptation and resistance than prokaryotic organisms [1]. Some develop highly resistant cyst forms that live outside hosts, and some are motile, using flagellae or pseudopods. As a result of millions of years of adaption, and by acquiring the ability to vary their antigenic presentation, several of the most important protozoa are difficult to treat because they have become resistant to many drugs. So far, successful vaccine development progress has been, at best, painfully slow and yet to be fully realized. Many of these organisms are so well adapted that they eagerly consume the very macrophages intended for their destruction. Toxic drugs such as arsenicals and antimonials still are relied on for treatment in a large part of the world. Also, occurring as protozoa do, largely in poverty-stricken areas, drug funding for the protozoal diseases that cause the most problems worldwide has lagged compared with that for other diseases.

Readers will soon understand that the best approach for these illnesses is prevention. Effective drug treatment is often so expensive that it is essentially unavailable to the vast numbers of individuals affected in many developing countries.

Malaria, one such protozoal illness that has the ability to cause death in a formerly healthy person in as short as a day, has assumed so much importance that it is covered in its own chapter in this edition. Malaria will not be covered here. See Chapter 25.

While diseases owing to helminthes have been known for centuries, it required the development of the microscope by Leeuwenhoek toward the end of the seventeenth century to identify protozoa. A significant advance came with the electron microscope in the 1950s, with which the internal structure of microscopic organisms was further studied.

For most primary care physicians in the relatively protected United States, parasitology was, until recently, limited to a few endemic protozoan diseases (e.g., amebiasis, giardiasis, and trichomoniasis) and the occasional roundworm infestation (e.g., hookworm, ascaris, trichuris, and strongyloidiasis). Since the onset of the AIDS epidemic, the number of parasitic pathogens recognized and the frequency with which they are encountered in clinical practice have increased. Four intestinal protozoa that have been identified increasingly in patients with AIDS are Cryptosporidia, Microsporidia, *Isospora,* and *Cyclospora.* These organisms also have been implicated as important pathogens in otherwise healthy persons. Each has unique features that have been reviewed recently, but they also have many common characteristics [2].

Even the most commonly encountered protozoal infections seen in the United States can be severe occasionally and challenging to treat. Microsporidial and cryptococcal infections were practically unknown until clinical HIV infections appeared in the past 20 years. Amebiasis, the sleeping sicknesses, leishmaniasis, and Chagas' disease are for most practitioners distant subjects, but these illnesses lie in wait for those who work and travel in distant lands unless there is special awareness of the need for prevention and early diagnosis and treatment. The African sleeping sickness disorders are no further under control now than they were three decades ago, and if anything, the situation has worsened.

Many protozoa, especially the *Entamoeba, Giardia,* and *Trichomonas* organisms, depend on the availability of host cholesterol, creating interesting possibilities for treatment options. This growth feature explains why *Entamoeba,* in particular, sometimes favors cholesterol rich organs such as liver and brain [3].

This chapter will serve to update a subject on which many have not given much thought since their early medical training, and it is hoped that practitioners of occupational medicine in particular may find the information useful.

The continued unrest in parts of the world decimated by ongoing wars, especially in the tropics, has diverted resources vital to public health efforts for control of diseases and further facilitated the spread of protozoal infections, helped in no small degree by the enormous growth in travel of all kinds and by global warming.

As Table 31-1 shows for the most common travel-related parasitic illnesses, the majority are protozoan infections. Transmission is either by vectors or by contaminated food and water. A discussion of each of these major travel diseases follows, including those considered to be "emerging" protozoan illnesses (e.g., Microsporidian infection and acathamebiasis).

The true prevalence of many of these diseases is not known because many are subclinical in healthy persons. One will see both giardiasis and amebiasis stated as the most common protozoal gastrointestinal (GI) illnesses, and in certain areas of the world, either may be the case. The taxonomy is still evolving, and for this reason, this chapter will stress the clinical aspects of these diseases.

Table 31-1
Most Common Travel-Related Parasitic Diseases

Related to:	Organisms:
Contaminated Food and Water	
	Giardiasis*
More Common	Cryptosporidiosis*
	Cyclosporiasis*
	Amebiasis*
Less Common	Trichinosis
	Taenia Infection
	Facioliasis
Vector-borne	
More Common	Malaria*
	Leishmaniasis*
	Chaga's Disease*
Less Common	Lymphatic filiariasis
	African Sleeping Sickness*
	Onchceriasis

*Denotes protozoal diseases
Source: Adapted from: Parasitic Diseases, Travel/Travelers, Some of the Parasitic Illness That Can Be Acquired During Travel (not a comprehensive list). Centers for Disease Control and Prevention (www.cdc.gov/ncidod/dpd/travel.htm).

Clinicians should keep in mind that protozoan infections, unlike helminthic infections, rarely induce eosinophilia [4]. Advances in diagnostic testing have been impressive, with sophisticated (but, unfortunately, not always available where they are most needed) antigen, antibody, and molecular methods that help to overcome a lack of skilled microscopists. A reference to a very helpful U.S. Centers for Disease Control and Prevention (CDC) website for diagnostic assistance is included. Advances in treatment have, to the contrary, been painfully slow to date.

While blood-sucking vectors transmit blood-borne pathogens including malaria, leishmaniasis, and the sleeping sicknesses, nonbiting insects such as flies and cockroaches also can be important in the transfer of food-borne protozoal diseases [5].

One factor that receives scant mention in articles on parasitic infections is gender differences that have an impact on the immune system and, through them, the incidence and severity of these diseases. Not only do males and females have differing exposure opportunities, but variations in sex hormones during the luteal cycle and in pregnancy occur that can affect immunity. Local immunologic changes favor an infection-free environment prior to ovulation, followed by a more permissive immunity that does not kill sperm or inhibit implantation. Variations in corticosteroid hormones also play a role. Experiments in female mice have shown that gonadectomy increases resistance to toxoplasmosis and administered estrogen exacerbates disease. Females appear to have slightly higher malarial mortality rates than males, and pregnancy clearly makes females more susceptible. Roberts, Walker, and Alexander have presented an intriguing discussion of gender-related susceptibilities [6].

The relevance of protozoal diseases to occupational medical practitioners, as well as to other providers interested in this subject, should be clear. All workers sent on assignments to other countries, including members of the military and their large contract support staffs, should be cognizant of the cautions needed to avoid these illnesses. A few of them are difficult to treat or come with a high price to pay in terms of toxic side effects and a tendency to recurrence. A virtual army of military and supporting contract workers is now stationed in countries with poorly developed infrastructures. From troops, to travelers, to day-care workers, to food handlers, to veterinarians, to health care personnel, the risk of either transmitting or contracting protozoal infections is ever-present.

The most common and important protozoal infections are discussed in this chapter. Doubtless, more will emerge as environmental changes and organismal adaptation occur, just as they have in the past.

Protozoan Illnesses Spread by Contaminated Food and Water

GIARDIASIS

Of those protozoal infections spread by food and water rather than by vectors, giardiasis is discussed first because it is a common travel illness and easily acquired by individuals who eat from street vendors, drink questionable water, and/or use recreational water facilities in lesser-developed areas of the world. Many countries have substandard water supplies that facilitate easy transmission. *Giardia lamblia* was the first protozoal infection to be shown microscopically by Leeuwenhoek from his own loose stools. It is a relatively simple organism, and few paid little attention to it until 1902, when the American parasitologist Stiles suspected it was associated with diarrhea. This was further observed in 1914–1918 in World War I, when soldiers with diarrhea were found to be passing the typical *Giardia* cysts that caused similar symptoms in laboratory animals. It was not until 1954, however, that Rendtorff produced evidence that definitely linked the organism to human disease. Since then, it is a common subject among travelers and known by various local names. It is not known how many separate species infect humans or if there is any role for reservoir hosts for human infection [7]. *G. duodenalis* (also called *G. intestinalis*) is the most common human intestinal parasite worldwide and is ranked in the top 10 parasites of humans [8].

G. lamblia is a binucleated flagellate that causes intestinal infection in mammals, birds, and amphibians. After its discovery by Leeuwenhoek, it was further studied by Lamblia, who gave it its name. It has been placed in the phylum Sarcomastigophora and class Zoomastigophorea, along with the other flagellated parasites, *Trypanosoma*, *Leishmana*, and *Dientamoeba*. On the basis of a small subunit rRNA, it has been proposed as one of the most primitive eukaryotes described to date. *G. lamblia* (or *G. intestinalis*) more recently has been further divided into several more species on the basis of electron microscopy. As few as 10 cysts can infect humans. Water is the most common form of transmission, followed by food [9].

The organism grows in the human intestine, where, like most other protozoa, it depends on cholesterol it cannot synthesize [10]. In the United States, giardiasis appears to be most prevalent in children younger than 5 years of age and women of childbearing age [11]. The organism is a pear-shaped flagellated organism that can cause a variety of GI complaints. It is spread by fecal-oral contamination, and as a result, the prevalence is highest in population with poor sanitation, close contract, and anal-oral sexual practices. Being resistant to the usual levels of chlorine used to treat water, and being common in mountain streams, it infects people who spend much time backpacking, camping, or hunting unless special precautions are taken. Because of this, in some areas, the illness produced is termed *backpacker's diarrhea* and *beaver fever*. Rarely, patients with giardiasis also present with reactive arthritis of asymmetric synovitis, usually of the lower extremities, and rashes and urticaria also may be present [12].

T-lymphocyte–mediated pathogenesis is common in giardiasis, as well as in a variety of enteropathies, including cryptosporidiosis, bacterial enteritis, celiac disease, food anaphylaxis, and Crohn's disease. In giardiasis, as well as in these other disorders, a diffuse loss of microvillous brush border, combined with villous atrophy, is responsible for disaccharidase insufficiencies and malabsorption of electrolytes, nutrients, and water that ultimately cause diarrheal symptoms. Other mucosal changes may include crypt hyperplasia and increased infiltration of intraepithelial lymphocytes. Recent studies using models of giardiasis have shed new light on the immune regulation of these abnormalities. Studies using an athymic mouse model of infection have found that these epithelial injuries are T-cell-dependent. The loss of brush-border surface area, reduced disaccharidase activities, and increase crypt:villus ratios are mediated by CD8+ T cells, whereas both CD8+ and CD4+ small mesenteric lymph node T cells regulate the influx of intraepithelial lymphocytes. Future investigations need to characterize the CD8+ T-cell signaling cascades that ultimately lead to epithelial injury and malfunction in giardiasis and other malabsorptive disorders of the intestine [8].

Giardiasis may be asymptomatic or may cause either acute or chronic intestinal symptoms. Acute symptoms are the most easily recognized and include diarrhea, abdominal pain, nausea, and weight loss. Some or all of these symptoms occur in 50–70% of individuals who are infected. Chronic infection can cause chronic diarrhea and steatorrhea, with an inordinate amount of malabsorption and weight loss, and severe hypothyroidism can result from chronic infection in patients using thyroid replacement drugs [11]. Diarrhea caused by *Giardia* does not contain blood or cause an increase in polymorphonuclear leukocytes, as would be expected in patients with other dysenteries [13]. The incubation period is from 3–25 days, with a median of 7 days [14]. Recalcitrant cases of irritable bowel syndrome should trigger a check not only for giardiasis but also for other enteropathies of infectious origin [15].

Diagnosis of giardiasis can be made by microscopic examination of stools or by more sophisticated antigen or antibody tests. Giardiasis is usually diagnosed by the identification of cysts or trophozoites in the feces using direct mounts as well as concentration procedures. Because *Giardia* infections can be difficult to diagnose, repeated samplings may be necessary (i.e., several stool specimens over several days). In addition, samples of duodenal fluid or duodenal biopsy may demonstrate trophozoites. Alternate methods for detection include antigen detection tests by enzyme immunoassays and detection of parasites by immunofluorescence [16].

The updated 2007 *Medical Letter* recommendations for giardiasis include metronidazole or tinidazole and some alternatives [17]. The user is urged to consult an authoritative source for the most current treatment recommendations of the diseases considered here because indications and reported side effects may change.

Diagnosis-related online links and treatment resources for protozoal infections are discussed in a separate section below.

AMEBIASIS

In the second century AD, both Galen and Celsus described liver abscesses that were probably amebic. As amebiasis became established in the Middle

Ages in the more developed world as a result of increased travel, there were records of "bloody flux" in Europe, Asia, Persia, and Greece. An authoritative report by William Thomas Councilman and Harry Lafleur, working at Johns Hospital in 1891, represents what was known about amebiasis at the end of the nineteenth century, and much is still valid today [18].

Humans harbor nine species of intestinal amebae, of which only one, *Entamoeba histolytica*, is a pathogen. Initially, *E. histolytica* was thought to be a single species, but it has been subdivided into two morphologically identical species—the pathogenic *E. histolytica* and the nonpathogenic *E. dispar*. Without appropriate clinical suspicion and laboratory examination, the diagnosis easily may be missed, with harmful consequences [19].

E. histolytica is 10–20 μm in length and moves by way of finger-like pseudopods. Spread is via the fecal-oral route, usually by poor hygiene by food workers or by the use of "night soil" (human waste fertilization), as well as by oral-anal sexual practices. Spread is frequent in persons with compromised immune systems. Crowding and poor sanitation contribute to its prevalence in Asia, Africa, and Latin America. It is estimated that 10% of the world's population is infected, but only 10% of them are symptomatic. Of 50 million symptomatic cases each year, up to 100,000 are fatal. It is second (by some reports, third) only to malaria as a leading protozoan cause of death [12].

The life cycle is simple, with the amebae living and multiplying in the gut, forming cysts that are passed in the feces, which infect new hosts when they ingest contaminated food or water. Most infections cause no or minor symptoms, but some strains of *E. histolytica* can invade the gut wall, causing severe ulcerations and dysentery with bloody stools. They may invade damaged blood vessels and, as noted earlier, may accumulate in the liver to create pus-filled cysts. Rarely, the trophozoites may cause a brain abscess [20].

Trophozoites hatch from ingested cysts and, like *Giardia*, pass in the stools and remain viable for weeks in a moist environment. Infection can be mistaken for inflammatory bowel disease. However, as would be expected, steroids given for presumed inflammatory disease only aggravate amebic infections. Treatment always should include a luminal agent to eradicate colonization, prevent spread, and/or reduce the risk of invasive disease. Medical therapy can cure invasive disease, including amebic liver abscesses [21].

About 10% of the world's population is infected with *Entamoeba*, the majority with the noninvasive *E. dispar*. Amebiasis results from infection with *E. histolytica* and is by some accounts the third most common cause of death from parasitic diseases after malaria and shistosomiasis. Most asymptomatic carriers, including homosexual men and AIDS patients, harbor *E. dispar* and have self-limited infections. Of the cases that become symptomatic, colitis develops about 2–6 weeks after ingestion of infective cysts. Cecal involvement may mimic appendicitis. More fulminant infection tends to occur in children. Extraintestinal infections usually are in the liver, and of travelers who develop an amebic abscess after travel, 95% do so within 5 months [22].

Diagnosis can be made by microscopy and commercially available enzyme immunoassay (EIA) kits, and polymerase chain reaction (PCR) tests can differentiate *E. histolytica* and *E. dispar*. These are fully described in a CDC link provided below.

Treatment of intestinal and extraintestinal disease is covered by the updated (2007) *Medical Letter* supplement noted earlier and includes iodoquinol and metronidazole, as well as other options [17].

INFECTION WITH FREE-LIVING AMEBAS

Free-living amebas of the genera *Acanthamoeba*, *Naegleria*, and *Balmamuthia* are found widely throughout the world. They are found in fresh and brackish water, including lakes, hot springs, and inadequately treated swimming pools that allow the protozoa to feed on bacteria and proliferate. Improperly maintained eyewash stations can even post risks. Contact lens cases, domestic tap water, and bottled water all have been implicated as sources. These organisms are also associated with sinusitis and cutaneous lesions in AIDS patients. *Acanthamoeba* species cause granulomatous amebic encephalitis (GAE), whereas the term *primary amebic meningoencephalitis* has been reserved for CNS infections caused by *Naegleria fowleri*. Until recently, these organisms have been regarded as pathogenic but not parasitic, depending on being in the right place at the right time to induce human disease. But now, *Acanthamoeba* and *Naegleria* have been termed *amphizoic organisms* because they have the ability to exist as free-living as well parasitic organisms [23].

The GAE (amebic encephalitis) form is generally found in individuals with underlying diseases such as malignancies, immune system disorders, alcoholism, diabetes, renal failure, and Hodgkin's disease or after organ transplantation. The route of entry may be from a skin wound, via the nose, or from a primary lung site spread through the bloodstream. The GAE form tends to turn chronic and to lead to slow deterioration [21].

The *Naegleria* form of primary amebic meningoencephalitis (PAM) can occur in healthy teenagers and adults owing to contaminated water entering the nose, usually via water being splashed or inhaled. The organism travels along olfactory nerves to the brain, where the amebae cause extensive damage to neural tissue. Diagnosis is difficult, and amebae found in CNS fluid are easily mistaken for white cells. Given the rapid onset, difficulty in diagnosis, and lack of effective treatment, the outcome is usually rapidly fatal, a good reason to avoid swimming in ponds and poorly maintained recreational waters, especially in warmer areas [24].

A severe keratitis is another form of infection by several species of *Acanthamoeba*. Individuals suffering corneal trauma first experienced the condition, but it occurs more commonly in contact lens users when, owing to poor sanitary conditions or practices, amebae proliferate in ophthalmic solutions and are transferred to the eye when the lens is inserted. Although potentially very serious to the eyesight, these infections are usually localized, and CNS spread has not been reported [22]. This should caution all who use prescription and nonprescription eye drops and lens care solutions to be aware of appropriate handling of these preparations. Just as for the intestinal form of amebiasis, the injudicious use of steroids in eye drops can be especially hazardous, so it is essential to establish the diagnosis as soon as possible [25].

For amebic meningoencephalitis from *Naegleria*, the drug recommended by *The Medical Letter* 2007 supplement is parenteral amphotericin B, with a caution that it is not currently an approved Food and Drug Administration (FDA) indication. The same supplement mentions in footnotes that several patients with GAE have been treated successfully with combinations of pentamidine, sulfa-diazine, flucytosine, and either fluconazole or itraconazole (noted in footnotes). Treatment for these conditions is complicated, and consultation with the appropriate specialists is urged in all cases [17].

COCCIDIA AND MICRORSPORIDIA

The Coccidia include three genera—*Cryptospridium*, *Isospora*, and *Cyclospora*. The latter two are of lesser importance in terms of morbidity and mortality. The Microsporidia include the genera *Enterocytozoon* and *Encephalitozoon*, only recently recognized as important agents of disease. Unlike the Coccidia, these organisms are more restricted to the immunocompromised population. Increased incidence and numbers of patients with prolonged diarrhea owing to these forms indicate the need for increased clinical vigilance with regard to prevention, diagnosis, and treatment [26]. Each of these three coccidian infections will be discussed briefly below.

Cryptosporidiosis

The CDC indicates that this coccidian organism is the next most common cause of water-borne travel illness behind giardiasis. Over the past two decades, *crypto* (the term often used for both the organism and the illness) has become recognized as one of the most common causes of water-borne disease (recreational water and drinking water) in humans in the United States. Cryptosporidiosis is a diarrheal disease caused by microscopic protozoa of the genus *Cryptosporidium*. Once an animal or person is infected, the parasite lives in the intestine and passes in the stool. The parasite is protected by an outer shell that allows it to survive outside the body for long periods of time and makes it very resistant to chlorine-based disinfectants.

Probably originally described by Clark in 1895, knowledge of *Cryptosporidium* was greatly expanded by the American parasitologist Tyzzer beginning about 12 years later. The parasite is found in every region of the United States and throughout the world [27].

C. parvum is relatively new on the public health front. In 1993, national attention was focused on an outbreak in Milwaukee that sickened more than 400,000 persons and thousands more in Las Vegas, Nevada. It has quickly become a major threat to HIV-infected persons because conventional water treatment fails to eradicate this organism. Even low doses of organisms are capable of inducing illness even in healthy persons. While dramatic outbreaks have earned the most attention, it is now realized that traditional disease reporting is greatly underestimating the burden of epidemic or endemic diarrheal diseases caused by food and drinking and recreational waters. Cryptosporidiosis has earned a great deal of respect as a potentially serious disease in recent years [28].

In healthy persons, the organism may cause a form of traveler's diarrhea that, while profuse and watery, rarely contains blood or leukocytes. It is commonly associated with temporary weight loss and, on occasion, fever, myalgia, and vomiting. AIDS patients, however, often experience a devastating and prolonged cholera-like illness. Four categories of AIDS-related cryptosporidiosis has been described: a cholera-like illness requiring intravenous rehydration (33%), a chronic diarrheal illness (36%), an intermittent diarrheal illness (15%), and a transient diarrheal illness (15%). However, since the advent of highly active antiretroviral therapy (HAART), the overall morbidity and mortality from cryptosporidiosis and other opportunistic infections have been greatly reduced [29].

The illness has been identified in some infants who present as failure to thrive, and those infected can become seriously malnourished. The spread is by highly environmentally resistant oocysts. This is an example of a recent emerging illness. Prior to 1980, infection with Cryptosporidium was considered rare in animals, and in humans, such infections were thought to be the result of a little-known opportunistic pathogen outside its usual host range. Since 1982, however, these infections have been seen as anything but rare. Fewer than 30 papers existed on the organism prior to 1980, but by 1991 they numbered over 950. While many early infections in rural areas were found to be due to zoonotic transmission from calves, they are now a persistent water-borne hazard. They have been found in urban areas where exposure to animal feces is minimal, and it also has been shown that person-to-person transmission is common [27]. For nonimmunocompromised persons, the drug of choice is nitazoxanide [17].

Cyclosporiasis

Although Cyclospora is a relatively newly described human pathogen, cyclosporiasis is now regarded as a common travel illness (see Table 31-1). Outbreaks in the United States and Canada in 1996 heralded the organism Cyclsporia into notoriety when it was associated with contaminated imported raspberries. A family physician reported the first cases in Ontario, and eventually, imported Guatemalan raspberries were implicated. Strawberries were implicated the following year. This established a source of infection aside from returning travelers [30].

Cyclospora are apicomplexians measuring 8–10 μm in diameter and are seen as nonrefractile spheres on wet-mount microscopic preparations. While relatively newly regarded as a human pathogen, they were first reported in the intestines of moles by Eimer and Schneider; the genus Cyclospora was introduced in 1881. Excreted oocysts are not infective, requiring days to weeks under favorable conditions to sporulate. For this reason, direct person-to-person transmission is not likely because only the sporulates are infectious. C. cayetanensis, the species that infects human, constitutes a significant cause of diarrhea, particularly in immune compromised patients. Both epidemiologic and environmental data have suggested that the organism is water-borne. Like Cryptosporiduim oocyts, Cyclospora are chlorine-resistant but can be removed more easily by filtration because they are larger, almost twice as big as Cryptosporidium oocysts and intermediate in size between C. parvum and Isospora belli. The zoonotic potential for C. cayetanesis is unknown, whereas C. parvum infects virtually all common wild and domestic animals. Fortunately, Cyclospora infections in healthy travelers have mostly responded well to trimethoprim-sulfamethoxazole. Cyclosporiasis should be considered in all cases of protracted or relapsing diarrhea [31].

In a recent study of 10,000 people involved in a total of 50 cruiseship food outbreaks, most outbreaks were of bacterial or viral origin. Cyclosporiasis was the only protozoal infection detected [32].

For both Cryptococcus and Cyclospora infections, diagnosis is by microscopy, EIA, or conventional PCR (see CDC link below).

Isospora Infections

The last coddician infection to be mentioned, parasites of the genus Isospora cause intestinal disease in several mammalian host species. These protozoal parasites have asexual and sexual stages within intestinal cells of their hosts and produce an environmentally resistant cyst stage, the oocyst. Infections are acquired by the ingestion of infective (sporulated) oocysts in contaminated food or water. Some species of mammalian *Isospora* have evolved the ability to use paratenic (transport) hosts. In these cases, infections can be acquired by ingestion of an infected paratenic host.

Human intestinal isosporiasis is caused by *I. belli*. Symptoms of *I. belli* infection in immunocompetent patients include diarrhea, steatorrhea, headache, fever, malaise, abdominal pain, vomiting, dehydration, and weight loss; blood is not usually present in the feces. The disease is often chronic, with parasites present in the feces or biopsy specimens for several months to years. Recurrences are common; symptoms are more severe in AIDS patients, with the diarrhea being more watery. Extraintestinal stages of *I. belli* have been observed in AIDS patients but not immunocompetent patients. Treatment of *I. belli* infection with trimethoprim-sulfamethoxazole usually results in a rapid clinical response, but maintenance therapy is often needed because relapses occur often once treatment is stopped [33].

Microscopic demonstration of the large, typically shaped oocysts is the basis for diagnosis. If stool examinations are negative, examination of duodenal specimens by biopsy or string test (Enterotest) may be needed. The oocysts can be visualized on wet mounts by microscopy with brightfield, differential interference contrast (DIC) and ultraviolet (UV) fluorescence. They also can be stained by modified acid-fast stain [34]. As with cyclosporiasis, trimethoprim-sulfamethoxazole is recommended by *The Medical Letter* [17].

Microsporidial Infections

Probably nothing better demonstrates an example of emerging diseases than micorsporidial infections. These organisms comprise more than 1,200 species, which parasitize a wide variety of invertebrate and vertebrate hosts. These organisms have long been known to be causative agents of economically important diseases in insects (e.g., silk worms and honey bees), fish, and mammals (e.g., rabbits, fur-bearing animals, and laboratory rodents), and they emerged as important opportunistic pathogens when AIDS became pandemic.

Microsporidia are unicellular obligate intracellular eukaryotes. Their life cycle includes a proliferative merogonic stage, followed by a sporogonic stage resulting in characteristically small (1–4 μm), environmentally resistant infective spores. The spores contain a most unique long, coiled tubular extrusion apparatus (*polar tube*), which distinguishes Microsporidia from all other organisms and has a crucial role in host cell invasion: On extrusion from the spore, it injects the sporoplasm along with its nucleus into the cytoplasm of a new host cell after piercing the host cell [27].

Before the onset of the AIDS pandemic, only eight cases of human microsporidial infection had been reported. In most cases, species identification of the causative agents was not conclusive. In 1985, as early as 2 years after identification of the human immunodeficiency virus (HIV) as the causative agent of AIDS, the microsporidial species *Enterocytozoon bieneusi* was discovered in HIV-infected patients with chronic diarrhea. Subsequently, several new genera and species of Microsporidia were found to be important opportunistic pathogens in humans, infecting virtually every organ in the body and a broad spectrum of cell types. Diarrhea is the most usual form of illness.

The most common microsporidial infections in humans are due to *E. bieneusi* and *Encephalitozoon intestinalis*. Both species have been found worldwide, mainly in HIV-infected patients with chronic diarrhea, but also in immunocompetent persons with acute, self-limited diarrhea. Owing to the administration of antiretroviral combination therapy, which restores immunity in HIV-infected persons, the number of clinically manifest microsporidial infections has decreased markedly in affluent countries. However, it is estimated that two-thirds of all HIV-infected persons live in sub-Saharan Africa, where antiretroviral therapy is not widely available owing to the costs, and consequently, opportunistic complications continue to cause severe morbidity and mortality. A recent study showed that 13% of HIV-positive diarrheic adults in Mali were positive for *E. bieneusi*, which thus was the most prevalent intestinal parasite in this African country. Furthermore, microsporidial infections are being diagnosed increasingly in affluent countries in immunosuppressed patients who undergo organ transplantation [27].

Ingestion of microsporidial spores is the most

probable mode of acquisition, and it is assumed that infection is most likely transmitted either directly from human to human via the fecal-oral route or indirectly via water or food. Although some epidemiologic studies indicated the possibility of human-to-human or water-borne infections, convincing epidemiologic results are still lacking. Transmission by the aerosol route also has been considered because spores have been found in the respiratory specimens of patients with *Encephalitozoon* and *E. bieneusi* infection. Patients who have severe cellular immunodeficiency appear to be at highest risk of developing microsporidial disease, but little is known about immunity to microsporidial infection. It is not understood whether microsporidial infection in these patients is primarily a reactivation of latent infection acquired before the state of suppressed immunity or whether microsporidial disease is caused by recently acquired infection. Based on the scarce current epidemiologic knowledge concerning transmission of Microsporidia, recommendations to prevent infections cannot be suggested at present [35].

Light microscopic examination of the stained clinical smears, especially fecal samples, is an inexpensive method of diagnosing microsporidial infections even though it does not allow identification of Microsporidia at the species level. The most widely used staining technique is the chromotrope 2R method or its modifications. This technique stains the spore and the spore wall a bright pinkish red. Often, a beltlike stripe, which also stains pinkish red, is seen in the middle of the spore. This technique, however, is lengthy and time-consuming. The CDC notes that a recently developed "quick-hot gram chromotrope technique," however, cuts down the staining time to less than 10 minutes and provides a good differentiation from the lightly stained background fecal materials so that the spores stand out for easy visualization. The spores stain dark violet, and the beltlike stripe is enhanced. In some cases, dark-staining gram-positive granules are also seen clearly. Chemofluorescent agents such as calcofluor white are also useful in the quick identification of spores in fecal smears. The spores measure from 0.8–1.4 μm in the case of *E. bieneusi* and 1.5–4 μm in *Brachiola algerae, Encephalitozoon* species, *Vittaforma corneae*, and *Nosema* species. Transmission electron microscopy (TEM) is still the "gold standard" and is necessary for identification of the Microsporidia species. However, TEM is expensive, time-consuming, and not feasible for routine diagnosis [36].

Immunofluorescence assays (IFAs) using monoclonal and/or polyclonal antibodies are being developed for identification of Microsporidia in clinical samples. Molecular methods (mainly PCR) are an alternative for the laboratory diagnosis of microsporidiosis. PCR is available only in research laboratories and has been used successfully for identification of *B. algerae, E. bieneusi, E. intestinalis, E. hellem,* and *E. cuniculi.* The principal drawback is that it does not work well on formalin-fixed samples stored for long term [36].

For treatment, *The Medical Letter* recommends albendazole with or without fumagillin depending on the individual type [17].

Vector Protozoan Diseases and Recent Influences

The following section discusses the important vector-borne protozoal diseases (e.g., leishmaniasis, trypanosomiasis, babesiosis, and Chagas' disease) that pose risks to all travelers and occupational groups. Malaria is covered in Chapter 25. Because these diseases are vector-spread, several important global factors influence their spread. In the tropics, the higher population densities, coupled with lack of effective infrastructure, leads to opportunities for vector spread owing to creation of breeding areas in accumulated water in pots, old tires, containers, and open garbage dumps. Deforestation has exposed humans to several infectious hazards, including the *Leishmania* vectors and an "edge effect" in western Africa, where humans occupying newly cleared lands has increased the spread of trypanosomiasis. The effects of increased trade and travel require little explanation, but concerns of such effects as chemical hormone disrupters are again attracting attention. Contamination of groundwater by industrial chemicals has been a concern. Of particular concern is the listing of not only dichlorodiphenyl-trichloroethylene (DDT) but also synthetic pyrethroid insecticides, and endocrine disrupting chemicals, termed EDCs, because they are being used so widely and are found in even the most remote areas. Their effect to suppress immunity, while not clear, is suspect. Even a minimal immunosuppressive effect spread over a very large and susceptible population could be significant and cumulative. Massive changes in travel and trade, changes in human population growth, and significant agricultural changes have made the pathway for human disease easier for a variety of infectious agents [37].

Descriptions of endocrine disruption largely have been associated with wildlife and driven by observations documenting estrogenic, androgenic, antiandrogenic, and antithyroid actions. These actions, in response to exposure to ecologically relevant concentrations of various environmental contaminants, have now been established in numerous vertebrate species. However, many potential mechanisms and endocrine actions have not been studied. For example, DDT and dichlorodiphenyl-dichloroethylene (DDE) are known to also disrupt prostaglandin synthesis in the uteruses of birds, providing part of the explanation for DDT-induced eggshell thinning. Few studies have examined prostaglandin synthesis as a target for endocrine disruption in humans, yet these hormones are active in reproduction, immune responses, and cardiovascular physiology [38]. If immune systems are shown to be consistently weakened by such persistent chemicals even by a very small amount, the public health impact still could prove to be significant, considering the numbers of potentially affected persons.

LEISHMANIASIS

Fortunately for most casual travelers, this vector-spread disease is not contracted nearly as frequently as are the food- and water-borne diseases, and leishmaniasis rarely sits in the limelight of prominent travel-related disease. However, this may be changing. More than 90% of the world's cases of visceral leishmaniasis occur in Bangladesh, northeastern India, Nepal, Sudan, and northeastern Brazil [22]. However, it has been present since antiquity, and while other diseases such as severe acute respiratory syndrome (SARS), HIV infection, and threats of pandemic H5N1 influenza attract the news, leishmaniasis continues as a neglected disease, producing misery and death in the countries where it is endemic, which include southern Europe, northern Africa, the Middle East, Central and South America, and India.

Leishmania species are obligate intracellular parasites in humans and reside in some other mam-

malian hosts. As a vector-spread disease, leishmaniasis is transmitted by mainly *Lutzomyia* in the Americas and by some 70 species of *Phlebotomus* sandflies elsewhere. Untreated visceral leishmaniasis carries a high mortality rate (up to 95%), but even the cutaneous form also can cause death by secondary infection. Drug resistance has become a problem in certain areas of the world, and despite understanding of the *Leishmania* genome, the organism has remained steadfastly vaccine-proof. The reservoirs of the disease are canines and rodents and, in some countries, humans. An amastigote develops into a promastigote in the sandfly's digestive tract and is injected into humans at the next bite [39].

From an historical standpoint, it is Old World leishmaniasis that is the most well known. This is an ancient disease, and there are descriptions of the conspicuous lesions on tablets in the library of King Ashurbanipal from the seventh century BC, some of which are thought to be from cases as early as 2500 BC. The search for the suspected vector was long, and it was not until 1921 that experimental transmission by sandflies was demonstrated by the Sergent brothers. However, the *actual* mode of transmission was not demonstrated until 1941. It was thought for a long time that the New World and Old World, leishmaniasis was one and the same, but in 1911 Vianna found that the parasites in South America were different, and he created a new species, *Leishmania braziliensis.* The vector in the New World is also now known to be a different sandfly of the genus *Lutzomyia.* In the New World, cutaneous and mucocutaneous leishmaniasis cause disfiguring conditions that have been recognized in sculptures since the fifth century and in the writings of Spanish missionaries of the sixteenth century [40]. Cutaneous and mucosal forms in the western hemisphere are typically related to *L. braziliensis* or *L. mexicana,* causing illness having common names of *Espundia* and *Chiclero* ulcer; in the eastern hemisphere, *L. tropiana, L. major,* and *L. aethiopica* are typically found, with common names of the illnesses including *oriental sore, Baghdad boil,* or *Delhi boil.*

Leishmaniasis is endemic in 88 countries. Cases are now being reported in Texas, and it is being seen in soldiers returning from the Middle East wars. Cutaneous leishmaniasis is a parasitic disease occurring throughout the Americas from Texas to Argentina and in the Old World, particularly the Middle East and North Africa. The condition is diagnosed every year in travelers, immigrants, and military personnel. Physicians in the United States must be alert to the diagnosis of leishmaniasis in travelers returning from endemic areas, and physicians working for short periods in endemic areas often must make the diagnosis and should be aware of local disease patterns. When faced with a possible leishmanial skin lesion, a skin scraping with microscopic analysis is the best test. Punch biopsies with tissue-impression smears also can be diagnostic. Needle aspiration of tissue fluid from the margin of a lesion can yield fluid for culture to isolate the organism and identify the species. Immunologic tests are being developed, including a highly sensitive PCR test. Not all patients require treatment; many lesions heal spontaneously. Traditionally used antimonials have a high incidence of toxic (but usually reversible) adverse effects [41].

The form of leishmaniasis termed *visceral leishmaniasis* or *kala azar* (*black disease*) is typically related to *L. donovani*, *L. infantum*, or *L. infantum/chagasi*. It has an incubation period of 3–8 months, and the features include fever, weight loss, hepatosplenomegaly (with the spleen usually being the larger of the two), lymphadenopathy, pancytopenia, and hypergammaglobulinemia. It sometimes is asymptomatic and self-resolving but usually runs an indolent, chronic course and may be fatal without treatment. Leishmania with HIV infection is considered to be an emerging disease in itself and a threat in several countries, according to World Health Organization data. The global experience, mainly in European countries, is marked by an increasing number of co-infection cases in this decade, leading to changes in the epidemiology, presentation, and clinical outcome of visceral leishmaniasis [42].

TRYPANOSOMIASIS

The genus *Trypanosoma* contains many protozoan species. There are three trypanosomal diseases in humans—Chagas' disease caused by *T. cruzi* in the Americas and two subspecies, *T. brucei gambiense* and *T. brucei rhodesiense,* that cause sleeping sickness. African trypanosomiasis, also known as *human African trypanosomiasis* (HAT) and *sleeping sickness,* comes in the two variants—the East African (rhodesiense) and West African (gambi-

ense) forms. While the average worker or tourist is not likely to encounter these diseases, they are too important to ignore given their seriousness and the lack of effective, nontoxic drug therapy.

The major difference between *T. cruzi* and the African forms is that the latter multiply in the bloodstream and perivascular tissues of the host and do not have a corresponding intracellular form. The annual incidence is about 300,000 cases that occur in a broad belt across the middle third of Central and West Africa. In the United States, cases are rare and have usually been seen in tourists who have visited African game parks [43].

Currently, the sleeping sickness diseases (e.g., HAT) occur in 36 countries in sub-Saharan Africa with some 60 million persons being at risk for it. After a decrease in cases from 1949–1965, wars and social unrest have diverted critical public health resources for its control. Adding to the problem are population movements, increasing drug resistance, changes in climate and vegetation, and the movements of animal reservoirs that have resulted in a resurgence of these diseases. In both types of trypanosomiases, the tsetse fly of the genus *Glossina* is the vector, with infected cattle and wild and domesticated animals acting as the reservoirs. The two forms are different in clinical presentation in that the rhodesiense form is more acute, and the gambiense form more chronic. In either case, there is an early hemolymphatic and late CNS stage, the latter with progressive degenerative signs and symptoms ending in coma, seizures, and systemic organ failure if untreated. Diagnosis is done in the earlier stage by demonstration of the parasites on blood films, but in the gambiense type, parasitemia is not continuous, and the difficulty of diagnosis by this method can contribute to the chronicity of the disease [44].

The characteristic sleep patterns in HAT are daytime somnolence and nighttime insomnia, but other symptoms also occur that do not differentiate the diseases from other CNS infections. The coexistence of other tropical diseases complicates diagnosis. Malarial drugs may improve symptoms initially but only delay and worsen the final outcome. A dilemma is that it is critical to start treatment as soon as it is needed, but treatments using arsenicals are themselves toxic, with a risk of posttreatment encephalopathy developing in about 10% of patients and with a case-fatality rate of about 50%

(this is a particular problem with melarsoprol; not all morbidity and mortality are from the drug itself but from cytokines, endotoxins, and antigens released as a result of the death of the parasites, among other possible causes). Better diagnostic and therapeutic regimens are needed for these diseases. While blood smears often may detect the rhodesiense form, an antibody test is in frequent use for the gambiense form [22].

For the hemolymphatic stage of the West African type, *The Medical Letter* recommends pentamidine and suramin. For late disease with CNS involvement, eflornithine and melarsoprol are recommended. In the East African form, suramin for the hemolymphatic stage and melarsoprol for CNS involvement are recommended [17].

CHAGAS' DISEASE

This disease, called *American trypanosomiasis,* is caused by the protozoa *T. cruzi.* This disease and the organisms that cause sleeping sickness are the only members of the genus that cause human disease. Chagas' disease is spread by the bite of reduvid bugs, called *kissing bugs* because they tend to bite around the face and lips. *T. cruzi* is found only in the Americas, usually from the vector that inhabits primitive wood, stone, and adobe houses. Human infection is primarily a problem in rural areas of Mexico, Central, and South America. An indurated "chagoma" often appears at the site of the bite. Characteristic pseudocysts accumulate in infected tissues, which are aggregates of multiplying parasites, and the first sign of disease is usually in a week after exposure. A classic Romano's sign may appear which is a unilateral painless periorbital edema with regional lymphadenopathy. Spread by blood transfusions has been a serious problem in some countries. In the minority of persons with chronic *T. cruzi* infections that develop related clinical manifestations, the heart is the organ most commonly and seriously affected, with conduction abnormalities and cardiomyopathy predominating. Chagas' disease of the esophagus and colon also may occur, creating varying degrees of dilatation [22].

Generalized lymphadenopathy and hepatosplenomegaly may develop, but most deaths are from heart failure. Much progress in control of the disease has been made in South America, especially the southern "cone" nations. Brain abscesses have developed in immunocompetent persons. Cur-

rently, it is estimated that 16–18 million people are infected with *T. cruzi* and that 45,000 deaths occur yearly, making it the most important parasitic disease burden in Latin America. Chronic Chagas' disease is diagnosed by antigen tests, of which some 20 commercial test kits are available. Detection of the parasite is not of absolute importance. The tests available have varying degrees of sensitivity and specificity, but PCR tests have not been shown to be better than other serologic tests, and none of the PCR tests are available commercially [36].

The Medical Letter recommends nifurtimox or benznidazole for Chagas' disease [17].

BABESIOSIS

Another vector-spread emerging disease that has been reported with increasing frequency in the United States is babesiosis, which often produces a malarial-like illness with similar fevers and chills. In the past decade, more cases of babesiosis in humans have been reported, especially in the northeastern United States. *Babesia microti* (in the United States) and bovine strains (in Europe) cause most infections in humans. Like malarial parasites, the parasites of babesiosis are intraerythrocytic and are commonly called *piroplasms* owing to the pear-shaped forms found within infected red blood cells. The spectrum of disease manifestation is broad, ranging from a silent infection to a fulminant disease not unlike the *falciparum* form of malaria, resulting in severe hemolysis and occasionally in death [45].

Most cases are tick-borne, although cases of transfusion-associated and transplacental or perinatal transmission also have been reported. Factors associated with more severe disease include advanced age, previous splenectomy, and immunodeficient states. Symptoms include high fever, chills, diaphoresis, weakness, anorexia, and headache. Later in the course of the illness, the patient may develop jaundice. Congestive heart failure, renal failure, and acute respiratory distress syndrome are the most common complications [46].

Babesia and its close relatives are members of a group of organisms called *piroplasms,* a name that comes from their pear-shaped outlines. Long associated with blood diseases of cattle and other mammals, members of the genus *Babesia* have been recognized since the 1950s as infectious agents in humans. Species of this protozoan blood parasite that have been isolated routinely from mice (*B. microti*) or cattle (*B. divergens*) also have been isolated from humans. In addition to these familiar species, new isolates that resist being placed in existing taxonomic categories are the basis for rethinking their phylogenetic relationships based on sequencing data. The parasite represents a threat to the safety of the blood supply in that blood from asymptomatic humans can transmit *Babesia* to blood recipients [47].

It is important for physicians to consider babesiosis when patients present with influenza-like symptoms and, instead of recovering in the usual time, go on to develop malarial-like fevers. Early, accurate diagnosis allows treatment that may help to prevent significant morbidity and possible mortality. Because 24–48 hours of attachment to the host is required for infection to occur, early tick removal can help to prevent disease. In patients with clinical findings suggestive of tick-borne disease, treatment should not be delayed for laboratory confirmation. The same tick may harbor different infectious pathogens and transmit several with one bite. Advising patients about prevention of tick bites, especially in the spring and summer months, may help to prevent exposure to dangerous vector-borne diseases [48]. Despite the superficial resemblance of babesiosis to malaria, these piroplasms do not respond to chloroquine or other similar drugs. However, the treatment of babesiosis using a clindamycin-quinine combination has been successful [49]. The most current *Medical Letter* recommendations are for clindamycin plus quinine or atovaquone plus azithromycin [17].

Trichomonas Infections

The sexually transmitted protozoal infection trichomoniasis is caused by the protozoal organism *Trichomonas vaginalis,* an organism about 9 by 7 μm in size; nondividing organisms have four anterior flagella. Unique energy-producing organelles, the hydrogenosomes, are evident as chromatic granules by light microscopy. Despite being readily diagnosed, being a treatable cause of sexually transmitted disease (STD), and being, in fact, the most common of these diseases, it is not a reportable disease. The incidence far surpasses that of *Chlamydia* and gonorrhea, with prevalence in inner-city STD clinics approaching 25%. Disease is transmitted by coitus and caused solely by a trophozoites stage, with no cyst stage being known. Humans are the only natural host. The World Health Organization estimates that this infection accounts for almost half of all curable infections worldwide [50].

Symptomatic women typically complain of vaginal discharge, pruritus, and irritation. Signs include vaginal discharge and odor with edema or erythema. Colpitis macularis (strawberry cervix) is a specific sign but is detected reliably only by colposcopy and rarely by routine examination. Nearly half the infected women are asymptomatic and thus, if not screened, will have a missed diagnosis. The spectrum of disease in males is less well characterized but also is often asymptomatic or an underlying cause of nongonococcal urethritis [50].

The most common means of diagnosis is by visualization of the motile *Trichomonas* in a saline preparation of vaginal fluid, but the test has limited sensitivity, ranging from 60–75%. Accompanying white blood cells in the fluid are often present. A Diamond's culture medium for inoculation is available, and newer tests using antigen detection have been licensed. In males, PCR appears to have far greater sensitivity. Long considered to be the cause of a minor STD with few complications, the organism has been implicated as a cause of preterm delivery in several studies [50].

Treatment traditionally has been with metronidazole, although reports of drug resistance are beginning to appear [51]. *The Medical Letter* recommends metronidazole or tinidazole for treatment [17].

Resources for Further Diagnostic and Therapeutic Information

Some excellent diagnostic and therapy information for these and other parasitic infections can be found at the CDC's designated parasitic diseases website [36]. The CDC also gives links to *The Medical Letter* for treatment of parasitic infections on pages that discuss diagnosis and treatment, as noted in the section on amebiasis [36]. The most recent treatment guidelines from the 2007 *Medical Letter* supplement on parasitic diseases is available in both handbook and downloadable formats. As noted earlier, these or some equally reliable sources should be consulted before instituting treatment because indications and side effects may change.

General Occupational Health Considerations

The vast array of occupational jobs, worksites, and exposure opportunities calls for caution for all workers involved in activities that pose risks for protozoal infections. Occupations at risk include day-care workers [52], health care workers [53], veterinarians and their staffs [54], crews on ships and airplanes (vehicles that may carry vectors), food service workers, travelers, workers residing in endemic areas, and persons working with human or animal wastes or in waters that are contaminated by such wastes [55]. Anyone with an immune deficiency or prior splenectomy should be aware of the increased risk of these infections (e.g., babesiosis, which is usually a mild disease, can be fatal in such patients [56]). The usual approach to worker safety for those working directly with these infectious agents, including first substitution of safer alternatives, administrative controls, and personal protective equipment (PPE), is no different in principle from that in other settings, such as for health care workers in general who face the continual risk of fecal contact and blood and airborne droplet-related diseases. Protection of travelers and residents in endemic areas is often a challenge. Some approaches and precautions are covered in more detail in Chapter 27.

The group of parasitic diseases discussed herein is by far the most important of those likely to be encountered by workers and travelers. A number of other protozoal diseases are still emerging or have not reached the level of concern as those in this chapter. Two very good reviews of parasitic diseases, the previously mentioned history of parasitic diseases by Cox [40] and an excellent book by Giles [57] on protozoal diseases, should prove rewarding as a starting point for any health care providers interested in pursuing further knowledge of these interesting and challenging diseases.

References

1. Talman AM et al. Gametocytogenesis: The puberty of *Plasmodium falciparum*. *Malar J* 2004;14:24.
2. Goodgame R. Understanding intestinal spore-forming protozoa: Cryptosporia, Microsporidia, *Isospora,* and *Cyclospora. Ann Intern Med* 1996;24: 429–41.
3. Bansal D, Singh B, Seghal R. Role of cholesterol in parasitic infections. *Lipids Health Dis* 2005;4:10.
4. Wolfe MS. Eosinophilia in the returning traveler. *Med Clin North Am* 1999;83:1019–32, vii.
5. Graczyk TK, Knight R, Tamang L. Mechanical transmission of human protozoan parasites by insects. *Clin Microbiol Rev* 2005;18:128–32.
6. Roberts C, Walker W, Alexander, J. Sex-associated hormones and immunity to protozoal diseases. *Clin Microbiol Rev* 2001;14:476–88.
7. Cox, FEG. History of human parasitology. *Clin Microbiol Rev* 2002;15:595–612.
8. Buret AG. Immunopathology of giardiasis: The role of lymphocytes in intestinal epithelial injury and malfunction. *Mem Inst Osweldo Cruz* 2005;100:185–90.
9. Adam R. The biology of *Giardia* spp. *Microbiol Rev* 1991;55:706–32.
10. Lujan HD, Mowatt MR, Byrd LC, et al. Cholesterol starvation induces differentiation of the intestinal parasite *Giardia lamblia. Proc Natl Acad Sci USA* 1996;93:7628–33.
11. Mahmoud AA. "New" intestinal parasitic protozoa. In Krausen RM (ed), *Emerging Infections.* San Diego: Academic Press, 1998.
12. Kucik C, Martin G, Sortor B. Common intestinal parasites. *J Fam Pract* 2004;69:1161–8.
13. Lindsay JA. Chronic sequelae of foodborne disease. *Emerg Infect Dis* 1997;3:443–52.
14. Outbreaks of cyclosporiasis—United States, 1997. *MMWR* 1997;46:451–2.
15. Stark D, van Hal S, Marriott D, et al. Irritable bowel syndrome: A review on the role of intestinal protozoa and the importance of their detection and diagnosis. *Int J Parasitol* 2007;37:11–20.
16. Centers for Disease Control and Prevention (CDC), www.dpd.cdc.gov/dpdx/HTML/Diagnostic Procedures.htm.
17. *The Medical Letter* 2007;5(suppl):1–15.
18. Councilman WT, Lafleur HA. Amebic dysentery. *Johns Hopkins Hosp Rep* 1891;2:395–548.
19. Hal S, et al. Amebiasis: Current status in Australia. *Med J Aust* 2007;187:412–6.
20. Morishita A, Yamamoto H, Aihara H. A case of amebic brain abscess. *No Shinkei Geka.* 2007;35:919–25.
21. van Hal SJ, Stark DJ, Fotedar R, et al. Amoebiasis: Current status in Australia. *Med J Aust* 2007;186: 412–6.
22. Kasper D, Fauci A, Longo D, et al (eds). *Harrison's Principles of Internal Medicine,* 16th Ed. New York: McGraw-Hill, 2005.
23. Marciano-Cabral F, Cabral G. *Acanthamoeba* spp. as agents of disease in humans. *Clin Microbiol Rev* 2003;16:273–307.
24. Schuster F. Cultivation of pathogenic and opportunistic free-living amebas. *Clin Microbiol Rev* 2002; 15:342–54.
25. McClellan K, Howard K, Niederkorn JY, Alizadeh H. Effect of steroids on *Acanthamoeba* cysts and trophozoites. *Invest Ophthalmol Vis Sci* 2001;42: 2885–93.
26. Collins R. Protozoan parasites of the intestinal tract:

A review of Coccidia and Microsporida. *J Am Osteopath Assoc* 1997;10:593.

27. Current W, Garcia L. Cryptosporidiosis. *Clin Microbiol Rev* 1991;4:325–58.

28. Gostin L, Lazzarini Z, Neslund V, Osterholm M. Water quality laws and waterborne diseases: *Cryptosporidium* and other emerging pathogens. *Am J Pub Health* 2000;90:847–53.

29. Clark D. New insights into human cryptosporidiosis. *Clin Microbiol Rev* 1999;12:554–63.

30. Manuel DG, et al. An outbreak of cyclosporiasis in 1996 associated with consumption of fresh berries—Ontario. *Can J Infect Dis* 1997;11:86–92.

31. Yazar S, Yalcin S, Shahin Y. Human cyclosporiasis in Turkey. *World J Gastroenterol* 2004;10:1884–7.

32. Rooney R, et al. A review of outbreaks of foodborne disease associated with passenger ships: Evidence for risk management. *Public Health Reps* 2004;119: 427–34.

33. Lindsay DS, Dubey JP, Blagburn BL. Biology of *Isospora* spp. from humans, nonhuman primates, and domestic animals. *Clin Microbiol Rev* 1997;10:19–34.

34. Centers fro Disease Control and Prevention (CDC), www.dpd.cdc.gov/dpdx/HTML/Isosporiasis.htm.

35. Mathis A, Weber R, Deplazes, P. Zoonotic potential of the Microsporidia. *Clin Microbiol Rev* 2005;18: 423–45.

36. www.dpd.cdc.gov/dpdx/Default.htm.

37. Porter WP, Jaeger JW, Carlson IH. Endocrine, immune, and behavioral effects of aldicarb (carbamate), atrazine (triazine) and nitrate (fertilizers) mixtures at groundwater concentrations. *Toxicol Ind Health* 1999;15:133–50.

38. Guillette L. Endocrine disrupting contaminants: Beyond the dogma. *Environ Health Perspect* 2006;114: 9–12S.

39. Piscopo T, Azzopardi. Leishmaniasis: Review. *Postgrad Med J* 2006;82:649–57.

40. Cox F. History of human parasitology. *Clin Microbiol Rev* 2002;15:595–612.

41. Markle WH, Makhoul K. Cutaneous leishmaniasis: Recognition and treatment. *Am Fam Physician* 2004;69:1455–60.

42. Ada R, et al. Microscopy and polymerase chain reaction detection of *Leishmania chagasi* in the pleural and ascitic fluid of a patient with AIDS: Case report and review of diagnosis and therapy of visceral leishmaniasis. *Can J Infect Dis Med Microbiol* 2004; 15:231–4.

43. Wallace R, Kohatsu N, Last J (eds). *Maxey-Rosenau-Last Public Health & Preventive Medicine*, 15th Ed. New York: McGraw-Hill, 2008.

44. Kennedy K. Human African trypanosomiasis of the CNS: Current issues and challenges. *J Clin Invest* 2004;113:496–504.

45. Homer MJ, et al. Babesiosis. *Clin Microbiol Rev* 2000;13:451–69

46. Mylonakis E. When to suspect and how to monitor babesiosis. *Am Fam Physician* 2001;63:1969–74.

47. Schuster FL. Cultivation of *Babesia* and *Babesia*-like blood parasites: Agents of an emerging zoonotic disease. *Clin Microbiol Rev* 2002;3:365–73.

48. Bratton RL, Corey R. Tick-borne disease. *Am Fam Physician* 2005;71:2323–30.

49. Weiss LM. Babesiosis in humans: A treatment review. *Exp Opin Pharmacother* 2002;3:1109–15.

50. Schwebke J, Burgess D. Trichomoniasis. *Clin Microbiol Rev* 2004;17:794–803.

51. Cudmore SL, Delgaty KL, Hayward-McClelland ST, et al. Treatment of infections caused by metronidazole-resistant Trichomonas vaginalis. *Clin Microbiol Rev* 2004;17:783–93.

52. DuPont HL, Chappell CL. The infectivity of *Cryptosporidium parvum* in healthy volunteers. *N Engl J Med* 1995;332:855–9.

53. Guerrant RL. Cryptosporidiosis: An emerging, highly infectious threat. *Emerg Infect Dis* 1997;3:51–7.

54. Schnurrenberger PR, Grigor JK, Walker JF, Martin RJ. The zoonosis-prone veterinarian. *J Am Vet Med Assoc* 1978;173:373–6.

55. Dutkiewicz J, Jablonski L, Olenchock SA. Occupational biohazards: A review. *Am J Ind Med* 1988;14: 605–23.

56. Cunha BA, Nausheen S, Szalda D. Pulmonary complications of babesiosis: Case report and literature review. *Eur J Clin Microbiol Infect Dis* 2007;26:505–8.

57. Giles H. *Protozoal Diseases*. London: Arnold, 1999.

32

Fungal Travel-Related Infections

Robert S. Rhodes

Fungal and other related diseases, until recently, were not considered important or significant health problems in the United States and other highly developed Western nations with advanced public health systems. Many studies reporting results of investigations of health problems in travelers did not include fungal diseases. In a 1996 study of 10,000 Swiss travelers, fungal diseases were not mentioned as a cause of significant health problems [1]. Travel publications, including those put out by the Centers for Disease Control and Prevention (CDC), private publishers, and the World Health Organization (WHO), made only passing reference to fungal skin infections of the feet [2–4]. By the end of the second millennium and the beginning of the third, this had begun to change. Endemic and opportunistic fungal infections have grown in incidence and importance internationally [5–7].

The expanding globalization of business and industry in recent years has brought with it significant concerns for business travelers and their families about a variety of health issues. Fungal infections and fungus-related diseases, as well as other health problems, must be included as concerns for the business traveler. The key to managing travel-related health problems is prevention, which requires a thorough understanding of the diseases that may cause these problems. Fungal and mold-related health problems, including those associated with both systemic and other mycoses, are addressed in this chapter [5, 8, 9].

Occupational medicine specialists and other occupational health professionals must become cognizant of implications for all traveling individuals for whom they may be called on to provide counsel and services in diverse parts of the world. They must use demonstrated successful methods to keep employees and their families healthy.

Concerns with skin and respiratory problems related to fungal agents or their spores vary significantly from the deserts of Mongolia to the villages and cities of China, the jungles of Central and West Africa, and the island nations of the Pacific. These concerns also vary significantly among the countries of South and Central America, Southeast Asia, Australia, and the various American states. The needs of specific individuals and their family members also vary depending on many factors, including current health status, potential predisposition to certain types of health problems, immune status, environmental considerations, personal habits, and recreational factors.

This chapter provides a global focus that stresses recognition of the increased volume and mix of travelers at risk. It is not intended to provide in-depth, comprehensive coverage of all fungal diseases. Many excellent resources cover these areas.

Work-related fungal respiratory infections are covered in Chapter 13 of this textbook. This chapter discussion is divided into systemic mycotic infections and superficial mycoses.

Epidemiology

Fungal pathogens are outnumbered by their bacterial, viral, and parasitic counterparts as primary etiologic agents producing infections. Despite this, they continue to be responsible for an increasing number of emerging infectious diseases. At present, individuals with suppressed immune function, such as acquired immune deficiency syndrome (AIDS) and transplant recipients, represent increasingly large numbers of persons worldwide who are becoming infected with fungal agents [5–16]. A growing number of these are nosocomial (hospital-acquired) infections. Worldwide, significant isolated outbreaks of various fungal diseases continue to occur in persons with normal immune systems. Increasing numbers of travelers, including many in business, along with their family members, fall into some of these risk categories or behave, through their recreational and other activities, in ways that bring them in contact with agents that put them at risk [7, 9, 17, 18].

During the 20-year period between 1985 and 2005, the U.S. National Institute of Allergy and Infectious Diseases more than quadrupled its funding of studies of mycoses. The actual funding increased from about $6.5 million in 1985 to almost $30 million annually from 1995–2005 [18]. In 2000, a working group sponsored by the institute recommended targeted investment in (1) diagnostic/awareness, with particular emphasis on aspergillosis, enabling improved therapeutic development, (2) basic science, blending genomics, pathogenesis, and target discovery, (3) clinical infrastructure, (4) development of animal models for studying the complexity of opportunistic fungal diseases, and (5) development of in vitro susceptibility tests to better correlate with in vivo activity in the host [19, 20].

In a U.S. nationwide hospital survey, fungal-related disorders were found to be responsible for approximately 10.4% of nosocomial infections, 5.1% of surgical wound infections, 5.7% of lung infections, 18.7% of urinary tract infections, and 9.9% of all bloodstream infections [21]. A study of 814 heart transplant recipients revealed that 12% developed fungal or protozoal infections. Patients with invasive fungal infections had a 36% fatality rate, nearly three times higher than that for bacterial or viral infections (13%) [22].

Many fungi found on the skin or in the environment rarely cause infections except in individuals who are compromised immunologically (e.g., *Aspergillus* among individuals receiving bone marrow transplants). One study reported that some 20% of 275 such individuals had developed nosocomial pneumonia secondary to *Aspergillus* and had a 95% fatality rate [23].

Pneumocystis jiroveci pneumonia (previously called *Pneumocystis carinii* pneumonia) is caused by an organism of changing taxonomy, the organism's classification being a point of continuing debate. It is classified as a fungus but shares biologic aspects with protozoa. It has been the most frequently recognized opportunistic infection in patients with AIDS, presenting as the AIDS-defining illness in about half these patients. However, fungal infections are increasingly being seen as the presenting infection in these patients [24].

Disease-causing fungi are characterized as either primary or opportunistic pathogens. Primary pathogens can, but do not always, cause disease in healthy people. Opportunistic pathogens, on the other hand, generally are harmless to healthy persons, causing serious disease only in people whose immune systems have been weakened or suppressed. The most common primary pathogens include *Coccidioides immitis*, *Histoplasma capsulatum*, *Sporothrix schenckii*, and *Blastomyces dermatitidis*. Opportunistic pathogens include *Candida* species, *Cryptococcus neoformans*, *Aspergillus* species, *Penicillium marneffei*, and *Trichosporon beigelii* [15, 16].

Most systemic fungal diseases are not transmitted from person to person. These disorders are usually acquired by individuals coming in contact with the fungal spores through inhalation when they are aerosolized and scattered from the soil or other habitats (e.g., in dust). Some opportunistic fungi, however, are normally present on human skin and in the gastrointestinal tract and therefore present the potential for person-to-person transmission, particularly in hospital settings.

On a global basis, there are numerous reports from medical centers worldwide of increasing occurrence of fungal infections. These involve a variety of cases, mostly in individuals with suppressed immune systems. Increasingly, however, there are many instances in which a fungal infection of a serious nature—life threatening or fatal—occurs when this is not the case. On the other hand, there are also frequent reports of fungal infections caused by organisms not usually associated with fungal infections [25, 26].

Worldwide, the most common systemic fungal diseases in the noncompromised individual are blastomycosis, coccidioidomycosis, and histoplasmosis; also common but to a lesser extent, primarily in the immunocompromised, are infections caused by C. albicans or S. schenckii. Until recently, these latter two have been more often associated with localized infections of the skin and mucous membranes [27–30]. A 2-year study involving over 13,000 transplant patients in 19 U.S. centers, reported in 2004, revealed that yeasts (mainly Candida species) were still the most frequent cause of invasive fungal infection. Aspergillus species were the predominant molds. Agents of zygomycosis and fusariosis followed these. Solid-organ transplant patients were more likely to develop candidiasis, and stem cell transplant recipients were at higher risk for infection by opportunistic molds [31].

Patients with invasive mold infections may acquire their infections in the hospital or in the community from different sources, particularly air and water. Opportunistic molds, including Aspergillus species and Fusarium species, are present in the air, hospital water, and water-related surfaces. Hospital water should be considered a potential source of nosocomial invasive mold infections [32–34]. Other potential sources of pathogenic fungi include the probiotic Ultralevura (a formulation of Saccharomyces boulardii) used for the treatment and prevention of Clostridium difficile–associated diarrhea [35], contaminated commercially bottled mineral water [36], and the synthetic fiber overalls worn by medical personnel [37].

The most common fungal diseases occurring among travelers are those associated with skin and nail disorders. Systemic infections occur much less often but are being reported more frequently as individuals at risk become better able to travel because of improved medical management of immunocompromised and related disorders.

As noted in the preceding paragraphs, Candida and Aspergillus species are significant, primarily causing skin problems and, in some instances, allergic phenomena, in the intact individual, but they rarely produce invasive disease in the absence of some type of preinjury (as a secondary contaminant) or in persons with a defect in their immune response.

SYSTEMIC MYCOTIC INFECTIONS

Coccidioidomycosis, blastomycosis, and histoplasmosis share a number of characteristics in their production of systemic mycotic infections. In countries where they are found, they all occur in relatively circumscribed geographic areas. Usually, their spores are present in soil, and aerosolization of this dry soil and their spores in moist areas makes the respiratory tract their usual route of entry. These organisms are dimorphic and exist in their natural state as mold/mycelium bearing infectious spores, which in the host evolve into yeastlike organisms that are pathogenic to tissue. The common route of entry is, as noted, the respiratory tract, although there have been reported cases with no obvious respiratory involvement, the initial lesion being present in deep soft tissue wounds or internal organs other than the lungs. The most common characteristic of these infections is production of a granulomatous inflammatory response. These disorders all share manifestations and pathologic features that are similar to those of other granulomatous disorders such as tuberculosis and are frequently misdiagnosed initially as tuberculosis infection. Individuals with intact or normal cell-mediated immune response only rarely develop clinical findings or overt evidence of clinical infection. The disease is often contained and consists of focal or localized suppurative granulomatous lesions. These infections tend to be of greatest danger in individuals with poor immune response. In these persons, the disseminated disease occurs very readily. In most individuals who contract systemic blastomycosis, coccidioidomycosis, histoplasmosis, or involvement by Aspergillus or, rarely, C. albicans, the most common route of entry is the respiratory tract [10, 28, 30–38].

Coccidioidomycosis

Coccidioidomycosis, also known as San Joaquin Valley fever, desert fever, and desert bumps, is caused by C. immitis. This dimorphic organism's natural habitat is desert soil and geologic and climatic areas with semiarid conditions and moderate rainfall. It occurs in California's San Joaquin Valley, southern Arizona, Utah, New Mexico, Nevada, southwestern Texas, areas of Mexico near the U.S. border, and Central and South America. The dust containing the spores can be airborne and thus transported many miles from areas in which it is usually endemic. Individuals handling such things as packages or other items containing the dust can be affected. Dust storms may carry the organism's spores many hundreds of miles from endemic areas. There is an increased incidence of this disorder associated with the rising incidence of AIDS and other immunocompromising disorders. Human-to-human transmission is not thought to occur. The disease's highest prevalence is in field and construction workers.

The health care systems in California and other southwestern states have begun to require reporting of coccidioidomycosis infections. During the 1980s, fewer than 500 cases of coccidioidomycosis were reported in the state of California each year. In 1991, that number jumped to 1,200. The following 2 years saw an even greater increase, with 4,516 and 4,137 cases reported in 1992 and 1993, respectively [38, 39]. In 2005, this number was 1,505 cases [40].

Blastomycosis

Blastomycosis is a systemic mycotic infection caused by the fungus *B. dermatitidis*. This disease is endemic in the southeastern and central portions of the United States and along some sections of the Mississippi and Ohio River valleys, as well as in central Canada, with the central United States being the most heavily endemic area in the world. It is also seen in Central America and many African nations. There has been no major effort at mapping this zone using large skin testing groups, as was done with histoplasmosis. Distribution plotting has been based on individual case findings and case reports. In other parts of the world, scattered cases of infection in individuals who have never traveled to one of the endemic areas are reported. Blastomycosis occurs in persons of all ages but most often in young and middle-aged adults. Individuals who work outdoors or participate in extensive outdoor recreation are in the greatest danger of contracting this infection. Its natural habitat is moist soil, particularly near waterways where there are large

amounts of organic matter, especially animal excreta [41]. Infection generally occurs after inhalation of the organism's conidia, which have become airborne as a result of disturbance of soil or the materials containing the organism. The incubation period is approximately 45 days. There have been significant problems in developing a sensitive and specific skin-test antigen, thus making it difficult to do accurate mapping of subclinical disease occurrences. The absence of acceptable immunologic markers of remote subclinical disease means that the size of the subclinical case "iceberg" remains uncertain relative to clinically apparent and diagnosed pulmonary and extrapulmonary cases [10, 28–30, 41–44].

Histoplasmosis

Histoplasmosis, also called *Darling's disease* and *reticuloendotheliosis,* is caused by the dimorphic fungus *H. capsulatum.* This agent is found worldwide in soil, particularly soil that is contaminated by droppings from starlings, chickens, other birds, and bats. There are endemic areas in various parts of the world. The greatest endemicity in the United States occurs in the eastern parts of the country, the Ohio and Mississippi River valleys, and Virginia and Maryland. Histoplasmosis is also endemic in other areas of North America and throughout Latin America. There are reported outbreaks of histoplasmosis particularly in those areas contaminated with droppings from birds and bats. Several incidents have involved outbreaks among cave explorers in bat-infested caves; there also has been a widespread epidemic involving over 100,000 persons in Indianapolis, Indiana, that was associated with construction. In Japan, *H. capsulatum* has rarely been isolated from the natural environment. Prior to 1993, only seven cases of histoplasmosis had been reported in Japan, and these included cases that were contracted in foreign countries. In 1994, histoplasmosis was diagnosed in a group of eight Japanese travelers who had been exposed to bat guano while exploring a cave in Manaus, Brazil, in March 1993. All eight had developed respiratory symptoms about 12–20 days after exposure. The total length of time in the cave for the eight persons was approximately 2 hours, and seven of the eight developed abnormal symptoms, whereas five also developed nodular pulmonary infiltrates. All had serologic evidence of histoplasmosis. Travelers therefore should be aware of the significant threat of histoplasmosis infection when exploring bat-inhabited caves in any part of the world. Persons particularly at risk are those who vacation or work in areas such as caves, forests, or buildings heavily populated by birds and bats. This disease is seen frequently in farmers and construction workers. It is contacted by inhalation. Infection is usually of the lung and is preventable [18, 27, 29, 43, 45, 46].

Sporotrichosis

Sporotrichosis is the fourth of the invasive endemic fungal infections and is caused by the agent *S. schenckii*. This dimorphic fungus is found worldwide in soil and decaying vegetation such as sphagnum moss, rose thorns, old rotted wood, and garden soils. It most often enters the body through direct contact with the skin, usually after having been inoculated into the lymphatic system following penetration by wood splinters or other similar woody substances, such as rose thorns containing the spores. This then produces the infection sporotrichosis. This systemic mycotic infection differs from coccidioidomycosis, blastomycosis, and histoplasmosis in that it is much wider in international distribution. Although it may infect other organs of the body, it occurs most commonly as a granulomatous skin infection in nonimmunocompromised individuals [47–49].

NONENDEMIC FUNGAL INFECTIONS

Almost all the nonendemic fungal infections are opportunistic infections that occur primarily in individuals with compromised immune systems. A number of fungal infections are seen in susceptible individuals at risk, and travelers are no exception. In over two-thirds of human immunodeficiency virus (HIV)–infected individuals with clinical disease, some type of pulmonary disorder is present. Fungal infections play a key role in producing infections in this group [50].

Opportunistic disorders include such conditions as aspergillosis, producing nonclostridial necrotizing soft tissue infections with gangrenous necrosis of the skin and associated tissue. Other opportunistic infections, caused by organisms such as the dimorphic fungus *Penicillium marneffei*, also have been reported. This organism has emerged as a significant agent particularly among patients with immunodeficiencies in Southeast Asia and is also

being seen in individuals who have traveled to this region as well as those who reside there. *P. marneffei* infection clinically may resemble tuberculosis, *Moluscum contageosum*, cryptococcosis, or histoplasmosis. This infection is also reported in increasing numbers of patients in southern China and the Middle East. *P. marneffei* infection causes a disseminated progressive disease and is the third most common opportunistic infection in HIV-infected patients in the reported areas [51–53].

Scytalidium dimidiatum and *Lecythophora hoffmannii* are also rare agents reported in recent years as involved in a number of infections in immunocompromised individuals in Australia and other countries. These pathogens have caused such disorders as chronic sinusitis, common skin lesions, lymphangitis, and lymphadenitis [26].

Scedosporium prolificans has been involved in cases of infection, trauma, or surgery in immunosuppressed individuals. Many of these patients have been reported from medical institutions in Spain; however, the infection has been noted in diverse areas of the world [54].

Travel-related fungal infections occur not only in adults but also in children. Travelers who have children must be aware of this. Children who are at risk, as well as normal, healthy children, may be susceptible not only to endemic fungal infections but also to opportunistic ones. Children may be infected at any age, from infancy to the teenage years. In some studies, many of these infections have been reported in patients in intensive care units, following surgery or chemotherapy, or in those with important underlying diseases, including malignancies, prematurity, and congenital anomalies. Medical procedures that commonly put patients at risk include parenteral nutrition, endotracheal incubation, central venous cathetertization, and surgical procedures. In many of these cases, the individuals have received antibiotics. The infectious organism seen most often is *C. albicans* [55]. The aggressive treatment of these invasive fungal infections since the early 1990s has resulted in a steady decrease in *C. albicans* bloodstream infections globally [56, 57]. This has resulted in an increase by non-*albicans* species including *C. galbrata, C. parapsilosis,* and *C. tropicalis* [58]. Recent studies also indicate that *C. albicans* remains the most frequent cause of nosocomial candidiasis in Brazil, Norway, and Italy [58].

Invasive fungal infections have become an increasing problem in older adults. Infections with opportunistic fungi have increased because older patients are more likely to be considered for transplantation, receive aggressive regimens of chemotherapy for cancer, and take immunosuppressive drugs for nonmalignant diseases. In addition, healthy older adults are now more likely to travel extensively and to indulge in outdoor activities that put them at risk for exposure to endemic mycoses. Although many of the clinical manifestations of fungal infections in older and younger adults are similar, there are aspects of histoplasmosis, aspergillosis, and cryptococcosis that are unique to older patients [59].

SUPERFICIAL MYCOSES (DERMATOPHYTES)

Epidemiologically, fungal skin infections have the highest incidence of all fungal infections. Although the skin is generally resistant to infection and has many inherent protective mechanisms, including the tough barriers of protein and lipid in the stratum cornea and the underlying epidermis, some organisms have the ability to attach to skin cells and reproduce, resulting in infection under certain conditions. This is especially true when environmental conditions such as excessive moisture or skin inflammation cause, for unknown reasons, breakdown of the skin's protective mechanisms [60].

The most common skin infections worldwide are those caused by dermatophytes. These fungi can infect keratinized tissues such as skin, nails, and hair. This group includes three genera—*Microsporum*, *Trichophyton*, and *Epidermophyton* species. These fungi are classified depending on whether the source is human, animal, or soil as *anthropophilic* (i.e., humans as primary hosts), *zoophilic* (i.e., animals as primary hosts), or *geophilic* (i.e., soil saprophyte). As of this publication, at least 40 dermatophytes have been identified and classified, but just 11 have been commonly associated with diseases in humans. The most common cause of these fungal skin infections in humans is contact with anthropophilic dermatophytes. These include *Tricophyton tonsurans*, *T. rubrium*, *T. mentagrophytes*, *Microsporum canis*, and *Epidermophyton flaccosum*. *M. gypseum* is a geophilic organism, consisting of a complex of three species, that has been associated with human ringworm infections on infrequent occasions. In addition, there are 17 other species of geophilic organisms. The most common routes of transmission are direct contact with an infected person or exposure to infected skin cells disseminated in the environment. The fungal spores from these agents can survive for many months in the environment. When the spores are inoculated directly into breaks in the skin, they can germinate and subsequently invade the cutaneous layers. As for other fungal infections, the most easily infected individuals are those with impaired immune systems [60–65].

The infections caused by various species of anthropophilic dermatophytes are unique in their geographic distribution patterns. In Southeast Asia and the Middle East, *T. violaceum* is the most common cause of scalp infections, whereas in the United States, the agent most commonly associated is *T. tonsurans*.

Dermatophytosis is more commonly referred to as *ringworm* and is classified according to the site at which fungal involvement occurs. Areas include the scalp (tinea capitis), the body (tinea corporis), bearded areas, (tinea barbae), the face in general (tinea faciei), the groin area (tinea cruris), the feet (tinea pedis), the nails (tinea unguium), and the skin of the hands (tinea manum). Dermatophytic skin lesions are characteristically circular scaly patches that are usually dry in appearance.

The zoophilic dermatophytes are those associated with exposure to animals commonly infected with *Microsporum* as well as *Trichophyton* species. They rarely affect humans, although human infection with zoophilic species has occurred after exposure to dogs, cats, horses, cattle, pigs, rodents, poultry, hedgehogs, and some other animals [60–65].

Zoophilic fungi (i.e., those with animal reservoirs) may specifically infect handlers of animals. Travelers should be cautious about adopting pets whose hygiene and general state of health are unknown. Zoophilic *T. mentagrophytes* may be carried by a wide range of animals, and these frequently produce an intense inflammatory cutaneous reaction with pustule formation. Lesions caused by *M. canis* (dogs and cats) typically have a ringworm-like appearance. *T. verrucosum* is acquired from infected cattle and may produce a deep inflammatory reaction on the neck, beard, or scalp. Diagnosis is established by demonstrating fungal hyphae on KOH examination of scales or hair from infected skin. Warm, moist environments may nonspecifically predispose travelers to several types of infections owing to *C. albicans*. As with dermatophyte infections, *Candida* infections may develop in intertriginous body surfaces (e.g., the groin, axilla, and inframammary skin). Infection of the fingernail folds (paronychia) can appear in virtually anyone whose hands are constantly exposed to moisture, and paronychia is often caused by *Candida*. The clinical appearance is a red, swollen, mildly to moderately painful nail fold that does not suppurate with local destruction of cuticle. Erosive dermatitis from *Candida* infections occasionally occurs in the web spaces between the fingers. *Candida* in the form of groin infection and vaginitis also may occur as an infection in travelers who had sexual contact during their time away [64, 66].

It is important to confirm the clinical diagnosis of onychomycosis and other tinea infections prior to commencing therapy. The identity of the fungal organism may provide guidance in choosing an appropriate topical or systemic antifungal agent. Special techniques that assist in obtaining the best yield of fungal organisms from a given site, especially the scalp and nails include

- Clean the suspected area with 70% alcohol to remove bacteria. Use sterile techniques and standard precautions.
- Scrape the peripheral erythematous margin of lesions with a sterile scalpel or wooden spatula, and place the scrapings in a covered sterile container.
- Clip samples of infected scalp or beard hair, and place them in a covered sterile container.
- Pluck hair stubs out with tweezers because the fungus is usually found at the base of the hair shaft. A Wood's light in a darkened room can assist in identifying infected hairs for examination. Infected hairs fluoresce a bright yellow-green.
- Procure samples of infected nails from beneath the nail plate to obtain softened material from the nail bed or collect shavings from the deeper portions of the nail, and place them in a covered sterile container [63, 64].

Other common superficial fungal skin infections of concern are those caused by the *Malassezia* genus of yeasts and tinea nigra. The *Malassezia* genus of yeasts is now thought to be composed of several different species, including

- *M. dermatis*
- *M. equi*
- *M. furfur*
- *M. globosa*
- *M. obtusa*
- *M. pachydermatis*
- *M. restricta*
- *M. slooffiae*
- *M. sympodialis*
- *M. ovalis* (also known as *Pityrosporum ovale*)

Malassezia species inhabit the skin of many adults without causing harm. Unfortunately, in some people the yeast proliferates, resulting in a skin disorder. The cause is not usually known. However, predisposing factors include humidity, sweating and oily skin. There is some controversy as to whether specific species cause different skin diseases.

Skin conditions caused or aggravated by infection by *Malassezia* include

- *Pityriasis versicolor*—most often owing to the subspecies *M. globosa*
- *Malassezia folliculitis*
- *Seborrhoeic dermatitis, dandruff, and sebopsoriasis*
- *Neonatal cephalic pustulosis*—a pustular eruption on young babies that resembles infantile acne
- *Gougerot-Carteau disease* (confluent and reticulated papillomatosis)—a pigmented eruption occurring mainly on the chest, back, and neck of adolescent girls
- *Invasive pityrosporosis*
- *Some facial atopic dermatitis*

Malassezia species are difficult to grow in the laboratory, so scrapings may be reported as "culture negative." The yeast grows best if olive oil is added to the culture medium [64–66].

Tinea nigra is a superficial dermatomycosis caused by *Hortaea werneckii* (formerly named *Phaeoannellomyces werneckii* and *Exophiala werneckii*). It usually occurs in tropical or subtropical areas, including Central and South America, Africa, and Asia. It is infrequent in the United States and

Europe. Of the cases reported in North America since 1950, the majority was associated with tropical travel. However, endemic foci exist in the coastal southeastern United States and Texas. Person-to-person transmission is rare. Tinea nigra is found on otherwise healthy people and presents as an asymptomatic, mottled brown to greenish black macule with minimal to no scale. Of noted concern is that it is frequently misdiagnosed as acral lentiginous melanoma. The macule is painless and discrete and often is darkest at the advancing border [63].

Prevention and Control

Prevention of the endemic mycoses continues to be a matter of great concern, particularly because of the increasing numbers of travelers who may be in an immunocompromised state. The same applies to opportunistic fungal infections. The most effective way to prevent infection with any of the described fungal agents is to avoid contact with and inhalation of conidia from the environmental source. Prevention of infection by S. schenckii involves protecting the skin through the use of gloves and other mechanisms to prevent contact with potentially infected woody or fibrous material.

The traveler must be aware of the risk of visits to endemic areas. These include areas of Canada, the United States, Mexico, and Central and South America. Recreational or tourist areas, including caves and forests inhabited by large flocks of birds, must be treated with appropriate caution. Respiratory protection as well as other means of contact avoidance should be used as indicated [18].

Health care institutions are potential sources of opportunistic fungal infections, particularly for immunocompromised individuals. High-risk travelers must be aware of environmental risks, take particular note of the status of care available at their destination(s), and understand risk-containment measures.

Prevention of dermatophytosis requires knowledge of the conditions predisposing to infection and the maintenance of strict personal hygiene, particularly in areas that have a hot, humid climate. If a person is known to be infected, coworkers and health care workers should avoid contact with potentially infected material and, again, exercise strict hygienic practices and isolation, if necessary. Hygiene involves both the skin in general and the feet

and scalp in particular when outbreaks of tinea pedis or tinea capitis are likely. Topical foot powders assist in drying, and certain antifungal shampoos may be helpful in the prevention of these disorders. Education of at-risk individuals about avoidance of contact with sources of infectious organisms is crucial [60, 62, 63].

Medical surveillance for systemic travel-related fungal diseases involves testing individuals who live in or have traveled from endemic areas. Medical surveillance for the dermatophytoses and other skin infections and superficial mycotic infections in travelers involves history taking, inspection of the involved skin, and diagnostic testing for the suspected pathogen when appropriate. In regard to travelers, biologic testing for fungal infections is often constrained by a lack of knowledge as to all the places where the person has traveled and is somewhat limited to the clinical testing that is done as a part of the diagnostic process. The exception to this is evaluation of soil and environmental samples from suspected areas and soil, dust, and avian and bat droppings from suspected areas harboring the fungal spores [27, 45, 67–69].

The prevention of any of the fungal diseases requires education of the traveler about

- The area to which the individual will be traveling
- The potential for various exposures
- The individual's susceptibility
- Mechanisms for prevention and information about means of managing simple problems early if they cannot be completely avoided

IMMUNIZATION AND PROPHYLACTIC MEASURES

At present, there are no immunizations available to prevent any of the known fungal diseases, either systemic or cutaneous. Infection by some of the agents induces immune responses that provide some level of immunity. Immunization against dermatophytosis has been investigated, but to date, no wholly effective vaccine has been developed for general use.

The prevention of opportunistic mycoses is extremely difficult because these infections are facilitated by the compromised immunity of individuals usually infected. Attempts have been made to use oral or systemic antifungal agents to reduce the occurrence of some of the infections, particularly candidiasis. Success with this approach has been mixed, however. For example, one of the more common opportunistic infections in immunocompromised individuals (travelers included) is aspergillosis. There has been limited success in prophylaxis by using controls in the environment of the individual exposed to aspergillosis (in the hospital environment in particular laminar airflow). However, to date, there has been no significant success with the use of antifungal drugs. In the case of zygomycosis, similar problems and results as those associated with attempts to prevent aspergillosis have occurred [60, 64]. In the case of the superficial mycoses tinea pedis and tinea capitis, the use of antifungal agents in creams and powders, along with maintaining good skin hygiene and other modalities, has been successful in helping to prevent occurrence in areas of high endemicity.

METRICS

Most mycotic infections are not reportable diseases in the public health sector, except for coccidioidomycosis in California and several other western states. It is estimated that there are at least 100,000 cases in the United States. The widespread public health data do not exist to allow accurate assessment of the adequacy of preventive measures other than in specific clinical studies reported in the literature [21, 39, 62].

Symptoms and Signs

In the immunologically competent host, blastomycosis, cryptococcosis, and histoplasmosis (the three most common of the primary systemic mycoses) all exhibit a similar presentation, namely, one resembling acute respiratory infection with influenza-like symptoms. The affected individual, and frequently the physician, often mistake these fungal diseases for the flu or a respiratory illness. If a traveler who lives in an endemic area or has visited or vacationed in one of those areas presents with these types of symptoms, systemic mycosis should be included in the differential diagnosis [18]. Each of the endemic systemic mycoses also may present with other types of clinical findings.

BLASTOMYCOSIS

Blastomycosis, with low frequency, may present as

* An illness resembling bacterial pneumonia, with acute onset, high fever, lobular infiltrates, and productive cough
* Subacute or chronic respiratory illness resembling active pulmonary tuberculosis or lung cancer, with masslike lesions or fibronodular granulomatous infiltrates
* Rapidly progressive adult respiratory distress syndrome (ARDS), with high fever, diffuse infiltrates, and progressive respiratory failure [10, 12, 28]

In almost 60% of cases of acute pulmonary blastomycosis, lung consolidation is the most consistent finding on chest radiographs. Other findings on chest radiographs include the presence of a mass lesion, intermediate-sized nodules, a miliary pattern, solitary cavitation, fibrotic and cavitary changes, a pattern of interstitial fibrosis, diffuse alveoli involvement, and mixed alveoli and interstitial infiltration. Other radiographic findings include hilar adenopathy, postinfectious calcification, chest wall invasion, and pleural effusion [70, 71].

Cutaneous disease is the most common form of extrapulmonary involvement and may present as raised verrucous, encrusted lesions with serpiginous borders, most often located on the face or upper extremities. These lesions have small abscesses that are apparent when the superficial crusting is removed. Atrophic scarification is sometimes present. Bacterial superinfection may change the appearance of these lesions, but characteristically they are not painful, nor is pruritus significant. Chronic draining fistulas also may be associated with blastomycosis, but these are rare [30, 69]. In most cases, cutaneous manifestations occur as a result of metastatic spread from the lungs. Primary cutaneous infection, when it occurs, is usually seen in laboratory workers or other individuals who come in contact with the fungus by direct skin contact, such as veterinary workers or autopsy staff [72].

Osseous, prostatic, and central nervous system (CNS) complications are the next most frequent presentations in descending order. From 50–75% of patients with active clinical blastomycosis have multiple-organ-system involvement.

CNS infection does not occur commonly in immunocompetent patients with blastomycosis. In immunocompromised hosts, however, it is a much more common presentation, and intracranial blastomycomas and other CNS manifestations are not uncommon in these individuals [11, 14, 30].

COCCIDIOIDOMYCOSIS

Coccidioidomycosis tends to develop into the previously described influenza-like illness approximately 7–28 days after exposure to the arthrospores. This occurs in approximately 40% of immunologically intact individuals and in a much higher percentage of individuals with compromised immune systems. In most immunocompetent individuals, there are no symptoms; the only sign of infection is a positive skin test. Those who develop progressive disease often have a generalized macular erythematous rash that is particularly prominent on the inguinal folds and the palms and soles. This rash is especially common in young children. Clinical disease is said to be more common among individuals of African or Philippino descent, Native Americans, and white females. There are, however, no significant data to determine if this is related to some racial or gender differences or if there are socioeconomic, nutritional, or other factors that account for it. In most of the literature in which statistics are quoted, the information is not discussed in relationship to these factors [39, 73–75].

Most individuals who develop clinical coccidioidomycosis present with erythema nodosum or erythema mutiforme, as well as flulike illness. These skin signs appear to occur as a result of the development of cell-mediated immunity and are often considered to be positive prognostic indicators. Other findings include the presence of generalized joint pain, conjunctivitis, episcleritis, and pharyngitis. These findings in individuals who work, live in, or have recently visited areas where coccidioidomycosis is known to be endemic dictate diagnostic testing for this disorder. Other common findings include severe pleuritis; about 5–10% of individuals with acute disease have pleural effusions. Early in the disease, the acute pneumonitits that appears is often associated with cavitary and cystic lesions in the lungs, usually followed in a short time by complete healing of all lesions. Seri-

ous long-term or permanent lung injury occurs in only about 5% of patients with symptomatic pulmonary disease. There have been some cases of coccidioidomycosis in which patients exhibit fulminate lung disease characteristic of ARDS. Another concern is individuals with AIDS or other disorders, in whom corticosteroid therapy has been started as adjuvant therapy for control of their disease. In these individuals, conversion of the coccidioidal infection into a rampant, progressive disorder often occurs and is fatal. The same is true for patients who have coccidioidomycosis but are misdiagnosed as having some other disorder and placed on corticosteroids. The disease then becomes rapidly progressive, leading to severe complications or death. There is evidence to suggest that when coccidioidomycosis becomes a disseminated disease, the primary factor governing this occurrence is the individual host's ability to develop an adequate cell-mediated immune response. If this is absent, the disease frequently becomes progressive, resulting in a poor response to therapy and, ultimately, death of the individual [39, 72, 74, 76].

The most serious extrapulmonary manifestation of coccidioidomycosis is the occurrence of meningitis. This occurs in approximately 30% of individuals who develop disseminated disease. The characteristic finding is a granulomatous meningitis completely encasing the brain with extensive involvement of the base of the brain, resulting in hydrocephalus and cranial nerve palsies. On occasion, aneurysms occur as a result of an associated vasculitis. These can rupture and result in subarachnoid hemorrhage. None of these CNS features is common in patients with coccidioidomycosis, however. As with other fungal disorders, skeletal problems can occur, although they are infrequent. They tend to be present in about 10–20% of individuals who develop disseminated disease [39, 77].

HISTOPLASMOSIS

Histoplasmosis occurring as a primary disorder results from the inhalation of *H. capsulatum* spores, and 60–90% of such patients exhibit either no symptoms or a complex of mild respiratory symptoms resembling those of the common cold. The next most serious group of symptoms are those that have been described for other primary fungal disorders. Usually, the presentation resembles an influenza-like syndrome. As with other fungal disorders, *erythema nodosum* and *erythema mutiforme* also may occur occasionally in the early stages. Individuals who develop significant symptoms resulting in laboratory workup may have bilateral bronchial pneumonia–like changes on chest radiographs, or there simply may be a single solitary pulmonary nodule or multiple pulmonary nodules. Regional lymphadenopathy is also a common finding, but pulmonary effusions are uncommon. Rarely, patients develop active cavitary lesions, with healing and scarring and other changes resulting in a process very much like tuberculosis. Some individuals have healed pulmonary lesions, which may be confused with lung carcinoma and result in surgery if the correct diagnosis cannot be established by other means.

Disseminated histoplasmosis develops in an extremely small number of individuals (estimated at less than 1 per 50,000 cases of primary histoplasmosis). Clinical disseminated histoplasmosis may have multiple-organ-system involvement, including hepatosplenomagly, generalized lymphadenopathy, fever, night sweats, anorexia, weight loss, anemia, and leukopenia. These findings also may be confused with tuberculosis. In some individuals, adrenal insufficiency occurs as a result of adrenal gland involvement and subsequent development of full-blown Addison's disease. In most individuals with disseminated disease, there is also concomitant immunodeficiency of some type. This disorder can be extremely serious in individuals with AIDS because often there is rapid development of rapidly progressive histoplasmosis and CNS involvement. Occasionally, histoplasmosis may be the prominent finding on presentation in patients with AIDS. Other individuals with impaired immune systems, including those with childhood leukemia and those who have had organ transplantation or have a disorder for which they are receiving long-term immunosuppressive therapy, may be particularly predisposed to the development of disseminated histoplasmosis. Again, histoplasmosis should be suspected in individuals who have returned from travel into areas known to be endemic or who have been involved in activities such as recreation in areas suspected to be infested by bats or heavily populated by birds [18, 22, 28, 46, 78–80]. It also should be suspected in an immuno-compromised individual who previously lived in an endemic area and develops findings compatible with disseminated histoplasmosis [81].

SPOROTRICHOSIS

Sporotrichosis, a fungal infection caused by the organism *S. schenckii*, differs from other systemic mycosis in that it is acquired most commonly through spore implantation in the skin, resulting in a painless ulcer or a subcutaneous nodule that is raised and surrounded by pink to purplish discoloration. This lesion then often breaks down to become a necrotic chancre–like lesion. There is usually extensive involvement of the draining lesional lymph nodes. These become swollen, and some suppuration may occur. Most of these patients have localized pain or serious disability. A systemic response presenting as fever, night sweats, or weight loss may occur in some patients. In an extremely small number of patients, disseminated pulmonary infections have occurred. In this group, the infection commonly mimics tuberculosis and resembles the other systemic mycoses, with manifestations such as hilar adenopathy and cavitary disease. There is often an associated persistent pulmonary infiltrate. It is assumed that this occurs when the spores are inhaled via the respiratory route of entry. In individuals who develop disseminated sporotrichosis, the onset is usually insidious and is characterized by low-grade fever and other symptoms mimicking tuberculosis. The major targets of these infections seem to be bones and joints rather than other organs of the body. There is sometimes a multifocal form of arthritis, with knee, ankle, wrist, and elbow involvement being most common. It is extremely rare to see widespread dissemination, although involvement of skin, mouth, nasal mucosa, and CNS may occur, especially in individuals with immune system deficiencies or advanced metastatic cancer, diabetes, alcoholism, or lymphoproliferative diseases [48–50].

Differential Diagnosis

SYSTEMIC MYCOSES

Infections caused by endemic fungi or other opportunistic organisms have been studied increasingly over the past 30 or more years. With increasing emphasis has come the recognition of significant differences between the various types of infections, the pathology associated with the specific causative organisms, and consequently, the ability to differentiate among them.

Just 30+ years ago, some medical textbooks still referred to cryptococcosis and blastomycosis as the same disorder [72]. As pointed out earlier, there are in fact many similarities between the endemic mycotic infections in their clinical presentations, and in most instances, they all may present with minimal clinical findings and transient respiratory symptoms, with the only evidence of infection in the form of serologic evidence or a positive skin test. When the diseases become manifest, there are clinical similarities among them, but there are also some distinctive differences. Diagnosis requires suspecting their presence and, most often, first differentiating between infection owing to one of these agents and pulmonary tuberculosis using a combination of radiography, skin testing, and culture of tissue samples. Often these fungal infections also must be distinguished from cancer of the lung or other organs because they are frequently misdiagnosed, sometimes resulting in unneeded surgery. It is also critical that a distinction be made, particularly in the presence of cryptococcosis and blastomycosis, so that treatment with corticosteroids does not ensue for a mistaken diagnosis of some other condition. Such improper treatment aids in the production of widespread dissemination and aggressive behavior of the infection.

It is important to be aware of a traveler's exposure, potential susceptibilities, and risks. Risk behavior among travelers is important because this sometimes may determine the likelihood of their acquiring a fungal or mycotic disorder. In instances in which the agent is demonstrated, as, for instance, in blastomycosis, the exact strain is of importance, and distinctions can be made, for example, between the African *B. dermatitidis* strain and those found in the United States and other parts of the world [71].

Definitive diagnosis of blastomycosis is made by successful growth of the organism in culture. Sputum or pus from cutaneous lesions, biopsy material, or prostatic secretions usually is used in the culture process and inoculated into Sabouraud's dextrose agar. The process usually requires approximately 30 days of growth at room temperature (30°C). The growth samples then are treated, and diagnosis is made by examination using the appropriate techniques and the light microscope. Exfoliative cytology using Papanicolaou's method is useful in the examination of pulmonary secretions from patients with respiratory involvement. Immunologic methods are also helpful in the diagnosis. These are addressed in more detail in the section on biologic testing below [10, 28, 82, 83].

C. immitis may be diagnosed if the characteristic spherules can be demonstrated on direct wet-mount preparation of pus or sputum. The endospores are classic and, if demonstrated, confirm the diagnosis. In addition, this agent is also easily cultured on Sabouraud's dextrose agar. Immunologic response to the organism is usually demonstrated within 2–21 days after symptoms appear, and skin testing with the antigen and the DNA probe can confirm the presence of infection. Appropriate precautions should be taken with skin testing because of the potential for severe reaction, particularly if testing is done during a time when the lesions of erythema nodosum are present. Other laboratory tests, including testing for the presence of antibodies in the spinal fluid and cytology of the spinal fluid, are also helpful. In many patients with mild or asymptomatic disease, complement-fixation IgG antibodies may develop. If they do, they are also useful in confirming the diagnosis [38, 75].

The diagnosis of histoplasmosis depends on the isolation of *H. capsulatum* in culture. The usual specimens to be cultured are sputum, blood, and urine. In disseminated disease, bone marrow and/or lymph node biopsy culture and tissue sections are useful. Culture of blood from involved organs and particle sections from marrow aspirates also may be helpful. Serologic tests probably are more useful than *Histoplasma* skin tests. Additional discussion of serologic implications may be found in the following section on biologic testing [33, 45, 46, 82, 84–86].

The usual clinical presentation of sporotrichosis is an ulcerated nodule on the dorsal hand, followed by the appearance of similar cutaneous nodules that spread in a linear fashion along lines of lymphatic drainage. The definitive diagnosis of sporotrichosis requires isolation of the organism on culture and subsequent microscopic examination for confirmation. Direct microscopic examination of pus and biopsy material from cutaneous lesions is not usually helpful in making this diagnosis, and other demonstration of the characteristic cigar-shaped organisms in infected tissue is difficult. Biopsies of the lesions may hinder the healing process and spread the organism. Material should be aspirated from the suspected lesions and cultured on glucose neopeptone argar. This results in the growth of a brownish black mycelium within a few days of inoculation if the patient has this infection. Antibody to *S. schencii* appears in the serum and CSF and is useful for confirmation. Sporotrichosis must be distinguished from atypical microbacterial infections caused by *M. marinum*, which it may mimic [53].

SUPERFICIAL MYCOSES

Skin infections are prevalent worldwide but particularly in warm, tropical climates. Various bacteria cause the most common and potentially harmful skin infections; however, a significant number are caused by fungi and molds. Effective management requires differentiation between bacterial and fungal etiology and then identification of the specific type of fungus. The cutaneous lesions of secondary syphilis are quite varied and often affect the palms and soles. In the tropics, yaws, caused by *Treponema pertenue* or *T. carateum,* must be considered in evaluating many skin infections. Fungal infections may be superficial or deep, and they are most common in hot, humid climates. The majority of superficial fungal skin infections are caused by dermatophytes and develop in a nonspecific fashion (particularly involving the groin and feet) because the presence of moisture, sweat, and heat promotes fungal growth. Dermatophytes may infect the fingernails and hands of those with frequent wet exposures. Superficial infections of the body or the groin are common; they appear as reddish, flat, ring-shaped lesions that are dry and scaly or moist and crusty. Deep fungal infections are more serious and should be treated promptly by a physician.

Tricophyton rubrum typically causes a dry, scaly, sometimes painful eruption of the palms, which for some unknown reason is characteristically present on only one hand of the affected individual, sparing the other. Evidence of *T. rubrum* infection usually can be found elsewhere on the body, particularly the toenails and soles. Wet work dries the skin of the affected palm even further, exacerbating the symptoms, and the individual often notices improvement when the wet exposure is discontinued. A scaling eruption confined to the palm of one hand should immediately prompt examination of the feet and a search for fungus.

Specific points to keep in mind when evaluating suspected skin infections are as follows:

- If the skin has tiny bumps or sores, with much itching between the fingers and the wrist, the individual may have scabies, not a fungus.
- If the skin has red scaly patches, with itching between the toes or on the bottom of the feet, the individual may be suffering from a fungal infection such as candidiasis.
- If the skin has pimples or sores, the individual may be suffering from a bacterial infection, not a fungus.
- If you cannot classify a skin infection into a specific category, then take biopsy samples of the skin and send them to a laboratory for examination and culture. Skin scrapings also may be used in some cases.

A diagnostic questionnaire may be useful in differentiating among skin infections. When used, it should include these questions:

- Where are the lesions?
- How big are they, and how many are there?
- Are the lesions symmetric?
- What shape are the lesions, and what did the first one look like?
- What color are the lesions?
- Are the lesions flat or raised? Are they solid or fluid-filled?
- Are the lesions wet or dry?
- What do the borders of the lesions look like?
- Do the lesions itch?
- How fast did the lesions develop?

Biologic Testing

Culture of body fluids and tissue for fungus continues to be the diagnostic mainstay for identifying specific systemic fungal diseases. It is important to note, however, that definitive identification by culture may require as long as 4 weeks. A presumptive diagnosis frequently is made on the basis of the characteristic histopathology and special tissue stains, including periodic acid–Schiff (PAS) and

Gomori–methenamine silver (GMS). Skin tests with antigens such as *H. spherulin* generally have no role in the diagnosis of active disease. Serologic tests have limited value for most fungal diseases because of low specificity and sensitivity; however, there are exceptions, which include the latex agglutination test for cryptococcal antigens in patients with suspected cryptococcosis. The complement fixation and immunodiffusion tests for coccidiomycosis and paracoccidiomycosis are also useful. Serologic tests for the diagnosis of blastomycosis have had improved results with the use of immunoassay (EIA) with the A antigen of *B. dermatitidis*. The standard serologic tests for diagnosis of histoplasmosis include the complement fixation (CF) test, which is quite sensitive, and the immunodiffusion (ID) test, which is fairly specific. Neither of these tests allows for rapid early confirmation of diagnosis. Early diagnosis can guide appropriate treatment and prevent mortality, and considerable effort has been made in developing nonculture approaches to diagnosing fungal infections. These include detection of specific host immune responses to fungal antigens, detection of specific macromolecular antigens using immunologic reagents, amplification and detection of specific fungal nucleic acid sequences, and detection and quantitation of specific fungal metabolite products. At present, highly specific and sensitive serologic tests using DNA probes are available for early and rapid diagnosis of many of the clinically important opportunistic fungal diseases [29, 62, 87–94].

Investigational approaches that show promise in improving the diagnosis and monitoring of systemic mycoses include

- Detection of unique fungal metabolites by gas-liquid chromatography or antigen/antibody-based methods.
- Detection of immunodominant fungal antigens by radioimmunoassay, ELISA, latex agglutination, or immunoblot test.
- Use of molecular probes, e.g., PCR, to detect fungal DNA [77].

Drug Therapy

SYSTEMIC MYCOSES

At present, the five licensed antifungal drugs that are the most important and commonly used agents against the systemic fungal diseases are amphotericin B, flucytosine, and the three azole drugs (i.e., ketoconazole, itraconazole, and fluconazole). Ergosterol, the principal sterol in the fungal cytoplasmic membrane, is the target site of action of amphotericin B and the azoles. Amphotericin B, a polyene, binds irreversibly to ergosterol, resulting in disruption of membrane integrity and ultimately cell death. The azole drugs inhibit synthesis of ergosterol through an interaction with the cytochrome P450–dependent enzyme 14α-demethylase necessary for the conversion of lanosterol to ergosterol. By contrast, flucytosine, an oral fluorinated pyrimidine, inhibits both fungal DNA and RNA protein synthesis.

While these drugs are effective therapies for many of the systemic mycoses, including blastomycosis, candidiasis, cryptococcosis, histoplasmosis, and sporotrichosis, they are only minimally or moderately effective for aspergillosis, coccidioidomycosis, non-*albicans* candidiasis, and phaeohyphomycosis caused by diatomaceous molds. Moreover, these drugs may involve other problems. Amphotericin B, considered by some authorities to be the "gold standard" because of its broad spectrum of activity and fungicidal action, is available only as an intravenous formulation in the United States, requiring continuous intravenous access, and is associated with significant dose-limiting toxicity, especially nephrotoxicity. Flucytosine also has the potential for considerable toxicity, especially affecting the bone marrow, liver, GI tract, and skin. As a result, this drug has never been used optimally. Although development of the azole class of drugs is an important advance and offers effective and safe alternatives to amphotericin B and flucytosine for many of the systemic mycoses, the azoles are not ideal drugs. Only fluconazole is available as both an oral and an intravenous formulation. Amphotericin B, flucytosine, and the azoles are potentially hepatotoxic. They may inhibit steroid hormone synthesis in humans and also may have the potential to interact with many classes of drugs (e.g., oral hypoglycemics, oral anticoagulants, phenytoin, cyclosporine, H_1 and H_2 receptor antagonists, and rifampin) with serious sequelae. *Candida* species resistant to fluconazole are an increasing cause of concern in AIDS patients and other immunocompromised hosts exposed to fluconazole as a prophylactic drug over extended periods.

The toxicity and other problems associated with the currently available antifungal drugs make development of new treatment approaches critical. Current efforts in antifungal drug development are focused on

- Drugs with novel fungal cell targets
- Investigational azole and allylamine drugs
- Novel formulations of currently licensed drugs

With regard to novel fungal cell targets, an important difference between fungi and mammalian cells is that the fungal cell envelope consists of a cell wall, consisting primarily of three carbohydrates—glycan, chitin, and mannoproteins—and the cytoplasmic membrane. By contrast, cell walls are not found in mammalian cells and other eukaryotic cells. Available evidence indicates that drugs that target fungal cell wall structures do not adversely affect mammalian cells; thus the potential for toxicity of such drugs in humans is reduced.

Examples of investigational drugs that interrupt formation of the unique fungal cell walls include

1. Nikkomycins, which inhibit chitin synthesis
2. The echinocandin/pneumocandin/lipopeptide class, which inhibits glycan synthesis
3. Pradimicins, which exhibit calcium-dependent binding to mannan (mannoprotein).
4. The investigational azole drugs, under development by several pharmaceutical companies, which have the potential to outperform the currently licensed azoles, ketoconazole, itraconazole, and fluconazole in terms of broader spectrum of activity, increased efficacy, and less toxicity
5. The allylamines, a new class of drugs, which inhibit squalene epoxidase, another enzyme in the biosynthetic pathway of ergosterol

Novel formulations of currently licensed drugs are aimed at enhancing the efficacy and reducing the toxicity of the parent compound. There are two classes of drugs in this group. The first class is lipid formulations of amphotericin B, including liposomal amphotericin B (AmBisome), amphotericin B colloidal dispersion (Amphocil), and amphotericin B lipid complex (ABLC). Enveloping amphotericin B in liposomes or complexing the drug with lipids offers several advantages of the novel formulations over conventional amphotericin B, which is complexed in desoxycholate, a bile salt.

These potential advantages include

- Up to a 5- to 10-fold increase in daily dose of amphotericin B, thereby increasing the therapeutic index
- Less nephrotoxicity, the major limiting toxic effect of conventional amphotericin B
- Tropism for reticuloendothelial organs such as lymph nodes, liver, and spleen, where fungi typically are in contrast to the tropism of conventional amphotericin B for kidneys
- Preferential binding of lipid-formulated drugs to fungal cell membranes, which may have efficacy in some patients who have failed or cannot tolerate conventional amphotericin B

New oral and intravenous preparations of itraconazole represent a second class of novel formulations. Itraconazole, currently available only for oral administration, is a weak base that requires an acid environment for optimal solubilization and absorption. The bioavailability of itraconazole is increased when it is formulated in hydoxypropyl-β-cyclodextrin, a cyclic oligosaccharide carrier molecule that increases the solubility of lipophilic compounds in aqueous solutions. Hydroxypropyl-β-cyclodextrin itraconazole may be especially helpful in selected clinical situations, such as for AIDS patients with achlorhydria or receiving concurrent drugs that impair absorption or critically ill hospitalized patients who cannot take oral medications [79, 84–89].

Invasive fungal diseases are observed increasingly in immunocompromised patients, especially those with protracted granulocytopenia secondary to neoplastic disease or cytotoxic chemotherapy, transplant recipients receiving immunosuppressive drugs such as high-dose corticosteroids and cyclosporine, and AIDS patients with progressively declining CD4+ T cells and other perturbations in immune function. Current evidence indicates that an adequate number and function of granulocytes, as well as intact cell-mediated immunity, are key to a successful outcome in patients with opportunistic yeast and mold diseases. Cellular immunity also plays an important role in the host's containment of the endemic mycoses. Far and away the most common fungal infection associated with HIV infection is candidiasis. This tends to produce mucosal topical infections, and local treatment may be enough to control them (generally, a course of 1–2 weeks rather than chronic suppression, for fear of eliciting resistance). Fluconazole-resistant *Candida* species may be an increasing problem. For cryptococcosis, the problem is complicated. Fluconazole is highly effective for chronic suppression but not effective for initial therapy. A short course of amphotericin B for 2 weeks should be followed by long-term azole suppression. Fluconazole appears excellent, but itraconazole also may be effective. For histoplasmosis, itraconazole appears to be the most advantageous drug, producing an excellent clinical response within 2 weeks [79, 90, 95–101].

Immunomodulators may become important adjuncts to therapy for systemic mycoses. Recent in vitro and animal in vivo data suggest a role in the management of fungal diseases for the expanding array of recombinant cytokines, especially interferon-γ, the colony-stimulating factors, the various interleukins or interleukin antagonists, and monoclonal antibodies passive immunotherapy. Trials of these agents performed in humans with fungal disease have been limited [79].

SUPERFICIAL MYCOSES (FUNGAL SKIN DISEASES)

Skin infections often can be treated by topical (surface) treatments alone. Sometimes it is necessary to take systemic (internal) medications. The following major rules apply:

1. If the lesion is wet, treat it with a dry dressing; if the lesion is dry, treat it with a cream or ointment.
2. If the lesion oozes, itches, or stings, treat it with cold compresses; if the lesion is hot, treat it with elevation and warm compresses.
3. Begin with the least potent treatment; work up to the most potent treatment only if necessary.

Since the advent of effective systemic antifungal agents, many have used them empirically for a broad range of skin diseases diagnosed as fungal disorders. It is important that dermatologic fungal conditions be diagnosed before they are treated so as to avoid use of an inappropriate drug. A systemic antifungal agent is of no value in treating a nonfungal condition. In general, most fungal der-

matoses are treated effectively using topical antifungal agents except in immunocompromised patients. In these individuals, the disease, while manifested in the skin, is often more extensive and severe. Multiple systemic and topical antifungals are available with efficacy against the dermatophytes. Infections involving hair-bearing skin necessitate oral antifungals because the dermatophytes penetrate the hair follicles.

Topical antifungal agents may be broadly divided into specific and nonspecific agents. The former have mechanisms of action against specific cell wall constituents or cellular enzyme systems, etc. They include the polyenes, azoles, allylamines, amorolfines, ciclopirox, and butenafine. The latter often act by increasing epidermal exfoliation and by less well defined antifungal metabolic mechanisms and include such agents such as selenium sulfide, keratolytic agents such as Whitfield's ointment (2% salicylic acid), tincture of iodine, undecylenic acid, potassium permanganate, silver nitrate, and benzoic acid. Various formulations of all these agents are available as creams, gels, powders, lacquers, solutions, and sprays.

This section is not intended as a specific therapeutic guide for managing fungal infections. For that purpose, I would refer you to any of a number of excellent textbooks and therapeutic guides that specifically address this in far greater detail than can be done here.

Several general principles should be kept in mind [102–105]:

- Candidal infections, which may occur as intertrigo of the groin or paronychias, should not be treated with oral griseofulvin because this is a penicillin-related agent and will actually aggravate and make these infections worse.
- Most true fungal infections are noticeably improved after 1–2 weeks of oral antifungal therapy (except for scalp and nails).
- Tinea versicolor does not respond to oral griseofulvin therapy.
- Selenium sulfide remains the least expensive effective treatment for tinea versicolor.
- Most external ear diseases are not caused by a fungus.
- Superficial dermatophyte infections (on the general body surface) may be treated with topical imidazole antifungal preparations.

- Fungal infections of the palms, soles, and the nails and deep inflammatory reactions on hair-bearing surfaces do not generally respond well to topical agents. Oral therapy with an appropriate systemic antifungal agent is preferred for these infections unless contraindicated.
- Chronic paronychia may need to be treated for months.
- Sulconazole nitrate has been used effectively for the treatment of skin infections in tropical Africa.
- The standard treatment of tinea capitis in the United States has been and continues to be griseofulvin. The oral triazole (e.g., *itraconazole* or *fluconazole*) and allylamine (*terbinafine*) antifungals also appear to be safe and effective and have the advantage of shorter treatment durations.
- With markedly inflammatory tinea capitis, oral glucocorticoids may reduce the incidence of scarring. The usual dose of prednisone is 1–2 mg/kg each morning for the first week of therapy.
- Like tinea capitis, oral antifungals are essential in the treatment of tinea barbae. Griseofulvin at 1 g daily, itraconazole, 200 mg daily for 2–4 weeks, terbinafine, 250 mg daily for 2–4 weeks, and fluconazole, 200 mg daily for 4–6 weeks, are all effective treatment plans.

Preventive health advice and first aid travel kits for individuals traveling to areas where fungal skin infections are of significant risk should include specific information on prevention of dermatophytoses and other skin infections. Fungal infections on the skin are contagious. They can be passed from one person to the next by direct skin-to-skin contact or by contact with contaminated items such as combs, unwashed clothing, and shower or pool surfaces. You also can catch ringworm from pets that carry the fungus. Some general advice that may be helpful includes [63–65]:

- Keep skin and feet clean and dry.
- Use drying powder in moist areas.
- Apply powder containing *miconazole* or *tolnaftate* to areas prone to fungal infection after bathing.
- Shampoo regularly, especially after haircuts.

- Do not share clothing, towels, hairbrushes, combs, headgear, or other personal care items. Such items should be thoroughly cleaned and dried after use.
- Wear sandals or shoes at gyms, lockers, pools, and beaches.
- Avoid touching pets. Wash your hands if you should have contact.
- Use hand sanitizer.

In summary, adequate knowledge and preparation are critical to ensuring that health problems do not interfere with travel for either the businessperson or family members. Even those who are healthy need to make plans to safeguard their health and that of all others accompanying them. Proper preparation is inexpensive relative to the costs of illness while traveling.

References

1. Steffen R, Raeber PA. Risks for travelers. *Med Trop* 1997;54:423.
2. Centers for Disease Control and Prevention. *Health Information for International Travel 1997–98.* Atlanta: CDC, 1998.
3. Rose SSR. *International Travel Health Guide.* London: McNaughton and Gunn, 1993.
4. Wolf MS. Preparing employees for international travel. *J Occup Med* 1977;19:671.
5. Groll AH, Shah PM, Mentzel C, et al. Trends in the postmortem epidemiology of invasive fungal infections at a university hospital. *J Infect* 1996;33:23–32.
6. Friedkin SK, Jarvis WR. Epidemiology of nosocomial fungal infections. *Clin Infect Dis* 1996;9:499–511.
7. Wilson ME, von Reyn CF, Fineberg HV. Infections in HIV-infected travelers: Risks and prevention. *Ann Intern Med* 1991;114:582–92.
8. Yamazaki T, Kume H, Murase S, et al. Epidemiology of visceral mycoses: Analysis of data in annual of the pathological autopsy cases in Japan. *J Clin Microbiol* 1999;37:1732–8.
9. Rosen GP, Neilsen K, Glenn S, et al. Invasive fungal infections in pediatric oncology patients: 11-year experience at a single institution. *J Pediatr Hematol Oncol* 2005;27:135–40.
10. Bradshear RW. Blastomycosis. *Clin Infect Dis* 1992; 14:SA2.
11. Wheat J. Endemic mycoses in AIDS: A clinical review. *Clin Microbiol Rev* 1995;8:146.
12. Myer KC, McManus DJ, Makai DG. Overwhelming pulmonary blastomycosis associated with the adult respiratory distress syndrome. *N Engl J Med* 1993; 329:1231.

13. Sarosi GA, Davies SF. Endemic mycosis complicating human immunodeficiency virus infection. *West J Med* 1996;164:335.
14. Pappas PG. Blastomycosis in the immunocompromised patient. *Semin Respir Infect* 1997;12:243.
15. Cooper CR Jr, McGinnis MR. Pathology of *Penicillium marneffei:* An emerging acquired immunodeficiency syndrome–related pathogen. *Arch Pathol Lab Med* 1997;121:798.
16. Duong TA. Infection due to *Penicillium marneffei*, an emerging pathogen: Review of 155 reported cases. *Clin Infect Dis* 1996;23:125.
17. Nittayananta W, Chungpanich S. Oral lesions in a group of Thai people with AIDS. *Oral Dis* 1997;3: S41–5.
18. Suzaki A, Kimura M, Kimura F, et al. An outbreak of acute pulmonary histoplasmosis among travelers to a bat-inhabited cave in Brazil. *Kansen Shogaku Zasshi* 1995;69:444.
19. National Institute for Allergy and Infectious Diseases. *Fungal Diseases—A Public Health Problem*, Fact Sheet. Bethesda, MD: NIAID, 1996.
20. National Institute for Allergy and Infectious Diseases. *Summit on Development of Infectious Disease Therapeutics: Report of the Anti-Fungal Working Group*, Bethesda, MD: NIAID, 2000.
21. Beck-Sague CM, Jarvis WR, and the NNIS. Secular trends in the epidemiology of nosocomial fungal infections in the United States, 1980–1990. *J Infect Dis* 1993;167:1247–51.
22. Miller LW, et al. Infection after heart transplantation: A multi-institutional study. Cardiac Transplant Research Database Group. *J Heart Lung Transplant* 1994;13:381–92.
23. Pannuti CS, et al. Nosocomial pneumonia in adult patients undergoing bone marrow transplantation. *J Clin Oncol* 1991;9:77–84.
24. *AIDS Surveillance Quarterly Update for Cases Reported through September 1994.* Albant: NY State Department of Health, 1995.
25. Marriott DJ, Wong KH, Harkness JL, et al. *Seytalidium dimidiatum* and *Lecthophora hoffmanni:* Unusual causes of fungal infections in a patient with AIDS. *J Clin Microbiol* 1997;35:2949–52.
26. Marriott DJ, Huang KH, Aznar E, et al. *Scytalidium dimidiatum* and *Lecythophora hoffmanni:* Unusual causes of fungal infections in a patient with AIDS. *J Clin Microbiol* 1997;35:2949.
27. Taylor ML, Perez-Mejia A, Yamamoto-Furusho JK, et al. Immunologic, genetic and social human risk factors associated to histoplasmosis: Studies in the state of Guerrero, Mexico. *Mycopathologia* 1997; 138:137.
28. Davies SF, Sarosi GA. Epidemiological and clinical features of pulmonary blastomycosis. *Semin Respir Infect* 1997;12:206.
29. Gueho E, Leclerc MC, deHoog GS, et al. Molecular taxonomy and epidemiology of *Blastomyces* and *Histoplasma* species. *Mycoses* 1997;40:69.
30. Bradsher RW. Clinical features of blastomycosis. *Semin Respir Infect* 1997;12:229.
31. Morgan J, Alexander B, Wannemuehler K, et al. Quantification of risk for invasive fungal infections among transplant recipients. Abstracts of the 44th interscience conference of antimicrobial agents and chemotherapy. Washington, 2004, abstract M-1058.
32. Anaissie EJ, Stratton SL, Dignani MC, et al. Pathogenic *Aspergillus* species recovered from a hospital water system: A 3-year prospective study. *Clin Infect Dis* 2002;34:780–9.
33. Anaissie EJ, Kuchar RT, Rex JH, et al. Fusariosis associated with pathogenic *Fusarium* species colonization of a hospital water system: A new paradigm for the epidemiology of opportunistic mold infections. *Clin Infect Dis* 2001;33:1871–8.
34. Anaissie EJ, Stratton SL, Dignani MC, et al. Cleaning patient shower facilities: A novel approach to reducing patient exposure to aerosolized *Aspergillus* species and other opportunistic molds. *Clin Infect Dis* 2002;35:E86–8.
35. Munoz P, Sanchez-Somolinos M, Perez M, et al. Outbreak of *Saccharomyces cerevisiae* infection in a heart surgery intensive care unit (HSICU). In Program and Abstracts of the Interscience Conference on Antimicrobial Agents and Chemotherapy, October 30–November 2, 2004. Washington, 2005; abstract K-877.
36. Klont R, Rijs A, Warris A, et al. Bacterial and fungal contamination of commercial bottled mineral water from 16 countries. In Program and abstracts of the Interscience Conference on Antimicrobial Agents and Chemotherapy, October 30–November 2, 2004. Washington, 2005; abstract K-1603.
37. Pavie J, Bouakline A, Feuilhade M, et al. Fungal contamination of hospital healthcare workers' overalls. In Program and Abstracts of the Interscience Conference on Antimicrobial Agents and Chemotherapy, October 30–November 2, 2004. Washington, 2005; abstract M-1031.
38. Stevens DA. Coccidioidomycosis. *N Engl J Med* 1995;332:1077–82.
39. Centers for Disease Control and Prevention. Update: Coccidioidomycosis/California, 1991–1993. *MMWR*, 1994;43:421–3.
40. California Department of Health Services. Communicable Disease Summaries, 2005.
41. Baumgardner DJ, Burdick JS. An outbreak of human and canine blastomycosis. *Rev Infect Dis* 1991;13:898.
42. Vaaler AK, Bradshear RW, Davies SF. Evidence of subclinical blastomycosis in forest workers in northern Minnesota and northern Wisconsin. *Am J Med* 1990;89:470.
43. Bradsher RW. Histoplasmosis and blastomycosis. *Clin Infect Dis Suppl* 1996;2:8102.
44. Reder PA, Neil HB III. Blastomycosis in otolaryngology: Review of a large series. *Laryngoscope* 1993; 103:53.

45. Wheat J. Histoplasmosis: Experience during outbreaks in Indianapolis and review of the literature. *Medicine* 1997;76:339.

46. Wheat LJ, Kauffman CA. Histoplasmosis. *Infect Dis Clin North Am* 2003;17:19.

47. Winn RE. Systemic fungal infections: Diagnosis and treatment: I. Sporotrichosis. *Infect Dis Clin North Am* 1988;2:899.

48. Heller HM, Fuhrer J. Disseminated sporotrichosis in patients with AIDS: Case report and review of the literature. *AIDS* 1991;5:1243.

49. Vierira-Dias D, Sena CM, Orefice F, et al. Ocular and concomitant cutaneous sporotrichosis. *Mycoses* 1997;40:197–201.

50. Crampuz A, Zimmerli W. HIV-associated lung diseases. *Schweiz Med Wochenschr* 1997;127:1725–33.

51. Johnson MA, Lyle G, Hanley M, et al. *Aspergillus:* A rare primary organism in soft tissue. *Am Surg* 1998;64:122–6.

52. Cooper CR Jr, McGinnis MR. Pathology of *Penicillium marneffeii:* An emerging acquired immunodeficiency syndrome–related pathogen. *Arch Pathol Lab Med* 1997;121:798–804

53. Dong TA. Infection due to *Penicillium marneffei,* an emerging pathogen: Review of 155 reported cases. *Clin Infect Dis* 1996;23:125–30.

54. Baranguer J, Rodriguez-Tudela JL, Richard C, et al. Deep infections caused by *Scedosporium prolificans:* A report on 16 cases in Spain and a review of the literature. *Scedosporium prolificans* Spanish Study Group. *Medicine* 1997;76:256.

55. Chiu NC, Chung YF, Huang FY. Pediatric nosocomial fungal infections. *Southeast Asian J Prop Med Public Health* 1997;28:191.

56. Abi-Said D, Anaissie E, Uzun O, et al. The epidemiology of hematogenous candidiasis caused by different *Candida* species (erratum appears in *Clin Infect Dis* 1997; 25:352). *Clin Infect Dis* 1997;24:1122–8.

57. Trick WE, Fridkin SK, Edwards JR, et al. Secular trend of hospital-acquired candidemia among intensive care unit patients in the United States during 1989–1999 (abstract). *Clin Infect Dis* 2002;35:627–30.

58. Pfaller MA, Diekema DJ, and International Fungal Surveillance Participant Group. Twelve years of fluconazole in clinical practice: Global trends in species distribution and fluconazole susceptibility of bloodstream isolates of *Candida. Clin Microbiol Infect* 2004;10:11–23S.

59. Kauffman CA. Fungal infections in older adults. *Clin Infect Dis* 2001;33:550–5.

60. Roth RR, James WD. Microbiology of the skin: Resident flora, ecology, and infection. *J Am Acad Dermatol* 1989;20:367.

61. Bottoni U, Dianzani C, Rossi ME, et al. Skin diseases in immigrants seen as outpatients in the Institute of Dermatology at the University of Rome La Spaienza from 1989–1994. *Aur J Epidemiol* 1998;12:201.

62. DeVroey C. Epidemiology of ringworm. *Semin Dermatol* 1985;4:185.

63. Schwartz RA. Superficial fungal infections. *Lancet* 2004;364:1173.

64. Macura AB. Dermatophyte infections. *Int J Dermatol* 1993;32:313.

65. Weitzman I, Summerbell RC. The dermatophytes. *Clin Microbiol Rev* 1995;8:240–59.

66. Ashbee HR, Evans EG. Immunology of diseases associated with *Malassezia* species. *Clin Microbiol Rev* 2002;15:21–57.

67. Gupta AK, Einarson TR, Summerbell RC, et al. An overview of topical antifungal therapy in dermatomycoses: A North American perspective. *Drugs* 1998;55:645–74.

68. Abraham AG, Kulp-Shorten CL, Callen JP. Remember to consider dermatophyte infection when dealing with recalcitrant dermatoses. *South Med J* 1998; 91:349.

69. Wolf R, Movshowitz M, Brenner S. Supplemental tests in the evaluation of occupational hand dermatitis in soldiers. *Int J Dermatol* 1996;35:173.

70. Brown LR, Swenson SJ, VanScoy RE, et al. Roentgenologic features of pulmonary blastomycosis. *Mayo Clin Proc* 1991;66:29–38.

71. Winer-Muram HT, Reuben SA. Pulmonary blastomycosis. *J Thorac Imag* 1992;7:23.

72. Mercantini R, Marsella R, Moretto D, et al. Macroscopic and microscopic characteristics of an African *Blastomyces dermatididis* strain. *Macroscop Mycos* 1995;38:477.

73. Sondergaard J, Weismann K, Vithayasai P, et al. Ethnic and geographic differences and similarities of HIV/AIDS-related mucocutaneous diseases. Danida Study Groups. *Int J Dermatol* 1995;34:416.

74. Mahaffey KW, Hippenmeyer CL, Mandel R, et al. Unrecognized coccidioidomycosis complicating *Pneumocystis carinii* pneumonia in patients infected with the human immunodeficiency virus and treated with cortical steroids: A report of two cases. *Arch Intern Med* 1993;153:1496.

75. Masuda K, Kumamoto K, Machida TA. Surgical case of right coccidioidomycosis in the left wrist. *Nippon Kyobu Geka Gakkai Zafshi* 1997;45:1770–3.

76. Standaert SM, Schaffener W, Galgiani JN, et al. Coccidioidomycosis among visitors to a *Coccidioides immitis* endemic area: An outbreak in a military reserve unit. *J Infect Dis* 1995;171:1672–5.

77. Oudiz R, Mahaisavariya P, Peng SK, et al. Disseminated coccidioidomycosis with rapid progression to effusive-constrictive pericarditis. *J Am Soc Echocardiogr* 1995;8:947–52.

78. Vincent T, Galgiani JN, Huppert M, et al. The natural history of coccidioidal meningitis: VA–Armed Forces Cooperative Studies, 1955–1958. *Clin Infect Dis* 1993;16:247.

79. Wheat J. Histoplasmosis in the acquired immunodeficiency syndrome. *Curr Top Med Mycol* 1996;7:7.

80. Wheat LJ, Batteiger BE, Sathapatayavongs B. *Histoplasma capsulatum* infections of the central nervous system: A clinical review. *Medicine* 1990;69:244.

81. Wheat LJ, Connolly-Stringfield PA, Baker RL, et al.

Disseminated histoplasmosis in the acquired immune deficiency syndrome: Clinical findings, diagnosis and treatment, and review of the literature. *Medicine* 1990;69:361.

82. Hart FD. *French's Index of Differential Diagnosis*, 10th ed. Baltimore: Williams & Wilkins, 1973. P 327.
83. Davies SF, Sarosi GA. Serodiagnosis of histoplasmosis and blastomycosis (editorial). *Am Rev Respir Dis* 1987;136:254.
84. Davies SF, Sarosi GA. Role of serodiagnostic tests and skin tests in the diagnosis of fungal disease. *Clin Chest Med* 1987;8:135.
85. Davies SF. Serodiagnosis of histoplasmosis. *Semin Respir Infect* 1986;1:9–15.
86. Rosatelli JB, Machado AA, Roselino AM. Dermatoses among Brazilian HIV-positive patients: Correlation with the evolutionary phases of AIDS. *Int J Termalog* 1997;36:729.
87. Henseler T, Tausch I. Mycosis in patients with psoriasis or atopic dermatitis. *Mycoses* 1997;40:22S.
88. Schmeller W, Baumgartner F, Dzikus A. Dermatophytomycoses in children in rural Kenya: The impact of primary health care. *Mycoses* 1997;40:55.
89. The National Institute of Allergy and Infectious Diseases. The Second NIAID Workshop in Medical Mycology: Molecular and Immunological Approaches to the Diagnosis and Treatment of Systemic Mycoses, Status and Limitations of Diagnosis and Therapy of Systemic Fungal Infections, Baltimore, 1996.
90. Wheat J, Wheat H, Connolly P, et al. Cross-reactivity in *Histoplasma capsulatum* variety capsulatum antigen assays of urine samples from patients with endemic mycoses. *Clin Infect Dis* 1997;24:1169–71.
91. Bradshear W, Pappas PG. Detection of specific antibodies in human blastomycosis by enzyme immunoassay. *South Med J* 1995;88:1256–9.
92. Cunningham ET Jr, Seiff SR, Berger TG, et al. Intraocular coccidioidomycosis diagnosed by skin biopsy. *Arch Ophthalmol* 1998;116:674.
93. Mangiaterra M, Alonso J, Galvan M, et al. Histoplasmin and paracoccidioidin skin reactivity in infantile population of northern Argentina. *Rev Inspir Med Trop (Sao Paulo)* 1996;38:349.
94. Yeo SF, Wong B. Current status of nonculture methods for diagnosis of invasive fungal infections. *Clin Microbiol Rev* 2002;15:465.
95. Wheat J, Hafner R, Korzun AH, et al. Intraconazole treatment of disseminated histoplasmosis in patients with the acquired immunodeficiency syndrome. AIDS Clinical Trial Group. *Am J Med* 1995; 98:336–42.
96. Wheat J, Merichal P, Vanden Bossche H, et al. Hypothesis on the mechanism of resistance to fluconazole in *Histoplasma capsulatum*. *Antimicrob Agents Chemother* 1997;41:410–4.
97. Mirels LF, Stevens DA. Update on treatment of coccidioidomycosis. *West J Med* 1997;166:291.
98. Stevens DA. Adequacy of therapy for coccidioidomycosis (editorial): Comment. *Clin Infect Dis* 1997;25:1205–10.
99. Bradsher RW. Therapy of blastomycosis. *Semin Respir Infect* 1997;12:263.
100. Pappas PG, Bradsher RW, Kauffman CA, et al. Treatment of blastomycosis with higher doses of fluconazole. The National Institute of Allergy and Infectious Diseases Mycosis Study Group. *Clin Infect Dis* 1997;25:200.
101. Graybill JR. Treatment of systemic mycoses in patients with AIDS. *Arch Med Res* 1993;24:403.
102. Millikan LE. Role of oral antifungal agents for the treatment of superficial fungal infections in immunocompromised patients. *Cutis* 2001;68:6–14S.
103. Gugnani HC, Gugnani A, Malachy O. Sulconazole in the therapy of dermatomycosis in Nigeria. *Mycosis* 1997;40:139.
104. Brautigam M, Nolting S, Schopf RE, et al. Randomised, double-blind comparison of trebinafine and itraconazole for treatment of toenail tinea infection. *Br Med J* 1995;311:919.
105. Maertens J, Boogaerts M. The place for itraconazole in treatment. *J Antimicrob Chemother* 2005;56:133–8S.

Unique Problems
and Settings

33

Occupational Infections in Pregnant Employees

Edward Seidel

Although credited with founding aseptic policy for the prevention of nosocomial disease, the early observations of Ignaz Philip Semmelweis (1818–1865) are rooted in obstetrics as well as the practices of occupational and preventive medicine. In 1847, while working as a physician in the Maternity Department at the Vienna Lying-in Hospital, Semmelweis observed that puerperal fever could be reduced by hand washing. Semmelweis noticed a higher incidence of puerperal fever cases when doctors who had worked with necropsy material and who immediately treated pregnant patients did not wash their hands in between. Fever cases were greatly reduced with preventive hand washing. Unfortunately, despite over 14 years of work, writings, and lectures documenting this simple preventive medical practice, there was an overall failure of acceptance by the medical community. Ignaz died in 1865. Later, the germ theory of disease, rooted in these early scientific observations of obstetric patients and the occupational practices of physicians, was accepted. Ignaz Semmelweis had become recognized as a pioneer of aseptic policy in the prevention of infectious disease [1].

The specialty of obstetrics and gynecology has advanced significantly since the era of Ignaz Semmelweis. Concerns regarding infections and the pregnant worker continue. In most of the preceding chapters, the infectious diseases to which workers may be at risk are described and discussed.

In the unique setting of pregnancy, frequent questions include how a worker should be assigned if she is pregnant and what, if any, special precautions should be taken in the workplace. Also questioned are whether antimicrobial treatments, skin testing, preventive vaccinations, or other medications, including over-the-counter (OTC) medications, are safe during pregnancy. In the case of women who are breast-feeding, safety of the breast milk also is a concern.

This chapter will explore drug effects and safety in pregnancy and breast-feeding, review antimicrobial chemotherapy in pregnancy, discuss specific viral infections that pose a risk for the pregnant worker, review the three common bloodborne pathogen exposures in health care workers, and go over the prevention of workplace-related infections with preventive vaccinations. This will include discussion of influenza risk during pregnancy and travel medicine concerns, specifically malaria, that are part of today's global business environment.

Infections that include tuberculosis, toxoplasmosis, and the zoonoses and tick-borne illnesses (e.g., Q fever, psittacosis, brucellosis, leptospirosis, Lyme disease, and ehrlichiosis) are covered in other chapters.

Drug Effects and Drug Safety in Pregnancy and Teratogenicity

EARLY PREGNANCY

The pregnant worker is a subcategory in today's global workforce. Many pregnancies are not known during the first 4–6 weeks following conception, and estimates are that as many as 56% of pregnancies are not planned, so many women may be inadvertently exposed to medications or other agents before their pregnancy is recognized. This could be 4–6 weeks or longer following conception [2]. A substantial proportion of pregnancies also occur without prior planning, so unintentional fetal exposures can occur during part or all of the most critical periods in embryonic development for drug-induced or other malformations [3]. Once pregnancy is known, one should advise and manage the pregnant worker in consultation with the treating obstetrician and an infection specialist as applicable. Both clinicians should have current collective knowledge and experience.

DRUG EFFECTS AND SAFETY

During 1960 in Europe, it was discovered that thalidomide was causing serious birth defects. It had not yet been approved for use in the United States and was recognized as the cause of a characteristic pattern of severe congenital anomalies in many of the offspring whose mothers used the medication at critical time periods during their pregnancies. Following this devastating observation, pharmaceutical manufacturers, regulatory agencies, and various private and public entities faced the challenge and responsibility of assessing the safety of medications and the risk to the fetus during pregnancy [3].

However, several studies have demonstrated that pregnant women may use as many as 3–11 different drugs during pregnancy [4]. OTC medications used include drugs such as ibuprofen, acetaminophen, pseudoephedrine, and other drugs [5]. Both chronic and acute medical conditions may require treatment before, during, and following pregnancy. Depression, epilepsy, asthma, rheumatoid arthritis, and autoimmune disorders are examples of conditions requiring treatment. Failure to treat these conditions could be detrimental to the woman, the pregnancy, and the fetus [6–9].

BREAST-FEEDING

The presence of drugs and medications in the breast milk is also of concern. The concentrations of all medications and substances depend on their solubility in fat or water, the molecular weight of the drug, and the degree to which the drug or substance is ionized. Although the concentrations of antibiotics secreted into the breast milk are usually small, almost all antimicrobial agents do appear in breast milk in some measurable concentration when given in therapeutic doses to women who are nursing [10]. Although these concentrations are small, sulfonamides in breast milk may increase bilirubin and may predispose premature infants to kernicterus. Sulfonamides and nalidixic acid in breast milk also have caused hemolysis in infants with glucose-6-phosphate dehydrogenase (G6PD) deficiency [10].

Antimicrobial Chemotherapy in Pregnancy

FETAL RISK

Virtually all antimicrobial agents cross the placenta, and the degree to which fetal exposure occurs varies [10]. Data regarding the use of specific agents, teratogenicity, pharmacokinetics in pregnancy, and other factors are not clear. Following the exposure to any toxicant, infectious or chemical, a number of factors can affect whether or not there is abnormal fetal development as a result. Some of these factors include maternal susceptibility factors, such as age, genetic background, metabolic state, underlying diseases, nutritional status, and stress. Factors that affect the placenta include whether placental transfer occurs and to what degree and if placental insufficiency exists [11]. Pregnancy and fetal development are dynamic states, and most exposures represent differing levels of risk depending on the stage of pregnancy. Timing of the exposure is critical in determining fetal risk. Risk also changes with breast-feeding. Nearly all reported adverse effects in nursing infants have occurred in infants younger than 6 months of age. Risk assessments (categories A, B, C, D, and X) have been assigned by the U.S. Food and Drug Administration (FDA) to all drugs based on the level of risk the drug poses to the fetus. These alphabetical classifications do not refer to breast-feeding risk [12].

Although a few antimicrobials are considered safe, and a few are contraindicated in pregnancy, most are in category C [12, 13] (Table 33-1).

ANTIMICROBIALS

There is a track record for several agents related to long and frequent use and hence presumed relative safety. These agents include the penicillins and cephalosporins, the macrolides, and antituberculosis drugs such as isoniazid, rifampin, and ethambutol. On the other hand, metronidazole has teratogenicity data for use in rodents, but data on teratogenicity for a number of other antimicrobials in pregnancy, including the fluoroquinolones, pyrazinamide, and trimethoprim, are not known [10].

Tetracycline has deleterious effects on fetal dentition, as well as certain other toxic side effects, including potentially fatal necrosis or fatty necrosis of

Table 33-1
Fetal Risk Assessment Category Summary, U.S. Food and Drug Administration

Category A	Controlled studies in women fail to demonstrate a risk to the fetus in the first trimester (and there is no evidence of a risk in later trimesters), and the possibility of fetal harm appears remote.
Category B	Either animal reproduction studies have not demonstrated a fetal risk but there are no controlled studies in pregnant women or animal reproduction studies have shown an adverse effect (other than a decrease in fertility) that was not confirmed in controlled studies in women in the first trimester (and there is no evidence of a risk in later trimesters).
Category C	Either studies in animals have revealed adverse effects on the fetus (teratogenic or embryocidal or other) and there are no controlled studies in women or studies in women and animals are not available. Drugs should be given only if the potential benefit justifies the potential risk to the fetus.
Category D	There is positive evidence of human fetal risk, but the benefits from use in pregnant women may be acceptable despite the risk (e.g., if the drug is needed in a life-threatening situation or for a serious disease for which safer drugs cannot be used or are ineffective).
Category X	Studies in animals or human beings have demonstrated fetal abnormalities or there is evidence of fetal risk based on human experience or both, and the risk of the use of the drug in pregnant women clearly outweighs any possible benefit. The drug is contraindicated in women who are or may become pregnant.

Sources: Refs. 12, 13.

the liver, pancreatitis, and renal damage. There have been data to suggest that tetracycline can be given in doses of 1 g or less per 24 hours [10]. However, standard guidelines generally recommend against the use of tetracyclines and tigecycline, a derivative of minocycline, in pregnant women or children younger than 8 years of age [14].

Aminoglycosides cross the placenta. A mild fetal vestibular toxicity effect has been reported for streptomycin. There is an unconfirmed report of neurologic toxicity with isoniazid in a small series of children whose mothers were treated with isoniazid for tuberculosis during pregnancy [10].

In addition, it is possible that serum levels of antimicrobial chemotherapy may differ from those in individuals who are not pregnant [10]. For example, serum levels of ampicillin are lower in pregnant than in nonpregnant women. This is likely related to more rapid clearance and volume of distribution of the drug. Other drugs may have similar kinetics, although data generally are not available.

Viral Infections and the Pregnant Worker

Pregnancy is a risk factor for developing viral infection. This is related to several physiologic changes occurring during pregnancy. A shift away from cell-mediated immunity toward humoral immunity can render pregnant women more susceptible to certain viral pathogens [15]. Historically, viral infections during pregnancy that have potential detrimental effects are infections caused by the rubella virus (3-day "German measles"), cytomegalovirus (CMV), and the herpes family of viruses, which includes herpes simplex virus (HSV) and varicella-zoster virus (VZV). More recently, other viruses are known to be associated with congenital infections, and these viruses are parvovirus B19, human immunodeficiency virus (HIV), coxsackieviruses, measles virus, enterovirus, adenovirus, and lymphocytic choriomeningitis virus (LCMV), which has been implicated as a teratogenic rodent-borne arena virus [16].

RUBELLA

Congenital rubella in the first 16 weeks of pregnancy is associated with multiple effects, including effect on the cardiac and neurologic systems. During the first 12 weeks of pregnancy, up to 90% of children exposed to maternal infection while in utero will have some manifestation of the congenital rubella syndrome, and this decreases during the next 4 weeks so that by 16 weeks, the risk is about 20% [17].

CYTOMEGALOVIRUS (CMV)

CMV is also in the family of herpes viruses. CMV infection is the most common congenital viral infection. It can cause growth restriction, sensorineural hearing loss, intracranial calcifications, microcephaly, hydrocephalus, hepatosplenomegaly, delayed psychomotor development, and optic atrophy. Most infections, however, cause no symptoms [18].

HERPES SIMPLEX VIRUS (HSV)

About 60% of pregnant women who are receiving obstetric care have serologic evidence of past HSV infection. HSV type 2 (HSV-2) is responsible for 70% of neonatal herpes cases. This infection can disseminate and is associated with neonatal skin lesions, encephalitis, and neurologic disability. Ninety percent of infections are transmitted perinatally through virus in the birth canal, and about 10% are congenital as a result of de novo maternal infection during pregnancy and subsequent transplacental transmission or by way of ascending infection [19, 20].

VARICELLA-ZOSTER VIRUS (VZV)

VZV infection causes both chickenpox and herpes zoster infections (shingles) in individuals who have previously had chickenpox. Chickenpox is the disseminated form of VZV occurring in previously uninfected individual, usually during childhood. Chickenpox infection in pregnant women can lead to a severe maternal disease, and it appears about five times more likely to prove fatal in pregnant women than in nonpregnant women [21]. We may see some beneficial effects following improved immunization practices with the use of an efficacious varicella vaccine administered before susceptible women become pregnant [22].

Infectious with CMV, HSV, and VZV can lead to severe maternal and fetal illness in pregnancy and many other complications, including maternal and fetal death, severe malformations, and premature birth. For severe HSV and VZV infections, antiviral treatment is necessary with valacyclovir and acy-clovir. Both are drugs of choice. Primary or recurrent HSV disease in the genital tract may be an indication for cesarean section, although suppression of recurrence with antiviral medication has reduced this indication. If neonates show signs of either HSV or VZV infection, treatment with acyclovir is recommended [23]. Because of the severity of the illness caused by these and other viral infections, management should include consultation with the treating obstetrician and infectious disease consultant as applicable.

B VIRUS

Cercopithecine herpes virus type 1, commonly known as *B virus,* normally is found among macaque monkeys, including rhesus macaques, pig-tailed macaques, and cynomolgus monkeys. Monkeys infected with the virus have no or very mild symptoms. If humans become infected, a fatal encephalomyelitis can develop. Persons at greatest risk include veterinarians, laboratory workers, and others who have contact with monkeys or monkey cell cultures. Bites or scratches or exposure to the tissues or secretions of infected monkeys causes B virus infection. Though rare, exposure to primate secretions can transmit B virus, which can be fatal. Analysis of B virus cases among primate workers suggests that certain types of exposures may pose greater risks. These exposures include deep puncture wounds that are difficult to clean, inadequately cleansed wounds, and wounds on the face and neck and thorax, especially wounds to the eye. Because virus propagation occurs retrograde along peripheral axons, an exposure to the head or thorax can rapidly involve the central nervous system (CNS) without any preceding local symptoms. The most common local symptom is numbness or paresthesia at the site of exposure. Because this infection is still rare in humans, few data exist to assess postexposure prophylaxis. Oral valacyclovir is a favored recommendation for postexposure prophylaxis, but alternative regimens are also available. Review of the literature suggests that no cases have been reported in humans who received postexposure prophylaxis within 72 hours of exposure [24].

The number of persons with potential and possibly unidentified exposure to B virus is large, and the number of clearly documented infections is small. This may suggest that there are subsets of individuals who are exposed to B virus who do not develop the illness or who develop a mild form of it without having received antiviral prophylaxis [24]. Further study is needed. Pregnant workers exposed to B virus should be managed in consultation with an infectious diseases specialist because time is of the essence.

PARVOVIRUS

Parvovirus B19 is the causative agent of erythema infectiosum, known as *fifth disease* in children, which presents as an acute febrile illness with rash. In pregnancy, acute infection has been associated with fetal anemia, hydrops fetalis, myocarditis, and intrauterine fetal death. Transmission is by the respiratory route and by blood, and maternal-to-fetal transmission can occur. Arthritis and skin and bone marrow effects are most predominant in the mother. Acute infection during 11 and 23 weeks of gestation has the highest incidence of hydrops fetalis but occurs rarely, in only about 1.6% of pregnancies when acute maternal infection occurs. There is currently no specific antimicrobial therapy, and diagnostics and preventive interventions rely on the presence of IgM and IgG antibodies to parvovirus in the mother. If IgG is positive at the time of the outbreak, the mother is immune, and there is little risk. Interestingly, rheumatoid factor can be positive in B19 infection. Pregnant women who work in outbreak settings (e.g., teachers and child-care workers) should be sent home [25]. Infectious diseases or public health consultation should be obtained. Treatment is symptomatic, and specific obstetrics recommendations should be followed.

Assessing viral and other infection risks during pregnancy is not an exact science, so the astute clinician always must rely on helpful input from the consulting obstetrician or infectious disease specialist.

Occupational Exposures to Blood in Health Care Workers

Occupational exposures of health care workers to blood necessitates addressing the probability of infection, immune status, and need for preventive treatment for hepatitis B virus (HBV), hepatitis C virus (HCV), and human immunodeficiency virus (HIV) infection. Recommendations for the management of occupational exposures to HBV, HCV,

and HIV are frequently updated and publicized by the U.S. Public Health Service [26].

"WHO DO I CALL?"

An excellent resource for special circumstances when there is a delay in the exposure report, an unknown source person, pregnancy in the exposed health care worker, resistance of the source virus to antiretroviral agents, or toxicity of the postexposure prophylaxis regimen is the National Clinicians' Post-Exposure Prophylaxis (PEP) Hotline, which is staffed by infectious disease consultants. The PEP line can be reached at 1-888-448-4911 and is based at San Francisco General Hospital, in San Francisco, California.

HEPATITIS B

Recommendations for HBV postexposure management include initiation of the hepatitis B vaccine series to any susceptible or previously unvaccinated person who sustains an occupational blood or body fluid exposure. For an unvaccinated person, the risk from a single needle stick or a cut exposure to HBV infected blood ranges from 6–30% depending on the e antigen status of the source individual [26].

Hepatitis B vaccine is an engineered product and is generally safe in pregnancy. PEP with hepatitis B hyperimmune globulin (HBIG) and/or the hepatitis B vaccine series should be considered for occupational exposures after evaluation of the hepatitis B surface antigen status of the source and the vaccination and vaccine-response status of the exposed person.

HBIG is not the same serum as gamma globulin. It is a biologic product of pooled sera, so consultation with an infectious disease consultant and/or the patient's obstetrician may be a consideration when HBIG is indicated. HBIG should be administered within 48 hours.

Hepatitis B surface antibody can be undetectable in the exposed individual in several scenarios. If the exposed individuals did not complete the hepatitis B vaccination series, or if he or she completed the series but did not respond to the vaccine, then hepatitis B surface antibody may not be present. Individuals who are nonresponders may be given a second hepatitis B vaccination series and tested for antibody response after completion of the second series. If there is still no detectable antibody response, these individuals should follow precautions for prevention of hepatitis B and should not be vaccinated with a third series. Presumed nonresponders also should be tested for hepatitis B surface antigen because chronic hepatitis B is a frequent reason for absence of detectable hepatitis B surface antibody.

Once hepatitis B surface antibody is detected or is known or verified to have been detected previously at any time, neither boosting nor revaccination is necessary. This is so because sufficient T-cell memory exists to provide a booster (anamnestic) response should HBV exposure result in presentation of hepatitis B antigen at a later time, even if antibody levels are low or not detectable.

HEPATITIS C

For HCV postexposure management, the HCV status of both the source and the exposed individual should be determined, with follow-up testing in health care workers who have been exposed to an identified HCV source. Although studies are limited, the risk of infection after a needle stick or cut exposure to HCV-infected blood is about 1.8%. Preventive treatments and vaccines for HCV are not currently available, but a pregnant woman who develops detectable HCV antibody following a negative baseline test should be referred to an infection specialist and/or her obstetrician.

HIV

In situations where a pregnant woman has a moderate- to high-risk exposure to HIV, PEP regimens should be determined in conjunction with the woman's obstetrician and/or an infection specialist. The average risk of HIV infection after a needle stick or cut exposure to HIV-infected blood is 0.3%, or about 1 in 300. About 99.7% of needle stick/cut exposures do not lead to infection. The risk after exposure to the eye, nose, or mouth to HIV-infected blood is estimated to be, on average, 0.1% or 1 in 1,000. The risk after exposure of blood on intact skin is estimated to be less than 0.1% and probably is no risk. There have been no documented cases of HIV transmission owing to an exposure involving a small amount of blood on intact skin, defined as a few drops of blood on skin for a short period of time.

When a source is identified and available for testing, and source testing is negative for HBV, HCV, and HIV, further follow-up may not be necessary.

In summary, occupational exposures should be considered urgent concerns to ensure timely postexposure management and administration of HBIG, hepatitis B vaccine, and/or HIV PEP [26].

Vaccinations in Pregnancy

Misconceptions and fear of vaccination safety and benefits are generally prevalent and are magnified during pregnancy, and adult immunization rates also have fallen short of national goals partly because of misconceptions regarding vaccine safety [27]. Routine vaccinations such as tetanus, diphtheria, influenza, and hepatitis B generally are safe. One can even consider giving other vaccines such as meningococcal and rabies vaccines. Administration in the second and third trimesters is preferred if the vaccination is given electively.

Live-virus vaccines, which include measles, mumps, and rubella (MMR), varicella, and bacille Calmette-Guérin (BCG), are contraindicated because of the theoretical risk of transmission, according to the Centers for Disease Control and Prevention (CDC) [28] (Table 33-2).

If a live-virus vaccine is given inadvertently to a pregnant woman, or if the woman becomes pregnant within 4 weeks of vaccination, she should be advised of potential effects on the fetus. Inadvertent administration of live vaccines is not considered an indication for termination of the pregnancy [27]. Breast-feeding is also a concern, and women should be reassured that no vaccines are contraindicated during breast-feeding [27].

Women who are breast-feeding always should consult with their obstetrician and/or pediatrician about whether live-virus vaccination, either for themselves or for the breast-feeding infant, is recommended.

Special recommendations are in place for other vaccines not administered routinely in the primary care setting, which include anthrax, smallpox, rabies, Japanese encephalitis, yellow fever, BCG vaccine, typhoid (oral and parenteral), cholera, and plague [27].

Tuberculin Skin Testing in Pregnancy

The diagnostic evaluation for active tuberculosis or for latent *Mycobacterium tuberculosis* infection (LTBI) is not changed during pregnancy. Tuberculin skin testing with purified protein derivative (PPD) or interferon-γ-based assays (Quantiferon or Quan-

Table 33-2
Immunizations during Pregnancy

Considered Safe if Otherwise Indicated	Contraindicated during Pregnancy or Safety Not Established	Special Recommendations Pertain
Tetanus and diphtheria toxoids (Td)	BCG[a]	Anthrax
Hepatitis B	Measles[a]	Hepatitis A
Influenza	Mumps	Japanese encephalitis
Meningococcal	Rubella	Pneumococcal
Rabies	Varicella	Polio (IPV)
Influenza		Typhoid (parenteral and Ty21a[a])
		Vaccinia[a]
		Yellow fever[a]

BCG = bacille Calmette-Guérin; IPV = inactivated polio virus.
[a]Live or attenuated vaccine
Source: Ref. 28.

tiferon Gold), chest radiography, and special sputum stains and cultures for acid-fast bacilli all should be used as applicable diagnostic tools in both the pregnant and the nonpregnant patient. Treatment for active tuberculosis is recommended as soon as the diagnosis is established. Treatment for LTBI should be based on the risk of progression to active disease [29].

Influenza Diagnosis, Prevention, and Treatment

EPIDEMIOLOGY

Pregnant women are at an increased risk for influenza-associated illness and death. The effects on the fetus of maternal influenza infection with its associated fever and medications used for prevention and treatment should be considered. As is the case with vaccinations, pregnant women might be reluctant to follow public health recommendations during an outbreak of pandemic influenza owing to fear of the effect of medications or vaccines on the fetus, and special challenges may come about owing to a conflict regarding guidelines for nonpharmaceutical interventions (e.g., voluntary quarantine) and routine prenatal care and hospital delivery [30]. Mortality rates among pregnant women in the influenza pandemics of 1918 and 1957 were abnormally high [30]. Among pregnancy-related mortality in the state of Minnesota during the 1957 pandemic influenza epidemic, influenza accounted for nearly 20% of deaths associated with pregnancy during the period, and half of women of reproductive age who died were pregnant [31]. The effects of maternal influenza infection on the fetus are not

well understood, but associations between maternal influenza and child hood leukemia [32], schizophrenia [33], and Parkinson's disease [34] are suggested in some studies.

NONPHARMACEUTICAL INTERVENTION IN PREGNANCY

A major component of health care response in the event of an influenza pandemic will be nonpharmaceutical interventions, such as social distancing and use of personal protective equipment. Pregnant women may be in the position of being care givers for children and family members who become ill, and health care facilities will need to develop plans to ensure that pregnant women the receive necessary prenatal and obstetric care, but with minimal exposure to ill patients. Experience with obstetrics services during the severe acute respiratory syndrome (SARS) epidemics in Hong Kong, China, and Toronto, Canada, may provide some examples of how to accomplish these goals [35, 36].

SEASONAL INFLUENZA VACCINATION

Pregnant women are recommended to have seasonal influenza vaccination. Although data on influenza vaccination safety in pregnancy are limited, a few published studies report no serious side effects in women or their infants, including no indications of harm from vaccination even during the first trimester. Vaccine recommendations do vary widely from country to country, mainly related to vaccination administration in the first trimester. The overwhelming evidence of excess morbidity and mortality during seasonal influenza annually and in the two previous pandemics supports vaccinating those with comorbidities during any trimester [37].

ANTIVIRAL MEDICATIONS IN PREGNANCY

Since vaccine likely will not be immediately available in a pandemic influenza outbreak, antiviral medications will be used to reduce the expected illness and death during a pandemic. Antiviral medications currently recommended for treatment and prophylaxis of influenza in humans are the neuraminidase inhibitors oseltamivir (Tamiflu) and xanamivir (Relenza). Two additional medications, the M_2 ion channel blockers amantadine and rimantidine, are not currently recommended owing to high rates of resistance among circulating community influenza A viruses, and this pattern also has been noted in some avian strains. Insufficient information on oseltamivir and zanamivir is available to assess potential risks to the fetus. This is reflected in the category C designation from the FDA (see Table 33-1). Animal studies have shown no evidence of increased risk of adverse effects. In 61 women exposed to oseltamivir in postmarketing studies, most pregnancies had normal outcomes. Single cases of trisomy 21 and anencephaly have been reported but are not believed to be causally related to oseltamivir exposure. The bioavailability of zanamavir is lower than that of oseltamivir, leading to the suggestion that it may be the preferred drug in pregnancy [30].

In conclusion, there is high risk for both the fetus and the mother in pandemic influenza. Although information is limited, pregnant women who become ill with influenza will require aggressive treatment of fever and should adhere to standard recommendations for folic acid consumption [38]. Pandemic influenza will require strategies, planning, research, communication, and careful assessments of local, regional, national, and international resources.

Travel Medicine and Malaria

International travel has increased in recent years as a result of global business opportunities, immigration, and recreational travel. There is likely an increase in travel during pregnancy as well [39]. A wide array of diseases associated with travel that can occur in utero or in the early neonatal period includes malaria, yellow fever, tuberculosis, leish-maniasis, toxoplasmosis, filariasis, Japanese encephalitis, typhoid fever, leptospirosis, dengue fever, and trypanosomiasis. When travel and exposures cannot be avoided, preventive measures through careful pretravel consultation should include discussion of length of travel, antimalaria prophylaxis, insect avoidance, food and water hygiene, and body fluid precautions [40].

MALARIA AND PREGNANCY

Adverse effects on the mother and fetus can occur when there is malaria infection during pregnancy. Of greatest concern is *Plasmodium falciparum* malaria. Maternal anemia, fetal loss, premature delivery, intrauterine growth retardation, and delivery of low-birth-weight infants (<2,500 g) can occur. The risks of these adverse outcomes are worse for women in their first and second pregnancies and for women who are HIV-positive. The World Health Organization (WHO) recommends a three-pronged approach to preventing these adverse effects in areas of Africa with high levels of *P. falciparum* malaria [41] (Table 33-3).

Pregnant women traveling to malaria risk areas in South America, Africa, the Indian subcontinent, Tajikistan, Asia, and the South Pacific should take mefloquine as their antimalarial drug. People with depression; those with a history of psychosis, other psychiatric disorders, or seizures; and people with cardiac conduction abnormalities or allergy to mefloquine should not take mefloquine [56].

Pregnant women traveling to malaria risk areas in Mexico, Haiti, the Dominican Republic, and certain countries in Central America, the Middle East, and eastern Europe should take either chloroquine or hydroxychloroquine sulfate as their antimalarial drug.

The CDC travel health website offers helpful information on malaria and travel during pregnancy (www.cdc.gov/travel/contentMalariaPregnantPublic.aspx).

Table 33-3
WHO Recommendations for Preventing Transmission of *P. falciparum* Malaria

1. Intermittent preventive treatment (IPT) with antimalarial drugs
2. Insecticide-treated bed nets (ITN).
3. Febrile malaria case management

Source: Ref. 41.

References

1. Bellis M, *History of Antiseptics*, About.com.
2. Forrest JD. Epidemiology of unintended pregnancy and contraceptive use. *Am J Obstet Gynecol* 1994: 170:1485–9.
3. Chambers CD, Andrews EB. Drug safety in pregnancy. In *Pharmacovigilance*, 2d ed. Englewood Cliffs, NJ: Wiley, 2007.
4. Bonati M, Bortolus R, et al. Drug use in pregnancy: An overview of epidemiological drug utilization studies. *Eur J Clin Pharmacol* 1990;38:325–28.
5. Werler MM, Mitchell AA, et al. First trimester maternal medication use in relation to gastroschisis. *Teratology* 2005;45:361–7.
6. Kessler RC, McGonagie KA, et al. Sex and depression in the National Comorbidity Survey. *J Affect Dis* 1993;29:85–96.
7. Kwon HL, Belanger K, et al., Asthma prevalence among pregnant and child bearing aged women in the United States: Estimates from national health surveys. *Ann Epidemiol* 2003;13:317–24.
8. Holmes LB, Wyszynski DF. The antiepileptic drug pregnancy registry: A 6-year experience. *Arch Neurol* 2004;61:673–78.
9. Belilos E, Carsons S, Rheumatologic disorders in women. *Med Clin North Am* 1998;82:77–101.
10. Moellering RC, Eliopoulos GM. Principles of anti-infective therapy. In Mandell GL, Bennett JE, et al. (eds), *Principles and Practices of infectious Diseases*, New York: Churchill-Livingstone, 2005, Chap 16.
11. Rogers JM, Kavlock RJ. Developmental toxicology. In Klassen CD (ed), *Casarett and Doull's Toxicology the Basic Science of Poisons*, 7th Ed. New York: McGraw Hill, 2007. Pp 430–3.
12. Briggs GG, Freeman RK, et al. Introduction. In *Drugs in Pregnancy and Lactation*, 7th ed. Philadelphia: Lippincott, 2005. Pp xii–xxvi.
13. Food and Drug Administration Fetal Risk Factors Summary. *Fed Reg* 1980;44:37434–67, 1980.
14. Choice of antibacterial drugs. *Treatment Guidelines from the Medical Letter* 2007;5:33–50.
15. Jamieson DJ, Theiler RN, et al. Emerging infections and pregnancy. *Emerg Infect Dis* 2006;12:1638–43.
16. Laartz B, Gompf G, et al. Viral infections and pregnancy. *Emedicine*, March 29, 2006.
17. Miller E, Craddock-Watson JE, et al. Consequences of confirmed maternal rubella at successive stages of pregnancy. *Lancet* 1982;2:781–4.
18. Gaytant MA, Steegers EA, et al. Congenital cytomegalovirus infection: Review of epidemiology and outcome. *Obstet Gynecol Surv* 2002;57:245–56.
19. Brown ZA, Selke S, et al. The acquisition of herpes simplex virus during pregnancy. *N Engl J Med* 1997; 337:509–15.
20. Corey L. Herpes simplex virus. In Mandell GL, Bennett JE, Dolan R (eds), *Mandell, Douglas, and Bennett's Principles and Practice of Infectious Diseases*, 5th Ed. Philadelphia: Churchill-Livingstone, 2000. Pp 1564–79.
21. *Drug Ther Bull* 2005;43:69–72.
22. Hollier LM, Grissom H. Human herpes viruses in pregnancy: Cytomegalovirus, Epstein-Barr virus, and varicella-zoster virus. *Clin Perinatol* 2005;32: 671–96.
23. Marculescu R, Richter L, et al. Infections with herpes simplex and varicella-zoster viruses during pregnancy. *Hautarzt* 2006;57:207–16.
24. Cohen JI, Davenport DS, et al. Recommendations for prevention and therapy for exposure to B virus (cercopithecine herpesvirus 1). *Clin Infect Dis* 2002; 35:1191–203.
25. Ghanem K. Parvovirus B19, Johns Hopkins poc-it center, antibiotic guide, http://prod.hopkins-abxguide .org, 2007.
26. Updated U.S. Public Health Service Guidelines for the Management of Occupational Exposures to HBV, HCV, and HIV, and Recommendations for Postexposure prophylaxis, *MMWR* 2001;50:1–52.
27. Sur DK, Wallis DH, O'Connell TX. Vaccinations in pregnancy. *Am Fam Physician* 2003;68:299–304.
28. Guidelines for Vaccinating Pregnant Women. Recommendations of the Advisory Committee on Immunization Practices (ACIP). Atlanta: Centers for Disease Control and Prevention, 2002.
29. Effren LS. Tuberculosis and pregnancy. *Curr Opin Pulm Med* 2007;13:205–11.
30. Rasmussen SA, Jamieson DJ, Bresee JS. Pandemic influenza and pregnant women. *Emerg Infect Dis* 2008 (in press); available from *www.cdc.gov/EID/ content/14/1/95.htm*.
31. Freeman DW, Barno A. Deaths from Asian influenza associated with pregnancy. *Am J Obstet Gynecol* 78:1172–1175, 1959.
32. Kwan ML, Metayer C, et al, Maternal illness and drug/medication use during the period surrounding pregnancy and risk of childhood leukemia among offspring. *Am J Epidemiol* 2007;165:27–35.
33. Ebert T, Kotler M. Prenatal exposure to influenza and the risk of subsequent development of schizophrenia. *Isr Med Assoc J* 2005;7:35–8.
34. Takahashi M, Yamada T. A possible role of influenza A virus infection for Parkinson's disease. *Adv Neurol* 2001;86:91–104.
35. Jamieson DJ, Ellis JE, et al. Emerging infectious disease outbreaks: Old lessons and new challenges for obstetrician-gynecologists. *Am J Obstet Gynecol* 2006;194:1546–55.
36. Owolabi T, Kwolek S. Managing obstetrical patients during severe acute respiratory syndrome outbreak. *J Obstet Gynecol Can* 2004;26:35–41.
37. Mak TK, Mangtani P, et al. Influenza vaccination in pregnancy: Current evidence and selected national policies. *Lancet Infect Dis* 2008;8:44–52.
38. Acs N, Banhidy F, et al. Maternal influenza during pregnancy and risk of congenital abnormalities in offspring. *Birth Defects [A]* 2005;73:989–96.
39. Samuel BU, Barry M. The pregnant traveler. *Infect Dis Clin North Am* 1998;12:325–54.
40. McGovern LM, Boyce TG. Congenital infections associated with international travel during pregnancy. *Travel Medicine* 2007;14:117–28.
41. CDC Travelers Health. Diseases: Malaria: Prevention, Pregnant Women; available at wwn.cdc.gov/ travel/contentMalariaPregnantPublic.aspx.

34

Occupational Infections in Research Laboratory Workers

Gregg M. Stave

Biologic laboratory research is conducted in academic, industrial, and governmental research settings. Scientists, technicians, and other personnel employed in these settings are potentially at risk for exposure to infectious agents and organisms. Exposures of concern include

- The agent or organism being studied
- Agents and organisms used in the course of the work
- Recombinant viruses and organisms
- Infectious hazards present in human- or primate-derived materials (including bloodborne pathogens)
- Zoonoses in research animals
- Transmission of infection by use of shared equipment (e.g., conjunctivitis transferred by a microscope eyepiece)

This chapter addresses the epidemiology, prevention, and control of infections in research laboratories. Zoonotic infections are covered in Chapter 36.

Epidemiology

The diversity of settings and types of biologic research mean that there is no broadly applicable epidemiology of risk. A substantial amount of laboratory research is conducted to study organisms such as *Escherichia coli* K-12 that have limited ability to cause illness or survive outside the laboratory; by contrast, other research is conducted specifically to study highly contagious and hazardous viruses and organisms, including bioterrorism defense research.

There are no broadly based population studies of laboratory-acquired infections. Instead, the literature contains reviews, case series, case reports, and findings from surveillance programs at specialized facilities [1–4]. Some published studies also fail to clearly differentiate between the research and clinical laboratory settings. Nonetheless, the literature contains sobering reports of thousands of cases of laboratory-acquired infections that have occurred during the twentieth century. An overwhelming percentage of the infections were reported prior to the past 25 years, although recent case reports clearly demonstrate that continuing vigilance is required. The most commonly reported laboratory-acquired infections are brucellosis, Q fever, typhoid, hepatitis, and tularemia. It is important to note that a documented laboratory accident had occurred in fewer than 20% of cases [4]. Determination of mechanisms of known or suspected exposure is instructive in developing prevention strategies and procedural guidelines for laboratories. Documented routes of exposure have included needlesticks, aerosol spray from syringes, lacerations from sharps and glassware, conjunctival exposure, mouth pipetting, and equipment failure. It is important to keep in mind that infections acquired through occupational exposure may have different presentations than the natural infection because the route of exposure may be different. While it is likely that many laboratory-acquired infections are not reported, there have been several notable publications. Recent case reports are illustrative.

SABIA VIRUS

In 1994, a virologist working at the Yale Arbovirus Research Unit developed a serious illness following exposure to Sabia virus [5–9]. Sabia is an arenavirus that was discovered after an agricultural engineer in Brazil died from hemorrhagic fever. Subsequently, a laboratory technician in Brazil developed a severe nonfatal illness during efforts to isolate and characterize the agent. The physician-scientist at Yale was most likely exposed following a centrifuge accident. After opening the centrifuge, the investigator noted liquid on the outside of one of the centrifuge bottles and also saw fluid at the bottom of the rotor. During decontamination and cleanup, he wore two pairs of gloves but did not use respiratory protection, even though a powered air purifying respirator (PAPR) was available. During his hospital stay, substantial precautions were taken in an effort to prevent secondary spread. This incident received extensive coverage in the media and resulted in a threat to shut down the research facility. Improvements in laboratory procedures were implemented following the incident.

HANTAVIRUS

A less well-publicized laboratory exposure (to hantavirus) occurred in the United Kingdom [10]. The case presented as hemorrhagic fever with associated renal syndrome. The hantavirus infection resulted from the handling of immunocytomas propagated in laboratory rats. In addition to the risk of infection presented by the rats, rat immunocytomas and anti-immunocytoma serum should be recognized as potentially infectious.

BRUCELLA

A 1994 report from Spain provides another reminder of the importance of adhering to standard microbiologic practice [11]. Acute brucellosis occurred in four technicians handling strains of *Brucella* and the blood cultures from which they were isolated. No accidents had been reported; however, blood culture bottles were handled without use of a biologic safety cabinet.

SIMIAN IMMUNODEFICIENCY VIRUS

Another topic of current concern is simian immunodeficiency virus (SIV) [12–17]. SIV is a lentivirus that causes an acquired immune deficiency syndrome (AIDS)–like illness in macaque monkeys and is used in the study of AIDS. SIV is genetically and antigenically related to human immunodeficiency virus type 2 (HIV-2), and HIV-2 is now considered to consist of a strain or strains of SIV that have become endemic in some regions of Africa.

The first case of laboratory-acquired SIV infection most likely occurred through skin exposure [13, 14]. A worker performed serology testing on clinical specimens from SIV-infected monkeys without wearing gloves while suffering from a severe dermatitis of the forearms and hands. There was no history of percutaneous or mucous membrane exposure. Antibody testing demonstrated persistent seroreactivity to SIV and HIV-2, although no clinical illness was described.

Another reported case of possible SIV infection in a laboratory worker occurred in 1990 [12, 14]. A technician in a research laboratory experienced a needlestick injury while drawing blood from an SIV-infected macaque. Antibodies to SIV were first detected 3 months following the exposure, and titers declined 5 months after exposure. No clinical illness developed. An effort to fulfill Koch's postulate by injecting blood from the exposed technician into a previously uninfected macaque failed to produce any evidence of SIV infection. It is possible that this worker experienced a transient infection with SIV. Alternatively, this incident may have occurred because of exposure to viral antigens, resulting in an increase in antibody titers but not an actual infection.

An anonymous survey conducted in 1992 by the National Institutes of Health (NIH) and the Centers for Disease Control and Prevention (CDC) to evaluate SIV seropositivity among SIV laboratory researchers determined that 3 of 472 samples were positive [14]. Because of the anonymous approach and use of stored serum samples, it is not known whether either of the cases of SIV described earlier was represented in the study. More recently, Sotir and colleagues reported a similar study involving 550 workers who handled nonhuman primates and nonhuman primate materials at 13 North American research institutions [17]. Two participants were seropositive, one of whom had been reported previously in the literature. The other was known to have experienced a needlestick injury with an inoculum of SIV. Possibly of more concern than the reports of seroconversion was the description of their frequency of exposures. Of the 378 workers handling nonhuman primate–derived material in the laboratory, 66 (18%) reported an injury with needlesticks or sharps, and 64 (18%) reported a skin or mucous membrane exposure. Among the 257 who performed laboratory work with SIV, 15 (6%) reported a needlestick, and 19 (7%) sustained a skin or mucous membrane exposure.

SYSTEMIC LUPUS ERYTHEMATOSUS

An intriguing paper provides a reminder that risk of infection may arise in the laboratory under unexpected circumstances [18]. A national study was conducted to evaluate the presence of antinuclear antibodies in female laboratory workers handling blood from patients with systemic lupus erythematosus (SLE). Antibodies to double-stranded DNA (anti-dsDNA) were higher in the high-exposure group than in the low-exposure group. No differences were found in anti-ssDNA or anti-poly(dA-dC)poly(dG-dT). This finding led the study authors to postulate that a transmissible agent may exist in blood from patients with SLE.

RECOMBINANT VACCINIA VIRUS

There have been several published reports of laboratory workers becoming infected with recombinant forms of vaccinia [19–23]. The first report is from early work on recombinant vaccinia in 1986. A researcher was injecting mice with a recombinant virus expressing the VSV serotype Indiana N protein. A small cut on the (ungloved) right ring finger was accidentally inoculated with a drop containing virus particles [19]. Another infection occurred

when a researcher accidentally injected his left thumb with recombinant virus [20]. A more recent report is concerning in that the route of exposure was not determined. A researcher with 10 years' experience working with genetically modified vaccinia strains developed a vesicular lesion at the distal phalanx of the second finger of his right hand that slowly progressed to a 15-mm infiltrated inflammatory nodule with central hemorrhagic necrosis. A second inflamed vesicular lesion developed at the third finger of the left hand 2 days later. The immunomodulating nature of the inserted construct thus might have added to the infectivity of the virus [21]. A Canadian researcher also developed an infection with recombinant vaccinia. She had eczema on both hands and did not wear gloves because they exacerbated her skin condition. She had noted a cut on the dorsal surface of her index finger at the second distal interphalangeal joint and subsequently developed a vesicular rash on the finger with yellowish fluid draining from some of the vesicles. She went on to develop marked swelling and redness in her hand as well as a reactive axillary lymph node and lymphangitis [22]. A case of ocular vaccinia infection occurred in an unvaccinated immunology graduate student who conducted some work outside a biologic safety cabinet. A review of work practices at that facility identified several breaches of established biosafety precautions. Staff infrequently wore eye protection while performing experiments with vaccinia. Laboratory coat sleeves were not elasticized and did not always cover the wrist. Waste pipettes were not disinfected before removal from the biosafety cabinet. Instances occurred in which samples with low titers of live virus were removed from the biosafety cabinet, transported to other parts of the facility, and manipulated. In addition, laboratory staff routinely vortexed tubes containing live virus outside the biosafety cabinet. The diagnosis was delayed because the worker did not mention her laboratory work until day 5 of her symptoms. Her lesions resolved after several weeks following hospitalization and treatment [23]. Additional reports come from the Health and Safety Executive (HSE) in the United Kingdom, including a case of a postgraduate student inoculating mice with a recombinant virus strain [24]. He had recently had an eyebrow pierced and developed a high fever and severe inflammation and swelling of the face. Although he

wore gloves and was not aware of an exposure incident, it was presumed that he had unintentionally
inoculated the open eyebrow wound. In all these reports, the lesions and symptoms resolved completely following supportive care and treatment.

Infections also have occurred in researchers with
nonrecombinant laboratory strains. In one case, a
laboratory worker experienced pain followed by the
appearance of erythema and a pustule on the left
thumb 3 days after an accidental needlestick while
working with material from a vaccinia virus (strain
WR)–infected cell culture during a virus purification procedure. Local symptoms worsened, and on
the days 5 and 6, respectively, she noticed new pustules on the fourth and fifth fingers of the same
hand Axillary lymphadenopathy was noticed on the
day 6, and on day 8, there were necrotic areas
around the lesions, and a large erythematous lesion
appeared on the left forearm. She was treated with
antibiotics, and the hand lesions were surgically excised to remove the necrotic tissue [25]. She made
a full recovery.

POTENTIAL AGENTS OF BIOTERRORISM

A recent article from the U.S. Army Medical Research Institute of Infectious Diseases (USAM-
RIID) on military researchers described their
experience with research on potential agents of
bioterrorism [26]. Between 1989 and 2002, 234
persons were evaluated for exposure to 289 infectious agents. Confirmed infections included
glanders, Q fever, vaccinia, chikungunya, and
Venezuelan equine encephalitis [26, 27]. A separate
publication described a military researcher studying anthrax who apparently became infected when
a contaminated paper towel was removed from a
biologic safety cabinet and the spores aerosolized
[28].

Prevention and Control

Development of a program to address occupational
infections in laboratory research necessitates a hazard assessment for the specific workplace. Prevention of laboratory-acquired infection should be
considered to be a component of a comprehensive
approach that addresses all workplace hazards, including chemical use and animal allergens. A prevention program should use a standard control
strategy to prevent exposure through inhalation,

ingestion, or skin penetration. Exposure can be
eliminated through a combination of administrative, work practice, and engineering controls, along
with the use of personal protective equipment. Employee education and training are essential, and
medical surveillance may be advisable. Under some
circumstances, immunization should be considered. Finally, a prevention program must incorporate postexposure evaluation and treatment.
Specific management guidelines for potential laboratory exposures to agents of bioterrorism have
been published recently [29].

ADMINISTRATIVE CONTROLS

Administrative systems need to be in place to ensure that hazard evaluations are performed and
control strategies are in place. For all but the most
innocuous settings, there should be a general
inventory of potential biologic hazards that is reviewed by occupational health and safety professionals.

Substitution is a sometimes neglected strategy
for control of hazards. Whenever possible, a less
hazardous substance or agent should be used in
place of a more hazardous one.

Work involving recombinant DNA should be
conducted according to the *Guidelines for Research
Involving Recombinant DNA Molecules* (NIH
Guidelines) [30]. While the guidelines must be followed by organizations receiving federal (NIH)
funding to conduct recombinant DNA work, the
guidelines represent "best practice" and should be
considered in all settings. From the administrative
oversight perspective, the guidelines make use of an
institutional biosafety committee (IBC) to review,
approve, and oversee research.

SAFE WORK PRACTICES

Good microbiologic technique is the cornerstone
of preventive work practices. The standard recommendations for work practices are described in the
CDC/NIH publication *Biosafety in Microbiological
and Biomedical Laboratories,* 4th edition [1], generally referred to by its acronym, *BMBL.* Laboratory
work is divided into four biosafety levels (BSLs).
The higher the level, the greater is the risk of exposure by the aerosol route. Each level has an associated set of recommendations for work practices,
engineering controls (including facility design),
and protective equipment, and each level builds on

the requirements of the previous level. Basic work practices for all laboratory work include (1) avoidance of mouth pipetting, (2) decontaminating work surfaces daily, (3) regular hand washing, (4) prohibition of eating, drinking, smoking, handling contact lenses, and applying cosmetics, and (5) restricting access to the laboratory. Anyone working in a microbiology laboratory should be familiar with all the relevant recommendations in BMBL.

In some circumstances, particularly with recombinant DNA work, a higher level of work practices is used without using a higher-level facility. Thus, for example, some work may be conducted using Biosafety Level 3 (BSL-3) practices in a BSL-2 facility.

ENGINEERING CONTROLS

Engineering controls are the preferred method to prevent exposure to biologic hazards. The handling of potentially infectious agents should take place in a biologic safety cabinet (BSC). BSCs can be class I, class II (A or B), and class III. The correct cabinet must be chosen to prevent exposure depending on the type of work being done. Class I cabinets are needed for work with low- to moderate-risk agents. In a class I cabinet, room air flows into the cabinet and is ducted through a high-efficiency particulate air (HEPA) filter. Class II cabinets are the most commonly used in microbiologic and biomedical applications. The air circulating inside the cabinet has already passed through a HEPA filter, protecting the materials inside from contamination. With class IIA cabinets, the filtered air is recirculated in the work zone. Class IIB cabinets are connected directly to the exhaust system and can be used when the work requires use of volatile or toxic chemicals or radioisotopes. Class III cabinets provide total enclosure and are used for the most hazardous organisms.

Another form of engineering controls is designing room ventilation systems so that the laboratory is maintained at negative pressure relative to adjacent rooms. In the event of a spill, aerosols in a negative-pressure environment will not contaminate surrounding facilities.

PERSONAL PROTECTIVE EQUIPMENT

The use of personal protective equipment (PPE) is necessary when hazards cannot be eliminated through other control strategies. The most common forms of PPE include gloves and laboratory coats. Respirators are not used for most routine work, except with highly hazardous agents. However, respirators may be necessary for clean-up activities following a spill.

EMPLOYEE EDUCATION AND TRAINING

Laboratory employees must receive both general and specific training. General training should address principles of biosafety and waste handling. Specific education and training of employees should lead to a full understanding of the hazards of the materials with which they will be working and procedures for working safely with specific agents or organisms. Training also should incorporate the appropriate responses to a spill, contamination, or exposure.

MEDICAL SURVEILLANCE

Medical surveillance begins with the preplacement evaluation. Specific areas of concern for biologic research include medical conditions that may make exposure more likely, such as dermatitis, or may result in heightened consequences from exposure, such as an immunocompromised state. While conditions identified at preplacement are not necessarily contraindications to work, they may require special precautions.

Periodic medical surveillance may be useful to detect the same types of conditions that are of interest at the preplacement evaluation. For some types of work, there may be value in performing testing for specific antibodies to agents being used in the laboratory. Testing can be done either at a periodic interval or at the completion of a specific work activity involving high titers of infectious material. While worth considering, periodic testing has limitations, including a lack of time specificity for the exposure. The value of periodic testing depends to some degree on the type of research being conducted. Antibody testing also raises sensitive issues, which may make some employees perceive the surveillance process as too invasive. For example, testing for herpes simplex virus or other viruses that may be considered to be sexually transmitted diseases may be disquieting. Decisions about antibody testing should be made after considering the broad range of issues, and employees should be educated about the purpose of any testing program.

Antibody testing may be more acceptable as a voluntary component of medical surveillance. However, once an exposure incident occurs, postexposure assessment is essential. Standing protocols should be developed so that immediate postexposure treatment can be initiated when appropriate.

A topic closely related to antibody testing is the use of serum banking. Serum banking is recommended for employees handling nonhuman primates and working with nonhuman primate–derived materials. In the event of an exposure incident or illness, frozen stored serum can be thawed and tested. In other settings, the value of serum banking is less clear. Efforts to maintain and track a serum bank should not be underestimated. Consent of the patient is necessary for tests conducted on stored samples, just as it is required for tests done on fresh samples, but may not be required if the tests are part of an anonymous survey.

IMMUNIZATIONS AND PROPHYLACTIC MEASURES

The most common vaccines administered to laboratory workers protect against tetanus and hepatitis B. Generally, when a vaccine is available to protect workers from a specific hazard, it is recommended as a component of the prevention program. However, the use of vaccinia vaccine for workers handling the vaccinia virus has been the subject of some debate [31–37]. Advantages of vaccination include (1) protection from inadvertent inoculation, (2) protection against serious infection from exposure through the eye, and (3) protection against seroconversion to a foreign antigen expressed by a gene inserted into a recombinant vaccinia virus. Disadvantages include (1) adverse effects of vaccination, including the risk of autoinoculation in the eye, (2) the need to prevent secondary infection for a 2-week period after inoculation, (3) false reassurance, causing workers to be less careful in their work, and (4) the possibility that immunized workers would not be able to take advantage of future vaccinia-based vaccines or gene therapy.

Another controversial issue is whether workers who decline recommended vaccinations or do not mount an adequate antibody response following immunization should be excluded from work with a specific agent. Some contend that exclusion is ap-

propriate because of the increased risk to the individual from potential exposure. However, it should be recognized that immunization is only one component of a comprehensive prevention approach and that avoidance of exposure is the most critical issue. Additionally, the lack of availability of vaccines for most infectious agents that are used in laboratory research does not preclude working with these agents. Ultimately, in these circumstances, recommendations will depend on the specific facts and risks, and the employee should be a fully informed and active participant in discussions. Final recommendations also must be consistent with the requirements of the Americans with Disabilities Act (ADA).

References

1. Centers for Disease Control and Prevention, National Institutes of Health. *Biosafety in Microbiological and Biomedical Laboratories,* 4th Ed. HHS pub no CDC 93-8395. Washington: Department of Health and Human Services, 1999.
2. Pike RM. Past and present hazards of working with infectious agents. *Arch Pathol Lab Med* 1978;102: 333–6.
3. Pike RM. Laboratory-associated infections: Incidence, fatalities, causes and prevention. *Annu Rev Microbiol* 1979;33:41–66.
4. Sullivan JF, Songer JR, Estrem IE. Laboratory-acquired infections at the National Animal Disease Center 1960–1976. *Health Lab Sci* 1978;15:58–64.
5. Barry M, Russi M, Armstrong L, et al. Treatment of a laboratory-acquired Sabia virus infection. *N Engl J Med* 1995;333:294–6.
6. Gandsman EJ, Aaslestad HG, Ouimet TC, et al. Sabia virus incident at Yale University. *Am Ind Hyg Assoc J* 1997;58:51–3.
7. Murphy FA, Johnson KM. An exotic viral disease acquired in a laboratory. *N Engl J Med* 1995;333:317–8.
8. Anonymous. Scientist tests the public trust. *Nature* 1994;371:1.
9. Ryder RW, Gandsman EJ. Laboratory-acquired Sabia virus infection (letter). *N Engl J Med* 1995; 333:1716.
10. Lloyd G, Jones M. Infection of laboratory workers with hantavirus acquired from immunocytomas propagated in laboratory rats. *J Infect* 1986;12:117–25.
11. Martin-Mazuelos E, Nogales MC, Florez C, et al. Outbreak of *Brucella melitensis* among microbiology laboratory workers. *J Clin Microbiol* 1994;32: 2035–6.
12. Khabbaz RF, Rowe T, Murphy-Corb M, et al. Simian immunodeficiency virus needlestick accident in a laboratory worker. *Lancet* 1992;340:271–3.

13. Khabbaz RF, Heneine W, George JR, et al. Infection of a laboratory worker with simian immunodeficiency virus. *N Engl J Med* 1994;330:172–7.

14. Anonymous survey for simian immunodeficiency virus (SIV) seropositivity in SIV-laboratory researchers—United States, 1992. *MMWR* 1992;41:814–5.

15. Essex M. Simian immunodeficiency virus in people. *N Engl J Med* 1994;330:209–10.

16. Langley RL. Simian immunodeficiency virus (SIV). In Wald PH, Stave GM (eds), *Physical and Biological Hazards of the Workplace.* New York: Wiley, 1994. Pp 311–2.

17. Sotir M, Swtzer W, Schable C, et al. Risk of occupational exposure to potentially infectious nonhuman primate materials and to simian immunodeficiency virus. *J Med Primatol* 1997;26:233–40.

18. Zarmbinski MA, Messner RP, Mandel JS. Anti-dsDNA antibodies in laboratory workers handling blood from patients with systemic lupus erythematosus. *J Rheumatol* 1992;19:1380–4.

19. Jones L, Ristow S, Yilma T, et al. Accidental human vaccination with vaccinia virus expressing nucleoprotein gene. *Nature* 1986;319:543–6.

20. Openshaw PJ, Alwan WH, Cherrie AH, Record FM: Accidental infection of laboratory worker with recombinant vaccinia virus. *Lancet* 1991;338:459.

21. Mempel M, Gisel I, Klugbauer N, et al. Laboratory acquired infection with recombinant vaccinia virus containing an immunomodulating construct. *J Invest Dermatol* 2003;120:356–8.

22. Loeb M, Zando I, Orvidas MC, et al. Laboratory-acquired vaccinia infection. *Can Commun Dis Rep* 2003;29:134–6.

23. Lewis FM, Chernak E, Goldman E, et al. Ocular vaccinia infection in laboratory worker, Philadelphia, 2004. *Emerg Infect Dis* 2006;12:134–7.

24. Accidental infection with vaccinia virus. *ACGM Newsletter* 32, June 2003; available at www.hse.gov.uk/biosafety/gmo/acgm/acgm32/paper8.htm.

25. Moussatche N, Tuyama M, Kato SE, et al. Accidental infection of laboratory worker with vaccinia virus. *Emerging Infect Dis* 2003;9:724–6.

26. Rusnak JN, Kortepeter MG, Aldis J, Boudreau E. Experience in the medical management of potential laboratory exposures to agents of bioterrorism on the basis of risk assessment at the US Army Medical Research Institute of Infectious Diseases (USAMRIID). *J Occup Environ Med* 2004;46:801–11.

27. Srinivasan A, Kraus CN, DeShazer D, et al. Glanders in a military research microbiologist. *N Engl J Med* 2001;345:256–8.

28. Rusnak J, Boudreau E, Bozue J, et al. An unusual inhalational exposure to *Bacillus anthracis* in a research laboratory. *J Occup Environ Med* 2004;46:313–4.

29. Rusnak JM, Kortepeter MG, Hawley RJ, et al. Management guidelines for laboratory exposures to agents of bioterrorism. *J Occup Environ Med* 2004;46:791–800.

30. National Institutes of Health. *Guidelines for Research Involving Recombinant DNA Molecules.* Washington, DC: Department of Health and Human Services, 2002; available at www4.od.nih.gov/oba/rac/guidelines_02/NIH_Guidelines_Apr_02.htm.

31. Centers for Disease Control and Prevention. Vaccinia (smallpox) vaccine: Recommendations of the Immunization Practices Advisory Committee. *MMWR* 2001;50:1–25.

32. Centers for Disease Control and Prevention. Recommendations for using smallpox vaccine in a pre-event vaccination program. Supplemental recommendations of the Advisory Committee on Immunization Practices (ACIP) and the Healthcare Infection Control Practices Advisory Committee (HICPAC). *MMWR* 2003;52:1–16.

33. Williams NR, Cooper BM. Counseling of workers handling vaccinia virus. *Occup Med* 1993;43:125–7.

34. Anonymous. Pros and cons of vaccinia immunization. *J Occup Med* 1992;34:757.

35. Jackson GW. Vaccinia. In Wald PH, Stave GM (eds), *Physical and Biological Hazards of the Workplace,* 2nd ed. New York: Wiley, 2002. Pp. 402–4.

36. Isaacs SN. Critical evaluation of smallpox vaccination for laboratory workers. *Occup Environ Med* 2002;59;573–4.

37. Fulginiti VA. The risks of vaccinia in laboratory workers. *J Invest Dermatol* 2003;120:viii.

35 Occupational Infections in Health Care Workers

Marian Swinker

The health care industry is one of the largest in the United States, employing over 12 million workers [1]. Hospitals employ about 50% of all health service personnel; 20% work in nursing homes and personal care settings and the remainder in outpatient and prehospital settings [2]. The majority (75–80%) of health care workers are women. The overall rate of work-related injury and illness for these employees is 11.8 per 100 for hospital workers and 17.3 for nursing home and personal care facilities, exceeding the average rate of 8.5 in private industry. Most of the injuries reported in health care workers are due to musculoskeletal injuries, not infectious diseases, but existing databases may not capture the incidence of infectious illness adequately in health care workers [3]. Seroconversion owing to bloodborne pathogens exposure or workplace infection with tuberculosis, including latent tuberculosis following exposure to a known case [4], should be recorded on the Occupational Safety and Health Administration's (OSHA's) 300 log record-keeping system. Other infections that are not unique to the health care setting or that do not follow a recognized exposure event may not be attributed to occupation.

Individuals who work in health care are exposed to a variety of infections from patients (Table 35-1) and may spread their own infections to patients (Table 35-2). Routes of infection include direct contact with infected persons, respiratory or airborne spread, transmission via fomites, and percutaneous sticks, cuts, or abrasions. The OSHA initiatives of the 1990s to protect health care workers from bloodborne pathogens and tuberculosis received considerable attention and carry the force of law, mandating hepatitis B immunization, surveillance, and postexposure procedures. The routine infection control policies and procedures that health care workers follow are less well publicized but just as important in preventing infection. These include isolation precautions, appropriate handling of materials, disinfection and sterilization practices, waste disposal, other immunizations (Table 35-3), and especially, proper hand washing, which contribute to the protection of workers and patients [5]. This chapter reviews some infections commonly of concern in the health care workplace. Recognition of the possibility of nosocomial spread of infection and prompt institution of control measures are critical to counteract spread.

In the hospital setting, prevention requires cooperation among various departments. Infection control, employee health services, administration, and human resources all have an important role. In smaller institutions or the outpatient setting, similar principles apply. The employer is ultimately responsible for ensuring that personnel are safe and productive and that regulatory requirements are met.

624

Table 35-1
Occupationally Acquired Infections Encountered in Specific Groups of Healthcare Workers

Groups Affected	Infections
Laboratory workers	*Neisseria meningitidis* infections, brucellosis, Q fever, hepatitis, typhoid fever, tularemia, tuberculosis, dermatomycosis, Venezuelan equine encephalitis, psittacosis, coccidioidomycosis, rickettsiosis, arenavirus infection
Pregnant healthcare workers[a]	Rubella, parvovirus B19 infection, cytomegalovirus infection, varicella, echovirus infection, coxsackievirus infection
Pathology workers	Tuberculosis, human immunodeficiency virus (HIV) infection (?), hepatitis B, Creutzfeldt-Jakob disease, legionnaires' disease, Lassa fever, anthrax, group A streptococcal infection, tetanus, typhoid fever
Surgery workers	Hepatitis B, other infections caused by bloodborne pathogens
Dentists	Hepatitis B, hepatitis C, herpetic whitlow, mumps, tuberculosis
Anesthesia workers	Hepatitis B, rhinovirus infection
Laundry workers	Smallpox, salmonellosis, hepatitis A, scabies, Q fever

[a]Incidence of infection is not increased, but infection poses a potential risk to fetal development.
Source: Adapted from Sepkowitz KA. Occupationally acquired infections in healthcare workers. Part II. *Ann Intern Med* 1996;125:917–28.

Table 35-2
Guidelines for Work Restrictions for Personnel with Infectious Diseases

Disease Problem	Relieve From Direct Patient Contact	Partial Work Restriction	Duration
Conjunctivitis, infections	Yes		Until discharge ceases
Cytomegalovirus infections	No		
Diarrhea[a]			
Acute stage (diarrhea with other symptoms)	Yes		Until symptoms resolve and infection with *Salmonella* is ruled out
Convalescent stage *Salmonella* (nontyphoidal)	No	Personnel should not take care of high-risk patients	Until stool is free of the infecting organism on two consecutive cultures not less than 24 hours apart
Other enteric pathogens[b]	No		
Enteroviral infections	No	Personnel should not take care of infants and newborns	Until symptoms resolve
Group A streptococcal disease	Yes		Until 24 hours after adequate treatment is started
Hepatitis, viral hepatitis A	Yes		Until 7 days after onset of jaundice
Hepatitis B, acute	No	Personnel should wear gloves for procedures that involve trauma to tissues or contact with mucous membranes or nonintact skin	Until antigenemia resolves
Chronic antigenemia	No	Same as acute illness	Until antigenemia resolves
Hepatitis C	No	Same as hepatitis B	
Hepatitis non-A, non-B	No	Same as acute hepatitis B	Periodic infectivity has not been determined
Herpes simplex			
Genital	No		
Hands (herpetic whitlow)	Yes	(**Note:** It is not known whether gloves prevent transmission)	Until lesions heal
Orofacial	No	Personnel should not take care of high-risk patients	Until lesions heal

Table 35-2
Continued

Disease Problem	Relieve From Direct Patient Contact	Partial Work Restriction	Duration
HIV-Ab positive	Yes		Until their job activities have been reviewed to determine under what circumstances, if any, they may continue to perform exposure-prone procedures
Measles (active)	Yes		Until 7 days after the rash appears
Postexposure (susceptible personnel)	Yes		From the 5th through the 21st day after exposure and/or 7 days after the rash appears
Mumps			
Active	Yes		Until 9 days after onset of parotitis
Postexposure	Yes		From the 12th through the 26th day after exposure or until 9 days after onset of parotitis
Pertussis (active)	Yes		From the beginning of the catarrhal stage through the 3rd week after onset of paroxysms or until 7 days after start of effective therapy
Postexposure (asymptomatic personnel)	No		
Postexposure (asymptomatic personnel)	Yes		Same as active pertussis
Rubella (active)	Yes		Until 5 days after the rash appears
Postexposure (asymptomatic personnel)	Yes		From the 7th day through the 21st day after exposure and/or 5 days after rash appears
Scabies	Yes		Until treated
Staphylococcus aureus (skin lesions)	Yes		Until lesions have resolved
Tuberculosis, pulmonary	Yes		Until receiving adequate therapy, proof of three consecutive daily negative acid-fast bacilli smears, cough is resolved
Upper respiratory tract infections[c] (high-risk patients)	Yes	Personnel with upper respiratory tract infections should not take care of high-risk patients	Until acute symptoms resolved
Zoster (shingles), active	No	Appropriate barrier desirable; personnel should not take care of high-risk patients	Until lesions dry and crust
Postexposure (asymptomatic personnel)	Yes		From the 10th through the 21st day after exposure or if varicella occurs, until all lesions dry and crust
Varicella (chickenpox)			
Active	Yes		Until all lesions dry and crust
Postexposure	Yes		From the 10th through the 21st day after exposure or if varicella occurs, until all lesions dry and crust

[a]Various agents may cause diarrhea.
[b]Generally, personal hygiene, particularly hand washing before and after all patient contact, will minimize risk of transmitting enteric pathogens to patients.
[c]High-risk patients with upper respiratory tract infections are neonates, young infants, patients with chronic obstructive pulmonary disease, and immunocompromised patients.
Source: Adapted from CDC guidelines for infection control in healthcare personnel. *Infect Control Hosp Epidemiol* 1998;19:407–63.

Table 35-3
Immunizing Agents Strongly Recommended for Healthcare Workers

Agent	Dosage Schedule	Indications
Hepatitis B (HB) recombinant vaccine	Two doses IM 4 weeks apart; third dose 5 months after second; booster doses not necessary.	**Pre-exposure:** HCWs at risk for exposure to blood or body fluids. **Postexposure:** See Table 35-5.
Influenza vaccine (inactivated whole-virus and split-virus vaccines)	Annual vaccination with current vaccine. Administered IM.	HCWs who have contact with patients at high risk for influenza or its complications.
Measles live-virus vaccine	One dose SC; second dose at least 1 month later.	HCWs born during or after 1957 who do not have documentation of having received 2 doses of live vaccine on or after the first birthday *or* a history of physician-diagnosed measles or serologic evidence of immunity. Vaccination should be considered for all HCWs who lack proof of immunity, including those born before 1957.
Mumps live-virus vaccine	One dose SC; no booster.	HCWs believed to be susceptible can be vaccinated. Adults born before 1957 can be considered immune.
Rubella live-virus vaccine	One dose SC; no booster.	HCWs who do not have documentation of having received live vaccine on or after their first birthday *or* laboratory evidence of immunity.
Varicella-zoster live-virus vaccine	Two 0.5-mL doses SC 4–8 weeks apart if ≥13 years of age.	For HCWs who do not have either a reliable history of varicella or serologic evidence of immunity.
Adult acellular pertussis vaccine (Tdap) with tetanus and diphtheria	One dose every 10 years anticipated	For healthcare workers with last tetanus booster at least 2 years ago or who require tetanus toxoid-containing vaccine for wound management.

Source: Adapted from Immunization of healthcare workers. *MMWR* 1997;46(suppl):3–37, and Preventing Tetanus, Diphtheria, and Pertussis among adults *MMWR* 2006;55(RR17);1–33.

Tuberculosis

Tuberculosis (TB), caused by *Mycobacterium tuberculosis,* is typically characterized by pulmonary or disseminated caseous lesions. Infected sites may include the meninges, bones, genitourinary tract, larynx, skin, pleura, and peritoneum. The disease course may be indolent or acute depending on host characteristics. Hospitals may be settings for nosocomial transmission of infection, especially when persons infected with human immunodeficiency virus (HIV) are treated in ward settings [6]. Data on TB transmission in health care overall are limited; most reports come from large, urban, acute care hospitals [6, 7]. Historically, TB was an expected hazard for health care providers. Today, the incidence of TB infection in health care workers varies widely depending on local prevalence and patient population served.

EPIDEMIOLOGY

In health care workers, the baseline prevalence of past TB infection (latent infection) ranges from 1–28% [7]. After a known exposure, 4–70% of exposed workers may develop a positive skin test; the higher risk is related to the performance of bronchoscopy [7, 8]. Without a known exposure, the yearly conversion rate for health care workers averages 0.1–5.0% [7]. From 1985–1993, the number of reported TB cases in the United States increased by 14%. This increase was associated with TB outbreaks in health care facilities and health care–associated transmission, frequently affecting HIV-infected health care personnel or patients (Figure 35-1). Rigorous emphasis on infection control measures in health care and public health settings and other control measures led to a decline in TB cases by 1997 [9]. The national TB rate continued to decline to 4.6 cases per 100,000 persons in 2006 primarily owing to a decline in incidence in U.S.-born persons. Incidence rates among foreign-born persons remain high [10]. Seven states (i.e., California, Florida, Georgia, Illinois, New Jersey, New York, and Texas) accounted for 60% of all TB cases in 2004, with wide variation by racial and ethnic group. This geographic variation persists because the incidence of TB in some geographic areas (Figure 35-2) is nearly double the national rate [11]. The CDC guidelines for preventing the transmission of TB in health care facilities, published in

Figure 35-1
Number of persons with reported cases of tuberculosis by country of birth—United States, 1996–1997.

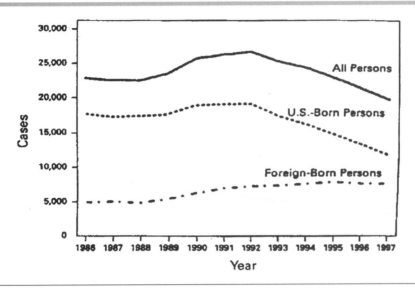

Source: From Tuberculosis morbidity—United States, 1997. *MMWR* 1994;43(Suppl):1–132.

Figure 35-2
Reported TB cases, United States, 1982–2006. The resurgence of TB in the mid-1980s peaked in 1992. Case counts began decreasing again in 1993, and 2006 marked the fourteenth year of decline.

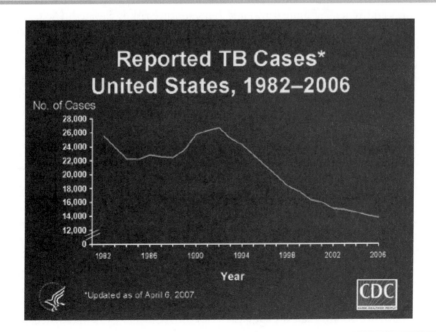

October 1994, were adopted by OSHA to guide its inspections [11]. The CDC guidelines were updated in 2005 and are expected to be similarly adopted by OSHA in the future.

PREVENTION AND CONTROL

Using CDC guidelines, OSHA mandates that health care facilities conduct a risk assessment, perform skin testing for TB at least yearly [12], and develop isolation procedures for potentially infectious TB patients in hospitals and in some outpatient settings. Patients are to be screened for symptoms of active TB and removed to isolation rooms as quickly as possible, using surgical masks on patients to contain their secretions during transport.

In hospitals and high-risk outpatient areas, respiratory protective devices, such as high-efficiency particulate (HEPA) filter masks, approved N-95 series filtering face masks, or helmet-type powered air purifying respirators (PAPRs), are to be worn by health care personnel when caring for patients with known or suspected tuberculosis. With the exception of PAPRs, the masks must be individually fitted to the worker. Respiratory protection for TB is now regulated under the same rules as all other OSHA respiratory protection programs, using a standard OSHA health questionnaire for the initial medical evaluation and requiring annual training and fit tests [13]. Even health care workers who are positive for the tuberculin skin test should use respiratory protection because reinfection with a different genotype of *M. tuberculosis* is possible, comprising 4% of recurrent TB cases in one study [14].

Multidrug-resistant (MDR) strains of TB are seen frequently in HIV-infected individuals and are associated with a high mortality rate. In 1997, 7.6% of isolates were resistant to isoniazid (INH) and 1.3% to both INH and rifampin [9]. Nearly half of MDR cases were reported from New York and California. It is recommended that four drugs be used in the initial management of active TB if the frequency of INH resistance in the state exceeds 4%; in 1998, the majority of states exceeded that threshold. By 2003–2004, the prevalence of MDR TB declined by over half to 1.1% [11].

Where INH resistance occurs, there are implications for employee health practice. If a health care worker is exposed to MDR TB and experiences a skin test conversion, the typical INH or rifampin treatment regimen for latent TB should be modified or supplemented using a drug(s) to which the infecting organism will be susceptible.

Recognition of infectious tuberculosis may be difficult in HIV-infected patients. HIV infection with low CD4 lymphocyte counts can lead to atypical presentations of TB. The tuberculin skin test may be nonreactive. Disease may have extrapulmonary presentations, such as meningitis or abscesses. Negative sputum smear results may occur in the presence of pulmonary disease [15], delaying recognition and institution of appropriate precautions.

Bacille Calmette-Guérin (BCG) vaccine, used in many high-prevalence countries, is 52–100% effective in preventing dissemination or development of active disease in children following latent infection. The protective effect is less in adults; efficacy in preventing adult forms of disease ranges from 0–17% up to 50% [16]. Under normal circumstances, BCG vaccine is not recommended routinely for preventive use in U.S. health care workers [17].

MEDICAL SURVEILLANCE

Currently, the CDC recommends that all health care workers with potential exposure (other than known reactors) be screened yearly and more often if exposure risk is elevated. The traditional screening mechanism is the tuberculin skin test (TST), also known as the *purified protein derivative* (PPD) *test*. Interpretation guidelines for PPD skin tests in health care personnel are given in Table 35-4.

Screening should include individuals who have previously received BCG vaccine, for whom testing is contraindicated only if the individual has experienced a large necrotic reaction to a past skin test. This represents a change in practice because many BCG-vaccinated health care workers previously have been advised not to participate in skin testing. Skin test reactions owing to prior vaccination typically decline in size with time, and the vaccine does not effectively prevent infection. If a TST response (induration) increases in size by 10 mm compared with the previous year's test, this suggests acquisition of new infection rather than past vaccination effect. Essentially, skin test results are interpreted no differently in BCG-vaccinated persons than in nonvaccinated individuals.

The 5-tuberculin-unit dose used in skin testing represents a compromise between sensitivity and

Table 35-4
Tuberculosis Skin Test Interpretation

1. An induration of ≥5 mm is classified as positive in:
   - Persons who have human immunodeficiency virus (HIV) infection or risk factors.
   - Persons who have had recent close contact[a] with persons who have active tuberculosis (TB).
   - Persons who have fibrotic chest radiographs (consistent with healed TB lesions).
2. An induration of ≥10 mm is classified as positive in all persons who do not meet any of the criteria above but who have other risk factors for TB, including high-risk groups[a] and high-prevalence populations.
3. An induration of ≥15 mm is classified as positive in persons who do not meet any of the above criteria.

[a]PPD skin-test results in healthcare workers (HCWs):
- The prevalence of TB in the facility should be considered when choosing the appropriate cutoff point for defining a positive PPD reaction. In facilities where there is essentially no risk for exposure to *Mycobacterium tuberculosis* (i.e., minimal- or very low-risk facilities, an induration ≥15 mm may be a suitable cutoff for HCWs who have no other risk factors. In facilities where TB patients receive care, the cutoff point for HCWs who have no other risk factors may be ≥10 mm.
- A recent conversion in a HCW should be defined generally as a ≥10-mm increase in size of induration within a 2-year period. For HCWs who work in facilities where exposure to TB is very unlikely (e.g., minimal-risk facilities), an increase of ≥15 mm within a 2-year period may be more appropriate for defining a recent conversion because of the lower positive-predictive value of the test in such groups.
Source: Adapted from Guidelines for preventing TB transmission in healthcare facilities. *MMWR* 1994;43(suppl):1–132.

specificity. The predictive value of a positive test is related to the prevalence of *M. tuberculosis* in the population tested. In a population with a low prevalence of infection, that is, 5–10%, the predictive value of a 10-mm skin test reaction (induration) is low, and the reaction is as likely to be due to nontuberculous mycobacteria as to TB. A 10-mm reaction is defined as a positive test in health care personnel owing to their increased likelihood of exposure to TB to maximize the sensitivity of the testing process. The area of cellular infiltration (induration) reflects the delayed, cell-mediated hypersensitivity response. Erythema, acute inflammation, vasodilatation, and capillary congestion alone, without induration, do not constitute a positive skin reaction [18]. Use of a 1-tuberculin-unit "test dose" owing to concern about allergy/humeral immunity is not standardized or recommended by the American Thoracic Society [19]. Yearly surveillance for previous TST reactors is by symptom reporting; repeat chest radiography is reserved for those experiencing symptoms of chronic cough, fever, night sweats, and/or weight loss.

In addition to annual surveillance, any workers who experience a recognized exposure to infectious TB in a clinical setting or pathology laboratory should receive a baseline skin test within 2 weeks and a follow-up at 8 weeks postexposure to detect latent infection [11]. If the baseline test cannot be obtained so soon, it may be eliminated because skin test reactions related to the exposure may be detected as early as 2 weeks.

For health care workers with organ transplants, HIV infection, corticosteroid use (15 mg/day of prednisone or equivalent), or other immune suppression, a skin test reaction of 5 mm or more of induration is considered positive [17]. Anergy testing is not recommended routinely for all HIV infected persons being skin tested for TB owing to reported selective nonreactivity to PPD; however, use in health care personnel with other causes of potential immune impairment is not addressed [20]. Of patients with active TB, 10–25% are nonresponders to TSTs; other infections, malnutrition, drugs, and general debility (including HIV infection with CD4 lymphocyte counts lower than 200/mm^3) may contribute to false-negative results [18].

OSHA's current enforcement directives for inspectors mandate the use of two-stage testing for TB in all new employees who have not had a PPD skin test in the past year [21]. This procedure is used to detect a possible "boosting" effect. This results when the first (negative) PPD in a person with previous latent infection leads to "recall" of the immune response. A larger skin test reaction occurs if the test is repeated in 1–3 weeks, indicating past infection. This boosting effect can persist for over a year and lead to falsely considering the individual to be a recent seroconverter when enrolled in yearly surveillance. One Canadian study found the incidence of boosting to be 10% in BCG recipients and 2.5% in others [22]. In a group of U.S. medical students at the Uniformed Services University of Health Sciences, the incidence of boosting effect was 4.8%, but the BCG history was not obtained [23]. The boosting effect is also reported to be more common in areas with frequent crossreactions owing to nontuberculous mycobacteria [22].

Boosting may be more common in males, individuals over age 55, persons born outside the United States, and BCG recipients [24]. The overall incidence of the boosting effect in health care workers is not known. In a high-prevalence area, a New York City hospital found that 40% of new hires were PPD positive, and an additional 10% were discovered by the two-step procedure [25]. In other settings, the prevalence of the booster effect may be much lower. In a tertiary care center in eastern North Carolina, 0.6% of preplacement skin tests were newly positive, and an additional 0.4% were detected with two-step testing [26]. While rare, this boosting effect would falsely elevate the low yearly skin test conversion rate of 0.1–0.2% if not recognized. CDC guidelines allow for decisions on the use of the two-stage test to be based on institutional data on the incidence of boosting in the facility, but OSHA has chosen to enforce use of the two-step procedure for new employees regardless of age, immune status, or facility experience.

Use of the TB skin test during pregnancy may generate unnecessary controversy. There is no evidence that pregnancy affects the accuracy of the test. The test is safe and valid throughout pregnancy and has no known teratogenic effects [8], yet pregnant employees frequently refuse the PPD test based on the recommendations of their personal physicians.

The TST has several limitations; reactions can be nonspecific, and interpretation is somewhat subjective, leading avid interest in the development of blood assays for MDR TB. A whole-blood interferon-γ release assay is available in the United States that can be used in health care worker screening and surveillance programs under the CDC 2005 guidelines (11). The blood assay does not require a two-step test at baseline and is more specific for *M. tuberculosis.* A positive test result indicates probable MTB infection. A negative result means infection is unlikely. Table 35-5 gives interpretation guidelines for use of the blood test. Table 35-6 compares its results with the TST.

Table 35-5

Interpretations of Tuberculin Skin Test (TST) and QuantiFERON®-TB Test (QFT) Results According to the Purpose of Testing for *Mycobacterium Tuberculosis* Infection in a Health-Care Setting

Purpose of Testing	TST	QFT
1. Baseline	1. ≥10 mm is considered a positive result (either first- or second-step)	1. Positive (only one-step)
2. Serial testing without known exposure	2. Increase of ≥10 mm is considered a positive result (TST conversion)	2. Change from negative to positive (QFT conversion)
3. Known exposure (close contact)	3. ≥5 mm is considered a positive result in persons who have a baseline TST result of 0 mm; an increase of ≥10 mm is considered a positive result in persons with a negative baseline TST result or previous follow-up screening TST result of ≥0 mm	3. Change to positive

Source: From Centers for Disease Control and Prevention. Guidelines for Preventing the Transmission of *Mycobacterium tuberculosis* in Health-Care Setting, 2005. *MMWR* 2005:54(No. RR-17) 1–89.

Table 35-6

Interpretation of QuantiFERON®-TB Gold Test (QFT-G) Results

QFT-G Result	Interpretation
Positive	
ESAT-6 or CFP-10* responsiveness detected	*Mycobacterium tuberculosis* infection probable
Negative	
No ESAT-6 and CFP-10 responsiveness detected	*M. tuberculosis* infection unlikely, but cannot be excluded, especially when
	1. any illness is consistent with TB disease, and
	2. the likelihood of progression to TB disease is increased (e.g., because of immunosuppression)
Indeterminate	Test not interpretable

*ESAT-6 is a 6-kDa early secretory antigenic target, and CFP-10 is 10-kDa culture filtrate protein.

Source: From Centers for Disease Control and Prevention. Guidelines for Preventing the Transmission of *Mycobacterium tuberculosis* in Health-Care Setting, 2005. *MMWR* 2005:54(No. RR-17) 1–89.

DIAGNOSIS AND TREATMENT

A new skin test or blood test converter should be questioned about symptoms and undergo chest radiography to rule out active disease. Persons with active infection are treated for 6–9 months using four drugs for the first 2 months, tapering the number of drugs as bacterial sensitivity results and clinical response are obtained. Those with no symptoms and negative chest x-ray have latent infection. What was previously termed *preventive therapy* is now called *treatment of latent TB* [17]. Treatment of latent TB should be considered for any health care worker who converts during yearly surveillance, regardless of age. These workers typically would meet the criteria for high risk: recent conversion and potential contact with active TB [12]. The risk of developing active (infectious) TB is about 3–5% during the first year after initial infection; another 3–5% may develop active disease at a time remote from acquisition. The ability of the host to contain the disease is diminished by conditions such as silicosis, HIV infection, diabetes mellitus, corticosteroid or immunosuppressive drug use, and gastrectomy [18]. Treatment of latent TB uses INH for 9 months optimally or 6 months at minimum. Rifampin for 4 months is another option. The combination of rifampin and pyrazinamide is not recommended owing to the hepatotoxicity observed [27]. Treatment of latent TB in an HIV-infected health care worker may lead to drug interaction with the antiretroviral drug treatment. For latent infection, a course of INH is 93–98% effective in preventing active TB. INH is frequently supplemented with pyridoxine, 25–50 mg, to prevent neurotoxicity. In states where MDR TB is common, alternative latent treatment regimens use drugs to which the organisms are likely to be sensitive. Individuals who are skin-test-positive are usually considered to be at very low risk for subsequent reinfection with TB, but there are reports of reinfection with a different strain of *M. tuberculosis*. Whether previous infection offers any degree of protection from reinfection is unclear [28].

The CDC 1994 guidelines suggest comparing the yearly skin test conversion rates of clinical employees with those of non–patient care employees (representing the community baseline) to assess the adequacy of preventive measures. Any skin test conversions occurring in clusters or resulting from a known exposure should trigger a review of the adequacy of existing control measures.

Use of the TST is complicated by sensitivity and specificity issues. In ill persons with active infection, the test is frequently negative. The 10-mm reaction that defines a positive test for a health care worker may reflect exposure to nontuberculosis environmental mycobacteria species; 30–50% of reactions in the 10- to 14-mm range are positive owing to *M. avium* exposure [29]. (The 15-mm cut point used for the general public is more specific but less sensitive to *M. tuberculosis*.) The skin test response may vary by about 15% in the same individual when a TST is applied to each arm simultaneously. There is variation (about 15%) in measuring induration among experienced TST readers [18] and a higher degree of measurement variability among less experienced readers [29]. The CDC 2005 guidelines advise that only trained designated individuals administer and read the surveillance skin tests for health care workers and prescribe a defined training program for test readers (11) to improve quality control of the surveillance testing.

Severe Acute Respiratory Syndrome (SARS)

In 2003, SARS was recognized in China and eventually spread to 29 countries, causing more than 8,000 cases and 780 deaths [30]. In the United States, there were 8 laboratory-confirmed cases and no significant local spread. The initial spread of the disease in health care settings in Asia and Toronto, Canada, was attributed to lack of optimal infection control practices. Global travel played a major role in its spread beyond the borders of China.

The overall SARS case-fatality rate is 10%, higher in the elderly and lower in children. SARS-associated corona virus (SARS-CoV) is related to the common cold virus and has an incubation period of 4–6 days. Most patients become ill within 2–10 days of exposure with fever, headache, and myalgias. Respiratory complaints follow symptom onset and typically consist of a nonproductive cough and dyspnea. Radiographic evidence of pneumonia develops by 7–10 days; 70–90% of patients manifest a lymphopenia. The nonspecific symptoms of SARS commonly include diarrhea, rigors, and chills; sore throat or rhinorrhea also may occur. Spread of infection is generally person to person; however, laboratory-related transmission occurred in 2004 in China.

Case detection for SARS is largely based on epidemiologic factors—the presence of radiologically confirmed pneumonia or acute respiratory distress syndrome in a person who has traveled to an area of the world where SARS was present or who has had close contact with an ill person who traveled there. Employment as a health care worker with direct SARS patient contact or in a laboratory working with live SARS-CoV is also a risk factor [30]. A cluster of atypical pneumonia in health care workers in the same facility without an alternative diagnosis may raise the suspicion for SARS.

Patients admitted to the hospital with radiologically confirmed pneumonia should be placed into droplet isolation and risk factors for SARS-CoV reviewed. If there is a high suspicion for SARS, SARS-CoV laboratory diagnostics can be obtained through the local health department while full SARS isolation is maintained and contacts identified. During the first week of illness, nasopharyngeal and oropharyngeal swabs are used for diagnosis, supplemented by stool tests after the first week. Serologic tests are rarely positive during the first week and usually become positive during the second week, but antibody detection may be delayed as late as day 29 [31].

The U.S. Centers for Disease Control and Prevention (CDC) recommends that hospitals develop contingency plans to be used if person-to-person transmission of SARS recurs. The level of anticipated response depends on the proximity of SARS; triage, surveillance, and other infection control activities would be increased according to the proximity of the risk [31]. Measures could include daily screening of all visitors and employees for fever or symptoms before entry, excluding visitors from the premises, furloughing any ill employees, and other contingencies. Quarantine measures would be invoked by the local health department if SARS is identified in the community.

Airborne and droplet isolation and contact precautions are used when caring for patients with known or possible SARS-CoV disease for the duration of infectivity. Health care workers should wear a standard isolation gown, gloves, respiratory protection (at minimum, an N-95 filtering face piece respirator), and eye protection before entering a SARS patient's room. It is unclear whether routine eye protection is needed to prevent SARS-CoV transmission, but it is recommended when within 3 ft of the patient or when performing procedures that spray or splash respiratory secretions [31]. A powered air purifying respiratory provides a greater degree of protection from respiratory contact with the virus.

During hospitalization, SARS patients should be placed in airborne isolation rooms, wear a mask and clean gown during transport, and have limited contact with others in hallways and elevators. Recovering patients should remain at home for at least 10 days even if fever and symptoms have resolved [32]. There is no specific treatment for SARS; care is supportive, with no prophylactic treatment or immunization available. Infection control practices are relied on to prevent nosocomial transmission.

High-risk procedures associated with transmission in Hong Kong included intubation and use of jet nebulizers and assisted ventilation [33]. In Singapore, both direct and indirect contact with respiratory or body fluids was considered a risk factor for transmission. Institution of personal protective measures against droplet spread and contact with body fluids was reported to be effective in preventing nosocomial spread [34]. SARS focused the attention of health care personnel on the use of personal protective equipment (PPE). In contrast to use for TB, the risk of SARS led to greater acceptance of PPE. Health care workers wearing an N-95 mask *together* with a powered air purifying respirator to treat SARS patients found this combination to be acceptable despite some interference with communication [35].

In Canada, N-95-equivalent respirators had been recommended for TB and other potentially infectious aerosols, but fit testing was not widely applied in health care settings until the SARS outbreaks. Studies comparing the use of N-95 respirators with and without fit testing reported conflicting results [36]. Based on theoretical models, the N-95 or equivalent filtering facepiece should provide an order of magnitude better protection than a surgical mask, which is better than no mask. An elastomeric (cartridge) HEPA respirator provides more protection than the disposable N-95 filtering facepiece but is less protective than the powered air purifying respirator [36]. The spread of SARS in health care settings focused attention on how airborne agents are spread and the need for active implementation of infection control practices. In the absence of recurrent SARS outbreaks, hospital SARS contingency plans can be adapted for other emerging airborne infections that may occur, such as pandemic influenza.

Bloodborne Pathogens

HUMAN IMMUNODEFICIENCY VIRUS

HIV is a viral infection that progressively damages the immune system, eventually leading to AIDS. More than a dozen opportunistic infections and several cancers are considered relatively specific indicators of AIDS. The first report of HIV transmission via needlestick ushered in an era of concern about occupational hazards in health care [2].

Epidemiology

By 2001, the CDC had documented 57 confirmed cases of occupational HIV transmission and over 100 possible cases in health care workers [37]. Most cases were caused by percutaneous injuries with sharps and affected nurses, physicians, and laboratory technicians.

Prevention and Control

Procedures that limit exposure to bloodborne pathogens, such as universal precautions and use of personal protective equipment or safety devices, minimize exposure to HIV. When exposure does occur, postexposure prophylaxis (PEP) should be provided. The risk of seroconversion following a needlestick with HIV-positive blood is generally estimated to be about 0.3%; it is 0.09% after a mucous membrane splash and less than 0.09% for a cutaneous splash on nonintact skin. Among occupationally exposed health care workers, the risk of seroconversion increases in direct proportion to the quantity of blood with contact (e.g., a visibly bloody instrument or a hollow needle that had been removed from a vascular site), the depth of the wound (e.g., subcutaneous), especially if injection is involved, and the source patient's viral load (e.g., a patient with terminal AIDS) [38]. After exposure to HIV-infected blood or body fluids, surveillance for seroconversion should be continued for a minimum of 6 months, according to CDC guidelines. Rare instances of delayed seroconversion (up to 12 months) have been reported and

may be associated with simultaneous exposure to hepatitis C virus (HCV) and HIV [38].

The efficacy of zidovudine (AZT) in reducing the risk of HIV infection in health care workers is about 80% based on case-control studies [39]. The cost of preventing a single case of HIV conversion is quite high in a setting of low HIV prevalence [40], but PEP is justified owing to the dire consequences associated with HIV infection. Many recipients of prophylactic treatment experience side effects (frequently nausea, diarrhea, and myalgia; uncommonly, bone marrow suppression). Absences owing to the side effects of prophylaxis or symptom-relieving drugs are not uncommon, and the full 4-week course of PEP may be difficult to complete. All antiretroviral agents are associated with side effects, and the toxicity profile is an important consideration in selection of an HIV PEP regimen.

Current guidelines better define terms such as a *deep wound* or *large-bore needle* [38]; a *large bore-needle* is larger than 18 gauge, and a *high-risk patient* has terminal AIDS with death imminent. *Deep wound* is defined as a "deep puncture or wound with or without bleeding," as opposed to a "surface scratch without bleeding" or "moderate skin penetration." When infection occurs, a deep wound was found to be associated with the greatest likelihood for infection [odds ratio (OR) = 15], followed by visible blood on the object (OR = 10), vascular source (OR = 6), or terminal AIDS (OR = 4.8) [41].

Most documented seroconversions in health care workers have resulted from direct exposure to blood or virus concentrated in the laboratory, rarely to nonblood infectious body fluids. Eighty-seven percent of exposures were percutaneous and 10% mucocutaneous. While a low viral load in the source patient probably indicates a lower exposure risk, viral load has not been definitely established as a surrogate measure of viral titer. An undetectable viral load does not rule out any possibility of HIV transmission [38]. The viral load reflects the level of cell-free virus in peripheral blood but not the presence of latently infected cells that might transmit infection.

The postexposure treatment guidelines use a matrix to characterize the riskiness of the exposure and the source patient for percutaneous and splash exposures (Table 35-7). Table 35-8 lists PEP guidelines for mucous membrane exposures and

Table 35-7
Recommended HIV Postexposure Prophylaxis for **Percutaneous Injuries**

	Infection Status of Source				
Exposure Type	**HIV-Positive Class 1***	**HIV-Positive Class 2***	**Source of Unknown HIV Status†**	**Unknown Source§**	**HIV-Negative**
Less severe¶	Recommend basic 2-drug PEP	Recommend expanded 3-drug PEP	Generally, no PEP warranted; however, consider basic 2-drug PEP** for source with HIV risk factors††	Generally, no PEP warranted; however, consider basic 2-drug PEP** in settings where exposure to HIV-infected persons is likely	No PEP warranted
More severe§§	Recommend expanded 3-drug PEP	Recommend expanded 3-drug PEP	Generally, no PEP warranted; however, consider basic 2-drug PEP** for source with HIV risk factors††	Generally, no PEP warranted; however, consider basic 2-drug PEP** in settings where exposure to HIV-infected persons is likely	No PEP warranted

*HIV-Positive, Class 1—asymptomatic HIV infection or known low viral load (e.g., <1,500 RNA copies/mL). HIV-Positive, Class 2—symptomatic HIV infection, AIDS, acute seroconversion, or known high viral load. If drug resistance is a concern, obtain expert consultation. Initiation of postexposure prophylaxis (PEP) should not be delayed pending expert consultation, and, because expert consultation alone cannot substitute for fact-to-face counseling, resources should be available to provide immediate evaluation and follow-up care for all exposures.
†Source of unknown HIV status (e.g., deceased source person with no samples available for HIV testing).
§Unknown source (e.g., a needle from a sharps disposal container).
¶Less severe (e.g., solid needle and superficial injury).
**The designation "consider PEP" indicates that PEP is optional and should be based on an individualized decision between the exposed person and the treating clinician.
††If PEP is offered and taken and the source is later determined to be HIV-negative, PEP should be discontinued.
§§More severe (e.g., large-bore hollow needle, deep puncture, visible blood on device, or needle used in patient's artery or vein).
Source: From Updated US Public Health Service Guidelines for the Management of Occupational Exposures to HBV, HCW, and HIV and Recommendations for Postexposure Prophylaxis, *MMWR* 2005; 54:1–2.

Table 35-8
Recommended HIV Postexposure Prophylaxis for Mucous **Membrane Exposures and Nonintact Skin*** Exposures

	Infection Status of Source				
Exposure Type	**HIV-Positive Class 1†**	**HIV-Positive Class 2†**	**Source of Unknown HIV Status§**	**HIV-Unknown Source¶**	**Negative**
Small volume**	Consider basic 2-drug PEP††	Recommend basic 2-drug PEP	Generally, no PEP warranted; however, consider basic 2-drug PEP†† For source with HIV risk factors§§	Generally, no PEP warranted; however, consider basic 2-drug PEP†† In settings where exposure to HIV-infected persons is likely	No PEP warranted
Large volume¶¶	Recommend basic 2-drug PEP	Recommend expanded 3-drug PEP	Generally, no PEP warranted; however, consider basic 2-drug PEP†† For source with HIV risk factors§§	Generally, no PEP warranted; however, consider basic 2-drug PEP†† In settings where exposure to HIV-infected persons is likely	No PEP warranted

*For skin exposure, follow-up is indicated only if there is evidence of compromised skin integrity (e.g., dermatitis, abrasion, or open wound).
†HIV-Positive, Class 1–asymptomatic HIV infection or known low viral load (e.g., <1,500 RNA copies/mL). HIV-Positive, Class 2–symptomatic HIV infection, AIDS, acute seroconversion, or known high viral load. If drug resistance is a concern, obtain expert consultation. Initiation of postexposure prophylaxis (PEP) should not be delayed pending expert consultation, and because expert consultation alone cannot substitute for face-to-face counseling, resources should be available to provide immediate evaluation and follow-up care for all exposures.
§Source of unknown HIV status (e.g., deceased source person with no samples available for HIV testing).
¶Unknown source (e.g., splash from inappropriately disposed blood).
**Small volume (i.e., a few drops).
††The designation, "consider PEP," indicates that PEP is optional and should be based on an individualized decision between the exposed persona and the treating clinician.
§§If PEP is offered and taken and the source is later determined to be HIV-negative, PEP should be discontinued.
¶¶Large volume (i.e., major blood splash).
Source: From Updated US Public Health Service Guidelines for the Management of Occupational Exposures to HBV, HCW, and HIV and Recommendations for Postexposure Prophylaxis, *MMWR* 2005; 54:1–2.

nonintact skin exposures. If there is high risk of transmission, an expanded three-drug or more regimen is recommended using AZT, lamivudine, and a protease inhibitor. In lower-risk situations, the basic two-drug regimen (AZT and lamivudine) is used. Most HIV exposures will warrant a two-drug PEP regimen [38] for 4 weeks. If data on the source patient's virus is available, the PEP medications should be chosen based on viral sensitivity. The availability of rapid HIV tests is obviating the common practice of instituting PEP for 48 hours pending results of source patient testing. Source patient HIV results are now available within about 30 minutes. These tests are highly sensitive and specific, but positive results should be verified by traditional tests. As with antibody tests in general, rapid test results may be negative during the first month after infection [42]. In low-risk situations, PEP may not be warranted. Exposure to tears, sweat, or nonbloody urine or feces is not considered HIV exposure and does not require evaluation for PEP.

If the individual source patient cannot be identified or tested, decisions about PEP should be based on exposure risk and the prevalence of HIV in the local patient population. For the untested source patient, a history of intravenous drug use, sexual contact with a known HIV-positive partner, unprotected sex with multiple partners, or transfusion before 1985 might lead to a decision to implement interim PEP pending source testing, if rapid testing is not available. For example, an unknown-source needle-stick in an AIDS clinic may justify PEP, whereas a similar event in a well-child clinic in a low-prevalence area may not. When PEP is prescribed, clinicians with experience in use of antiretrovirals should be consulted for their expertise in recognizing and handling drug side effects and interactions (Table 35-9). Prophylaxis is most effective if instituted within hours of exposure, before systemic infection has occurred. Animal studies suggest that treatment is most effective when started early, up to 24–48 hours postexposure [38, 43]. PEP may be less effective after 24–36 hours, but the interval after which it is of "no benefit" in humans is undetermined [38]. In animal studies, protection is incomplete when PEP is delayed 48–72 hours or if the duration of treatment is cut to 3–10 days. In practice, most authorities would not deny prophylaxis to persons with a high-risk exposure

Table 35-9
Situations for Which Expert Consultation for HIV Postexposure Prophylaxis is Advised

- Delayed (i.e., later than 24–36 hours) exposure report
  - the interval after which there is no benefit from postexposure prophylaxis (PEP) is undefined
- Unknown source (e.g., needle in sharps disposal container or laundry)
  - decide use of PEP on a case-by-case basis
  - consider the severity of the exposure and the epidemiologic likelihood of HIV exposure
  - do not test needles or other sharp instruments for HIV
- Known or suspected pregnancy in the exposed person
  - does not preclude the use of optimal PEP regimens
  - do not deny PEP solely on the basis of pregnancy
- Resistance of the source virus to antiretroviral agents
  - influence of drug resistance on transmission risk is unknown
  - selection of drugs to which the source person's virus is unlikely to be resistant is recommended, if the source person's virus is known or suspected to be resistant to ≥1 of the drugs considered for the PEP regimen
  - resistance testing of the source person's virus at the time of the exposure is not recommended
- Toxicity of the initial PEP regimen
  - adverse symptoms, such as nausea and diarrhea are common with PEP
  - symptoms often can be managed without changing the PEP regimen by prescribing antimotility and/or antiemetic agents
  - Modification of dose intervals (i.e., administering a lower dose of drug more frequently throughout the day, as recommended by the manufacturer), in other situations, might help alleviate symptoms

Source: From Guidelines for the Management of Occupational Exposures to HBV, HCV and HIV and Recommendations for Post-exposure Prophylaxis. *MMWR* 2001, 50; 1–42.

even after a 1- to 2-week delay based on the assumption that it may represent early treatment rather than pure prevention. If PEP is delayed, expert consultation should be obtained. The baseline and follow-up testing strategy may be adjusted to include HIV RNA or p24 antigen tests for acute infection rather than using HIV antibody (which appears later).

Treatment and Rehabilitation

In general, HIV-infected health care workers need not be restricted from routine or nonsurgical patient care activities (see "Nosocomial Bloodborne Pathogens Transmission" below). The Americans with Disabilities Act (ADA) covers people who have AIDS or who are infected with HIV. The ADA prohibits employers from discriminating against "physically handicapped" persons or those perceived to be handicapped. Its employment provisions apply to businesses with 25 or more employees. Besides prohibiting discrimination, the ADA also requires employers to make "reasonable accommodations" for workers with disabilities, defined as physical or mental impairment that substantially limits a major life activity. Such accommodations include flexible work schedules, restructuring the job, time off for medical appointments, more flexible sick leave, or job reassignment or transfer. Until immunosuppression occurs, as reflected by CD4 lymphocyte counts, the infected health care worker need not be routinely restricted; after the immune system begins to fail, it may be necessary to minimize exposure to potentially life-threatening infectious agents. If systemic illness or general debilitation occurs, the worker may request other accommodations comparable with those provided to employees with chronic illness such as cancer or heart disease. Confidentiality issues and questions about benefits, disability, job restrictions, or flex time may arise.

Hepatitis B

Hepatitis B virus (HBV) causes a spectrum of clinical illnesses ranging from malaise, anorexia, vague abdominal discomfort, nausea and vomiting to jaundice or fulminating liver necrosis [44]. One-third of infections are asymptomatic; most patients experience flulike symptoms, with or without jaundice, lasting weeks to months. Some may require hospitalization for acute symptoms.

EPIDEMIOLOGY

The risk factors for hepatitis B are well known, including intravenous drug use, sexual transmission, maternal-neonatal spread, exposure to blood or infectious body fluids via occupational blood exposure, or travel to endemic areas. In 30–40% of cases, the source of transmission is unknown [45]. The sequelae of hepatitis B are well documented: 5% of infected adults may develop chronic hepatitis with persistent infectivity, and 5–15% of those with chronic hepatitis eventually develop cirrhosis or hepatocellular cancer [44, 46].

It is estimated that 5% of the American population carries serologic evidence of past infection by HBV and that 0.1–0.5% of these are chronic carriers of the virus [44]. In the past, up to 30% of health care workers in high-risk areas such as dial-

ysis units were infected by HBV. In 1990, the CDC reported 12,000 cases of hepatitis B in health care workers [47].

PREVENTION AND CONTROL

While there has been a slight decline in the incidence of hepatitis B in the general population since 1985, there has been a 90% decrease in new cases in health care workers owing to the widespread adoption of preventive immunization, universal precautions, and use of personal protective equipment such as gloves, shields, and masks [46].

OSHA requires that hepatitis B vaccine be offered to all health care workers who are exposed to blood and body fluids as part of their job duties [48]. This protection also should be offered to persons who are not health care workers per se but who are also at risk—for example, hospital housekeeping personnel who clean up blood spills or encounter needlesticks from improperly disposed syringes or the plumbers and other maintenance personnel who dismantle drains where blood and body fluids are discarded. Overall, the risk of infection with percutaneous exposure is estimated at 20–30% [49], ranging from 2%, if the source patient is hepatitis B e-antigen (HBeAg)–negative, to 30–40% if HBeAg is positive [46]. In theory, hepatitis B vaccination is highly effective: 95% seroconversion rates were noted in initial studies [45]. In practice, 73–88% seroconversion is seen. Males, smokers, older individuals, and the very obese are less likely to develop protective titers [50–53]. Postvaccination testing is helpful and cost-effective [54] if performed within 1–6 months of completing the vaccination series and is expected by OSHA for health care workers with ongoing patient or body fluid contact [53].

While some employees fail to seroconvert after a three-shot series, most will respond after receipt of a second series of three doses. Up to 20% of individuals who do not respond to the original series will seroconvert when they receive a fourth dose, and 30–50% respond after a fifth or sixth dose [52]. If no antibody response occurs after six injections, no further vaccination is offered, but testing for the chronic carrier state with hepatitis B surface antigenemia (Table 35-10) or screening for alcoholism may be indicated [55]. In one study, alcoholics as a group required larger vaccine doses to seroconvert [56]. Vaccine is injected into the deltoid muscle;

Table 35-10
Interpretation of the Hepatitis B Panel

Tests	Results	Interpretation
HBsAg	Negative	
anti-HBc	Negative	Susceptible
anti-HBs	Negative	
HBsAg	Negative	
anti-HBc	Positive	Immune due to natural infection
anti-HBs	Positive	
HBsAg	Negative	
anti-HBc	Negative	Immune due to hepatitis B vaccination**
anti-HBs	Positive	
HBsAg	Positive	
anti-HBc	Positive	
IgM anti-HBc	Positive	Acutely infected
anti-HBs	Negative	
HBsAg	Positive	
anti-HBc	Positive	
IgM anti-HBc	Negative	Chronically infected
anti-HBs	Negative	
HBsAg	Negative	
anti-HBc	Positive	Four interpretations possible*
anti-HBs	Negative	

*Four Interpretations:
1. Might be recovering from acute HBV infection.
2. Might be distantly immune and test not sensitive enough to detect very low level of anti-HBs in serum.
3. Might be susceptible with a false positive anti-HBc.
4. Might be undetectable level of HBsAg present in the serum and the person is actually chronically infected.

**Antibody response (anti-HBs) can be measured quantitatively or qualitatively. A protective antibody response is reported quantitatively as 10 or more milliinternational units (≥10mIU/mL) or qualitatively as positive. Post-vaccination testing should be completed 1–2 months after the third vaccine dose for results to be meaningful.
Source: From CDC website www.cdc.gov/ncidod/diseases/hepatitis/b/Bserology.htm

gluteal muscle injection is associated with higher rates of failure to develop antibody. The vaccine is very safe, although anaphylactic reactions occurring once in 600,000 doses have been reported [57]. At present, there is no need for booster doses of hepatitis B vaccine after the initial series because protection has persisted for over 20 years since the vaccine was introduced. The vaccine contains no infectious material, and use in pregnant women is not contraindicated. Its elective administration for general prevention is often delayed during pregnancy but should be considered if an infectious exposure may occur [57]. An individual who is a documented seroconvertor need not receive hepatitis B immune globulin (HBIG) if exposed to a patient who is hepatitis B antigen–positive, even if his or her titer is undetectable at the time of the incident (Table 35-11). Antibody titers will predictably decline with time; 60% of immunized individuals lose circulating antibody over 12 years [46], but an individual who has previously seroconverted will generate antibody if exposed [54].

Hepatitis C

As HBV infection declined in health care workers, the relative proportion of cases of bloodborne hepatitis owing to hepatitis C virus (HCV) increased. Hepatitis C constitutes the majority of what was previously termed *non-A, non-B hepatitis*. Since institution of blood donor screening in 1990, the incidence of posttransfusion hepatitis C has fallen to less than 1%. Use of injected drugs is the major risk factor today [58]; use of nasal cocaine with shared straws also has been implicated.

HCV leads to persistent infection in 60–85% of patients or to chronic hepatitis in up to 70%. Disease progresses slowly over decades, with hepatocellular carcinoma as a late risk, developing after cirrhosis [59]. Acute infection causes clinically

Table 35-11
Recommended Postexposure Prophylaxis for Exposure to Hepatitis B Virus

Vaccination and Antibody Response Status of Exposed Workers*	Treatment		
	Source HBSAg[†] Positive	Source HBsAg[†] Negative	Source Unknown or Not Available for Testing
Unvaccinated	HBIG[§] × 1 and initiate HB vaccine series[¶]	Initiate HB vaccine series	Initiate HB vaccine series
Previously vaccinated			
Known responder**	No treatment	No treatment	No treatment
Known nonresponder[††]	HBIG × 1 and initiate Revaccination Or HBIG × 2[§]	No treatment	If known high risk Source, treat as if source were HBsAg positive
Antibody response unknown	Test exposed person for anti-HBs[¶] 1. If adequate,** no treatment is necessary 2. If inadequate,** administer HBIG × 1 and vaccine booster	No treatment	Test exposed person for anti-HBs[¶] 1. If adequate,[†] no treatment is necessary 2. If inadequate,[††] administer vaccine booster and recheck titer 1–2 months

*Persons who have previously been infected with HBV are immune to reinfection and do no require postexposure prophylaxis.
[†]Hepatitis B surface antigen.
[§]Hepatitis B immune globulin; dose is 0.06 mL/kg intramuscularly.
[¶]Hepatitis B vaccine
**A responder is a person with adequate levels of serum antibody to HBsAg (i.e., anti-HBs ≥ 10 mIU/mL).
[††]A nonresponder is a person with inadequate response to vaccination (i.e., serum anti-HBs < 10 mIU/mL).
[§]The option of giving one dose of HBIG and reinitiating the vaccine series is preferred for nonresponders who have not completed a second 3-dose vaccine series. For persons who previously completed a second vaccine series but failed to respond, two doses of HBIG are preferred.
[¶]Antibody to HBsAg.
Source: From Updated U.S. Public Health Service Guidelines for the Management of Occupational Exposures to HBV, HCV, and HIV and Recommendations for Postexposure Prophylaxis. *MMWR* 2001;50(RR11): 1–42.

overt disease in less than a third of patients. Serum alanine aminotransferase (ALT) levels begin to rise several weeks after infection and may remain elevated after acute symptoms, if any, have resolved [59]. One-third of patients with chronic infection have a normal ALT, but levels may fluctuate [60].

EPIDEMIOLOGY

Risk factors for infection include intravenous drug or nasal cocaine use and receipt of a blood transfusion before 1990 or of clotting factors manufactured before 1987. Use of intravenous drugs accounts for 60% of cases and sexual contact for 20%; other household, occupational, hemodialysis, and perinatal exposures account for about 10% [60]. At present, only 10% of cases have no reported exposure source. The estimated prevalence of HCV infection in health care workers is no greater than that in the general population, averaging 1–2% [60–63] despite contact with patients. Hepatitis C is more prevalent in the patient population because one-third of patients with alcoholic liver disease, 12–55% of patients with hepatitis B, 15–30% of renal dialysis patients, and 40% of transplant patients are infected

[58]. A New York City study found that among asymptomatic persons with mildly elevated transaminase levels, 58% were HCV-positive, but the paper cited references noting a 17% prevalence of HCV in similar circumstances in other locales [64]. The risk of HCV transmission from needlestick is roughly 2%, perhaps higher using the more sensitive RNA polymerase chain reaction (PCR) [65].

PREVENTION AND CONTROL

If lapses in technique or disinfection procedures occur, nosocomial transmission of HCV is possible. Most cases of transmission to health care workers occur because of accidental needlesticks or sharps cuts. Conjunctival splashes also have been reported to result in seroconversion [58]. Universal precautions and use of personal protective equipment are the primary preventive measures because no vaccine exists for HCV.

TREATMENT

There is no prophylactic treatment after exposure. Gamma globulin is ineffective, and interferon-ribavirin is used for treatment. There is some evidence that treatment begun early in the course of HCV infection is associated with a higher rate of resolution, but it is not clear if acute-phase treatment is more effective than treatment in the early chronic phase [60]. Viral RNA testing can detect viral antigen at 2–4 weeks after exposure to HCV. This is well before anti-HCV antibody develops at 8–10 weeks and allows for early referral. Surveillance for development of HCV via anti-HCV antibody should continue for 6–9 months after a verified blood or body fluid exposure incident. Anti-HCV antibody testing can be used for surveillance when the exposure source is not HCV-positive. Anti-HCV antibody is a mainstay of hepatitis C diagnosis but cannot distinguish between acute and chronic infection in the source patient. False-negative (5–10%) and false-positive results can occur, the later especially in low-prevalence populations. Supplementary testing with a more specific test such as the recombinant immunoblot assay (RIBA) or RNA PCR is used to confirm a positive anti-HCV antibody if a false-positive result is suspected (Table 35-12).

The conventional wisdom has been to counsel HCV-infected persons not to change sexual practices if they are in a monogamous relationship owing to the low risk (5–10%) of sexual transmission [65]. Household spread of both hepatitis C and B can occur by sharing articles such as toothbrushes, razors, etc. that may be contaminated with blood.

Nosocomial Bloodborne Pathogen Transmission

EPIDEMIOLOGY

Occupational exposure to blood is still frequent in health care activities. The rate of needlestick injuries among nurses is estimated to be 10–34%. Underreporting of such injuries is common—an estimated 30–60% of incidents are not reported [2].

Transmission of bloodborne pathogens from patient to health care workers is not uncommon, although there has been greater public concern about transmission from infected health care workers. There have been reports of transmission of HBV

Table 35-12
Interpretation of HCV Test Results

If Your HCV Test Result Is:			Interpretation		Action
Anti-HCV Supplemental Test					
Anti-HCV Screening Test*	RIBA[†] or HCV RNA		Anti-HCV	HCV Infection	Additional Testing or Evaluation
Negative	Not Needed	Not Needed	Negative	None	No
Positive	Not Done	Not Done	Not Known	Not Known	Supplemental Anti-HCV (RIBA) or HCV RNA
Positive	Not Done	Negative	Not Known	Not Known[▲]	Supplemental Anti-HCV (RIBA)
Positive (high s/co ratio[§])	Not Done	Not Done	Positive	Past/current	Evaluate for chronic infection and liver disease
Positive	Negative	Not Needed	Negative	None	No
Positive	Positive	Not Done	Positive	Past/current	Evaluate for chronic infection and liver disease
Positive	Positive	Negative	Positive	Past/current[▲]	Repeat HCV RNA
Positive	Positive/Not Done	Positive	Positive	Current	Evaluate for chronic infection and liver disease
Positive	Indeterminate	Not Done	Indeterminate	Not Known	Test for HCV RNA or repeat Anti-HCV testing
Positive	Indeterminate	Positive	Indeterminate	Current	Evaluate for chronic infection and liver disease
Positive	Indeterminate	Negative	Negative	None	No

*EIA-enzyme immunoassay or CIA-enhanced chemiluminescence immunoassay
[†]Recombinant immunoblot assay, a more specific anti-HCV assay
[▲]Single negative HCV RNA result cannot determine infection status as persons might have intermittent viremia
[§]Samples with high s/co ratios usually (>95%) confirm positive, but supplemental serologic testing was not performed. Less than 5 of every 100 might represent false-positives; more specific testing should be requested, if indicated.
Source: From: www.cdc.gov/NCIDOD/Diseases/Hepatitis/resource/PDFs/hcv_graph.pdf

from surgeons, even those who were HBeAg-negative [66]. Such reports support the use of postvaccination antibody titers to detect chronic carriers when they fail to seroconvert. In 1996, 34 cases of HBV transmission were reported from provider to patient and one case of HIV transmission from a dentist [67]. Most cases of hepatitis transmission could have been prevented by vaccination.

PREVENTION AND CONTROL

OSHA mandated the use of safety sharps with the Needlestick Safety and Prevention Act of 2001. Safety sharps such as needleless infusion sets, retractable-needle syringes, and puncture-resistant gloves should replace nonsafety devices with end-user input in the selection. As universal precautions and the use of safety devices effectively prevent percutaneous exposures, a relative increase in exposures owing to skin and mucous membrane splashes may be observed.

In response to public concern about bloodborne pathogens transmission in the health care setting, CDC made recommendations to limit some occupational activities of HIV- or HBV-infected health care workers [65], and Congress mandated that each state implement the CDC guidelines or their equivalent to receive federal public health funding [68]. All states have complied with a fair degree of state-to-state variation regarding specific provisions. Some states require that HIV- and HBV-infected surgeons or others who perform infection-associated procedures be reported to the state health officer for review and possible limitation of their work practices. High-risk procedures are defined as use of fingers, needles, or sharps in a poorly visualized, highly confined area during surgical, obstetric, or dental procedures. Local or state public health officials should be contacted to determine the applicable local regulations. These reporting requirements and recommended work restrictions have potential legal, ethical, risk management, and workers' compensation implications, leading some surgeons and health care workers to be reluctant to report their exposure incidents. The highly effective antiviral treatments for HIV used today have mitigated concerns about HIV transmission to some extent. At present, there are no recommendations from the CDC or other authorities to restrict health care workers with HCV because the risk of transmission appears to be very low [69].

Bite Wounds

Human bites may occur in health care and lead to skin infections or bloodborne pathogen transmission. Human bites can become infected with skin flora such as *Staphylococcus, Streptococcus,* anaerobes, and other mouth flora, such as *Eikenella corrodens* (associated with dental disease). Bite wounds of the hands are at increased risk for infection. A broad-spectrum antibiotic that will cover most potential pathogens (e.g., amoxicillin-clavulanate, ciprofloxacin, or cloxacillin) may be used for prophylaxis or treatment of infection [70].

Bite wounds raise questions about the risk of transmission of bloodborne pathogens to the bitten worker if the biter has bleeding gums or open mouth lesions. Although saliva is not generally considered an infectious body fluid (unless visibly contaminated with blood), transmission of HBV via saliva alone has been reported [71]. HIV rarely exists in saliva, but there have been isolated case reports of HIV transmission via bite wounds [72, 73]. While possible, the risk of transmission of HIV through saliva alone (or via biting) is considered so low as to be negligible. At present, CDC guidelines do not recommend postexposure prophylaxis for HIV when a health care worker is bitten by an HIV-positive source in the absence of bleeding gums, mucosal lesions, or other risk factor [38]. The risk for HCV infection via bite wound is considered to be very low but has not been well quantified. Detection of the presence of HCV in saliva varies depending on the study method, timing, and population [74–76]. In addition, if a bite results in an open wound, the biter is also exposed to the blood of the health care worker, resulting in a need to evaluate both parties as source and recipient, that is, a two-way exposure.

Skin Breaks, Lesions, and Infections

Health care workers with rashes or nonintact skin, regardless of cause, may present a staffing dilemma. These workers can spread infections to patients if their condition results from a systemic or local infection. Broken skin may preclude the scrubbing necessary for participation in sterile procedures or work in special units in the hospital. If serous fluid is weeping from broken skin and cannot be covered, patients may be exposed to the employee's body fluid. Employee skin breaks present an entry route for a variety of infectious agents in addition to bloodborne pathogens. The algorithm in Figure 35-3 presents an approach to dealing with the complexities of employee skin breaks and lesions and is intended for use by unit managers in a tertiary care center. The specific approach used in any situation should take into account actual work practices and estimation of employee and patient risk.

Patient skin infections may be a hazard to health care workers. While this chapter deals primarily with preventing transmission of infection to health care personnel, the health care worker may serve as vector for methicillin-resistant *Staphylococcus aureus* (MRSA) and vancomycin-resistant enterococci (VRE), which are capable of surviving on environmental surfaces for days or weeks in health care fa-

cilities. Personnel whose hands or gloves are contaminated by these surfaces may transmit the organisms to patients. There is an increasing body of evidence that cleaning or disinfection of the environment can reduce transmission of health care–associated pathogens such as MRSA, VRE, and *Clostridium difficile* [77].

Stethoscopes and otoscope handles used in an outpatient setting were found to be colonized 90–100% of the time, usually with *Staphylococcus* and 7–9% with MRSA. Cleaning with alcohol reduced the colony count by an average of 96% [78]. In a hospital setting, *Staphylococcus* was isolated from 33% of blood pressure cuffs, MRSA from 8%, and *C. difficile* from 33% [79]. Used tourniquets have been found to be colonized at a similar rate

Figure 35-3
Restrictions for Healthcare Workers with Skin Conditions (Rash or Nonintact Skin, i.e., Cuts, Sutures, Burns, Blisters, Deep Abrasions)

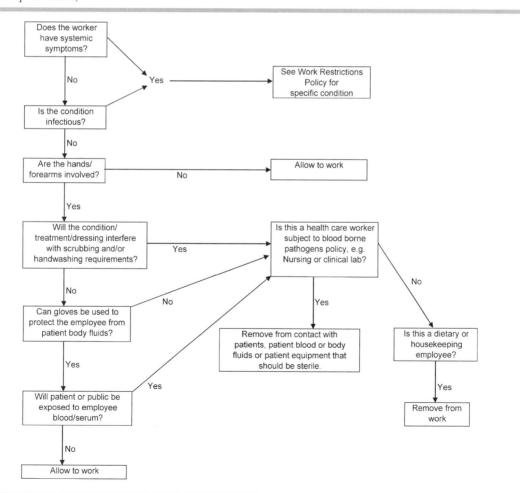

[80]. Physician's ties have been suggested to be frequently colonized and potential vectors [81]. National estimates from 2001–2002 suggest that 32% of all individuals are colonized with *Staphylococcus* and 0.8% with MRSA. Among the general population, including most health care workers, colonization rarely leads to disease. Health care workers have been identified as the source of MRSA spread in numerous outbreak investigations, and 30–60% of health care workers become colonized in wards where epidemics of MRSA occur [82].

Hand washing and infection control measures such as use of contact precautions in addition to standard precautions can protect the patient, worker, and environment. When cleaning surfaces, health care workers should closely follow the manufacturer's directions for disinfectant contact time to ensure adequate killing of microbes. Contact times can range from 2–30 minutes. Table 35-13 outlines some infection control measures indicated for MRSA in the outpatient setting.

Table 35-13
Stop the Spread of MRSA in our Clinics

Methicillin Resistant *Staphylococcus aureus*
- **Wash hands** with soap and water or use alcohol based hand sanitizers if not visibly soiled between all patients.
- Use **Contact Precautions** in addition to **Standard Precautions** for all patients with open or draining wounds and all patients known to be infected with MRSA.
  1. Wear gloves when providing care.
  2. Avoid touching own nose, or face while providing care.
  3. Change gloves after contact with infective material that may contain high concentrations of microorganisms (e.g., wound drainage or dressings).
  4. Remove gloves before leaving the patient's room and wash hands immediately. After glove removal and hand washing, do not touch potentially contaminated environmental surfaces or items in the exam room.
  5. Wear a gown when providing care if there will be substantial contact with the patient's wound. Remove the gown before leaving the exam room.
  6. Clean and disinfect exam room and equipment
     - Select EPA-registered disinfectants and use them according to the manufacturer's instructions.
     - Clean and disinfect non-critical medical equipment surfaces (e.g., stethoscopes, blood pressure cuffs) as well as high touch surfaces (e.g., door knobs, chair arms) between uses.
  7. Keep your own skin infections and open wounds covered with clean, dry bandages. Wash hands before and after dressing changes.

Patient Skin Infestations

Tinea corporis may spread from patients to staff. *Herpes simplex* virus type 1 is a potential hazard for nonimmune dentists, anesthetists, physical therapists, and nurses [5]. Patients can transmit ectoparasites such as lice (*Pediculus humanis, P. capitis, P. pubis,* or *P. corporis*) or scabies (*Sarcoptes scabei miti*) to health care workers.

The burrowing mites of scabies cause papular eruptions that itch, especially at night. In older children and adults, scabies lesions occur in interdigital folds and centrally in skinfolds. In children under age 2, the eruption is more likely to occur as vesicles on the head, neck, palms, and soles [83]. Scabies is readily spread by direct skin-to-skin contact, which may occur during bathing, lifting, or applying lotions. Minimal contact with crusted scabies can result in mite transmission, even before the source is symptomatic. Incubation time can be 4–6 weeks, but a previously infected, sensitized individual may develop symptoms within 1–4 days. A scabicide prescription is recommended for all health care workers after scabies exposure owing to the high risk of infestation. Permethrin 5% cream is the current topical medication of choice [83]. Other options are crotamiton 10% and lindane 1% lotions. Contact precautions should be instituted when caring for infested patients prior to application of topical scabicide to their lesions. Routine cleaning of bed linens and upholstered furniture will help to eliminate mites, but additional cleaning may be needed for crusted scabies [55]. The term *Norwegian scabies* is applied when the mite infests an immunocompromised host. The lesions are more numerous and crusted and contain a larger number of organisms; treatment is more difficult owing to decreased host defenses.

Head lice are spread by hair-to-hair contact with infested persons; body lice can be spread by manual contact with the bed linen or clothing of infested persons, necessitating the use of gloves for such activities. Lice stay alive while on the host; away from the host, their survival time ranges from 1–2 days for head lice to 10 days for body lice. Incubation time is 6–10 days from laying of eggs until hatching [83]. Health care workers are treated only if infested and should be restricted from work from the time of recognition until 24 hours after treatment [55]. Acquisition of pediculosis requires more intimate, direct, prolonged body contact than does scabies. Infestation may be treated with permethrin 1% cream or malathion 0.5% lotion or lindane 1% lotion.

Conjunctivitis

Infectious conjunctivitis in a health care worker can be an indication to restrict the worker from patient contact. There are many viral and bacterial causes of conjunctivitis (e.g., *Haemophilus influenzae, Streptococcus pneumoniae,* enterovirus, adenoviral pharyngeal conjunctival fever, and chlamydial neonatal conjunctivitis), but nosocomial outbreaks owing to such agents are rare [44]. In the health care setting, and in adults generally, adenovirus is of most concern because it can cause epidemic keratoconjunctivitis (EKC).

EPIDEMIOLOGY

EKC is spread by direct contact with infected eye secretions. Outbreaks have been reported in eye clinics and medical offices [44]. The incubation time for adenoviral conjunctivitis averages 5–12 days. The virus is typically communicable from late in the incubation period to 14 days after symptom onset; viral shedding may be prolonged beyond 14 days [55].

PREVENTION AND CONTROL

To prevent the spread of EKC in clinics, thorough hand washing and high-level disinfection of instruments that come into contact with the conjunctiva or eyelids are recommended. Gloves should be worn to examine the eyes of patients with possible or confirmed EKC. Single-use strips, droppers, or applicators for ophthalmic medications should be used. Health care workers with infectious conjunctivitis, whether EKC or purulent conjunctivitis, should be restricted from patient care while symptoms are present.

Varicella

Chickenpox (varicella) is an acute viral disease characterized by sudden onset of fever, mild constitutional symptoms, and skin eruption. The rash, which occurs in crops, is maculopapular for a few hours and then vesicular for 3–4 days, leaving scabs. Varicella-zoster virus (VZV) is spread from person to person by direct contact with vesicular fluid or respiratory secretions or by articles freshly soiled by these fluids or by the airborne route. The incubation period is about 2–3 weeks, typically 14–16 days [44].

EPIDEMIOLOGY

Varicella infection is most severe in adults, with a case-fatality rate of 30 per 100,000 in the United States; viral pneumonia is a frequent complication [44]. Children with acute leukemia, even those in remission, are at increased risk of disseminated infection, which is fatal in 5–10% of cases. Premature or low-birth-weight infants and individuals with immune suppression or malignancy are at greatest risk for nosocomial infection. Although rare, congenital varicella syndrome can cause low birth weight, cutaneous scarring, limb hypoplasia, chorioretinitis, cataracts, and other anomalies in newborns. If infected in utero, the risk for development of congenital varicella syndrome is 0.7–2.0% [84]. Nonimmune pregnant women who develop chickenpox near term also can transmit varicella to the newborn, resulting in severe or fatal infection, because insufficient maternal antibody will have developed to protect the infant.

Herpes zoster, or shingles, a localized outbreak of skin vesicles, results from reactivation of varicella virus, which lies dormant in the dorsal root ganglia, years after the primary chickenpox infection. Varicella virus is highly contagious, especially in the early stages of cutaneous eruption; herpes zoster has a lower rate of transmission than systemic infection, but both can cause chickenpox in seronegative contacts [44].

Exposure to varicella can be problematic for the nonimmune health care worker because nosocomial spread is well recognized. If infected, the worker will be contagious for 1–2 days prior to onset of the rash, at which time the virus can be spread to nonimmune or immunocompromised individuals [44]. For these reasons, it is recommended that the nonimmune employee be removed from work following exposure from days 10–21 [85] or days 8–21 [84]. Most adults have developed immunity to varicella. A clinical history of overt chickenpox disease is a very reliable indicator of immunity; 97–99% will be positive for antibody. Of adults with a negative or uncertain history, 71–93% are actually seropositive [84, 86]. On the other hand, prior infection and the presence of circulating antibody to VZV is not 100% protective against reinfection with chickenpox or against recurrence as herpes zoster. Cellular immunity plays an important role. When chickenpox reoccurs in immune persons, disease may be mild and slightly atypical, with few lesions and minimal fever. The immune response to vaccine appears to be shorter-lived than that resulting from natural infection.

The CDC's Advisory Committee on Immunization Practices recommends that all health care providers have evidence of immunity to varicella. In the past, a history of chickenpox disease was considered adequate evidence, and for the general public, birth before 1980 is still considered adequate evidence of varicella immunity [87]. With the use of varicella vaccine, fewer cases of overt, typical disease and more mild, subclinical breakthrough infections in vaccinated persons have been observed.

For health care providers, adequate evidence of immunity now includes either documentation of two doses of varicella vaccine, serologic evidence of immunity, or provider-diagnosed chickenpox or herpes zoster (shingles), regardless of age. Serologic screening of personnel who have a negative or uncertain history of varicella disease before vaccination is still a cost-effective strategy [87].

PREVENTION AND CONTROL

Since the 1995 introduction of childhood vaccination, the incidence of varicella infection has declined by about 90% and mortality by about 66% [88]. Varicella vaccine is recommended in health care workers with no history of chickenpox disease or immunization who have tested negative for varicella antibodies. Two shots are delivered 4–8 weeks apart. Vaccine is reported to be 100% effective in preventing moderate or severe disease and 85% effective in preventing all varicella [89]. Vaccine effectiveness wanes over time, declining from 97% the first year to 84% through 8 years postvaccination [88]. Other studies document antibody persistence to some degree for up to 20 years [89]. Vaccine-induced immunity (like natural immunity) may allow "breakthrough" infection to occur, but disease will be mild and shorter in duration with fewer lesions [90]. Removal of newly vacci-

nated workers from work is not recommended unless a rash develops, occurring in up to 5% of vaccinated adults within 2–6 weeks and averaging two to five lesions that last 2–3 days and shedding of virus at a low titer [91]. The employee with postimmunization lesions should be evaluated, and removal from patient contact may be recommended after considering whether the lesions can be covered by clothing, the nature of his or her patient contacts, or institutional policy [46]. While the incidence of secondary transmission of the attenuated viral strain is very low, immunocompromised patients are at greatest risk [84].

Despite demonstrable circulating antibody to VZV, 20–40% of vaccinated adults may develop breakthrough varicella following household exposure [89]. Occupational exposure in health care is considered less intense and may result in boosting of vaccine-inducted immunity without disease. Immunity to VZV is complex and not fully understood. Antibodies can be directed against a number of viral components [90]. The relationship between seroconversion and protection is imprecise. It is unclear whether breakthrough varicella is the result of primary or secondary vaccine failure [92]. Most investigations of outbreaks have shown 80–85% vaccine effectiveness, but some show rates as low as 45–55%. The most sensitive antibody demonstrates seroconversion in 96% of vaccinated health care workers, but one-third lose this antibody over time. Commercially available antibody tests are less sensitive (70–80%) even immediately after vaccination [93]. Routine postvaccination titers are not recommended by the Advisory Committee on Immunization Practices (ACIP), which cites the 99% rate of seroconversion after two doses and the insensitivity of commercial antibody tests [85].

Postexposure immunization of nonimmune workers with two doses 4 weeks apart may prevent disease or reduce its severity if provided within 3–5 days [87]. Exposed health care workers who have received two doses of vaccine are monitored daily during days 10–21 for fever, skin lesions, and systemic symptoms, and they are removed from work if symptoms develop [87]. Unvaccinated exposed employees are furloughed from work during this incubation period [86, 92].

Varicella vaccine contains live virus and is not recommended for pregnant women, HIV-positive individuals, or those with immune suppression or malignancy. Vaccination should be delayed at least 5 months after receipt of blood, plasma, immune globulin, or varicella-zoster immune globulin (VZIG) [86]. VZIG receipt after exposure can prolong the incubation time for chickenpox to 28 days and is not recommended for immunocompetent health care workers. If used, VZIG should be given within 96 hours of exposure [85]. There is no evidence that VZIG will prevent congenital varicella if given after exposure to a pregnant woman; the primary indication in pregnancy is to protect the mother, not the baby. VZIG is not recommended for immunocompromised patients exposed to vaccine.

Health care workers with chickenpox should not care for immunocompromised patients until all lesions are dry and crusted. Workers with localized herpes zoster should not care for such patients unless lesions can be well covered by clothing or bandages. Both contact and airborne precautions should be observed by health care workers caring for infected patients, who should be in a negative-pressure room.

Pertussis

Pertussis is an endemic disease with periodic outbreaks among young children. The incidence of pertussis (Figure 35-4) has increased over recent decades in the United States [94], possibly owing to increased recognition and testing or increased reporting [95]. Pertussis, or whooping cough, can be a life-threatening infection in infants, but childhood immunization has eliminated much of the morbidity and mortality in young children. Until recently, pertussis vaccine was not given to children older than 7 years of age, and immunity from vaccination wanes with time. Previously immunized adolescents and adults lose their protective immunity, become susceptible to infection, and serve as a reservoir of infection for younger children. In 1994 it was estimated that 50 million adults were susceptible to pertussis [97]. In adults, pertussis presents as a mild, atypical respiratory illness, usually without the characteristic whooping cough. Up to 25% of coughs lasting over 1–2 weeks are attributed to pertussis [96].

Figure 35-4
Pertussis (whooping cough) by year—United States, 1966–1996.

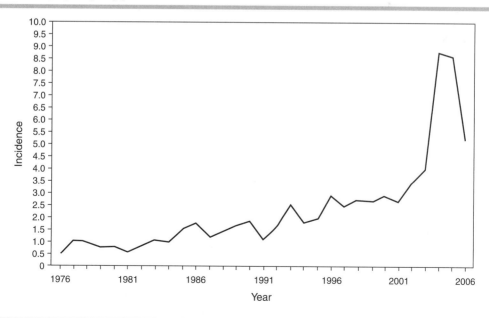

Source: Adapted from Selected notifiable disease reports. *MMWR* 1996;46:1021.

EPIDEMIOLOGY

In 2002, 23% of cases were in adults aged 20 years or older. Infection in adults and adolescents is less likely to manifest as the classic pertussis symptoms, with milder symptoms and a mild or moderate cough [98]. The nonspecific symptoms may be attributed to generic "bronchitis." Pertussis is frequently not diagnosed in adults owing to the need for specific testing of nasopharyngeal secretions. While health care workers are not at substantially greater risk of infection than the general population [44], pertussis can result in miniepidemics in hospitals, where adult health care workers have transmitted it to pediatric patients. The causative organism, *Bordatella pertussis,* a gram-negative bacillus, is spread by direct contact with respiratory secretions. The incubation period for pertussis is 6–20 days, and infection can last for 4–8 weeks if untreated [44].

PREVENTION AND CONTROL

Infected inpatients should be placed on isolation precautions to control respiratory droplet spread until 5 days of therapy are completed. If an outbreak occurs in a health care setting, prophylactic treatment for direct care providers and booster pertussis immunizations can break the cycle of spread. For asymptomatic individuals, PEP consists of a 14-day course of erythromycin or trimethoprim-sulfamethoxazole started within 3 weeks of exposure [97]. The treatment dose and the prophylactic dose are the same. Azithromycin for 5 days is an alternative; the new macrolides may have fewer side effects, but there are fewer studies on their use. In one report, 7 days of erythromycin estolate was as effective as a 14-day course of a macrolide [99]. After paroxysmal cough develops, antibiotics may not affect the course of the illness but will eradicate nasopharyngeal carriage and thus limit transmission.

Nasopharyngeal culture for *B. pertussis* on Bordet-Gengou or Regan-Lowe medium is helpful if positive, but organisms can be difficult to recover, especially in the later phase of paroxysmal cough. Direct fluorescent antibody testing of secretions is an alternative for making a presumptive diagnoses but is not especially sensitive or specific. Polymerase chain reaction (PCR) testing and enzyme-linked immunosorbent assay (ELISA) for antibodies are more accurate but less widely available.

If a worker is symptomatic, a nasopharyngeal swab specimen is cultured, and the employee is removed from work and started on an antibiotic regimen. After at least 5 days of treatment, the worker may return to work if symptoms have resolved. The nonspecific symptoms of pertussis in adults are similar to those of various other respiratory infections.

Two adult formulations of acellular pertussis vaccine combined with diphtheria and tetanus toxoids (Tdap) are now available. Use of a single dose in adolescents or adults is reported to be about 95% effective in preventing pertussis, and no increase in vaccine-associated side effects are reported from the addition of the acellular pertussis antigens to the dT [98]. Pertussis vaccine is especially recommended for adults who have close contact with infants younger than 12 months of age and health care providers.

A single dose of Tdap is now recommended for all adults in place of the dT when a routine tetanus booster is due, or for postinjury wound management in adults aged 19–64 years, Tdap may be given even if less than a 10-year interval has passed since receipt of the last tetanus toxoid–containing vaccine in order to accelerate protection [100].

Immunization of health care personnel eventually may obviate the need to provide prophylactic antibiotic treatment to exposed personnel, but the CDC continues to recommend antibiotic prophylaxis for immunized exposed health care workers [100].

Measles

Measles is an acute viral disease characterized by fever, conjunctivitis, coryza, cough, and a red blotchy rash. The rash begins on the face and becomes generalized, lasting 4–7 days [44]. In the United States, measles generally occurs in children too young to be vaccinated or in older individuals. Pneumonia and encephalitis are potential complications. Outbreaks have occurred in immunized school populations prior to adoption of the two-dose regimen for children.

Measles is transmitted by large respiratory droplets and airborne virus or by direct contact with respiratory secretions and is highly transmissible during close contact. The incubation time is 5–21 days. Virus is shed from the nasopharynx during the prodrome and for 3–4 days after the rash appears—longer if the infected individual is immunocompromised.

EPIDEMIOLOGY

Although transmission of measles in the health care setting accounts for less than 5% of total cases, the risk for measles infection in medical personnel is 13 times greater than in the general population [44]. Individuals born before 1957 are generally assumed to be immune to measles, but serologic studies show that 5–10% of these older workers lack measles antibodies. In epidemic situations, up to one-fourth of measles cases among health care workers have occurred in persons born before 1957. Of adults with measles, 40% had previously received a single immunization [67], suggesting possible waning of vaccine-induced immunity.

PREVENTION AND CONTROL

Nosocomial spread can be minimized by verifying employee immunity or providing vaccine, isolating patients with fever and rash, and adopting precautions against airborne transmission when measles is suspected or proven. If exposed, a nonimmune health care worker should be furloughed from work from day 5 after first exposure until day 21 after the last exposure. If rash develops, the worker should be restricted from work for at least 4 days after eruption.

The CDC recommends a single dose of vaccine for workers born before 1957 if they lack evidence of immunity, for example, are unvaccinated, have no history of disease, or lack serologic evidence of immunity (see Table 35-3); for those born in or after 1957, documentation of physician-diagnosed measles, *two* doses of vaccine after age 1, or serologic evidence of immunity is required [55]. Many adults immunized during childhood will need a second vaccine dose. Persons who received killed measles virus prior to 1968 should receive a second dose to protect against atypical measles [44], although they may have more frequent local or systemic reactions on repeat vaccination. During measles outbreaks, vaccination should be given within 72 hours of exposure, without prior sero-

logic testing, to any adult who has not received two doses of vaccine regardless of age or serologic status [46]. Some hospitals require two doses for all employees, preplacement, in anticipation of such an event. Contraindications to the live attenuated measles virus vaccine include pregnancy (based on theoretical grounds) and immunosuppression, regardless of cause. Asymptomatic HIV infection is not a contraindication unless CD4 lymphocyte counts are suppressed. To be fully effective, administration of this live-virus vaccine should be delayed for at least 5 weeks after receipt of IgG. Anaphylaxis is a rare reaction to measles vaccine, with 30 reported cases of anaphylaxis per 70 million doses; urticaria and wheal and flare reactions are more common [57]. Egg allergy is a contraindication only when associated with anaphylactic reaction; skin testing for egg allergy has not been useful in predicting reactions [46]. Vaccine efficacy is 95% with one dose and 99% with two. Measles vaccine prevents subacute sclerosing panencephalitis (SSPE) and does not increase its risk, even in those previously infected or vaccinated with live virus. Rarely, the combined measles-mumps-rubella (MMR) vaccine has been associated with thrombocytopenia within 2 months, at a rate of 1 in 30,000–40,000; a prior history of idiopathic thrombocytopenic purpura (ITP) is associated with increased risk of recurrence [57].

Mumps

The age group at greatest risk for mumps infection is shifting from childhood to adolescence. This viral infection of the salivary and other glands can cause orchitis in 20–30% of postpubertal males and oophoritis in 5% of postpubertal females, with sterility as a rare complication [44]. Aseptic meningitis is a relatively common complication of infection. Encephalitis occurs less often, at 1–2 cases per 10,000; pancreatitis occurs in 4% of cases [44].

EPIDEMIOLOGY

Outbreaks of mumps involving adolescents and young adults have occurred in hospitals and long-term care facilities [46]. Mumps virus is spread by contact with saliva or other respiratory secretions; the incubation period is 12–25 days, generally 16–18 days. Virus can be present in saliva for 6–7 days prior to observable parotitis and for 9 days after its onset. Infection is asymptomatic in about one-third of cases.

PREVENTION AND CONTROL

Droplet precautions should be implemented and continued for 9 days for inpatients when infection is recognized. Health care workers are considered immune if they have had physician-diagnosed mumps or have serologic evidence of immunity. Most persons born before 1957 are considered immune; those born after 1957 should receive two doses of MMR (measles-mumps-rubella) vaccine. During outbreaks in health care settings, unvaccinated older employees may be immunized if documentation of immunity is missing or questionable. Nonimmune employees exposed to mumps should be restricted from patient care or furloughed from days 12–26 and for 9 days after the onset of parotitis [46]. Vaccine is about 95% effective.

Rubella

Rubella is a mild febrile illness; it is associated with a diffuse, punctate, maculopapular rash in over half of cases. Encephalitis and arthralgia/arthritis are occasional complications in adults. Rubella is most important because of its teratogenic effect on the developing fetus. Congenital rubella syndrome occurs in up to 90% of infants born to women infected during the first trimester. Fetal risk falls to 10–20% by the sixteenth week of gestation and is rare after week 20. Rubella during pregnancy is associated with intrauterine death, spontaneous abortion, or congenital malformations resulting in deafness, cataracts, congenital glaucoma, microphthalmia, mental retardation, cardiac defects, or insulin-dependent diabetes [44].

EPIDEMIOLOGY

Transmission of rubella from both male and female workers has occurred in the hospital setting. Rubella is less infectious than measles, but 10–15% of young adults may be susceptible, and about 6% of health care workers lack detectable antibody [46]. Transmission occurs through direct contact and nasopharyngeal droplets. The incubation period ranges from 12–23 days, with rash usually appearing at 14–16 days. Virus is shed from 1 week before to 5–7 days after appearance

of the rash; individuals are most contagious while it is erupting.

PREVENTION AND CONTROL

Because of the frequency of subclinical, inapparent infections and the nonspecific nature of the illness, the clinical diagnosis of rubella is unreliable, and a history of vaccination or serologic immunity must be obtained even in health care workers born prior to 1957. Serologic screening prior to vaccination is not needed because prior immunity does not increase the incidence of adverse reactions. Pregnancy is a contraindication to vaccination, and women are counseled to avoid pregnancy for 3 months following administration of vaccine, primarily on theoretical grounds. In cases in which pregnant women were immunized inadvertently, congenital defects have not been observed, so vaccination need not be considered an indication for abortion. The live, attenuated virus vaccine elicits an antibody response in 98–99% of recipients. Rubella vaccine is grown in human diploid cells, not in eggs; it may contain a trace of neomycin and thus so may be contraindicated in persons with anaphylactic allergy [101]. The CDC recommends that health care workers be immunized with MMR vaccine if any single component is indicated unless there is a specific contraindication to the combination. Owing to successful immunization programs in the United States, congenital rubella has become a rarity, although sporadic cases of rubella are reported [102].

Meningococcal Infection

Neisseria meningitidis is an aerobic gram-negative diplococcus that is spread by droplets of respiratory secretions. Meningococcal infection can lead to a wide spectrum of disease, including sepsis, meningitis, and pneumonia. Up to 5–10% of people in countries with endemic disease carry *N. meningitidis* asymptomatically in the nasopharynx [44]. A small minority of individuals colonized with the bacteria develop invasive disease.

EPIDEMIOLOGY

Group A organisms are found in sub-Saharan Africa and the Asian subcontinent. Group B has been the most common cause of disease in the Americas, with group C equally common in the

United States. Presently, serogroups B and C constitute 90% of endemic cases in this country [55]. Infection is ubiquitous, and disease occurs commonly in children and young adults, frequently among newly aggregated adults in crowded conditions such as barracks, dormitories, and institutions.

During sporadic endemic episodes, the incidence of secondary transmission cases is low at 0.5 case per 100,000 per year. During outbreaks, this may rise to over 10 per 100,000 [103, 104]. Persons at greatest risk include household contacts, with a transmission rate of 7 per 1,000, and day-care contacts, with a transmission rate of 4 per 1,000. Risk is fostered by close personal contact and direct exposure to oral secretions. The secondary transmission rate has been reported to be as high as 7% when individuals are exposed in a small, closed space [105].

Nosocomial transmission from patients is uncommon. At-risk health care workers are those who have intimate, direct contact with oropharyngeal secretions of infected persons, for example, during intubation, resuscitation, suctioning the airway, or examining the throat of a coughing patient in a small examination room or enclosed space, such as an ambulance. After 24 hours of appropriate antibiotic therapy, patients are considered noninfectious.

The risk of transmission and disease for health care workers with close contact with airway secretions is considered very low. Workers who are not directly exposed to nasopharyngeal secretions are at negligible risk [106]. An overall (secondary) attack rate of 0.8 per 100,000 in health care workers has been estimated by one author [107].

PREVENTION AND CONTROL

Droplet precautions should be implemented where caring for patients with meningococcal meningitis or pneumonia, using masks and gloves for the high-risk procedures involving oropharyngeal secretions. These precautions also should be considered during the evaluation of any noninfant patient suspected of having meningitis pending laboratory diagnosis. Patients with pneumonia or a productive cough have the greatest potential for spreading infection. Casual contact with infected persons, such as during the cleaning of rooms or the delivery of trays, involves negligible risk of infection [46]. Pharyngeal colonization alone is not a risk factor for dissemination.

For health care workers who are intimately exposed to nasopharyngeal secretions without using mask protection, postexposure prophylaxis should be administered, ideally within 24 hours, to eradicate possible pharyngeal colonization. *N. meningitidis* has a short incubation time, typically 3–5 days; by 14 days following exposure, prophylaxis is of limited to no value [103]. Rifampin is the traditional prophylaxis but cannot be used in pregnant women and may decrease the effectiveness of oral contraceptive medications. Ciprofloxacin can be used in adults, but not pregnant women, and is reported to be 90% effective. Ceftriaxone, given intramuscularly, is 97–100% effective and may be used in pregnancy [104].

Laboratory personnel also may be at risk through handling respiratory secretions or blood specimens. Laboratory aerosolization of a specimen can transmit infection; precautions should continue in the laboratory and with specimen handling. Prophylaxis for laboratory personnel should be considered after significant laboratory exposures. Laboratory personnel who routinely culture for *N. meningitidis* (or create aerosols in the laboratory) are at highest risk of infection and may be considered for vaccination with the quadrivalent vaccine available in the United States. This vaccine provides immunity against serogroups A, C, Y, and W-135, but not to serogroup B, which caused 33% of disease in the United States between 1995 and 1998 [108].

Other types of bacterial meningitides do not have the same implications for health care workers. With *H. influenzae* meningitis, only children who are household or day-care contacts require prophylaxis [104]; adult contacts are not at risk.

Influenza

Influenza is transmitted primarily by respiratory secretions via large airborne droplets or contact with contaminated surfaces. The incubation time is 1–5 days. Individuals are most infectious during the first 3 days of illness; virus is shed prior to the onset of symptoms and for 7 days thereafter.

EPIDEMIOLOGY

Individuals over age 65, those living in nursing homes or chronic care facilities, and those with chronic conditions such as diabetes, pulmonary or cardiovascular disease are at greatest risk [55]. In these groups, influenza can lead to secondary pneumonia and mortality, which can be reduced significantly by vaccination [109]. Nosocomial transmission can occur during community outbreaks, spreading among patients and staff and resulting in widespread absenteeism that may disrupt the effective operation of the health care facility [55].

PREVENTION AND CONTROL

Nosocomial infection can be prevented by annual vaccination of health care personnel, including pregnant women after the first trimester. Health care personnel should wear a mask when providing care within 3–6 ft of persons with known or suspected influenza who are coughing or sneezing, in addition to the use of standard precautions to avoid hand contact with respiratory secretions.

While vaccination reduces influenza infection and absenteeism among health care workers and prevents mortality in their patients, only 40% of health care workers typically avail themselves of the vaccine [110]. Employee incentives or mobile immunization carts have been used to improve vaccination rates. The optimal time for vaccination is mid-October to mid-November because it takes 2 weeks for immunity to develop in anticipation of the peak flu season. Too-early vaccination may result in waning of protection by late spring. Work-restriction policies should remove infected personnel from the delivery of patient care, especially in high-risk areas such as intensive care, neonatal, and transplant units.

During community epidemics, it may become necessary for health care facilities to isolate or cohort patients with influenza in negative-pressure rooms, restrict hospital visitors with febrile respiratory illness, and postpone elective surgery [109]. During an outbreak, obtaining culture specimens from employees via nasopharyngeal swabs or washings may be useful if there is not adequate community characterization of the influenza strains responsible for the epidemic. Culture and characterization of the virus may take 5–7 days and usually will not change management of the illness in the individual. Rapid influenza tests can be used to confirm the diagnosis of influenza in patients or ill staff; some rapid tests can detect and/or distinguish

between influenza A and B. Because of the lower sensitivity of the rapid tests, negative tests should be verified by culture [110].

The neuraminidase inhibitors oseltamivir and zanamivir can be used to treat both influenza A and B [110]. If instituted within 48 hours of symptom onset, treatment may reduce the duration of illness by 1–2 days [111]. Central nervous system side effects may occur in 5–10% of young, healthy adults using amantadine or rimantadine; fewer CNS side effects are seen with the neuraminidase inhibitors. If nosocomial transmission of influenza A is documented, prophylaxis with the antiviral agents amantadine, rimantadine, or oseltamivir can be given to healthy unvaccinated staff, preferably in conjunction with vaccination. These drugs are 70–90% effective in preventing illness in healthy individuals, less in those who are elderly or have chronic medical problems [109]. Prophylaxis for the duration of a flu epidemic may be considered for workers at high risk of serious complications for whom vaccination is contraindicated or for those who are immune suppressed and expected to have poor antibody response. In 2004–2005, the CDC recommended using amantadine or rimantadine for chemoprophylaxis of influenza A and reserving oseltamivir and zanamivir for treatment of influenza A or B, giving priority to those with high-risk personal factors or occupational contacts [111].

Influenza vaccine is offered annually to reduce the transmission of influenza in health care settings and to prevent staff illness and absenteeism and influenza-related morbidity and mortality among persons at increased risk for severe influenza illness. Higher vaccination rates among health care staff are associated with a lower incidence of nosocomial influenza cases [111].

Overall, flu vaccine is about 70–90% effective. Occasionally, the vaccine virus and the virus occurring in the community do not match closely. In such circumstances, vaccination still appears to reduce death rates, even when it does not prevent illness [112]. Flu vaccine may reduce overall rates of respiratory illness and absenteeism when compared with placebo [113–115], justifying its use on a cost-effectiveness basis even in healthy, low-risk workers. Side effects of the vaccine include mild local reaction in 25–50% lasting 1–2 days. Systemic reactions are less frequent; 6% of adults have fever, chills, malaise, and myalgia with onset within 6–12 hours and lasting 1–2 days. Guillain-Barre syndrome has not been clearly associated with influenza vaccination since 1976. Anaphylactic hypersensitivity to eggs is a contraindication to flu vaccination [116].

The shortage of inactivated injectable influenza vaccine in 2004–2005 resulted in a delay in immunizing both health care personnel and patients at risk. The new live influenza virus vaccine, administered nasally, was widely offered to healthy health care workers. The nasal vaccine contains a temperature-sensitive attenuated virus that replicates in the nasopharynx but not in the lower airway and is recommended for healthy, nonpregnant personnel under age 50. Nasal shedding of the vaccine virus may occur, usually during the first 2–3 days after receipt and at low titers. The CDC recommends that nasally immunized health care workers refrain from contact with severely immunosuppressed patients, such as those requiring care in a protective environment (e.g., bone marrow transplant patients or the severely neutropenic), for 1 week owing to a theoretical risk of transmission of vaccine virus [116]. There is some suggestion that the nasal vaccine may be slightly more effective than the injected vaccine by inducing mucosal as well as circulating immunity.

NOVEL INFLUENZA

Since 2003, there have been over 300 confirmed cases of human infection with avian influenza A (highly pathogenic H5N1 strain), seen primarily in Asia and in persons with direct contact with sick or dead infected poultry [117]. Several isolated instances of possible human-to-human transmission were observed, raising the specter of an avian influenza epidemic on the scale of the 1918–1919 pandemic. The case-fatality rate of H5N1 bird flu in humans can be 50–70%. Some avian flu viruses isolated in Asia in 2004 were resistant to amantadine and rimantadine, reinforcing the recommendation to reserve the newer drugs for treatment of very ill patients [118]. The potential for flu viruses to mutate and spread between species has stimulated research to develop an avian flu vaccine for humans.

Although the seasonal flu vaccine would not cover an emerging pandemic strain, annual vaccine for health care workers is advocated to increase their residual immunity to influenza and to obtain some potential for partial protective immunity against a new strain. The extensive public health and health care preparation and planning recommended for SARS are now being focused on pandemic influenza, which is spread primarily by droplets and to a lesser intent by contact and/or aerosol.

Rabies

Rabies is an acute viral encephalomyelopathy presenting with headache, fever, malaise, and other localized sensory changes and progressing to delirium, convulsions, and death. Routes of infections other than bites are frequently involved in the spread from zoonotic sources; 40% of cases have no identified source of exposure [119].

EPIDEMIOLOGY

In the United States, human rabies occurs infrequently but is almost always fatal. The incubation period is 3–8 weeks but can be as short as 9 days or as long as several years [44]. In 1996, three cases of rabies were reported in humans and 6,982 cases in animals [120].

Rabies virus may be present in a variety of human fluids and tissues during the first 5 weeks of illness. In a majority of cases, virus is usually found in saliva or respiratory secretions, but not in urine, blood, or serum [121]. Cerebrospinal fluid, brain tissue, skeletal muscle, skin, and peripheral nerve tissue also are frequent sites for virus isolation. Exposure of an open wound or mucus membrane to infected saliva is especially risky.

PREVENTION AND CONTROL

Although transmission of rabies from patients to health care personnel has not been documented, personal protective equipment (e.g., gloves, gowns, and masks) should be used to avoid contact with saliva of patients who are coughing or unable to control secretions. A health care worker should be given prophylaxis if bitten, scratched, or stuck or if mucous membranes or broken skin is splashed with infected fluid. Prophylaxis consists of immediate administration of human rabies immune globulin, half infused into the wound and the other half given intramuscularly, and initiation of the rabies vaccine series. Rabies vaccination consists of one dose injected into the deltoid muscle on days 1, 3, 7, and 14 and followed by one dose anytime from day 28 to day 35. If the recipient has been immunized previously, only two booster doses of vaccine are needed after exposure.

Theoretically, a bite or nonbite exposure to saliva could result in human-to-human infection, although there are no documented cases of such spread. The need for PEP for health care workers caring for a patient with rabies should be assessed on a case-by-case basis to ascertain the level of actual risk. High-risk contact is percutaneous or mucus membrane contact with saliva, respiratory secretions, corneal tissue or tears, cerebrospinal fluid, or urinary sediment, especially associated with a bite, skin break, or percutaneous injury. Strategies to minimize exposure of health care workers include early consideration of rabies in the differential diagnosis of progressive neurologic disease of unknown etiology or febrile encephalopathy, followed by prompt implementation of standard barrier precautions [120].

Preexposure prophylaxis is indicated for veterinarians and animal researchers using dogs, cats, or other carrier animals and for laboratory personnel involved in production of or research using rabies virus. Standard precautions and proper biosafety equipment should be used in the laboratory setting. Airborne spread does not occur unless there is centrifugation or other aerosolization of infected fluid or tissue. In these situations, respiratory and eye protection, as well as gloves and gowns, should be used, and a biosafety hood should be used if an aerosol is generated [44].

Gastrointestinal Infection

Nosocomial transmission of agents that cause gastrointestinal infection (Table 35-14) can occur through contact with infected individuals; consumption of contaminated food, water, or beverages; or exposure to contaminated objects or environmental surfaces. Spread of infection to health care workers can occur via inadequate hand washing or inadequate disinfection or sterilization

of patient care equipment and environmental surfaces.

EPIDEMIOLOGY

Person-to-person direct contact or contact with infected surfaces is the route of exposure for most agents, but airborne spread of Norwalk virus is postulated [122, 123]. Laundry workers have been noted to be at increased risk for *Salmonella* infection; *Helicobacter pylori* has a higher seroprevalence in endoscopists compared with general internists [5]. *Clostridium difficile* can cause hospital-acquired diarrhea and may be found on the hands of 14–50% of asymptomatic health care workers [5].

PREVENTION AND CONTROL

Personnel with acute gastrointestinal illness (i.e., vomiting, diarrhea, nausea, fever, and abdominal pain) should be excluded from work in patient care or food handling. Return to work is appropriate after symptoms resolve or, if a specific pathogen is involved, when cultures are negative [46]. Good personal hygiene is essential before and after contact with patients or food. Observance of standard contact precautions minimizes the risk of transmission.

Pregnant Health Care Workers

Occupational acquisition of infection is of special concern to female health care workers of childbearing age (Table 35-15). During pregnancy, there are some cell-mediated immune system changes that permit fetal development, but these generally do not increase maternal susceptibility to infectious diseases [55]. Women health care workers should be encouraged to receive immunizations prior to becoming pregnant and to adhere to appropriate infection control practices.

EPIDEMIOLOGY

Varicella infection may be more severe during pregnancy. Transplacental infection with parvovirus, varicella, or rubella may affect the fetus. Agents such as cytomegalovirus, hepatitis B, influenza, and measles are transmissible to the fetus. Some drugs used to treat or prevent infections, such as TB, may be contraindicated during pregnancy or require a risk/benefit assessment by the treating physician.

Cytomegalovirus (CMV) frequently causes a

Table 35-14
Occupationally Acquired Infections Resulting from Airborne, Bloodborne, and Oral-Fecal Transmission

Infection	Attack Rate (%)[a]	Healthcare Workers Most Affected
Airborne transmission		
Tuberculosis	20–50	Nurses, pathologists, laboratory workers, housekeepers
Varicella	4.4–14.5	All
Measles	NA	Physicians, nurses
Influenza	3.8–4.5	Nurses, physicians
Rubella	13	All
Mumps	NA	Pediatricians, dentists
Pertussis	43	All
Parvovirus	27–47	Nurses
Respiratory syncytial virus	42–56	All
Adenovirus	22–39	Workers in ophthalmology clinics, intensive care units, long-term care facilities
Bloodborne transmission		
Human immunodeficiency virus	0.1–0.4 (per needlestick)	Nurses, laboratory workers
Hepatitis B	2 to 20–40[b]	Nurses, laboratory workers, surgeons, dentists, dialysis unit workers
Hepatitis C	1.2–10.0 (per needlestick)	Oral surgeons
Cytomegalovirus	Very low	None
Ebola virus	High	Nurses
Oral-fecal transmission		
Salmonella	5–20	Nurses, laundry workers
Hepatitis A	20	Neonatal nurses
Helicobacter pylori	Seroprevalence rate twice that of the general population	Endoscopy personnel
Clostridium difficile	Very low	None, serve as vectors
Norwalk virus	30–50	Nurses, care attendants

[a]For airborne transmission, the attack rates are as reported for outbreaks; for bloodborne transmission, exposure-associated attack rates are given.
[b]Higher rate if source is positive for Hepatitis B early antigen.
NA = Not available.
Source: Adapted from Sepkowitz K. Occupationally acquired infections in healthcare workers. *Ann Intern Med* 1996;125:826–34, 917–28.

mononucleosis-like illness in students or young adults. CMV infection is most severe in infants infected perinatally and may result in central nervous system or liver impairment. Most fetal infections occur because of primary maternal infection but can be caused by reinfection or reactivation in the seropositive mother [55]. Women of childbearing age should be counseled regarding their occupational and nonoccupational risks. Infants, young children, and immunocompromised individuals may serve as reservoirs of infection. Virus is secreted primarily in urine, saliva, and respiratory secretions and may be found in blood. Patient care personnel have no greater risk of acquisition of CMV than personnel who do not care for patients. Personnel who provide care to high-risk patients have a rate of primary CMV infection similar to that in other health care workers at 2–3%. The CDC concludes that the risk of occupational transmission of CMV to pregnant health care workers is no greater than the general public's risk [55]. Pregnant health care workers who care for infants and young children should follow standard precautions, including thorough hand washing; work transfer is not indicated. Likewise, if a health care worker is infected with CMV, work restriction is not required when standard precautions are used consistently.

Human parvovirus B19 is also of concern to pregnant health care workers. In a nonimmune woman, there is a possibility of fetal parvovirus infection and subsequent hydrops fetalis. An increase in the fetal death rate of 2–10% may be seen if parvovirus is acquired before the twentieth week of

Table 35-15
Pregnant Healthcare Personnel and Risk Due to Occupational Exposures to Infectious Agents

Agent	Potential Effect on Fetus	Rate of Perinatal Transmission	Maternal Screening	Prevention
1. CMV	Hearing loss; congenital syndrome[a]	15% after primary material infection; symptomatic 5%	Antibody protects against clinical disease; routine screening not recommended	Standard Precautions
2. Hepatitis B	Hepatitis; hepatocellular cancer as adult	HBeAg pos. 90% HBeAg neg. 25%	Anti-HBsAg Anti-HBeAg	Vaccine (safe during pregnancy); Standard Precautions
3. Hepatitis C	Hepatitis	0%–15%	Anti-HCV; HCV RNA in reference labs	IgG no longer contains anti-HCV and is not recommended; Standard Precautions
4. Herpes simplex	Mucocutaneous lesions, sepsis, encephalitis; congenital malformations (rare)	Unlikely from nosocomial exposure; primary 33%–50%, recurrent 4%	Antibody testing not useful; inspection for lesions at delivery	Standard Precautions
5. HIV	AIDS by 2–3 years of age	8%–30%	Antibody by ELISA, Western blot; PCR	Avoid high-risk behaviors; consider postexposure prophylaxis following high-risk needlestick; zidovudine
				Intrapartum and postnatal for HIV-positive mothers and their babies; Standard Precautions
6. Influenza	Inconsistent	Rare	None	Vaccine (safe during pregnancy); Droplet Precautions
7. Measles	Prematurity; abortion	Rare	History, antibody	Vaccine;[b] Airborne Precautions
8. Parvovirus B19	Hydrops, stillbirth	Rare, 3%–9% maximum adverse outcome	IgM, IgG antibody prepregnancy; antibody protective	Droplet Precautions
9. Rubella	Congenital syndrome[a]	45%–50% overall; 90% in first 12 weeks	Antibody	Vaccine;[b] Droplet Precautions for acute infection; Contact Precautions for congenital rubella
10. Tuberculosis	Hepatomegaly, pulmonary, CNS	Rare	Skin test	INH ± ethambutol; Airborne Precautions
11. Varicella-zoster virus	Malformations (skin, limb, CNS, eye); chickenpox	Total 25%; congenital syndrome (0–4%)	Antibody	Vaccine;[b] VZIG within 96 hours of exposure if susceptible; Airborne and Contact Precautions

[a]Congenital syndrome: varying combinations of jaundice, hepatosplenomegaly, microcephaly, CNS abnormalities, thrombocytopenia, anemia, retinopathy, skin and bone lesions.
[b]Live-virus vaccines are given routinely prior to pregnancy.
Source: From *CDC Guidelines for Infection Control in Healthcare Personnel,* 1998.

gestation; the highest risk of fetal infection occurs during the first 10 weeks. The virus infects erythroid precursors in the fetus, leading to severe anemia, hypoxia, and high-output cardiac failure. This can result in generalized edema and death. Parvovirus infection is common; half of adults have serologic evidence of past infection [124]. Exposure to human parvovirus B19 is common during community outbreaks, but 20% of adult and childhood infections are asymptomatic [125].

Parvovirus is associated with erythema infectiosum (EI), or Fifth's disease. The characteristic slapped-cheek rash is an immune manifestation that occurs after the constitutional symptoms and fever. By the time the rash appears, the patient is no longer infectious. Immunosuppressed anemic patients frequently can carry chronic infection with parvovirus. Most patients with hematologic disease (e.g., spherocytosis or sickle cell anemia) who present in transient aplastic crisis are infected with parvovirus [125] and represent potential sources of infection; the transmission rate ranges from 0–37% [124].

Current data on infection and fetal risk in health care workers suggest less cause for alarm than previously reported. In one hospital outbreak, rates of positive serologic tests (presence of IgM to B19) were similar in affected wards, control wards, and community controls, with a high rate of asymptomatic acquisition [126]. Nontransmission to susceptible health care workers from a chronically infected patient, even in the absence of isolation precautions, was reported. Overall, transmission in the hospital or laboratory is reported infrequently [127].

When viral infection is recognized in a patient, health care workers can decrease their risk of acquiring parvovirus by instituting droplet precautions (using masks) to avoid contact with respiratory secretions. EI is noninfectious, and there is no need for isolation. Patients with transient anemic crisis or chronic anemia and immunosuppression, such as in patients with AIDS or leukemia, should be considered infected and placed in isolation until serologic studies can be obtained [127]. Aplastic crisis is infectious for 7 days after onset; chronic infection may persist for years. When acute infection occurs, IgM production begins within 3 days in 90% of those infected and declines after 2–3 months [125]. IgG appears in the blood of an infected person about 10 days after IgM.

The CDC recommends ensuring that pregnant personnel are aware of the risks associated with parvovirus infection and procedures to prevent transmission but states that pregnant personnel should not be excluded routinely from caring for patients with B19. The 1997 *Pediatric Red Book* concludes: "In view of the high prevalence of B19, low incidence of ill effects on the fetus and the fact that avoidance of child care or teaching can only reduce and not eliminate the risk of exposure," exclusion of the pregnant woman from the workplace where EI occurs is not recommended [128]. The *Red Book* does recommends that pregnant health care workers be informed of the potential risks and preventive measures to reduce infection, which include "nonparticipation" in the care of high-risk patients.

Laboratory-Acquired Infections

The clinical pathology laboratory represents a unique health care environment where potentially infectious specimens are manipulated in various ways. In the microbiology laboratory, pathogens are propagated and handled in concentrated form.

Aerosol-generating procedures include pouring liquid cultures or supernatants, using automatic pipettes, mixing liquids with a pipette, spilling or breaking specimen containers, cutting or sawing through unfixed tissue, and homogenizing infected tissue. Aerosols may be inhaled directly or settle on environmental surfaces and be spread by direct contact.

EPIDEMIOLOGY

The laboratory worker may be at elevated risk for hepatitis B, brucellosis, Q fever, typhoid fever, and *Chlamydia*. Rare infections may be encountered, such as simian herpes B virus in primate research laboratories and the Creutzfeldt-Jakob disease prion in autopsy specimens. Potential exposure routes include percutaneous inoculation, skin breaks, inhalation, and mucous membrane or skin contact; however, only 18% of probable laboratory infections involve a known or identifiable incident [129].

Clinical diagnostic laboratories appear to have a lower incidence of laboratory-acquired infection than research laboratories, especially when the volume of specimens handled is considered; however, laboratory workers do have a higher risk of infection than other hospital personnel. Not only are scientific and technical personnel at risk, but also the laboratory support—clerical staff, dishwashers, janitors, and maintenance personnel. Among public health and hospital clinical laboratory personnel, the overall annual incidence of laboratory-acquired infections has been calculated as 1.4 per 1,000 in public health, 3.5 per 1,000 in hospitals, and 2.7 and 4.0 per 1,000, respectively, for the persons who work directly with infectious agents in those laboratories [129].

In a review of laboratory-acquired infections, over 4,000 laboratory-acquired infections were documented in the United States by 1978. The 10 most commonly reported infections were brucellosis, Q fever, hepatitis (especially hepatitis B), typhoid fever, tularemia, TB, dermatomycosis, Venezuelan equine encephalitis, psittacosis, and coccidioidomycosis [130].

PREVENTION AND CONTROL

Standard laboratory procedures can generate respirable particles, and some agents, such as *Francisella tularensis*, *Coxiella burnetii*, measles, and coxsackievirus A21, have a very low infectious dose for humans. Inhalation of a small number of such organisms can lead to laboratory-acquired infection (Table 35-16). Generally, clinical laboratories operate at Biosafety Level 2 (BSL-2), which is appropriate for handling most specimens and for inactivated specimens or fixed tissue. If aerosol-generating procedures are performed on potentially infectious materials, especially those containing respiratory pathogens, additional precautions should be used to protect against airborne diseases, including gowns and respiratory protection (e.g., HEPA masks or PAPRA), working under biological safety cabinates, or adopting full BSL-3 containment.

Because the infectious dose of 1–10 TB bacilli can be contained in only 1- to 3-droplet nuclei, aerosol transmission of TB in the laboratory is possible. Specimens that can transmit the bacilli include sputum, gastric aspirate, bronchial lavage fluid, cerebrospinal fluid, urine, and unfixed caseous tissue lesions. Laboratory workers have a rate of TB infection 100 times that of the general population, and workers in TB laboratories have an incidence three to five times that of other laboratory workers [129].

Table 35-16
Infectious Dose for Humans

Disease or Agent	Dose[a]	Route of Inoculation
Scrub typhus	3	Intradermal
Q fever	10	Inhalation
Tularemia	10	Inhalation
Malaria	10	Intravenous
Syphilis	57	Intradermal
Typhoid fever	10	Ingestion
Cholera	10	Ingestion
Escherichia coli	10	Ingestion
Shigellosis	10	Ingestion
Measles	0.2[b]	Inhalation
Venezuelan equine encephalitis	1[c]	Subcutaneous
Poliovirus 1	2[d]	Ingestion
Coxsackie A21	18	Inhalation
Influenza A2	790	Inhalation

[a]Dose in number of organisms.
[b]Median infectious dose in children.
[c]Guinea pig infective dose.
[d]Median infectious dose.
Source: From Fleming D, Richardson J, Tulis J, et al. (eds). *Laboratory Safety,* 2nd Ed. Washington, DC: American Society for Microbiology, 1995, with permission.

There have been case reports of laboratory-acquired meningococcemia [131]. The CDC recommends that work involving high concentrations or aerosolization of *N. meningitidis* should be performed in a BSL-3 laboratory [130]. The tetravalent vaccine (covering types A, C, Y, and W135) can be administered to laboratory workers who routinely deal with concentrated specimens or large quantities of meningococcal organisms, such as in research laboratories or vaccine production facilities. Exposure in clinical laboratories is typically sporadic and involves small quantities of meningococcus. In 1991, the CDC recommended use of penicillin as prophylaxis for percutaneous exposure and rifampin for mucosal exposures in the laboratory [131].

Laboratory personnel are at greater risk of *Salmonella typhi* infection than other health care workers. The incidence of infection has decreased in recent decades, but the occurrence of *S. typhi* infection continues, especially in laboratories involved in proficiency testing or research. The typhoid vaccine is suggested for microbiology workers who regularly work with *S. typhi*. Either the oral or parenteral vaccine can be used, with boosters given at appropriate intervals [55].

Malaria can be spread via needlestick or infected blood from open wounds. *Leishmania* is found in infected tissue and less commonly in blood. *Trypanosoma* can be acquired from handing cultures or blood specimens [132]. Toxoplasmosis can be acquired by a seronegative woman working with live organisms via percutaneous or mucus membrane exposure or by handling infected human tissues, with potential for congenital problems in the fetus.

Because some exposure risks are unique to laboratories, health care institutions must ensure that laboratory personnel have adequate information regarding their risks and are supplied with appropriate personal protective equipment and biosafety cabinets. Separate laboratory safety policies and procedures detailing the safety equipment and precautions to be used should be developed [130].

Summary

The diseases discussed in this chapter are just a few of the many infections that may cause problems in health care settings. Compared with the general adult population, health care workers have not been considered to be at increased risk for diphtheria, pneumococcal disease, or tetanus, and the ACIP recommends that these immunizations be obtained from the individual's primary care provider rather than considered in routine employee health programs [55]. Laboratory personnel and animal researchers, however, may have a work-related indication for routine tetanus boosters.

Hand washing/hand hygiene still plays a major role in infection control and as new organisms such as methicillin-resistant *Staphylococcus aureus* (MRSA) and *Acinetobacter baumannii* emerge in health care settings. In order to improve handwashing/hand hygiene practices, the CDC has recommended use of alcohol-based hand rubs by personnel in patient care [133]. Hand rubs take less time to use than traditional hand washing and have some residual antibacterial activity on the skin after use. Alcohol-based products are somewhat more effective than medicated or nonmedicated soaps in reducing levels of most bacteria and some viruses on the hands, but the alcohols have very poor activity against bacterial spores, protozoan oocytes, and certain nonenveloped viruses. For this reason, the use of alcohol-based hand rubs and antimicrobial soap and water may be viewed as complementary. Hand washing with antimicrobial soap and water is the method of choice for hands that are visibly soiled or exposed to spore formers such as *Bacillus anthracis* or *Clostridium difficile*. Staff compliance with hand hygiene practices in general is reported to range from 25–70%, leaving room for improvement [133]. Safety concerns were raised about installation of dispensers for potentially flammable alcohol-based hand rubs in hospital corridors; while national guidelines for installation are being developed, local fire codes may vary and should be consulted [134].

Reducing the morbidity and mortality from some work-related infections became a federal issue with OSHA's initiatives regarding TB and bloodborne pathogens. Control measures can protect health care workers and their patients and include immunization, work removal, work practices and use of personal protective equipment, and administration of prophylactic antibiotics postexposure. Hand washing, vaccination, and prompt isolation of potentially infectious patients are cost-effective strategies to prevent occupationally ac-

quired infection [5]. Effective infection control for the health care worker can be accomplished only when the employer and employee cooperate to use the full spectrum of administrative, educational, organizational, medical, physical, and behavioral measures to best advantage.

References

1. National Institute of Occupational Safety and Health (NIOSH). Safety and Health Topic: Health Care Workers, 2008; available at www.cdc.gov/niosh/topics/health care.
2. Rogers B. Health hazards in nursing and health care. *Am J Infect Control* 1997;25:248–61.
3. Perry J, Parker G, Jagger J. 2002 Percutaneous injury rates. EPI Net Report. *Adv Exp Prevent* 2004;7:18–19.
4. US Department of Labor, Occupational Safety and Health Administration. Recording Criteria for Work-Related Tuberculosis Cases. Standards 20 CFR-1904.11 (66 FR 6129, Jan 19, 2001); available at www.osha/gov.
5. Sepkowitz K. Occupationally acquired infections in health care workers. *Ann Intern Med* 1996;125:826–34, 917–28.
6. Frieden T, Sherman L, Maw K, et al. A multi-institutional outbreak of highly drug-resistant tuberculosis. *JAMA* 1996;276:1229–35.
7. Bowden K, McDiarmid M. Occupationally acquired tuberculosis: What's known. *J Occup Med* 1994;36:520–4.
8. Sbarbaro J. Tuberculosis: Yesterday, today and tomorrow (editorial). *Ann Intern Med* 1995;122:955–6.
9. Tuberculosis morbidity—United States, 1997. *MMWR* 1998;47:253–7.
10. Trends in Tuberculosis—United States, 2004. *MMWR* 2005;54:245–9.
11. Centers for Disease Control and Prevention. Guidelines for preventing the transmission of *Mycobacterium tuberculosis* in health care settings, 2005. *MMWR* 2005;54:1–89.
12. Guidelines for preventing TB transmission in health care facilities. *MMWR* 1994;43:1–132.
13. US Department of Labor, Occupational Safety and Health Administration. Standard Interpretations: 7/30/2004—Tuberculosis and Respiratory Protection; available at www.osha.gov.
14. Jasmer RM, Boxeman L, Schwartzman K et al. Recurrent tuberculosis in the United States and Canada: Relapse or reinfection. *Am J Respir Crit Care Med* 2004;170:1360–6.
15. Sepkowitz K, Raffalli J, Riley L, et al. Tuberculosis in the AIDS era. *Clin Microbiol Rev* 1995;8:180–99.
16. The role of BCG vaccine in the prevention and control of tuberculosis in the United States. *MMWR* 1998;45:5–7.

17. American Thoracic Society. Targeted tuberculosis testing and treatment of latent tuberculosis infection. *Am J Crit Care Med* 2000;161:S221–47.

18. Huebner R, Schein M, Bass J. The tuberculin skin test. *Clin Infect Dis* 1993;17:968–75.

19. American Thoracic Society. Diagnostic standards and classification of tuberculosis. *Am Rev Respir Dis* 1990;142:725–35.

20. Anergy skin testing and preventive therapy for HIV-infected persons: Revised recommendations. *MMWR* 1997;46:1–10.

21. Enforcement procedure and scheduling for occupational exposure to tuberculosis. OSHA Instruction CPL 2.106, February 9, 1996.

22. Menzies R, Belkes V, Rocher I, et al. The booster effect in two-step tuberculin testing among young adults in Montreal. *Ann Intern Med* 1994;120:190–8.

23. Manusov E, Bradshaw D, Fogarty J. Tuberculosis screening in medical students. *Fam Med* 1996;28:645–9.

24. Sepkowitz K, Fella P, Rivera P, et al. Prevalence of PPD positivity among new employees at a hospital in New York City. *Infect Control Hosp Epidemiol* 1995;16:344–7.

25. Sepkowitz K, Feldman J, Louther J, et al. Benefit of two-step PPD testing of new employees at a New York City hospital. *Am J Infect Control* 1997;25:283–6.

26. Swinker M. Prevalence of positive PPD skin tests in two-step testing program at a teaching hospital in eastern North Carolina. *Infect Control Hosp Epidemiol* 2000;21:39–40.

27. Update: Adverse event data and revised American Thoracic Society/CDC recommendation against the use of rifampin and pyrazinamide for treatment of latent tuberculosis infection—United States, 2003. *MMWR* 2003;52:735–6.

28. Stead W. Management of health care workers after inadvertent exposure to tuberculosis. *Ann Intern Med* 1995;122:906–12.

29. Marsh BJ, San Vincente J, Von Reyn CF. Utility of dual skin tests to evaluate tuberculin skin test reactions of 10 to 14 mm in health care worker. *Inf Control Hosp Epidemiol* 2003;24:821–4.

30. In the Absence of SARS-CoV Transmission Worldwide: Guidance for Surveillance, Clinical and Laboratory Evaluation and Reporting, Version 2, January 21, 2004; available at CDC:SARS homepage: www.cdc.gov/ncidod/sars/clinicians/html 3/1/05 and www.cdc.gov/ncidod/sars/word/absenceofsars.doc.

31. Public Health Guidance for Community-Level Preparedness and Response to Severe Acute Respiratory Syndrome (SARS), Version 2, January 8, 2004, Supplement C: CDC: Preparedness and Response in Health Care Facilities, and Supplement I: Infection Control in Health Care, Home and Community Settings, CDC:SARS homepage.

32. Kare R, Wachter D, Barnosky HR. SARS in the workplace. *Occup Environ Med Rep* 2004;18:9–12.

33. Chan-Yeung M. Severe acute respiratory syndrome (SARS) and health care workers. *Int J Occup Environ Health* 2004;10:421–7.

34. Teleman MD, Boudville IC, Hen BH, et al. Factors associated with transmission of severe acute respiratory syndrome among health care workers in Singapore. *Epidemiol Infect* 2004;132:797–803.

35. Khoo KL, Leng PH, Ibrahamin IB, Lim TK. The changing face of health care worker perceptions on powered air-purifying respirators during the SARS outbreak. *Respirology* 2005;10:107–10.

36. Yassi A, Moore D, Fitzgerald JM, et al. Research gaps in protecting health care workers from SARS and other respiratory pathogens. *J Occup Environ Med* 2005;47:41–9.

37. National Center for HIV, STD and TB Prevention. Fact Sheet: Preventing Occupational HIV Transmission to Health Care Personnel, 2005; available at www.cdc.gov/nchstp/od/nchstp.html.

38. Updated US Public Health Service guidelines for the management of occupational exposures to HBV, HCW, and HIV and recommendations for postexposure prophylaxis. *MMWR* 2005;54:1–17.

39. Case-control study of HIV seroconversion in health care workers after percutaneous exposure to HIV infected blood. *MMWR* 1995;44:929–35.

40. Forst L, Fletcher B. HIV prophylaxis for health care workers. *J Occup Environ Med* 1997; 39:1212–8.

41. Cardo D, Culver D, Cielsielski C, et al. A case-control study of HIV seroconversion in health care workers after percutaneous exposure. *N Engl J Med* 1997;337:1485–90.

42. Centers for Disease Control and Prevention. Rapid HIV Testing, 1998; available at www.cdc.gov/ncidod.

43. Centers for Disease Control and Prevention. Management of Occupational Exposure to HIV, 1998; available at www.cdc.gov/ncidod.

44. Heymann D (ed). *Control of Communicable Diseases Manual*, 18th ed. Washington: American Public Health Association, 2004.

45. Update on Hepatitis B prevention. *MMWR* 1987;36:355.

46. Immunization of health care workers. *MMWR* 1997;46:3–37.

47. Protection against viral hepatitis: Recommendations of the Immunization Practices Advisory Committee. *MMWR* 1990;30:1–25S.

48. OSHA Final Standard for Occupational Exposure to Bloodborne Pathogens, December 6, 1992. 29 CFR 1910.1030:64175–82.

49. Guidelines for prevention of transmission of human immune deficiency virus and hepatitis B virus to health care and public safety workers. *MMWR* 1989;38:1–37S.

50. Roome A, Walsh S, Cartter M, et al. Hepatitis B vaccine responsiveness in Connecticut public safety personnel. *JAMA* 1993;270:2931–4.

51. Wood R, MacDonal K, White K et al. Risk factors for lack of detectable antibody following hepatitis B

vaccination of Minnesota health care workers. *JAMA* 1993;270:2935–9.

52. Havlichek D, Rosenman K, Simms M, Guss P. Age-related hepatitis B seroconversion rates in health care workers. *Am J Infect Control* 1997;25:418–20.

53. US Department of Labor, Occupational Safety and Health Administration. Enforcement Procedures for the Occupational Exposure to Bloodborne Pathogens, CPL 2-2.44D, November 5, 1999.

54. Alimonas K. Prediction of response to hepatitis B vaccine in health care workers. *Clin Infect Dis* 1998; 26:566–71.

55. CDC guidelines for infection control in health care personnel. *Infect Control Hosp Epidemiol* 1998;19: 407–63.

56. Rosman AS, Basu P, Galvin K, et al. Efficacy of a high and accelerated dose of hepatitis B vaccine in alcoholic patients: A randomized clinical trial. *Am J Med* 1997;103:217–22.

57. Update: Vaccine side effects, adverse reactions, contraindications and precautions. *MMWR* 1996;45:8S.

58. Rosen H. Acquisition of hepatitis C by a conjunctival splash. *Am J Infect Control* 1997;25:242–7.

59. *Hepatitis C* (monograph). Cedar Grove, NJ: American Liver Foundation, 1997.

60. Centers for Disease Control and Prevention. Hepatitis C: What Clinicians and Other Health Professionals Need to Know, 2005; available at www.cdc.gov/ncidod/hepatitis/ctraining/edu.

61. Koff R, Wright T, Liang J. *Finding the Answers to Hepatitis B and C.* Cedar Grove, NJ: American Liver Foundation, 1996; available at *http://gi.ucsf.edu/ALF/pubs.*

62. Centers for Disease Control and Prevention. *Hepatitis: Surveillance Issues and Answers.* Report 14. Atlanta: CDC, April 1996.

63. Davis G. Hepatitis C among health care workers. *JAMA* 1996;275:1474.

64. Salazar A, Hermogenes P, Yens D. Incidence of hepatitis C in patients with chronic elevations of aminotransferases. *J Am Board Fam Practice* 1996;9: 157–61.

65. Centers for Disease Control and Prevention. *Hepatitis C: Recommendations for Medical Evaluation and Counseling.* Atlanta: CDC, July 1994.

66. Heptonstall J. Transmission of hepatitis B to patients from four infected surgeons without hepatitis B antigen. *N Engl J Med* 1997;336:178–84.

67. Gerberding J. The infected health care provider. *N Engl J Med* 1996;334:594–5.

68. Lombardo L, Meyer J. Should hepatitis B–infected health care workers perform invasive procedures? *Occup Environ Med Rep* 1997;11:41–3.

69. Centers for Disease Control and Prevention. *Frequently Asked Questions about Hepatitis C.* Atlanta: National Center for Infectious Diseases, 2005; available at www.cdc.gov.

70. Carr MM. Human bites to the hand. *J Can Dent Assoc* 1995;61:782–4.

71. Richman K, Rickman L. The potential for transmis-

sion of human immunodeficiency virus through human bites. *J Acq Immun Defic Synd* 1993;6:402–6.

72. Khajatia R. Transmission of human immunodeficiency virus through saliva after a lip bite (letter). *Arch Intern Med* 1997;157:1901.

73. Anonymous. HIV transmission by a human bite (news). *Infect Control Hosp Epidemiol* 1996;117:707.

74. Numata N, Ohori H, Hayakawa Y, et al. Demonstration of hepatitis C virus genome in saliva and urine of patients with type C hepatitis. *J Med Virol* 1993; 41:120–8.

75. Figueredo J, Borges A, Martinez R, et al. Hepatitis C virus but not HIV transmitted by a human bite (letter). *Clin Infect Dis* 1994;19:547–8.

76. Detection of hepatitis C virus RNA in the cell fraction of saliva before and after oral surgery. *J Med Virol* 1995;43:223–6.

77. Boyce JM. Environmental contamination makes an important contribution to hospital infection. *J Hosp Infect* 2007;65:50–4.

78. Cohen HA, Amir J, Matalon A, et al. Stethoscopes and otoscopes: A potential vector of infection? *Family Pract* 1997;14:446–9.

79. Walker N, Gupta R, Cheesbrough J. Blood pressure cuffs: Friend or foe? *J Hosp Infect* 2006;63:167–9.

80. Sacar S, Turgut H, Kaleli I, et al. Poor hospital infection control practice in hand hygiene, glove utilization and usage of tourniquets. *Am J Infect Control* 2006;34:606–9.

81. Dixon M. Neckties as vectors for nosocomial infection (letter). *Intensive Care Med* 2000;26:250.

82. Johnston CP, Stokes AK, Ross T, et al. *Staphylococcus aureus* colonization among health care workers at a tertiary care hospital. *Infect Control Hosp Epidemiol* 2007;28:1404–7.

83. Herwaldt L, Pattinger J, Carter C, et al. Exposure workups. *Infect Control Hosp Epidemiol* 1997;18: 850–71.

84. Recommendations for the use of live attenuated varicella vaccine. *Pediatrics* 1995;95:791–6.

85. Centers for Disease Control and Prevention. Prevention of varcella. *MMWR* 2007;56:1–40.

86. Prevention of varicella. *MMWR* 1996;45:1–27S.

87. National Center for Immunization and Respiratory Diseases. Varicella Vaccine: Q&As About Health Care Providers, 2008; available at www.cdc.gov/vaccine/vpd-vac/varicella/vac-faqs=clinichep.htm.

88. Vazquez M, Shapero ED. Varicella vaccine and infection with varicella-zoster virus. *N Engl J Med* 2005; 352:439–40.

89. Varicella-related deaths among children—United States, 1997. *MMWR* 1998;47:365–7.

90. Wurtz R, Check IJ. Breakthrough varicella infection in a health care worker despite immunity after varicella vaccination. *Infect Control Hosp Epidemol* 1999;20:561–2.

91. Hambelton S, Gershon AA. Preventing varicella-zoster disease. *Clin Microbiol Rev* 2005;18:70–7.

92. Gershon AA. Varicella-zoster virus infections. *Pediatr Rev* 2008;29:5–10.

93. Saiman L, LaRussa P, Steinbery SP, et al. Persistance of immunity to varicella-zoster virus after vaccination of health care workers. *Infect Control Hosp Epidemiol* 2001;22:279–83.

94. Selected notifiable disease reports. *MMWR* 1996; 46:1021.

95. Tanaka M, Vitek C, Pascual B, et al. Trends in pertussis among infants in the United States, 1980–1999. *JAMA* 2003;290:2968–75.

96. Weber D, Rutala W. Management of health care workers exposed to pertussis. *Infect Control Hosp Epidemiol* 1994;15:411–5.

97. Herwaldt L. Pertussis in adults. *Arch Intern Med* 1991;151:1510–2.

98. Swinker M. Adult pertussis: An occupational concern. *Clin Care Update* 2006;12:17.

99. Halperin S, Bortolussi R, Langley J, et al. Seven days of erythromycin estolate is as effective as fourteen days for the treatment of *Bordetella pertussis* infections. *Pediatric* 1997;100:65–71.

100. Preventing tetanus, diphtheria and pertusses among adults. *MMWR* 2006;55:1–33.

101. Advisory Committee on Immunization Practices. Immunizations in medical education. *Am J Prevent Med* 1995;10:60–80S.

102. Centers for Disease Control and Prevention. Rubella No Longer Major Public Health Threat in the United States. Press release, March 23, 2005; available at www.cdc.gov/oc/media/pressel/r050321.html.

103. Control and prevention of serogroup C meningococcal disease. *MMWR* 1997;46:1–8S, 13–21S.

104. Schwartz B. Chemoprophylaxis for bacterial infections. *Rev Infect Dis* 1991;13:170–3S.

105. Harrison L, Armstrong L, Jenkins S, et al. A cluster of meningococcal disease on a school bus following epidemic influenza. *Arch Intern Med* 1991;151; 1005–9.

106. Begg N. Meningococcal disease and health care workers (editorial). *Br Med J* 1999;319:1147–8.

107. Gilmore A, Stuart J, Andrews N. Risk of secondary meningococcal disease in health-care workers. *Lancet* 2000;356:1654–5.

108. Danzig L. Meningococcal vaccines. *Pediatr Infect Dis J* 2004;23:285–92S.

109. Centers for Disease Control and Prevention. Guidelines for Prevention of Nosocomial Pneumonia and Prevention and Control of Influenza, January 1998; available at www.cdc.gov/ncidod.

110. Prevention and control of influenza: Recommendations of the Advisory Committee on Immunization Practice (ACIP). *MMWR* 2004;53:1–40.

111. Centers for Disease Control and Prevention. Information for Health Care Professionals: Antivirals. Influenza Antiviral Recommendations: 2004–2005 Interim Chemoprophylaxis and Treatment Guidelines, 2004; available at www.cdc.gov.

112. Pearson ML, Bridges CB, Harper SA. Influenza vaccination of health-care personnel. *MMWR* 2006;55: 1–16.

113. Nichol K, Lind A, Margolis K, et al. The effectiveness of vaccination against influenza in healthy working adults. *N Engl J Med* 1995;333:884–93.

114. Campbell D, Rumley M. Cost-effectiveness of the influenza vaccine in a health working-age population. *J Occup Envir Med* 1997;39:408–14.

115. LaForce M, Nichol K, Cox N. Influenza: Virology, epidemiology, disease and prevention. *Am J Prevent Med* 1994;10:31–41.

116. Centers for Disease Control and Prevention. Live, attenuated influenza vaccine recommendations. In *Information for Health Care Professionals: Vaccination, www.cdc.gov.*

117. Avian Influenza A Virus Infections of Humans CDC, 2008; available at http://virusus.cdc.gov/flu/avian/gen-info/avian-flu-humans.htm.

118. Antiviral agents for influenza in prevention and control of influenza: Recommendations of the Advisory Committee on Immunization Practices (ACIP). *MMWR* 2003;53:1–34.

119. Human rabies—Michigan. *MMWR* 1983;32:159–60.

120. Human rabies and postexposure prophylaxis in health care workers. *MMWR* 1996;45:353–6.

121. Helmick C, Tauxe R, Vernon A. Is there a risk to contacts of patients with rabies? *Rev Infect Dis* 1987;9: 511–8.

122. Evans MR, Meldrum R, Lane W, et al. An outbreak of viral gastroenteritis following environmental contamination at a concert hall. *Epidemiol Infect* 2002;129:355–60.

123. Hutson AM, Atmar RL, Estes MK. Norovirus disease: Changing epidemiology and host susceptibility factors. *Trends Microbiol* 2004;12:279–87.

124. Dowell S, Turok T, Thorp J, et al. Parvovirus B19 infection in hospital workers. *J Infect Dis* 1995;172: 1076–9.

125. Turok T. Parvovirus B19 and human disease. *Adv Int Med* 1992;37:431–54.

126. Koziol D, Kurtzman G, Ayrib J, et al. Nosocomial human parvovirus B19 infection: Lack of transmission from a chronically infected patient to hospital staff. *Infect Control Hosp Epidemiol* 1992;13:343–8.

127. Guerina N. Management strategies for infectious disease in pregnancy. *Semin Perinatol* 1994;18:305–20.

128. Georges P (ed). *Red Book,* 24th ed. Elk Grove Village, IL: American Academy of Pediatrics, 1997.

129. Fleming D, Richardson J, Tules J, Vesley D (eds). *Laboratory Safety,* 2d ed. Washington: American Society for Microbiology, 1995.

130. US Department of Health and Human Services. *Biosafety in Microbiological and Biomedical Laboratories,* 5th ed. Washington: US Government Printing Office, 2007; available at www.cdc.gov/od/ohs/biosfty/bmbl5/bmbl5toc.htm.

131. Laboratory-acquired meningococcemia—California and Massachusetts. *MMWR* 1991;40:46–55.

132. Herwaldt B, Juranek D. Laboratory-acquired

malaria, leishmaniasis, trypanosomiasis and toxo-plasmosis. *Am J Trop Med Hyg* 1993;48:313–23.

133. Guideline for hand hygiene in health care settings. *MMWR* 2002;51:9–42.
134. Centers for Disease Control and Prevention. Alcohol-Based Hand Rubs and Fire Safety. Update: Hand Hygiene in Health Care Settings, September 15, 2003; available at www.cdc.gov.od/oc/media/pressed/fs021025.html.

Additional Resources

- For information on the type and duration of isolation precautions needed for selected infections and conditions, please consult the CDC at www.cdc.gov/ncidod/hip/isolat/isoapp_a.htm.
- For recommendations on work restrictions for infected health care workers, refer to *Am J Infect Control* 1998;26:289–354.
- For more information on hepatitis, contact the American Liver Foundation at 1-800-GO-LIVER (465-4827) for the public; 1-888-4HEP-ABC (443-7222) for professionals.
- For more information on the Americans with Disabilities Act, contact the Office of the Americans with Disabilities Act, U.S. Department of Justice at 202-514-0301.
- For consultation regarding occupational HIV exposure, contact the National Clinician's Post-Exposure Prophylaxis Hotline or PEP line at 1-888-448-4911.

For additional information on methicillin-resistant *Staphylococcus*, see CDC. Information about MRSA for Health Care Personnel at www.cdc.gov/ncidod/dhqp/ar_mrsa_healthcareFS.html.

36 Occupational Zoonoses

Roy L. DeHart

By tradition, zoonoses are diseases and infections that are naturally transmitted between vertebrate animals and humans. Afflictions caused by vertebrate-produced toxins or venoms, such as those of snakes and fish, are not within this definition [1].

For the purposes of this chapter, a broader definition of *zoonoses* has been developed that includes other pathogens and modes of transmission. For example, in order to be more inclusive, viral transmission from animals to humans by insect vectors (arbovirus) are included in this discussion. The four arbovirus families included are Bunyaviridae, Reoviridae, Togaviridae, and Flaviviridae.

A classification system, based on the life cycle of the infectious organism, has been devised:

- *Direct zoonoses.* Transmission between an infected vertebrate host and a susceptible host via direct or fomite contact or by mechanical factors. Examples are brucellosis, rabies, and tularemia.
- *Cyclozoonoses.* Requires more than one vertebrate host but no invertebrate hosts. Examples include echinococcosis, pentastomiasis, and taeniasis.
- *Metazoonoses.* An agent multiplies, develops, or both in an invertebrate host before transmission to a vertebrate host is possible. Examples include arbovirus, plague, and schistosomiasis.
- *Saprozoonoses.* For these infections to be transmitted, a nonanimal development site or reservoir, such as food, plants, soil, or other organic material, is required. Examples include larva migrans and mycotic diseases.

Using the broader definition of *zoonoses,* there are nearly 200 organisms that produce a zoonotic disease [2]. These include prions, viruses, rickettsiae, bacteria, fungi, protozoa, helminths, and arthropods. Tables 36-1 and 36-2 illustrate the infections that are categorized as zoonoses [2–5]. Those that are more common and those with greater potential for adverse health outcome are described in more detail elsewhere in this textbook. Most zoonotic diseases occur in the general population and are not limited to the work setting. For example, rabies, tularemia, plague, and hantavirus infection have a higher incidence owing to activities of daily living than to exposures at work.

Epidemiology

Information on the actual incidence of these diseases in the general population is not available. However, Taylor and colleagues catalogued 1,415 known human pathogens and identified 62% as being of zoonotic origin [6]. It appears that as time passes,

Table 36-1
Bacterial and Viral Zoonotic Diseases Acquired from Animals

Disease	Mode of Transmission	Source
Anthrax	Contact	Cattle
	Airborne	Sheep
		Goats
		Donkeys
		Wild herbivores
		Animal by-products
		Hides and furs
		Contaminated soil
Arbovirus encephalitis	Blood-sucking insects	Birds
	Mosquitoes	Horses
	Mites	Mules
	Lice	
	Ticks	
St. Louis encephalitis (SLE)		
Western equine encephalitis (WEE)		
Eastern equine encephalitis (EEE)		
Powassan encephalitis (POW)		
Bovine spongiform encephalopathy	Ingestion	Cattle
	Contact (?)	
Brucellosis (bangs, undulant fever)	Contact	Cattle
	Airborne	Swine
	Ingestion (milk, cheese)	Goats
		Canines
		Buffalo
		Yaks
Cat-scratch disease	Contact	Felines
		Canines
Ebola hemorrhagic fever	Contact (?)	Unknown
	Inhalation (?)	
Erysipeloid	Contact	Cattle
		Chickens
		Ducks
		Fish
		Pheasants
		Sheep
		Shellfish
		Swine
		Turkeys
		Crabs
Fish tank granuloma	Contact	Fish
		Fish tanks
		Crustacea
Hantavirus	Airborne	Deer mice
		Cotton rats
Infectious diarrhea	Fecal-oral	Cattle
		Felines
		Canines
		Chickens
		Rodents
		Sheep
		Swine

(continued)

Table 36-1   Continued

Disease	Mode of Transmission	Sourc
Influenza	Airborne	Swine
		Horses
		Birds
Leptospirosis	Contact	Cattle
	Waterborne	Rats
	Inhalation	Foxes
	Ingestion	Raccoons
		Marsupials
Lyme disease	Tick bite	Deer
		Dogs
		Mice
		Squirrels
Lymphocytic choreomeningitis	Airborne	Mice
		Hamsters
Marburg virus	Contact	Monkeys
	Inhalation (?)	
Newcastle disease	Airborne	Poultry
		Other birds
Orf	Contact	Sheep
		Goats
Ornithosis (psittacosis)	Airborne	Parrots
	Contact	Poultry
		Other birds
		Sheep
		Goats
		Cattle
Plague	Airborne	Rats
	Flea bite	Prairie dogs
		Ground squirrels
		Chipmunks
		Mice
		Rabbits
Q (Query) fever	Airborne	Cattle
	Contact	Sheep
	Ingestion (milk)	Goats
		Rabbits
		Felines
Rabies	Contact (animal bite)	Canines
		Skunks
		Bats
		Raccoons
		Cattle
		Monkeys
		Felines
		Horses
		Most animals
Tularemia	Contact	Rabbits
	Bite	Hares
	Insect vector	Rodents
		Squirrels
		Birds

Table 36-2
Fungal and Parasitic Zoonotic Diseases Acquired from Animals

Disease	Mode of Transmission	Source
Cryptosporidiosis	Water	Cattle
	Fecal-oral	Sheep
		Rodents
		Fowl
Cutaneous larva migrans	Contact	Canines
		Fish
		Cattle
		Sheep
Echinococcosis	Ingestion	Canines
	Contact	Sheep
		Goats
		Camels
		Horses
Histoplasmosis	Airborne	Poultry
		Birds
		Bats
		Soil
Ringworm	Contact	Canines
		Felines
		Poultry
		Swine
		Rodents
		Horses
		Cattle
Taeniasis	Ingestion	Beef
		Pork
Toxoplasmosis	Ingestion	Felines
		Birds
		Sheep
		Goats
		Some cattle
Trichinosis	Ingestion	Swine
Tuberculosis	Inhalation	Cattle
	Ingestion	

more human pathogens will be discovered to be of animal origin. Most current emerging infectious diseases are proving to be zoonoses [7]. Although the true overall incidence of zoonoses among workers is unknown, a survey conducted in 1990 in Great Britain among farm workers reports that 15% indicated at least one infectious episode [5]. Approximately 800 cases of psittacosis were reported to the Centers for Disease Control and Prevention (CDC) from 1987–1996 [8]. However, not all states require physicians to report cases of psittacosis. Most of these cases resulted from exposure

to pet birds; 43% were among owners and bird fanciers, with only 10% reported to be among pet shop operators.

In the United States, 102 cases of brucellosis were reported in 2007 [9]. Most of these cases involved workers who became infected as part of their job. Farmers and ranchers may be victims, but nearly 50% are abattoir workers. The National Brucellosis Eradication Program has nearly eliminated *Brucella abortus* infections from U.S. cattle herds. A 25-year review of laboratory workers who acquired infections at the National Animal Disease Center illustrated the risk of zoonoses. During the review period, 128 cases caused by transmission from animals occurred. The investigations focused on 70 strains of bacteria, viruses, and mycotic agents. Infections are in descending order of frequency: brucellosis, Q fever, typhoid, hepatitis, tularemia, tuberculosis, dermatomycoses, Venezuelan equine encephalitis, typhus, and psittacosis [10].

Leptospirosis was first described in 1983 among sewer workers. It continues to be work-related, particularly among farmers and ranchers. Approximately 100 cases occur each year in the United States and between 1,500 and 2,000 cases worldwide [11].

The U.S. reported incidence of selected zoonoses for 2007 is given in Table 36-3 [9]. However, not all

Table 36-3
Selected Zoonotic Diseases Reported in the United States, 2007

Disease	Number of Reported Cases
Anthrax	0
Brucellosis	122
Encephalitis	
California	44
Eastern equine	4
St. Louis equine	7
Western equine	0
Hantavirus	32
Lyme disease	1,296
Plague	6
Psittacosis	11
Rabies	
Human	0
Animal	175
Rocky Mountain spotted fever	146
Trichinellosis	6
Tularemia	113

Source: From Provisional cases of selected notifiable diseases, U.S., cumulative, week ending January 18. *MMWR* 2008;57:61–5.

states require reporting for each of these diseases, nor are there any data on the percent that may represent occupationally related disease. Fauci and coworkers have noted that recently (1994–2004), many new and reemerging zoonoses have challenged the public health communities worldwide. Among those emerging organisms are severe acute respiratory syndrome–associated coronavirus (SAR-CoV), henspaviruses, avian flu viruses, and in the United States, West Nile fever. Further, previously established illnesses have reemerged, such as human monkey pox, dengue, and Lyme disease [12]. During this period, we had our own home-grown spread of an infectious organism—the bioterrorism with anthrax that resulted in 22 infections and 5 related deaths in 2001.

Although some data are available on the epidemiology of zoonoses among workers, they are limited and may be misleading. The actual rate of these diseases among workers is unknown. Many of the infections are mild for most infected individuals or are mistaken for another illness (e.g., Q fever, Newcastle disease, leptospirosis, or histoplasmosis). Because the symptoms may mimic other, more common infections, such as the flu, zoonotic diseases may be misdiagnosed. The reporting system, both in the United States and worldwide, is inconsistent, and rarely are the existing systems designed to identify occupational relevance. Without a comprehensive reporting system, the available incidence data are minimal at best. In order for a zoonotic disease to be reported, it must be entered in the surveillance system, but many of those infected, such as farmers and ranchers, are stoic and seek health care only when an illness becomes life-threatening.

When considering the epidemiology of zoonotic diseases over time, the evidence supports the conclusion that the rate of human disease is decreasing. Improved sanitation in both the workplace and the community has reduced the opportunity for spread to humans. Vaccination programs for domestic animals (e.g., brucellosis and bovine tuberculosis) and the introduction of vaccine programs for wild animals (e.g., rabies) has increased herd immunity, lessening animal infection and thus reducing human exposure. Improved worker education and bloodborne pathogen training have reduced exposure for animal handlers, laboratory technicians, and veterinary personnel. In-house animal husbandry practices to reduce cross-infection have had a major role in the successful downward trend in the incidence of zoonotic diseases in agricultural workers.

Occupations at Risk

Risk of zoonotic disease is highest among those occupations with direct and frequent contact with animals. Table 36-4 lists the most common occupations in which risk is increased [4, 5]. Most episodes of zoonotic diseases are not unique to specific jobs but occur in situations of casual, infrequent, or unrecognized contact or exposure. Examples include rabies, arthropod-spread infections, hantavirus infection, and tapeworms. Workers in close contact

Table 36-4
Selected Occupations with Exposure to Zoonotic Disease Classification

Agriculture	Health Services	Animal Products	Miscellaneous
Animal transporters	Animal control officers	Abattoir workers	Animal trainers
Breeders	Laboratory technicians	Butchers	Circus, carnival, and fair operators
Dairy workers	Refuge collectors	Furriers	Foresters
Farmers	Veterinarians	Hide processors	Game wardens
Animal groomers		Meat packers	Grass cutters
Poultry keepers		Rendering plant workers	Hunters
Ranchers		Stockyard workers	Line maintenance workers
Sheep shearers		Tanning workers	Military personnel
Shepherds		Wool workers	Pet shop workers
			Transport workers
			Trappers
			Wild life managers
			Wood cutters

with animals have the highest risk for exposure to zoonotic diseases; these are farmers, ranchers, veterinarians, animal research personnel, pet shop operators, and animal-product workers. Some workers, such as transport workers, out-of-doors workers, and sanitation employees, have only occasional but time-intensive exposure. A final group of individuals has only occasional or distant exposure: sports hunters, hikers, campers, tourists, and those who are simply in the wrong place at the wrong time.

Case Studies

BRUCELLOSIS

Worldwide, it is estimated that 500,000 cases of brucellosis occur in humans annually [13]. In six Middle East countries, there are nearly 100,000 human cases of brucellosis annually. The cost of current control activities for people and animals approaches $400 million yearly [14]. Ingestion of unpasteurized dairy products manufactured in developing countries continues to be a primary source of brucellosis. Cheese made from raw goat's milk is a particular problem. Brucellae are potential agents of bioterrorism because the infecting dose for humans is low and the organisms may enter the body via the respiratory mucosa, conjunctivae, gastrointestinal tract, or abraided skin. However, person-to-person transmission does not occur, nor do infected persons pose a threat to their surroundings [15].

LYME DISEASE

The 1975 epidemic of juvenile inflammatory arthropathy in Old Lyme, Connecticut, implicated the spirochete *Borrelia burgdorferi*. Surveillance for this disease began by the CDC in 1982 as it developed into the most common vector disease in the United States [16]. By 2003, a total of 21,273 cases were reported, with over 90% reported from the northeastern and north-central United States. The large proportion of these cases occurs in two age groups, under 15 years and 45–59 years, and may reflect less use of personal protective measures. During the period 2003–2005, nearly 60,000 cases were reported from 10 reference states (Connecticut, Delaware, Maryland, Massachusetts, Minnesota, New Jersey, New York, Pennsylvania, Rhode Island, and Wisconsin). With approximately 20,000 new cases reported each year, Lyme disease is the most common vector-borne disease in the United States [17].

HANTAVIRUS PULMONARY VIRUS SYNDROME

In May 1993, the New Mexico Department of Health was notified that two persons died within a week of each other from similar respiratory symptoms. In early June 1993, the CDC proved that a new hantavirus was the cause [18, 19]. From May 1993 through July 1994, the CDC reported 83 confirmed cases, with 45 deaths. At least three viruses have been identified: Sin Nombre, Black Creek, and Bayou [20]. The primary rodents in the United States that play host to hantaviruses include the deer mouse, the cotton rat, the rice rat, and the white-footed mouse [21].

RABIES

Although only several cases of human rabies occur in the United States annually, the disease is of far greater concern worldwide. Each year, approximately 50,000 humans and millions of animals die from rabies worldwide. Respiratory transmission was implicated when two men who had been working in a bat cave died of rabies [22]. In the United States, the four wild animal groups responsible for dissemination are skunks, raccoons, foxes, and bats. In October 2004, a 15-year-old girl was diagnosed with rabies after being bitten by a bat. This was the sixth known recovery following a diagnosis of rabies; however, it is the first recovery without vaccination therapy [23]. An estimated 10 million people undergo postexposure treatment each year following exposure to rabies-suspect animals. [24].

ANTHRAX

The work of Davaine, Koch, Pasteur, and others identified anthrax as the first disease recognized to be caused by a microorganism. Anthrax also was the first bacterial disease to be prevented by a vaccine. Causes of human cases have been reported to be commercial products of animal origin, such as fur, shaving brushes, yarn, and lanolin oil [25]. Anthrax in humans is secondary to the disease in animals, except for the recent case of bioterrorism in the United States. There are three types of anthrax in humans: *cutaneous,* acquired when a spore enters through the skin via a cut or abrasion;

gastrointestinal, from eating contaminated food; and *pulmonary,* from breathing airborne spores [27].

Q FEVER

In a European country, a shipment of cotton received from another nation was the source of the disease among those who handled the shipment. Evidence suggests that the cotton was contaminated by rodents during storage. In moving the shipment, the workers were exposed to cotton dust heavily contaminated with *Coxiella burnetii* [1]. Although most outbreaks have been associated with farms or farm animals, other urban outbreaks have been described. In the summer of 2002, Q fever struck a factory that produced cardboard packing materials, causing 95 cases [26].

TULAREMIA

A large outbreak of tularemia involving over 100 workers occurred in a sugar factory. This was related to mechanical washing of sugar beets that had been contaminated with field soil containing the causative organism, the bacillus *Francisella tularensis.* The beet-cleaning process suspended the infective organisms in an aerosol [1]. In most situations, transmission occurs by direct contact with an infected animal or by an insect bite from a tick, fly, or mosquito.

ARBOVIRUSES

This group of viruses causes a number of diseases, including encephalitis. The virus is transmitted primarily by mosquitoes; however, other biting insects, including ticks, have been implicated. This group includes Japanese encephalitis, West Nile encephalitis, and dengue.

WEST NILE VIRUS (WNV) INFECTION

West Nile virus entered the United States in 1999 and began the continuing epizootic in birds with spillover infections in equines and humans. By 2003, nearly 10,000 human cases were reported in 45 states. A third of the cases were classified as neuroinvasive [28]. The attempt to control WNV has been inhibited by the lack of accurate knowledge regarding the mosquitos' vector. Work by Kilpatrick and colleagues employing a risk assessment technique identified two species not previously considered important in transmitting WNV to humans that may be responsible for up to 80% of infections. Control efforts focused on these vectors may reduce infections significantly in the northeastern United States [29].

LEPTOSPIROSIS

As with many zoonotic diseases, there has been a reduction in cases of leptospirosis owing in large part to improved sanitation and better animal control. However, it remains a concern for sewage workers and others who work in water along rivers or estuaries. In Great Britain, employers usually provide workers with an information card to show to a physician if they develop symptoms [5]. Recreational water enthusiasts, such as water skiers and canoers, are considered at risk, although minor, owing to their increased exposure. Human infection is contracted through skin abrasions or the mucosa of the nose, mouth, and eyes. The most common route for infection is from exposure to contaminated urine from infected animals [30].

ROCKY MOUNTAIN SPOTTED FEVER

The infection is caused by *Rickettsia rickettsii* that is transmitted to humans by several tick species, most commonly the American dog tick. The tick becomes infected from a blood meal taken from a natural wild animal reservoir, typically dogs, coyotes, and goats. The annual incidence is approximately 2.2 cases per 1 million persons. More than half (56%) of reported cases are from only five states: North Carolina, South Carolina, Tennessee, Oklahoma, and Arkansas. Outdoor activities during April to September in areas of high grass, weeds, and low brush increase the risk for tick bites. Activities that increase risk include hiking, hunting, forestry, and surveying. The diagnosis requires a high index of suspicion [31].

Emerging Occupational Zoonoses

For most animal infections, transmission to humans does not occur or is rare. In some cases, although the human is infected, the result is a dead-end host, and there is no further transmission. On rare occasions, although it has occurred more frequently recently owing to greater human encroachment into the remaining jungles and rain forests of the world, the rate of species' jumping to humans has increased [32]. So has the severity of health effects on humans. The infections in humans caused by human immunodeficiency virus (HIV) and Ebola hemorrhagic fever virus are examples. There has been an upward trend in new emerging zoonotic diseases that have a potentially serious impact on human health and economic growth. *Emerging zoonosis* is defined as an event that is newly recognized or newly evolved or shows an increase in incidence or expansion in geographic host or vector range [33].

SEVERE ACUTE RESPIRATORY SYNDROME (SARS)

On March 12, 2003, the World Health Organization (WHO) issued a global health alert in response to clusters of SARS in Hong Kong, Vietnam, and China [34]. Before the WHO declared the global epidemic of SARS had been contained on July 5, 2003, approximately 8,500 cases in 29 countries with 800 deaths were reported [35]. Investigators remain unsure of the exact natural reservoir of the SARS virus, but strong evidence suggests the live meat markets, "wet markets," and restaurants in Guangdong, China, where small carnivores and several species of civet cat, raccoon, dog, and ferret badger captured in China, Laos, Vietnam, and Thailand were brought into close human proximity. It is clear, however, that some of the palm civet cats were infected with SARS-related viruses, but it is still uncertain whether these represent the original source species [36, 37].

The respiratory symptoms of SARS were a critical factor in the person-to-person spread of this disease among primary contacts and health care workers. This factor also played a major role in the international spread of the epidemic globally. This is the first time that a major epidemic spread by commercial aircraft has been so well documented [35, 38, 39].

Of interest in the SARS literature and reports are the occupational health and medicine responses. During the height of the epidemic in Singapore, occupational health professionals and industrial hygienists were invited to visit hospitals and make recommendations to reverse institutional shortcomings [40]. An occupational health and medical monitoring protocol was developed by the New York Department of State as a prospective step to prevent spread [41].

AVIAN INFLUENZA (H5N1)

Avian flu H5N1 appears to have made the initial jump from poultry to people in 1997 in Hong Kong. The outbreak involved occupational exposure to poultry and was controlled by culling stocks. In 2004, this influenza strain swept through Asian poultry flocks and resulted in the death of at least 22 people in Vietnam and an additional 12 in Thailand. It is feared that should the virus evolve to become easily transmittable between humans, a pandemic could result [42]. During 2004, 35 avian influenza A virus H5N1 human-to-human transmissions were reported from Vietnam, as well as 2 from Thailand, and it is strongly suspected to have occurred in the earlier outbreak in 1997 in Hong Kong [43]. Although Thailand culled an estimated 66 million chickens and ducks in 2004, Vietnam has only recently announced that it would begin to control the bird population in 2005. A visit by this author to Vietnam in the spring of 2005 found chickens and ducks ubiquitous from Hanoi to Ho Chi Minh City. Particularly in rural areas, fowl are numerous and free-roaming on most farms. By the end of December 2006, it was reported that the virus had infected 263 people in 10 countries from Asia to Turkey, resulting in 158 deaths. The international health community has two principal tasks: (1) reduce the opportunity for the H5N1 virus to enhance its human-to-human infectivity and (2) prepare for a potential pandemic. The geographic spread of N5H1 in animals in 2006 has been the most rapid recorded since the disease was first detected [44].

VIRAL HEMORRHAGIC FEVER

A new family of viruses has been identified—the Filoviridae. This family includes Marburg virus, Reston virus, and two types of Ebola virus. Each produces a form of hemorrhagic fever. Marburg virus first appeared in 1967 among laboratory workers in Marburg, Germany, and nearly simultaneously in Bulgaria, Yugoslavia; these workers had been exposed to blood and tissue from African green monkeys. This outbreak produced 25 primary cases and 6 secondary cases of hemorrhagic fever. In subsequent years, further cases have occurred in African nations [45]. More recently, in the fall of 2004, the Marburg virus again appeared in Africa, causing at least 214 cases with 194 reported deaths [46].

Ebola fever first appeared in two major outbreaks in 1976, which also occurred nearly simultaneously: one in Zaire and the other in Sudan. Over 500 cases, with exceptionally high mortality (88% in Zaire and 53% in Sudan), were identified. Although there have been extensive investigations, there is no convincing evidence of an association with monkeys. Marburg and Ebola viruses are identified with Africa, but the third, Reston virus, originated in the Philippines and was isolated from cynomolgus monkeys. The virus can infect humans, as was demonstrated when an animal caretaker working in a primate facility in Reston, Virginia, developed antibodies. This occurred during a devastating spread among the primates in the holding facility. Although a species jump occurred, the victim experienced few symptoms, and no secondary human cases were identified. This outbreak became the centerpiece for Richard Preston's 1994 best-seller, *The Hot Zone*. The CDC announced in April 1996 that two monkeys developed Reston fever at a primate quarantine facility in Texas. No human disease was reported, however.

Secondary transmission of Ebola virus infection to humans appears to be caused only by direct contact with infected patients [47]. However, the primary route of transmission to humans remains speculative. The evidence suggests human contact with infected monkeys as a primary source of infection. Revised standards issued by the CDC recommend eye and oral nasal mask protection for health care workers treating viral hemorrhagic fever patients [48].

MONKEYPOX

Because of the similarities between smallpox and monkeypox, there is intense interest in the natural history of this disease. The first case of monkeypox was identified in 1970, and over the next decade, only 55 cases were confirmed by the WHO in the forested areas of central and western Africa. It was believed initially that human-to-human transmission would die out by the tenth generation or so. However, new case reports from the Democratic Republic of the Congo have been increasingly reported by the WHO [49]. Smallpox vaccination provides cross-protection from monkeypox; however, with the increasing number of young people who have never been vaccinated, there is a growing population susceptible to monkeypox. In 2003, there were 35 cases in the United States with a common source, pet prairie dogs. These animals had been housed with Gambian giant rats recently shipped from Africa.

SPONGIFORM ENCEPHALOPATHIES

Since the identification of bovine spongiform encephalitis (BSE) in Great Britain in 1986, there has been renewed interest in the spread of spongiform encephalopathies (SEs) to humans. Several forms of SE have occurred in humans, including occupationally related infections. The two main forms are kuru and Creutzfeldt-Jakob disease (CJD). Occupational transmission of CJD from corneal grafting and neurosurgery has been related to cases of the disease in laboratory technicians, a neurosurgeon, an orthopedic surgeon, and a pathologist [5]. More recently, exotic ruminants in zoos in Great Britain were diagnosed with BSE around the time the disease was first identified, and later the disease also appeared in domestic cats. The risk to human health from BSE has been carefully monitored. In 1995, a variant of CJD was first diagnosed in Great Britain. Studies of additional variant cases have subsequently established that these cases can be regarded as human BSE [50]. To date, the route of transmission appears to be limited to the food chain, that is, from ingestion of contaminated animal products. Other forms of contact with animals or animal products do not appear to represent an occupational hazard for contracting BSE, but the potential remains.

Prevention

In the industrial world, control of zoonoses is proving effective for most related diseases, but it continues to present major problems for developing countries. The expenses associated with vaccination and immunization programs, sacrifice of diseased animals, improved sanitation, and other control measures are not just barriers; without international assistance, they also may be impossible for developing nations. Expenses related to animal reservoir controls can be expected to increase further.

The methodologies used in occupational medicine to control toxic or bloodborne exposures are applicable to protection from zoonotic diseases. Whenever possible, hazard should be reduced or eliminated. Whenever appropriate, vaccination should be provided for employees who are at risk. Personal protective equipment should be provided to those exposed to direct contact or aerosol spread of the zoonotic organism. Strict hygiene practices and work environments that are hygienically maintained reduce the opportunity for exposure. As always, training and education are the foundation for effective preventive strategies. Finally, a continuous improvement program will help both the employer and employee to cross-check program implementation, be sensitive to a breakdown in procedures, and be vigilant for the introduction of a new "sentinel case."

During the height of the SARS epidemic in China, I had the opportunity to witness the responses of individuals, commerce, and government in both Beijing and Hong Kong to this epidemic. An extensive educational campaign was marshaled, emphasizing personal hygiene and case isolation with contact management. Paper masks were ubiquitous on transport systems, at public gatherings, and frequently on the streets and in the malls. Hand-cleaning packets were freely available as one entered department stores and shops. Common surfaces were washed frequently by special cleaning crews, and items such as elevator floor selector pads were covered with plastic sheeting to facilitate cleaning. The government was slow to respond, but once the international community was involved, China corrected the denial policies and engaged the epidemic with vast resources, building isolation hospitals, curtailing large gatherings, and closing schools. Worldwide, the epidemic was contained by applying traditional public health and occupational medicine measures [51].

Fortunately, most zoonotic transfers or species jumps do not result in sustainable infections because the disease is usually species-specific. However, there is no current method to predict the next new zoonotic pathogen or its virulence in humans.

For research and technical personnel who are working with zoonotic organisms, established work procedures, as prescribed by the degree of infectious hazard, need to be observed. These include the facility's isolation design, biohazard disposal methods, care of any cut or skin lesions, safe practices when working with sharps, scrupulous personal hygiene, and appropriate immunizations.

When zoonotic disease is suspected in humans, public health resources must be committed to investigate the source for the index case and to maintain surveillance for secondary cases. In the occupational setting, an index case should be considered a sentinel and require an investigation similar to the response of safety professionals following an accident or industrial hygienists after a toxic exposure.

The CDC is engaged in the development of a strategy for preventing emerging infectious diseases [52]. In part, this is driven by recent outbreaks of zoonotic diseases. It was recognized that many emerging diseases are acquired from animals or are transported by arthropods. The prevention strategy includes (1) improved surveillance and response, (2) applied research, (3) enhanced training, and (4) prevention and control.

In the future, zoonotic diseases can be expected to continue to challenge humankind both in the workplace and in the larger community. Occupational health professions, especially, must be well versed in the prevention and identification and management of zoonotic diseases. Animal disease reporting and oversight are split among agencies in many states. This occurs at the federal level and recently was the subject of a report from the National Academy of Sciences. The study recommended the establishment of a centralized coordinating system to enhance collaboration and cooperation among all stakeholders [53].

References

1. Abdussalem M. Zoonoses. In Parmeggian L (ed), *Encyclopedia of Occupational Health and Safety,* 3rd Ed. Geneva: International Labor Office, 1985. Pp 2344–6.
2. Merchant JA, Thorne PS, Reynolds SJ. Animal exposure. In Rosenstock L et al. (eds), *Textbook of Clinical and Environmental Medicine,* 2nd Ed. Philadelphia: Elsevier Saunders, 2005. Pp 917–23.
3. Snashall D. Occupational infections. *Br Med J* 1996;313:551–4.
4. Dieckhous KD, Garibaldi RA. Occupational infections. In Rom WN (ed), *Environmental and Occupational Medicine,* 3rd Ed. Philadelphia: Lippincott-Raven, 1998. Pp 755–74.
5. Heptonstall J, Cockcroft A, Smith RMM. Occupation and infectious disease. In *Hunter's Diseases of*

Occupations, 9th Ed. London: Arnold, 2000. Pp 489–520.

6. Taylor LH, Latham SM, Woodhouse ME. Risk factors for human disease emergence. *Philos Trans R Soc Lond [B]* 2001;356:983–9.

7. Kruse H, Kirkemo AM, Handeland K. Wildlife as source of zoonotic infections. *Emerg Infect Dis* 2004;10:2067–72.

8. Compendium of measures to control *Chlamydia psittaci* infection among humans (psittacosis) and pet birds (avian chlamydiosis), 1998. *MMWR* 1998; 47:1–9.

9. Centers for Disease Control and Prevention. Summary of notifiable diseases—United States, 2007. *MMWR* 2008;57:61.

10. Miller CD, Songer JR, Sullivan JF. A twenty-five year review of laboratory-acquired human infections at the National Animal Disease Center. *Am Ind Hyg Assoc J* 1987;48:271–5.

11. Kaufmann AF, Perkins Bradley. Leptospirosis. In Wallace RB (ed), *Public Health and Preventive Medicine,* 14th Ed. Stanford, CT: Appleton & Lange, 1998. Pp 360–2.

12. Fauci SA, Touchette NA, Folker GK. Emerging infectious diseases: A 10-year perspective from the National Institute of Allergy and Infectious Diseases. *Emerg Infect Dis* 2005;11:519–25.

13. Joint FAO/WHO Expert Committee on Brucellosis. *Sixth Report.* Tech Report Series No 740. Geneva: World Health Organisation, 1986.

14. Corbel MJ. Brucellosis: An overview. *Emerg Infect Dis* 1997;3:213–17.

15. Yagupsky P, Baron EJ. Laboratory exposures to brucellae and implications for bioterrorism. *Emerg Infect Dis* 2005;11:1180–95.

16. Centers for Disease Control and Prevention. Lyme disease. *MMWR* 2001;50:182–4.

17. Centers for Disease Control and Prevention. Lyme disease—United States, 2003–2005. *MMWR* 2007; 55:573–6.

18. Marshall E. Hantavirus outbreak yields to PCR. *Science* 1993;262:832–6.

19. Duchin JS, Koster FT, Peters CJ, et al. Hantavirus pulmonary syndrome: A clinical description of 17 patients with a newly recognized disease. *N Engl J Med* 1994;330:949–55.

20. Centers for Disease Control and Prevention. Hantavirus pulmonary syndrome. *MMWR* 1994;43: 548–9.

21. Centers for Disease Control and Prevention. Rodents that Carry the Types of Hantavirus that Cause HPS in the United States; available from www.cdc.gov/ncidod/diseases/hanta/hps/noframes/rodents.

22. Constantine DG. Rabies. In Wallace RB (ed), *Public Health and Preventive Medicine,* 14th ed. Stanford, CT: Appleton & Lange, 1998. Pp 349–53.

23. Centers for Disease Control and Prevention. Recovery of a patient from clinical rabies. *MMWR* 2004; 53:1171–3.

24. World Health Organization. Factsheet no 099, November 21, 2007; available at www.who.int/mediacentre/factsheets/fs099.en.

25. Anthrax vaccine. *Med Newslett* 1998;40:52–3.

26. Van Woerden HC, Mason BW, Nehaul LK, et al. Q fever outbreak in industrial setting. *Emerg Infect Dis* 2004;10:1282–9.

27. World Health Organization, Factsheet no 264, December 17, 2007; available at www.who.int/mediacentre/factsheets/fs264/en.

28. Komar N. West Nile virus: Epidemiology and ecology in North America. *Adv Virus Res* 2003;61:185–234.

29. Kilpatrick MA, Kramer LD, Campbell SR et al. West Nile virus assessment and the bridge vector paradigm. *Emerg Infect Dis.* 2005;11:425–9.

30. World Health Organization. *Recommended Standards and Strategies for Surveillance, Prevention and Control of Communicable Diseases.* Geneva: WHO, 2007.

31. Centers for Disease Control and Prevention. Diagnosis and Management of Tickborne Rickettsial Disease, January 6, 2008; available at www.cdc.gov/mmwr/preview/mmwehtml/rr550al.

32. Murphy FA. Emerging zoonoses. *Emerg Infect Dis* 1998;4:429–35.

33. World Health Organization. Zoonoses, January 12, 2008; available at www.who.int/zoonoses/emerging_zoonoses/en.

34. World Health Organization. Issue of a Global Alert about Cases of Atypical Pneumonia. Press release on the Internet, March 12, 2003.

35. Olsen SJ, Chang HL, Cheung YY, et al. Transmission of the severe acute respiratory syndrome on aircraft. *N Engl J Med* 2003;349:2416–22.

36. Weiss RA, McMichael AJ. Social and environmental risk factors in the reemergence of infectious diseases. *Emerg Infect Dis* 2004;10:570–6.

37. Peiris JSM, Guan J, Yuen KY. Severe acute respiratory syndrome. *Nature* 2004;10:588–97.

38. Breugelmans JG, Zucs P, Porten K, et al. SARS transmission and commercial aircraft. *Emerg Infect Dis* 2004;10:1502–3.

39. Flint J, Burton S, Macey JF, et al. Assessment of inflight transmission of SARS: Results of contact tracing, Canada. *Can Commun Dis Rep* 2003;29:105–10.

40. Koh D, Lim MK, Ong CN, Chia SE. Occupational health response to SARS. *Emerg Infect Dis* 2005;11: 167–8.

41. Centers for Disease Control and Prevention. SARS coronaviruses and highly pathogenic influenza viruses: Safety and occupational health for laboratory workers. *Emerg Infect Dis* 2005;11:1–5.

42. Aldhouse P. Vietnam's war on flu. *Nature* 2005;433: 102–4.

43. Schultsz C, Dong VC, Chau NVV, et al. Avian influenza H5N1 and healthcare workers (letter). *Emerg Infect Dis* 2005;11:1158–9.

44. World Health Organization. WHO Activities in

Avian Influenza and Pandemic Influenza Preparedness, 2007; available at www.who.int/csr/disease/avian_influenza/WHOactivitiesavianinfluenza/en.

45. Childs J, Shope RE, Fish D, et al. Emerging zoonoses. *Emerg Infect Dis* 1998;4:453–4.

46. Centers for Disease Control and Prevention. Outbreak of Marburg viral hemorrhagic fever. *MMWR* 2005;54:1–2.

47. Johnson KM, Scribner CL, McCormick JB. Ecology of Ebola virus: A first clue? *J Infect Dis* 1981;143:749–51.

48. Jaax N, Jahrling P, Geisbert T, et al. Transmission of Ebola virus (Zaire strain) to uninfected control monkeys in a biocontainment laboratory. *Lancet* 1995;346:1669–71.

49. Breman JG, Henderson DA. Poxvirus dilemmas: Monkeypox, smallpox, and biological terrorism. *N Engl J Med* 1998;339:556–9.

50. Pattison J. The emergence of bovine spongiform encephalopathy and related diseases. *Emerg Infec Dis* 1998;4:390–4.

51. Centers for Disease Control and Prevention. Compendium of measures to prevent disease associated with animals in public settings. *MMWR* 2005;54:1–20.

52. Centers for Disease Control and Prevention. Preventing emerging infectious disease: a strategy for the 21st century. *MMWR* 1998;47:1–19.

53. Kahn LH. Confronting zoonoses, linking human and veterinary medicine. *Emerg Infect Dis* 2006;12:556–61.

37

Globally Emerging Occupational Infections

Marc Croteau and Marcia Trapé

The twentieth century revolutionized infectious disease health care through advanced research, vaccinations, antibiotics, improved sanitation, and other public health measures. By the 1960s, a number of experts anticipated that the human burden of infectious disease was coming to an end. Unfortunately, they were mistaken [1]. The World Health Organization (WHO) reports that infectious disease accounted for 26% of the 57 million worldwide deaths in 2002 and 30% of all disability-adjusted life-years [1].

Emerging/reemerging infectious diseases are defined as infections that have recently appeared in a population, or are rapidly increasing in incidence or geographic range, or are threatening to increase in the foreseeable future [2–6]. The appearance of new antimicrobial-resistant forms of diseases is often included within this category. Despite continued advances in diagnostic techniques, antibiotics, vaccines, and public health, new infectious diseases continue to emerge, and old diseases, once regarded as controlled, reemerge [7–9]. Intact ecosystems function in controlling transmission of infectious diseases [6]. Population growth, coupled with current development, production, and consumption practices, is changing the geographic, environmental, and behavioral barriers that limit contact to agents and potential disease transmission [10]. The emergence and spread of infectious diseases in the early twenty-first century are driven by several factors: poverty, crowding, and urbanization; global movement across boundaries by workers, immigrants, refugees, tourists, and products; changing animal habitats; high-intensity food processing and distribution; and increasing numbers of immunocompromised persons [7–9, 11]. Complex disasters, war, famine, political instability, and social inequities resulting in widening health disparities between the developing and developed parts of the world increase the risk further. The specter of intentional release of infectious agents presents yet another concern. Whether intentional or natural in origin, the prevention and control of infectious disease is increasingly recognized as vital to social and economic security throughout the globe [8].

Sustainable solutions depend on a better understanding and control of the complex interactions among the biologic, environmental, social, economic, and political factors that contribute to disease emergence [8]. Solutions must be multidisciplinary and multilayered, addressing global macroeconomic drivers as well as local and individual factors. This recognition is encouraging collaborations with clinical and veterinary medicine, public health, academia, industry, government, and private partners [8].

Factors Contributing to Emerging Infections and the Public Health Response

In 1992, the Institute of Medicine (IOM) published a landmark report entitled, "Emerging Infections: Microbial Threats to Health in the United States" [4]. This report identified six factors that contribute to disease emergence. The factors identified were (1) ecologic changes secondary to agricultural or economic development and/or climate anomalies, (2) changes in human demographics and behavior, (3) increased international travel and commerce, (4) advances in technology and industry, (5) microbial adaptation and change, and (6) breakdown in public health infrastructure.

This report led to the development of better systems for the identification, control, and prevention of emerging infectious disease. In 1994, the Centers for Disease Control and Prevention (CDC) launched a strategic plan to address emerging infectious disease threats within a global context [5]. *Enhanced surveillance* became a key component of public health control of infectious disease. This plan advocated increased surveillance; international outbreak assistance; the implementation of applied research, including the integration of laboratory science and public health practice; communication improvement; the enhancement of databases; and the development of increased public health capacity [5, 9]. In 2000, the WHO launched the Global Outbreak Alert and Response Network, thereby expanding preparedness and response mechanisms for international outbreaks. The U.S. government worked to strengthen its public health infrastructure further in response to the World Trade Center disaster and the anthrax attacks in 2001. In 2003, IOM reconvened and updated its report to include additional factors that promote the emergence of infectious diseases. Some of these overlapping factors reflect the ways of nature, but the majority reflects ways of life. Any of these factors alone can trigger problems, but their convergence creates especially high-risk conditions where infectious diseases may readily emerge or reemerge. Thirteen factors were cited (Table 37-1). Ultimately, these derive from complex interactions of genetic and biologic factors, physical environmental factors, ecological factors, and social, political, and economic factors in a globalized community [8]. Preventive and control measures require evaluating values and balancing tradeoffs between the beneficial and harmful effects of human activities on a global scale as well as locally.

Relationships among infectious diseases of wildlife, domestic animals, and humans are increasingly recognized for their relevance in emerging disease [12]. In fact, zoonoses account for approximately 75% of emerging pathogens [1, 3, 6]. Zoonotic infections may cross species as a consequence of changes to the natural environment. Animals can serve as amplifying hosts, and animal die-offs may function as important sentinel events. In 1999, the emergence of West Nile virus in the western hemisphere was heralded by a large avian die-off primarily affecting crows. This die-off preceded the human outbreak by several weeks [13]. Crows, jays, and magpies are particularly significant as sentinel species because infections within these species lead to high mortality rates [12]. In fact, public health officials assumed that the West Nile virus outbreak was caused by St Louis encephalitis (SLE) until a veterinary pathologist, realizing that birds are resistant to SLE, linked the avian and human outbreak [14]. Surveillance of other species can have similar value. In 2005, swan die-offs heightened concerns about the appearance of avian influenza in Europe [15]. Prairie dog die-offs have heralded human cases of tularemia, and rodent die-offs in the southwestern United States may indicate an outbreak of plague. These phenomena highlight the advantages that closer communication and collaboration among physicians, veterinarians, and public health officials have to strengthen prevention and control efforts [2, 14]. At present, only a minority of states require that veterinarians contact local public health agencies directly about reportable zoonotic disease [14]. Nevertheless, current efforts at joint surveillance between animal and human disease outbreaks are already yielding benefits [14]. In 1999, the CDC established ArboNet, which monitors West Nile virus in humans, mosquitoes, birds, and other animals. Since then, ArboNet has provided an effective system for detecting arboviral disease activity within the environment and targeting mosquito control [14, 16–18]. The Canary Database (http://canarydatabase.org/) represents another innovative approach to improve access to animal sentinel data for early recognition of human environmental health hazards, including infectious disease.

The Consequences of Ecologic Changes

Many emerging pathogens already exist in the environment but surface when provided with opportunities to infect new hosts [3]. Ecologic changes related to economic development and land use are some of the most frequently cited reasons for disease emergence (see Table 37-1). Specific risk factors related to ecology include agricultural processes, changes in water ecosystems from dams and irrigation, deforestation/reforestation, and climate change resulting in drought [3]. Frequently, the underlying cause of the emerging disease relates to increasing contact between humans and animal reservoirs. For example, the emergence of Lyme disease in New England may be related to suburban sprawl and its encroachment into forest habitats [1]. At other times, changes in the environment promote selective pressures that alter the organism itself.

Agricultural and food processing are among the most significant ways in which human activity alters the environment [3]. Every year, an estimated 76 million cases of food-borne illness occur within the United States, resulting in 5,000 deaths [19]. Traditional small farms have been replaced by large systems [11]. High-risk food production practices include concentration and consolidation of production, transportation across long distances, centralized processing of food from many sources, and use of low-dose antibiotics and low-fiber feeds to promote animal growth [3, 11, 20]. Clearly, ensuring the safety of food requires an understanding of the relationship between food and

Table 37-1
Examples of Promoting Factors in the Emergence of Infectious Diseases

Factors in Emergence	Examples of Factor	Examples of Agents/Diseases
1. Microbial adaptation and change	Drug resistance Antigenic drift	*Salmonella, Campylobacter*, HIV, malaria influenza A
2. Human susceptibility to infection	Malnutrition Immunosuppression	
3. Climate and weather changes	Flooding Global warming Heavy rainfall El Niño	Malaria, Rift Valley fever, hantavirus
4. Changing ecosystems	Agricultural industry Dams Irrigation Deforestation	Nipah virus, *Escherichia coli* O157:H7-contaminated produce, Rift Valley fever, malaria, Japanese encephalitis
5. Economic development and land use	Encroachment into wildlife habitat Suburban sprawl	Argentine hemorrhagic fever (agriculture) Lyme disease
6. Human demographics and behavior	Urbanization crowding Wet markets Haj	Dengue Avian influenza, SARS Meningitis
7. Technology and industry	Food production practices	Resistant *Salmonella, Campylobactor, E. coli* hemolytic syndrome, *Cyclospora*, VJC
8. International travel and commerce	Air travel	SARS, influenza
9. Breakdown of public health measures	Poor sanitation	Dengue Anthrax in Zimbabwe
10. Poverty and social inequality	Lack of resources	Tuberculosis, malaria
11. War and famine	Crowding, loss infrastructure	Tuberculosis
12. Lack of political will	Inadequate funding	Malaria, tuberculosis
13. Intent to harm	Development of weaponized anthrax	2001 anthrax attack

Source: Adapted from Refs. 3, 6, and 8.

pathogen from farm to consumption [21]. The consolidation of animal food production concentrates large numbers of animals for production, transportation, slaughter, and processing [11]. These practices create high-density animal populations that promote opportunities to amplify point-source contamination. Hamburger production and distribution provides a clear example. To grind beef for hamburger, processors take beef from multiple sources, mix it, and grind it. Packers regrind it, and grocers sometimes grind it again. One investigator once traced the origin of a single lot of hamburger meat at one processing plant to 443 individual animals originating from slaughterhouses in six different states [11]. Health officials estimate that one infected carcass has the potential to contaminate eight tons of beef. Another example of the effect of amplification involved an outbreak of *Salmonella* linked to packaged ice cream. In 1994, 220,000 people in 41 states were affected by an outbreak of *Salmonella* that was traced to cross-contamination of a *single* tanker delivery truck. The ice cream was produced from a pre-mixed liquid base that had been delivered in a tanker truck. Investigation of this incident revealed that the tanker truck had previously delivered liquid eggs, resulting in cross-contamination of the liquid ice cream base [11, 22]. In collaboration with the Food and Drug Administration (FDA) and the U.S. Department of Agriculture (USDA), the CDC has established FoodNet, the principal food-borne component of the CDCs Emerging Disease Program. FoodNet provides active surveillance of food-borne disease in order to better identify trends and provide interventions to reduce the burden of disease. Another network coordinated by the CDC is PulseNet, a molecular subtyping network designed to help recognize point-source outbreaks and enhance real-time responses.

Another noteworthy group of evolving food-related diseases involves prion-associated diseases, sometimes referred to as *transmissible spongiform encephalopathies* (TSEs). The infectious agent in prion diseases is believed to be composed of a single protein. Prion-associated diseases are adapting to an increasing variety of species. Variant Creutzfeldt-Jakob disease (vCJD) caused by the human form of the prion is associated with bovine spongiform encephalopathy (BSE), better known as *mad cow disease*. BSE has been detected within cattle in the United Kingdom and other countries. Disease has been transmitted to humans through the consumption of contaminated beef, resulting in variant Creutzfeldt-Jakob disease (vCJD), an incurable neurodegenerative disease that slowly results in death. There is an extended incubation period between exposure to the agent and manifestation of clinical symptoms. Exposure to BSE prions in Europe from eating contaminated beef has resulted in at least 170 cases of vCJD. The epizootic outbreak among cattle probably originated from a previous practice of supplementing cattle feed with the pulverized meat and bones of previously slaughtered cattle. BSE itself is suspected to have emerged because of even earlier use of cattle feed containing the agent of sheep scrapie [23]. Clearly, addressing food production practices as they relate to the emergence of infectious disease is an important public health priority. Although no occupational exposures to prions have ever been documented, strict infection control practices in laboratories and health care settings are of upmost importance [24–26].

Traditional practices also can increase the risk of infectious disease emergence. Despite the widespread availability of refrigeration, many Asians prefer to purchase live animals for fresh meat. Live-animal markets, known as *wet markets*, are common in tropical and subtropical regions of the world. Wet markets are implicated in the genetic transformation of organisms. Wet markets sell live poultry, fish, reptiles, and mammals of every kind. Wet markets bring a wide range of animals and humans in close contact to each other, often under unhygienic conditions. Conditions within wet markets represent environments prone to selective pressures for evolution and transfer of infectious disease. Stalls containing live poultry (mostly chickens, pigeons, quail, ducks, geese, and a wide range of exotic wild-caught and farm-raised fowl) often sit in close proximity to fish, reptiles, or red-meat animals with little physical separation [6, 27]. Wet markets may be regarded as hot zones for disease emergence related to zoonoses. Targeting surveillance of animal viruses in wet markets may provide early warning for the reappearance of severe acute respiratory syndrome (SARS) and the evolution of avian influenza.

Lessons from the Emergence of SARS

SARS is caused from a novel single-stranded RNA coronavirus named *SARS-coronovirus* (SARS-CoV) [28, 29]. SARS gained international attention in 2003 during the course of a costly and rapidly spread outbreak. However, the first known cases of SARS occurred in 2001.

The original cases probably resulted from animal-to-human transfer from contact with wild game food animals caged in the wet markets located in Guangdong China [6, 27–29]. A retrospective analysis of the early cases before 2003 revealed that more than one-third represented food handlers (i.e., persons who handled, killed, and sold food animals or those who prepared and served food) [30]. The finding of SARS-CoV-like viruses among live wild animals in wet markets suggests that conditions in these markets provided a venue for the animal SARS-CoV-like viruses to amplify and be transmitted to new hosts, including humans, a critically important finding from the point of view of public health [31]. The palm civet is considered to be the most likely amplification host and a likely introductory host [29].

SARS arrived in Hong Kong in February 2003, where the index case, a professor attending a wedding, infected 14 people during his stay at the Metropole Hotel [1, 32, 33]. These infected but still asymptomatic hotel guests carried the disease around the world. Since SARS-CoV was a novel virus, there existed essentially no herd immunity. Within 1 week, SARS spread to 11 countries and 3 continents, reflecting the high mobility of world travel associated with globalization [33]. The rapid spread of SARS led to panic that adversely affected the travel-dependent global economy. By the end of the outbreak in June 2003, SARS had spread across 30 countries and 5 continents worldwide. In 2004, the WHO reported 8,096 cases and 774 deaths (a case-fatality rate of 9.6%) from SARS across 30 countries and 5 continents worldwide [6, 33–35].

Toronto, Canada, experienced the largest SARS outbreak outside Asia [36]. SARS in Toronto was primarily a nosocomial and occupational illness, infecting persons who were exposed in affected hospitals and then transmitting the infection to their household contacts [36]. During the 2003 outbreak, occupationally exposed health care workers comprised 43% of SARS cases in Canada and

21% globally. Risk factors for infection included a lack of awareness and preparedness when the disease first struck, lack of training in infection control procedures, and poor compliance in the use of personal protective equipment. Performance of certain medical procedures such as endotracheal intubation augmented the risk of transmission [33].

Most contagious respiratory agents are transmitted by a combination of mucosal inoculation from contaminated hands, large-droplet mucosal contact (3–6 ft from the source), or inhalation of long-range airborne droplet nuclei. In common with more typical person-to-person respiratory infectious diseases, the most important route of transmission for SARS involved direct or indirect contact with infectious respiratory droplets or fomites with the mucous membranes of the eyes, mouth, or nose [31]. In addition, airborne transmission to health care workers may have occurred during the performance of procedures such as patient airway by suction, intubation, bronchoscopy, and cardiopulmonary resuscitation or administration of medications via nebulization.

Data from Toronto indicate that emerging infectious diseases such as SARS can be controlled in a major North American urban center if there is a robust and responsive public health infrastructure [36]. Once implemented, compliance with infection control measures and community containment measures (i.e., tracing and quarantine of contacts) worked well. Effective health care worker control measures included strict adherence to droplet and contact precautions, including hand hygiene, and systematic procedures for donning and removal of personal protective equipment, including gowns, gloves, eye protection, and use of fitted N-95 respirators. Another strategy that was applied involved cohorting workers in order to limit exposure potential to specialized teams. Nevertheless, within hospitals, restrictions owing to SARS resulted in delays in treatments for cancer and other surgeries. The continuous, universal use of N-95 respirators and strict, but necessary, forms of personal protection proved stressful for health care workers [36].

Prior to the SARS outbreak, there was virtually no literature available to guide expectations of how an emerging infection would affect the psychological well-being of health care workers. Since then, the psychological consequences of SARS among health care workers have been widely studied. Significant emotional distress was present in up to 57% of health care workers and was associated with quarantine, fear of contagion, concern for family, job stress, interpersonal isolation, perceived stigma, and conscription of nonspecialists into infectious disease work. Studies continue to reveal long-term consequences among health care workers involved in the SARS outbreak. Toronto health care workers report significantly higher levels of burnout, psychological distress, and posttraumatic stress. These workers are more likely to have reduced patient contact and work hours and to report behavioral consequences of stress. Perceived adequacy of training and support is associated with a protective effect. These findings reinforce the general belief that effective staff support and training are key components of preparation for future disease outbreaks [37].

The rapid spread and high morbidity and mortality rates associated with SARS affected trade, travel, and societal interactions. The overall economic cost of the SARS epidemic worldwide has been estimated to be US$30 billion [38]. The SARS experience also highlighted larger concerns about the potential for the emergence of pandemic influenza from avian influenza. Both SARS and avian influenza are respiratory infections with high mortality and little herd immunity. In general, influenza is more easily transmissible from person to person than the 2003 SARS-CoV. Despite nationwide vaccination campaigns against influenza in the United States, an average of 36,000 U.S. residents die annually from seasonal influenza infections—nearly 50 times more people than the number killed by SARS worldwide. Furthermore, epidemiologic studies of influenza indicate that transmission occurs commonly within schools and at workplaces. Protecting workers, particularly responders and essential service workers, within the workplace in the face of a severe pandemic is an important strategy for maintaining infrastructure and the continuity of society [39].

Concerns about Pandemic Influenza

Pandemics represent global disease outbreaks. Severe pandemics may occur when a novel, highly pathogenic virus subtype emerges under conditions where the virus spreads easily from person to person, people have little or no immunity, and there is no available vaccine. Pandemics may sweep across the country and around the world in a very short time, providing little opportunity to implement effective control measures. In so doing, pandemics have the potential of disrupting the functional integrity of communities. It is therefore appropriate that the word *pandemic* is derived from the Greek meaning "of all the people." The name implies that we are all stakeholders. As stakeholders, we have shared responsibilities in advancing preparedness and response activities related to pandemics.

In 1918, a virulent strain of influenza A caused the most deadly pandemic in recorded history. In 1918, 500,000–675,000 Americans died from influenza at a time when the population of United States was only about 100 million people. This number of deaths is greater than the number of U.S. military deaths from World War I, World War II, and the Korean and Vietnam wars combined. Worldwide, the 1918 influenza death estimates range between 40 million and 100 million. The 1918 pandemic affected those between the ages of 20 and 40 years in particular, integral members of productive societies. Global conditions today may be even more vulnerable to a severe and disastrous pandemic outbreak such as the one that occurred in 1918. Global populations are larger and increasingly urbanized. Much of modern living clusters people within indoor environments. International travel is much greater. Populations consist of increasing numbers of elderly and persons with chronic medical conditions. Planning for a potential disaster on the scale of the 1918 pandemic involves multidisciplinary expertise in disaster preparedness [39–42].

A thorough understanding of any hazard is a critical early step in preparedness. As such, an important early step in influenza pandemic preparedness involves a thorough understanding of the dynamics of seasonal influenza. Seasonal influenza characteristically spreads rapidly from person to person. Infected people may shed virus for 1–2 days before becoming symptomatic. Some flu-infected individuals remain asymptomatic. Asymptomatic individuals infected with influenza also may shed virus. Symptoms are nonspecific. The clinical syndrome consists of an abrupt onset of fever, headache, body aches, and malaise following a short incubation (2–4 days). Respiratory symptoms consisting of cough, coryza, and tracheobronchitis typically follow. There are no pathognomonic signs [39, 42].

Common sites for person-to-person transmission of seasonal influenza include schools, households, and workplaces. Children pose a particular challenge in terms of control because they are at greater risk for infection, shed virus longer than adults, and spread infection more than adults. Evidence indicates that children are the most likely conduits of the virus both to adults and to other children. The highest attack rates typically occur among school-age children. Twenty-one percent (21%) of child-to-child spread occurs within schools, and child-to-adult spread accounts for 17% of household cases. Similarly important, 22% of adult-to-adult cases occur within workplaces [40, 44, 45].

Person-to-person spread of seasonal influenza occurs mainly via droplet transmission, whereby contaminated droplets come into contact with a recipient's oral, nasal, or ocular mucosae. Droplet transmission is characterized by large droplets (e.g., >5 μm) expelled by coughing and sneezing. Such droplets travel through the air for no more than 3–6 ft from the source. Transmission typically requires close physical contact. Large droplets do not remain suspended in the air and do not typically require special air handling and ventilation systems to control spread. Contact transmission may account for some spread of influenza. Influenza A can survive for 24–48 hours on nonporous surfaces and less than 12 hours on porous surfaces. Hands can become contaminated and transfer the virus to oral, ocular, or nasal mucosae. The proportion of influenza transmission caused by contaminated hand contact is unknown [43–45].

Influenza A viruses are characterized by an inherent variability, a dynamic capacity to change, and an ability to cross species barriers and adapt to new hosts. Biologically, influenza A is a round, single-stranded RNA virus enclosed in a helical protein shell. Eight segments of single-stranded RNA provide the genetic information. The virus is covered by a lipid envelope from which spikes a symmetric layer of the surface proteins hemagglutinin (H) and neuraminidase (N) as shown in Figure 37-1. Viral subtypes are based on these highly immunogenic surface proteins. In nature, 16 different

Figure 37-1
Influenza A Virus.

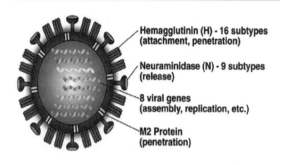

Source: www.fda.gov/CbER/summaries/nfid051806jg.htm.

H proteins and 9 different N proteins are known to exist, all of which have been isolated from birds. In fact, influenza A is primarily a bird virus. For millions of years, the virus has existed in wild aquatic birds such as ducks and shore birds and does not typically harm them. In fact, only three H subtypes (H1, H2, and H3) and two N subtypes (N1 and N2) are known to have circulated among humans via human-to-human transmission. These human virus subtypes evolved and adapted to humans from avian virus predecessors [43, 46–49].

Understanding the evolution of antigenic changes and adaptations among influenza A viruses is important to understanding the evolving epidemiology of influenza and the emergence of pandemics. In general, RNA viruses are typically associated with many mutations. Minor changes in the antigenicity of circulating influenza occur continuously owing to frequent point mutations and copying errors. These changes, known as *antigenic drift*, result in new viral variants and are one reason why influenza vaccines are updated and administered yearly. Predominant variants typically circulate for a few years before being supplanted by a newly predominant variant. In contrast, an antigenic shift represents a significant evolutionary change within the influenza A virus. An antigenic shift results when an influenza A virus bears a novel H, N, or both and has succeeded in adapting to human-to-human transmission.

Antigenic shift may occur when two viruses of different subtypes simultaneously infect the same host, resulting in a reassortment of their genetic material. Pigs have been implicated in reassortment. Host attachment is mediated via the H protein attaching to a specific mucoprotein (e.g., silaic acid) receptor. Avian species contain 2,3-galactose-linked receptors, whereas human receptors are 2,6-galactose-linked [48, 49]. Pigs contain receptors for both avian and human viruses. In locations such as wet markets, where chickens, humans, and pigs live in close proximity, pigs may function as virus "mixing bowls." If a pig is infected with circulating avian and human influenza viruses simultaneously, the two types of virus may exchange genes. A novel human-to-human virus with the capacity to attach to human receptors may emerge.

Pandemics result from antigenic shifts when a novel virus can be easily transmitted among an immunologically naive human population. Antigenic shift is a sporadic event occurring approximately every 20 years. Historically, these have occurred every 11–42 years [46]. In the past century, pandemics occurred in 1918–1919, 1957–1958, and 1968–1969. Not all influenza A pandemics strike with equal severity. In 1957, reassortment led to the emergence of a novel H2N2 virus consisting of three genes from the avian viral pool circulating among ducks and five genes from the human circulating pool. In the United States, 68,800 people died from the 1957–1958 pandemic. A novel H2N2 strain emerged in 1968 following the reassortment of two genes from avian influenza circulating among ducks combined with six genes from the human viral pool. The N2 antigen was unchanged. The 1968 strain was associated with 33,800 deaths in the United States, a lower death rate than with the 1967 strain.

In February 2007, the U.S. Department of Health and Human Services released the Pandemic Severity Index (PSI) as a way to grade pandemics. The evidence suggests that the pandemic severity level is initially based on its case-fatality ratio (CFR), a single criterion that likely will be known even early in a pandemic when small clusters and outbreaks are occurring [44]. The PSI is well illustrated in Figure 37-2.

According to the PSI, the pandemics of 1957 and 1968 both fit into category 2, whereas the 1918 pandemic qualifies as a category 5. This knowledge may help to guide the level of control measures that

Figure 37-2
Pandemic Severity Index.

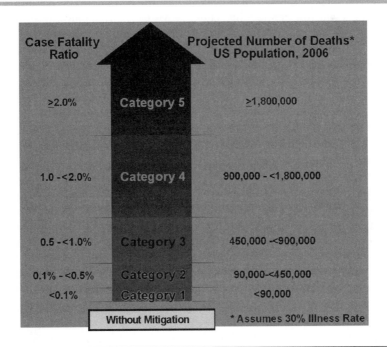

Source: CDC. Interim Prepandemic Planning Guidance: Community Strategy for Pandemic Influenza Mitigation in the United States—Early, Targeted, Layered Use of Nonpharmaceutical Interventions, February 2007 [44].

government may impose on society. Workplaces will need to coordinate their control efforts within the context of these broader government controls. However, in order to be effective, planning must begin long before even these risk categories are known.

Avian influenza is an ecologic designation intended to describe influenza A subtypes among birds. In recent years, there have been growing concerns about the emergence of a particularly pathogenic strain of avian influenza, H5N1. The H5N1 strain has widespread prevalence among migratory birds. It is endemic in Asia, and there have been outbreaks among commercial poultry in expanding geographic locations. In fact, live poultry markets serve as the primary reservoir for the maintenance, amplification, and dissemination of avian influenza viruses. Although migratory birds may spread H5N1 viruses to different geographic regions, the geographic spread of H5N1 appears to be primarily via movement of poultry and poultry products. As a result, H5N1 has already had serious economic consequences. As of May 2006, there have been deaths in 140 million domesticated birds by infection or culling. Documented mammalian infections also have occurred. Significantly, H5N1 has been isolated in pigs in China in an area where human H3N2 is endemic among pigs. The H5N1 virus has infected new species such as cats. At the time of this writing (March 2008), the epizootic avian influenza H5N1 is causing human disease associated with high mortality rates. There have been 340 human cases worldwide as of December 2007. The estimated case-mortality rate is greater than 50%. Ninety percent of the human cases are in persons 40 years of age and younger. Handling of sick or dead poultry is the most commonly recognized risk factor for infection. H5N1 continues to evolve and is becoming more genetically diversified into a number of clades and subclades. H5N1 viruses pose a pandemic threat should they develop characteristics enabling efficient human-to-human transmission. There has been no *sustained* human-to-human transmission documented as of early 2008. However, isolated cases of human-to-human spread have occurred [50–53]. A mutation enabling H5N1 avian influenza virus to recognize viral cell receptors found in human upper airways could enhance person-to-person transmission by allowing easier viral attachment, replication, and transmission through the upper respiratory tract [49].

Ironically, the widespread use of over-the-counter amantadine in China as a response to SARS in 2003 may have precipitated widespread M2 ion channel inhibitor–resistant influenza. Prior to 2003, influenza resistance to M2 ion channel inhibitors (e.g., amantadine and rimantadine) among influenza isolates ranged from 1–3%. During the 2004–2005 influenza season, approximately 70% of the influenza virus isolates from China and nearly 15% of those from the United States were resistant strains. The incidence of M2 inhibitor resistance among human influenza A (H3N2) viruses in the United States during the 2005–2006 season was 97% [54].

Influenza Pandemic and Workplace Response Planning

Severe pandemics represent true public health emergencies that likely would evoke the implementation of government disaster plans. However, the desired outcomes and responsibilities in pandemic influenza planning are shared among private and public entities. In fact, 85% of the U.S. critical infrastructure rests in the hands of the private sector (www.osha.gov/Publications/influenza_pandemic .html). Common desired outcomes include limiting sickness and death, maintaining essential services and infrastructure, minimizing damage to stakeholders, reducing economic losses, easing strain on vital essential services, and maintaining the functional continuity of society. All organizations must plan in order to become more resilient to the consequences of a pandemic. Effective plans are tested, modified, and then retested. They remain dynamic. Perfunctory plans shelved in a case are unlikely to work during a time of need [55].

The first step in any disaster preparedness involves establishing a multidisciplinary planning team with a clear mission and an appropriate level of authority and funding. Buy-in among the various stakeholders across all levels of the organization is crucial to operationalization and effectiveness. The Federal Emergency Management Agency (FEMA) advocates that disaster planning teams include members from upper management, line management, labor, human resources, engineering and maintenance, industrial hygiene, safety, health and environmental affairs, a public information officer, security, community relations, sales and marketing, legal, and finance and purchasing sectors. In so doing, the organization will be better positioned to anticipate the consequences of decision making (www.fema.gov/business/guide/section1a.shtm).

Government and nongovernment agencies, as well as many other workplace organizations, are actively developing and testing dynamic continuity of operation plans (COOP) in preparation for the next pandemic influenza outbreak. In planning, each phase of an outbreak must be anticipated and considered as part of the COOP. Adequate preparation must include advancing preevent measures focused on primary prevention, event measures focused on response and secondary mitigation, and recovery measures focused on consequence management. To a large degree, all these measures must be anticipated and planned for in advance so that resources are allocated appropriately and staff receives the necessary training.

In general, the planning process begins by identifying and characterizing the hazard. In the case of influenza A, the hazard is well known in principle, although certain critical specifics cannot be known far in advance. Advanced planning relies on well-established industrial hygiene and infection control measures and reasonable premises. The PSI is essentially a means of anticipating and adjusting for unknowns. It assumes rapid person-to-person transmission and a 30% illness rate in the absence of control measures. Planning includes a menu of graded responses to relatively mild outbreaks, as well as worst-case-scenario responses [44]. Once the hazard has been characterized, the next step in the planning process is to analyze the organization's capabilities and vulnerabilities, including both the human impact and the service impact. This step includes consideration of the stability and resiliency of the workforce; a determination of critical core services, operations, and personnel; cross-training needs; service and contractual obligations; the reliability of supply requirements; and access to available internal and external resources. Response organizations such as hospitals also must assess surge capacity. Important codes and regulations must be considered. Plans will need to be cohesive with government response efforts.

A critical component of any COOP includes worker health and safety. Plans for front-line essential service workers, including health care workers, utility workers, emergency responders, police, firefighters, and so on, must have an internal focus as well as an external response focus. Organizations must plan to safeguard workers' mental health needs as well as their physical needs. Planning may include provisions for food, rest, ability to contact family during prolonged shifts, recuperation (including breaks from personal protective equipment), and psychosocial support. Advanced training in appropriate infection controls not only helps to maintain operations by enhancing safety but also builds confidence and reduces stress among staff. Nevertheless, in anticipation of losses and absenteeism, core services and personnel also require cross training for a minimum of three-deep backup. Not only may staffing levels be affected by high illness rates, but further reductions also may occur secondary to conflicting family needs and government-mandated school closures. Many organizations are preparing for 10%, 20%, 30%, 40%, or more loss of staff. In many ways, cross training can be viewed as another safety measure by reducing the risk of errors, miscommunication, and mishaps. Remaining workers are more likely to engage and experience less psychological stress if they sense organizational support for themselves and their families. Despite these efforts, however, organizations may be required to scale back to a prioritized set of core services.

Specific Control Strategies

Vaccination represents the key infection containment strategy, but an effective vaccine is not expected to be available until a minimum of 6 months following the onset of a pandemic. Furthermore, at current production capacities, experts do not expect to vaccinate more than 14% of the world's population within a year of a pandemic. Other control strategies will need to be applied. These alternative measures are attempts to buy time by slowing the epidemic curve in order to develop, produce, and distribute an effective vaccine (Figure 37-3) [44].

Relevant government agencies and experts are reviewing a menu of potential control measures. These include selective use of antiviral medication, isolation of sick people in hospital or at home,

Figure 37-3
Interim Goals for Control Strategies Pending Effective Vaccine Availability

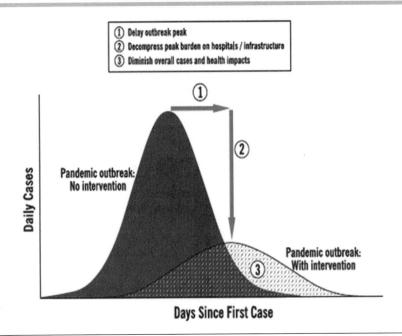

Source: CDC. Interim Prepandemic Planning Guidance: Community Strategy for Pandemic Influenza Mitigation in the United States—Early, Targeted, Layered Use of Nonpharmaceutical Interventions, February 2007[44].

quarantine of people believed to have been exposed, widespread application of hand washing and respiratory etiquette, travel restrictions, prohibition of social gatherings, school closures, maintaining personal distance, and use of personal protective equipment such as N-95 respirators and disposable masks [44, 55]. During an outbreak, specific public health measures will be driven by a consideration of the PSI (Table 37-2) and the availability of resources. Community mitigation strate-gies will be implemented early (e.g., perhaps while the virus is circulating in Asia), targeted, and layered. Strategies will remain dynamic, continuously assessed, and modified based on experience, new information, and additional resources.

Two key questions arise: How will proposed public health control measures affect your workplace? Can any of these community control measures be adapted and applied to your workplace? Government mandates will affect businesses and

Table 37-2
Pandemic Severity Index

Interventions by Setting	1	2 and 3	4 and 5
Workplace/CommunityAdult social distancing			
—decrease number of social contacts (e.g., encourage teleconferences, alternatives to face-to-face meetings)	Generally not recommended	Consider	Recommend
—increase distance between persons (e.g., reduce density in public transit, work-place)	Generally not recommended	Consider	Recommend
—modify, postpone, or cancel selected public gatherings to promote social distance (e.g., stadium events, theater performances)	Generally not recommended	Consider	Recommend
—modify workplace schedules and practices (e.g., telework, staggered shifts)	Generally not recommended	Consider	Recommend

Source: CDC. Interim Prepandemic Planning Guidance: Community Strategy for Pandemic Influenza Mitigation in the United States—Early, Targeted, Layered Use of Nonpharmaceutical Interventions, February 2007 [44].

workers. Specifics will depend, in part, on your organization's functions and level of preparedness. Advanced knowledge, training, and ongoing communication and coordination among all stakeholders, including government agencies and businesses, are paramount.

The U.S. Department of Health and Human Resources is currently stockpiling antiviral medication for potential use in prophylaxis and treatment in the event of an influenza A pandemic. Viral sensitivities to these medications are yet to be determined. Currently, resistance to medications such as oseltimir is developing [44, 56, 57].

Availability of antiviral medications will be limited and tightly controlled. At present, the plan limits use only to maintain critical workforce and to treat the most severely ill. However, under consideration is a plan to use antiviral medications to dampen the outbreak in order to make it more manageable. This approach would prompt treatment of all initial cases and give prophylaxis to all household contacts.

The remaining mitigation strategies involve the application of administrative controls and work hygiene practices, the selective use of personal protective equipment, and perhaps the use of engineering controls in special circumstances. Since workplaces pose a significant environmental risk for transmission, perhaps the next most effective workplace mitigation strategy involves the enforcement of a policy that the sick stay home. In fact, voluntary isolation of the ill at home (both adults and children), combined with use of antiviral treatment as available and indicated, is expected to be a basic public health recommendation in a pandemic of any magnitude. Work policies should be enabling in order to help ensure compliance with these recommendations. Action items include a review of work restriction policies, clear guidance for staff to stay home if symptoms occur, the development of policies for exposed workers (e.g., family leave), clear guidance on returning to work (7–10 days), and plans for extended health care costs, lost time, sick leave, short-term disability insurance, and the means to track and communicate with out-of-work staff. Community outbreaks are expected to come in waves. Persons who become sick and recover from the first wave of a pandemic will have some immunity in the second wave and thus may be critical for the workforce.

Depending on state statutes, a category 4 or 5 pandemic could evoke a public health state of emergency. In a state of emergency, governors, on the advice of public health authorities, may advise voluntary quarantines or impose mandatory quarantines on those with substantial contact with infected persons. Quarantines for 7 days from the time that the last family member becomes ill could be combined with provisions for antiviral medication. Implementation of quarantines could significantly reduce an already stressed workforce. Compensatory preparedness action items include building telecommuting, teleconferencing capabilities, providing safety guidance for home care, and cross-training staff. Concerns about a severe category 4 or 5 pandemic also could prompt workplace/community social distancing measures in an attempt to reduce population density. Workplace measures might include more telecommuting, respacing work stations, teleconferencing, and staggered shifts.

Because children are inherently "risky" for acquiring and spreading infection, school closings are regarded as an important early step to control a severe outbreak [44]. Preschool children are also a concern. A recent study of children between the ages of 25 and 36 months found that children in group care with six or more children were 2.2 times as likely to have an upper respiratory tract illness than children reared at home or in small-group care (defined as fewer than six children). Early public health interventions not only could close schools but also could limit day care and social gatherings. Thirty-four percent (34%) of households include young children. Single parents make up 9% of these households. Five percent (5%) of households state that they have no additional child support (www.hsph.harvard.edu/panflu/1OM_Avian_flu.ppt) [44, 55]. Organizational preparedness should include the impact that closures of schools and day-care facilities would have on the workforce. Preparedness action items may include plans for flexible work hours and/or small-group (i.e., fewer than 6 children) shared day-care support.

Any measures that effectively reduce workplace transmission not only help to maintain operations but also reduce the outbreak within the community at large. Instituting workplace hygiene practices for respiratory illness transmission has benefits under any circumstances. Hand hygiene is a simple but

effective tool. Hand-washing programs implemented at a Navy training center among navy recruits demonstrated a 45% reduction in outpatient
visits for respiratory illness. Frequent hand washers
had fewer respiratory illnesses [58]. Use of 70%
ethanol–based hand rubs is also thought to be effective.

Providing seasonal influenza vaccine within the
workplace offers a number of potential advantages.
Yearly influenza vaccines are proven to reduce absenteeism. This practice encourages and helps to
build a vaccine market. During a pandemic, it may
reduce the number of false-positive respiratory
conditions and help to unload the health care system. In theory, a pandemic influenza strain may
occur concurrently with seasonal strains, and vaccination may reduce the risk of reassortment. Table
37-3 provides a summary of basic recommendations for employees that can be readily implemented.

Certain jobs may require workers to be in close
proximity to infected persons. Health care workers
and other responders are at high risk for exposure.
Limiting the number of employees at risk of exposure is an important measure. Cohorting workers
in teams who take care of infected patients represent one approach. As much as possible, support
staff such as receptionists should remain out of
harm's way (e.g., behind a protective glass barrier).

Table 37-3
Summary of Employee Recommendations

Start now; Make it part of culture

1. **Get influenza shot annually**
2. **Wash hands**
—Wash hands often with a soap and warm water (15 seconds)
  or use an alcohol based hand sanitizer (70% ethanol)
3. **Avoid touching eyes, nose or mouth**
4. **Cover mouth when coughing or sneezing**
—Never cough in the direction of someone else. Cough or
  sneeze into a tissue. Dispose of tissue in a covered container.
5. **Clean things that are touched often**
—Clean things that are touched often (computer key
  boards/mouse, phone and doorknobs)
6. **Avoid close contact with others who are ill.**
7. **Avoid crowded conditions. Practice social spacing.**
8. **Prepare your home** (essential supplies, alternative daycare,
  preserve sick leave, daycare)
9. **Stay home when you are ill.**
—If you have flu symptoms, stay home from work or school
  and avoid public activities for a least 5 days (7 days for children), probably 7–10 days in a pandemic.

Source: Adapted from www.cdc.gov/flu/about/qa/preventing.htm.

Compliance with the appropriate use of personal
protective equipment such as properly fitted N-95
respirators is an important adjunctive protective
measure for health care workers. Additionally, regular surgical masks can be used on patients to help
contain infectious droplets. The broader use of
masks is more controversial. Masks are used much
more liberally among the public in Asia, and this is
considered part of respiratory etiquette there.
Seventy-six percent (76%) of Hong Kong residents
wore masks during the 2003 SARS epidemic. Although no control studies were performed, there
was an apparent decrease in influenza and other
upper respiratory tract infections during this period. In general, the level of appropriate personal
protective equipment that is used should match the
exposure risk.

Occupational Safety and Health Administration
(OSHA) guidance for preparing workplaces for a
pandemic flu can be found at www.osha.gov/
Publications/influenza_pandemic.html. Additional
up-to-date information can be obtained at www
.pandemicflu.gov.

Tuberculosis: A Current Pandemic

EPIDEMIOLOGY

Tuberculosis (TB) represents a current and ongoing pandemic. It remains a leading cause of worldwide morbidity and mortality. In 2000, an
estimated 8.3 million people became ill with TB
[59]. Indeed, TB is the infectious disease that causes
the highest morbidity and mortality in the world,
with over 30% (2 billion people) of the world population infected and 2 million deaths annually [60].
Globally, the active TB incidence rate is expected to
increase, with a rate approximating 150 active cases
per 100,000 population, resulting in 10 million new
cases of disease per year [61]. Countries where the
incidence of human immunodeficiency virus
(HIV)/acquired immune deficiency syndrome
(AIDS) is higher carry a larger burden of active TB
as well as drug-resistant TB.

The burden of TB is closely related to the burden of AIDS. Yet, like AIDS, TB is preventable. The
spread and control of TB are affected by immigration, international travel, poverty, stigmatization,
war, overcrowding, mass migration, and the loss of
public health infrastructure. The overall goals for
treatment of TB are (1) to cure the individual patient and (2) to minimize transmission to other

persons. Thus, successful treatment of tuberculosis benefits both the individual patient and the larger community [62]. Tragically, mismanagement of TB cases has led to the emergence of multidrug-resistant disease. Control measures depend on early diagnosis of active disease, compliance with a full course of multidrug treatment for active cases, identification and treatment of high-risk latent cases, and ongoing education and support. The cornerstone of these measures depends on active surveillance among high-risk groups [63]. Intact health care systems and public health infrastructures are important to ensure appropriate disease management and prevention of antibiotic resistance owing to noncompliance.

Surveillance is an important tool for control of TB. It is estimated that each individual with an active TB infection will contaminate at least another 10 persons who then will develop active disease or latent TB infection (LTBI). [64]. In the United States, the incidence rate for TB has decreased to 4.6 per 100,000 population in 2006, approximately a 3% decline from 2005 [65]. However, the proportion of active TB cases among foreign-born individuals within the United States has increased yearly since 1993. Most patients with active disease progressed from LTBI, which was acquired before

entering the United States. Commonly, these individuals have arrived from countries with a high prevalence of TB [65].

There is no surveillance for LTBI in the United States, so rates are estimated from WHO reports [66]. Although active TB cases and positive cultures are reportable diseases in all the U.S. states, a positive tuberculin skin test (TST) or a positive serologic test such as the interferon-γ release assay is usually not reportable except in special circumstances [67]. LTBI is usually only reportable to public health agencies (i.e., state and local health districts) in the presence of HIV infection or in children under age 13.

Data from the CDC for 2006 show that over 50% of the reported active TB cases are among foreign-born individuals from five countries: Mexico, the Philippines, Vietnam, India, and China [65]. Continued surveillance of workers at the point of entry into the United States, such as those working in health care professions and students at universities and professional training programs, is essential to control TB. Early identification of active TB, rapid cultures with determination of drug sensitivity, and HIV results have been important measures to control the incidence of active TB [68]. Figures 37-4 and 37-5 illustrate the rate of TB in

Figure 37-4
Rate of TB Cases by State, United States, 2006.

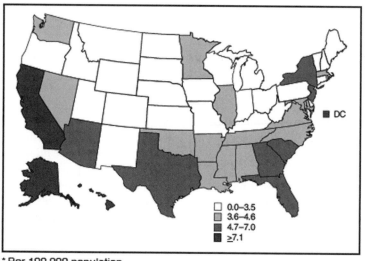

* Per 100,000 population.
† Data are provisional.

Source: CDC. Extensively drug-resistant tuberculosis—United States, 1993–2006. *MMWR* 2007;56:250–3.

Figure 37-5
Number and Rate of TB Cases among U.S.- and
Foreign-Born Persons, by Year Reported, United States,
1993–2006.

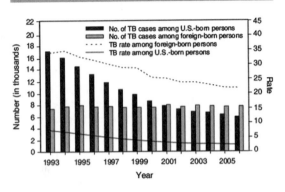

* Per 100,000 population.
† Data for 2006 are provisional.

Source: CDC. Extensively drug-resistant tuberculosis—United States,
1993–2006. *MMWR* 2007;56:250–3.

U.S. states and the rate and number of cases of active TB among U.S.-born and non-U.S.-born individuals, respectively.

In the United States, the incidence rate for TB has been decreasing yearly. However, some groups still present higher levels of active TB, such as the homeless, the incarcerated, and immigrants. Data from the CDC about homelessness and TB have shown that from 1994–2003, there were over 185,000 cases of TB reported among homeless individuals. For the homeless, a higher proportion of patients with active disease occurred among (1) those incarcerated (9% versus 3% on nonhomeless incarcerated), (2) those infected with HIV/AIDS, and (3) those with alcohol or chemical dependency [69]. Social agency workers and public health professionals dealing with the homeless or prisoners have increased risk for TB infection and should have periodic monitoring program designed for them.

RESURGENCE OF TB, AN AIRBORNE DISEASE

The occupational spread of TB is well recognized epidemiologically. However, this spread can go undetected in specific instances because TB is transmissible via the airborne route and results in a long, slowly progressive course. Active surveillance in high-risk settings is important to ascertain the presence of disease and institute effective preventive measures. Active TB rates increased from

1985–1992 owing to decreased funding for public health preventive programs, relaxation of active surveillance in hospitals, and the AIDS epidemic. Health care institutions have been able to reverse the 20% increase in transmission of TB that was observed among health care workers in the United States between 1985 and 1992 [65].

Cases of drug-resistant TB have become more common as resources for the appropriate treatment and follow-up of individuals with active disease have become less available, particularly in countries with severe economic difficulties. For example, resistant TB strains became prevalent in Russian prisons and in Central and South America among the poor. In Russia, previous imprisonment has been identified as a risk factor significantly associated with resistant strains but not HIV/AIDS co-infection [70]. The WHO reports that currently in the world, 1.1% of the new cases of active TB are multidrug resistant [66].

The magnitude of resistant TB varies from country to country. According to a WHO report, the prevalence of resistance to at least one antituberculosis drug ranges from 0% in some western European countries to 57.1% in Kazakhstan. The prevalence of multidrug-resistant (MDR) TB was exceptionally high in almost all former Soviet Union countries surveyed, including Estonia, Kazakhstan, Latvia, Lithuania, the Russian Federation, and Uzbekistan. Proportions of isolates resistant to three or four drugs also were significantly higher in this region. High prevalences of MDR TB also were found among new cases in China (Henan and Liaoning provinces), Ecuador, and Israel. The exact burden may be underappreciated, particularly in countries such as China and India. Increases in the prevalence of resistance is associated with poor or worsening TB control, immigration of patients from areas of higher resistance, outbreaks of MDR disease, and variations in surveillance methodologies. WHO surveillance findings include significant increases in the prevalence of any resistance in Botswana, New Zealand, Poland, and Tomsk Oblast (Russian Federation). Cuba, Hong Kong, and Thailand reported significant decreases over time. Tomsk Oblast (Russian Federation) and Poland reported significantly increased prevalences of MDR TB. Decreasing trends in MDR TB were observed in Hong Kong, Thailand, and the United States [66, 71].

In the United States, the number of active TB cases with resistant strains has declined from 1994–2003 from 486 to 114 cases, respectively. Pockets of MDR strains within this country persist mostly in regions where large numbers of individuals reside for less than 5 years [68, 72]. In California, Granich and colleagues found that 84% of active MDR TB was among foreign-born persons [73]. Table 37-4 lists the characteristics of individuals in the United States with MDR TB.

Table 37-4

Reported cases of TB, MDR TB, and Extensively Drug-Resistant (XDR) TB, U.S. National TB Surveillance System, 1993–1999 and 2000–2006

Characteristics	1993–1999		2000–2006	
	No.	(%)§	No.	(%)§
Total number of culture-confirmed TB cases with initial drug-susceptibility test (DST) results reported for at least isoniazid and rifampin	111,758	—	78,554	—
No. of cases with initial resistance to at least isoniazid and rifampin (i.e., MDR TB¶) (% of total-TB cases)	2,005	(2)	922	(1)
No. of cases with reported initial DST results sufficient to rule in XDR TB** (% of MDR-TB cases)	1,069	(53)	596	(65)
No. of cases with reported initial DST results sufficient to rule out XDR TB** (% of MDR-TB cases)	360	(18)	291	(32)
No. of XDR-TB cases under revised definition (% of MDR-TB cases)	32	(2)	17	(2)
Country of origin (% of XDR-TB cases)				
U.S. born	19	(59)	4	(24)
Foreign born	12	(38)	13	(76)
Unknown	1	(3)	0	—
Human immunodeficiency virus (HIV) status†† (% of XDR-TB cases)				
HIV positive	14	(44)	2	(12)
HIV negative	5	(16)	8	(47)
HIV test not administered or status unknown	13	(40)	7	(41)
Age group (yrs) (% of XDR-TB cases)				
0–14	1	(3)	0	—
15–24	1	(3)	4	(24)
25–44	21	(66)	6	(35)
45–64	3	(9)	6	(35)
≥65	6	(19)	1	(6)
Race/ethnicity (% of XDR-TB cases)				
Hispanic	11	(34)	5	(29)
Asian, non-Hispanic	3	(9)	7	(41)
Black, non-Hispanic	9	(28)	2	(12)
White, non-Hispanic	8	(25)	3	(18)
Other race, non-Hispanic	1	(3)	0	—
Sex (% of XDR-TB cases)				
Female	9	(28)	9	(53)
Male	23	(72)	8	(47)
TB history (% of XDR-TB cases)				
Previous TB§§	4	(13)	3	(18)
No previous TB	27	(84)	14	(82)
Unknown	1	(3)	0	—
Results of sputum microscopy for acid-fast bacilli (% of XDR-TB cases)				
Positive	15	(47)	12	(71)
Negative	9	(28)	3	(18)
Not done/Unknown	8	(25)	2	(12)

(continued)

Table 37-4
Continued

Characteristics	1993–1999		2000–2006	
	No.	**(%)§**	**No.**	**(%)§**
Treatment outcome (% of XDR-TB cases)				
Completed treatment	11	(34)	6	(35)
Died during treatment	10	(31)	2	(12)
Outcome not yet reported	3	(9)	5	(29)
Moved, lost to follow-up, or other	8	(25)	4	(24)

*Defined as resistance to at least isonaizid, rifampin, any fluoroquinoione, and to at least one second-line injectable drug (amikacin, capreomycin, or kanamycin)

† On the basis of cases reported from 50 states and the District of Columbia (DC), through February 8, 2007. Cases reported from U.S.-affiliated island territories excluded.

§ Percentage might not add to 100% because of rounding.

¶ Defined as resistance to at least isoniazid and rifampin.

**On the basis of DST results in the U.S. National TB Surveillance System for drugs included in the definition of XDR TB; isoniazid, rifampin, ciprofloxacin, ofloxacin, kanamycin, amikacin, and capreomycin.

†† HIV reporting for California, which only reports HIV-positive results, completed through 2004; no HIV positives were reported from California. HIV reporting for 49 states other than California and DC completed through 2005, provisional for 2006.

§§ Persons who had verified TB disease in the past, were discharged (e.g., completed therapy) or lost to supervision for > 12 consecutive months, and had verified disease again.

Source: CDC. Extensively drug-resistant tuberculosis—United States, 1993–2006. *MMWR* 2007;56:250–3.

Poor compliance with a full course of treatment and use of lower doses of first-line antituberculous drugs are two of the reasons for appearance of MDR TB strains. Homelessness, substance abuse, mental health disorders, and lack of social supports are risk factors for nonadherence. Up to 90% of the homeless fail to comply with self-administered treatment. Migrant workers may pose a particular challenge owing to cross-border seasonal mobility and instability of resources. Cultural factors and stigmatization also play a role in nonadherence. Directly observed therapy programs have helped to ensure better adherence and reduce the risk of emergence of multidrug resistance. The responsibility for successful treatment is assigned to the public health system and the medical provider, not simply the patient. Success is best achieved within a framework that addresses social as well as clinical circumstances [62]. Occupational medicine in partnership with employers and public health officials can play an important role in tracking and ensuring compliance.

TB AMONG U.S. HEALTH CARE WORKERS

Health care workers in the United States first encountered drug-resistant TB between 1985 and 1992. Nosocomially acquired drug-resistant strains of TB resulted in five deaths among health care workers. Several factors contributed to these occur-

rences: (1) delayed diagnosis, (2) inadequate use of engineering controls such as negative-pressure isolation rooms within hospitals and infirmaries, (3) cross-air communication from isolation rooms with other areas of the ward, and (4) generation of aerosols during procedures (such as suction of tracheostomies, bronchoscopies, and sputum induction) with no personal protective TB respirators readily available for workers to use [74]. Early identification of possible cases of active TB and isolation of these patients with prompt diagnosis and treatment were important factors for TB control in health care institutions. Improved environmental controls, including properly functioning negative-pressure isolation rooms, adequate timely monitoring of these rooms, and high-efficiency particulate filters to recirculate air from isolation rooms to other areas, were essential for the prevention of TB transmission to health care workers and other patients. The use of appropriate personal protective equipment (PPE), after adequate training and fit testing, also was important [74–78].

Reluctance to undergo treatment for latent TB infection continues to be a problem among health care workers in the United States, which is particularly important owing to the increased numbers of health care workers who are immigrants from countries with high rates of TB. Driver and colleagues [79] report that in New York State, the number of non-U.S.-born health care workers has increased by 17% between 1990 Census and the 2000 Census. The proportion of TB cases among foreign-born health care workers in New York State increased from 50% to close to 78% from 1994–2002 following the increase in the proportion of non-U.S.-born health care workers. In health care institutions, initial screening of all health care workers for latent or active TB is crucial to control TB. Physicians' perceptions about the importance of treating latent TB infection must improve. Frequently, the treatment needed for LTBI is minimized by physicians or infected health care workers. These beliefs undermine the recommended CDC guidelines for treatment of LTBI as one of the important steps to control TB within the United States [80, 81]. Although health care workers and many other non-U.S.-born workers are currently screened for LTBI during preplacement evaluation at their employment sites, they frequently opt out of receiving treatment [67, 82].

RESPIRATORY PROTECTION FOR ACTIVE TB

The CDC/National Institute for Occupational Safety and Health (NIOSH) continues to study the proper respiratory protection for health care workers, social workers, and public health officers dealing with patients with active TB. Willeke and Qian have demonstrated that N-95 particulate respirators (95% efficiency or higher for filtering 0.1- to 0.3-μm particles) are effective in preventing TB infection. When fitted properly, N-95 respirators collect 99.5% or higher of aerolized particles of 0.8 μm (the approximate size of TB bacteria) or larger [83]. Laboratory tests indicate negligible reaerolization (0.1% or less) with low humidity and high airflow, such as may occur during violent coughing or sneezing. Today, N-95 particulate NIOSH-certified respirators constitute the standard PPE for employees who fall under respiratory TB protection programs. When workers cannot be fit tested with an N-95 mask, then other respirator options with the same or higher protection factor are available and should be used.

GLOBALIZATION: TB AND AIR TRANSPORTATION

Recently, the CDC was involved in the investigation of a high-profile incident involving one airflight traveler with an active case of extensively drug resistance (XDR) TB strain (defined as resistance to first- and second-generation antituberculous drugs, isoniazid, rifampin, and any fluoroquinolone, and to at least one second-line injectable drug such as amikacin, capreomycin, or kanamycin) in a person who traveled extensively [84, 85]. Another case was identified when a traveling woman sought care for hemoptysis and was found to have a MDR TB disease (resistance to first generation of antituberculous drugs, isoniazid and rifampin) [86].

Air travel presents a setting where the spread of a disease potentially could go unrecognized. The WHO has developed tuberculosis and air travel guidelines. Guidance is provided for customers, crew members, public health officers, and physicians on handling investigation of contacts with an active case of TB disease during an air flight [87]. Today, commercial airplane cabins have several safeguards to protect the passengers and crew. These include engineering safeguards such as laminar airflow, where air circulates from the top of the cabin downward exiting close to the floor. Directional laminar airflow results in little longitudinal airflow from the front of the plane to the back, or vice versa. Additionally, most commercial airplanes recirculate air through high-efficiency particulate air (HEPA) filters. These engineering controls also improve air circulation and humidity required for passenger comfort [88]. In the event of TB concerns, the WHO recommends investigation of those passengers with seats two rows in front and two rows behind the row of the index case, together with all those in the same row of the index case [87]. Also, for exposure to an active case of TB, the WHO recommends investigation of contacts only for flights lasting 8 or more hours. No cases of active TB have been documented following an in-flight exposure to an index case of TB. However, there were 2 TB skin test conversions following in-flight exposure when the active TB index case was a flight attendant who exposed 271 individuals, including 212 crew members, during a 5-month period [89–91]. TB skin test conversions also occurred among 4 passengers who sat two rows from the individual with active disease. No crew members were infected in this incident.

Other Airborne Diseases and Air Travel

Prior to the engineering control instituted in 2005, there were well-documented cases of various in-flight transmitted infections. Before smallpox eradication in 1963, a passenger with smallpox transmitted the illness to 24 other individuals causing 4 deaths. In this incident, it was unclear if the transmission was during the flight or at the airport terminal [92, 93]. Other documented in-flight related outbreaks have involved influenza, measles, meningococcal meningitis, and most recently, SARS. There have been three well-documented outbreaks of influenza associated with transmission during air flights, all before 2000. These outbreaks were associated with departure delays while passengers sat on board for hours without active ventilation [94] and probable contact between passengers both on the ground and aboard in the two other cases (a military squadron returning from duty [95] and mine workers traveling in a small 75-seat airplane [96]). Although the CDC has received 21 reports of suspected air flight index cases with meningococcal disease from 1999–2001, no secondary cases were identified [97]. Today, commercial airplane cabins have the added safeguards described earlier.

Other Multidrug-Resistant Organisms

In addition to MDR and XDR M. tuberculosis strains, there exists a growing problem with the emergence of many other organisms that have developed drug resistance. An increasing number of resistant organisms are found among bacteria, viruses, and parasites. Ironically, the emergence of resistance is often related to selection pressures created by human activities intended to control infection. Even insect vectors are demonstrating resistance to pesticides used for their control. Industrial agricultural practices have been implicated in bacterial resistance. Widespread use of low-dose antibiotics in animal feed in the 1990s has resulted in fluoroquinolone-resistant *Campylobacter* among poultry and cephalosporin-resistant *Salmonella* among cattle [11]. Fortunately, the routine use of antibiotics in poultry feed has been curtailed by major agricultural suppliers within the United States. Nevertheless, these resistant organisms continue to cause human disease from cross-

contaminated, poorly processed food products. The widespread use of over-the-counter amantadine in China as a response to SARS in 2003 may have precipitated widespread resistant influenza strains. There are new concerns that the seasonal use of vaccines for influenza also leads to viral selection pressures for viral drift and the emergence of vaccine-resistant strains. Resistant organisms are not only increasing in numbers but are also spreading across wider geographic ranges and social environments. Among parasites, malaria chloroquine resistance is a major concern given its worldwide disease burden.

The lack of strict infection control practices has contributed to the spread of MDR germs inside and outside health care institutions. Control and prevention of infections caused by MDR organisms (MDROs) is a priority in the United States. MDROs are frequently resistant to several antibiotics. Methicillin-resistant *Staphylococcus aureus* (MRSA) emerged as a nosocomial infection in the 1960s. Some other examples include vancomycin resistant enterococcus (VRE); some of the gram-negative bacteria (GNB), which include those producing extended-spectrum beta-lactamases (ESBLs); and other bacteria resistant to multiple classes of antibiotics. Strains of *Streptococcus pneumoniae* resistant to penicillin, macrolides, and fluoroquinolones have been reported in long-term care facilities. Also, *S. aureus* with intermediate vancomycin sensitivity (VISA) and resistance to vancomycin have been described in dialysis patients [98,99].

VRE prevalence has increased among hospitalized patients from fewer than 1% in 1990 to approximately 15% in 1997 [100]. VRE was responsible for 28.5% of enterococcal isolates in the National Nosocomial Infection Surveillance in ICUs report from 2003 [101]. Judicious use of antibiotics and avoidance of transmission inside health care institutions by following strict infection control practices are essential to curb this trend.

METHICILLIN-RESISTANT *STAPHYLOCOCCUS AUREUS*

MRSA became a major problem for hospitals and long-term care facilities before its emergence into the wider community. Survey of members of the Association for Professionals in Infection Control and Epidemiology (APIC) in 2006 covering 1,237 hospitals throughout the country found that MRSA in hospitals is primarily hospital-acquired (HA-MRSA) rather than community-acquired MRSA infection (CA-MRSA) [102]. CA-MRSA has been defined as that involving predominantly skin/soft tissues, having occurred in 48 hours from admission or lesser time, and being susceptible to selected antimicrobials, mostly to non-beta-lactam agents, such as trimethoprin-sulfamethoxazole, clindamycin, and rifampim [103–115]. Resistance to three or more different classes of non-beta-lactam antibiotics based on susceptibility to erythromycin, clindamycin, chloramphenicol, levofloxacin, tetracycline, trimethoprin-sulfamethoxazole, and rifampin has been identified in several inpatient and outpatient outbreaks [112,116]. MRSA infections have been associated with prior admission to a health care institutions and prior exposure to other risk factors, such as intravenous drug use, surgery, catheterization, and device implantation during the previous year [117]. Figure 37-6 demonstrates the classic picture of a community-acquired MRSA infection.

COMMUNITY-ACQUIRED MRSA

Initiatives to control and prevent outbreaks in health care institutions rely on strict contact precautions and standard precautions. Inadequate compliance by health care workers with hand hygiene practices has been documented by many researchers [118–122]. Training and reinforcement regarding the importance of proper hand hygiene

Figure 37-6
Community-Acquired MRSA Infection.

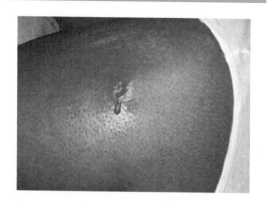

among health care workers cannot be overemphasized. Family and visitors also require education before visiting the MRSA-infected or -colonized patient. Hand hygiene posters and dispensers availability throughout the institution help to reinforce disease control [123].

Additionally, segregation of infected or colonized patients to private rooms or with other similar patients has been an effective way to control spread of this infection in hospital settings [123–125]. It is still unclear if the benefits of contact precautions outweigh those of standard precautions for the care of colonized MRSA patients. However, strict contact precautions, with the use of gowns and gloves by all in contact with high-risk patients, have been shown to reduce nosocomial transmission [126] and are essential for outbreak control.

When MRSA cases continue to present despite targeted contact isolation, the possibility of a health care worker carrier functioning as a disease vector must be considered. Active surveillance, including nasal cultures, among workers may identify the colonized worker. Decolonization with intranasal mupirocin and/or oral antibiotics (usually rifampin and trimethoprim-sulfamethoxazole or rifampin and doxycycline or rifampin and minocycline) and skin antiseptics for daily baths has been recommended [127]. Additional measures may be appropriate in certain high-risk conditions. Nasal colonization in a health care nurse was associated with a nosocomial outbreak in a patient burn unit. Despite successful decolonization, the incidence of new cases was curtailed only after the application of universal preemptive barrier methods in all burn unit patients. Staff was required to use a new clean gown and gloves for any contact with patients or their environment [126].

MRSA screening for all newly admitted patients to services where a MRSA infection case has been identified [128] has been described by some investigators as an additional way to control an outbreak. However, the associated costs of this approach may be prohibitive. In Canada, where the prevalence rate of MRSA and other MDRO infections continue to be low, most teaching hospitals surveyed by the Canadian Nosocomial Infection Surveillance Program (CNISP) in 2003 were conducting admission screenings for MRSA (27 of 28, or 96.4%) and VRE (25 of 28, or 89.3%). Also, all these facilities flagged patients with a previous history of MRSA or VRE [129].

Decolonization of patients and health care workers identified as carriers has been successful in outbreak situations but may enhance the appearance of antibiotic resistance [130]. MRSA screening of health care providers has been used only during outbreak situations when other practices failed to stop the transmission of MRSA. Contact precautions with use of gloves and gowns before entering the room of the patient have been shown to increase the hand hygiene frequency from health care workers [131].

Emerging Zoonoses

Animals serve as potential reservoirs for human disease. Animal pathogens can jump species to infect susceptible humans. Such infections are known as *zoonoses*. Increasingly, zoonotic infectious agents are expanding their geographic and host ranges. Diseases such as pandemic influenza, SARS (discussed earlier), and even HIV/AIDS can be regarded as zoonoses. Disruption of natural ecosystems can bring humans into contact with these pathogens. Conversely, anthropogenic disturbances affect the life history dynamics of pathogens, vectors, and hosts and can significantly alter the prevalence of pathogens in the natural environment [132]. Focusing on the geographic ranges of reservoir hosts may provide a means of predicting spillover events. In general, the geographic distribution of a virus is limited by the geographic distribution of its reservoir host, whereas the geographic distribution of a viral disease results from the combined effect of the reservoir host's distribution, the location of the spillover host (or hosts), and the environmental conditions in which they interact [38]. Emergence of zoonoses can be viewed as a three-step process. First, environmental, ecologic, or demographic factors alter host-pathogen dynamics within the reservoir host. These changes lead to increased transmission rates within or between populations or set up new transmission routes from reservoir to human populations. Selective pressures allow the emergence of the strains that are able to survive in the altered environment or new host [133]. Social, ecologic, climatic, and economic activities all play a role in the emergence of zoonoses.

In the fall of 1992, the second of two successive El Nino events led to exceptionally heavy precipitation in the Four Corners region of the southwestern United States. This change in climate led to an abundance of food supplies for deer mice. Consequently, the deer mice population flourished and encroached on human domestic environments. A cluster of unexplained deaths in humans in May 1993 led to the discovery of the Sin Nombre virus, a previously unrecognized subtype of hantavirus [134]. Infected humans developed characteristic hantavirus pulmonary syndrome (HPS), characterized by severe pulmonary illness and a case-fatality ratio of 30–40%. Infected deer mice shed this virus in urine, saliva, and possibly feces. Hantavirus infection can occur in humans after exposure to infectious virus in rodent saliva or excreta. The CDC confirmed 438 cases of HPS reported from 30 states between 1993 and 2006. Deer mice populations continue to factor into risks of infection. Since 1994, CDC has sponsored continuous monitoring of rodent populations at study sites in Arizona, Colorado, New Mexico, and Montana. Potential occupational exposure to rodent excreta exists in a number of work settings [135]. However, most humans with HPS are thought to have been infected in and around their homes, therefore limiting opportunities for peridomestic exposure to rodents and their excreta is an important control measure. Public health education regarding risk-reduction measures can be found on the CDC website [136].

International trade in exotic animals led to a monkeypox outbreak among commercialized prairie dogs and humans in the midwestern United States. Monkeypox, an orthopoxvirus (as is smallpox), was recognized initially among captive nonhuman primates in 1958. Monkeypox also occurs in several species of African rodents. The first cases in humans were reported in 1970 in what is now the Democratic Republic of Congo. Since then, monkeypox has occurred rarely in humans throughout that region. Prior to 2003, monkeypox had not been reported outside Africa [137]. In 2003, there occurred the first cluster of human monkeypox cases ever reported in the United States. Human infection was transmitted from contact with ill pet prairie dogs. The prairie dogs had become infected with the monkeypox virus while housed in a distribution center along with various exotic African rodents that had been shipped from

Ghana to the United States. Trace-back culture and polymerase chain reaction (PCR) tests demonstrated monkeypox virus in two rope squirrels, one Gambian rat, and three dormice. This outbreak resulted in 72 human cases from 6 midwestern states. The 2003 monkeypox outbreak was large compared with outbreaks of 23–88 cases reported in African areas of endemic disease. Enhanced surveillance owing to bioterrorism concerns may have helped identify the outbreak. The U.S. monkeypox virus outbreak demonstrates how new diseases can emerge owing to facile movement of species from one location to another. On June 11, 2003, the CDC and the FDA banned the import of all rodents from Africa. Additionally, state and federal bans have curtailed further sale and transport of prairie dogs. Whether monkeypox virus may have spread to North American rodents remains unknown [137,138].

Changes in traditional agricultural practices led to a human outbreak of Nipah virus in Malaysia in 1998–1999. Agricultural intensification and expansion into pristine forests in Malasia led to a spillover emergence of Nipah virus from *Pteropus* fruit bats, host reservoirs, to domestic pigs. These forests served as natural habitats for the *Pteropus* bats. Slash-and-burn deforestation resulted in a severe haze that blanketed much of Southeast Asia in the months directly preceding the Nipah virus disease outbreak. Environmental conditions were further exacerbated by a drought driven by the 1997–1998 El Nino southern oscillation (ENSO) event. Combined, these events led to an acute reduction in flowering and fruiting forest trees for foraging. *Pteropus* fruit bats were already facing a shrinking wildlife habitat. Bats became attracted to orchards of fruit trees abutting overcrowded pig farms in the area leading to a host spillover [139]. Pigs became infected via aerosolation of contaminated bat droppings. The disease presented as a respiratory illness among pigs. It spread rapidly from pig to pig. The outbreak of Nipah virus infection in Malaysia was costly in terms of human morbidity and mortality and the country's economy. Infections in humans presented with encephalitis. The outbreak resulted in 265 human cases and 105 fatalities [38]. Seventy percent (70%) of the human patients had direct occupational exposure to sickened pigs, including pig farmers and workers [139]. Eleven million pigs were culled. The closure of pig farms resulted in a loss of

36,000 jobs. The Malaysian economy suffered owing to the costs associated with the culling of pigs, the closure of farms, the loss of trade, and government subsidies related to control measures. The Malaysian outbreak provides another example of how poorly regulated intensification of food production practices can lead to the emergence of infectious disease. Several outbreaks of Nipah virus have occurred recently in India and Bangladesh, where during a period of 5 years a total of 123 people have died, with case-fatality rates of 37.5–75%. Nipah virus in Bangladesh appears to have occurred from direct contact between humans and bats. Human-to-human transmission also has been documented [140].

Even once remote zoonoses that jump species can adapt and become devastatingly entrenched if conditions are favorable. HIV may be illustrative. HIV has infected more than 60 million people worldwide. HIV is thought to have jumped to humans about 60–70 years ago secondary to the consumption of "bush meat" from nonhuman primates. However, the broader emergence of HIV/AIDS followed disruptions in the economic and social infrastructure in postcolonial sub-Saharan Africa. Increased travel, the movement of rural populations to large cities, urban poverty, and a weakening of family structure encouraged sexual practices facilitating HIV emergence [23].

Vector-Borne Diseases

Vector-borne diseases cause millions of deaths worldwide per year. Important vectors include mosquitoes and ticks. Important hosts include birds, rodents, and domesticated animals. Poverty is strongly associated with vector-borne diseases. Not only does poverty increase the risk of disease, but disease contraction also contributes to poverty. Vector-borne diseases are particularly influenced by the ecologic environment, including the availability of suitable habitats and hosts. Human activities that alter natural ecosystems have an impact on the transmission cycles of vector-borne infectious diseases. Changes within the environment may contribute to the spread of vector-borne diseases by altering the geographic range and/or affecting human contact. Human settlement and deforestation patterns; the development of dam, drainage, and agricultural irrigation systems; and climate change all influence the patterns of disease, disease emergence, and distribution. Policies that influence population demographics, living conditions, migration, energy production/consumption, agricultural food production, and overall demand for natural resources have significant effects on transmission of these infectious agents and their disease consequences [141].

Expansive global trade may provide a means for viruses to become established in new locations where a lack of herd immunity can lead to epidemics. West Nile virus was introduced to the western hemisphere in 1999 when it caused a few cases of encephalitis in New York City. Since then, West Nile virus has spread across the continent. In fact, West Nile virus is currently the most common arboviral cause of encephalitis in the United States. Unlike most viruses, which typically adapt to narrow host reservoirs, West Nile virus infects more than 30 North American mosquito species, which together transmit infection to at least 150 North American bird species. Many of these birds migrate to distant locations, potentially spreading the virus to rural and urban ecosystems throughout North and Central America [38]. Other vector-borne diseases that are actively reemerging globally are malaria and dengue.

MALARIA AND DENGUE: GLOBAL PUBLIC HEALTH THREATS
Malaria

Malaria is the most prevalent infectious disease on the globe. More than 500 million people are infected with malaria every year, and 2 million die from this illness annually [141]. Every 40 seconds a child dies of malaria [142]. Children under age 5 and pregnant women are more vulnerable to poor outcomes from this illness, including death. The economic and social toll of malaria in populations is tremendous owing to medical costs for acute illness and personal expenditures on preventive measures such as insecticide-impregnated bed nets, skin insecticides, and prophylactic treatments. An increasing distribution of drug-resistant strains of malaria, as well as the spread of insecticide-tolerant mosquito vectors, contributes to the malaria problem.

The expanding geographic range of mosquitos from global warming [143] and the increasing resistance to antibiotics and insecticides make this vector-borne disease very difficult to control [144].

Although usually occurring in rural communities, increased urbanization and population migration from the country to the cities have resulted in its emergence in the cities, causing an enormous drain in public health efforts in underdeveloped countries. Deforestation, changes in agricultural practices, and building of dams and irrigation systems have resulted in an expansion of mosquito vectors [142]. Gallup and Sachs have demonstrated how malaria and poverty predominate in the same regions of the world, mostly in the tropical and subtropical zones [145].

The increase in travel to endemic areas and emigration from malaria-endemic regions has highlighted concerns about malaria in occupational settings. About 500 million individuals will cross international borders this year. It is estimated that 10,000–30,000 travelers from industrialized countries develop malaria each year after traveling to endemic regions. Kain and colleagues [146] reported seven fatal cases of malaria owing to *Plasmodium falciparum* in Canada or in Canadian travelers. Two of these patients acquired the illness while working in Africa for a temporary period of time. Measures that were identified as promoting the disease were (1) inadequate prophylactic therapy before, during, and after going to endemic areas, (2) delay in diagnosis, and (3) incorrect initial treatment. In 1996, there were 744 cases of malaria reported in Canada, a 73% increase from 1994. In the United States, approximately 1,000 case are reported annually [147, 148].

The *Anopheles* mosquito is responsible for the transmission of malaria. Humans are the intermediate host of the parasites, and the mosquito is the definitive host and vector. There are four types of malarial parasites from the genus *Plasmodium* that cause disease in humans: *P. vivax, P. ovale, P. malariae,* and *P. falciparum.* When the female anopheline mosquito becomes infected after a blood meal from a human with mature male and female stages of the protozoa (parasite called *gametocytes*), the cycle in the vector host begins with the union of the male and female in the stomach of the mosquito and production of sporozoites in their salivary glands [148]. The time needed for these parasites to mature (sporogonic phase) in the mosquito depends on the environmental temperature and on the *Plasmodium* species. When the temperature is below 16°C for *P. vivax* and 18°C for *P. falciparum,* the sporogonic cycle cannot be completed, and transmission to humans cannot occur. The highest temperature compatible with the sporogonic phase is 33°C. The protozoa will require longer period of time as the temperature lowers: At 27°C, *P. vivax* and *P. falciparum* will need 8–13 days to complete the cycle. *P. vivax* will require 20 days at 20°C and 30 days at 18°C. *P. falciparum* will require 30 days at 20°C to complete the sporogonic phase. The gametocytes develop at different times after infection by a feeding, infectious mosquito: For *P. vivax*, gametocytes develop in the initial days after infection. On the other hand, *P. falciparum* gametocytes will take 10–14 days to appear. *P. vivax* and *P. ovale* may form dormant liver stages, and gametocytemia may occur months to years after exposure. Malaria transmission depends on adequate breeding sites and large number of mosquitos, weather conditions allowing for the completion of the sporogonic phase of the mosquito cycle, and gametocytemic humans to infect the mosquitos [149].

The anopheline mosquito has been found in the 48 states of the contiguous United States. Malaria was endemic in the United States in the late nineteenth and early twentieth centuries. Eradication of mosquito vectors and malaria within the United States resulted from the use of DDT to control mosquito larvae combined with appropriate sanitation and effective treatment of the disease [149]. Since the 1980s, several countries have experienced a resurgence of malaria following a decrease or elimination of the use of DDT as an insecticide and subsequent increases in mosquito populations [150].

In the United States, several malaria outbreaks occurred during the 1980s and 1990s in urban areas in California, New Jersey, and Houston, Texas. They all occurred in densely populated areas with large numbers of immigrants from countries with malaria and hot and humid weather conditions propitious to the completion of the sporogonic phase of the parasite's life and to the survival of the mosquito. Most cases involved workers in agriculture activities, including many migrant rural workers living with substandard housing and unsanitary conditions [149].

Dengue

Dengue, caused by flaviviruses (as are West Nile encephalitis, Japanese encephalitis, and yellow fever virus), has been considered to be among the most important reemerging infectious diseases in the world, with an estimated 50–100 million cases per year, 500,000 hospitalizations, and over 20,000 deaths per year [151, 152]. Dengue can be caused by any of four serotypes of related but distinct viruses. Infection with one serotype induces lifelong immunity to only that serotype. Subsequent infection with a second serotype may result in more serious disease, including dengue hemorrhagic fever and dengue shock syndrome.

Dengue constitutes a significant occupational concern as business travel to dengue-endemic areas such as Central and South America, Africa, and Asia becomes more common. There have been an increasing number of cases diagnosed in the United States among workers who have traveled abroad. Also, dengue has been steadily returning into the United States with an epidemic in Hawaii in 2001 and in Puerto Rico during the 1990s. Moreover, the CDC has reported increased number of cases in the Texas-Mexico border area [153].

Dengue is transmitted via *Aedes* mosquitoes [*A. aegypti* or *A. albopictus* (tiger mosquito)]. Dengue occurs primarily in tropical urban areas. However, dengue-carrying *Aedes* mosquitoes have been adapting to different climates and are responsible for the rapid spread of dengue since the cessation of DDT use [154, 155]. Many infections may be asymptomatic. The incubation period ranges from 3–14 days. Clinically know as *breakbone fever,* symptoms may include fever, headache, prostration, and myalgias. The more severe forms of the disease, dengue hemorrhagic fever (DHF) or dengue shock syndrome (DSS), have been shown to occur more often in individuals who become reinfected with a second serotype. Also, DHF can be caused by more pathogenic strains of dengue virus (dengue-1/dengue-2 sequence and dengue-3/dengue-2 sequence) [156–158].

Physicians should consider dengue in any worker returning from a business trip to endemic areas who presents with hemorrhagic fever or severe viral illness with shock. However, illness onset that occurs more than 14 days after returning from a dengue-endemic region is unlikely to be dengue fever. Aggressive supportive therapy in intensive care units is the main focus of therapy, with particular attention to fluid replacement and maintenance of electrolytes balance. The capacity to transfer U.S. workers who become ill overseas to U.S. health care facilities should be planned for in anyone traveling to endemic regions.

As with all arboviral infections, dengue is prevented mainly by elimination or control of mosquito vectors and the avoidance of insect bites [159]. Personal methods of prevention when workers are in the field include protective clothing and use of mosquito repellent and mosquito netting. DEET (N,N-diethylmethyltoluamide) is the most effective mosquito repellent available for use on the skin. Use of permethrin-impregnated clothes, tents, and netting provides additional protection [160]. Currently, there is no vaccine approved for dengue, although research continues in this area.

CONTROL OF VECTOR-BORNE DISEASES

As indicated earlier, the control of vector-borne diseases depends on active surveillance of viral activity among insect and animal populations. Preventive measures are based on vector control programs coupled with public health education. Integrated vector management programs combine source reduction with chemical and biologic vector control. These programs target vector-breeding sites, disrupt vector life cycles, and minimize vector-human contact while attempting to preserve ecosystems. Source reduction can be achieved by addressing breeding habitats such as freestanding water, sanitation, and regional water management. For instance, better engineering designs for reservoirs and dams that include alterations in flow, periodic flushing of reservoirs, and weed removal may reduce breeding habitats for malarial vectors. Biologic controls targeting mosquito larvae including larvivorous fish and biolarvicides such as *Bacillus thurengieneasesis, B. israelensis,* and *B. sphaericus* also have been applied to malarial vectors. Regulations discouraging human settlements near potential mosquito breeding sites also may reduce disease transmission. As already discussed, rapid unplanned urbanization associated with a proliferation of water-retaining containers has driven a resurgence of dengue. Models suggest that within specific locales, less than 1% of the containers (e.g., old tires and discarded water drums) may produce more than 95% of the outbreak-triggering adult mosquitoes. Specific knowledge of local conditions enables a more manageable targeted environmental clean-up effort. Biologic controls to reduce dengue transmission are being applied in Vietnam. Mesocyclops, which feed on the larvae of *A. aegypti,* have been introduced into household water tanks and water jars. In Cambodia, the WHO is testing a simple engineering control consisting of long-lasting insecticide-impregnated net mesh water tank covers [6]. Nevertheless, regulation of rapid urbanization is ultimately the most important measure in controlling a resurgence of dengue. In fact, regulating growth and human settlement has general applicability in vector-borne diseases. Human settlements that are close to natural systems serve as frequent sites for the transmission of vector-borne pathogens. Even within wealthy countries such as the United States, suburban encroachment of forest habitats contributes to transmission of Lyme disease and West Nile virus. In general, better regulation of housing development may have a significant role in the control of vector-borne disease. Insecticides may be required when source-reduction attempts are inadequate and the application of biologic controls is unavailable. The use of insecticides may lead to resistance and potential toxic effects. Resistance management programs are now integrated into the use of insecticides. Public health education is another important component of prevention. Public health education, applicable to workers as well as to the general public, disseminates information regarding vector and bite avoidance, use of protective clothing, use of insect repellants, and recognition of symptoms. In certain settings, education regarding the protection of pets and domestic animals also may be important. Vaccine use among domestic animals and humans does have a role in certain vector-borne diseases such as yellow fever and Japanese encephalitis.

Summary

Emerging infectious disease results primarily from human activities interfacing with and affecting the environment. Social and work conditions, as well as commercial practices, also can have an impact on disease emergence. Outbreak response systems have been strengthened in recent years. These systems incorporate measures such as enhanced surveillance, more robust communication, stockpiling, and the timely mobilization of targeted resources. Coordinated collaboration among key stakeholders is also critical to effective preparedness and response. At every level, efforts must include the protection of workers, particularly responders and essential workers, in a time of crisis. Root causes of infectious disease emergence also must be addressed. Primary preventive measures that address fundamental risk factors are only now being considered. Research investigating the long-term risks and benefits of economic development, commercial activities, food production, energy, land use, and water management are needed. Moreover, responsible action means adherence to Principle 15 of the 1992 Rio Declaration on Environment and Development. This principle states: "Where there are threats of serious or irreversible damage, lack of full scientific uncertainty shall not be used as a reason for postponing cost-effective measures to prevent environmental degradation" [6]. The current division of responsibilities among organizations means that assessment and programmatic actions fall within narrow disciplinary frameworks. Sustainable solutions depend on better understanding and control of the complex interactions among the biologic, environmental, social, economic, and political factors that contribute to disease emergence [8]. The adoption of a coordinated long-term multidisciplinary view of the interactions between ecosystems and infectious diseases would help to ensure sustainable benefits to human well being. A more comprehensive approach examines strategies from a multidisciplinary perspective and considers not only direct and immediate effects on disease but also long-term and indirect effects that may occur via alterations to ecosystems. Ultimately, the integration of health and well-being into growth and development strategies is more sustainable and provides better security for everyone. This approach can help to guide policymakers in balancing competing values regulating development and commerce [6]. Nevertheless, many workers will continue to assume higher risks because they must function within various environments under variably hazardous conditions. Applying sound industrial hygiene and infection control practices is critical to protecting susceptible workers against infections as well as other occupational diseases.

Resources

Open Access to Emerging Infectious Diseases, published monthly by the National Center for Infectious Diseases, Centers for Disease Control and Prevention (CDC), www.cdc.gov/ncidod/EID/index.htm.

National Institute of Allergy and Infectious Disease, www.niaid.nih.gov/dmid/eid/.

World Health Report Changing History, www.who.int/whr/2004/en/report04_en.pdf.

References

1. Fauci AS. Emerging and re-emerging infectious diseases: The perpetual challenge. *Acad Med* 2005;80: 1079–85.
2. Morse SS. Factors in the emergence of infectious diseases. *Emerg Infect Dis* 1995;1:7–15.
3. Morse SS. Factors and determinants of disease emergence. *Rev Sci Technol* 2004;23:443–51.
4. Lederberg J, Shope RE, Oakes SC Jr (eds). *Emerging Infections: Microbial Threats to Health in the United States.* Institute of Medicine. Washington: National Academy Press, 1992.
5. Centers for Disease Control and Prevention. Addressing emerging infectious disease threats: A prevention strategy for the United States—Executive summary. *MMWR* 1994;43:1–18.
6. Hassan R, Scholes R, Ash N (eds). *Ecosystems and Human Well-being: Current State and Trends,* Vol 1. Washington: Island Press, 2005.
7. Centers for Disease Control and Prevention. Preventing emerging infectious diseases: A strategy for the 21st century overview of the updated CDC plan. *MMWR* 1998;47:1–14.
8. Institute of Medicine, Board on Global Health Institute. *Microbial Threats to Health: Emergence, Detection, and Response.* Washington: National Academy Press, 2003.
9. Institute of Medicine. *The Impact of Globalization on Infectious Disease Emergence and Control: Exploring the Consequences and Opportunities.* Washington: National Academy Press, 2006.
10. Kuiken T, Holmes EC, McCauley J, et al. Host species barriers to influenza virus infections. *Science* 2006;312:394–7.
11. Nestle M. *Safe Food: Bacteria, Biotechnology, and Bioterrorism.* Los Angeles: University of California Press, 2003.
12. Reed KD, Meece JK, Henkel JS, et al. Birds, migration and emerging zoonoses: West Nile virus, Lyme disease, influenza A and enteropathogens. *Clin Med Res* 2003;1:5–12.
13. Fine A, Layton M. Lessons from the West Nile viral encephalitis outbreak in New York City, 1999:

Implications for bioterrorism preparedness. *Clin Infect Dis* 2001;32:277–82.

14. Kahn LH. Confronting zoonoses, linking human and veterinary medicine. *Emerg Infect Dis* 2006;12: 556–61.

15. Olsen B, Munster VJ, Wallensten A, et al. Global patterns of influenza A virus in wild birds. *Science* 2006; 312:384–8.

16. O'Leary DR, Marfin AA, Montgomery SP, et al. The epidemic of West Nile virus in the United States, 2002. *Vector Borne Zoonotic Dis* 2004;4:61–70.

17. Centers for Disease Control and Prevention. Assessing capacity for surveillance, prevention, and control of West Nile virus infection—United States, 1999 and 2004. *MMWR* 2006;55:150–3.

18. Nash D, Mostashari F, Fine A, et al. The outbreak of West Nile virus infection in the New York City area in 1999. *N Engl J Med* 2001;344:1807–14.

19. Mead PS, Slutsker L, Dietz V, et al. Food-related illness and death in the United States. *Emerg Infect Dis* 1999;5:607–25.

20. Altekruse SF, Cohen ML, Swerdlow DL. Emerging foodborne diseases. *Emerg Infect Dis* 1997;3:285–93.

21. Batz MB, Doyle MP, Morris G Jr, et al. Attributing illness to food. *Emerg Infect Dis.* 2005;11:993–9.

22. Hennessy TW, Hedberg CW, Slutsker L, et al. A national outbreak of *Salmonella enteritidis* infections from ice cream. The Investigation Team. *N Engl J Med* 1996;334:1281–6.

23. Morens DM, Folkers GK, Fauci AS. The challenge of emerging and re-emerging infectious diseases. *Nature* 2004;430:242–9.

24. Jarvis WR. Precautions for Creutzfeldt-Jakob disease. *Infect Control* 3:238–9.

25. Gajdusek DC, et al. 1977. Precautions in the medical care and in handling materials from patients with transmissible virus dementia (Creutzfeldt-Jakob disease). *N Engl J Med* 1977;297:1253–8.

26. Centers for Disease Control and Prevention, National Institutes of Health, and Wilson DE, Chosewood LC (Eds). *Biosafety in Microbiological and Biomedical Laboratories*, 5th ed. Washington: US Government Printing Office, 2007.

27. Webster RG. Wet markets: A continuing source of severe acute respiratory syndrome and influenza? *Lancet* 2004;363:234–6.

28. Drosten C, Gunther S, Preiser W, et al. Identification of a novel coronavirus in patients with severe acute respiratory syndrome. *N Engl J Med* 2003;348:1967–76.

29. Ksiazek TG, Erdman D, Goldsmith CS, et al. A novel coronavirus associated with severe acute respiratory syndrome. *N Engl J Med* 2003;348:1953–66.

30. Breiman RF, Evans MR, Preiser W, et al. Role of China in the quest to define and control severe acute respiratory syndrome. *Emerg Infect Dis* 2003;9: 1037–41.

31. Wong SS, Yuen KY. The severe acute respiratory syndrome (SARS). *J Neurovirol* 2005;11:455–68.

32. Tsang KW, Ho PL, Ooi GC, et al. A cluster of cases of severe acute respiratory syndrome in Hong Kong. *N Engl J Med.* 2003;348:1977–85.

33. Chan-Yeung M. Severe acute respiratory syndrome (SARS) and healthcare workers. *Int J Occup Environ Health* 2004;10:421–7.

34. Wang JT, Sheng WH, Fang CT, et al. Clinical manifestations, laboratory findings, and treatment outcomes of SARS patients. *Emerg Infect Dis.* 2004;10: 818–24.

35. Yu WC, Hui DS, Chan-Yeung M. Antiviral agents and corticosteroids in the treatment of severe acute respiratory syndrome (SARS). *Thorax* 2004;59:643–5.

36. Svoboda T, Henry B, Shulman L, et al. Public health measures to control the spread of the severe acute respiratory syndrome during the outbreak in Toronto. *N Engl J Med* 2004;350:2352–61.

37 Maunder RG, Lancee WJ, Balderson KE. Long-term psychological and occupational effects of providing hospital healthcare during SARS outbreak. *Emerg Infect Dis* 2006;12:1924–32.

38. Halpin, K, Hyatt AD, Plowright RK, et al. Emerging viruses: Coming in on a wrinkled wing and a prayer. *Clin Infect Dis* 2007;44:711–7.

39. Smith DJ. Predictability and preparedness in influenza control. *Science* 2006;312: 392–4.

40. World Health Organization. WHO Interim Protocol: Rapid operations to contain the initial emergency of pandemic influenza, October 2007; available at www.who.int/csr/disease/avian_influenza/ guidelines/RapidContProtOct15.pdf.

41. Stimola AN, Ross GL. *Avian Influenza, or "Bird Flu": What You Need to Know.* New York: American Council on Science and Health, 2006.

42. Beigel JH, Farrar J, Han AM, et al. Avian influenza A (H5N1) infection in humans. *N Engl J Med* 2005; 353:1374–85.

43. Ferguson NM, Cummings DA, Fraser C, et al. Strategies for mitigating an influenza pandemic. *Nature* 2006;442:448–52.

44. Centers for Disease Control and Prevention. Interim Prepandemic Planning Guidance:Community Strategy for Pandemic Influenza Mitigation in the United States—Early, Targeted, Layered Use of Non-pharmaceutical Interventions, February 2007; available at www2a.cdc.gov/phlp/docs/community _mitigation.pdf.

45. Bartlett JG. Planning for avian influenza. *Ann Intern Med* 2006;145:141–4.

46. Blaser, MJ. Pandemics and preparation. *J Infect Dis* 2006;194:S70–2.

47. Stevens J, Blixt O, Tumpey TM, et al. Structure and receptor specificity of the hemagglutinin from an H5N1 influenza *Virus Science* 2006;312:404–10.

48. Gerberding JL. Pandemic preparedness: Pigs, poultry, and people versus plans, products, and practice. *J Infect Dis* 2006;194:S77–S81

49. Shinya K, Ebina M, Yamada S, et al. Avian flu: in-

fluenza virus receptors in the human airway. *Nature* 2006;440:435–6.

50. Ungchusak K, Auewarakul P, Dowell SF, et al. Probable person-to-person transmission of avian influenza A (H5N1). *N Engl J Med* 2005;352:333–40.

51. World Health Organization, Writing Committee of WHO Consultation on Human Influenza A/H5. Avian influenza A (H5N1) infection in humans. *N Engl J Med* 2005;353:1374–85.

52. Wong SSY, Yuen KY. Avian influenza virus infections in humans. *Chest* 2006;129:156–68.

53. World Health Organization Writing Group. Non-pharmaceutical public health interventions for pandemic influenza, national and community measures. *Emerg Infect Dis* 2006;12:88–94.

54. Hayden FG. Antiviral resistance in influenza viruses—Implications for management and pandemic response. *N Engl J Med* 2006;354:785–8.

55. Perry RW, Lindell MK. Preparedness for emergency response: Guidelines for the emergency planning process. *Disasters* 2003;27:336–50.

56. Regoes RR, Bonhoeffer S. Emergence of drug-resistant influenza virus: Population dynamical considerations (Perspective). *Science* 2006;312:389–91.

57. de Jong, MD, Thanh TT, Khanh TH, et al. Oseltamivir resistance during treatment of influenza A (H5N1) infection. *N Engl J Med* 2005; 353:2667–72.

58. Ryan MAK, Christian RS, Wohlrabe J. Handwashing and respiratory illness among young adults in military training. *Am J Prevent Med* 2001;21:79–83.

59. Corbett EL, Watt CJ, Walker N, et al. The growing burden of tuberculosis global trends and interactions with the HIV epidemic. *Arch Intern Med* 2003;163:1009–21.

60. Angelis CD, Flanagin A. Tuberculosis: A global problem requiring a global solution. *JAMA* 2005; 293:2793–4.

61. Dye C, Watt CJ, Bleed DM, et al. Evolution of tuberculosis control and prospects for reducing tuberculosis: Incidence, prevalence and deaths globally. *JAMA* 2005;293:2790–3.

62. American Thoracic Society/Centers for Disease Control and Prevention/Infectious Diseases Society of America. *Treatment of Tuberculosis*. Official Joint Statement of the ATS, the CDC, and the IDSA approved by the ATS Board of Directors, the CDC, and the Council of the IDSA in October 2002. *Am J Respir Crit Care Med* 2003;167:603–62.

63. Walker PF, Barnett ED (eds). *Immigrant Medicine*. Philadelphia: Saunders/Elsevier, 2007.

64. Horsburgh CR Jr. Priorities for the treatment of latent tuberculosis infection in the United States. *N Engl J Med* 2004;350:2060–2067.

65. Centers for Disease Control and Prevention. Trends in tuberculosis incidence—United States, 2006. *MMWR* 2007;56:246–50.

66. WHO. Global tuberculosis control: Surveillance, planning, financing. World Health Organization Report, 2005. Geneva, WHO, 2005 (WHO/HTM/TB/2005.349).

67. Jensen PA, Lambert LA, Iademarco MF, et al. Guidelines for preventing the transmission of *Mycobacterium tuberculosis* in health care settings, 2005. *MMWR* 2005;54;1–141.

68. Centers for Disease Control and Prevention. Extensively drug-resistant tuberculosis—United States, 1993–2006. *MMWR* 2007;56:250–3.

69. Haddad MB, Wilson TW, Ijaz K, et al. Tuberculosis and homelessness in the United States, 1994–2003. *JAMA* 2005;293:2762–6.

70. Drobniewski F, Balabanova Y, Nikolayevsky V, et al. Drug-resistant tuberculosis, clinical virulence, and the dominance of the Beijing strain family in Russia. *JAMA* 2005;293:2726–31.

71. World Health Organization. *Anti-Tuberculosis Drug Resistance in the World*. Report no 3. Global Project on Anti-Tuberculosis Drug Resistance Surveillance. Geneva: World Health Organization, 2003.

72. Moore M, Onorato IM, McCray E, Castro KG. Trends in drug-resistant tuberculosis in the United States, 1993–1996. *JAMA* 1997;278:833–7.

73. Granich RM, Oh O, Lewis B, et al. Multidrug resistance among persons with tuberculosis in California, 1994–2003. *JAMA* 2005;293:2732–9.

74. Menzies D, Fanning A, Yuan L, FitzGerald M. Tuberculosis among health care workers. *N Engl J Med* 1995;332:92–98.

75. Jarvis WR, Bolyard EA, Bozzi CJ, et al. Respirators, recommendations and regulations: The controversy surrounding protection of health care workers from tuberculosis. *Ann Intern Med* 1995;122:142–6.

76 Jarvis WR. Nosocomial transmission of multidrug-resistant *Mycobacterium tuberculosis*. *Res Microbiol* 1993;144:117–22.

77. Pearson ML, Jereb JA, Frieden TR, et al. Nosocomial transmission of multidrug-resistant *Mycobacterium tuberculosis* A risk to patients and health care workers. *Ann Intern Med* 1992;117:191–6.

78. Maloney SA, Pearson ML, Gordon MT, et al. Efficacy of control measures in preventing nosocomial transmission of multidrug-resistant tuberculosis to patients and health care workers. *Ann Intern Med* 1995;122:90–5.

79. Driver CR, Stricof RL, Granville K, et al. Tuberculosis in health care workers during declining tuberculosis incidence in New York State. *Am J Infect Control* 2005;33:519–26.

80. Salazar-Shicchi J, Jedlovsky V, Ajayi A, et al. Physician attitudes regarding bacilli Calmette-Guérin vaccination and treatment of latent tuberculosis infection. *Int J Tuberc Lung Dis* 2004;8:1443–7.

81. LoBue PA, Moser K, Catanzaro A. Management of yuberculosis in San Diego County: A survey of physicians' knowledge, attitudes and practices. *Int J Tuberc Lung Dis* 2001;5:933–8.

82. Sterling TR, Haas DW. Transmission of *Mycobacterium tuberculosis* from health care workers. *N Engl J Med* 2006;355:118–21.

83. Willeke K, Qian Y. Tuberculosis control through respirator wear: Performance of National Institute for Occupational Safety and Health–regulated respirators. *Am J Infect Control* 1998;26:139–42.

84. Centers for Disease Control and Prevention. Health Alert Network, 00261-2007-05-29-ADV-N, Investigation of US Traveler with Extensively Drug Resistant Tuberculosis (XDR TB), 2007.

85. Centers for Disease Control and Prevention. Health Alert Network, 00262-2007-05-29-UPD-N, Corrected: Investigation of US Traveler with Extensively Drug Resistant Tuberculosis (XDR TB), 2007.

86. Centers for Disease Control and Prevention. Health Alert Network, 00267-2007-12-29-ADV-N, Investigation on International Traveler with Multidrug-Resistant Tuberculosis (MDR-TB), 2007.

87. *Tuberculosis and Air Travel: Guidelines for Prevention and Control,* 2nd ed. Geneva: World Health Organization, 2006 (WHO/HTM/TB/2006.363).

88. Mangili A, Gendreau MA. Transmission of infectious diseases during commercial air travel, *Lancet* 2005;365:989–96.

89. Driver CR, Valway SE, Morgan WM, et al. Transmission of *Mycobacterium tuberculosis* associated with air travel. JAMA 1994;272:1031–35.

90. Centers for Disease Control and Prevention. Exposure of passengers and flight crew to *Mycobacterium tuberculosis* on commercial aircrafts, 1992–1995. *MMWR* 1995;44:137–40.

91. Kenyon TA, Valway SE, Ihle WW, et al. Transmission of multidrug resistant *Mycobacterium tuberculosis* during a long airplane flight. *N Engl J Med* 1996;334:933–8.

92. Ritzinger F. Disease transmission by aircraft. *Aeromed Rev* 1965;4:1–10.

93. Centers for Disease Control and Prevention. International Notes: Smallpox—Stockhom. *MMWR* 1963;12:56.

94. Moser MR, Bender TR, Margolis HS, et al. An outbreak of influenza aboard a commercial airline. *Am J Epidemiol* 1979;110:1–6.

95. Klontz KC, Hynes NA, Gunn RA, et al. An outbreak of influenza a/taiwan/1/86 infections at a naval base and its association with airplane travel. *Am J Epidemiol* 1989;129:341–8.

96. Marsden AG. Influenza outbreak related to air travel. *Med J Aust* 2003;179:172–3.

97. Centers for Disease Control and Prevention. Exposure to patients with meningococcal disease on aircrafts—United Sates, 1999–2001. *MMWR* 2001; 50:485–9.

98. Fridkin SK. Vancomycin-intermediate and -resistant *Staphylococcus aureus* What the infectious disease specialist needs to know. *Clin Infect Dis* 2001; 32:108–15.

99. Centers for Disease Control and Prevention. *Staphylococcus aureus* resistant to vancomycin—United States, 2002. *MMWR* 2002;51:565–7.

100. Jones RN. Resistance patterns among nosocomial pathogens: Trends over the past few years. Chest 2001;119:S397–404.

101. National Nosocomial Infection Surveillance in ICUs, Report 2003. *Am J Infect Control* 2003;31: 481–98.

102. Jarvis WR, Schlosser JA, Chinn RY, et al. National prevalence of methicillin-resistant *Staphylococcus aureus* in inpatients at US health care facilities, 2006. *Am J Infect Control* 2007;35:631–7.

103. Moran CA, Hadler JL. Population-based incidence and characteristics of community-onset *Staphylococcus aureus* infections with bacteremia in 4 metropolitan Connecticut areas, 1998. *J Infect Dis* 2001; 184:1029–34.

104. Rosario-Rosado RV, Rene AA, Jones B. Descriptive analysis of patients with community-onset and hospital-onset methicillin-resistant *Staphylococcus aureus* infections. *Infect Control Hosp Epidemiol* 2004; 25:171–3.

105. King MD, Humphrey BJ, Wang YF, et al. Emergence of community-acquired methicillin-resistant *Staphylococcus aureus* USA 300 clone as the predominant cause of skin and soft-tissue infections. *Ann Intern Med* 2006;144:309–17.

106. File TM Jr. Impact of community-acquired methicillin-resistant *Staphylococcus aureus* in the hospital setting. *Cleve Clin J Med* 2007;74:S6–11.

107. Furuya Y, Cook HA, Lee MH, et al. Community-associated methicillin-resistant *Staphylococcus aureus* prevalence: How common is it? A methodological comparison of prevalence ascertainment. *Am J Infect Control* 2007;5:359–66.

108. Popovich K, Hota B, Rice T, et al. Phenotypic prediction rule for community-associated methicillin-resistant *Staphylococcus aureus*. *J Clin Microbiol* 2007;45:2293–5.

109. Tsuji BT, Rybak MJ, Cheung CM, et al. Community and health care-associated methicillin-resistant *Staphylococcus aureus* A comparison of molecular epidemiology and antimicrobial activities of various agents. *Diagn Microbiol Infect Dis* 2007;58:41–7.

110. Skiest DJ, Brown K, Cooper TW, et al. Prospective comparison of methicillin-susceptible and methicillin-resistant community-associated *Staphylococcus aureus* infections in hospitalized patients. *J Infect* 2007;54:427–34.

111. Huang H, Flynn NM, King JH, et al. Comparisons of community-associated methicillin-resistant *Staphylococcus aureus* (MRSA) and hospital-associated MRSA infections in Sacramento, CA. *J Clin Microbiol* 2006;44:2423–7.

112. Frank AL, Marcinak JF, Mangat PD, Schreckenberger PC. Community-acquired and clindamycin-susceptible methicillin-resistant *Staphylococcus aureus* in children. *Pediatr Infect Dis J* 1999;18:993–1000.

113. Herold BC, Immergluck LC, Maranan MC, et al. Community-acquired methicillin-resistant *Staphylococcus aureus* in children with no identified predisposing risk. *JAMA* 1998;279:593–8.

114. Gorak EJ, Yamada SM, Brown JD. Community-acquired methicillin-resistant *Staphylococcus aureus* in hospitalized adults and children without known risk factors. *Clin Infect Dis* 1999;29:797–800.

115. Sattler CA, Mason EO Jr, Kaplan SL. Prospective comparison of risk factors and demographic and clinical characteristics of community-acquired, methicillin-resistant versus methicillin-susceptible *Staphylococcus aureus* infection in children. *Pediatr Infect Dis J* 2002;21:910–7.

116. Martinez-Aquilar G, Hammerman WA, Mason EO Jr, Kaplan SL. Clindamycin treatment of invasive infections caused by community-acquired, methicillin-resistant versus methicillin-susceptible *Staphylococcus aureus* in children. *Pediatr Dis J* 2003;22:93–8.

117. Pillar CM, Draghi DC, Sheehan DJ, Sahm DF. Prevalence of multidrug resistant, methicillin-resistant *Staphylococcus aureus* in the US: Findings of the stratified analysis of the 2004–2005 LEADER Surveillance Program. *Diagnos Microbiol Infect Dis* 2007; available at www.sciencedirect.com.

118. Larson EL, Quiros D, Lin SX. Dissemination of the CDC's Hand Hygiene Guidelines and impact on infection rates. *Am J Infect Control* 2007;35:666–75.

119. Larson E. A tool to assess barriers to adherence to hand hygiene guidelines. *Am J Infect Control* 2004; 32:48–51.

120. Boyce JM, Pittet D. Guidelines for hand hygiene in health-care settings. Recommendations of the Healthcare Infection Control Practices Advisory Committee and the HIPAC/SHEA/APIC/IDSA Hand Hygiene Task Force. *Am J Infect Control* 2002; 30:S1–46.

121. Pittet D. Compliance with hand disinfection and its impact on hospital-acquired infections. *J Hosp Infect* 2001;48:S40–6.

122. Misset B, Timsit JF, Dumay MF, et al. A continuous quality improvement program reduces nosocomial infection rates in the ICU. *Intensive Care Med* 2004;30:395–400.

123. Muto CA, Jernigan JA, Ostrowsky BE, et al. SHEA guidelines for preventing nosocomial transmission of multi-drug-resistant strains of *Staphylococcus aureus* and enterococcus. *Infect Control Hosp Epidemiol* 2003;24:362–86.

124. Seigel JD, Rhinehart E, Jackson M, Chiarello L, and the Healthcare Infection Control Practices Advisory Committee. 2007 Guidelines for isolation precautions: Preventing transmission of infectious agents in healthcare settings. Available at www.cdc.gov/ncidod/dhqp/gl.isolation.html.

125. Association for Professionals in Infection Control and Epidemiology. *Guide to the Elimination of Methicillin-Resistant Staphylococcus aureus (MRSA) Transmission in Hospital Settings.* Washington: APIC, 2008; MRSA Implementation Guide; available at www.apic.org/Content/NavigationMenu/GovernmentAdvocacy/MethicillinResistantStaphylococcusAureusMRSA/Resources/MRSAguide.pdf.

126. Safdar A, Marx J, Meyer NA, Maki DG. Effectiveness of preemptive barrier precautions in controlling nosocomial colonization and infection by methicillin-resistant *Staphylococcus aureus* in a burn unit. *Am J Infect Control* 2006;34:476–83.

127. Simor AE, Phillips E, McGeer A, et al. Randomized, controlled trial of chlorhexidine gluconate for washing, intranasal mupirocin, and rifampin and doxycycline versus no treatment for eradication of methicillin-resistant *Staphylococcus aureus* colonization. *Clin Infect Dis* 2007;44:178–85.

128. Trautmann M, Pollitt A, Loh U, et al. Implementaiton of an intensified infection control program to reduce MRSA transmission in a German tertiary care hospital. *Am J Infect Control* 2007;35:643–9.

129. Ofner-Agostini A, Varia M, Johnston L, et al, Canadian Nosocomial Infection Surveillance Program, and Gravel D. Infection control and antimicrobial restriction practices for antimicrobial-resistant organisms in Canadian tertiary care hospitals. *Am J Infect Control* 2006;35:563–8.

130. Garner JS. Hospital Infection Control Practices Advisory Committee, Centers for Disease Control and Prevention. Guideline for isolation precautions in hospitals. *Infect Control Hosp Epidemiol* 1996;17:53–80.

131. Bearmann GML, Marra AR, Sessier CN, et al. A controlled trial of universal gloving versus contact precautions for preventing the transmission of multidrug-resistant organisms. *Am J Infect Control* 2007;35:650–5.

132. Lehmer EM, Clay CA, Pearce-Duvet J, et al. Differential regulation of pathogens: The role of habitat disturbance in predicting prevalence of Sin Nombre virus. *Oecologia* 2007; available at www.springerlink.com.

133. Olival KJ, Daszak P. The ecology of emerging neurotropic viruses. *J Neurovirol* 2005;11:441–6.

134. Engelthaler DM, Mosley DG, Cheek JE, et al. Climatic and environmental patterns associated with hantavirus pulmonary syndrome, Four Corners Region, United States. *Emerg Infec Dis* 1999;5:87–94.

135. Zietz PS, Graber JM, Voorhees RA, et al. Assessment of occupational risk for hantavirus infection in Arizona and New Mexico. *J Occup Environ Med* 1997; 39:463–7.

136. Centers for Disease Control and Prevention. Hantavirus pulmonary syndrome—Five States, 2006. *MMWR* 2006;55:627–9.

137. Reed, KD, Melski JW, Graham MB, et al. The detection of monkeypox in humans in the western hemisphere. *N Engl J Med* 2004;350:342–50.

138. Guarner J, Johnson BJ, Paddock CD, et al. Monkey-pox transmission and pathogenesis in prairie dogs. *Emerg Infect Dis* 2004;10:426–31.

139. Chau, KB. Nipah virus outbreak in Malaysia. *J Clin Virol* 2003;26:266–75.

140. Epstein JH, Field HE, Luby S, et. al. Nipah virus: Impact, origins, and causes of emergence. *Curr Infect Dis Rep* 2006;8:59–64.

141. Campbell CC. Malaria: An emerging and re-emerging global plague. *FEMS Immunol Med Microbiol* 1997;18:325–31.

142. Sachs J, Malaney P. The economic and social burden of malaria. *Nature* 2002;145:680–5.

143. Martens WJM, Niessen LW, Rotmans J, et al. Potential impact of global climate change on malaria risk. *Environ Health Perspect* 1995;103:458–64.

144. van Lieshout M, Kovats RS, Livermore MTJ, Martens P. Climate change and malaria: Analysis of the SRES climate and socioeconomic scenarios. *Global Environ Change* 2004;14:84–99.

145. Gallup JK, Sachs JD. The economic burden of malaria. *Am J Trop Med Hyg* 2001;64:85–96S.

146. Kain KC, MacPherson DW, Kelton T, et al. Malaria deaths in visitors to Canada and in Canadian travelers: A case series. *Can Med Assoc J* 2001;164:654–9.

147. Kain KC, Keystone JS. Malaria in travelers: Epidemiology, disease, and prevention. *Infect Dis Clin North Am* 1998;12:267–84.

148. Speil C, Mushtaq A, Adamski A, Khardori N. Fever of unkwnown origin in the returning traveler. *Infect Dis Clin North Am* 2007;21:1091–113.

149. Zucker JR. Changing patterns of autochthonous malaria transmission in the United States: A review of recent outbreaks. *Emerg Infect Dis* 1996;2:37–43.

150. Roberts DR, Laughlin LL, Hsheih P, Legters L. DDT, global strategies, and malaria control crisis in South America. *Emerg Infect Dis* 1997;3:295–302.

151. World Health Organization. Dengue and Dengue Hemorrhagic Fever, 2008; available at www.who.int/mediacenter/factsheets/fs117/en/.

152. Morens DM, Fauci AS. Dengue and hemorrhagic fever. *JAMA* 2008;299:214–216.

153. Centers for Disease Control and Prevention. Dengue hemorrhagic fever—US–Mexico border, 2005. *MMWR* 2007;56:785–9.

154. Benedict MQ, Levine RS, Hawley WA, Lounibos LP. Spread of the tiger: Global risk of invasion by the mosquito *Aedes albopictus*. *Vector Borne Zoonotic Dis* 2007;7:76–85.

155. Hales S, de Wet N, Maindonald J, Woodward A. Potential effect of population and climate changes on global distribution of dengue fever: An empiric model. *Lancet* 2002;360:830–4.

156. Halstead SB. Dengue. *Lancet* 2007;370:1644–52.

157. Morens DM. Antibody-dependent enhancement of infection and the pathogenesis of viral disease. *Clin Infect Dis* 1994;19:500–12.

158. Sangkawibha N, Rojanasuphot S, Ahandrik S, et al. Risk factors in dengue shock syndrome: A prospective epidemiological study in Rayong, Thailand: I. The 1980 outbreak. *Am J Epidemiol* 1984;120:653–9.

159. Pan American Health Organization. *Dengue and Dengue Hemorrhagic Fever: Guidelines for Prevention and Control*, vol 12, no 3. Washington: PAHO, 1994.

160. Schreck CE. Protection from blood-feeding arthropods. In Aurebach PS (ed), *Wilderness Medicine*, 3rd ed. St Louis: Mosby, 1995. Pp 813–30.

38 Microbial Diseases of the Indoor Environment

Jeanne M. McGregor

Microbial contamination has been a problem of indoor spaces since the dawn of human history. Through the centuries, the development of civilization was inseparably connected with an expansion of microbial colonization in places and abodes in which humans have dwelled. Prehistoric times (confirmed by the analyses of rock paintings from Paleolithic caves) [1–4], archeological investigations [5–8], and conservation studies [9–12] have revealed that the destruction of organic and inorganic materials was mainly connected with fungal and actinomycetal biodeterioration activities. Perhaps the first known literary reference to the destructive influence of fungal flora on human dwellings and clothes is found in the third book of the Bible, Leviticus [13].

The hazards posed by exposure to microbiologic aerosols in the indoor environment are of increasing concern in modern times. This issue pertains to exposure in residential, commercial, and occupational settings. Epidemiologic and case studies have revealed that 33% of indoor air quality problems are related to microbial contamination [14, 15]. The potential for indoor air microbial toxin exposure has increased as people in industrial nations have been found to spend at least 90% of their time indoors, often with sole reliance on mechanical ventilation in airtight buildings [16].

American investigations reveal that 27–56% of homes have problems with visible fungal contamination of surfaces and/or bad quality of indoor air [17–20]. In Europe, this percentage ranges from 12–80% [21–33].

The major important indoor air microbial contaminants that cause disease include fungi, bacteria, viruses, and less frequently, protozoa. In addition to intact microorganisms, their cell wall constituents [endotoxin and β-(1,3)-D-glucan] and metabolites (mycotoxins and volatile organic compounds) are often the etiologic agents of disease. These bioaerosols, which are airborne particles that are living on or in or originate from living organisms, are ubiquitous in the natural environment. However, they can pose health risks when problematic environmental conditions (such as wetted porous building materials) provide an appropriate substrate for growth of mold and gram-negative bacteria. Additionally, building systems and occupant activities may further foster their amplification and dissemination.

Microbiologic and epidemiologic studies have shown that sources of indoor moisture, including elevated relative humidity and mold growth on walls, in heating, ventilation, air-conditioning, and refrigeration (HVACR) systems and within wall cavities are associated with bioaerosol contamination and adverse health effects in building occupants [34–42]. Indoor moisture sources have been found to be significant factors in mold levels and dust-mite contamination [43]. Building dampness and flooding have been associated with respiratory, dermal, neurologic, and constitutional symptoms, asthma, hypersensitivity pneumonitis, and other immunologic abnormalities [44–50].

Physicians and industrial health professionals are called on to provide assistance when concerns regarding potential building-related health problems arise and/or indoor sources of microbial growth are recognized. Multiple complex challenges then must be approached. The microbial source, route of transmission, and associated health outcomes must be identified. This challenge is often complicated by the societal, technologic, and environmental conditions affecting human hosts, each of whom has individual susceptibilities. It is essential that the physician have an appreciation of the dynamic interactions of these factors to have a true understanding of indoor air quality problems and be able to help those affected and prevent or mitigate illness in those who have yet to have exposure to toxins in the affected building(s). It is also necessary for the physician to understand the multidisciplinary approach that is used in handling building-related illness.

To most effectively address the issue, a team consisting of human resources personnel, industrial hygienists, microbiologists, engineers, remediation specialists, and occupational and environmental medicine physicians must work together to correctly identify specific etiologies for illness within a building, perform proper clean-up and removal of offending agents, correct or improve conditions that may have predisposed the contamination conditions to prevent recurrence, and render appropriate health care to affected persons. An open and honest disclosure of findings is imperative to help prevent the social fears and hysteria that can spread among a group of people who cohabitate a building. How human resources personnel handle these situations can greatly affect the outcome of the problem. Psychosocial issues associated with indoor air quality not only may affect the reliability of subjective information obtained during problem characterization but also may interfere with problem resolution even after appropriate remediation/control measures have been carried out. Implementing administrative controls to prevent occupation of contaminated areas until remediation is completed is crucial.

The evolving knowledge base of this field has many limitations that pose a challenge to those entrusted to address microbe-related indoor environmental illness. Building occupants are often simultaneously exposed to multiple offending environmental agents, both microbial and nonmicrobial, and the effect of this mixture of exposures (i.e., synergistic, additive, or antagonistic) is not yet fully known. Clinically, dose-response data are limited, and interpretation of sampling data for bioaerosols can be difficult.

Microbes in the indoor environment can be a cause or aggravator of certain medical conditions. Microbial bioaerosol exposure to molds, bacteria, and viruses has been shown to be associated with an increased risk of sarcoidosis [51, 52]. Asthma and allergies can be caused or aggravated by indoor allergens [53]. Domestic mites, which are deposited in floors and buried deep within carpets, mattresses, and soft furnishings, are a major cause of asthma worldwide [54]. Sensitization to cockroach allergens is a risk factor for asthma, especially among lower socioeconomic groups and minority populations. Pets create allergens from secretions (saliva), excretions (urine and feces), and danders. Cat allergens are liberated as small respirable particles, chiefly from the saliva, pelt, and sebaceous secretions. Many children keep pet rodents in their bedrooms, which can be a source of airborne allergens. Additionally, there are innercity areas where wild mice or rats are present and represent an important animal allergen pool. Molds and yeast are indoor airborne allergens, especially *Alternaria*, which is a known risk factor of asthma and is associated with the risk of asthma death in the United States. Pollens and fungi are common allergens that have been associated with asthma. Many of the literature reports of occupational asthma and pollens have occurred in florists and greenhouse workers.

Research into the formation of indoor bioaerosols has yielded knowledge regarding the role of filamentous microorganisms (i.e., fungi and actinomycetes) and their submicrometer propagules (fragments) [55]. Their release from contaminated surfaces and aerosolization have been shown to be influenced by such factors as air velocity, colony structure, moisture conditions, vibration of the surface, and time factors. The immunologic reactivity of these fragments has been studied. They can be at least partially responsible for the symptoms observed among inhabitants of buildings with mold problems and/or water damage.

This chapter discusses the predominant pathogenic indoor microorganisms, with specific focus on fungi and bacteria, and their impact on health. It provides an overview of the important issues in identifying and treating microbial-related illness, as well as identification of hazardous indoor environmental conditions containing or condusive to hazardous microbial contamination. At the end is a listing of resources and Web sites that are available to assist physicians in treating affected patients and in helping to prevent or mitigate microbial-related illness in populations of building occupants.

Microbial Sources, Agents, and Effects

Fungi and bacteria are ubiquitous in the natural environment. After becoming airborne, they may enter the indoor building environment. They also may enter by seepage, flooding, carriage on shoes, clothing, and personal items, delivered products including food and other organic matter, vermin, entry or housing of animals, or animal products. The commonly encountered indoor fungi include *Cladosporium, Penicillium, Aspergillus, Alternaria,* basidiomycetes, and less often *Acremonium, Trichoderma, Drechslera,* and *Epicoccum* [56–59]. If conditions allow (e.g., water damage of a building material substrate or excessive humidity), some fungal spores and bacteria, principally gram-negative, may grow and develop into active colonies. These colonies then may release more spores and bacteria, as well as microbial volatile organic compounds (MVOCs). Fungal spores are particularly problematic because they are known allergens [60, 61] and may contain mycotoxins in both viable and nonviable states [1, 13]. Several fungi commonly found indoors have been reported to produce mycotoxins, including immunosuppressive chemicals, such as cyclosporine [2] and stachybotrylactones [3, 4], and carcinogens, such as aflatoxins. Additionally, gram-negative bacteria are known to release endotoxins, which are lipopolysaccharide components of their outer cell wall.

RESERVOIRS, AMPLIFIERS, AND DISSEMINATORS

Airborne microbial populations depend on the presence of a source or reservoir of the microorganism, a means for the microorganism to multiply (amplify), and a mechanism for dissemination [62]. Fungi and bacteria that grow indoors are saprophytes—that is, they may feed on organic nutrients in the environment or on building materials of an organic nature. The available moisture content is also a critical factor affecting fungal growth indoors [63].

Paper and wood products are particularly susceptible to the cellulolytic fungi and bacteria. Species of Basidiomycetes, *Chaetomium, Chrysosporium, Stachybotrys,* and *Trichoderma,* all known producers of cellulases, are frequently detected and identified in water-damaged building materials. Fast-growing colonizers, such as species of *Acremonium, Aspergillus, Cladosproium, Penicillium,* and *Uloclaium,* are also found commonly on water-damaged materials. In addition, gram-negative bacteria, including species of *Acinetobacter, Methylobacterium, Pseudomanoas,* and *Stenotrophomonas,* are common contaminants of water-damaged materials or stagnant water in building systems. Filamentous bacteria (actinomycetes) occasionally grow indoors in wet and damp conditions. Fungi, bacteria, and mite presence also has been found to be increased by the presence of building flooding, chronically damp carpets, poor exhaust of bathrooms, and appliances that collect water, such as humidifiers, dehumidifiers, air conditioners, drip pans, and ventilation systems.

Extensive water damage after major hurricanes and floods increases the likelihood of fungi/mold contamination in buildings. This causes three primary adverse effects: (1) damage to buildings, (2) the rendering of buildings unpleasant to live in by looking and smelling bad, and (3) the possibility of causation of adverse health effects in sensitive individuals. In 1997, a major flood in Poland damaged 680,000 dwellings and several thousand factories and institutions [64]. In Germany, the costs caused by mold damage in buildings are estimated to amount to more than 200 million Euro per year [65]. Most recently, on August 29 and September 24, 2005, hurricanes Katrina and Rita, respectively, made landfall along the Gulf Coast of the United States. After both storms, levees were breached, leading to massive flooding in New Orleans and surrounding parishes. An assessment of homes in New Orleans (Orleans Parish) and the surrounding parishes of St. Bernard, East Jefferson, and West

Jefferson (excluding the ninth ward) identified more than 100,000 homes with some mold contamination, and approximately 40,000 homes had heavy mold contamination [66]. After the 1999 flood in North Carolina after Hurricane Floyd, a reported increase in persons presenting with asthma symptoms was postulated to be caused by exposure to mold [67]. Finally, in 2001, flooding and subsequent mold growth on the Turtle Mountain reservation in Belcourt, North Dakota, was associated with self-reports of rhinitis, rash, headaches, and asthma exacerbation [68].

The Centers for Disease Control and Prevention (CDC) *Morbidity and Mortality Weekly Report (MMWR) Recommendations and Reports* dated June 9, 2006, indicated that in the aftermath of major hurricanes or floods, buildings wet for more than 48 hours generally will support visible and extensive mold growth and should be remediated. It also reported that excessive exposure to mold-contaminated materials can cause adverse health effects in susceptible persons regardless of the type of mold or the extent of contamination.

Finally, mechanical devices or structures in a problem building, such as contaminated humidifiers, water towers, or heating, ventilating, and air-conditioning (HVAC) ducts, may serve as both reservoirs and amplifiers or amplifiers and disseminators of indoor microorganisms. Further dissemination of spore and bacteria may occur via mites and insects attracted to the fungal growth, disturbances in a room caused by occupant activities, or building renovation.

SPORE RELEASE, LONGEVITY, AND VIABILITY

Fungal spores can survive for a period until suitable ambient conditions provide an environment for germination, growth, and continued spore production and dissemination. Spore release is extremely variable, thus affecting the usefulness of air sampling. Spores of some fungal species, such as *Penicillium* and *Aspergillus*, have been reported to be viable for over 12 years, whereas some other spores are viable but not culturable. Finally, although not all airborne fungal spores are viable, they are potentially allergenic and may contain mycotoxins. It is generally recognized that this potential allergenicity depends on an individual's genetic composition and previous sensitization.

MYCOTOXINS

Concern has arisen about exposure to certain molds that produce substances called *mycotoxins*. It is thought that these toxins are produced as protection against competing organisms. Since these toxins are not essential for growth, they are classified as *secondary metabolites*. Because they require extra work on the part of the organism, production does not occur at all times or with all types of mold [69].

Mycotoxins are principally nonvolatile and of low molecular weight. As such, exposure via inhalation is most likely associated with spore inhalation. Many case studies of bioaerosol inhalation exposures have focused on one particular mycotoxin group, the trichothecenes. Several fungi, including *Memnoniella echninata*, *Stachybotrus chartarum*, and some species of *Trichoderma*, *Aspergillus*, and *Penicillium* are commonly found in water-damaged materials and have been documented to produce trichothecenes. Although associations of health outcomes with exposure to toxin-producing strains of certain fungi have been drawn, the actual role for exposures to fungus and their mycotoxins or to them in combination with other fungal and bacterial contaminants continues to require further investigation [70].

Health effects related to mycotoxins are generally linked to ingestion of large quantities of fungal-contaminated material [71, 72]. No conclusive evidence exists of a link between indoor exposure to airborne mycotoxins and human illness [73–76]. Although the potential for health problems is an important reason to prevent or minimize indoor mold growth and to remediate any indoor mold contamination, evidence is inadequate to support recommendations for greater urgency of remediation in cases where mycotoxin-producing fungi have been isolated.

MICROBIAL VOLATILE ORGANIC COMPOUNDS

Microbial metabolism produces not only mycotoxins but also microbial volatile organic compounds (MVOCs). Actively growing fungi and bacteria (including actinomycetes) produce various MVOCs both by primary metabolism, which extracts energy from nutrient molecules for essential cell component use, and by secondary metabolism, which is not essential to maintaining the life of an organism and requires extra energy. Current interest in MVOCs is based on use of their moldy odors and specific compounds as markers of microbial growth (even when not visible) and their potential adverse health effects [77].

Many types of MVOCs are produced and typically include aldehydes, alcohols, ketones, and hydrocarbons. When one smells a "musty moldy" odor, it is generally the MVOCs that one is noticing. MVOCs are often considered irritants to mucous membranes and are capable of short-term and possible long-term adverse health effects. The presence of these MVOCs suggests that mold is consuming and growing.

The health effects associated with exposures to MVOCs have remained a topic of ongoing study. However, there have been suggestions that MVOCs contribute to the symptoms and complaints of some building occupants, such as mucous membrane and respiratory tract irritation, exacerbation of asthma, cacosmia, and central nervous system symptoms of headache, inability to concentrate, and dizziness [77, 78].

β-(1,3)-D-GLUCANS

Microbial cell wall constituents, such as β-(1,3)-D-glucan and endotoxin, have been associated with health problems of occupants of water-damaged indoor environments. β-(1,3)-D-Glucan is a polyglucose polymer found in the cell walls of plants, fungi, and certain bacteria [79], and it is an immunomodulator [79–81]. Epidemiologic studies have linked glucan exposure with airway inflammation, headaches, and fatigue in occupants of damp buildings [79, 82, 83]. However, it remains unclear whether these building-related health effects are specifically due to glucan exposure versus exposure to a mixture of fungi and bacteria and their cell wall constituents and metabolites.

ENDOTOXIN

Endotoxin is derived from the cell walls of gram-negative bacteria. It contains lipopolysaccharide as part of the complex, with protein and other lipids, and may be released from the bacterial cell wall in various complex forms during active cell growth, division, or death [84]. Elevated levels of indoor endotoxin have been associated with contaminated humidifiers, water-damaged building materials,

and industrial settings where organic dust or recirculated water-based or metal-working fluids have been aerosolized [85].

In summary, regarding microbial sources and agents, in a water-damaged environment, various species of fungi and bacteria (particularly gram-negative bacteria) may proliferate. It is very likely that building occupants are exposed to mixtures of fungi (and their spores) and bacteria of various species, as well as to mycotoxins, MVOCs, endotoxin, and glucans. Health effects therefore should be assessed with recognition of this complex exposure mixture. Recent studies have shown that there is a synergistic interaction in the simultaneous exposure to *Streptomyces californicus* and *Stachybotrys chartarum* and *Stachybotrys chartarum* and *Aspergillus versicolor* [86–88].

Health Effects

SPECIFIC HEALTH ENDPOINTS

The adverse health effects associated with fungal and gram-negative bacterial cell wall constituents and metabolites have already been discussed, that is, toxic and irritant effects. This section addresses specific health endpoints related to bioaerosol exposure in the indoor environment. These disorders, which have diverse pathophysiologic mechanisms and clinical manifestations, include hypersensitivity diseases, inhalation fever, and infections. There have been some reports of inflammatory joint symptoms in association with exposure to moisture damage in workplace buildings [89].

Hypersensitivity Diseases

Hypersensitivity disorders, including allergic rhinitis/sinusitis and asthma and hypersensitivity pneumonitis, are among the most common bioaerosol-related diseases. Allergic rhinitis and asthma are both type I (IgE-mediated) hypersensitivity diseases. Hypersensitivity pneumonitis, also known as *extrinsic allergic alveolitis,* is a spectrum of inflammatory, granulomatous, interstitial, bronchiolar, and alveolar pulmonary disease [90]. It is caused by continuous or repeated inhalation exposures and sensitization to bioaerosols [e.g., bacteria, fungi, and animal proteins (avian)], or certain low-molecular-weight chemicals (such as isocyanates). Onset of symptoms usually occurs 4–12 hours after exposure.

In its acute form, hypersensitivity pneumonitis may present as recurrent bouts of fever, chills, malaise, shortness of breath, cough, chest tightness, and myalgias. Physical findings may be normal, nonspecific, or those of bibasilar crackles on lung auscultation. Chest radiographs may reveal normal findings, diffuse patchy infiltrates, or a ground-glass appearance. Pulmonary function tests may reveal a restrictive pattern, with decreased diffusion capacity. Marked lymphocytosis, without eosinophilia or neutrophilia, is typically found on bronchoalveolar lavage. The results of lung biopsy reveal inflammatory infiltrates at sites distant from granulomas. In the chronic form of hypersensitivity pneumonitis, irreversible lung damage and associated gas-exchange impairment may occur. Several epidemiologic studies have linked hypersensitivity pneumonitis with exposure to microbial contamination of ventilation systems and to endotoxin-containing respirable bioaerosol exposures at an indoor swimming pool.

Inhalation Fever

Inhalation fever is an acute, short-term, benign, and self-limited reaction. Symptoms include fever, chills, myalgias, cough, headache, general malaise, and chest discomfort. Onset of symptoms usually occurs 4–8 hours after exposure, and symptoms typically subside within 12–48 hours if exposure does not continue. Tolerance (decreased symptoms with continued exposure) does occur, but after prolonged absence and then return to exposure, the symptoms do recur.

Physical findings, pulmonary function tests, and chest radiographs are usually normal, although an increased erythrocyte sedimentation rate and polymorphonuclear leukocytosis are common. In contrast to the lymphocytosis seen on bronchoalveolar lavage in patients with hypersensitivity pneumonitis, this test in patients with inhalation fever reveals an increase in neutrophils. Treatment is symptomatic, and there are no reported sequelae.

Infections

Infections owing to indoor microbial contamination principally include legionellosis, tuberculosis, other airborne bacterial infections, airborne viral infections, and systemic fungal infections. Both legionellosis and tuberculosis are fully discussed in other chapters in this text and thus are not ad-dressed here. Airborne viral infections and bacterial infections of pneumococcal origin are contagious diseases that are transmitted from person to person. The risk of their aerosol transmission is increased by recirculated air, low ventilation rates, and increased occupant density. Thus their prevention can be enhanced by mechanical HVAC delivery of adequate ventilation that is appropriate to occupant density, as well as by appropriate use of immunizations.

The health endpoint of systemic fungal infection is determined by the immune status of the host. An immunocompromised host is at increased risk for severe infection by many fungi, including the thermotolerant fungus *A. fumigatus* [91, 92]. The geographic location tends to determine what fungal sources are available and the size of the fungal innoculum. *Histoplasma capsulatum* is a soil-borne fungus that flourishes in moist environments such as the Mississippi River Valley, whereas *Coccidioides immitis* is associated with dry soil, mainly in the southwestern United States. *Cryptococcus neoformans* and *H. capsulatum* have been recovered from bird droppings and bat excrement.

Evaluation

Microbial contamination of the indoor environment presents unique and complex issues that require a systematic problem-oriented approach for their complete assessment and resolution. It is important that there is involvement of qualified professionals who are experienced in the investigation of microbial issues. A multidisciplinary collaboration of industrial hygienists, engineers, microbiologists, and environmental and occupational health professionals is essential for such evaluations. It is also important to check the background and references of such parties because there continues to be much variation in how microbial contamination is handled.

The essential details of this problem-oriented approach are as follows:

- Review of the presenting problem and available records
- Characterization of the complaint (health and building conditions)
- Site investigation (including evaluation of potential sources of biologic agents)

- Hypothesis formation
- Evaluation of bioaerosol and environmental conditions
- Medical evaluation
- Interpretation of data
- Recommendation of corrective measures
- Remediation
- Validation of effectiveness

An indoor air quality task force composed of all involved parties, including management and employees of commercial buildings, should be formed for the purpose of defining the current problem and planning remediation collectively. Full disclosure of all information improves the opportunity to resolve the indoor air quality problem and fosters trust and credibility between employees and management.

MEDICAL EVALUATION

Environmental and occupational medicine physicians are challenged with the unique complexities related to indoor microbial contamination when asked to evaluate potentially related health effects. It is often difficult to characterize exposure, document disease, identify causal linkages, and intervene and manage disease. This applies to the evaluation of individuals as well as assessment of health risks of cohorts in a public health setting. Nevertheless, these limitations in knowledge and the technical difficulties related to exposure mixtures, dose-response data, characterization of health endpoints, and diagnostic testing must not impede physicians' assistance of their patients. Clinical decisions must be made based on the currently available evidence, professional judgment, commonsense, and a true sense of caring for the patient's physical and mental well-being.

The occupational and environmental medical history is the cornerstone of the evaluation. A comprehensive, detailed physical examination is also imperative. Diagnostic testing should be individualized to the outcome of the history and physical and the suspect target organ possibly affected by the exposure. Regarding specialized laboratory tests, there are concerns with the clinical use of tests with inadequately defined sensitivity, specificity, and predictive value. Referral to subspecialists should be carried out as needed for further diagnostic testing and treatment. Data obtained in the

building investigation, such as bioaerosol sampling results, should be reviewed. After all these steps have been accomplished, the physician should define the diagnosis and establish whether a casual association between the disease and the building environment exists.

If a causal linkage between disease and exposure has been established, decisions about medical removal of the individual, and possibly other building occupants, need to be made on a case-by-case basis. In making these decisions, the following factors should be considered:

1. Character and severity of the health problem
2. Extent and type of microbial contamination
3. Specific risk factors of the individual, such as immunocompromised health status, age (infants younger than 12 months old and the elderly), pregnancy, and past history of hypersensitivity disease or chronic inflammatory respiratory disease
4. If remediation is planned, assessment regarding occupancy should depend on whether methods of containment would be adequate to prevent building occupant exposure.

Finally, after both remediation and reoccupancy have occurred, surveillance of individuals with building-related illnesses should be conducted. Protocol components and surveillance duration should be uniquely determined to address the specific clinical issue.

Summary

Excess moisture and elevated humidity in indoor environments clearly have been shown to be associated with microbial contamination and adverse health effects, particularly respiratory problems. This microbial contamination is typically composed of a mixture of fungi and their spores and gram-negative bacteria and their cell wall constituents and metabolites. As knowledge in this area of science evolves, it is essential for investigators to accurately and responsibly draw conclusions regarding associations between exposure to mixtures and resulting disease. *S. chartarum* has become well known as a mycotoxin producer and was blamed initially for a cluster of cases of acute idiopathic pulmonary hemorrhage among infants. It was later shown that this was not the case. Nevertheless, this mold is now blamed for a diverse array of maladies when it is found indoors. There remains a need for continued study to advance the knowledge base concerning microbial contaminants in the indoor environment, as well as implementation of environmental controls to prevent and mitigate the presence of such contaminants and thus their adverse effect on human beings.

Resources

American Conference of Governmental Industrial Hygienists, www.acgih.org.

Centers for Disease Control and Prevention, National Center for Environmental Health, www.cdc.gov/mold.

The Council of State and Territorial Epidemiologists, www.cdc.gov/nceh/airpollution/indoor_air.htm.

EPA Indoor Air Quality Information, www.epa.gov/mold.

Federal Emergency Management Agency, www.fema.gov.

References

1. Ciferi O. Microbial degradation of paintings. *Appl Environ Microbiol* 1999;65:879–885.
2. Cunningham KI, Northup DE, Pollastro RM, et al. Bacteria, fungi, and biokarst in Lechuguilla Cave. Carlsbad Caverns National Park New Mexico. *Environ Geol* 1995;25:2–8.
3. Groth I, Vettermann R, Schuetze B, et al. *Actinomyces* in Karstic Caves of northern Spain (Altamira Tito Bustillo). *J Microbiol Methods* 1999;36:115–22.
4. Sarbu SM, Kane TC, Kinkle BK. A chemoautotrophically based cave ecosystem. *Science* 1996;272:1953–5.
5. Blanchette RA. A review of microbial deterioration found in archeological wood from different environments. *Int Biodeterior Biodegrad* 2000;46:189–204.
6. Giacobini C, De Cicco MA, Tiglie I, et al. Actinomyces and biodeterioration in the field of fine art. In Houghton DR, Smith RN, Eggins HOW (eds), *Biodeterioration.* New York: Elsevier Applied Science, 1987.
7. Janinska B. Historic buildings and mould fungi: Not only vaults are menacing with "Tutankhamen's curse." *Found Civil Environ Eng* 2002;2:43–54.
8. Valentin N. Preservation of historic materials by using inert gases for biodeterioration control. In

Maekawa S (ed), *Research in Conservation: Oxygen-Free Museum Case.* Los Angeles: Getty Conservation Institute, 1998. Pp 17–29.
9. Gorbushina AA, Heyrman J, Kornieden T, et al. Bacterial and fungal diversity and biodeterioration problems in mural painting environments of St. Martins church (Greene-Kreiensen, Germany). *Int Biodeterior Biodegrad* 2004;53:13–24.
10. Krumbein WE. Patina and cultural heritage: A geomicrobiologist's perspective. In Proceedings of 5th EC Conference: *Biodeterioration and Its Control—Biotechnologies in Cultural Heritage Protection and Conservation.* Krakow: Polska Akademia Nauk, 2002. Pp 39–47.
11. Nugari MP, Roccardi A. Aerobiological investigations applied to the conservation of cultural heritage. *Aerobiologia* 2001;17:215–23.
12. Sampo S, Luppi Mosca AM. A study of the fungi occurring on 15th century frescoes in Florence, Italy. *Int Biodeterior* 1989;25:343–53.
13. *Bible,* Leviticus, chap 14, verses 34–45.
14. Yang CS. Understanding the biology of fungi found indoors. In Johanning E, Yang CS (eds), *Fungi and Bacteria in Indoor Air Environments: Health Effects, Detection, and Remediation.* Latham, NY: Eastern New York Occupational Health Program, 1995. Pp 131–7.
15. Lewis FA. Regulating indoor microbes. In Johanning E, Yang CS (eds), *Fungi and Bacteria in Indoor Air Environments: Health Effects, Detection, and Remediation.* Latham, NY: Eastern New York Occupational Health Program, 1995. Pp 5–9.
16. *Report to Congress on Indoor Air Quality, Vol II: Assessment and Control of Indoor Air Pollution.* EPA-400-89-001C. Washington: U.S. Environmental Protection Agency, 1989. Pp 1, 4–14.
17. Crandall MS, Sieber WK. The National Institute of Occupational Safety and Health indoor environmental evaluation experience: I. Building environmental evaluations. *Appl Occup Environ Hyg* 1996;11:533–9.
18. Dales RE, Burnett R, Zwanenburg H. Adverse health effects among adults exposed to home dampness and molds. *Am Rev Respir Dis* 1991;143:505–9.
19. Ellringer PJ, Boone K, Hendrickson S. Building materials used in construction can affect indoor fungal levels greatly. *Am Ind Hyg Assoc J* 2000;61:895–9.
20. Spengler JD, Neas L, Nakai S, et al. Respiratory symptoms and housing characteristics. *Indoor Air* 1994;4:72–84.
21. Adan OCG. On the fungal defacement of interior finishes. Ph.D. thesis, Technical University, Eidhoven, 1994.
22. Becker R. Condensation and mould growth in dwellings: Parametric and field study. *Build environ* 1984;19:243–50.
23. Brunekreef B. Damp housing and adult respiratory distress symptoms. *Allergy* 1992;47:498–502.
24. Burr ML, Mullins J, Merret TG, et al. Asthma and indoor mould exposure. *Thorax* 1985;40:688.

25. Hunter CA, Lea RG. The airborne fungal population of representative British homes. In Samson RA, Flannigan B, Flannigan ME, et al. (eds), *Air Quality Monographs*, Vol 2: *Health Implications of Fungi in Indoor Environments*. Amsterdam: Elsevier Science, 1994. Pp 141–53.

26. International Energy Agency. Energy Conservation in Buildings and Community Systems Programme: Annex XIV: *Condensation and Energy*, Vol 1, *Source Book*. Leuven, Belgium. International Energy Agency, 1991.

27. Martin CJ, Platt SD, Hunt SM. Housing conditions and ill health. *Br Med J* 1987;294:1125–7.

28. Nevalainen A, Partanen P, Jaaskelainen E, et al. Prevalence of moisture problems in Finnish houses. *Indoor Air* 1998;4:45–9.

29. Pirhonen I, Nevalainen A, Husman T, et al. Home dampness, moulds and their influence on respiratory infections and symptoms in adults in Finland. *Eur Respir J* 1996;9:2618–22.

30. Platt SD, Martin CJ, Hunt SM, et al. Damp housing, mold growth, and symptomatic health state. *Br Med J* 1989;298:1673–8.

31. Sanders CH, Cornish JP. *Dampness: One Week's Complaints in Five Local Authorities in England and Wales*. London: Report Building Research Establishment, 1982.

32. van der Laan PCH. Moisture problems in the Netherlands: A pilot project to solve problem in social housing. In Samson FA, Flannigan B, Flannigan ME, et al (eds), *Air Quality Monographs, Vol 2: Health Implications of Fungi in Indoor Environments*. Amsterdam: Elsevier Science, 1994. Pp 507–16.

33. Verhoeff AP, van Wijnen JH, Boleij JS, et al. Enumeration and identification of airborne viable mould propagules in houses. *Allergy* 1990;45:275–84.

34. Smoragiewicz W, Cossette B, Boutard A, et al. Trichothecene mycotoxins in the dust of ventilation systems in office buildings. *Int Arch Occup Environ Health* 1993;65:113–7.

35. Andersson MA, Nikulin M, Koljalg U, et al. Bacteria, molds, and toxins in water-damaged building materials. *Appl Environ Microbiol* 1997;63:387–93.

36. Croft WA, Jarvis BB, Yatawara CS. Airborne outbreak of trichothecene toxicosis. *Atmos Environ* 1986;20:549–52.

37. Verhoeff AP, van Wijnen JH, Brunekreef B, et al. The presence of viable mould propagules in indoor air in relation to home dampness and outdoor air. *Allergy* 1992;47:83–91.

38. Hunter CA, Grant C, Flannigan B, et al. Mould in buildings: The air spora of domestic dwellings. *Internat Biodeterior* 1988;24:81–101.

39. Platt DP, Martin CJ, Hunt SM, et al. Damp housing, mould growth, and symptomatic health state. *Br Med J* 1989;298:1673–8.

40. Hodgson MJ, Morey P, Leung W-Y, et al. Building-associated pulmonary disease from exposure to *Stachybotrys chartarum* and *Aspergillus versicolor*. *J Environ Occup Med* 1998;40:241–9.

41. Bernstein RS, Sorenson WG, Garabrant D, et al. Exposures to respirable, airborne *Penicillium* from a contaminated ventilation system: Clinical, environmental and epidemiological aspects. *Am Ind Hyg Assoc J* 1983;44:161–9.

42. Outbreaks of respiratory illness among employees in large office buildings—Tennessee, District of Columbia. *MMWR* 1984:33:506–13.

43. Lawton MD, Dales RE, White J. The influence of house characteristics in a Canadian community on microbiological contamination. *Ind Air* 1998;8:2–11.

44. Dales RE, Burnett R, Zwaneburg H. Adverse health effects among adults exposed to home dampness and molds. *Am Rev Respir Dis* 1991;143:505–9.

45. Strachen DP. Damp housing and childhood asthma: Validation of reporting of symptoms. *Br Med J* 1988;297:1223–6.

46. Hodgson MJ, Morey PR, Attfield M, et al. Pulmonary disease associated with cafeteria flooding. *Arch Environ Health* 1985;40:96–101.

47. Brunekreef B. Damp housing and adult respiratory symptoms. *Allergy* 1992;47:498–502.

48. Brunekreef B, Dockery DW, Speizer FE, et al. Home dampness and respiratory morbidity in children. *Am Rev Respir Dis* 1989;140:1363–7.

49. Waegemaekers M, Van Wageningen N, Brunekreef B, et al. Respiratory symptoms in damp homes. *Allergy* 1989;44:1–7.

50. Johanning E, Biagini R, Hull D, et al. Health and immunology study following exposure to toxigenic fungi (*Stachybotrys chartarum*) in a water-damaged office environment. *Int Arch Occup Environ Health* 1996;68:207–18.

51. Newman LS, Rose CS, Bresnitz MD, et al. A case control etiologic study of sarcoidosis: Environmental and occupational risk factors. *Am J Respir Crit Care Med* 2004;170:1324–30.

52. Department of Veteran's Affairs, Veterans Health Administration. Under Secretary for Health's Information Letter: Sarcoidosis. Washington, 2007; IL 10-2007-001.

53. Hamilton RG. Assessment of indoor allergen exposure. *Curr Allergy Asthma Rep* 2005;5:394–401.

54. Brooks SM, Truncale T, McCluskey J. Occupational and environmental asthma. In Rom WN (ed), *Environmental and Occupational Medicine*, 4th ed. Philadelphia: Lippincott Williams & Wilkins 2007. Pp 418–63.

55. Gorny RL. Filamentous microorganisms and their fragments in indoor air: A review. *Ann Agric Environ Med* 2004;11:185–97.

56. Lewis FA. Regulating indoor microbes. In Johanning E, Yang CS (eds), *Fungi and Bacteria in Indoor Air Environments: Health Effects, Detection, and Remediation*. Latham, NY: Eastern New York Occupational Health Program, 1995. Pp 5–9.

57. Dungy CI, Kozak PP, Gallup J, et al. Aeroallergen exposure in the elementary school setting. *Ann Allergy* 1986;56:218–24.

58. Strachen DP, Flannigan B, McCabe EM, et al. Quantification of airborne moulds in the homes of children with and without wheeze. *Thorax* 1990;45:382–7.

59. VerHoeff AP, van Wijnen JH, Boleij B, et al. Enumeration and identification of airborne viable mould ropagules in houses. *Allergy* 1990;45:275–84.

60. Pope AM, Patterso R, Burge H. *Indoor Allergens; Assessing and Controlling Adverse Health Effects.* Washington: National Academy Press, 1993.

61. Gravesen S. Fungi as a cause of allergic disease. *Allergy* 1979;34:135–54.

62. Burge HA, Feeley JC. Indoor air pollution and infectious diseases. In Samet JM, Spengler JD (eds), *Indoor Air Pollution: A Health Perspective.* Baltimore: John Hopkins University Press, 1991. Pp 273–84.

63. Yang CS, Johanning E. Airborne fungi and mycotoxins. In Hurst CJ, Knudsen GR, McInerney MJ, et al. (eds), *Manual of Environmental Microbiology.* Washington: ASM Press, 1996. Pp 651–60.

64. Portnoy JM, Kenney K, Barnes C. *Sampling for Indoor Fungi: What the Clinician Needs to Know.* Kansas City, MO: Children's Mercy Hospitals and Clinics, 2005.

65. Majewski W. Powodz lipiec 1997. *Pismo PG* 1998;4.

66. Sedlbauer K. Prediction of mould fungus formation on the surface of and inside building components. Ph.D. thesis, Fraunhofer Institute for Building Physics, Stuttgart 2001.

67. Centers for Disease Control and Prevention. Health concerns associated with mold in water-damaged homes after Hurricanes Katrina and Rita—New Orleans, Louisiana, October 2005. *MMWR* 2006;55:41–4.

68. Centers for Disease Control and Prevention. Morbidity and mortality associated with Hurricane Floyd—North Carolina. *MMWR* 2000;49:369–72.

69. Stock AL, Davis K, Brown CM, et al. An investigation of home dampness and adverse health effects on a Native American reservation. *J Soc Toxicol* 2005;84:1–5.

70. Bennett JW, Klich M. Mycotoxins. *Clin Microbiol Rev* 2003;16:497–516.

71. Centers for Disease Control and Prevention. Mold prevention strategies and possible health effects in the aftermath of hurricanes and major floods. *MMWR* 2006;55(RR-8): 1–27.

72. American Conference of Governmental Industrial Hygienists. *Bioaerosols Assessment and Control.* Cincinnati, OH: American Conference of Governmental Industrial Hygienists, 1999.

73. Institute of Medicine, Committee on Damp Indoor Spaces and Health. *Damp Indoor Spaces and Health.* Washington: National Academy Press, 2004.

74. Centers for Disease Control and Prevention. *State of the Science on Molds and Human Health.* Atlanta: US Department of Health and Human Services, CDC, 2002.

75. Hardin BD, Kelman BJ, Saxon A. Adverse human health effects associated with molds in the indoor environment. *J Occup Environ Med* 2003;45:470–8.

76. Chapman JA, Terr AI, Jacobs RL, et al. Toxic mold: Phantom risk vs science. *Ann Allergy Asthma Immunol* 2003;91:222–32.

77. Ammann HM. Microbial volatile organic compounds. In Macher J (ed), *Bioaerosols: Assessment and Control.* Cincinnati, OH: American Conference of Governmental Industrial Hygienists, 1999. Pp 26-1–26-17.

78. Flannigan B, McCabe EM, McGarry F. Allergenic and toxigenic microorganisms in houses. *J Appl Bacteriol* 1991;79:61–73S.

79. Rylander R. Microial cell wall constituents in indoor air and their relation to disease. In Seppanen O (ed), *Indoor Air and Health: Causative Agents, Health Hazards and Risk Assessment.* 10th Medical Symposium of the Yrjo Jahnsson Foundation Porvoo, Finland, August 1996. Copenhagen: Munksgaard, 1998. Pp 59–65.

80. DiLuzio NR. Update on the immunomodulation activities of the glucans. *Springer Semin Immunopathol* 1985;8:387–400.

81. Fogelmark B, Sjostrand M, Rylander R, et al. Pulmonary inflammation induced by repeated inhalations of (1,3)-β-D-glucan and endotoxin. *Int J Exp Pathol* 1994;75:85–90.

82. Rylander R. Investigations of the relationship between disease and airborne (1,3)-β-D-glucan in buildings. *Mediators Inflam* 1997;6:275–7.

83. Rylander R, Norrhall M, Engdahl U, et al. Airways inflammation, atopy, and (1,3)-β-D-glucan exposures in two schools. *Am J Respir Crit Care Med* 1998:158:1685–7.

84. Rylander R, Snella MC. Endotoxins and the lung: Cellular reactions and risk for disease. *Prog Allergy* 1983;33:332–44.

85. Milton DK. Endotoxin and other bacterial cell wall components. In Macher J (ed), *Bioaerosols: Assessment and Control.* Cincinnati, OH: American Conference of Governmental Industrial Hygienists, 1999. Pp 23-1–23-14.

86. Huttunen K, Pelkonen J, Nielsen KF, et al. Synergistic interaction in simultaneous exposure to *Streptomyces californicus* and *Stachybotrys chartarum.* *Environ Health Perspect* 2004;112:659–65.

87. Penttinen P, Huttunen K, Pelkonen J, et al. The proportions of *Streptomyces californicus* and *Stachybotrys chartarum* in simultaneous exposure affect inflammatory responses in mouse REW264.7 macrophages. *Inhal Toxicol* 2005;17:79–85.

88. Murtoniemi T, Penttinen P, Nevalainen A, et al. Effects of microbial cocultivation on inflammatory and cytotoxic potential of spores. *Inhal Toxicol.* 2005;17:681–93.

89. Luosujarvi RA, Husman TM, Seuri M, et al. Joint

symptoms and diseases associated with moisture damage in a health center. *Clin Rheumatol* 2004;22: 381–5.

90. Rose C. Hypersensitivity pneumonitis. In Harber P, Schenker MB, Balmes JR (eds), *Occupatonal and Environmental Respiratory Disease.* St Louis: Mosby, 1996. Pp 201–15.

91. Hajjeh RA. Disseminated histoplasmosis is persons infected with human immunodeficiency virus. *Clin Infect Dis* 1995;21:108–10S.

92. Ampel NM. Emerging disease issues and fungal pathogens associated with HIV infection. *Emerg Infec Dis* 1996;2:109–16.

39 Biologic Agents Applied to Warfare and Terrorism

Tee L. Guidotti, Marina S. Moses, Harold E. Hoffman

Biologic threats in warfare and terrorism are regrettably of interest in occupational and environmental health because workforce protection, individual worker protection, emergency management, and coordination with public health agencies are essential duties of the occupational physician. The threat of bioterrorism has led to a reinvestment in public health, a greater appreciation of public and occupational health practitioners as first responders, and an emphasis on coordination with emergency response and security agencies. [1] The threat of biological weapons is likely to continue well into the future. These weapons pose a particular threat in the hands of small, unpredictable terrorist groups and countries with limited resources that feel under extreme military pressure [2].

Occupational health practitioners are part of the response team, whether they like it or not. Many lives might be saved following an assault if occupational health care providers understand the biologic agents, their associated syndromes, preventive measures, modes of weaponization and deliver, hazard identification, immunization, early surveillance, principles of isolation and precautions, and early treatment. Considerable preparation among civilian health providers is required for adequate education, training, and response in the event of biological warfare [3].

Occupational physicians and preventive medical officers in the military have long been trained in the characteristics of weaponized biologic agents and the diseases they cause when intentionally disseminated. Occupational physicians in civilian life in the United States have been systematically trained in this field only relatively recently, beginning in the late 1990s, when bioterrorism emerged as a credible threat. The version of this chapter in the first edition of this book was one of the first efforts to make this important information available to occupational health professionals. In 2000, the American College of Occupational and Environmental Medicine undertook an urgent program to prepare occupational physicians by providing training sessions at its annual meetings and in its basic curriculum, which were well attended. Following the anthrax assaults in 2001 and the lethal demonstration of dissemination of anthrax in the workplace, occupational physicians and other occupational health professionals almost universally have had some introduction to this topic. Unfortunately, the training continues to be relevant and necessary [4, 5]. Fortunately, the training is also relevant to other applications, in particular surveillance and contingency planning for similar common-source outbreaks, as was demonstrated in surveillance during the outbreak of West Nile virus in 1999 [6] and the management of the SARS outbreak in 2003 [7].

Biological warfare and bioterrorism are closely related but distinct problems of security and health risk. Both are intentional uses of biologic agents, perverting the principles of public health. Both are crimes against humanity. Biological warfare is the use of biologic agents (1) to kill or disable combatants and targeted noncombatant people for strategic purposes in war, (2) as a strategic weapon to threaten people, or (3) to deny the use of terrain to opposing forces in warfare. Crude forms of biological warfare have been deployed and used throughout history. In the twentieth century, taking advantage of the scientific revolution in biology and, later, biotechnology, most of the world's great armies and several lesser forces developed arsenals of biological weapons and at times were prepared to use them. Because of its horror, the risk of suffering for noncombatants, the risk of infecting large populations beyond combatants, and perhaps decisively, opinions on its impracticality in battlefield tactics, biological warfare was outlawed by international treaty, which may have slowed but did not stop its proliferation. Biological warfare, therefore, is the conduct of warfare by means that are assumed in civilian opinion to be unconventional only because they have not been prominent historically in actual battles in recent times. In the past, biologic agents were not considered practical for modern warfare because they were indiscriminate, difficult to control, and delayed in their effect. In that sense, biological warfare, like nuclear war, has been a threat more than a battlefield reality [3, 8].

Bioterrorism is an assault using biologic agents, or the threat of using them, against civilian populations or against military personnel outside combat in the context of terrorism, which is discussed further below. In recent years, however, small groups, whose apparent aim is to cause fear and confusion, have used them for indiscriminate urban terrorism. Since these efforts are likely to continue, health professionals need to consider biological warfare in disaster planning and in the evaluation of unusual or suggestive outbreaks of disease.

Terrorism is an elusive concept. Since 1937, when the League of Nations and later the United Nations began to debate the matter, there has been no agreement on an internationally accepted definition of terrorism despite debates resulting in the passage of 12 conventions on the suppression of terrorism. This is so because acts widely viewed as terrorism have played a role in numerous liberation movements and are selectively viewed by some as legitimate tools of resistance. The closest approximation to an internationally recognized legal definition of terrorism is that incorporated in United Nations General Assembly Resolution 51/210 (1992), which states: "criminal acts intended or calculated to provoke a state of terror in the general public, a group of persons or particular persons for political purposes are in any circumstance unjustifiable, whatever the considerations of a political, philosophical, ideological, racial, ethnic, religious or other nature that may be invoked to justify them" [9]. Under this resolution, acts of terrorism are considered under international law to be the peacetime equivalent of war crimes. The definition has been further elaborated by Schmidt [10] as follows:

> Terrorism is an anxiety-inspiring method of repeated violent action, employed by (semi-) clandestine individual, group or state actors, for idiosyncratic, criminal or political reasons, whereby—in contrast to assassination—the direct targets of violence are not the main targets. The immediate human victims of violence are generally chosen randomly (targets of opportunity) or selectively (representative or symbolic targets) from a target population, and serve as message generators. Threat- and violence-based communication processes between terrorist (organization), (imperiled) victims, and main targets are used to manipulate the main target (audience(s)), turning it into a target of terror, a target of demands, or a target of attention, depending on whether intimidation, coercion, or propaganda is primarily sought.

Federal agencies use the definition of terrorism contained in Title 22 of the U.S. Code, Section 2656f(d): "[P]remeditated, politically motivated violence perpetrated against noncombatant targets by subnational groups or clandestine agents, usually intended to influence an audience." This definition does not include the use of terrorist tactics by states or groups sponsored by states. Bioterrorism exists on the boundary of this definition because some terrorist groups may access biologic materials originally developed for biological warfare, and some countries may have encouraged or permitted development of biologic agents by terrorists groups on their territory.

Bioterrorism incidents are (and, one hopes, will remain) exceedingly rare. There have been several attempts and at least two known successful assaults in the United States (The Dalles, Oregon, in 1984 [11] and the anthrax assault in the fall of 2001 [8, 12]). However, frequent outbreaks of "emerging infections" in the United States are now common, recently including West Nile virus, severe adult respiratory syndrome (SARS), mad cow disease, monkeypox, many antibiotic-resistant strains of bacteria, and measles (because of scandalously low—frankly negligent—immunization rates among American children). At the time of this writing, public health agencies are on guard against a potentially devastating threat of avian influenza (H5N1). All this new activity has taken place against the backdrop of the numerous small outbreaks of food-borne, water-borne, and airborne diseases that, in the aggregate, already kill thousands of Americans each year.

History

The antecedents of biological warfare and terrorism run deep in history. In biblical times, the Egyptians were said to have been visited by a series of plagues by God in order to force them to free the enslaved Israelites. Regardless of the historical events that gave rise to this passage, it is vivid and speaks to the intentional use of a biologic threat. In ancient history, the Greeks and Romans condemned biological warfare. Toxins were considered inhumane in warfare and were forbidden by the Manu Law of India around 500 BC. Biologic threats were used in the Middle Ages as tactics to break sieges. Bodies of plague victims were catapulted into the city of Kaffa (now Feodosia) by the besieging Mongols in the fourteenth century. The ensuing flight of refugees is thought by scholars to have spread the Black Plague across Europe [2]. In 1763, blankets from a smallpox hospital were given to Native Americans on orders of a British army officer with the intention of creating an epidemic of smallpox, a deliberate act of genocide that appears to have killed thousands [13, 14].

The modern history of biological warfare began in 1919, when the Bolsheviks, who were losing the Russian Civil War, adopted a policy of weaponizing pathogens as a desperate measure to counter superior Menshevik and invading forces, leading directly to the subsequent Soviet effort to produce biological weapons. The 1925 Geneva Protocol forbade the use of bacterial agents in war. However, at one time or another over subsequent decades, most of the great armies of Europe tried to develop some capability in biological weapons, and biological warfare research has been conducted throughout the twentieth century, often for defensive purposes but sometimes covertly for offensive purposes. The greatest commitment between the two World Wars was that of Japan, which in 1937 developed a widespread and elaborate program with laboratories scattered throughout China and occupied Southeast Asia, directed by the infamous Unit 731 in Manchuria and led by Ishii Shiro, a distinguished public health scientist who turned war criminal. Research on biologic agents was conducted on human subjects in Japanese-occupied Manchuria and elsewhere in China and Southeast Asia, most notably by the infamous "731 battalion." The degradations of human experimentation and intentional epidemics continue to haunt survivors to this day [13–15]. These events are documented in a museum dedicated to the incident near Harbin, in Heilongjiang Province.

Biological warfare research continued and even accelerated during the Cold War despite the availability of nuclear weapons because biologic agents were seen as one rung below nuclear in the stepladder of escalation. Military doctrine initially held that they could be used without provoking nuclear retaliation when the use of nuclear weapons would be blocked by the risk of mutual annihilation. Later, this doctrine changed with the declaration in the 1960s that NATO reserved the right to use nuclear weapons to repel Soviet aggression using overwhelming force by conventional weapons, which rendered the issue of escalation involving biological weapons moot [16]. The Soviet weaponization program, Biopreparat, became both a major force in the military industry and a distorting force in scientific research in the Soviet Union. Concern over this escalation and the risk of uninhibited proliferation of biologic agents prompted a small group of advocates, mostly scientists, to press for biological weapons disarmament, especially after 1954, when an early treaty imposed an obligation on Germany not to produce biological weapons. This movement, largely pushed by the British, crested in an effort to revisit and strengthen the

Geneva Convention of 1925 and resulted in the Biological Weapons Convention of 1971. The United States refused to sign this new treaty, however, because it was thought to restrict measures necessary for defensive research. In 1969, however, after pressure from Matthew Meselson and other prominent scientists, President Richard Nixon announced that the United States was unilaterally renouncing biological weapons and would destroy its stockpiles, except for small quantities needed for research to ensure adequate defense. In 1975, the United States ratified both the Biological Weapons Convention and the 1925 Geneva Protocol and rapidly carried out the destruction of stocks [17].

Until 1990, just before the Gulf War, scientific knowledge regarding the possible effects of an attack using anthrax and botulism agents was limited largely to reconstruction of an event of uncontrolled release of anthrax that had occurred in a Biopreparat facility in Sverdlovsk (now and historically Ekatrinburg) in 1979. The major risks to combatants in the Gulf War were thought to be anthrax spores and *Clostridium botulinum* toxin [18]. In the invasion of Iraq in 2002, the use of biological weapons in combat was anticipated but never materialized, and weaponization facilities have not been found.

On the other hand, a series of assaults using anthrax occurred in the fall of 2001, following only 2 weeks after the September 11 attack on the World Trade Center and the Pentagon. The targets for these assaults were communications facilities (print media and television) and the U.S. Congress. These assaults featured anthrax carried in the mail in letter envelopes, resulting in five deaths and several infections [19]. The perpetrator and motive are still not known. The incident pointed out the vulnerability of occupational groups handling mail, a group previously not recognized to be at risk. Studies conducted using simulants just months earlier at the Canadian Forces Base Suffield had already demonstrated the effectiveness of paper mail envelopes (which act as bellows when compressed) to disseminate weaponized spores, but this information was not immediately available at the time of the crisis.

Weaponization

Biological weapons require some technologic expertise but are easy to conceal, require small quan-

tities of starting material, and are difficult to detect in real time. Dispersion of biologic agents requires relatively low levels of technology, modest financial resources, and minimal training [2, 20, 21].

The most likely biological warfare tactic is release of an agent into the air as a biologic aerosol, which would create a persistent cloud of suspended microscopic droplets or dry particles of bacteria or viruses. For optimal attack advantage, the aerosol particle size would be approximately 1–20 μm, generating particles that can remain suspended in the air for hours. When inhaled, these particles penetrate into the lower respiratory tract efficiently. Because the aerosol would be undetectable by the human senses and requires special, locally placed instrumentation to detect, the target population would not identify an attack until health effects occurred. Agents also might be introduced into air-conditioning systems or, conceivably, into the water supply, especially if infection controls are inadequate.

Tactically, a biological warfare attack is not very efficient in the battlefield. The effects are delayed, whether mediated by infection or toxins, and this allows time for retaliation. The agents dispersed in air may expose the attacker's own troops or population centers if there is a change in the direction of the wind. Highly communicable agents would interfere with the occupation of enemy positions and territory after the attack, even if occupying troops were immunized. However, these tactical limitations are less of a drawback for acts of terrorism, wherein randomness of position and the horrific effects on a population are used to foster confusion, fear, and distrust.

Biologic Agents of Terrorism

Many biologic agents could be used for warfare or terrorism: bacteria, viruses, rickettsiae, and the toxins of microbes, plants, or animals. Toxins are high-molecular-weight compounds produced by organisms; they tend to act much faster than infectious agents. The diseases of primary concern include anthrax, smallpox, plague, tularemia, viral hemorrhagic fevers, viral encephalitis, and the botulinum toxin. Agents of secondary concern include brucellosis, Q fever, and staphylococcal enterotoxin B (SEB) [2, 4, 14, 21].

A sophisticated, especially state-sponsored terrorist group could easily engineer a pathogen with special characteristics. These might include drug resistance, toxin production, and characteristics to make it more infectious or more easily dispersed. It is therefore conceivable that the usual presentations of disease and the natural history may be quite different in a bioterrorist assault. However, it remains most likely that perpetrators will use wild-type agents or pathogens that otherwise follow the usual clinical pattern [3, 4, 8].

The descriptions and treatment recommendations outlined below are for general preparation and briefing purposes for general readers. In the event of an actual event or patient management issue, the reader is advised to consult the recommendations of the Centers for Disease Control and Prevention (www.cdc.gov) or, in Canada, the Public Health Agency of Canada. Most of the information below on biologic threats is summarized from a series of reviews prepared by the so-named Working Group on Civilian Biodefense, which was published in the *Journal of the American Medical Association,* and pathogen-specific information available on the CDC website with periodic updating. References cited below should be considered to be supplemental to these primary sources. Another source useful for the occupational physician is a special issue of *Clinics in Occupational and Environmental Medicine* in 2003 [22].

ANTHRAX

The anthrax bacillus is the biologic agent considered to be the greatest threat to civilian populations owing to its relative ease of manufacture, the favorable dispersion characteristics of its spores, and its lethality [2, 12, 23]. Anthrax is noncommunicable. Outbreaks resulting directly or indirectly from intentional use have occurred at least twice.

In the Russian Urals in 1979, an outbreak occurred in Yekatrinburg (then known by its Soviet name of Sverdlovsk) owing to an unintentional release in the early morning resulting from a failure to replace a filter on an exhaust vent in a secret military compound devoted to producing biological weapons. The resulting outbreak caused 79 cases and 68 fatalities among humans (and many more among animals) and remains the source of most clinical information on the human natural history of the inhalational form of the disease [2].

In the United States, in September 2001, a series of letters containing processed (weaponized) an-

thrax spores was mailed from Trenton, New Jersey, ultimately infecting 22 people and killing 5, including 2 postal workers, and causing several cases of cutaneous anthrax. The perpetrator has never been identified. Because most of the exposures took place in the victim's place of work and were incurred in the course of doing his or her job, anthrax clearly is an occupational health risk, although public health authorities were late in recognizing this aspect of the problem. The occupational health issues that arose involving the Washington, DC, postal workers in particular played out as frantic exaggerations of the response to more typical health hazards in the workplace, with all the attendant lack of communication and uncertainty [12, 24].

Anthrax is caused by *Bacillus anthracis,* an exceptionally large gram-positive spore-forming bacillus that is a soil saprophyte. Anthrax spores can survive adverse environmental conditions and remain viable for many decades. Naturally occurring in cattle, sheep, and wildlife, anthrax is widespread in the soil. Natural human infection is exceedingly rare today but was once a common and feared occupational disease in the wool industry and in occupations involving contact with raw hides and goat- and horsehair.

Anthrax produces three clinical syndromes in human beings, none of them spread by person-to-person transmission. Gastrointestinal anthrax is a rare infection caused by eating contaminated meat, causing massive bowel necrosis, and will not be discussed further. Cutaneous anthrax and inhalational anthrax are the greater risks following an assault with anthrax.

Cutaneous anthrax occurs when the anthrax spore enters through a wound or break in the skin. A vesicle is formed initially, followed within a few days of infection by a characteristic necrotic eschar surrounded by a brawny, nonpitting edema. Cutaneous anthrax was observed among several victims during the anthrax assaults of 2001 [25, 26].

Inhalational anthrax occurs when spores are dispersed through aerosolization and inhaled. In the lungs, the spores are phagocytized and transported to hilar and mediastinal lymph nodes. The spores germinate into vegetative (live bacteria) bacilli, producing a necrotizing hemorrhagic mediastinitis. Inhalational anthrax begins with a nonspecific prodrome, lasting a few days, of fever, malaise, and fatigue, after a latency of 3 to as long as 43 days or possibly longer, reflecting delayed germination of the spores [3]. Within 2–3 more days, there is often a period of apparent recovery, followed by a rapid downhill course characterized by hemorrhagic shock, vascular collapse, respiratory failure, and septicemia. A pathognomonic sign of the disease is an acutely widening mediastinum on the chest film, a manifestation of the edema and inflammation extending beyond the draining nodes [27, 28].

The pathophysiology of the disease reflects the release of three bacterial products: protective antigen (a highly specialized protein that inserts the other factors into cells), edema factor (which floods the cell with cAMP), and lethal factor (which interferes with cell signaling). The anthrax bacillus is protected by a poly-D-glutamic acid capsule that makes it difficult for macrophages to clear.

If untreated, inhalational anthrax has a mortality rate of about 95% from multiple-organ failure [3]. Recommended treatment includes life support, intravenous quinolone antibiotics (such as ciprofloxacin), and immunization against anthrax in order to produce an immune response that will protect against late-germinating spores untouched by antibiotic treatment. As the anthrax assaults of 2001 demonstrated, treatment does not prevent high mortality if it is started after symptoms appear in the second phase [12].

In contrast to the dire prognosis of advanced inhalational anthrax, prophylaxis is highly effective and can be efficacious for some days after infection. If anthrax exposure or early infection can be recognized before major symptoms appear, the prognosis is good. The CDC recommends a course of doxycycline for 60 days. In 2001, ciprofloxacin was recommended initially, but it is associated with many side effects. There appears to be no advantage to it in prophylaxis, and widespread use, as might be required if a population were subject to airborne assault, carries a risk of emergent multiorganism resistance at a time when the quinolones may be needed as antibiotics of last resort. If available, immunization is also highly effective in the early days following infection.

The anthrax vaccine currently in use is not practical for civilian use for prophylaxis, requiring six administrations: at 0, 2, and 4 weeks and at 6, 12, and 18 months [3]. A protective antibody response does not develop until 7 days after the second dose [3].

The vaccine has a nuisance side effect of soreness and nodules at the site of injection but, despite controversy, no evidence of serious side effects [29, 30].

Evaluation of the patient suspected of exposure to anthrax rests on the assessment of exposure opportunity. In a typical "white powder" incident, in which a material claimed to be anthrax has been sent through the mail or otherwise delivered, there is time to identify the agent before initiating treatment with potentially significant side effects. Nasal swabs are very useful for recovering the agent in situations where aerosolization has occurred in the presence of the patient and are used for defining the perimeters of exposure. Nasal swabs are used for the purpose of mapping exposure but are not considered to be reliable indicators of infection in the individual patient.

Several products have appeared for rapid confirmation of anthrax, some of which are overly sensitive and not very specific and so lead to many false-positive results. Culture takes about 2 days. Polymerase chain reaction (PCR) analysis has become the method of choice for early identification. As the disease progresses, the bacteremia becomes obvious and may even be visible on a Gram stain of a blood smear.

Weaponizing anthrax involves producing spores in large quantities, drying them, and milling them in the presence of a coating, which reduces electrostatic charge and the tendency of small particles to aggregate. A delivery system that disperses the spores, which are of respirable dimensions (about 2 μm in diameter), requires more sophisticated engineering than an unconverted crop duster (a frequently mentioned scenario) but can be constructed readily by someone with appropriate engineering expertise. The dry aerosol would be easily spread in a conventional plume from the source, exposing many people in densely populated urban areas.

Further complicating the very real threat of assault, hoaxes involving anthrax have been very common. Fear of delivery by mail has been a particular concern. Numerous anthrax scares have been perpetrated by sending letters or packages that included an unidentified or falsely identified white power in the envelope. Suspicious mail should be opened inside clear plastic bags, by persons wearing gloves, in order to prevent aerosolization in the event that the envelope contains anthrax spores [30]. Unfortunately, the original recommendation specified latex gloves, but any impermeable glove material will do. Latex is unnecessary and presents a risk of latex allergy, which can be a serious health risk and a career-limiting condition for health and laboratory professionals.

SMALLPOX

Smallpox is one of many similar diseases affecting many species that are caused by poxviruses, a family of large capsulated DNA viruses. The variola virus causes smallpox in human beings [31–35].

Smallpox is highly communicable through droplet aerosols. First responders and health providers would be at risk if the virus were released in a bioterrorism incident. Persons who have been immunized in the past are partially protected, but since 1972, immunization against smallpox for the general population ceased in the United States because the risk of the vaccine exceeded the risk of contracting the disease. This means that most Americans born since have no immunity.

Historically, there have been many devastating smallpox outbreaks. Several severe outbreaks occurred in the late-middle decades of the twentieth century, notably in Kosovo in 1972, in India in 1972, in Bradford (UK) in 1962, and in an incident thought to be directly related to weapons testing, in Soviet Kazakhstan in 1971 [2]. Smallpox was the first disease to be preventable by a vaccine, by Edward Jenner in 1796, and vaccination provided the instrument for eradicating the disease in 1977. Global eradication was officially declared by the World Health Organization (WHO) in 1979. Subsequent to that, however, there have been laboratory accidents resulting in fatalities. Reintroduction of the virus would go beyond terrorism and should be considered a crime against all humanity.

There are several forms of the disease, as listed in Table 39-1, with different prognoses [34]. Because of its eradication, few practicing physicians have actually seen a case, and so there is a reduced capacity to identify smallpox in all its variety. Ordinary smallpox begins about 12 days after infection with a spiking fever, which is an invariant feature of the disease, associated with severe prostration, severe headache, and backache, and accompanied in most patients with chills and vomiting and in some with delirium, abdominal pain, diarrhea, and convulsions. Shortly thereafter, an enanthem appears

Table 39-1
Forms of Smallpox and Case-Fatality Rates With and Without Immunization

Variety	Naive	Vaccinated
Ordinary smallpox, all	30	3
Ordinary, confluent	62	26
Ordinary, semiconfluent	37	8
Ordinary, discrete	9	<1
Modified (accelerated), v. minor	0	0
Flat type	97	67
Hemorrhagic, early (into skin)	100	100
Hemorrhagic, late (into pustules)	97	90

Source: Rao AR. *Smallpox.* Bombay: Kothari Book Depot, 1972.

in the oropharynx, visible as tiny petechial spots on the tongue and soft palate and severe pharyngeal pain. The appearance of the enanthem signals the release of the virus into oral secretions and the risk of person-to-person transmission. Within a few days, the skin rash, or exanthema, appears, first as maculopapular, erythematous "herald spots" on the face and progressing to shotty, indurated pox lesions similar at first to that of other pox diseases but later umbilicated. Although smallpox resembles other pox diseases, such as chickenpox, monkeypox, camelpox, and cowpox, it has distinguishing characteristics: The pustules begin and are more dense on the extremities rather than the trunk, sit on an erythematous skin lesion, may involve soles and palms, and are of uniform maturity.

Smallpox has a high mortality rate in all its forms except the uncommon variola minor form. The disease also causes dread complications, including a scarring conjunctivitis and keratitis, osteomyelitis, and encephalitis (which has a good prognosis if the patient survives). Severe, permanent facial scarring may occur. The vesicles may become superinfected. Respiratory infection may occur but is characteristically without a cough [34].

Management is not currently satisfactory, although there are antiviral agents under investigation (without the possibility of clinical trials). Immunization up to the first few days of the prodromal symptoms is effective in preventing smallpox after exposure. Supportive care and infection control procedures (type C in the CDC definition) impose a heavy burden on health care facilities and place unimmunized caregivers at an unacceptable risk. Confinement should be restricted to dedicated isolation facilities, which raises obvious issues of identification, isolation, and safe transport. Fortunately, the poxvirus is relatively easily disinfected.

A sufficient quantity of smallpox vaccine, which is based on live vaccinia virus (the virus originally associated with cowpox), now exists to protect the U.S. population in the event of mass immunization. However, the vaccine carries a relatively high risk of serious side effects (about 3×10^{-6}), 40% of which are fatal. There are also many contraindications to the vaccine, including such common conditions as acute inflammatory skin diseases, a history of eczema, pregnancy, and immunosuppression. These contraindications are absolute for prevent prophylaxis but following an actual event would be ignored for persons exposed in the interests of giving them the best chance of survival. Because it is a live virus, there are a number of unpleasant but benign side effects to the vaccine and several complications, some of them potentially serious but rare. The live virus also presents a risk to intimate, household contacts, who are at risk owing to pregnancy or immunosuppression after inadvertent secondary infection [33, 35].

Immunization against smallpox is the primary strategy for protecting the population. The first public health response presumably would be "ring immunization," attempting to "surround" the case by immunizing all contacts to prevent transmission. However, models have come to a consistent conclusion that ring immunization would work only for a small outbreak in a population of low density. An urban outbreak would, almost inevitably, require mass immunization [34–37].

An effective program would require a cadre of qualified, immunized, and specially trained vaccinators because the bifurcated applicator and puncture method of application are unique to smallpox immunization. In 2002, the federal government launched a program to prepare such a cadre of vaccinators, but it fell far short of goals and foundered on issues of compensation for adverse effects and liability issues [34].

PLAGUE

Plague is one of the great scourges of humankind, called the "Black Death" in the Middle Ages. It is caused by a small gram-negative coccobacillus, *Yersinia pestis*. The pathogen is transmitted by fleas and is endemic in the United States and central Asia [38–40].

There are three major clinical forms of the disease and several minor forms. Bubonic plague, the most familiar, is characterized by sudden onset of fever, chills, and prostration, accompanied by visibly erupting, painful inflamed lymph nodes 2–8 days after infection. Plague septicemia is sometimes a primary manifestation of the disease but usually occurs as a sequela of the bubonic form. Pneumonic plague, likewise, may occur as a primary manifestation when infection occurs by the inhalation route or may be an end stage of bubonic plague. Although historically some patients with bubonic plague survived, the great majority who do not receive treatment die, as do all patients with septicemia and pneumonic plague. In modern times, the fatality rate of all types is 14% for bubonic, 22% for septicemic, and 57% for pneumonic plague, all of which improve with early identification and treatment.

Plague is easily weaponized and was considered to be the Soviet Union's main biological weapon. Following an airborne biologic assault, widespread, rapidly progressive primary pneumonic plague would be the most likely presentation after an incubation of 2–4 days. A vaccine against plague has been developed, but it was not very protective, failed to prevent pneumonic plague, and was discontinued in 1999. Fortunately, the plague bacillus is very sensitive to antibiotics. Streptomycin is the antibiotic therapy of choice for treatment, with alternate choices for women during pregnancy. During mass casualties, recommendations change to doxycycline or ciprofloxacin. Postexposure prophylaxis with doxycycline or ciprofloxacin is also recommended. Isolation of patients is required, and medical personnel should take appropriate precautions.

TULAREMIA

Tularemia (also known as *rabbit fever* or *deer fly fever*) is a serious but usually not lethal (15% case-fatality rate) systemic bacterial infection with *Francisella tularensis*, a small gram-negative nonmotile coccobacillus. In most forms, this illness is characterized by an unusual "chancriform" lesion resembling a syphilitic chancre that is a painful, persistent ulcer with a black necrotic base, usually at the point of inoculation and variably elsewhere. It is similar to plague and as incapacitating in the short term but generally less severe, and like plague, it may present in several variants, with or without ulcers (e.g., ulceroglandular, oculoglandular, oropharyngeal, pneumonic, and typhoidal, the latter two being disseminated forms of the disease). Each form may result in prostration and pulmonary involvement, with an incubation period of 1–10 days [39, 40].

Tularemia is common and widespread over much of the northern hemisphere, including the United States, Canada, Scandinavia, northern Japan, and especially Russia. It is an occupational disease of hunters and trappers. Tularemia is transmitted by ticks, deer flies, and fleas, but the latter are inconsequential for human transmission. Tularemia also may be transmitted through contact with mucous membranes and by ingestion, in which cases the characteristic primary ulcer may not be seen. The minimum infectious dose of tularemia organism is very low, possibly as low as 10 organisms, making it among the most infectious bacterial disorders known.

Fortunately, tularemia is relatively easy to treat. Streptomycin is the antibiotic treatment of choice, although tetracyclines and chloramphenicol also can be used. Because person-to-person transmission is not thought to occur, standard precautions are considered sufficient. There is an effective vaccine available.

VIRAL HEMORRHAGIC FEVER

The viral hemorrhagic fevers (VHFs) are a heterogeneous group of highly communicable disorders that could be more lethal than anthrax in a biologic assault but are difficult to culture [39]. They are readily dispersed by aerosolization or water contamination. The VHFs caused by filoviruses, especially Ebola and Marburg viruses, are of greatest concern, followed by Rift Valley fever, a much milder disease that is caused by a bunyavirus but which sometimes causes blindness. Only the Marburg strain has been effectively weaponized (by the former Soviet Union), although it is theoretically possible to weaponize both Rift Valley fever and Ebola, and the Soviet Union was working on an Ebola weapon as late as the 1980s. Other VHFs include machupo (endemic in Bolivia, an arenavirus), junin (endemic in Argentina, also an arenavirus), and Congo-Crimean hemorrhagic fever (caused by a bunyavirus).

The common features of the VHFs include an incubation period of about 4–16 days, a nonspecific prodromal illness resembling malaria, with a high fever, and a rapidly fatal course thereafter owing to shock associated with vascular leak and third-spacing, disseminated intravascular coagulation, hemorrhage, and multiple-organ-system failure. There is no specific treatment or vaccine for any disease in the group.

The spread of an outbreak is effectively prevented by strict barrier techniques, and the viruses are easily decontaminated.

TOXINS
Botulinum Toxin

Botulinum toxins are proteins produced by the anaerobic bacteria *C. botulinum*, a spore-forming gram-positive bacillus under anaerobic conditions at pH levels above 4.5. Botulinum toxin is the most toxic compound known: 1 pg is lethal to human beings. The toxin exists in seven distinct antigenic types, all of which are heat-sensitive. It acts by binding to the presynaptic nerve terminal at neuromuscular junctions and at cholinergic autonomic sites, irreversibly blocking acetylcholine release. This interrupts neurotransmission, causing bulbar palsies and skeletal muscle weakness. Bulbar palsies begin with dysarthria, dysphonia, dysphagia, and ocular symptoms such as blurred vision. Skeletal muscle paralysis progresses from a symmetric, descending weakness to respiratory failure. Symptoms appear 12–72 hours after ingestion or inhalation of contaminated food. Initial symptoms are nausea and diarrhea, followed by weakness, dizziness, and progressive respiratory paralysis. Mental status, cruelly, is preserved. Care is supportive. A pentavalent vaccine is available as an investigational new drug. Antitoxin sometimes can arrest the process [39].

The use of this agent actually would be a form of chemical attack. Botulism toxin can be "weaponized" by aerosol generators, including simple spray cans, or contamination of food. The Soviet Union attempted to introduce genes that would produce botulinum toxic into weaponized bacteria to increase the lethality of the bioweapon.

Staphylococcal Enterotoxin B

Staphylococcal enterotoxin B (SEB) is produced by *Staphylococcus* bacteria and has its major effects on the gastrointestinal tract. SEB is extremely toxic, rendering a high proportion of exposed people very ill within a few hours. In biological warfare, dispersion would most likely be through aerosolization; SEB may incapacitate humans many miles downwind from release. SEB also might be used to sabotage food or water supplies [39].

BRUCELLOSIS

Brucellosis is caused by small, slow-growing, gram-negative, non-spore-forming coccobacilli of the genus *Brucella*. Brucellosis is not generally transmitted from person to person, although rare transmission by sexual contact or breast milk has been noted. Natural transmission of *Brucella* occurs primarily through contact with infected animals and unpasteurized milk. Brucellae are highly infectious through aerosolization and may survive for 6 weeks in dust and 10 weeks in soil or water. Weaponized organisms could be delivered in slurry by bombs or as a dry aerosol. No vaccine is available. Isolation of patients is not considered necessary [39].

Q FEVER

Q fever is caused by *Coxiella burnetii*, which is an intracellular rickettsia-like bacteria. The sporelike form can withstand heat and drying and can survive on inanimate surfaces for weeks or months. A single organism is sufficient to cause the disease in humans. This organism can be disseminated by wind, inducing infection miles from the source. The acute disease is self-limited. Chronic disease develops in less than 1% of acute infections, but fatigue may occur for months, and an endocarditis may result. The case-fatality rate of acute Q fever is low, even without treatment. A vaccine is available in Australia [39].

ENCEPHALITIDES

Equine encephalitis viruses are highly infectious by aerosolization. These viruses can be produced in large amounts in inexpensive and unsophisticated systems, and they are relatively stable during storage. No vaccine is available [39].

Countermeasures

Prevention of biological warfare is ultimately possible only by limiting the development and production of biological weapons. The use of biologic agents would be a crime against humanity, and full deterrence must be adopted by the international community. Education is a vital factor because it increases awareness of the threat.

Countermeasures for biological warfare include intelligence and appropriate intervention, detection devices, epidemiologic identification of biologic attacks, and use of personal protective equipment, vaccines, diagnostic modalities, and treatments.

Defense against biological warfare requires early and, preferably, advance knowledge of the organism used in an attack. For countermeasures to be effective, the organism needs to be vulnerable to medical intervention. Immunization and treatment requirements need to be anticipated.

Immunization can be performed against certain agents. Active immunization may be useful for military forces, but civilian populations probably cannot be protected adequately in this manner before an event. If vaccines are available, the causative agents must be determined quickly so that relief workers can prepare and administer these agents. Unfortunately, vaccines are not available for many agents.

Prophylactic medications such as antibiotics are effective against some bacterial agents but are not effective against viruses. To prevent infectious disease, appropriate antibiotic therapy must begin within a few hours of exposure, before symptoms appear. Obviously, this is not possible in the event of a massive attack.

Personal protective equipment needs to be available to protect relief workers. Respirators or gas masks require filter canisters that have activated charcoal to remove simple organic molecules, such as nerve gas, by adsorption. The paper filter in the canister removes particulates larger than 0.3 μm in size. Large populations will not wear gas masks for long periods of time. Some people feel claustrophobic in them, and others with respiratory disorders cannot use them. In hot weather, people are not able to tolerate a facemask for more than a few minutes at a time.

Clothing protects against contact with open wounds or broken skin. Protective shelter, in a closed room insulated with plastic and ventilated with filtered air, may be effective in airborne attacks but requires substantial preparation. Although sunlight and ambient temperatures destroy most agents, and surfaces can be decontaminated with disinfectants, anthrax spores survive for decades and are not easily killed.

Early detection systems are needed, but only rudimentary field units for a few specific agents are currently available. Electronic detection devices, when available, should be placed in high-risk locations, where an attack is likely. Medical detection involves the identification and reporting of suspicious diseases. Epidemiologic evaluation will determine a pattern of disease but is likely to come too late to affect the course of the biologic effects of attack.

Although clinical tests can reliably detect and identify a biologic agent, they are dependent on optimal procedures. During an attack, it is unlikely that there will be time for such tests or that the equipment will always be operational. In warfare or terrorist conditions, substances such as engine exhaust, dust, dirt, chemical fumes, and fuel residue may interfere with the tests.

Most diseases resulting from biological warfare present nonspecific signs and symptoms that could be misinterpreted as natural occurrences. Initially, a point-source outbreak of disease likely would occur. Individuals in the attacked population would come into contact with the agent at approximately the same time, with a peak incidence for the most likely agent occurring within hours or at most days. The incubation period for a virus, bacterium, or toxin could be several days, but toxins require no incubation period.

In the event of an assault, a likely scenario would be the unnoticed release of a biologic agent. When widespread effects on the attacked population become apparent, the health system would need to quickly detect the disease outbreak and begin prompt treatment for large numbers of exposed people. The immediate task for health personnel would be to confirm the existence of an outbreak.

In addition to the adverse health effects on the general population, biological warfare agents would have an impact on the health care system. A biological terrorist attack could cause thousands of casualties requiring prompt medical attention. The biologic agent also could contaminate air, water, and food supplies, and the local health resources could be overwhelmed. An act of overt biological warfare could result in hundreds of thousands or even millions of casualties. Patients would present in unprecedented numbers, overwhelming the medical resources.

After the onset of illness from biological warfare, diagnosis of the disease, specific medical treatment, and general supportive care over the long term will be required. Health care workers need the protection of personal protective equipment and education about work practices, including the psychological reactions of survivors and health professionals, as well as the medical management of victims.

The immediacy of the threat of bioterrorism has prompted federal agencies, led by the Department of Homeland Security, to introduce a variety of purpose-built and highly targeted programs for the detection of potential biological threats and assaults [41]. Public health leaders would prefer a policy of "dual use" or "dual benefit," in which systems are designed to enhance the operation of the public health system in general while adding new capabilities in emergency response [42]. Such a policy would ensure benefit from the investment even if no bioterrorism event ever occurred locally and would enhance the reliability of the system. For example, a single-purpose surveillance program for bioterrorism is likely to have an unacceptably high risk of failure and unreliability in any rare true bioterrorism event if it is not regularly tested by the type of outbreak that occurs many times a week in every metropolitan health department.

Surveillance

Surveillance against a bioterrorism event rests on three strategies: rapid detection of an assault in progress, rapid identification of the organism, and rapid identification of the consequences. Identification of an assault in progress requires means of detecting the biologic agent. At present, the state of the art involves "sniffers," which are automated devices for sampling relatively large volumes of air in a given location and isolating and identifying pathogens. These machines are based on technology to detect molecules or reactions unique to life forms (such as ATP or NADP). The organism is then recovered and isolated for PCR amplification and DNA analysis, culture, and further identification. Sniffers are very expensive, often produce irrelevant false-positive results (especially for tularemia, which is more often airborne than previously realized), and are not widely deployed.

Identification of the organism requires extensive backup facilities. Since 2001, systems have been put into place by state laboratories and the CDC to provide rapid screening, PCR amplification, and strain typing when required. The state of the art of field testing remains weak, with available hand-held and field devices performing unreliably.

Rapid identification of the consequences rests on *syndromic surveillance,* the early recognition of characteristic features of the disease by physicians and other health care providers who are first responders on the scene or first receivers of sick patients in emergency rooms. However, the utility of syndromic surveillance as an early-detection strategy is limited. Characteristic syndromes, such as the widening mediastinum in anthrax or the distribution of pox lesions in smallpox, tend to be late rather than early signs in the evolution of an illness. More commonly, for many of the agents of interest, the first indication of disease is malaise and symptoms that resemble influenza, which is not helpful.

Conclusion

The lack of preparedness evident in 2001 was not solely due to a failure in antiterrorism planning. It is as much the result of many years of indifference and disinvestment in the public health system in the United States. Public health agencies, which are devoted to prevention, control, and tracking of disease rather than individualized medical care, are mostly the responsibility of state and local governments in this country. Investment in public health–oriented research and the budgets of public health agencies have been inadequate for many years.

The initial response of the federal government has been to stress security measures and homeland defense. This is necessary but only addresses half the problem where bioterrorism is concerned. A bioterrorist attack represents a risk of low probability in any one location (perhaps higher in Washington, DC, and New York City) but potentially devastating consequences should it occur. Investment in special-purpose national programs to deal with bioterrorism would spend much money to build a local capacity that would sit idly when the threat recedes. However, it may be possible to use that investment to rebuild the public health system. Emerging infections, food-borne illness, air pollution, and water contamination require the same technologies of prevention, disease surveillance, and outbreak investigation.

A strengthened public health system would protect workers and community residents all the time and would be there, tested and in readiness, when needed to respond to bioterrorism. This policy of "dual use" would benefit everybody whether or not another bioterrorist assault occurs. Because it would be tested frequently, people would know that the system works and is in a state of readiness.

In any event, what happened in the initial anthrax assault in Florida (the index case of the 2001 assault in the United States) [43] may represent the best possible scenario one could reasonably hope for in a first incident. It was a given that the first case would be recognized too late to save the victim; although tragic, this was not unexpected. However, the assaults to date have been inept. The fact that the delivery to date has been so incompetent is actually encouraging with respect to the capacity of perpetrators to deliver the agents. However, if a future terrorist act is state-sponsored and has the (relatively modest) resources required to conduct genetic modification, all bets are off. Bioengineered anthrax may not behave like a wild strain. The Soviets reportedly engineered at least one antibiotic-resistant strain that may have been widely disseminated to allies [44].

Acknowledgment

H. M. Mottl of Dycor R&D provided insight and technical information on biological warfare.

References

1. Franz DR, Jahrling PB, Friedlander AM, et al. Clinical recognition and management of patients exposed to biological warfare agents. *JAMA* 1997;278: 399–411.
2. Lederberg J (ed). *Biological Weapons: Limiting the Threat.* Cambridge, MA: MIT Press, 1999.
3. Guidotti TL, Hoffman H. Terrorism and the civilian response. *Clin Occup Environ Med* 2003;2:169–80.
4. Institute of Medicine. *Chemical and Biological Terrorism: Research and Development to Improve Civilian Medical Response.* Washington: National Academy Press, 1999.
5. Guidotti TL. Occupational medicine: An asset in time of crisis. In *Disaster Medicine.* New York: Elsevier, 2005, Chap 23.
6. Crupi RS, Asnis DS, Lee CC, et al. Meeting the challenge of bioterrorism: Lessons learned from West Nile virus and anthrax. *Am J Emerg Med* 2003;21: 77–9.
7. Herceg A, Geysen A, Guest C, Bialkowski R. SARS and biothreat preparedness: A survey of ACT

general practitioners. *Commun Dis Intell* 2005;29: 277–82.

8. Zilinkas RA (ed). *Biological Warfare: Modern Offense and Defense.* Boulder, CO: Lynne Rienner, 2000.

9. United Nations General Assembly Resolution 51/210 (1992): Measures to eliminate international terrorism.

10. Schmidt AP, Jongman AI, et al. *Political Terrorism.* Amsterdam: Transaction Books, 1988. P 5.

11. Torok TL, Tauxe RV, Wise RP, et al. A large community outbreak of salmonellosis caused by intentional contamination of restaurant salad bars. *JAMA* 1997; 278:389–95.

12. Thompson MW. *The Killer Strain: Anthrax and a Government Exposed.* New York: HarperCollins, 2003.

13. Christopher GW, Cieslak TJ, Pavlin JA, et al. Biological warfare: A historical perspective. *JAMA* 1997; 278:412–7.

14. Mangold T, Goldberg J. *Plague Wars: The Terrifying Reality of Biological Warfare.* New York: St Martin's Press, 1999.

15. Geissler E, Moon JE v C. *Biological and Toxin Weapons: Research Development and Use from the Middle Ages to 1945.* Stockholm International Pease Research Institute (SIPRI) Chemical and Biological Warfare Studies no 18. Oxford, UK: Oxford University Press, 1999.

16. Baylis J. NATO strategy: The case for a new strategic concept. *Int Affairs* (Royal Institute of International Affairs, London) 1987;64:43–59.

17. Wheelis M, Rozssa L, Dando M (eds). *Deadly Cultures: Biological Weapons since 1945.* Cambridge, MA: Harvard University Press, 2006.

18. Zilinskas RA. Iraq's biological warfare program: The past as future? *JAMA* 1997;278:418–24.

19. Cole, LA. *The Anthrax Letters: A Medical Detective Story.* Washington: Joseph Henry Press, 2003.

20. Dando M. *The New Biological Weapons: Threat, Proliferation, and Control.* Boulder, CO: Lynne Reinner, 2001.

21. Kadlec RP, Zelicoff AP, Vrtis AM, et al. Biological weapons control prospects and implications for the future. *JAMA* 1997;278:351–6.

22. Upfal MJ, Krieger GR, Phillips SD, et al. (eds). *Clinics in Occupational and Environmental Medicine: Terrorism: Biological, Chemical, and Nuclear,* Vol 2, No 2. Philadelphia: Saunders, 2003.

23. Ingelsby TV, Henderson DA, Bartlett JG, et al. Anthrax as a biological weapon: Medical and public health management. *JAMA* 1999;281:1735–45.

24. Bresnitz EA, DiFernando GT Jr. Lessons from the anthrax attacks of 2001: The New Jersey experience. *Clin Occup Environ Med* 2003;2:227–52.

25. Godyn JJ, Reyes L, Siderits R, Hazra A. Cutaneous anthrax: Conservative or surgical treatment? *Adv Skin Wound Care* 2005;18:146–50.

26. Shieh WJ, Guarner J, Paddock C, et al. The critical role of pathology in the investigation of bioterrorism-related cutaneous anthrax. *Am J Pathol* 2003; 163:1901–10.

27. Gair R. Clinical predictors of bioterrorism-related inhalational anthrax. *Lancet* 2005;365:214–5.

28. Cuneo BM. Inhalational anthrax. *Respir Care Clin North Am* 2004;10:75–82.

29. Committee to Assess the Safety and Efficacy of the Anthrax Vaccine, Institute of Medicine. *The Anthrax Vaccine: Is It Safe? Does It Work?* Washington: National Academy Press, 2002.

30. Friedlander AM, Phillip R, Parker GK. Anthrax vaccine: Evidence for safety and efficacy against inhalational anthrax. *JAMA* 1999;282:2104–6.

31. Matsumoto G. Anthrax powder: State of the art? *Science* 2003;302:1492–7.

32. Henderson DA, Inglesby TV, Bartlett JG, et al. Smallpox as a biological weapon: Medical and public health management. *JAMA* 1999;281:2127–37.

33. Murane ET. Vaccinia: The vaccine that protects against smallpox. *CME Res (Sacramento, CA)* 2004; 118:1–26.

34. Committee on Smallpox Vaccination Program Implementation, Institute of Medicine. *The Smallpox Vaccination Program: Public Health in an Age of Terrorism.* Washington: National Academy Press, 2005.

35. Kuritsky JN, Massoudi MS, Deitchman SD, Urquhart G. Smallpox: Brief review and update. *Clin Occup Environ Med* 2003;2:207–26.

36. Lane M, Goldstein J. Evaluation of 21st-century risks of smallpox vaccination and policy options. *Ann Intern Med* 2003;138:488–93.

37. Kaplan EH, Craft DL, Wein LM. Emergency response to a smallpox attack: The case for mass immunization. *Proc Nat Acad Sci USA* 2002;99:10935–40.

38. Ingelsby TV, Dennis DT, Henderson DA, et al. Plague as a biological weapon: Medical and public health management. *JAMA* 2000;283:2281–90.

39. Sullivan JB Jr, Steward C, Phillips S. Weapons of mass destruction: Biologic agents. *Clin Occup Environ Med* 2003;2:191–206.

40. Guidotti TL, Naidoo K. Hunting, trapping, and wilderness-related work. In Weissman DN, Huy JM (eds), *Occupational Infectious Diseases: Clinics in Occupational and Environmental Medicine.* Orlando, FL: Elsevier Science, 2002. Pp 651–61.

41. Meadows M. Project Bioshield: Protecting Americans from terrorism. *FDA Consum* 2004;38:32–3.

42. Guidotti TL. Why do public health practitioners hesitate? *J Homeland Security & Emergency Management* (online) 2004;1:art. 403.

43. Maillard J-M, Fischer M, McKee KT, et al. First case of bioterrorism-related inhalational anthrax, Florida, 2001: North Carolina investigation. *Emerg Infect Dis* 2002;10:2–389.

44. Alibek K. Many countries have smallpox. Newsmax.com, October 22, 2001, http://archive.newsmax.com/archives/articles/2001/10/21/204923.shtml.

40 Occupational Infections in Sewage Workers

Robert P. Hurley

The sewage worker's occupational environment consists of large, open sewer drains, medium-sized pipes, collection systems, and several sewage treatment processes that present a myriad of exposures. Sewage, compost, and wastewater workers are exposed to multiple biologic, chemical, metallic, and radioactive agents [1–3]. Concentrations of these agents vary widely depending on the environment, season, country, local health events, and completeness of processing wastes [4]. The potential for many infectious diseases is present at all times based on the inability of workers to fully protect themselves or avoid all sewage exposure during the course of employment. Despite this potential, sewage work has few clearly associated infectious diseases. In the 1960s, the lack of defined infectious relationships was cited as owing to the constraints of human experimentation [5]. Since that time, risk characterization has improved, yet not to the extent that the occupational physician may become clinically lax when approaching an ill sewage worker. In addition to understanding pathogen burden, the physician also must understand the waste stream and processes of treatment when assessing the causative nature and treatment of infections in this population.

There are two classes of pathogens in sewage. The primary pathogens consist of bacteria, viruses, protozoa, and helminthes. The second class consists of molds and fungi, particularly *Aspergillus* species. The presence, concentration, and ability of these pathogens to cause disease are determined by several factors:

- Prevalence of the pathogens in the population connected to the sewer system
- Pathogen characteristics, such as virulence, resistance to destruction during the sewage treatment processes, and the ability of these organisms to survive and grow in sewage and sludge after treatment
- Host factors, such as immune competence and resistance

Exposures to these pathogens have been associated with acute gastrointestinal, dermatologic, and pulmonary syndromes or chronic disease such as liver cancer [6]. Inhalation of moist or dried bioaerosols may produce immune system dysfunction via allergic responses or direct toxic action [7]. Zoonoses alone comprise over 160 diseases that, if present in the waste stream, are transmissible from vertebrate animals to humans [8]. Although the prospects of well-controlled human studies pose unacceptable risks, quantification of worker risk for these infectious agents is improving. This is due to improved surveillance measures and the advent of genetic laboratory techniques. This chapter focuses on the typical exposures, risks, and infections experienced by individuals employed in the varied processes of sewage work.

Phases of Sewage Treatment

The first phase of waste treatment is traditionally called *pretreatment,* a process that involves bar racks, grit chambers, and equalization chambers. These are used primarily to protect the wastewater treatment plant itself. The bar racks and grit chambers remove large objects such as rags, logs, and glass. Equalization chambers improve the plant's efficiency by modulating wastewater flow variation throughout the day. After the initial phase, *primary treatment* occurs. In this process, solids such as grease, grit, human waste, tampons, sanitary napkins, and condoms are separated out from the wastewater stream by screens, mechanical rakes, or sedimentation or settling tanks. The *secondary treatment* processes reduce the biologic oxygen demand (BOD) and remove additional solids. The biologic material is degraded or converted to solid mass during aerobic or anaerobic bacterial digestion using trickle filters or a process known as *activated sludge. Tertiary treatment* involves further filtration, aeration, and/or disinfection with ozone, chlorine, or ultraviolet (UV) light [9].

Primary, secondary, and tertiary phases of treating the waste stream expose workers to microorganisms that may be splashed on intact or abraded skin, mucous membranes, or clothing. Immersion of the body in wastewater for short or prolonged periods of time increases the risk of disease from pathogenic and nonpathogenic organisms. Later stage treatment of sewage such as aeration places sewage workers at risk of inhalation of bioaerosols. Handling of biosolids, which are spread on land for irrigation, fertilization, or composting, increases the risk of ingestion, inhalation, or absorption of bacteria, viruses, helminthes, fungi, protozoa, heavy metals, and solvents.

Epidemiology

Sewage workers are exposed to a number of infectious agents. Bacteria, viruses, helminthes, protozoa, fungi, and toxic substances derived from vertebrate animals are all found in the waste stream. Workers are exposed not only to the known human reservoir of pathogens but also to zoonotic

infections (e.g., *Leptospira interrogans*) and water-residing organisms (e.g., *Legionella pneumophila*) that are associated with significant morbidity. Sewage compost workers are routinely exposed to several major pathogens such as gram-positive/negative and endotoxin-producing bacteria. Viruses potentially in the waste stream include hepatitis A, B, C, D, and E and other human enteric viruses, such as poliovirus, coxsackievirus, echovirus, and rotavirus. Other primary and secondary pathogens, such as *Helicobacter pylori, Aspergillus,* helminthes, and protozoa have a known presence in the work environment of sewage workers.

The concentrations of pathogens vary by the endemicity of disease in the community, season, wastewater treatment schemes, geography, and climate [10]. In the United States, concentrations from facility to facility vary according to the process with which the waste is treated. To date, clear dose-response relationships have not been established for many of these pathogens. Improved methods of study need to be employed, and existing methods require validation [11]. Table 40-1 summarizes the relative concentrations of major pathogens in waste during the various stages of treatment [12, 13].

BACTERIA
Leptospirosis

Leptospirosis, first recognized as an occupational disease of sewer workers in 1883, is a zoonosis or anthrozoonosis. The reservoirs of leptospirosis, nonhuman mammal carriers, excrete the bacteria in their urine and transmit the bacteria to humans throughout the world. Disease severity ranges from an unnoticed subclinical condition to an acute pulmonary infection with septicemia that can be fatal. The infection, originally thought to be more common in tropical climates, is reported more often in temperate zones. Incidence in the United States has remained stable in the past 10 years. During the years 1987–1993, 43–93 cases were reported annually [14]. In 1995, the Council of State and Territorial Epidemiologists and the Centers for Disease Control and Prevention (CDC) removed leptospirosis from the U.S. list of notifiable diseases [14, 15]. Adding to the difficulty in characterizing leptospirosis is the fact that there has been a shift in the prevalence of the different infectious serotypes.

Table 40-1

The Relative Concentrations of Several Important Human Pathogens Found in Sewage. Density Levels of Organics in Raw Sludge and Septage [12] ($\times$ Average mean of organisms per gram of dry weight [13].)

Organism	Primary	Secondary	Mixed	Septage
Total coliform count	1.2×10^8	7.1×10^8	1.1×10^8	1.4×10^8
Fecal coliform count	2.0×10^7	8.3×10^6	1.9×10^5	1.2×10^6
Fecal streptococci	8.9×10^5	1.7×10^6	3.7×10^{16}	6.6×10^5
Bacteriophage	1.3×10^5	NR	NR	NR
Salmonella sp.	4.1×10^2	8.8×102	2.9×10^2	5.1×10^{-1}
Shigella sp.	NR	NR	ND	NR
P. aeruginosa	2.8×10^3	1.1×10^4	3.3×10^3	2.6×10^1
Parasites: ova/cysts $\times$ total	2.1×10^2	NR	$<5.0 \times 10^1$	NR
Ascaris sp.	7.1×10^2	1.4×10^3	2.9×10^2	NR
Trichuris trichiura	1.0×10^2	$<1.0 \times 10^1$	0	NR
Trichuris vulpis	1.1×10^2	$<1.0 \times 10^1$	1.4×10^2	NR
Toxocara sp.	2.4×10^2	2.8×10^2	1.3×10^3	NR
Hymenolepis diminuta	6.0×10^0	2.0×10^1	0	NR
Enteric viruses	3.9×10^2	3.2×10^2	3.6×10^2	NR

NR = no data available; *ND* = none detected.

In 1948, 90% of cases of leptospirosis were reported to be caused by *L. icterohaemorrhagiae,* compared with 1978–1987, when only 32% were ascribed to that serotype [16]. At present, many serovars may cause the myriad symptoms of this biphasic disease. Table 40-2 lists many of the serovars associated with leptospirosis in the sewer workers' environment.

Leptospirosis, including the severe form called *Weil's disease,* traditionally was attributed to infection by *L. icterohaemorrhagiae.* However, leptospirosis is now recognized as a disease caused by various species of *Leptospira,* which comprise both pathogenic and saprophytic strains on the basis of DNA relatedness.

The genus *Leptospira* has at least 12 genospecies. Any one of a large number of serologic types (serovars) can cause disease. Historically, the taxonomic classification of serovars and serogroups was based on serology using cross-agglutination with rabbit antisera and microscopic identification. This older taxonomic classification grouped pathologic species serologically as *L. interrogans.* Nonpathogens were grouped as *L. biflexa.* Based on this older serologic classification, the significant reservoirs of *Leptospira* infecting humans were thought to be the serovars *canicola,* found in dogs; *icterohaemorrhagiae,* associated with Norway rats; and *pomona,* found in cattle and swine.

The modern classification of *Leptospira* is based on genetic relationships of distinct species (genospecies). *Leptospiral serogroup* is the collective term for antigen-related serovars. Members of any serogroup may belong to multiple species with DNA relatedness. At least 22 serogroups are based on or share major agglutinogens, and 250 different serotypes of *Leptospira* have been identified. The species *interrogans, borgpetersenii, alexanderi, kirschneri, santarosai, weilii,* and *noguchii* are known pathogenic strains. *Inada, faineii,* and *meyeri* are strains that present pathogenic uncertainty. *Biflexa, wolbachi, parva,* and *illini* represent a saprophyte class of the organism. There are also unnamed genomospecies as yet not fully characterized [15].

The spirochetes of *Leptospira* are finely coiled, thin, motile, obligate, slow-growing anaerobes. Their flagella allow them to burrow into tissue, which places sewer workers at particular risk. The primary reservoir of leptospires is usually wild, warm-blooded vertebrates, although some serovars appear to have adapted to domestic and potentially domesticated animals as hosts. For the sewer worker, the urine of infected rats or other wild mammals is the most common source of *Leptospira.* These animal shedders remain asymptomatic or have subclinical disease. The *Leptospira* organisms become lodged in the mammal's renal

Table 40-2
Common World Wide Infectious Serotypes of *Leptospira*: Animal Hosts [17]

Serovar	Human	Domestic	Wild
autumnalis		D	HH, R, RA, SK
australis		D	BA, FM, M[a]
ballum		S	HH, HM, SR
balcanica		C,	PO[a]
bratislava		D, H[b], P, S	B, HH, R, RA, SK
bulgaica		D	
canicola	+	D[a], H, P, C, S	R, RA, SK
copenhageni	+	C, D, H, S	A, M, R, RA
cynopteri		D	
djasiman		D	
grippotyphosa		C, P, H	F, FM, L, M, MO, PO, RA, SK, V[c]
georgia	+	PO, RA, SK	
hardjo	+	C, D, H, S[a]	
hebdomadis			BA, FM
icterohaemorrhagiae	+	D, P, C	AP, F, HH, HM, M, PO, R, RA, SK,
javanica			BA, FM, R, V
kennewicki			SK
kremastos		D	
lora		P	M
mendanesis		D	
muenchen		H, P	B
mozdok		P	FM, R
pomona	+	C,[a] P,[a] D, H, G, S	A, DE, F, HM, RA, SK, SL, PO, V, W
robinsoni		D	
shermani		P	
saxkoebing			M
swajizak		C, D	
tarassovi		D, C, P	

[a]Known major maintenance host.
[b]Known major maintenance host in Ireland.
[c]Possible maintenance host.
M = man; A = armadillo; AP = ape (zoo); B = boar; BA = badger; C = cattle; D = dog; DE = deer; F = fox; FM = field mice; G = goat; H = horse; HH = hedgehog; HM = house mouse; L = leopard; M = muskrat; MO = mole P = pig; PO = possum; R = rat RA = racoon; S = sheep; SK = skunk; SL = sea lion; SR = ship rat; V = vole; W = woodchuck.

tubules and may remain there for long periods of time without causing objective evidence of disease. The infected mammal then serves as a reservoir that produces large quantities of host-adapted serovars into the environment via excreted urine. This leptospiruria in mammals may persist for many months. Humans and other nonadapted mammals are considered incidental hosts, and human-to-human transmission is considered rare.

The moisture, warmth, and alkaline to neutral pH of sewer environments favor rapid growth of *Leptospira*. Increasing numbers of *Leptospira* may come in contact with sewer workers' skin via their partial or total immersion in contaminated waters.

This intimate, prolonged, chronic contact facilitates infection by either direct or indirect contact with the urine of infected animals. The major routes of transmission to humans are by immersion in or ingestion of urine-contaminated soil, food, or water. Breaks in skin surfaces or abraded, macerated mucosal membranes facilitate but are not necessary for infection. Occasionally, the sewer worker may be become infected via intact skin or from animal or rat bites.

Leptospirosis is an important disease for sewage workers that can result in both an acute and prolonged incapacity for work as well as loss of productivity. The costs of medical care, workers' compensation payments, and preventive measures to reduce these losses place financial strains on municipalities in which there are outbreaks of leptospirosis [16].

Legionella

There are more than 39 species in the Legionellaceae family and more than 61 serogroups [17, 18]. *L. pneumophila* is responsible for about 90% of infections caused by members of this family. Other species include *L. micdadei, L. longbeachae, L. dumoffi,* and *L. bozemanii. L. pneumophilia* alone contains 14 serogroups, but the important pathogenic members are 1, 4, and 6, which account for most human infections. The natural habitats for *L. pneumophila* appear to be rivers, streams, and polluted waters. The pathogen can survive wide ranges in temperature (0–63°C), a pH of 5.0–8.5, and reduced oxygen concentrations. The bacteria are chlorine-resistant and therefore pass through the water-treatment process and into the distribution system [19, 20]. In natural aquatic environments, symbiotic relationships with amebas and water bacteria are necessary for optimal growth of *Legionella* [21, 22]. *Legionella* infect and then multiply within amebas and ciliated protozoa. When the protozoan host ruptures, large numbers of *Legionella* are released [23, 24].

The occurrence of legionnaires' disease depends on the concentration of the organism, susceptibility of the individual, and intensity of exposure. Cigarette smoking, chronic lung disease, advanced age, and immunosuppression have been implicated as risk factors. Sewer systems, treatment plants, composting, and land dispersion provide *Legionella* species an excellent environment in which to breed and aerosolize. The major mode of *Legionella* transmission is inhalation of aerosols, and sick individuals can have severe diarrhea. However, there is little documentation in the literature to support increased risk of infection from *Legionella* in the sewer worker population. *Legionella* is further addressed in Chapter 10.

VIRUSES
Enteric Viruses

The enteric viruses may be divided into two groups of pathogens. The first can be grown in culture yet only infrequently causes disease. The second group, of which Norwalk-like viruses, astroviruses, and hepatitis A and E viruses belong, grows poorly in culture yet causes sporadic outbreaks throughout the year [25].

Hepatitis A. Hepatitis A virus (HAV), by the nature of its transmission, places sewage treatment workers at risk. As a small RNA virus of the Picornaviridae family, its genomic organization and replication are similar to those of polio. HAV is heat-stable and can live for 2 weeks in feces [26]. It is viable at a pH as low as 3 and can live for many years at −20°C. Formalin and heating to 100°C will deactivate HAV, but it is resistant to chlorine, hence its risk for sewage workers. Individuals who work in sewage treatment plants are theoretically at increased risk for HAV infection, but documented increased risk of infection has not been demonstrated consistently [27, 28].

The fecal-oral mode of transmission, coupled with the inability of sewage workers to protect themselves from all contamination, presents significant risk. Sewers provide an ideal environment that enhances the capacity of viruses to remain viable for long periods of time. HAV is endemic in the United States and remains the most reported vaccine-preventable diseases in the United States [29]. Although there are periodic outbreaks, the number of new cases reported in 2003 (61,000) was down significantly from 1989 (380,000) [29]. The decline has been attributed to the increased rate of vaccination for hepatitis A in infants and children. Still, there are groups with higher incidences of HAV infection, such as Native Americans, Alaskan natives, and the Hispanic and Hasidic communities.

HAV antibodies found in sewer workers have been shown to increase with age, yet this trend does not differ markedly from the general population [30]. Sewer workers older than age 40 do have a statistically significant seropositivity rate compared with matched controls. The strongest correlation appears to be an association between seropositive status and the duration of sewage exposure. Among HAV-positive sewer workers, it has been shown that sewage exposure, increasing age, stay in an endemic area, or increased number of siblings were significant risk factors. Regression analysis of these data reveals an adjusted odds ratio (OR) of 2.15 for seropositivity to HAV among sewer workers compared with those not exposed to sewage [31].

Hepatitis B. At one time, Greece had a high burden of hepatitis B virus (HBV) infection. Recently, HBV infection there has declined to an intermediate endemnicity. A recent cross-sectional study suggests a possible association with exposure to sewage and subsequent contraction of hepatitis B [32].

Hepatitis C (previously known as non-A, non-B hepatitis). A few studies have suggested that work exposures in sewers is associated with risk for hepatitis C (HCV) infection. Although there have been reported outbreaks of hepatitis C in Algeria, India, and Nepal, there has been only a few case reports of transmission in the United States related to sewage work [33–35].

Hepatitis E. Outside the United States, hepatitis E virus (HEV) is a major cause of enteric non-A, non-B hepatitis. In endemic areas, it may be the causal agent in as many as 60% of cases of sporadic viral hepatitis [36]. In 1980, Khuroo and Wong first described epidemics of non-A, non-B hepatitis contracted by exposure to contaminated water [37, 38]. In the 1980s, Balayan demonstrated that the entity now known as *hepatitis E* shared many of the viral characteristics of hepatitis A. Hepatitis E is a nonenveloped, single-stranded RNA virus and shares other HAV characteristics, such as having a fecal-oral route of transmission, point-source infectiousness, absence of persistent antibodies, and a chronically active state. First identified in India, HEV now can be found in Mexico, the Middle and Far East, northern and western Africa, and Asia. Recently, it has been noted that there is an association of hepatitis E and the human polyomavirses. Thought of as environmental contaminants with complex interactions, there are a number of diverse strains that infect populations in industrialized societies [39]. The virus may cause a fatal fulminant hepatitis in gravid females, especially in the third trimester.

Other Viruses

Hantavirus. Hantavirus, first isolated in 1976, is not known to be occupationally related to sewage work. Nevertheless, mouse and rat droppings are ubiquitous in the sewer worker environment, and thus the potential for transmission exists. In one case-control study, entering buildings rarely opened or inhabited was associated with hantavirus pulmonary syndrome (HPS) [40]. The uncommonness of the disease makes risk assessment difficult. Transmission to humans is from the saliva, urine, or feces of infected rodents. Hantavirus diseases, initially known as *Korean hemorrhagic fever,* are now known to comprise two distinct syndromes in humans. These syndromes are hemorrhagic fever with renal syndrome (HFRS) and HPS. The hantaviruses are RNA viruses that belong to the family Bunyaviridae, of which there are currently at least eight types associated with HPS. The CDC data indicate an overall HPS case-fatality rate of 40% [40, 41]. Clinically, the early presentation can be confused with leptospirosis (Weil's syndrome), although laboratory testing can differentiate between the two. Hantavirus syndromes are covered in Chapter 16.

Human Polyomaviruses. Recently, concentrations of human polyomaviruses BKV and JCV have been found in urban sewage. These viruses carry the potential for oncogenic gene transmission and therefore requires improvement in detection and surveillance measures [39].

PARASITES

Parasitic diseases are a major health problem in the developing world. Many infections are acquired by eating feces-contaminated food or water. Others are acquired by arthropod vectors. The parasitic diseases are divided into two categories, the protozoa and the helminths.

Protozoa

These single-cell organisms can be considered in two classes: the systemic protozoa and the intestinal protozoa. Major systemic diseases such as malaria, sleeping sickness, leishmaniasis, and toxoplasmosis have been described as possible in sewage workers in India but are not proven to be associated with sewage work generally [42]. In countries where parasites are endemic, sewer workers are assumed to be at risk for *Toxoplasma gondii* infection because it can be transmitted by the fecal-oral route. Protozoa that are primarily known to cause intestinal disease and diarrhea and that can be present in the sewage worker's environment in specific countries include *Giardia,* Cryptosporidia, *Cyclospora, Isospora,* and Microsporidia.

HELMINTHS

In countries where solid waste and sewage are often mixed or handled together, there are significant increases in parasitic infections in sewage workers. Stool samples taken from Indian sewage workers revealed that 98% were positive for parasites. In comparison, the control group revealed a prevalence of 33%. Of those infected, the most prevalent parasites were *Trichuris trichuria* (human whipworm) and *Ascaris lumbricoides* (human roundworm) [42]. In the United States, sewer work has not been found to predispose workers to helminthic infections [43].

MOLD AND FUNGI

Aspergillus fumigatus and other fungi can be secondary or opportunistic pathogens that colonize individuals under certain circumstances. People who are immunocompromised or otherwise debilitated by a preexisting medical condition, such as severe viral infection or chemotherapy, are prone to such colonization. Occasionally, *A. fumigatus* may cause widespread invasion of lung tissue, yet severe infections usually occur only in individuals lacking a competent immune system. Sewage workers who have immunodeficiencies are likely to be subject to more severe and opportunistic infections.

BIOSOLIDS AND THE SEWAGE WORKERS' WORK PROCESSES

The exposure to biosolids in sewage work depends on the treatment processes at the facility. Recommended treatment guidelines for biosolids can be found in the *Federal Register,* Appendix B, 40 CFR, Part 503. There are five types of secondary sewage treatment processes that reduce microorganism load and biologic oxygen demand:

- Aerobic digestion
- Drying
- Anaerobic digestion
- Composting
- Lime stabilization

In aerobic digestion, biosolids are agitated with air or oxygen often in open or closed containers or lagoons to maintain aerobic conditions. Using high-temperature operations to 55°C produces increased biosolid mass with reduced pathogen content. The agitation of liquid, slurry, or desiccated material generates carbon dioxide, water, nitrogen, and varying concentrations of bioaerosols.

Drying of biosolids can be accomplished by placing them in sandbags or in basins that may be paved or unpaved. This process generally takes a minimum of 3 months. Another method, heat drying, uses active or passive dryers to remove or dewater the biosolids. This process eliminates most of the water content and pathogens. Whether air or heat drying methods are employed, the storage of biosolids in an open basin results in little release of pathogens or organic material. If biosolids are left in a powder state, significant amounts of bacteria, viruses, and bacterial toxins can be dispersed by the wind for considerable distances. Sewage workers without masks may inhale high concentrations of dust and thus be exposed.

Heat-drying methods used on primary treatment stage biosolids result in material that retains objectionable odors even in dried form. When heat-drying methods are applied to secondary treatment stage biosolids the resulting material is essentially free of objectionable odors and acceptable for long-term storage. This secondary-stage dried product has been sold to consumers successfully as a home and garden fertilizer in pelletized form for well over 80 years.

Anaerobic digestion is relatively safe because the sewage is kept in containers under anaerobic conditions in order to reduce organic content, mass, odor, and pathogen content. Organisms consume part of the organic content and convert it to carbon dioxide, methane, and ammonia. Anaerobic digestion is typically done at 35°C but can be operated at higher temperatures to ensure reduction in solids or pathogens. However, when containers are opened and this material is transported, sewage workers are at risk for exposure.

Composting facilities typically use any of three different processes: within-vessel, static-aerated pile, or windrow composting. Each of these processes raises the temperature of the biosolids to 55–60°C or higher and maintains this state for 3–4 weeks, followed by a less active period of 1 month called *curing.* Composting requires piles of biosolids to be turned repeatedly, often by machine, in order to introduce oxygen and expose the entire pile to temperatures of at least 55°C. Whether done in the open air or in closed vessels, when turned, high airborne concentrations of bioaerosols can occur, especially within a closed composting facility. Outside, high concentrations of bioaerosols may be generated by wind and can expose workers and those living nearby the facility.

Lime stabilization is a crude process in which sufficient lime is added to biosolids to raise the pH to 12 after 2 hours of contact. Lime is the most common compound used, but other materials, such as cement kiln dust, lime kiln dust, Portland cement, and fly ash, sometimes are used. Newer technologies involving additional chemicals, higher doses, and/or supplemental drying are also employed.

Sewage workers are at the highest risk of inhaling aerosolized pathogens when they are engaged in work near aerobic digestion, air-drying, and composting sewage-processing sites. To better characterize worker risk, industrial hygiene air sampling data should be collected near these processes. The most useful representative sample of airborne organic content is volumetrically based data [44].

BIOAEROSOLS AND BIOSOLIDS IN THE WASTEWATER SETTING

Bioaerosols are airborne particulates that are comprised of living materials, their toxic products, or both. The major airborne pathogens are bacteria, viruses, fungi, and endotoxins. Wastewater treatment workers who process biosolids such as sludge are exposed primarily to microbes, especially gram-negative rods. These exposures have been associated with symptoms such as fever and chest tightness [45]. Exposure to fungi such as *A. fumigatus,* which proliferates during wastewater treatment, has been shown to be pathogenic to workers with impaired immune systems.

In wastewater treatment plants, aerosols are created during phases in which materials are agitated. There are three forms of aerosols: liquid, moist, and dry. The concentrations of airborne biologic materials depend on facility design and prevailing environmental conditions. Sewage treatment workers may be exposed not only when participating in sewage treatment processes but also when working nearby, in unrelated job activities. In some communities, biosolids are dumped on the land for fertilization and disposal purposes [46, 47]. Irrigation or dumping of solid waste often occurs at night, ostensibly to maintain water content. Without the benefits of solar radiation, desiccation and decrease of the biologic load does not occur, and heavy concentrations of all three forms of bioaerosols may be spread into respirable air. Buildings can become contaminated by these aerosols if biosolids are dumped nearby. Sewage workers and people in nearby facilities may become exposed to sewage plant bioaerosols from the carpets, drapes, and ventilation systems of these contaminated structures.

Dermal exposure to bioaerosols may cause irritant contact dermatitis. Bioaerosols also can result in respiratory tract inflammation [48]. The nasal passages and upper airways usually filter out large-sized bioaerosol particles, those ranging from 30–60 μm in diameter. Large particles typically are organic and inorganic dirt, fibers, pollens, and mold spores. Smaller particles in the 5-μm range can include hyphal fragments, pollen, and mold spores, which have the capacity to be respired deeply into the lower airways. The smallest pathogens, such as bacteria, fungal spores, and viruses, can be carried by inorganic matter as small as 1–5 μm and are considered truly respirable. Immune competent sewage workers are capable of inhaling very high numbers of spores or microorganisms without systemic effect or infection. Studies examining workers' exposure to sewage sludge and waste water in the United States and Sweden have revealed no increased risk of infection, except under extreme exposure conditions, such as total-body immersion in sewage water tanks with inhalation of water [49–51]. Nevertheless, the Environmental Protection Agency (EPA) has enacted Part 503, The Biosolids Rule, which sets strict standards, including process treatment parameters, in order to reduce the threat of pathogen transmission. This rule divides biosolids into class A and class B based on pathogen content. Class A biosolids must be treated so that pathogenic bacteria, enteric viruses, and viable helminth ova are below detectable levels. Class B biosolids have reduced pathogen levels that do not present a risk to public health or the environment if handled and used in specific fashions. Class B biosolids cannot be sold or given away. Typically, they are used for municipal solid-waste landfill cover. This is governed by Part 258, MSW Landfill Requirements [52, 53].

BIOAEROSOLS AND BIOSOLIDS IN THE COMPOST SETTING

When processed properly, compost bioaerosols contain less than 20% moisture and are very friable. During normal handling, some of the biologic components may be released into the air [54]. Depending on the process or stage of waste treatment, workers may be exposed to a multitude of pathogenic organisms that are not destroyed in the sewage treatment process. Compost bioaerosols may contain *Actinomyces,* other bacteria, fungi, arthropods, protozoa, and organic constituents of feedstock materials. Microbial products include endotoxins, microbial enzymes, β-1,3-glucans, and mycotoxins [54]. The compost contains not only biologically active organisms but also chemicals and heavy metals [55–61]. These primary and secondary pathogens are summarized in Tables 40-3 through 40-6.

The most important biologically active material is *A. fumigatus. A. fumigatus* is one of the most prevalent *Aspergillus* species on Earth. It is able to grow within a wide range of temperatures (12–50°C), relative humidity, and growth media [62]. Individual spores (conidia) are small (2 μm in diameter) and, if inhaled, can enter the lungs [54]. *A. fumigatus* can cause dermal and mucosal irritation as well as inflammation and infection [13, 63]. It is a common organism in the general environment, with levels up to several hundred spores per cubic meter having been reported [64]. In the aeration tank or compost row, the growth of *A. fumigatus* can be impressive. However, studies show that 250–500 ft from compost sites, the airborne concentrations of *A. fumigatus* are at or below background concentration levels [65–66].

The microorganisms present in bioaerosols represent human pathogens and opportunistic human pathogens. Although there is concern that airborne microbes may cause disease from inhaled mists or dried organic dusts, documented infections are rare [54, 65, 67]. Currently, the data do not support the contention of elevated risk in immunocompetent individuals who handle or have ambient exposure to biosolid waste material.

Municipalities are increasingly looking to compost solid waste from their sewage treatment plants for use as fertilizer or for other uses. With this increase in municipal composting, the exposure to bioaerosols of workers and residences nearby will increase, as will health and safety concerns. Case studies from Silver Springs, Maryland, Westbrook, Maine, and Windsor, Ontario, support European data indicating that with current technology *A. fumigatus* reaches background levels at less than 500 ft from compost sites. Furthermore, at the Silver Springs site, an employee surveillance program instituted in 1987 failed to reveal any adverse health effects related to *A. fumigatus* during a 5-year period [68]. Studies outside the United States have documented small numbers of workers who experienced subjective symptoms such as nausea, headaches, and diarrhea. In these workers, endotoxins were thought to be the causative agent [65]. In 1983, Clark studied airborne gram-

Table 40-3
Principal Bacterial Infectious Agents of Concern in Sewage

Bacteria	Reservoir	Disease/Comments
Acinetobacter calcoaceticus	FL, W	Tracheobronchitis, pneumonia
Aeromonas hydrophilia	M, F, SF, W	Gastoenteritis, gangrenous wound infections, pneumonia
Campylobacter jejuni	B, C, D, DA, R	Gastroenteritis
Enterobacter agglomerans cloacae	M	Opportunistic skin, respiratory, and urinary tract infections
Escherichia coli	M, DA, WA	Gastroenteritis, pathogenic strains
Klebsiella pneumoniae	P, A, W	Endocarditis, LRT infections, ear infections
Legionella pneumophila	S, W, PZ, AM	Pontiac fever, pneumonia
Leptospira	R, DA, D, SW	Myocarditis, hepatitis, meningitis, conjunctivitis, lymphadenitis, pneumonia
	S, W, P, A, PR	Endocarditis, respiratory infections
Pseudomonas aeruginosa	M	Skin and soft tissue infections: osteomyelitis: pneumonia; toxic shock syndrome; gastroenteritis; endocarditis
Staphylococcus		
Streptococci	M, SW	Scarlet fever, pharyngitis, pneumonia; streptococcal toxic shock syndrome
Salmonella sp.	M, DA, WA, B, RP	Enteric fever, enterocolitis (over 1,700 types)
S. typhi	M, WA, SF	Typhoid fever
Shigella	M, I	Shigellosis, bacillary dysentery
Vibrio cholerae	M	Cholera

A = animals; AM = amoebae; B = bird; C = chicken; D = dog; DA = domestic animal; F = fish; FL = free living; I = insects; M = man; P = plants; PZ = protozoa; R = rat; RP = reptiles; S = soil; SW = swine; SF = shellfish; W = water; WA = wild animals.

Table 40-4
Viral Infectious Diseases Found in Sewage

Viruses	Disease	Reservoir	Comments
Adenovirus	Respiratory disease, conjunctivitis, gastroenteritis	M	31 types
Astroviruses	Gastroenteritis	M, T	
Coxsackie A, B	Myopericarditis B 1–5	M	23 group A (A1–A24, except type A23)
	HFM disease A16 +		6 group B (B1–B6)
	Entero 71[a]		
	AHC disease A24 +		
	Entero 70[b]		
Echovirus	Petechial exanthem, meningitis	M	31 types (1–34, except 10, 28, and 34)
Enteroviruses (nonpolio)	Gastroenteritis, heart anomalies, meningitis	M, WA	4 types (68–71)
	Entero 71 encephalitis		Polio-like paralysis
Hantavirus	Sin Nombre virus	R	Pneumonitis with hemorrhage and shock
Hepatitis A	Hepatitis	M, P	Myocarditis (rare)
Hepatitis E	Hepatitis	M	Not endemic in Europe or North America
Parvovirus[c]	Gastroenteritis	M	
Poliovirus	Paralysis, meningitis	M	Poliomyelitis
Reovirus	Respiratory disease, gastroenteritis	M, DA	Orthoreovirus, Coltivirus, Rotavirus, Orbivirus
Rotavirus	Gastroenteritis	M, DA	Acute gastroenteritis, diarrhea

[a]Hand foot and mouth disease.
[b]Acute hemorrhagic conjunctivitis.
[c]Parvovirus-like agents.
DA = domestic animal; M = man; P = primates; R = rat; T = turkey; WA = wild animals.

Table 40-5
Fungal Infectious Diseases Found in Sewage

Organism	Disease	Comments
Aspergillus fumigatus	Bronchitis, endocarditis, aspergilloma, aspergillosis allergy	
Bronchopulmonary *Aspergillus candidus, A. flavus, A. niger, A. terreus*	ABPA	Rare; usually occurs among immunosuppressed or immunocompromised
Cladosporium cladospoidies	Asthma, hyperactive airways	
Eurotimea amstelodam		
Histoplasma capsulatum	Histoplasmosis, pneumonia, disseminated disease, skin lesions	
Penicillium spinulosum	Organic dust toxic syndrome	Implicated

negative bacteria, endotoxins, and *A. fumigatus*. Indoor as well as outdoor bioaerosol concentrations were assessed related to mixing biosolid waste and sludge. Airborne levels of gram-negative bacteria ranged from $0.0–3.7 \times 10^5$ CFU/m³. Refuse hoppers, waste-processing areas, and screening areas had the highest mean airborne levels. Over half the bioaerosols was respirable, and endotoxin levels ranged from 0.001–0.042 µg/m³. Rylander has studied exposure to aerosols of biologically active agents and endotoxins. In compost facilities, respirable dust levels ranged from 0.1–12.0 mg/m³.

The compost screening areas generated the highest mean levels: 10.6 mg/m³. The lowest levels were associated with the areas of storage for compost piles. Respirable proportions of bacteria ranged from 50–60%, but the data could not establish a dose-response relationship between respirable bacteria and illness. Until safe standards are set, it would be prudent to limit individuals working with aerosolized biosolid waste to concentrations no greater than 0.02–0.1 µg/m³ because this is the level sufficient to stimulate the mucociliary response of the upper and lower airways [66]. For

Table 40-6
Protozoan and Helminths Found in Sewage

Organism	Disease	Reservoir	Comments
Protozoa			
Balanitidum coli	Balantidiasis	M, S	
Cryptosporidia spp.	Cryptosporidiosis	B, C, D, DA, F, RP, W, S, P	Gastroenteritis, may be chronic in immuno-compromised
Entaomoeba histolytica	Amebiasis	M	
Giardia lamblia	Giardiasis	B, F, RP, R, W, WA, M, DA	Diarrhea
Helminths			
Nematodes (roundworms)			
Ascaris lumbricoides	Ascariasis	M, SW	Abdominal pain
Ascaris suum	Ascariasis	M, SW	Coughing, chest pain
Ancyclostoma duodenal	Ancyclostomiasis	M	Wakana disease Chronic anemia
Necator americanus	Necatoriasis	M	Mild CLM symptoms[a]
Ancylostoma braziliense	CLM[a]	C	Cat hookworm
Ancylostoma caninum	CLM[a]	D	Dog hookworm
Enterobius vermicularis	Enterobiasis	M	Pin worm
Strongyloides stercoralis	Strongloidiasis	M, D	Threadworm
Toxocara cati	VLM[b]	CA	Cat roundworm
Toxocara canis	VLM[b]	CA	Dog roundworm
Trichuris trichiura	Trichuriasis	M	Whip worm
Cestodes (tapeworms)			
Taenia saginata	Taeniasis	M	Beef tapeworm
Taenia solium	Taeniasis	M	Pork tapeworm
Hymenolepis nana	Taeniasis	M, R	Dwarf tapeworm
Echinococcus granulosis	HCD[c]	C, D, DA	Dog tapeworm (larval cysts)
Echinococcus multiocularis	ACD[d]	D, CA	Infected canines (larval cysts)

[a]Cutaneous larva migrans.
[b]Visceral larva migrans.
[c]Hydatid cyst disease.
[d]Alveolar cyst disease.
B = bird; C = cat; CA = carnivores; D = dog; DA = domestic animal; F = fish; FA = farm animals; M = man; P = plants; R = rat; RP = reptiles; S = soil; SW = swine; W = water; WA = wild animals.

case definitions and evaluation protocols, please refer to Table 40-7.

BACTERIAL ENDOTOXIN, GLUCANS, AND MYCOTOXINS

Sewage processing and sewage composting are known to be occupations in which workers are exposed to endotoxins, glucans, and mycotoxins [63]. Gram-negative bacteria and their endotoxins are found in high concentrations in areas of biosolid processing. Studies support the notion that dust in and of itself can cause changes in respiratory responsiveness and lung function [69]. Within the outer layer of the gram-negative bacterial cell wall resides endotoxin. This cell wall constituent forms a heat-stable complex that is released into the environment during cell growth and after cell death

[70]. In the airways, the bacterial cell walls are capable of stimulating macrophage activity, thus causing release of endotoxins. The endotoxins, in turn, increase the activity of the macrophages and escalate the inflammatory response [71, 72]. Interestingly, endotoxin inhalation has been reported to have a statistically significant protective effect against lung cancer based on reduced rates in populations with known exposures [73].

Fungal cell walls contain the polymer β-1,3-glucan, a polysaccharide composed of glucose units. In the lung, these glucans depress macrophages, inhibiting their ability to function in response to endotoxins and other antigens [74, 75]. Another toxic metabolite of fungi are the mycotoxins, which are excreted into sewage by either the mycelium or the spore. Generally speaking, the toxins are heat-stable

Table 40-7
Case Definitions for Diseases Caused by *Aspergillus Fumigatus*

I. Invasive aspergillosis
  A. *Aspergillus:* isolated by culture from a normally sterile site (blood or tissue); culture of sputum is not acceptable.
  B. Mycetoma (aspergilloma): diagnosed by sputum culture and chest or sinus radiography or CT scan.
II. Allergic bronchopulmonary aspergillosis
  A. Definitive diagnosis requires that *all* seven of the following criteria be met:
  B. Identification of possible cases requires that *five* of seven criteria be met:
    1. Asthma (evidence of reversible airflow obstruction defined by $FEV_1/FVC < 0.70$).
    2. Evidence of immediate skin reactivity, i.e., wheal and flare reaction, to *Aspergillus fumigatus* antigen using intradermal injection or "prick" test.
    3. The presence of *Aspergillus*-specific IgE in serum.
    4. Quantitative serum IgE > 400 IU/mL or IgE > 250 IU/mL plus evidence of titer fluctuation with disease activity.
    5. IgG or precipitating antibody to *Aspergillus.*
    6. History of peripheral eosinophilia (absolute eosinophil count > 500 cells/mm^3).
    7. History of pulmonary infiltrates documented by chest radiography.
III. Acute allergic alveolitis (hypersensitivity pneumonitis)
  A. Fever and severe dyspnea 4–6 hours after exposure to a source of *Aspergillus* or episodic fever and dyspnea and high serum IgG precipitating antibodies to *Aspergillus.*
  B. At the time of symptoms, either diffuse micronodular infiltrates on chest radiograph or restrictive ventilatory defect documented by pulmonary function testing.
  C. A positive response to an inhalation-provocation test, using *Aspergillus* as the antigen.
  D. Lung histopathology with mononuclear inflammatory cell infiltrates in alveoli and interstitial spaces documented by lung biopsy.
IV. Asthma induced by *Aspergillus:* criteria A, B, C, and D must be met for a definite case; criteria A, B, and E must be met for identification of a possible case.
  A. Recurrent or intermittent symptoms consistent with asthma, including wheezing, dyspnea, cough, or chest tightness.
  B. Documentation of reversible or variable airway obstruction (improvement of at least 10% in FEV_1 with use of a bronchodilator); at least 20% variability in serial peak expiratory flow rate (PEFR) measurements in a 24-hour period; positive inhalation challenge testing with methacholine or histamine (20% decrease in FEV_1 produced by five inhalations of 8 mg/mL or less).
  C. Temporal association between episode of asthma and known exposure to *Aspergillus.*
  D. Positive wheal/flare to *Aspergillus* or positive *Aspergillus*-specific IgE radioallergosorbent test (RAST) in absence of reaction to other allergens.
  E. Positive wheal/flare to *Aspergillus* or positive *Aspergillus*-specific IgE RAST.
    Note: Allergic asthma due to *Aspergillus* exposure usually occurs in atopic persons and is rarely due solely to such exposure. Allergic asthma occurs less often in individuals with *Aspergillus* exposure than those with hay fever.
V. *Aspergillus* sinusitis: criteria A and B must be met.
  A. Isolation of *Aspergillus* species from sinus culture.
  B. Severe abnormalities on sinus CT scan.
VI. Allergies: While persons with sensitivity to aspergillus may have a skin test reaction or IgE levels to *Aspergillus* antigens, these tests alone are not definitive and the contribution to fungal exposure to allergy is difficult to evaluate. IgE skin testing correlates with biologic activity. RAST testing is an immunoassay and is less sensitive than skin testing. MAST testing evaluates antibody levels to a panel of antigens. Detection of antibodies in sera indicate exposure and are not diagnostic of an adverse health response.

and of a low molecular weight and exhibit cytotoxic, mutagenic, teratogenic, carcinogenic, and/or immunologic properties [76].

INFLAMMATION AND INFECTION FROM BIOAEROSOLS

Organic dusts affect the upper and lower respiratory tract, as well as the dermal surfaces. Individual responses vary, possibly based on polymorphism in genes, particularly affecting TLR-4 receptors, CD14 cell surface proteins, and lipopolysaccharide-binding proteins [77]. Understanding of the exact mechanisms of symptom development is evolving, but the clinical picture suggests an immunologic or allergic response. Repeated exposures irritate the mucous membranes of the eyes, ears, nose, and throat [78]. Hyperreactivity of the airways and chronic bronchitis are the sequelae of heavy, repeated exposures. In the lung, increased activity of the macrophages and migration of neutrophils characterize the initial inflammatory response. Neutrophil activity and leakage from nearby capillaries, if severe, result in *organic dust toxic syndrome* (ODTS). This nonallergic syndrome is characterized by fever, influenza-like symptoms, general malaise, and fatigue. Acute hemorrhagic pneumonitis has been associated with inhalation of high levels of fungal spores (10^{9-10}/m^3) [79]. Asthma, although by definition an immunologic response, may well be mediated by antigenic properties associated with these agents. The most common fungal allergen spores are the saprophytic microfungi *Mucor, Rhizopus, Cladosporium,* and *Aspergillus.* Experimentally, it has been shown that 100 *Alternaria* and 3,000 *Cladosporium* per cubic meter of air can evoke allergic symptoms [80].

Infections caused by airborne microbial agents in or on organic dusts may occur. Pathogenic and opportunistic organisms may invade tissue disrupted by irritants. Genetically sensitive individuals are at higher risk. Studies to date have not supported an increased risk of infection related to organic dust inhalation in individuals in the United States, and Sweden [63, 81, 82].

Secondary pathogens such as *A. fumigatus* may colonize and infect individuals who are immunocompromised or have underlying debilitating medical conditions. Diagnosis is not made easily. The organism is so common and readily inhalable that isolation in the sputum is not considered diagnostic. Blood tests for circulating *Aspergillus* antibodies have detected elevated levels in healthy adults. Positive serologic testing is considered to be a marker of past exposure (see Table 40-7). Further allergy testing via skin prick, patch, or scratch testing is often unreliable because commercially available antigenic extracts are often contaminated with *A. fumigatus.*

When evaluating the ill sewage worker, it is important to keep in mind that there is little supportive evidence that *A. fumigatus* and related species pose a risk to immunocompetent individuals. This is not the case for immunocompromised individuals. This difference emphasizes the necessity of performing a thorough history during initial and annual surveillance examinations. The immune

competent individual is capable of clearing *Aspergillus* species by a combination of cellular defense and the mucocilliary transport system. Unchecked, the pathways of infection are from (1) outer ear to inner, (2) nasal mucosa to meninges and brain, and (3) lung to the bloodstream. Individuals with malignancies, those taking immunosuppressant medications, and those who have suffered trauma may be at increased risk for *A. fumigatus* colonization. Individuals with abnormal lung function, such as those suffering from tuberculosis or sarcoidosis, also may be at risk for colonization. Saprophytic growth leads to the formation of "fungus balls," also known as *aspergillomas* or *mycetomas.* Despite mounting an antibody response, patients have mild symptoms early in the disease.

The immunodeficient individual is particularly at risk for colonization and serious infections. Immune globulin disorders or immunodeficiency diseases occur in 1 in 500 individuals [83]. HIV increases the risk of contracting disease from both pathogenic and nonpathogenic organisms. Other at-risk individuals include those with genetically impaired immune system. Atopic individuals must be aware of the risks of sewage, both dry and moist. Bioaerosol concentrations in some settings may be sufficiently high to increase symptoms in atopic individuals and sensitize nonatopic workers.

The effects and reactions of sewer workers exposed to bioaerosols are often the same as those experienced by those in other environments. Under certain conditions, bioaerosol counts as high as 4.5×10^5 fungal spores/m^3 of air have been demonstrated in air samples from buildings [84]. It is difficult to correlate measured levels of bioaerosols and ascribe a particular health effect based on data alone. Investigation of illnesses and alleged exposures must include site surveys and air sampling of exposure concentrations. The route of exposure as well as the immune condition, antigen sensitivity, and underlying diseases of individuals must be considered. Although a subjective matter, "annoyance" is often a large component of sewage workers' complaints and can be quantified by questionnaire. Rylander has set a threshold of 10%, "very annoyed," as an upper limit for airborne sewage sludge emissions in densely populated areas. When the threshold has been exceeded, requests are made to reduce or eliminate airborne bioaerosols [45].

Prevention and Control

ADMINISTRATIVE CONTROLS

A thorough understanding of the current sewage collection and processing systems in the community is required to effect reductions in exposures. Prevention of exposure to potentially infectious agents can be kept to a minimum by administratively controlling factors that expose sewer workers to contaminated environment or animal hosts. Managers charged with ensuring the health and safety of workers need to provide support, leadership, training, and periodic assessment of worker understanding in order to protect the workers' health. All outbreaks of water-borne disease should be investigated to characterize a potential common or point source. Some recommend exclusion from work for individuals with a history of disorders of the liver or gallbladder or a past history of jaundice when the work involves potentially hepatotoxic agents, including HAV, HBV, HCV, HEV, *Leptospira,* protozoans, or organic chemicals [85]. However, in the United States, consideration must be given to specific workplace hazard evaluations, effectiveness of protective measures, and the Americans with Disabilities Act (ADA), including addressing direct threat analysis and the concept of imminent harm (see Chapter 6).

For new sewage or sewage-composting facilities, preplanning and public involvement in the process are necessary for successful control. A large number of indoor air quality complaints, as well as illnesses, stem from external or outdoor sources. Preplanning of sewage facilities should consider their proximity to residencies and public facilities. Cities should regulate construction through the building inspection department to ensure that new buildings near sewage treatment areas are not constructed with "closed" ventilation systems. Those presently in operation should have periodic sampling to ensure that contamination has not occurred. Environmental studies of the meteorologic and topographic characteristics of the site and nearby the facility should be analyzed. New, upgraded or expanded sewage facilities require evaluation and installation of buffer zones or enclosures. Good management practices defined by state and federal legislation are concerned primarily with operational efficiency, pathogen reduction, and dust and odor control. In order to minimize bioaerosols and odors, current technology dictates the mechanization of sewage treatment and the method of handling materials.

Municipal solid-waste streams change over time, so working with local industries and the board of health, periodic sampling of local biologic agents should be instituted. Although stationary and personal sampling measurements are typically low at indoor worksites performing agitation of wastewater, high values can be obtained [86]. Illegal dumping of toxic wastes by industry, although banned by local, state, and federal statute, nevertheless occurs. Periodic unannounced sampling of all forms of sewage waste products is necessary to reduce the risk to workers and ensure safe working conditions.

SAFE WORK PRACTICES AND ENGINEERING CONTROLS

The occupational physician must understand the nuances of the job description of sewage workers in order to encourage and help to ensure safe work practices. Workers in *main drainage* are exposed to large intercepting sewers, pumping stations, and sewage disposal units. *Sewage systems* consist of pipes 20–60 cm in diameter. Brick and concrete sewers are generally 80–150 cm in height. *Compost systems,* open and closed, have special risks, as described earlier in this chapter.

Evaluating engineering controls requires an understanding not only of the composting process but also of the environment. Physical and meteorologic characteristics have an impact on workers and nearby public sectors, as well as on the operation of the compost facility. Some compost facilities are designed to distribute aerosols over large areas in order to decrease atmospheric concentrations. A wind map or information on daily prevailing winds should be used to schedule high release points to minimize concentrations of bioaerosols. If the plan is to keep the aerosols close to the facility, composting operations should be shielded from wind, and emission of aerosols should be kept below grade or at low release heights [87]. An undisturbed compost pile does not generate a significant amount of aerosolized microbes; therefore, those working in sewage composting or air drying of sludge should avoid churning piles during windy conditions. Mechanical agitation, as well as bulk movement, has been shown to be a major source of airborne emissions. Reducing the size of the loads being moved or agitated, as well as vigilance in dust control, can minimize bioaerosol releases. Downdrafts onto dust-laden surfaces, as well as the mechanical agitation of wheels and tires of machines handling this material, increase bioaerosol releases. Attempts to reduce emissions may include changing the time of biosolid agitation and enclosing the facility to minimize site and off-site contamination. Monitoring of the temperature and moisture concentrations of bulking agents will help to minimize formation of bioaerosols. Consideration of the amount of time that the compost "cures" may reduce the levels of pathogens, especially those of *Aspergillus.* The use of filters has been suggested for odor control, but because of low emissions from static waste piles, there has not been adequate study of their effectiveness.

Dose-response modeling or quantitative risk assessment to assign safe levels of bioaerosol exposure has been done, but the differences in the responses of the human immune system limit the ability to promulgate a minimum safe level. Dose-response literature regarding endotoxins is available, but the issue of testing humans for microbial proteins may not be feasible yet. Because there are no widely recommended exposure levels for endotoxins, setting a time-weighted average (TWA) or threshold limit for total airborne endotoxic proteins should be considered [88]. The lowest concentration of endotoxin at which a pulmonary response has been detected is 10 ng/m^3 [89]. Palchack has recommended an 8-hour TWA exposure limit of 30 ng/m^3 for periodic industrial hygiene monitoring. This incorporates a 10-fold safety factor based on the median exposure associated with a 5% decrease in FEV$_1$ [90]. Rylander has set a threshold limit of 100–200 ng/m^3 for exposures to endotoxins based on a documented decline in FEV$_1$ over one working shift [91].

Personal Protective Equipment and Practices

Although it is an admirable effort to institute environmental hygiene measures such as rodent control and work surface decontamination, the sewer environment is such that workers should assume that all waste and surfaces are contaminated. Since the environment is one in which exposure cannot be excluded by engineering and administrative procedures, preventive efforts center on education and measures to physically protect the individual [27]. Using personal protective equipment (PPE) for waste management and treatment and practicing proper hygienic habits are essential.

First, all workers should be educated on a yearly basis on how to avoid prolonged or direct contact with sewage. Eliminating prolonged immersion by requiring workers to wear rubber boots and gloves, long pants, and protective eyewear will decrease exposure to skin, mucous membranes, and eyes. PPE should include waterproof footwear, watershedding aprons worn outside and over the boots or other clothing, and clear plastic face masks. In sewers, hot climates, and areas requiring dexterity, impermeable protective equipment has been poorly accepted, but because pathogens often infect via wet, abraded or macerated skin, the use of waterproof boots by the sewer worker is an absolute minimum.

It is strongly recommended that sewage workers wash their hands prior to eating, smoking, or touching facial areas such as the eyes, nose, and mouth. After exposure to sewage, sewage products and processes, and bioaerosols, contaminated articles should be disposed of in an appropriate receptacle or cleaned in an appropriate manner. Showering after the work shift also should be required. Laundering of work garb using enzyme cleansing methods will eliminate pathogens and reduce complaints of dermatitis caused by traditional soaps and cleaners.

Respirators of an appropriate design, capability, and protective factor should be used, especially when the worker is in confined spaces or when sampling has documented volatile chemicals in the waste stream. Regular worksite monitoring of benzene and other volatile organic solvents is recommended. For those working with compost sewage waste, protective facemasks, which filter particle sizes of 1–5 μm, are recommended. Periodic examination of this equipment is necessary to ensure adequate protection. For those with special risks, such as those working in biofilter towers, the OSHA respirator medical evaluation questionnaire and physical examination are required on assignment or transfer to a contaminated area. Fit testing and training in an American National Standards Institute (ANSI)/National Institute of Occupational Safety and Health (NIOSH)–approved and appropriate-for-use respirator is also required for workers prior to their entry into contaminated areas. Individuals performing fit testing and training must be experienced and knowledgeable; the occupational physician should know the credentials of the person or company providing this service if it is not performed by the physician.

Proactive Preventive Measures in Developing a Prevention Program

The most important element in minimizing potential adverse health effects is a site-specific assessment of the risk of exposure to infectious as well as physical and chemical agents. Preventive measures for control of human infections vary depending on risks present, sewage worker activity, and local animal reservoirs. There are three important factors to consider when developing a prevention program:

- *The exposed worker/individual.* Minimize skin contact with sewage sludge, compost, and incinerator exhaust-fan residue and fly ash [92].
- *The contaminated environment.* (1) Ensure adequate ventilation for all sewage workers, (2) implement measures to minimize workers' contact with bacterial aerosols, such as in aeration basins, especially if indoors, and (3) perform volumetric and biologic sampling around the sewage site at intervals determined based on known fluctuations and changes in pathogens. For *Legionella*, there are recommendations that a standard plate count be performed every month, and a *Legionella* bacterial count be performed every 3 months [93, 94].
- *The animal shedder.* The rodent is an important carrier of several diseases; it is the most common shedder of *Leptospira*. Rodent control and testing programs have never been able to eradicate the organism within the wild animal population. Ascertaining serovars via sampling of the shedder population and assessing shedder prevalence is recommended. Antibiotics to eliminate the shedder state have not proved successful in animals. In humans, prophylaxis with antibiotics has been demonstrated to be successful in exposure situations involving animals with high prevalence of carrier states. Chronic prophylaxis in humans has not been proven to be a successful strategy.

EMPLOYEE EDUCATION AND TRAINING

Individuals, whether working in a typical sewage treatment plant, state-of-the-art composting facility, or near or at the point source of sewage, should be educated about the risks associated with exposures to sewage and biologically active agents. Emphasis on personal hygiene practices is extremely important to the prevention of illness. Reinforcement of this information should take place on hire, annually during surveillance examinations, during personal protective equipment (PPE) fitting and training, or with job change or transfer. Emphasis should be placed on the following messages:

1. Clean all scratches or abrasions, and keep them covered while at work.
2. Avoid rubbing the eyes with contaminated hands or other items.
3. Use appropriate protective clothing and PPE when exposed to aerosolized, liquid, or dried sewage. This includes explanation of what constitutes appropriate work clothes, coveralls, and boots and, when appropriate, gloves and plastic face shields.
4. Remove protective clothing at the end of the shift, and leave it at work.
5. Bathe or shower daily, and wash hands and face prior to eating or smoking.
6. Avoid biting fingernails [95].

New employees should undergo training in the risks of exposure to *Leptospira, Legionella*, HAV, HEV, and other common pathogens as part of job orientation. Education about signs and symptoms of organic solvent exposure and industrial and radioactive wastes also should be included. Sewer line workers must understand the potential for gaseous and chemical hazards and should know procedures for safe sewer entry.

Individuals working in processing of open compost, with or without agitation, or aeration tanks and those working downwind from other workers performing these activities should know the prevailing wind patterns. Records of monthly wind arrows should be kept to limit the concentration of exposure of bioaerosols and other pathogenic materials. Workers involved in operations that generate bioaerosols should be educated about personal risks as well as risks to their fellow workers and the population near the worksite. Workers who accidentally fall into sewage should shower and clean themselves immediately. If complete immersion occurs, the individual should be taken for medical assessment. Basic life support (BLS) training should be a part of the new-hire orientation and annually thereafter so that workers overcome by immersion or other gaseous or chemical hazards can be helped immediately [95, 96].

PERIODIC MEDICAL SURVEILLANCE

An occupational and medical history should be obtained from all employees on hire and annually thereafter as long as they perform this type of work. Special attention should be paid to the medical history of the following conditions:

1. Individuals with a presence of joint problems or disorders that limit mobility.
2. Recurrent or long-term skin disorders that predispose to infection. Be aware that exposure to aerosolized, liquid, or dried sewage can result in contact dermatitis or skin irritation.
3. Chronic or recurrent asthma that may be exacerbated by exposure to aerosolized, liquid, or dried sewage.
4. Conditions such as epilepsy, stroke, or diabetes mellitus that might produce unconsciousness or loss of physical control. For these individuals, a reasonable accommodation may be working with a partner at all times.
5. A completed OSHA respirator medical evaluation questionnaire that assesses any condition that might affect the worker's ability to wear a respirator.

The preplacement examination should be directed toward organ systems that require assessment with regard to a codified task analysis. Examinations of grip strength, joint mobility, and visual acuity, as well as health concerns disclosed during the medical history, should be evaluated. The examiner should request reports from other treating physicians in these areas to clarify fitness-for-duty determinations [95, 96]. It should not be overlooked that sewage workers are engaged in a physically demanding trade. Particular care should be employed for individuals with a past or present history of liver disease. Immunosuppressed individuals or those afflicted with human immunodeficiency virus (HIV) infection are at risk for progressive infections, extrapulmonary complications, bacteremia, and lung abscesses owing to *Aspergillus* and *Legionella.*

After this initial assessment, a complete physical examination should be performed on an annual basis [95]. Individuals who have identified issues or difficulties on the OSHA respirator questionnaire or by history and examination may be at risk for pulmonary problems and should undergo pulmonary function testing. Individuals in compost facilities are at increased risk for occupational asthma. It is recommended that pulmonary function testing be performed on a periodic basis to assess loss of lung function in settings of wet, slurry, or dry bioaerosol exposure [97]. It is prudent to document personal habits or other behaviors that may contribute to lung disease, such as smoking or use of marijuana. Passive exposure to cigarette smoke should not be overlooked.

Routine or periodic blood and urine testing is not recommended for all individuals. For individuals with special risks, such as chronic liver disease, men who have sex with men, and the immunosuppressed or immunocompromised, appropriate testing should be performed on an individual basis.

IMMUNIZATION AND PROPHYLACTIC MEASURES

Pre- and Postexposure Measures

Eradication of bacterial pathogens in the sewage workers' environment is not possible. Yet there are other considerations to be made in this worker population based on known risks. All adults should be up to date on their Td immunization. During the initial and subsequent medical history, three doses of Td with booster doses administrated every 10 years should be documented. For *Leptospirosis,* there are vaccines available for both animals and humans. Transmission of infection to workers from immunized, asymptomatic animals shedding leptospires in their urine has occurred. Human leptospirosis vaccines have been used in Europe, Israel, Japan, and Italy; they are serotype-specific, require two or more doses 2–4 weeks apart, and must be repeated annually [99]. These vaccines are not used in the United States because they are serovar-specific, must be repeated annually, and are associated with painful swollen vaccination sites. Animal vaccines have been shown to prevent symptomatic disease, but infection, organism shedding, and transmission still may occur [15]. Because both human and animal vaccines are serovar-specific, knowledge of the prevalent type is paramount if one is to consider a vaccination program.

Prophylaxis for leptospirosis can be provided with doxycycline, 200 mg administered once weekly. Doxycycline has been shown by clinical study and the Cochrane database to be efficacious. and is indicated when the exposure is known to be of short duration and the attack rate is calculated to exceed 1%. The 200-mg weekly dose has a demonstrated efficacy of 95% against leptospirosis and may be given to help prevent the disease in short-term rather than long-term exposures.

Legionella is a known contaminate of the aquatic environment. The most cost-effective methods of primary and secondary prevention of legionellosis have not been identified. Development of preventive strategies is limited by the complex interaction of the environment, transmission, and animal hosts. The CDC has recommended culturing of environmental sources only in situations in which documented legionnaires' disease has occurred. Biocides and hyperchlorination have been ineffective in eradicating the organism from cooling towers and have been marginally effective in reducing pathogen counts [100]. Hyperchlorination of influent or effluent sewage is not recommended because the bacteria are relatively resistant to chlorine. Chlorine breaks down at higher temperatures and leads to corrosion of plumbing systems and the potential formation of chlorinated carcinogenic by-products [101]. Methods for destruction of *Legionella*, such as UV irradiation, copper-silver ionization, and superheat and flush, are not plausible in the sewer environment. *Legionella* immunization in guinea pigs has resulted in development of cell-mediated immunity, but there is no *Legionella* vaccine approved for human use as of 2007 [102–104]. For the immunosuppressed, erythromycin chemoprophylaxis has been protective against legionnaires' disease. However, owing to the low overall attack rate in workers in sewer environments, this strategy is seldom indicated.

There are numerous reports from around the world that identify the incidence and prevalence of hepatitis viruses among sewage workers. Studies both recent and historical have not revealed clear evidence that sewage workers are at increased risk for acquisition of viral hepatitis [98]. In Greek sewer workers, anti-HAV antibodies have been found at a rate twice that of controls [105]. In Singapore, a sharp decline in hepatitis A transmission was concomitant with improvements in environmental hygiene. In the United States, fewer than 1% of the population under 20 years of age possesses Ig antibodies to HAV (anti-HAV).

The CDC and Advisory Committee on Immunization Practices (ACIP) do not recommend routine HAV vaccination of sewage workers. These organizations do not list sewage work as an exposure indication for immunization. The ACIP recommends HAV vaccination for individuals working with HAV-infected primates or with the virus in a research laboratory setting. In addition, vaccination is recommended for persons traveling to or working in countries that have high or intermediate endemicity of hepatitis or any person seeking protection from HAV infection [106].

If vaccination is indicated based on recognized exposures in the community, it should be administered prior to exposure to point-source sewage or during a known community outbreak of HAV. Currently, follow-up titers are neither recommended nor required. For individuals who are not offered or who refuse hepatitis A vaccination, there is no recommended biologic monitoring. The decision to vaccinate sewer workers against hepatitis A ultimately will be made by the occupational physician exercising prudent practice that balances the inevitable contact with sewage fluid with the fact that the probability of contracting HAV from the workplace is low [27].

Case reports of sewer workers contracting hepatitis B after exposure in the workplace have been published. Typically, this occurs in countries with an epidemic or high endemic rates. There are no current recommendations that sewer workers be vaccinated against hepatitis B prior to exposure or work [105, 106]. In the United States, it is now a long-standing public health policy to vaccinate individuals under the age of 18 and those in high-risk occupations, such as health care workers. Many younger sewer workers may have had these hepatitis B vaccinations. The occupational physician may wish to perform hepatitis B serology and liver function tests prior to work or exposure because individuals with chronic liver disease are considered to be at increased risk for disease from hepatotoxins.

If the community has episodes of sporadic exposures to raw sewage owing to flooding or storm damage, the occupational physician may wish to consider preemployment HAV, HBV, and HCV antibody testing.

On notification by the local board of health of a current infectious disease outbreak in the community or toxic spill into the sewage system, appropriate surveillance and testing should be performed. Under these conditions, considerations should include how safe work situations can be provided for those with chronic liver disease, HCV, HBV, those not immunized against HAV, and those who are immunocompromised, taking into account the requirements of the ADA and concepts of direct threat and imminent harm covered in Chapter 6.

There presently is no hepatitis E (HEV) vaccination or specific treatment available. Experimental data with vaccine using baculovirus-expressed recombinant capsid protein has shown protection of mammals from hepatitis E and are promising [107]. No vaccine is currently available in the United States. In areas outside the United States, where HEV is endemic, pooled-serum immune globulin is sometimes used to protect individuals or modify the illness. In the United States, the processing of serum immune globulin excludes these antibodies, so this approach is not available to sewer workers or travelers to endemic areas.

The ACIP guidelines recommend a yearly influenza vaccination for all individuals [108]. Many employers, both public and private, provide for annual influenza vaccinations. Sewage workers have no recognized increased risk for influenza infection, but their being included in a worksite vaccination program under the general population recommendation and as essential infrastructure personnel is prudent.

It is no longer considered adequate to rely on a personal or family recall of infection with measles, mumps, or rubella to determine need for vaccination. A single injection of the measles-mumps-rubella (MMR) vaccine is also considered inadequate. It is recommended that documentation

of two MMR vaccinations are in the medical record prior to medical clearance [95, 108].

In countries with sporadic outbreaks of measles or rubella, documentation of titers is necessary prior to medical clearance to work with sewage.

Symptoms and Signs of Illness

Undiagnosed febrile illnesses in sewage workers should be reported to the local board of health or occupational physician for evaluation.

LEPTOSPIROSIS

Leptospires that cross the epithelium proliferate and may disseminate widely. Every major organ system may be affected, and *Leptospira* antigens can be detected in affected tissues. *Leptospira*-mediated injury characterizes the initial phase of the disease. A host immune response marks onset of the second phase of symptoms [16].

Leptospirosis has an incubation time that may range from 7–12 days, with a range of 2–20 days. The disease reveals biphasic tendencies, with the initial, or febrile, stage lasting around 7 days, followed by the second (or immune) stage, lasting 0–30 days or more [109, 110]. Many organ systems can be affected; therefore, the clinical presentation may vary. Mild flulike symptoms or a fulminant course may ensue. In the initial stage, fever (39–41°C) of a week's duration or more is common. Individuals complain of anorexia, myalgia, headache, prostration, and retroorbital pain. Often, there is profuse sweating. During the first 48 hours, bulbar conjunctival injection may be observed. Respiratory symptoms may be prominent. In the second stage, anorexia progresses to nausea and vomiting accompanied by either diarrhea or constipation. During this febrile period, ophthalmologic examination may reveal papilledema, optic neuritis, and oculomotor paresis. Late manifestations include uveitis, which may occur from 2 weeks to 1 year after infection. Other neurologic symptoms, such as stiff neck and nuchal rigidity, are present. Lymphadenopathy that mimics mononucleosis is noted in roughly 50% of patients. For the remainder of afflicted individuals, glandular swelling is not prominent. Hemorrhagic manifestations may occur. The occurrence of liver and spleen enlargement, as well as jaundice and kidney involvement, depends on the severity of the infection and its stage.

LEGIONELLOSIS

Diseases attributed to *Legionella* species are legionnaires' disease, a potentially fatal form of pneumonia, and Pontiac fever, a self-limited, nonpneumonic illness. In patients with legionnaires' disease, pneumonia is the predominant clinical finding; symptoms may be mild (e.g., slight cough and fever) or severe (e.g., pulmonary infiltrates and multisystem failure). The incubation period is 2–10 days. Mild cough may progress to a productive one that is occasionally streaked with blood. Pleuritic or nonpleuritic chest pain accompanied by hemoptysis suggests pulmonary embolus. Diarrhea, which is watery rather than bloody, occurs in 20–50% of patients. Nausea, vomiting, and abdominal pain are experienced by 10–20%.

Pontiac fever has an incubation period of 24–48 hours; its attack rate is often more than 95%. Prominent symptoms are malaise, myalgias, fever, chills, and headache. In some cases, a nonproductive cough, dizziness, and nausea are present. Findings of chest radiography are normal, and with supportive care, complete recovery is the norm.

HEPATITIS

Hepatitis A and E infections are acute self-limiting illnesses. Patients often present with complaints of fever, malaise, jaundice, anorexia, and nausea. In children, hepatitis A infection is often mild. The illness is usually several weeks in duration, but cases of relapsing disease lasting as long as 6 months may occur. Fulminant hepatitis is rare, and chronic infection is not known to occur. Hepatitis E infection is not distinguishable from other forms of hepatitis but may be fulminant in the third trimester of pregnancy.

ASPERGILLOSIS

The signs and symptoms of *Aspergillus* infection will vary with the type of infection.

Allergic Bronchopulmonary Aspergillosis

Sewer workers with asthma or cystic fibrosis have an increased chance to experience an allergic reaction to *Aspergillus* mold. Signs and symptoms of this condition, known as *allergic bronchopulmonary*

aspergillosis, include fever, general malaise, cough, wheezing, and a worsening of asthma.

Chronic pulmonary aspergillosis may cause cough, often with hemoptysis and shortness of breath or wheezing. Invasive pulmonary aspergillosis is the most severe form of aspergillosis. It usually causes rapidly progressive, ultimately fatal respiratory failure if untreated. A systemic disorder, it rapidly spreads via the bloodstream to the brain, heart, kidneys, or skin. Signs and symptoms depend on which organ system is affected, but in general, invasive aspergillosis can cause fever and chills, headaches, cough with bloody sputum, and shortness of breath. In later stages, chest or joint pain is prominent. End stages exhibit massive bleeding in the lungs.

Extrapulmonary invasive aspergillosis begins with skin lesions, sinusitis, or pneumonia and may involve the liver, kidneys, brain, and other tissues; it is often rapidly fatal. Aspergillosis in the sinuses can form an aspergilloma, an allergic fungal sinusitis, or a chronic, slowly invasive granulomatous inflammation with fever, rhinitis, and headache. Necrosing cutaneous lesions may overlie the nose or sinuses, palatal or gingival ulcerations may be present, signs of cavernous sinus thrombosis may develop, and pulmonary or disseminated lesions may occur.

Workers with emphysema or a history of tuberculosis or other diseases resulting in cavitations may develop a pulmonary aspergilloma. It is characterized by a tangled ball of fungus fibers that forms in these spaces. Initially, an aspergilloma may not produce symptoms, but over time, workers may complain of a productive cough with blood, chest pain, wheezing, shortness of breath, and unintentional weight loss.

Other Aspergillus Infections

Aspergillus may invade sinuses or ear canals locally. In the sinuses, it may cause a stuffy nose, drainage, inflammation, fever, facial pain, and headache. Ear canal infections can cause itching, drainage, and pain.

Differential Diagnosis

The history of medical problems related to work with sewage does not make the job of diagnosing disease any easier. Sewer workers suffer less from nausea than referent groups and exhibit no significant difference in the prevalence of diarrhea, dyspepsia, or irritable bowel syndrome. There is no evidence to support either increased gastrointestinal symptoms, elevated *H. pylori* antibody response, or peptic ulcer disease in sewer workers [54, 111, 112].

The clinical manifestations of leptospirosis are not pathognomonic and have been confused with many other diseases, such as influenza, poliomyelitis, dengue, Q fever, and viral meningitis. Unless a physician has considerable clinical experience with leptospirosis, the diagnosis is usually made by laboratory analysis. Of the greater than 1,000 cases registered by the CDC since 1949, leptospirosis had been included in the differential diagnosis in only 25% [113]. The difficulty in making a timely diagnosis is often due to a locale's lack of laboratory procedures that would rapidly confirm the diagnosis in the important first stage. Therefore, a high degree of suspicion is warranted when sewage treatment workers present with fever.

Legionella infections, both Pontiac fever and legionnaires' disease, present nonspecifically. The following signs should raise the clinician's suspicions as to the diagnosis:

- Sputum Gram stain with increased neutrophils but few organisms seen on microscopic examination
- Hyponatremia
- Failure to respond to β-lactams (i.e., penicillin or cephalosporin) or aminoglycoside antibiotics
- Exposure to potentially contaminated aquatic environments

In the sewer worker, exposure to HAV, HEV, or *Leptospira* may cause jaundice. When jaundice occurs in sewage workers, discharges of potent hepatotoxins from industrial sources must be considered in the differential diagnosis of workers who become ill. Releases by industry of certain chemicals in sufficient quantities can cause toxic hepatitis. It is important not only to ask coworkers about unusual smells that have their onset within several days to 2 weeks of the onset of jaundice but also to understand the types of industries and potential by-products of manufacturing that could be illegally dumped into the sewage system. Hospital emergency departments usually have the Material

Safety Data Sheets (MSDSs) of local industry. When these are not available, the health and safety or industrial hygiene officer at the local plant can be a valuable resource in understanding the etiology of jaundice in sewage workers.

Hantavirus infection presents in several phases: the prodrome, followed by the cardiopulmonary and convalescent phases. The nonspecific prodromal symptoms include fever and myalgia lasting 3–6 days, as well as headache, backache, and gastrointestinal symptoms. The disease becomes differentiated in the second stage, in which noncardiogenic pulmonary edema often accompanies shock. Those who have progressed to the second stage have a mortality rate that often reaches 50%.

Diagnostic Evaluation

Many diseases of sewer workers also afflict the general population. When confronted with an ill sewage worker, it is important to remember that sewage workers' illnesses often reflect the illnesses in the community at that specific period in time. If an early diagnosis is to be made, a high degree of suspicion must be maintained for the typical pathogens that inhabit the sewage worker's environment. A thorough occupational history and an understanding of the various processes and stages of the community's sewage treatment process and conditions of exposure are paramount in assessing an ill sewage worker.

LEPTOSPIROSIS

In patients with leptospirosis, routine laboratory testing reveals an elevated erythrocyte sedimentation rate, with either leukocytosis or leukopenia and a left shift. Aminotransferases, alkaline phosphatase, and serum bilirubin may be mildly elevated. Urine may contain protein with proteinaceous casts. Other urine sediment findings may include leukocytes, erythrocytes, or hyaline and granular casts. Increases in blood urea nitrogen (BUN) and creatinine also can be noted. With Weil's disease, patients may exhibit a mild thrombocytopenia often accompanied by azotemia and renal failure. Other laboratory findings in Weil's disease are a marked leukocytosis with elevated creatine phosphokinase and prothrombin times.

The diversity of symptoms in leptospirosis can make diagnosis difficult. Culture of blood and other body fluids is recommended. Culture media containing long-chain fatty acids, such as oleic acid or Tween with 1% bovine serum albumin as a detoxicant, are used. Optimal temperature for cultivation is 28–30°C. Most strains do not grow above 37°C. In culture, small amounts of growth may be seen within 2–3 days, but routinely, cultures should be examined weekly for up to 3 months. Blood cultures taken during the first acute phase of the infection (up to 10 days) usually are positive. Cultures also may be taken from cerebrospinal fluid (CSF), urine, and tissues, including autopsy specimens. Phase-contrast microscopy is of limited value, as is staining of the organisms. Serologic typing requires reference antisera or serogroup/serovar-specific monoclonal antibodies. Gene probes using PCR are capable of detecting $10–10^3$ leptospires in specimens [114]. This method is particularly useful in the diagnosis of acute illness and identification of leptospires in cultured isolates [115, 116]. Detection of antibodies in sera of infected individuals may be performed using agglutination or enzyme-linked immunosorbent assay (ELISA). There are two types of agglutination methods. The microscopic agglutination test (MAT) is considered positive when there is a four-fold rise in convalescent titers. A presumed diagnosis is made by observing an antibody titer greater than or equal to 1:1,000 in conjunction with symptoms consistent with the disease. The MAT uses a battery of live leptospiral strains and has the disadvantage that antibody responses are affected by treatment and are usually not detectable until the second week of the disease. The macroscopic slide agglutination test allows for a presumptive diagnosis. As with the MAT, clinical signs and symptoms of the disease need to be present to support the diagnosis. The test uses an antigen that is useful for screening but lacks specificity. Both tests share the drawback that few laboratories do the test. The practitioner is admonished not to delay treatment while awaiting the results [14, 15]. Other tests include an indirect hemagglutination test and immunoglobulin M (IgM) ELISA testing. ELISA technology has the advantages of precision, objectivity, ability to screen large numbers of sera specimens, reasonable cost, and ability to measure IgG and IgM antibodies. Commercial tests are now available, such as Dip-S-Ticks, that can detect Leptospira antibodies [14, 15]. In terms of making the diagno-

sis, practically speaking, MAT and ELISA are preferable to culture. To an experienced pathologist using dark-field microscopy and thin specimen preparations, the organisms appear as motile, bright, beaded, rotating, thin rods, usually with one or both ends curved, against a black background. Dark-field examination frequently leads to misdiagnoses and generally should not be used.

Imaging studies such as chest radiographs may reveal a patchy alveolar pattern consistent with hemorrhage. These changes take place most often in the peripheral and lower lobes. Electrocardiographic abnormalities are common during the leptospiremic phase. In severe cases, congestive heart failure and cardiogenic shock may occur.

LEGIONELLOSIS

Legionnaires' disease (LD) is recognized as a cause of community-acquired pneumonia (CAP). The disease may present with a wide spectrum ranging from mild cough and low-grade fever to high fever, altered mental status, and respiratory failure [117, 118]. The signs, symptoms, routine laboratory tests, and radiographic findings do not distinguish LD from other CAPs, so specific laboratory tests are necessary to establish the diagnosis of LD. Sewage treatment workers with potential exposures to Legionella who present with cough and fever should have chest radiography. By the third day of the disease, the majority of patients with LD will have an abnormal radiograph. Classic findings are that of a predominantly unilateral lower lobe infiltrate. The definitive method for diagnosis of Legionella infection is culture of respiratory secretions. Culture of secretions from both the infected individual and his or her environment is still considered the "gold standard" for diagnosis. Legionella organisms are best demonstrated by using buffered charcoal-yeast extract medium enriched with α-ketoglutarate (BCYE-α). They cannot be grown on routine clinical bacteriologic media. Laboratories in the United States and other countries may lack proficiency in culturing Legionalla organisms. A recent survey found that nearly two-thirds of laboratories were unable to culture a heavy growth of L. pneumophilia from sputum. Often, sputum that may have culturable Legionella present is routinely discarded because it has too many squamous cells and too few polymorphonuclear cells [119, 120].

Serologic tests have limitations in that a fourfold

rise in antibody titers by indirect immunofluorescent assay IFA occurs in 70–80% of patients, and seroconversion may take place 2–3 months after the onset of illness. A fourfold rise in titer does not confirm the diagnosis of LD in patients with CAP [121]. Acute- and convalescent-stage sera are required. Serology is therefore not helpful in making an early and immediate diagnosis. The sensitivity of direct fluorescent antibody DFA testing is 25–75%, and its specificity is less than 95%. The specificity of polyvalent DFA reagents is probably lower than that of monoclonal reagents, leading some laboratories to advocate their exclusive use [122]. DFA is more likely to be useful when there are diffuse, multilobar infiltrates on chest radiograph. Urinary radioimmunoassay (RIA) testing is available commercially for detection of *L. pneumophila* serogroup 1. In infected individuals, its sensitivity is 60–80%, and its specificity is nearly 100% [123]. Genus-specific DNA probe technology is available and is comparable in sensitivity and specificity with DFA testing. Using this technique exclusively has resulted in the erroneous identification of outbreaks as LD owing to false-positive test results. It is recommended that other confirmative methods be used in conjunction with this diagnostic method. PCR is a promising technology because it has the capability of identifying the organism in water [124]. LD is addressed further in Chapter 10.

VIRUSES

HAV and HEV quantifications can be obtained by monitoring IgM anti-HAV or IgM anti-HEV, respectively. Monitoring IgG antibody titers is also helpful. Hantavirus pulmonary syndrome (HPS) will reveal a progressive thrombocytopenia. This finding can be highly discriminatory when one is considering the diagnosis of febrile illnesses with pulmonary involvement in endemic areas. Renal impairment may be present in the pulmonary syndrome. Hypoalbuminemia and lactic acidosis are late manifestations of the disease. IgG and IgM antibody tests for the Sin Nombre virus (SNV) are available at most state public health laboratories.

HELMINTHS

The most common parasitic helminths found in sewage are *Ascaris lumbricoides, Trichuristrichura* (whipworm), *Necator americanus* (hookworm), and *Taenia saginata* (beef tapeworm). The poten-

tial sources of parasites in municipal sludge are untreated wastes from slaughterhouses, meat and poultry plants, and infected individuals. *Ascaris* ova (eggs) are extremely resistant to treatment processes and are used as indicator organisms of parasite contamination and the survival of parasites in sludge. The number present in the human host depends on the number of ova ingested because the worms do not reproduce in the body. Tapeworm infections can spread in livestock owing to grazing on soils containing sludge in which ova are present. Disease in humans can occur when ova are ingested. Evaluation of ill sewage workers with diarrhea should include analysis of stool samples for ova and parasites.

MOLD AND FUNGI
Screening and Diagnosis

Diagnosing aspergillosis can be difficult because *Aspergillus* is found in the saliva and sputum of healthy individuals, and *Aspergillus* infection can mimic other illnesses. A thorough occupational history may identify worksite sources of infection. To help arrive at a diagnosis, imaging with either a chest radiograph or a computed tomographic (CT) scan of the chest should be performed, which may show characteristic signs of aspergillomas or invasive disease. The medical history should include questions about allergic symptoms and symptoms of bronchospasm. A sputum stain to check for the presence of *Aspergillus* filaments and culture should be obtained if the worker has a productive cough or has radiographic findings suggestive of *Aspergillus*-related disease. If allergic bronchopulmonary aspergillosis is suspected, skin and blood tests (serology) may help to establish the diagnosis. In disseminated infection, skin lesions may be present, and skin biopsy may help to confirm the diagnosis. More invasive studies such as a biopsy of the lungs or sinuses requires referral to appropriate subspecialists. Pathologic evaluation of tissue can confirm a diagnosis of invasive aspergillosis.

Because *Aspergillus* species are common in the environment, positive sputum cultures may result from either environmental contamination or noninvasive colonization in patients with chronic lung disease. Positive cultures are clinically significant mainly when obtained from patients with increased susceptibility to opportunistic infection owing to immunosuppression or when typical imaging findings raise suspicions for *Aspergillus* infection. However, sputum cultures from patients with aspergillomas or invasive pulmonary aspergillosis are often negative; cavities are often walled off from airways, and invasive disease progresses mainly by vascular invasion and tissue infarction.

Chest radiographs and CT scan of the sinuses is usually done when sinus infection is suspected. A fungus ball within a cavitary lesion is characteristic on both images, although most lesions are focal and solid. Sometimes imaging detects a halo sign, a thin air shadow surrounding a nodule representing cavitation within a necrotic lesion. Diffuse, generalized pulmonary infiltrates occur in some patients.

Tissue sample for culture and histopathology is usually necessary for confirmation of the diagnosis. Most tissue samples are obtained from the lungs via bronchoscopy and the sinuses by anterior rhinoscopy. Large vegetations often release sizable emboli that may occlude blood vessels and provide specimens for diagnosis. Because cultures require significant time for growth to occur, may be negative, and histopathologic examinations may be falsely negative, most decisions to treat are based on strong presumptive clinical evidence. Various serologic assays exist but are of limited value for rapid diagnosis of acute, life-threatening invasive aspergillosis. Detection of antigens such as galactomannans can be specific but not sufficiently sensitive to identify most cases in their early stages. Blood cultures are almost always negative, even with rare cases of endocarditis.

Clinical Management and Rehabilitation

Recommendations for prevention and treatment are often predicated on the population and the type of sewer system in place. Occupational physicians may be asked to make recommendations regarding the health, safety, welfare, and treatment of these individuals. At present, a case-by-case approach is recommended because there are few consensus guidelines to follow.

LEPTOSPIROSIS

The treatment of leptospirosis should be started as soon as possible and may be effective even several days into the clinical illness. The Cochrane database has concluded that there is insufficient evidence to provide clear guidelines for the treatment of lep-

tospirosis [14]. Traditionally, penicillin, streptomycin, tetracycline, cephalosporins, and macrolides have been used with success. Tetracycline antibiotics, however, are leptospirostatic rather than leptospiricidal and are contraindicated in children, gravid women, and individuals with compromised renal function. For mild cases, doxycycline, 100 mg bid, ampicillin, 500–750 mg PO qid and 1 g if severe, and amoxicillin, 500 mg PO qid and 1 g if severe, can be used. For systemic febrile syndromes, penicillin G, 1.5 million units intravenously every 6 hours, or ceftriaxone, 1 g every 24 hours, is recommended for 7 days. Alternative regimens are doxycycline, 100 mg intravenously or PO every 12 hours, or ampicillin, 0.5–1 g intravenously every 6 hours. For pneumonia, erythromycin and ciprofloxacin are the preferred antibiotics. Alternatives are clarithromycin and azithromycin. The most extensive experience has been with erythromycin, 500 mg intravenously qid [14, 15, 125–127].

Antibiotics must be administered within 2–4 days for optimal outcome. Since the presentation may include myriad symptoms, a high level of clinical suspicion should be maintained in this population of workers with febrile illnesses. For those who present with severe infection, admission to a hospital for supportive care, with particular attention to fluid and electrolyte status, is required. Patients with renal failure may require dialysis, with normal function typically restored. Those with Weil's syndrome may require transfusions of whole blood or platelets. The patient should be monitored until afebrile for at least 1 week. Relapses are fairly common, especially in those who present late for treatment or diagnosis. Hemodialysis may be necessary for individuals with renal failure. For those traveling in areas where leptospirosis is endemic, doxycycline, 200 mg once weekly, appears to be protective.

LEGIONNAIRES' DISEASE

Legionella diseases traditionally have been treated with erythromycin, 2 g orally or 4 g intravenously daily. Early administration and appropriate dosage improve survival [128]. There is associated ototoxicity with the 4-g dose. Oral administration may be adequate for some patients, yet abrupt deterioration in "stable" patients with advanced disease may occur. The high percentage of patients with gastrointestinal symptoms makes oral administration and absorption of erythromycin difficult, however.

The Infectious Diseases Society of America (IDSA) has published evidence-based guidelines for the management of community-acquired pneumonia (CAP) [129, 130]. Newer macrolides such as azithromycin and clarithromycin have good activity against *Legionella* and are better tolerated than erythromycin, and they should be strongly considered if treatment is in the outpatient setting. The quinolones have shown superior in vitro activity compared with erythromycin, and given their low side effects, once-daily dosing, and excellent bioavailability both parenterally and orally, they too should be considered. If based on IDSA protocol the employee is admitted to the hospital, once stable (3–5 days), oral therapy with an appropriate agent may replace parenteral treatment for total treatment duration of 10–14 days in immunocompetent individuals.

Convalescence from *Legionella* infection may take several months. Lingering problems such as shortness of breath and weakness are common. Pulmonary diffusing capacity defects, as well as reinfection in the immunocompromised, have been noted [131, 132].

HEPATITIS

Based on numerous studies, routine HAV immunization for sewage workers is not recommended [133]. HBV immunization should have been accomplished during childhood and, if not, should be offered to all sewage workers. For adults with viral hepatitis, expedient diagnosis and established supportive protocols should be followed; supportive care is usually all that is needed in the acute stages.

Those with a history of liver disease or recent hepatitis should be evaluated for duty. Many sewer systems place the worker at risk for exposure to heavy metals, inhaled aflatoxins, and infections that can adversely affect the liver. Consideration of job safety related to these factors during current and future duties is important. Decisions about duties must take into account hazard evaluations, the ADA, and issues of direct threat and potential for imminent harm, as covered in Chapter 6.

HANTAVIRUS INFECTION

Hantavirus infection, whether the pulmonary (HPS) or hemorrhagic fever with renal syndrome (HFRS), is best managed by early recognition and aggressive cardiopulmonary and renal support.

Sewage workers with a high degree of exposure to rodent excrement should have hantavirus infection considered in the differential diagnosis of many illnesses because it can resemble many other viral conditions. When the diagnosis is made, admission of the infected individual to the hospital for monitoring and supportive care is required. Fluid and electrolyte management for shock is critical for the survival of patients with this disease. The use of intravenous ribavirin (Virazole), a guanosine analogue, has been suggested for treatment. It has not been shown to be effective for treatment of HPS despite its effects on HFRS. In vitro activity of ribavirin against SNV has been shown, but there have been no demonstrated clinical benefits in its use in HPS. Ribavirin is not recommended for treatment of HPS [134].

ASPERGILLUS

Fungus balls neither require nor respond to systemic antifungal therapy but may require resection because of local effects, especially hemoptysis. Invasive infections generally require aggressive treatment with intravenous amphotericin B used as salvage therapy. Generally, complete cure requires reversal of immunosuppression (e.g., resolution of neutropenia and discontinuation of corticosteroids). Recrudescence is common if neutropenia reoccurs. The role of combinations of antifungals as either primary or salvage therapy requires additional evaluation.

References

1. Nethercott JR, Holness DL. Health status of a group of sewage treatment workers in Toronto, Canada. *Am Ind Hyg Assoc J* 1988;49:346–50.
2. Dutkiewicz J. Occupational bio hazards: Current issues. *Med Pr* 2004;55:31–40. Review Polish PMID: 15156765.
3. Cyprowski M, Krajewski JA. Harmful agents in municipal wastewater treatment plants. *Med Pr* 2003;54(1):73–80. Review. Polish. PMID: 12731408.
4. Elia VJ, Clark CS, Majeti VA, et al. Hazardous chemical exposure at a municipal wastewater treatment plant. *Environ Res* 1983;32:360–71.
5. Jonstone RT, Miller SE. Infectious occupational diseases. In *Occupational Diseases and Industrial Medicine*. Philadelphia: Saunders, 1960. Pp 252–61.
6. Khuder SA, Arthur T, Bisesi MS, Schaub EA. Prevalence of infectious diseases and associated symptoms in wastewater treatment workers. *Am J Ind Med* 1998;33:571–7.

7. Hanson ES, Hilden J, Klausen H, Rosdahl N. Waste-water exposure and health: A comparative study of two occupational groups. *Occup Environ Med* 2003; 60:595–8.

8. Cohen SH, Hoeprich PD. Environmental factors in infectious diseases. In Hoeprich PD, Jordan MC (eds), *Infectious Diseases*, 4th Ed. Philadelphia: Lippincott, 1989. P 184.

9. Garvey DJ. Exposure to biohazards. *Professional Safety Magazine* 2005;50:26–31.

10. Godfree A, Farrell J. Processes for managing pathogens. *J Environ Qual* 2005;34:105–13.

11. Douwes J, Thorne P, Pearce N, Heederik D. Bioaerosol health effects and exposure assessment: Progress and prospects. *Ann Occup Hyg* 2003;47: 187–200.

12. Golueke CG. 1983 Epidemiology aspects of sludge handling and management. *Biocycle* 1983;24:52–8.

13. Epstein E. Neighborhood and worker protection for composting facilities: Issues and actions. In Hoitink AJ, Keener HM (eds), *Science and Engineering of Composting Design: Environmental, Microbiological, and Utilization Aspects.* Environmental Science and Engineering of Composting: International Symposium. Worthington, OH: Renaissance Publications, 1993. Pp 319–38.

14. Green-McKenzie J, Shoff WH, *Leptospirosis in Humans*, September 13, 2008; available at www.emedicine.com/emerg/TOPIC856.htm.

15. Hickey PW. *Leptospirosis*, March 31, 2006; available at. www.emedicine.com/ped/fulltopic/topic1298.htm.

16. Faine S. Leptospirosis. In Evans AS, Brachman PS (eds), *Bacterial Infections of Humans: Epidemiology and Control*, 3rd ed. New York: Plenum Publishing Company 1998, Chap 20. Pp 395–420.

17. Brenner DJ. Classification of Legionellae. *Semin Respir Infect* 1987;2:90–205.

18. Dennis PJ, Brenner DJ, Thacker WL, et al. Five new *Legionella* species isolated from water. *Int J Sys Bacteriol* 1993;43:329–37.

19. Kuchta JM, States SJ, McNamara AM, et al. Susceptibility of *Legionella pneumophila* to chlorine in tap water. *Appl Environ Microbiol* 1983;1134–9.

20. Muraca P, Stout JE, Yu VL. Comparative assessment of chlorine, heat ozone and UV light for killing *Legionella pneumophila* within a model plumbing system. *Appl Environ Microbiol* 1987;53:447–53.

21. Tison DL, Pope DH, Cherry WB, et al. Growth of *Legionella pneumophila* in association with blue-green algae (cyanobacteria). *Appl Environ Microbiol* 1980;39:346–59.

22. Stout JE, Yu VL, Best M. Ecology of *Legionella pneumophila* within water distribution systems. *Appl Environ Microbiol* 1985;49:221–8.

23. Rowbotham TL. Isolation of *L. pneumophila* from clinical specimens via amoebae, and the interaction of those and other isolates with amoebae. *J Clin Pathol* 1983;36:978–86.

24. Feilds BS. *Legionella* and protozoa: Interaction of a pathogen and its natural host. In Barbaree JM, Breriman RF, Dufour AP (eds), *Legionella: Current Status and Emerging Perspectives.* Washington: American Society for Microbiology, 1993. Pp 129–36.

25 Wyn-Jones P. Enteric viruses in sewage, recreational waters and rural drinking water supplies. *Occup Med* 2002;52:431–2.

26. Margolis HS. Diseases spread by close personal contact. In Last JM, Wallace RB, et al. (eds), *Public Health and Preventive Medicine.* East Norwalk, CT: Appleton & Lange, 1992. Pp 131–3.

27. Poole CJ, Shakespeare AT. Should sewage workers and careers for people with learning disabilities be vaccinated for hepatitis A? *Br Med J* 1993;306:1102.

28. Jilg W. Adult use of hepatitis A vaccine in developed countries. *Vaccine* 1993;11:S6–8.

29. Buggs AM, Lim JK. *Hepatitis*, July 12, 2006; available at www.emedicine.com/emerg/topic244.htm.

30. De Serres G, Levesque B, Higgins R, et al. Need for vaccination of sewer workers against leptospirosis and hepatitis A. *Occup Environ Med* 1995;52:505–7.

31. Cadilhac P, Roudot-Thoraval F. Seroprevalence of hepatitis A virus among sewage workers in the Parisian area, France. *Eur J Epidemiol* 1996;12: 237–40.

32. Dounias G, Kypraiou E, Rachiotis G, et al. Prevalence of hepatitis B markers in municipal solid waste workers in Keratsini (Greece). *Occup Med* 2005;55:60–3.

33. Belalabbes EH, Bougermouth A, Benatallah A, et al. Epidemic non-A, non-B hepatitis in Algeria: Strong evidence for its spreading by water. *J Med Virol* 1985;16:257–63.

34. Kane MA, Bradley DW, Shrestha SM, et al. Epidemic non-A non-B hepatitis in Nepal: Recovery of a possible etiology agent and transmission studies in marmosets. *JAMA* 1984;252:3140–5.

35. Risbaud AR, Chandha MS, Kushwah SS, et al. Non-A non-B hepatitis epidemic in Rewa district of Madhya Pradesh. *J Assoc Phys India* 1992;40:262–4.

36. Nanda SK, Ansari IH, Acharya SK, et al. Protracted viremia during acute sporadic hepatitis E virus infection. *Gastroenterology* 1995;108:225.

37. Khuroo MS. Study of an epidemic of non-A, non-B hepatitis: Possibility of another human hepatitis virus distinct from post-transfusional non-A, non-B type. *Am J Med* 1980;68:818–24.

38. Wong DC, Purcell RH, Sreenivasan MA, et al. Epidemic and endemic hepatitis A in India: Evidence for a non-A, non-B hepatitis virus etiology. *Lancet* 1980;2:876–9.

39. Bofill-Mas S, Clemente-Cesares P, Albinana-Gimenez NM, deMotes Porta CM, et al. Effects on health of water and food contamination by emergent human viruses. *Rev Esp Salud Publica* 2005;79: 253–69.

40. Zeitz PS, Butler JC, Cheek JE, et al. A case-control

study of hantavirus pulmonary syndrome during an outbreak in the southwestern United States. *J Infect Dis* 1995;171:864–70.

41. Warner GS. Hantavirus illness in humans: Review and update. *South Med J* 1996;89:264.

42. Bhide AD, Sundaresan BB. Street cleaning and waste storage and collection in India. In Holmes JR (ed), *Managing Solid Wastes in Developing Countries.* New York: Wiley, 1984.

43. Clark CS, Linnemann CC Jr, Clark JG, Gartside PS. Enteric parasites in workers occupationally exposed to sewage. *J Occup Med* 1984;26:273–5.

44. US Environmental Protection Agency. Biosolids Generation, Use and Disposal in the United States. EPA530-R-99-009, September 1999.

45. Rylander R, Andersson K, Belin L, et al. Studies on humans exposed to airborne sewage sludge. *Schweiz Med Wochenschr* 1977;107:182–4.

46. Linnemann CC Jr, Jaffa R, Gartside PS, et al. Risk of infection associated with a wastewater spray irrigation system used for farming. *J Occup Med* 1984; 26:41–4.

47. Mueller HE. [Hygienic aspects of agricultural land applications of wastewater and sewage sludge.] *Naturwissenschaften* 1985;72:238–48.

48. Nethercott JR. Airborne irritant contact dermatitis due to sewage sludge. *J Occup Med* 1981;23:771–4.

49. Clark CS, Rylander R, Larsson L. Levels of gram-negative bacteria, *Aspergillus fumigatus,* dust and endotoxin at compost plants. *Appl Environ Microbiol* 1983;5:1501–5.

50. Clark CS, Linnemann CC, Clark JG, et al. Enteric parasites in workers occupationally exposed to sewage. *J Occup Med* 1984;26:273–5.

51. Lundholm M, Rylander R. Work-related symptoms among sewage workers. *Br J Ind Med* 1983;40:325–9.

52. Environmental Protection Agency. Non-cancer health and discomfort effects of poor indoor air quality. In *Report to Congress on Indoor Air Quality,* Vol 2. EPA Publication 400/1-89/001C. Washington: EPA, Office of Air and Radiation, 1989.

53. Gerba CP, Pepper IL, Whitehead LF. A risk assessment of emerging pathogens of concern in the land application of biosolids. *3rd. Water Sci Technol* 2002;46:225–30.

54. Millner PD, Olenchock SA, Epstein E, et al. Bioaerosols associated with composting facilities. *Compost Sci Util* 1994;2:6–57.

55. Morse DL, Kominsky JR, Wisseman CL III, et al. Occupational exposure to hexachlorocyclopentadiene: How safe is sewage? *JAMA* 1979;241:2177–9.

56. Morgan RW, Kheifets L, Obrinsky DL, et al. Fetal loss and work in a waste water treatment plant. *Am J Public Health* 1984;74:499–501.

57. Martin JE, Fenner FD. Radioactivity in municipal sewage and sludge. *Public Health Rep* 1997;112:308–16.

58. Ikatsu H, Nakajima T, Okino T, et al. [Health care of workers engaged in waste water treatment: 1. The exposure conditions to organic solvents in workers engaged in waste water treatment.] *Sangyo Igaku* 1989;31:355–62.

59. Frost P, Camenzind R, Magert A, et al. Organic micropollutants in Swiss sewage sludge. *J Chromatogr* 1993;643:379–88.

60. Elia VJ, Clark CS, Majeti VA, et al. Hazardous chemical exposure at a municipal wastewater treatment plant. *Environ Res* 1983;32:360–71.

61. Baker EL Jr, Landrigan PJ, Glueck CJ, et al. Metabolic consequences of exposure to polychlorinated biphenyls (PCB) in sewage sludge. *Am J Epidemiol* 1980;112:553–63.

62. Millner PD. Effect of nutritional and non-nutritional factors on the growth of *Aspergillus fumigatus* (AF) and natural sources of airborne AF and thermophillic *Actinomycetes.* In Sikora LS, Millner PD, Burge WD (eds), *Chemical and Microbial Aspects of Sludge Composting and Land Application.* U.S. EPA Interagency Agreement Project AD-12-F-2-534. Cincinnati: EPA, 1985.

63. Mattsby I, Rylander R. Clinical and immunological finding in workers exposed to sewage dust. *Occup Med* 1978;20:690–2.

64. Aspergillosis and Composting Advisory Medical Panel, April 4, 1994. Santa Clara County Public Health Department, Division of Disease Control and Prevention, 1994.

65. Lundholm M, Rylander R. Occupational symptoms among compost workers. *J Occup Med* 1980;22:256–7.

66. Clark CS, Rylander R, Larsson L. Levels of gram-negative bacteria, *Aspergillus fumigatus,* dust and endotoxin at compost plants. *Appl Environ Microbiol* 1983;5:1501–5.

67. Clark CS, Linnemann CC, Clark JG, et al. Enteric parasites in workers occupationally exposed to sewage. *J Occup Med* 1984;26:273–5.

68. Chesapeake Occupational Health Services. *Health Surveillance Program for Compost Workers: An Epidemiological Review. WSSC Site II.* Silver Spring, MD: COHS, 1991.

69. Carvalheiro MF, Peterson Y, Rubenowitz E, et al. Bronchial reactivity and work-related symptoms in farmers. *Am J Ind Med* 1995;27:65–74.

70. Windholz M, Budvari S, Stroumstos LY, et al. (eds). *The Merck Index,* 9th Ed. Rahway, NJ: Merck and Company, 1976. P 469.

71. Duncan RL Jr, Hoffman J, Tash BL, et al. Immunologic activity of lipopolysaccharides released from macrophage after the uptake of intact *E coli* in vitro. *J Immunol* 1986:136:2924–9.

72. Rylander R, Snells M-C. Endotoxins and the lung: Cellular reactions and risk for disease. *Prog Allergy* 1983;33:332–44.

73. Lange JH, Mastrangelo G, Thomulka KW. Will sewage workers with endotoxin-related symptoms have benefit of reduced lung cancer? (Letter). *Occup Environ Med* 2003;60:142–9.

74. Rylander R. Experimental exposures to (1,3)-β-D-glucan. In: Building Design, Technology & Occupant Well-Being in Temperate Climates. Sterling E, Bieva C, Collett CW (eds), American Society of Heating, Refrigeration, Air Conditioning, and Engineering, New York, 1993. Pp 338–40.

75. Fogelmark B, Lacey J, Rylander R. Experimental allergic alveolitis after exposures to different microorganisms. *J Exp Pathol* 1991;72:387–95.

76. Ciegler A, Burnmeister HR, Vesonder RF, et al. Mycotoxins: Occurrence in the environment. In *Mycotoxins and N-Nitroso Compounds: Environmental Risks,* Vol 1. Boca Raton, FL: CRC Press, 1981.

77. Rylander R. Endotoxin in the environment: Exposure and effects. *J Endotoxin Res.* 2002;8:241–52.

78. Richerson HB. Unifying concepts underlying the effects of organic dust exposure. *Am J Ind Med* 1990; 17:139–42.

79. Creasia DA, Thurman JD, Wannemacher RW, et al. Acute inhalation toxicity of T-2 mycotoxin in the rat and guinea pig. *Fund Appl Toxicol* 1990;14:54–9.

80. Gravesen S. Fungi as a cause of allergic disease. *Allergy* 1979;34:135–54.

81. Clark CS, Bjoronson HS, Schwartz-Fulton J, et al. Biological health risks associated with the composting of wastewater treatment plant sludge. *J Water Poll Cont Fed* 1984;56:1269–76.

82. Clark CS, Rylander R, Larsson L. Levels of gram-negative bacteria, *Aspergillus fumigatus,* dust and endotoxin at compost plants. *Appl Environ Microbiol* 1983;5:1501–5.

83. National Institutes for Allergy and Infectious Disease. *Report of the NIAID Task Force on Immunology and Allergy.* Bethesda, MD: US Department of Health and Human Services, National Institutes of Health, 1991. P 84.

84. Hunter CA, Grant C, Flannigan B, et al. Mould in buildings: The air spores of domestic dwellings. *Int Biodeterioratino* 1988;24:81–101.

85. Stellman JM (ed). *Encyclopedia of Occupational Health and Safety,* 4th ed. Geneva: International Labour Organization, 1998.

86. Jorgen J, Beijer L, Jonsson T, Rylander R. Measurement strategies for the determination of airborne bacterial endotoxin in sewage treatment plants. *Ann Occup Hyg* 2002;46:549–54

87. Millner PD, Marsh PB, Snowden RB, et al. Occurrence of *Aspergillus fumigatus* during composting of sewage sludge. *Appl Environ Microbiol* 1977;34:764–72.

88. Laitinen S, Kangas J, Kotimaa M, et al. Workers' exposure to airborne bacteria and endotoxins at industrial wastewater treatment plants. *Am Ind Hyg Assoc J* 1994;55:1055–60.

89. Castellan RM, Olenchock SA, Kinsley KB, et al. Inhaled endotoxin and decreased spirometric values. *N Engl J Med* 1987;317:605–10.

90. Palchack RB, Cohen R, Ainslie M, et al. Airborne endotoxin associated with industrial scale production of protein products in gram-negative bacteria. *Am Ind Hyg Assoc J* 1988;49:420–1.

91. Rylander R. The role of endotoxin for reactions after exposure to cotton dust. *Am J Ind Med* 1987;12:687–97.

92. Nethercott JR. Airborne irritant contact dermatitis due to sewage sludge. *J Occup Med* 1981;23:771–4.

93. *Code of Practice for the Control of Legionella Bacteria in Cooling Towers,* 4th ed. Published by Institute of Environmental Epidemiology, Ministry of the Environment, Singapore, a World Health Organisation Collaborating Centre for Environmental Epidemiology, March 2001.

94. *Code of Practice for Water Treatment Service Providers (Cooling Tower Systems),* January 2002. Department of Human Services, Public Health Group. Published by Public Health Group, Victorian Government Department of Human Services Melbourne, Victoria.

95. Alberta Human Resources and Employment, Workplace Health and Safety. *Medical Monitoring of Workers Exposed to Sewage.* Medical guideline, revised July 2000; available at www.whs.gov.ab.ca.

96. Alberta Human Resources and Employment, Workplace Health and Safety. *Sewer Entry Guidelines: CH037–Confined Spaces.* Revised November 2006; available at www.whs.gov.ab.ca.

97. Lees PSJ, Tockman MS. *Evaluation of Possible Public Health Impact of WSSC Site II Sewage Sludge Composting Operations.* Report prepared for Maryland Department of Health and Mental Hygiene, Baltimore. Baltimore: John Hopkins University, School of Hygiene and Public Health, 1987.

98. Glas C, Hotz P, Steffen R. Hepatitis A in workers exposed to sewage: A systemic review. *Occup Environ Med* 2001;58:762–8.

99. Torten M, Marshall RB. Leptospirosis. In Beran GW (ed), *Handbook of Zoonoses,* Section A: *Bacterial, Rickettsial, Chlamydial and Mycotic Diseases,* Vol 1, 2nd Ed. Boca Raton, FL: CRC Press, 1994. Pp 245–64.

100. Muraca PW, Stout JE, Yu VL. Environmental aspects of legionnaires' disease. *J Am Water Works Assoc* 1988;80:78–86.

101. Morris RD, Audet AM, Angelillo IF, et al. Chlorination, chlorination by-products, and cancer: A meta-analysis. *Am J Public Health* 1992;82:955–63.

102. Blander SJ, Horwitz MA. Major cytoplasmic membrane protein of *L. pneumophila,* a genus common antigen and member of hsp family of heat shock proteins induces protective immunity in guinea pig model of legionnaires' disease. *J Clin Invest* 1993;91: 717–23.

103. Howitz MA, Marston BJ, Broome CV, et al. Prospects for vaccine development. In Barbaree JM, Breiman RF, Du Four AP (eds), *Legionella: Current Status and Emerging Perspectives.* Washington: American Society for Microbiology, 1993. Pp 296–7.

104. Centers for Disease Control and Prevention. Le-

gionellosis Resource Site (Legionnaires' Disease and Pontiac Fever), www.cdc.gov/legionella/, April 3, 2007.

105. Arvanitidou M, Mamassi P, Vayona A. Epidemiological evidence for vaccinating wastewater treatment plant workers against hepatitis A and hepatitis B virus. *Eur J Epidemiol* 2004;19:259–62.

106. Fiore AE, Wasley A, Bell BP. *Prevention of Hepatitis A Through Active or Passive Immunization,* Recommendations of the Advisory Committee on Immunization Practices (ACIP). May 19, 2006/55 (RR07): 1–23.

107. Twu J, Sherker AH, Fung K, et al. Inhibition of hepatitis E virus replication by ribavirin and human alpha-interferon in primary human hepatocyte explants. Presented at the 1993 International Symposium on Viral Hepatitis and Liver Disease, Tokyo, May 1993.

108. Kroger AT, Atkinson WL, Marcuse EK, Pickering LK. General Recommendation son Immunization: Recommendations of the Advisory Committee on Immunization Practices (ACIP). *MMWR* December 1, 2006;55(RR15);1–48.

109. Turner LH. Leptospirosis I. *Trans R Soc Trop Med Hyg* 1967;61:842–55.

110. Dutkiewicz J, Jablonski L, Olenchock S. Occupational biohazards: A review. *Am J Ind Med* 1988;14: 605–23.

111. Friis L, Engstrand L, Edling C. Prevalence of *Helicobacter pylori* infection among sewage workers. *Scand J Work Environ Health* 1996;22:364–8.

112. De Schryver A, Van Hooste W, Charlie A-Mr, et al. Helicobacter pylori infection in sewage workers at municipal wastewater treatment plants in Belgium. *Eur J Public Health* 2006;16:30.

113. Alexander A. Leptospirosis. In Hoeprich PD, Jordan MC (eds), *Infectious Diseases,* 4th ed. Philadelphia: Lippincott, 1989. P 816.

114. Letocart M, Baranton G, Perolat P. Rapid identification of pathogenic *Leptospira* species (*Leptospira interrogans, L. borgpetersenii,* and *L. kirschneri*) with species-specific DNA probes produced by arbitrarily primed PCR. *J Clin Microbiol* 1997;35:248–53.

115. Merien F, Perolat P, Mancel E, et al. Detection of *Leptospira* DNA by polymerase chain reaction in aqueous humor of a patient with unilateral uveitis. *J Infect Dis* 1993;168:1335–6.

116. Gravekamp C, van der Kemp H, Franzen M, et al. Detection off seven species of pathogenic leptospires by PCR using two sets of primers. *J Gen Microbiol* 1993;139:1691–700.

117. Stout JE, Yu VL. Legionellosis. *N Engl J Med* 1997; 337:682–7.

118. Bartlett J, Mundy L. Community acquired pneumonia. *N Engl J Med* 199524:1618–24.

119. Eldenstein PH. Legionnaires' disease. *Clin Infect Dis* 1993;16:741–9.

120. Ingram JG, Plouffe JF. Danger of sputum purulence screens in culture of *Legionella* species. *J Clin Microbiol* 1994;32:209–10.

121. Plouffe JF, File TM, Breiman RF, et al. Reevaluation of the definition of legionnaires' disease: Use of the urinary antigen assay. *Clin Infect Dis* 1995;20:1286–91.

122. Eldenstein PH. Legionnaires' disease. *Clin Infect Dis* 1993;16:741–9.

123. Ingram JG, Plouffe JF. Danger of sputum purulence screens in culture of *Legionella* species. *J Clin Microbiol* 1994;32:209–10.

124. Matsiota-Bernard P, Pitsounni E, Legakis N, et al. Evaluation of commercial amplification kit for detection of *Legionella pneumophila* in clinical specimens. *J Clin Microbiol* 1994;32:1503–5.

125. Gilbert D, Moellering R, Eliopoulos G, Sande M. *Sanford Guide to Antimicronbial Therapy 2008.* Arlington. VA: Antinmicrobial Therapy, 2008.

126. Guidugli F, Castro AA, Atallah AN. Antibiotics for preventing leptospirosis. *Cochrane Database Syst Rev* 2003;2:CD001305.

127. Guidugli F, Castro AA, Atallah AN. Antibiotics for Leptospirosis. Cochrane Database Syst Rev, 2003;2: CD001306.

128. Roig J, Carreres A, Domingo C. Treatment of legionnaires' disease: Current recommendations. *Drugs* 1993;46:63–79.

129. Thibideau K, Viera AJ. Atypical pathogens and challenges in community-acquired pneumonia. *Am F Pract* 2004;7:1699–706.

130. Bartlett JG, Dowell SF, Mandell LA, et al. Practice guidelines for the management of community-acquired pneumonia in adults. Infectious Diseases Society of America. *Clin Infect Dis* 2000;31:347–82.

131. Lattimer GL, Rhodes LV III, Salventi JS, et al. The Philadelphia epidemic of legionnaires' disease: Clinical, pulmonary and serologic findings two years later. *Ann Intern Med* 1979;90:522–6.

132. Leverstein–van Hall MA, Verbon A, Huisman MV, et al. Reinfection with *Legionella pneumophila* documented by pulsed-field gel electrophoresis. *Clin Infect Dis* 1994;19:1147–9.

133. Trout D, Mueller C, Venczel L, et al. Evaluation of occupational transmission of hepatitis A virus among wastewater workers. *J Occup Environ Med* 2000;42:83.

134. Centers for Disease Control and Prevention, Special Pathogens Branch, Division of Viral and Rickettsial Diseases. National Center for Infectious Diseases, CDC and P. Washington: DHHS, June 22, 2004.

Appendices

A | General Resources, World, Regional, and National

These appendices present useful internet Web resources and resources from other media that the occupational health practitioner can use to keep abreast of developments in the field of infectious diseases. The World Health Organization in its information on the revision of the International Health Regulations (IHR) stated: "The phenomenon of globalization has altered the traditional distinction between national and international health. Very few urgent public health risks stay solely within national boundaries." This textbook and these appendices have been written with this perspective in mind and to remind practitioners of the interrelatedness of humans, their shared interests, and shared fate.

William E. Wright, Editor

General Resources

World Health Organization (WHO, www.who.org)
    Communicable Disease Surveillance & Response (CRS)
    Epidemic and Pandemic Alert and Response (EPR)
    Water Sanitation and Health (WSH)
    International Health Regulations (IHR)
    Global Alert and Response Network (mentioned in IHR revision information)
    Emergency Preparedness and Response
    Specific health topics, pathogens, statistics
    Advice for travelers
        European Observatory on Health Systems and Policies, Health Care Systems in Transition (www.euro.who.int/Document/)-has country-specific "HiT" summaries

International Labour Organization (ILO, www.ilo.org; English, French, Spanish, and other languages), an agency of the United Nations
    International Occupational Safety and Health Information Centre (CIS)
    Programme on Safety and Health at Work and the Environment (SafeWork)
    Worker and Migration/Migrant Worker Standards, other programs and standards

International Society of Travel Medicine (ISTM, www.istm.org)
    Travel clinic directory and other resources
    Sponsors travel medicine listserve

Publications, education, and training; multilanguage handouts

GeoSentinel (www.istm.org/geosentinel/main.html)
Global surveillance network of the ISTM and CDC; worldwide information and data-collection network for the surveillance of travel-related morbidity
Surveillance and monitoring of travel-related diseases and migrating populations through a network of globally dispersed medical clinics on all continents
Site posts current advisories

United States Of America

GOVERNMENTAL

Centers for Disease Control and Prevention (CDC, www.cdc.gov), 1-800-CDC-INFO
Listings and updates for specific diseases; outbreak updates, country-specific information, emerging infections, pandemics, bioterrorism, food- and water-borne diseases, statistics
Travel health services (www.cdc.gov/travel)
CDC Traveler's Health Hotline: phone: 877-394-8747; fax: 888-232-3299
Private travel medicine clinic resources
State health department Web sites
Yellow fever vaccination clinic sources
Sanitation scores for specific cruise ships
Vaccinations, pandemic information, safe food and water, mosquito and tick protection, illness and injury abroad, specific disease and infectious disease topics
CDC Health Information for International Travel 2008 ("Yellow Book"), available online and in hard copy
Health care provider hotline for assistance with diagnosis and management of malaria (CDC Malaria Hotline): 770-488-7788, or after usual business hours: 770-488-7100
National Notifiable Disease Surveillance System
Case definitions for infectious conditions under public health surveillance, www.cdc .gov/ncphi/disss/hhdss/casedef/. Includes access/links to
Case definitions for conditions under public health surveillance 1990 report: *MMWR* 1990;39(RR-13)-uniform criteria for reporting cases

Case definitions for infectious conditions under public health surveillance 1997 report: *MMWR* 1997;46(RR-10)-includes definitions of nationally notifiable diseases and some that are not yet notifiable; has hot links to new and revised definitions developed after the 1997 report

National Institutes for Occupational Safety and Health (NIOSH, www.cdc.gov/niosh)
Information of respirators and protective equipment, diseases, specific industry and occupational hazards, emergency preparedness and response, statistics, safety and prevention

National Institutes of Health (NIH, www.nih.gov)
National Institutes for Allergy and Infectious Disease (NIAID, www3.niaid.nih.gov)
Biodefense and related programs, information about studies of experimental treatments and vaccines for infectious diseases, information on specific infectious diseases, food-borne diseases, antimicrobial resistance, emerging infectious diseases, minority populations/special populations, women's health

Department of State (www.state.gov)
Hotline for American Travelers: 202-647-5225
At www.travel.state.gov: travel alerts, travel warnings, worldwide caution (information on terrorist threats and violence against Americans and their interests throughout the world), country-specific information and country-specific health information, tips for travelers abroad, tips for living abroad, emergency assistance for American citizens abroad, search infectious disease topics, death overseas, evacuations, medical/health insurance overseas, vaccinations, pandemics, taking pets overseas, travel registration with U.S. embassies, other topics

Occupational Safety and Health Administration (OSHA, www.osha.gov)
Standards, regulations, compliance assistance, training, recordkeeping, statistics
Information on specific infectious diseases, indoor air quality, biologic agents, bloodborne pathogens, disaster recovery, food-borne diseases, hospitals and health care facilities, laboratories, personal protective equipment, international travel, other topics

Has Spanish-language versions of some information

Federal Emergency Management Agency (FEMA, www.fema.gov)

Information on emergency preparedness and response, training aids, emergency management guide for business and industry, standard checklist criteria for business recovery

Environmental Protection Agency (EPA, www.epa.gov)

Approaches to mold problems, moisture control, and clean-up (www.epa.gov/mold/moldresources.html)

Indoor Air Pollution: An Introduction for Health Professionals. EPA 204-R-94-007. Washington: US Government Printing Office, 1994. Includes sections on animal dander, molds, dust mites, other biologicals; tuberculosis, legionnaires' disease, allergic reactions, hypersensitivity pneumonitis, humidifier fever; nonbiologic issues

Mold Remediation in Schools and Commercial Buildings. EPA 402-K-01-001. Washington: US Environmental Protection Agency, 2001.

Indoor Air Quality Information Clearing House (IAQINFO, www.epa.gov/iaq/iaqinfo.html)

NONGOVERNMENTAL

Council of State and Territorial Epidemiologists (CSTE, www.cste.org)

Promotes effective use of epidemiology data to guide public health practice and improve health; includes members from Canada and Great Britain

Provides point-of-contact lists for epidemiologists, state epidemiologists, large city and urban epidemiologists; directory of designated state public health veterinarians; occupational health contacts

Lists occupational health indicators, occupational health position statements on surveillance and programs, publications, educational programs

Infectious Diseases Society of America (IDSA, www.idsociety.org)

Information on the Emerging Infection Network (EIN)

Infectious disease practice guidelines on many

topics; some available as PDA files for handhelds. Includes fact sheets and guidance on antimicrobial use, infections by organ system, opportunistic infections, hand hygiene in health care settings, fever and infections, specific organisms/diseases, bioterrorism, avian/pandemic flu, travel medicine

State and regional societies and resources, HIV Medicine Association

National Network for Immunization Information (NNii, www.immunizationinfo.org)

Society of Health Care Epidemiology of America (SHEA, www.shea-online.org)

SHEA/CDC Courses in Healthcare Epidemiology

Journal: *Infection Control and Hospital Epidemiology*

Guidelines and recommendations related to infectious disease topics

Association for Professionals in Infection Control & Epidemiology, Inc. (APIC, www.apic.org)

Hospital epidemiology, health care-associated infections, standards and guidelines, resources related to influenza, pandemics, surveillance technology, definitions, reports and recommendations, many other topics; infection control courses, Webinars, conferences

American Society of Tropical Medicine and Hygiene (ASTMH, www.astmh.org)

Travel clinic directory and other resources

American College of Occupational and Environmental Medicine (www.acoem.org)

Position statements on disaster preparedness and emergency management, molds in the indoor environment, influenza control programs for health care workers

Guidelines for Employee Health Services in Health Care Environments, 1998

ACOEM Guidelines for Protecting Health Care Workers from Tuberculosis, 2008

Publications, educational programs, practice guidelines

American Public Health Association (APHA, www.apha.org)

Various topics, educational programs, and publications including Heymann DL (ed), *Control of Communicable Diseases Manual,* 18th ed. Washington: American Public Health Association, 2004.

American Industrial Hygiene Association (AIHA, www.aiha.org)
Industrial hygiene, respiratory protection, molds, nanotechnology, pandemics, emergency response

American Conference of Governmental Industrial Hygienists (ACGIH, www.acgih.org)
Industrial hygiene information, published threshold limit values (TLVs) and biologic exposure indices (BEIs), recommended practices for operation and maintenance of industrial ventilation systems, sampling for biologic agents during emergency response, bioterrorism

Canada

Canada Centre for Occupational Health and Safety (CCOHS, www.ccohs.ca)
Information available in English, French, Spanish

Public Health Agency of Canada (PHAC, www.phac-aspc)
Information in English and French
Infectious Disease and Emergency Preparedness Branch (IDEP)
Centre for Infectious Disease Preparedness and Response (CEPR)
Pandemic Preparedness Secretariat (PPS)
Centre for Emergency Preparedness and Response (CEPR)
Counter-Terrorism Coordination and Health Information Networks Section (CTCHIN)
Global Public Health Intelligence Network (GPHIN)
Laboratory Centre for Disease Control
Travel Health Services
Information sheets on specific infectious diseases

Canadian Society for Epidemiology and Biostatistics (CSEB, www.cseb.ca)
Fosters epidemiologic and biostatistical research and training in Canada

Central And South America

Pan American Health Organization (a regional office of WHO, www.paho.org)

Great Britain/United Kingdom

(For Canada, see above; for Australia, see below.)

Health Protection Agency (HPA, www.hpa.org.uk)
Site for infectious diseases, emergency response, radiation, chemicals, poisons
Centre for Emergency Preparedness and Response
Training and Exercise Response Programmes
Deliberate and Accidental Releases
Clinical Management and Health Protection Guide
Centre for Infections
Local and Regional Services

Department of Environment, Food and Rural Affairs (DEFRA, www.defra.gov.uk)
Topics on specific infectious diseases, zoonoses, epidemic disease surveillance, disease control, veterinary surveillance, environmental issues, local waste management, notifiable diseases

The Royal Society for the Promotion of Health (RSPH, www.rsph.org)
Infectious disease topics, manuals, education programs
Climate change challenges for public health

The Royal Society of Medicine (RSM, www.rsm.ac.uk)
Online resources, continuing medical education, pandemic flu preparedness course, other topics

British Medical Association (BMA, www.bma.org/ap.nsf/)
Various topics, including health care-associated infections, optimal use of antimicrobials, sexually transmitted infections

London School of Hygiene & Tropical Medicine (LSHTM, www.lshtm.ac.uk)

European Centre on Health of Societies in Transition (ECOHOST, www.lshtm.ac.uk/ecohost/index.htm)

Australia

Australasian Society for Infectious Diseases (ASID, www.asid.net.au)

Special interest groups on mycology, healthcare infection control

Australian Government Department of Health and Ageing - www.health.gov.au

Pandemic flu guidelines, modeling, preparedness; travelers' health alerts, SARS guidelines

Australian Health Protection Committee (APHC) and Environmental Health Committee (enHealth)—deal with issues of biosecurity: health disaster management planning, response, preparedness, recovery related to terrorist events, natural or man-made mass-casualty situations, infections outbreaks, and other environmental health matters

Includes advice for medical practitioners, various emergency response guidelines (Bali bombings 10/12/02; "white powder" hoaxes and false alarms in Australia in late 2001 following 09/11/01)

Sweden

Swedish Institute of Infectious Disease Control (SMI, www.Smittskyddsinstitutet.se)

Centre for Microbiological Preparedness (KCB)

Southern Asia

International Health Organization (IHO, www.ihousa.org)

Focus on environmental health, community health, education in India, Nepal, Bangladesh

See also Australasian listings

B Specific Topics

This appendix lists a number of online and print resources, some of which are supplemental to the material in this book or latebreaking since the chapters were written. Additional resources are found in the chapters themselves.

Bioterrorism and Emergency Preparedness

Bioterrorism Emergency Number, CDC, Emergency Response Office, NCEH: 770-488-7100.

Emergency Preparedness and Response, CDC (www.bt.cdc.gov).

Guidance for Protecting Building Environments from Airborne Chemical, Biological, or Radiological Attacks. NIOSH publication no 2002-139. Available at www.cdc.gov/niosh/docs/2002-139.

Bioterrorism Readiness Plan: A Template for Healthcare Facilities, April 13, 1999. Association for Professionals in Infection Control and Epidemiology (APIC) Bioterrorism Task Force, CDC Hospital Infections Program Bioterrorism Working Group.

Sheltering in Place. Centers for Disease Control and Prevention. Available at http://emergency.cdc.gov/planning/Shelteringfacts.asp.

Emergency Preparedness for Business, Business Emergency Management Planning, National Institutes of Occupational Safety and Health (NIOSH), U.S. Centers for Disease Prevention and Control (www.cdc.gov/niosh/topics/prepared/).

Domestic Preparedness Helpline: 1-800-368-6498 (Office for Domestic Preparedness, U.S. Department of Homeland Security, www.ojp.usdoy.gov).

The Office for Domestic Preparedness Guidelines for Homeland Security, June 2003: *Prevention and Deterrence.* U.S. Department of Homeland Security, Office for Domestic Preparedness, Washington, 2003; available at www.ojp.usdoj.gov/odp/docs/.

National Response Center: 1-800-424-8802 (NRC, U.S. Coast Guard, www.nrc.uscg.mil).
- National point of contact for reporting of all oil, chemical, radiologic, biologic, and etiologic discharges into the environment anywhere in the United States and its territories

- For incident reporting of suspicious activity, terrorist or suspected terrorist activity, use the Domestic Preparedness Chemical/Biological Hotline: 1-800-424-8802 or 1-877-249-2824 (1-877-24WATCH)

Emergency Preparedness Management Planning (CDC), www.cdc.gov/niosh/topics/prepared/.

Federal Emergency Management Agency (FEMA, www.fema.gov)
- *Emergency Management Guide for Business and Industry*

CDC Emergency Preparedness and Response website
- Laboratory Information (www.bt.cdc.gov/ labissues/)

World Health Organization (www.who.org)
- Organisms, emergency preparedness and response
- Global Alert and Response Network

American Red Cross (www.redcross.org)
- *Shelter-in-Place in an Emergency* www.redcross .org/services/disaster/beprepared/shelterinplace .html
- *Business and Industry Preparedness Guide* www.redcross.org/services/disaster/beprepared/ busi_industry.html#fema

National Institute for Chemical Studies (NICS, www.nicsinfo.org)
- *Model Shelter-in-Place Plan for Businesses*

U.S. Army Medical Research Institute on Infectious Diseases (USAMRIID www.usamriid.army .mil)
- Medical management of chemical and biologic casualties, courses, publications
    "Blue Book"—*USAMRIID's Medical Management of Biologic Casualties Handbook*, 6th ed. Frederick, MD: Fort Detrick, 2005.

Bloodborne Pathogens

Model Plans and Programs for the OSHA Bloodborne Pathogens and Hazard Communication Standards, 2003 (www.osha.gov/Publications/osha3186.html)

Blood Donations and Infectious Disease Considerations

U.S. Food and Drug Administration (FDA, www .fda.gov)

Keeping Blood Transfusions Safe: FDA's Multi-layered Protections for Donated Blood, www.fda.gov/ opacom/factsheets/justthefacts/15blood.html

AABB User Brochure Flow Chart, in *Guidance for Industry: Implementation of Acceptable Full-Length Donor History Questionnaire and Accompanying Materials for Use in Screening Donors of Blood and Blood Components*, Food and Drug Administration, 2005, www.fda.gov/cber/dhq/dhq11/dhq11d.html

Blood: Frequently Asked Questions (FAQs), www.fda .govCber/faq/bldfaq.htm

American Red Cross (www.redcross.org)

Buildings—Water Systems

The American Society of Heating, Refrigeration, and Air Conditioning Engineers (ASHRAE)

Guideline 12-2000, *Minimizing the Risk of Legionellosis Associated with Building Water Systems;* available at www.ashrae.org and www.marleyct.com/ publications.asp and other sites

U.S. Environmental Protection Agency (EPA, www.epa.gov).

Disease Reporting and Surveillance (USA)

For the United States, state health departments can be contacted at their Internet Web sites or by other means. The CDC website at www.cdc.gov has a link to state health department Web sites. All reportable diseases from state and territorial health departments are received by the National Electronic Telecommunications System for Surveillance. Many government entities have Internet-accessible information. The CDC website has information on special reporting systems, which include

Epi-X, www.cdc.gov/epix/. CDC's Epidemic Information Exchange is a secure information exchange network that can be used to post a "call for cases." This is used to communicate information of public health importance, such as clusters of disease, including travel-related diseases and the possibility of legionnaires' disease cases associated with individual hotels or cruise ships.

Legionnaires Disease Reporting System. Elements include sites for informing CDC about travel-associated cases by e-mailing travellegionella@cdc.gov. In addition, a cruise ship—related case notification can be made to the CDC Division of Global Migration & Quarantine and the CDC Vessel Sanitation Program at VSP@cdc.gov and FMAO@cdc.gov.

ArboNET, www.cdc.gov/ncidod/dvbid/.CDC's surveillance data network maintained by 54 state and local public health agencies and the CDC.

HIV Antiretroviral Pregnancy Registry (for voluntary reporting of pregnant women exposed to antiretroviral agents), www.apregistry.com/index.htm.

Automated detection and reporting of notifiable diseases using electronic medical records versus passive surveillance—Massachusetts, June 2006–July 2007. *MMWR* 2008;57:373–6.

See Appendix I for sites related to notifiable diseases and disease definitions.

Occupational Disease Surveillance: Indicators for occupational health surveillance (Recommendations and Reports). *MMWR* 2007;56(RR-1):1–7.

Disease Reporting and Surveillance (Non-USA)

For non-U.S. reporting, please check with local, state, province, territory, or national health services and/or with regional offices of the World Health Organization.

The European Working Group for Legionella Infections (EWGLI) operates a surveillance system (EWGLINET) for legoinnaires' disease among European travelers that can be accessed at www.ewgli.org.

Disease Statistics

For the United States, disease statistics are published in the *Morbidity and Mortality Weekly Report*

and the *Annual Surveillance Summary,* available by subscription (mail) or on the website www.*cdc.gov.* State health departments may publish local, regional, and state statistics and alerts about common infections, outbreaks, or emerging infections.

GeoSentinel (www.istm.org/geosentinel/main.html)

FOOD- AND WATER-BORNE DISEASES

The "Bad Bug Book," *Foodborne Pathogenic Microorganisms and Natural Toxins Handbook,* 1992, with online updates. U.S. Food and Drug Administration, Center for Food Safety and Applied Nutrition, Washington (combines information from the FDA, CDC, USDA Food Safety Inspection Service, and NIH, www.cfsam.fda.gov/%7Emow/intro.html).

Surveillance for foodborne-disease outbreaks—United States, 1998–2002 (Surveillance Summaries). *MMWR* 2006;55(SS-10):1–42.

Appendix A: CDC Form 52.13: *Investigation of a Foodborne Outbreak*—used to report investigation of a food-borne outbreak.

Appendix B: *Guidelines for Confirmation of Foodborne-Disease Outbreaks.*

FoodNet (www.cdc.gov/foodnet/), U.S. Centers for Disease Prevention and Control

Sanitation on Ships: Compendium of Outbreaks of Food- and Water-Borne Disease and Legionnaires' Disease Associated with Ships 1970–2000. World Health Organization, Geneva, 2001 (available on Internet).

Rolling Revision of the WHO Guidelines for Drinking-Water Quality (draft), *Guide to Ship Sanitation.* World Health Organization, Geneva, October 2004 (available on Internet).

Suitor CW, Oria M. *Foodborne Disease and Public Health: Summary of an Iranian-American Workshop.* Office for Central Europe and Eurasia, Institute of Medicine and National Research Council. Washington: National Academy Press, 2008.

Surveillance for waterborne disease and outbreaks associated with recreational water—United States, 2003–2004. (Surveillance Summaries) *MMWR* 2006;55(SS-12):1–24.

The European Working Group for Legionella Infections (EWGLI) operates a surveillance system (EWGLINET) for legionnaires' disease among European travelers that can be accessed at www.ewgli.org.

HIV

National Clinician's Postexposure Hotline, University of California at San Francisco: 888-448-4911 (www.ucsf.edu/hivcntr/Hotlines/PEPline).

Guidelines for occupational exposure and postexposure prophylaxis (PEP): Updated U.S. Public Health Service guidelines for the management of occupational exposure to HIV and recommendations for postexposure prophylaxis. *MMWR* 2005; 54:1–17. Available at www.cdc.gov/hiv/resources/guidelines/index.htm#occupational.

CDC for reporting HIV infections in health care professionals and failure of postexposure prophylaxis: 800-893-0485.

HIV/AIDS Treatment Information Service (drug information, PDA guidelines, HIV information) at the U.S. National Institutes of Health, *http://aidsinfo.nih.gov.*

HIV Antiretroviral Pregnancy Registry (for voluntary reporting of pregnant women exposed to antiretroviral agents), www.apregistry.com/index.htm.

INDOOR AIR QUALITY (IAQ)

U.S. Environmental Protection Agency, IAQ Clearinghouse (IAQINFO, www.epa.gov)
Standards for IAQ, guidelines for mold remediation.

American Conference of Governmental Industrial Hygienists (ACGIH, www.acgih.org)
Information on nanotechnology, biologic monitoring, biologic hazards in the workplace, endotoxins, minimizing risks of pandemic influenza; many other topics.

American Industrial Hygiene Association (AIHA, www.aiha.ogr)
Determination of biologic contaminants in environmental samples, information on mold remediation and postremediation, laboratory quality assurance programs; many other topics; biologic exposure indices.

The American Society of Heating, Refrigeration, and Air Conditioning Engineers (ASHRAE)
Guideline 12-2000: *Minimizing the Risk of Le-gionellosis Associated with Building Water Systems;* available at www.ashrae.org and www.marleyct.com/publications.asp and other sites.

Federal Emergency Management Agency (FEMA, www.fema.gov)
Publications on floods and floodproofing.

Occupational Safety and Health Administration (OSHA, *www.osha.gov*)
Guidance on molds in buildings.

INFLUENZA

Antivirals for Pandemic Influenza: Guidance on Developing a Distribution and Dispensing Program. Committee on Implementation of Antiviral Medication Strategies for an Influenza Pandemic, Board on Population Health and Public Health Practice. Institute of Medicine. Washington: National Academy Press, 2008.

Prevention and control of influenza: Recommendations of the Advisory Committee on Immunization Practices (ACIP), 2007 (Recommendations and Reports). *MMWR* 2007;56(RR-6):1–54.

LABORATORY ISSUES

CDC Emergency Preparedness and Response Website (www.bt.cdc.gov)
Laboratory information (www.bt.cdc.gov/labissues/) for bioterrorism emergencies.

CDC Division of Laboratory Systems—information on best practices in laboratory medicine, nationwide laboratory system, good laboratory practices, Laboratory Medicine Sentinel Monitoring Networks, antimicrobial susceptibility testing, etc.

Public Health Guidance for Community-Level Preparedness and Response to Severe Acute Respiratory Syndrome (SARS), Version 2, May 3, 2005.

Laboratory Guidance and Laboratory Biosafety Guidelines for Handling and Processing Specimens Associated with SARS-CoV, www.cdc.gov/ncidod/sars/guidance/f/app5.htm.

Biosafety Levels (BSLs)—BMBL, includes laboratory biosafety level criteria, recommended BSLs for infectious agents, agent summary statements, etc. Office of Health and Safety (OHS), U.S. Centers for Disease Control and Prevention. Available online at www.cdc.gov/OD/ohs/biosfty/bmbl/.

College of American Pathologists (www.cap.org)
Information on laboratory accreditation, inspection, proficiency testing, quality assurance, quality management tools.

Clinical Laboratory Improvement Amendments (CLIA), U.S. Food and Drug Administration, Department of Health and Human Services (www.fda.gov/cdrh/clia)

Clinical and Laboratory Standards Institute (CLSI, formerly NCCLS, www.clsi.org) Guidelines, checklists, standards development, evaluation protocols, training, various documents.

LYME DISEASE

Infectious Diseases Society of America (IDSA; www.idsociety.org)
Information on the Emerging Infection Network (EIN); practice guidelines.

CDC sites (www.cdc.gov)
Stafford KC. Tick management handbook: An integrated guide for homeowners, pest control operators, and public health officials for the prevention of tick-associated disease. *Connecticut Agricultural Experiment Station Bulletin 1010* (revised), 2007.

MALARIA

Intavenous artensuate for severe malaria is available now from the CDC Malaria Branch (M–F, 8 am–4:30 pm Eastern Time, 770-488-7788, or after hours, 770-488-7100.
IV artensunate for severe malaria. *The Medical Letter on Drugs and Therapeutics*, 2008;50:37.

Travel Health Issues

World Health Organization (www.who.org)

CDC Traveler's Health Hotline: phone: 877-394-8747; fax: 888-232-3299 (also see www.cdc.gov/travel).

CDC Health Information for International Travel 2008 (Yellow Book). Atlanta: U.S. Centers for Disease Control and Prevention, 2008.

Heymann DL (ed.), *Control of Communicable Diseases Manual.* Washington: American Public Health Association, 2004.

Sanitation on Ships: Compendium of Outbreaks of Food- and Water-Borne Disease and Legionnaires' Disease Associated with Ships 1970–2000. Geneva: World Health Organization, 2001 (available on Internet).

Rolling Revision of the WHO Guidelines for Drinking-Water Quality (draft): *Guide to Ship Sanitation.* Geneva: World Health Organization, October 2004 (available on Internet).

Tuberculosis and Air Travel: Guidelines for Prevention and Control, 2nd ed. Geneva: WHO Press, 2006.

Therapeutics

Infectious Diseases Society of America, *Treatment Guidelines* (www.idsa.org)

Handbook of Antimicrobial Therapy, 18th ed. New Rochelle, NY: The Medical Letter, Inc., 2008 (www.medicalletter.org).

Choice of antibacterial drugs. *Treatment Guidelines from The Medical Letter* 2007;57:33–50.

Drugs for Parasitic Infections, 1st ed. New Rochelle, NY: The Medical Letter, Inc., 2007 (www.medical-letter.org).

The Medical Letter on Drugs and Therapeutics
Bimonthly publication covers updates on drugs and therapeutics; includes vaccines. Canadian version available in French and English.

Vaccines

Centers for Disease Control and Prevention. "The Pink Book"—Atkinson W, Hamborsky J, McIntyre L, Wolfe S (eds). *Epidemiology and Prevention of Vaccine-Preventable Diseases,* 10th ed. Washington: Public Health Foundation, 2008; available online at www.cdc.gov/vaccines/pubs/pinkbook/.

Centers for Disease Control and Prevention. Wharton M, Hughes H, Reilly M (eds). *Manual for* *the Surveillance of Vaccine-Preventable Diseases,* 3rd ed. Washington: National Immunization Program, 2002.

National Network for Immunization Information (NNii, www.immunizationinfo.org)

Advisory Committee on Immunization Practices (ACIP), U.S. Centers for Disease Control and Prevention

Various documents in print and online, including *MMWR* (www.cdc.gov).

Prevention and control of meningococcal disease: Recommendations of the Advisory Committee on Immunization Practices (ACIP) (Recommendations and Reports). *MMWR* 2005;54(RR-7): 1–21.

Guiding principles for development of ACIP recommendations for vaccination during pregnancy and breastfeeding. *MMWR* 2008;57:580.

The Medical Letter on Drugs and Therapeutics
Bimonthly publication covers updates on drugs and therapeutics; includes vaccines. Canadian version available in French and English.

Vector-Borne Diseases

ArboNET (www.cdc.gov/ncidod/dvbid/)

CDC's surveillance data network maintained by 54 state and local public health agencies and the CDC.

World Health Organization (www.who.org)

Information on diseases, specific vectors, epidemiology, emerging problems; Communicable Disease Surveillance & Response (CRS); Epidemic and Pandemic Alert and Response (EPR).

Stanley M, Lemon P, Sparling F, et al. *Vector-Borne Diseases: Understanding the Environmental, Human Health, and Ecological Connections* (Forum on Microbial Threats). Washington: National Academy Press, 2008.

Drugs for Parasitic Infections, 1st ed. New Rochelle, NY: The Medical Letter, Inc., 2007 (www.medicalletter.org).

Zoonoses

National Association of State Public Health Veterinarians, Inc. Compendium of animal rabies prevention and control, 2008. *MMWR* 2008;57(RR-2): 1–9.

National Association of State Public Health Veterinarians, Inc. Compendium of measures to prevent disease associated with animals in public settings, 2007 (Recommendations and Reports). *MMWR* 2007;56(RR-5).

National Association of State Public Health Veterinarians, Inc. Compendium of animal rabies prevention and control, 2007 (Recommnedations and Reports). *MMWR* 2007;56(RR-3).

WHO Expert Consultation on Rabies, *First Report, 2004.* (WHO Technical Report Series 931). Geneva: WHO Press, 2005.

Some General Infectious Disease Texts

Cook GC, Zumla AI (eds). *Manson's Tropical Diseases,* 21st ed. Philadelphia: Saunders, 2003.

Engelkirk PG, Duben-Engelkirk J. *Laboratory Diagnosis of Infectious Diseases: Essentials of Diagnostic Microbiology.* Philadelphia: Wolters Kluwer Health/Lippincott Williams & Wilkins, 2008.

Guerrant RL, Walker DH, Weller PF (eds). *Tropical Infectious Diseases,* 2nd ed. New York: Churchill Livingstone, 2006.

Heymann DL (ed). *Control of Communicable Diseases Manual,* 18th ed. Washington: American Public Health Association, 2004.

Jarvis WR (ed). *Bennett and Brachman's Hospital Infections,* 5th ed. Philadelphia: Lippincott, Williams & Wilkins, 2007.

Jong EC, Sanford CA. *The Travel and Tropical Disease Manual,* 4th ed. Philadelphia: Saunders, 2008.

Mandell GL, Bennett JL, Dolin R (eds). *Principles and Practice of Infectious Diseases,* 6th ed. New York: Elsevier (Churchill Livingstone), 2005.

Markle W, Fisher M, Smego R. *Understanding Global Health.* New York: Lange, 2007.

Mayhall CG (ed). *Hospital Epidemiology and Infection Control,* 3rd ed. Philadelphia: Lippincott,Williams & Wilkins, 2004.

Peters W, Pasvol G (eds). *Atlas of Tropical Medicine and Parasitology,* 6th ed. St Louis: Mosby, 2007.

Rose SR, Keystone JS (eds). *International Travel Health Guide,* 13th ed. St Louis: Mosby, 2006.

Tan JS, File TM, Salata RA, et al. (eds). *Expert Guide to Infectious Diseases,* 2nd ed. Philadelphia: ACP Press, 2008.

Wallace, RB (ed). *Maxcy-Rosenau-Last Public Health and Preventive Medicine,* 15th ed. New York: McGraw-Hill, 2008.

C Infectious Disease Issues Related to Blood Donations

The following issues apply to regular volunteer donations of blood in the United States. The autologous donation of blood is a medical procedure and has less strict rules for donation. There are noninfectious disease issues related to blood donation that are not covered here. For further information, the reader should consult the Food and Drug Administration, Center for Biologics Evaluation and Research (CBER, www.fda.gov/cber/blood), the American Red Cross (www.redcross.org), or the local hospital or agency involved in obtaining blood donations. This is a changing area of medicine, and the practitioner should consult current sources for updated guidance.

General Medical Conditions

FEVER AND INFECTIONS, GENERALLY

- If a fever [temperature above 99.5°F (37.5°C)] is present, wait until it has resolved completely.
- If taking antibiotics for a bacterial or viral infection, wait until 7 days after an antibiotic injection for an infection.
- If taking oral antibiotics, wait until the course of antibiotics is finished. Prophylactic antibiotics for dental procedures or other prophylactic antibiotic uses generally are not reasons to defer donation.

COLD OR FLU

- Don't donate if you are not feeling well on the day of donation.
- Don't donate if fever or productive cough is present.
- If treated with antibiotics for sinus, throat, or lung infection, wait until treatment is completed and you feel well.

SKIN DISEASE WITH RASH

- If infected, wait until the infection has cleared.
- Otherwise, if skin over the donation site is not affected, it is acceptable for donation.

Specific Medical Conditions

SEXUALLY TRANSMITTED DISEASES

- Wait 12 months after treatment for syphilis or gonorrhea.
- If other criteria are met, no deferral required for *Chlamydia*, venereal warts (HPV), or genital herpes if you are feeling well and healthy.

HEPATITIS OR JAUNDICE

Not acceptable if hepatitis caused by a virus or unexplained jaundice has occurred since age 11. Ineligibility includes any viral hepatitis, including that caused by cytomegalovirus or Epstein-Barr virus.

HEPATITIS EXPOSURE

- Wait 12 months after last contact if you've lived with or had sexual contact with someone who has hepatitis.
- If incarcerated in a juvenile detention facility, lockup, jail, or prison for more that 72 consecutive hours, defer donation for 12 months from the date of last occurrence.
- Wait 12 months after exposure to hepatitis if given hepatitis B immune globulin.

MALARIA

- Wait 12 months after returning from a malaria area.
- Wait 3 years after completing treatment for malaria.

TUBERCULOSIS

- No donation if active TB is present or is being treated. If being treated for TB, wait until treatment is completed successfully before donating.
- Can donate if TB skin test is positive but no active TB is present.
- Can donate if receiving antibiotics only for a positive TB skin test.

Medical Procedures

ACUPUNCTURE

No limitations.

CJD AND vCJD-RELATED CONCERNS

- No donation if a blood relative has CJD.
- No donation if ever had a dura matter transplant or human pituitary growth hormone.
- No donation if, since 1980, ever received an injection of bovine (beef) insulin made from cattle in the United Kingdom.

DENTAL PROCEDURES

- Delay donation for 3 days after oral surgery.
- Delay until finished antibiotics for dental infections.

- Acceptable after dental procedures if no infection is present.

ORGAN/TISSUE TRANSPLANTS OTHER THAN DURA MATTER

- Wait 12 months after kidney transplant or other tissue transplant from another person.
- Not eligible if taking medication to prevent rejection of kidney or other tissue.

AFTER RECEIVING A NONAUTOLOGOUS BLOOD TRANSFUSION

- Wait 12 months after the last transfusion prior to donation.
- Not eligible to donate if received a blood transfusion since 1980 in the United Kingdom owing to variant CJD (mad cow disease) or if received a blood transfusion in some African countries since 1977 owing to concern about rare strains of HIV not detectable on standard testing (e.g., HIV group O).

VACCINATIONS—WAITING PERIODS AFTER VACCINATIONS

- None: influenza, tetanus, meningitis, and HPV vaccines if free of symptoms and fever.
- One year deferral: received an unlicensed vaccine.
- Eight weeks: smallpox vaccination or development of symptoms or skin lesions after close contact with someone who received the vaccination. If complications after vaccination, wait either 8 weeks after the vaccination or 14 days after resolution of complications, whichever is the longer period of time. If close contact with a vaccinee in the last eight weeks but did not develop symptoms or skin lesions, eligible to donate.
- Four weeks: Rubella, MMR, chicken pox, and shingles vaccines.
- Two weeks: Rubeola, mumps, oral polio, yellow fever vaccines.
- Seven days: hepatitis B vaccine (if not given for exposure to hepatitis—see "Hepatitis" above).

Percutaneous Exposures and Nonsterile Piercings of the Skin

HUMAN BITES

Wait 12 months from date of bite if it broke the skin.

NONSTERILE NEEDLE STICK/BODY PIERCING/TATTOOING, OR EXPOSURE TO SOMEONE ELSE'S BLOOD

- Wait 12 months following the event, unless the tattoo was done by a state-regulated entity using sterile needles and ink that is not reused (only a few states currently regulate tattoo facilities).
- If any question about sterility of instruments, wait 12 months following ear piercing or electrolysis.

INTRAVENOUS DRUG USE

Not eligible to donate unless drugs were prescribed by a physician.

RECEIVED MONEY, DRUGS, OR OTHER PAYMENT FOR SEX

Defer donation for indefinite period.

SEXUAL CONTACT WITH ANYONE BORN OR LIVED IN AFRICA WHO LEFT AFRICA AFTER 1977 AND THE SEXUAL PARTNER WAS BORN IN CAMEROON, CENTRAL AFRICAN REPUBLIC, CHAD, CONGO, EQUATORIAL GUINEA, GABON, NIGER, OR NIGERIA

Defer donation for indefinite period.

Living and Travel Situations

LIVING ABROAD

Ineligible for donation if

- Visited or lived in the United Kingdom for 6 months or more between January 1, 1980 and December 31, 1996.
- U.S. military, civilian military employee, or dependent of a U.S. military member who spent 6 months or more on or associated with a military based in any of the following areas: Belgium, the Netherlands, or Germany (1980–1990) or Spain, Portugal, Turkey, Italy, or Greece (1980–1996).
- Visited or lived for a cumulative time of 5 or more years since January 1, 1980 in any combination of countries in Europe listed (33 countries listed—see American Red Cross Web site).
- Not eligible if born in or ever lived in Cameroon, Central African Republic, Chad, Congo, Equatorial Guinea, Gabon, Niger, or Nigeria since 1977 (owing to risk for HIV type O).

OTHER TRAVEL

Travel to a malaria zone (see "Malaria" under "Specific Diseases" above).

Other Life Settings

- CJD in a blood relative—not eligible to donate.
- Living with or close contact with someone who had a smallpox vaccination (see vaccinations above).

Abbreviations: CJD = Creutzfeldt-Jacok disease; HIV = human immunodeficiency virus; HPV = human papilloma virus; MMR = measles, mumps, rubella; TB = tuberculosis; vCJD= variant Creutzfeldt-Jacok disease.

Sources: Adapted from information from the U.S. Food and Drug Administration's AABB User Brochure Flow Chart, October 27, 2006 update (www.fda.gov/cber/dhq/dhq11d.htm) and American Red Cross, March 2008 (www.redcross.org/services/biomet/0,1082,0_557),00.html).

Index

Numbers followed by a *t* indicate a table, numbers followed by an *f* indicate a figure